TEXTBOOK OF

IN VITRO FERTILIZATION AND ASSISTED REPRODUCTION

Dedication

This book is dedicated with affection and respect to the memory of Patrick C. Steptoe,
who, together with Robert G. Edwards, founded Bourn Hall Clinic

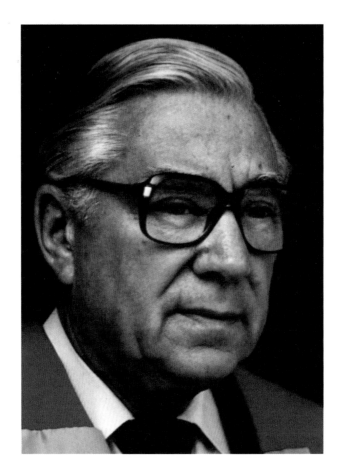

Third Edition

TEXTBOOK OF
IN VITRO FERTILIZATION AND
ASSISTED REPRODUCTION

The Bourn Hall Guide to Clinical and Laboratory Practice

Based upon the clinical and laboratory practices
and teaching courses at Bourn Hall Clinic,
with special guest contributions

Edited by

Peter R. Brinsden
Bourn Hall Clinic
Bourn
Cambridge, UK

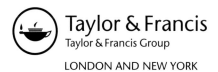

Taylor & Francis
Taylor & Francis Group

LONDON AND NEW YORK

© 2005 Taylor & Francis, an imprint of the Taylor & Francis Group

First published in the United Kingdom in 2005
by Taylor & Francis,
an imprint of the Taylor & Francis Group,
2 Park Square, Milton Park
Abingdon, Oxon OX14 4RN, UK

Tel: +44 (0) 20 7017 6000
Fax: +44 (0) 20 7017 6699
Website: www.tandf.co.uk

British Library Cataloguing in Publication Data

Data available on application

Library of Congress Cataloging-in-Publication Data

Data available on application

ISBN 1-84214-293-3

Distributed in North and South America by

Taylor & Francis
2000 NW Corporate Blvd
Boca Raton, FL 33431, USA

Within Continental USA
Tel: 800 272 7737; Fax: 800 374 3401
Outside Continental USA
Tel: 561 994 0555; Fax: 561 361 6018
E-mail: orders@crcpress.com

Distributed in the rest of the world by
Thomson Publishing Services
Cheriton House
North Way
Andover, Hampshire SP10 5BE, UK
Tel: +44 (0) 1264 332424
E-mail: salesorder.tandf@thomsonpublishingservices.co.uk

Composition by Parthenon Publishing
Printed and bound by T.G. Hostench S.A., Spain

Cover illustraions
Electronmicrograph reproduced with the kind permission of Pers Sundstöm, IVF Department, Curakliniken, Malmö, Sweden.
Picture of four-cell embryo reproduced with the kind permission of Dr Lucinda L.Veeck Gosden, Cornell University Medical College, New York, USA

Contents

Contributors

Mohamed Aboulghar
10 Geziret El Arab Street
Mohandessen
Cairo 12411
Egypt

Fidelis T. Akagbosu
Department of Obstetrics and Gynecology
Maimonides Medical Center
967 48th Street
Brooklyn, NY 11219
USA

Michael Alper
Boston IVF
40 Second Avenue, Suite 300
Waltham, MA 02451
USA

Tim Appleton
IFC Resource Centre
44 Eversden Road
Harlton
Cambridge CB3 7ET
UK

Awoniyi O. Awonuga
Department of Obstetrics and Gynecology
Maimonides Medical Center
967 48th Street
Brooklyn, NY 11219
USA

Adam H. Balen
Department of Obstetrics and Gynaecology
Leeds General Infirmary
Clarendon Wing
Leeds LS2 9NS
UK

Vera Baukloh
Fertility Center Hamburg
Speersort 4
20095 Hamburg
Germany

Guiseppi Benagiano
Department of Gynaecological Sciences,
    Perinatology, and Perinatal Care
University "La Sapienza"
Viale del Policlinico
00161 Rome
Italy

Martyn Blayney
Bourn Hall Clinic
Bourn
Cambridge CB3 7TR
UK

Peter R. Brinsden
Bourn Hall Clinic
Bourn
Cambridge CB3 7TR
UK

William M. Buckett
Department of Obstetrics and Gynecology
Division of Reproductive Endocrinology and
 Infertility
McGill University
Royal Victoria Hospital
687 Avenue des Pins Ouest
Montreal, Quebec
Canada H3A 1A1

Adam Burnley
Bourn Hall Clinic
Bourn
Cambridge CB3 7TR
UK

Jacques Cohen
The Institute for Reproductive
 Medicine and Science
101 Old Short Hills Road
West Orange, NJ 07052
USA

Jean Cohen
Clinique Marignan
8 rue de Marignan
75008 Paris
France

Salim Daya
Department of Obstetrics and Gynecology
McMasters University
1200 Main Street West, HSC-4D11
Hamilton, Ontario
Canada L8N 3Z5

Anick De Vos
Centre for Reproductive Medicine
University Hospital, Brussels Free University
Laarbeeklaan 101
1090 Brussels
Belgium

Klaus Diedrich
Klinik für Frauenheilkunde und Geburtshilfe
 des Universitätsklinikum
Ratzeburger Allee 160
23538 Lübeck
Germany

Sandra K. Dill
ACCESS
Box 959
Parramatta, NSW 2124
Australia

Geoffrey Driscoll
Faculty of Medicine
University of New South Wales
Randwick, NSW
Australia

Robert G. Edwards
Duck End Farm
Dry Drayton
Cambridge CB3 8DB
UK

Kay Elder
Bourn Hall Clinic
Bourn
Cambridge CB3 7TR
UK

Ricardo E. Felberbaum
Klinikum Kempten – Oberallgäu GmbH
Klinik für Frauenheilkunde und Geburtshilfe
Robert-Weixler-Strasse 50
87439 Kempten
Germany

Robert Fischer
Fertility Center Hamburg
Speersort 4
20095 Hamburg
Germany

Luca Gianaroli
S.S.Me.R
Reproductive Medicine Unit
Via Mazzini 123
40138 Bologna
Italy

Susan Golombok
Family and Child Psychology Research Centre
City University
Northampton Square
London EC1V 0HB
UK

Roger G. Gosden
Weill Medical College of Cornell University
Center for Reproductive Medicine and Fertility
505 East 70th Street (HT 340)
New York, NY 10021
USA

Rajat Goswamy
Harley Street Fertility Centre
122 Harley Street
London W1G 7JP
UK

Lars Hamberger
Department of Obstetrics and Gynecology
Sahlgrenska University Hospital
Bla Straket 6
413 45 Göteborg
Sweden

Hazel Harrison
Bourn Hall Clinic
Bourn
Cambridge CB3 7TR
UK

Lamia Haj Hassan
The Farah Hospital
Zahran Area
PO Box 5323
Amman 11183
Jordan

Johan Hazekamp
Volvat Medical Center
Postboks 5280 Majorstua
0303 Oslo
Norway

Anthony V. Hirsh
London Women's Clinic
115 Harley Street
London W1N 1DG
UK

Colin M. Howles
Serono International SA
15bis chemin des Mines
Case Postale 54
1202 Geneva
Switzerland

Julian Jenkins
Centre for Reproductive Medicine
Obstetrics and Gynaecology, CSSB
St Michael's Hospital
Bristol BS2 8EG
UK

Howard W. Jones, Jr
Department of Obstetrics and Gynecology
Eastern Virginia Medical School
601 Colley Avenue
Norfolk, VA 23507-1627
USA

Christoph Keck
Reproductive Health TA
Serono International S.A.
15bis chemin des Mines
Case postale 54
CH-1211 Geneva 20
Switzerland

Zaid Kilani
The Farah Hospital
Zahran Area
PO Box 5323
Amman 11183
Jordan

Janet Kirkland
Bourn Hall Clinic
Bourn
Cambridge CB2 7TR
UK

Anver Kuliev
Reproductve Genetics Research and
 Education Centre
2825 North Halsted Street
Chicago, IL 60657
USA

Amir Lass
Serono Pharmaceuticals Ltd
Bedfont Cross
Stanwell Road
Feltham
Middlesex TW14 8NX
UK

Suzi Leather
Human Fertilization and Embryology Authority
21 Bloomsbury Street
London WC1B 3HF
UK

Michael Ludwig
Centre for Gynaecological Endocrinology and
Reproductive Medicine
Endokrinologikum Hamburg
Lornsenstrasse 6
22767 Hamburg
Germany

Bruno Lunenfeld
Faculty of Life Sciences
Bar-Ilan University
Ramat Gan
52900 Israel

Henry Malter
The Institute for Reproductive
  Medicine and Science
101 Old Short Hills Road
West Orange, NJ 07052
USA

Samuel F. Marcus
Lead Fertility Services
Queen Elizabeth Hospital NHS Trust
Stadium Road
Woolwich
London SE18 4QH
UK

Karunakar Marikinti
Bourn Hall Clinic
Bourn
Cambridge CB3 7TR
UK

Thomas Matthews
Bourn Hall Clinic
Bourn
Cambridge CB3 7TR
UK

Peter Mills
Human Fertilization and Embryology Authority
21 Bloomsbury Street
London
WC1B 3HF
UK

Leila M. Mitchell
Bourn Hall Clinic
Bourn
Cambridge CB3 7TR
UK

David Mortimer
Oozoa Biomedical Inc
Box 93012
Caulfield Village RPO
West Vancouver
Canada BC V7W 3G4

Sharon T. Mortimer
Oozoa Biomedical Inc
Box 93012
Caulfield Village RPO
West Vancouver, BC
Canada V7W 3G4

Margaret A. Muirhead
Bourn Hall Clinic
Bourn
Cambridge CB2 7TR
UK

Neela Mukhopadhaya
Bourn Hall Clinic
Bourn
Cambridge CB3 7TR
UK

Botros Rizk
Department of Obstetrics and Gynecology
University of South Alabama
307 University Blvd, Suite 326
Mobile, AL 36688
USA

P. Sass
Fertility Center Hamburg
Speersort 4
20095 Hamburg
Germany

Mohammed Shaban
Faculty of Medicine
University of Jordan
Amman 11942
Jordan

Andrew M. Sharkey
Academic Department of Obstetrics and
Gynaecology
The Rosie Hospital
Robinson Way
Cambridge CB2 2SW
UK

Françoise Shenfield
Reproductive Medicine Unit
Elizabeth Garrett Anderson Obstetric Hospital
Huntley Street
London WC1E 6DH
UK

J. Robert A. Sherwin
University of Cambridge
Department of Obstetrics and Gynaecology
The Rosie Hospital
Cambridge CB2 2SF
UK

James Stachecki
The Institute for Reproductive
 Medicine and Science
101 Old Short Hills Road
West Orange, NJ 07052
USA

Alastair G. Sutcliffe
Centre for Community Child Health
Royal Free and University College Medical
 School
Rowland Hill Street
Hampstead
London NW3 2PF
UK

Seang Lin Tan
Department of Obstetrics and Gynecology
Women's Pavilion F4.29
Royal Victoria Hospital
687 Pine Avenue West
Montreal, Quebec
Canada H3A 1A1

André Van Steirteghem
Centre for Reproductive Medicine
University Hospital, Brussels Free University
Laarbeeklaan 101
1090 Brussels
Belgium

Lucinda L. Veeck Gosden
Weill Medical College of Cornell University
Department of Obstetrics and Gynecology
Center for Reproductive Medicine and Fertility
505 East 70th Street (HT 340)
New York, NY 10021
USA

Yury Verlinsky
Reproductive Genetics Institute
2825 N Halsted Street
Chicago, IL 60657
USA

Dagan Wells
The Institute for Reproductive Medicine
 and Science
101 Old Short Hills Road
West Orange, NJ 07052
USA

Preface

The original *Textbook of In Vitro Fertilization and Assisted Reproduction* was conceived after the first Bourn Hall (then also associated with the Hallam Medical Centre) foundation course in September 1989. The idea to produce a book owes a great deal to delegates on courses held regularly at Bourn Hall, initially designed by Bob Edwards, to teach the practice and principles of *in vitro* fertilization. They expressed a wish to have a textbook, so they would have to carry less paper in the form of protocols and reprints on the latest advances in assisted conception! Its success was a tribute to David Bloomer, of Parthenon Publishing, who prophesied correctly that it would be an immediate success. He also encouraged Peter to produce a second and now a third edition. The original co-editor, Paul Rainsbury, also deserves deepest thanks for collaborating so well in the initial issue of the book, which was delivered in 1992.

When Bourn Hall and the Hallam Medical Centre in London were originally merged in 1988, we were together, we believe, the largest assisted conception-treatment group in the world, carrying out at that time some 2500 *in vitro* fertilization and related treatment cycles each year. The Hallam Medical Centre ceased to be part of the Bourn–Hallam group in 1994 when it was taken over by another management group. From the founding of Bourn Hall by Patrick Steptoe and Robert Edwards in 1980 until now, Bourn Hall has been responsible for the birth of more than 6000 babies, conceived as a result of treatment by *in vitro* fertilization and related techniques.

This enormous accumulation of knowledge is reflected in the pages of this book, widely known as the 'Bourn Hall textbook'. They were written largely by our own clinical and scientific staff, plus a few experts from other clinics and laboratories, some of whom were trained or who practiced in Bourn Hall.

New authors and novel methods have been added to this third edition, to produce a vigorous text for clinicians, scientists and other professionals working in assisted conception. Contributors have been encouraged to use their own styles of writing and presentation, and the editorial hand has been applied sparingly. The intention is to encourage scientists and clinicians to work together, just as Steptoe, the clinician, and Edwards, the scientist, collaborated so closely. A shared understanding is bound to lead to still further improvements. Each chapter is intended to stand alone, while allowing the book to follow the theme of patient management and care through the whole spectrum of current assisted conception.

We do not maintain at Bourn Hall that we are, or were, the best in the world at assisted conception treatment, or that we possess all the answers. We do believe, however, that our unique experience over the past 24 years, since the Clinic first opened in September 1990, gives us an expertise and experience which is of interest and attractive to clinicians and scientists worldwide, and we welcome the large numbers of visitors we receive here each year.

David Bloomer and Jean Wright, who were so supportive in the production of the first two editions of this book, have been replaced by Nick Dunton and Oliver Walter, who unfailingly have been supportive with this, the third edition – thank you. Last, but not least, we sincerely thank all existing and previous members of staff who have done so much to make Bourn Hall successful, and who have contributed to making this book a success. In particular, we thank Helen Charman, Peter's personal assistant, who has been so supportive and encouraging over many years. Finally, we thank Dr Mike Macnamee, previously the Scientific Director at Bourn Hall, and now the Head of Pre-clinical Development, Serono International SA, for his help and support as a friend and colleague over many years.

Enjoy your reading, and let us know how we can improve and refresh our next edition!

Robert G. Edwards
Peter R. Brinsden
May 2005

1.1

An introduction to Bourn Hall: the biomedical background of Bourn Hall Clinic

Robert G. Edwards

This stately Jacobean mansion (Figure 1), still serene 400 years after its final reconstruction, became home to an *in vitro* fertilization (IVF) clinic in the late 1970s. It was the first and, throughout the 1980s, the largest the world had seen. This dramatic conversion from an ancient Hall depended on the introduction of human IVF which was carried out in its initial phases at Cambridge University, then in the Oldham and District General Hospital, and finally in the Hall itself.

Descriptions of the origins of its present inheritance must be provided by me, because I am the only one of the three original pioneers still living. Sadly, the others, namely Patrick Steptoe and Jean Purdy, passed away in the early years of Bourn Hall Clinic. Nevertheless, they bequeathed their mantle of our joint experience and collaboration, covering the first distant possibilities of human IVF, preimplantation genetic diagnosis and stem cells[1]. We shared successes, failures and even

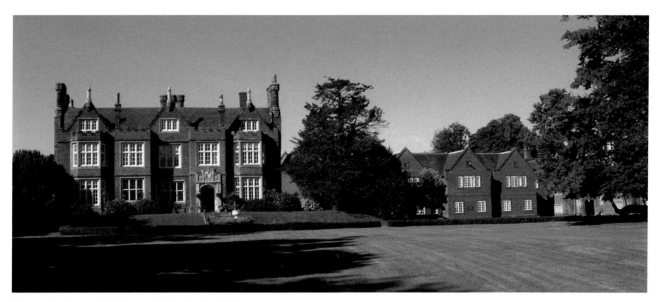

Figure 1   Bourn Hall Clinic in 2004. Photo: P. Brinsden

disasters over 20 years, and learned that it was essential to co-operate as a team at every stage, combining the best of science, medicine and nursing. Close co-operation was made simpler by being such a small team, sustained in Oldham by Muriel Harris, Patrick's senior nursing sister, over many years. It was essential during those hectic times to maintain a clear ethical stance, as defined in 1971[2], publish data at the first opportunity when verified scientifically, consult patients in detail, and work with the Press to ensure that our intentions and results were presented accurately and publicly.

We came from widely differing backgrounds. For me, the origins of human IVF lay fortuitously in the Institute of Animal Genetics in Edinburgh in the 1950s. Two Professors, Rogers-Brambell and Waddington, had contrived to send me there after a disastrous Agriculture degree in Bangor, North Wales. They still command my deepest respect. Virtually penniless, and an ex-soldier, my postgraduate course in the Institute organized by Waddington opened new vistas in science. And then, my PhD, supervised by Alan Beatty, taught me the fundamentals of a combination of genetics with mammalian reproduction in my postgraduate years when attempting to induce haploidy and triploidy in mouse embryos. This involved mastering the genetic control of oocyte maturation, fertilization and early embryonic development, and the formation of stem cells within blastocysts. As a new PhD, these years were succeeded by a very happy period of collaboration with senior colleagues, including my teachers and other graduate students. Opportunities in the Institute were endless, as we worked with radioactive tracers, immunological methods, the induction of superovulation and pregnancy in mice and, most important, a constantly advancing understanding of mammalian and human embryological genetics. These wonderful years taught me the basic principles of my field, provided me with many colleagues, and sowed the seeds of later work in several universities and led to 10 exciting years at Bourn Hall.

On leaving Edinburgh, a very different vista opened in the National Institute of Medical Research at Mill Hill, in London, with two senior colleagues, Professor Alan Parkes and Dr Bunny Austin. This widened my horizons from working only with animals to an involvement in the wide world of medical research. I soon learned about the opportunities and restrictions of medical research, and of the astonishingly high incidence of human infertility.

Work on the immunology of reproduction took most of my time, but my thoughts constantly returned to Edinburgh, and to oocyte maturation and the potential of fertilization *in vitro* in humans. Mastering maturation *in vitro* would provide opportunities of studying the meiotic events of diakinesis and metaphase I, and preparing oocytes for fertilization. It was clearly the first essential step to human embryology and clinical IVF, and the availability of morulae and blastocysts *in vitro* might just help in the understanding of normal embryonic growth, and, one day, understanding how to use human stem cells *in vitro* to repair tissues in sick recipients.

Gregory Pincus had worked on the spontaneous maturation of oocytes placed *in vitro*, and while his estimate of 12 h to mature rabbit eggs *in vitro* could be sustained by its similarity to maturation *in vivo*, it was incorrect in relation to humans. I followed similar lines, working with my first clinical colleague, Molly Rose of the Edgware and District General Hospital, London. After several years of failure, it became apparent that human oocytes did not mature after 12 h *in vitro*, unlike those of laboratory animals, rhesus monkeys and baboons. A period of 24 h in culture was essential before the onset of maturation became visible in human oocytes, as chromosomes in diakinesis, the last stage of prophase of meiosis I, could be seen and characterized by its wonderful chromosomal crossovers. Knowledge of this work spread to the press and to my colleagues in the Institute, and led to the first ethical dissensions to human IVF, including those made by the Director of the Institute. The arrival of a new Director, Peter Medawar, changed all this, as he encouraged me to proceed. Now, excited by the discovery of diakinesis, it was a simple matter to judge that the remaining stages to full maturation would require 36 h.

By an unusual coincidence, a letter from John Paul in Glasgow noted my work on embryos and suggested that we should work together for a year with Robin Cole to introduce the world's first mammalian embryo stem cells. This year proved to be really incredible, as John's superb tissue culture included using droplets of medium under paraffin oil and CO_2 incubators to culture embryos and cell lines derived from them, ideas which have spread throughout the world of IVF and stem cell biology. We prepared stem cell lines from disaggregates of the inner cell mass in rabbits, which were everlasting (immortal), were stable enzymically and morphologically and remained diploid. They passed through 200 or more generations and could be cryopreserved. When blastocysts were cultured intact, trophoblast formed a pavement of inner cells. These differentiated into blood islands, muscle, nerves and other tissues in whole-blastocyst cultures[3]. Such results strengthened thoughts of therapeutic human stem cells. A 5-year grant from the Ford Foundation took me to Cambridge, rejoining Alan and Bunny, to study the immunology of reproduction. The thought of working in Cambridge was irresistible. While working hard on immunology, oocyte maturation and fertilization and stem cells remained my major passions. Indeed, the alleviation of many forms of human infertility, the preimplantation genetic diagnosis of inherited human genes and therapeutic stem cells were totally dominating. They all relied on human IVF and the birth of a normal baby to bring them to fruition.

Meanwhile, Patrick Steptoe, who used to play supporting piano accompaniment for Chaplin movies, had decided as a young man to read either music or medicine at Oxford after his Navy service in the Second World War. Choosing medicine, he selected obstetrics and gynecology as his field, and sought a job in London. This was not forthcoming, so he settled in Rochdale, near Oldham, where he was appointed consultant at the nearby Oldham and District General Hospital (ODGH). At first, he had to deal with huge cancers in many of his patients. Very busy with these and other routine operations, he became disillusioned by the difficulty in diagnosing internal disorders in his patients, and the frequent false diagnosis made with the available methods. He was determined to develop a tool enabling him to view organs in the peritoneal and perhaps other body cavities, with highly specialized small instruments passed through small incisions in the abdominal wall. These would allow him to perform some operations and biopsies via laparoscopy, instead of laparotomy.

His search across the world led him to abandon culdoscopy, and to seek the advice of Palmer and Fragenheim in Europe on laparoscopy, then being carried out using hot lamps to illuminate the abdominal cavity. These European teachers taught him the fine details of operating instruments, the use of magnifying lenses and the risks of laparoscopy, especially the use of hot lamps in the abdominal cavity. He returned to Oldham determined to use these skills and end his

long period of failure in producing a safe laparoscope to simplify intra-abdominal approaches.

The introduction of carbon fiber technology to transmit light from a cold source outside the body to illuminate organs brilliantly in the peritoneal cavity did much to improve safety. He developed the use of the pneumoperitoneum, working on cadavers in the mortuary, and felt himself ready with his new diagnostic and perhaps operative laparoscopy by the early 1960s. One of his nurses volunteered to be his first patient. He recorded how he failed totally to visualize any internal organs, and his failure caused him endless misery. The same nurse then requested a second attempt, which succeeded, to the joy of everyone in the operating theatre. He was opening up the new world of endoscopy, yet his work attracted the opposition of many colleagues, who treated him shabbily, simply because they considered laparoscopy to be dangerous. This had been so at one time, but was no longer under Patrick's care. It was curious that both he and I were fighting our own difficult, ethical battles when we met!

Patrick was also disillusioned by the weak methods available to cure his patients' infertility. All he had in his armoury were basal body teperatures to establish the occurrence of ovulation, vaginal smears for diagnosing structure and disease, sperm analyses and surgery, often uncertain, in men and women, with little else. Yet he was liberal in establishing a clinic for sperm donation for infertile couples, and accepted without question his full duties in carrying out abortions at the ODGH, after the UK Abortion Act was passed in the mid-1960s.

Jean Purdy, the third of the trio, trained in Cambridge as a nurse, and often worked in Papworth Hospital near to Bourn Hall. After some time, she became ward sister. Seeking new ventures, she joined me in the Physiological Laboratory, Cambridge, having heard about my plans for a revolutionary new treatment for infertility. I had just completed the full program of oocyte maturation *in vitro* in monkeys, farm animals and humans, and confirmed that human oocytes did require 36–37 h for its completion[4]. Brief intervals in the USA, at Johns Hopkins with Victor McKusick and Howard and Georgeanna Jones, and at Chapel Hill with Robert McGaughey, had provided sufficient human oocytes for analysis of maturation and for initial studies on fertilization *in vitro*. Meanwhile, new scientific and clinical opportunities were emerging in Cambridge. Supervising a series of graduate students there, and encouraging them along specific lines of research, led to the opening study on the preimplantation genetic diagnosis of inherited factors in mammals, and the world's first chimeric mouse offspring, formed by injecting a single stem cell into the blastocoel of mouse blastocysts[5,6]. These discoveries helped to assess the properties of individual stem cells and are used widely today.

Human fertilization *in vitro* was finally achieved in Cambridge. Having noted occasional human eggs with two nuclei, a possible sign of fertilization, Barry Bavister, another graduate student, and I decided to apply his medium, successful already with hamster fertilization, to the attempted fertilization of human eggs *in vitro*[7]. Climbing over the gates to the laboratory late one evening, because I had forgotten to bring my keys, we examined the inseminated eggs one by one. We witnessed all pre- and post-insemination stages, photographed them and calculated the timing of successive events. The clinical application of human IVF was becoming a near certainty. The Press scented a story of secret intrigue when they heard of our climbing the gates, to be deeply disappointed when they found out the true reason! At this stage, while reading *The Lancet* in the Physiological Laboratory library, I discovered the nature of Patrick's work through one of his new papers. I realised that he would be invaluable to us, with his skills permitting the aspiration of mature oocytes from their follicles using his laparoscopy technique. I telephoned him and invited him to join the team. He was delighted to be involved, especially since he urgently wished for new approaches to assist his infertile patients.

Deciding to work together as a team with Patrick placed extreme pressures on me and my Cambridge colleagues. Patient care would obviously be devolved to Oldham in order to have the necessary facilities for the laparoscopic recovery of their oocytes. I would have to travel there to perform all the embryology, and then back to Cambridge for my university duties. All our media and equipment would be organized in Cambridge and then taken to Oldham on the day that oocyte aspirations had been planned. One of my assistants would have to come to help during oocyte collection. I remember with deepest gratitude how several of them volunteered. This duty was finally taken over largely by Jean, who was familiar with scientific and clinical disciplines. She could help both Patrick and me, and collaborate with Muriel Harris

and other members of Patrick's team. A model for stimulating several follicles in infertile patients, based on work on mice in Edinburgh, differed in the substitution of pregnant mare's serum (PMS) by purified human menopausal gonadotropin (hMG), prepared by Organon, on the basis of work by Lunenfeld and Donini. Low doses of hMG and a single injection of human chorionic gonadotropin (hCG) induced the maturation of many human follicles. Mature oocytes were aspirated successfully and rapidly from mature follicles by laparosopy at 36 h post-hCG. They were inseminated and fertilized, and grew through their cleavage stages to beautiful blastocysts at 5 days and wonderfully expanding blastocysts at day 9[8,9]. Their inner cell masses and embryonic disks were packed with stem cells. Several media seemed to be equally effective in sustaining growth to blastocysts, and we chose Ham's F10 with added patient's serum as our standard medium. All stages of the growth of human embryos to implantation had been revealed, to help alleviate certain forms of infertility, make human stem cells using the methods devised in rabbits and introduce human preimplantation genetic diagnosis.

We decided to transfer single blastocysts on day 5 to our patients, using a transcervical catheter. No one had done this before. Catheters were improvised from plastic transfusion cannulas, with smoothed tips. I loaded them with one blastocyst. Patrick inserted the catheter gently through the cervical cavity into the uterine cavity to a position below the tubo-uterine junction. I then gently expelled the embryo from the catheter. There were numerous potential risks of failure. Embryos might accidentally be expelled from the catheter, leak from the uterus after transfer or be infected as the catheter passed through the cervical canal. The endometrial surface might be scraped as the catheter was introduced, difficulties could arise in traversing the cervical canal and scraping the endometrium could block the catheter tip. Transfers were not easy in some patients. Previous sounding of the uterine cavity enabled Patrick to direct the catheter tip to a site just below the uterotubal junction. Plasma samples were collected from the patients on various days post-transfer, ready for pregnancy tests using hCG assays.

Our IVF routine was taking shape, but the first embryo transfers in the early 1970s were followed by disasters involving luteal phase disorders[10,11]. Treating cyclic women with gonadotropins induced an early estrogen-related luteolysis and a deficiency of progesterone. Many of the patients menstruated from as early as day 6 of their luteal phase. Progesterone supplements were obviously required, and would be needed until the placenta took over the endocrine functions of the ovary at approximately 9 weeks postfertilization. We decided to use Primulot Depot®, as the progestogen, since it was supposed to save threatened abortions. Giving it every 5 days from day 3 postaspiration, no patient menstruated until well after their expected time. None became pregnant, month after month. We tested different catheters, reduced uterine contractions, tested different media, varied stimulation protocols, meaured urinary estrogens throughout the entire follicular phase and found a correlation between higher estrogen excretion and early menstruation, and even tested a few transfers direct to the oviduct using laparoscopy, to no avail. This period of immense strain to us was a golden opportunity for our critics, who took full advantage! Patrick and I supported each other as failed transfers accumulated. Lecturing at conferences became much more difficult since we had to explain failure, yet we both remained determined to continue, intent on helping our patients if remotely possible.

Intensive checking of every stage in my procedures revealed nothing wrong with the embryos growing *in vitro*. Out of the blue, after 2 years of failure, Ken Bagshawe in London wrote to say he now had a β-hCG assay. I sent him all the blood samples we had collected from our patients after embryo transfer. He reported back: several of them displayed a blip of β-hCG over the implantation period. We called them biochemical pregnancies. We suspected good embryos had been transferred and then aborted by Primulot depot, and 2 disastrous years of using it led to our decision to reduce and then omit it from our work. A patient with a single transferred blastocyst and progesterone support now had a positive pregancy test. Our dreams of a first IVF baby were shattered when Patrick discovered that the pregnancy was ectopic and had to be removed. This was a disaster indeed, yet I had seen on ultrasound scans the first human fetus established *in vitro*[12]. My media and methods were correct, and our way was now clear. Another patient had a very long luteal phase, with a very long-delayed menstruation, but menstruated some weeks later. Patrick then developed prostatic cancer.

Now it was obviously necessary to work full-time on IVF; I took sabbatical leave from Cambridge to work continuously with Patrick and his team in Oldham. He only had a few months before his retirement at 65. It was essential to improve our control over the duration of the luteal phase. We had employed hMG and hCG consistently, yet their use opened up too many problems. It induced severely short luteal phases, especially in patients with higher levels of urinary estrogens. Working full-time with Patrick enabled different forms of ovarian stimulation to be tested and new forms of stimulation to be learned, guaranteeing a normal luteal phase. High levels of prolactin had become topical, so we combined bromocriptine with hMG. Embryo transfer to a non-stimulated uterus seemed obvious, so one trial was performed with a single blastocyst donated to another couple. Stimulation with clomiphene produced excellent luteal phases, so we combined it with hMG. Clomiphene/hMG was integrated with the transfer of spermatozoa and one or two oocytes to recipients' ampullae, i.e. the first gamete intrafallopian transfer (GIFT). Oocytes and embryos were cryopreserved and seemed to have a good morphology on thawing.

Could we use the natural menstrual cycle? We felt sufficiently skilled to handle single mature oocytes and grow them *in vitro*. It would be essential to find a very rapid assay to measure the onset of the luteinizing hormone (LH) surge to control the timing of oocyte maturation. Bridget Mason suggested using HiGonavis®, a simple sedimentation method for assaying LH, and I modified it to produce a very rapid assay. Urine samples were collected from patients before their rising body temperatures signified the onset of ovulation, and applying HiGonavis to urine samples collected eight times throughout the day, from about day 9 of their follicular phase, gave us a reasonably reliable indication of the onset of the LH surge. Lesley and John Brown were the second couple for natural cycle IVF. Their single egg was aspirated, inseminated and placed in overnight culture within 15 min, and led to the birth of Louise. Concentrating on this success led to more than 30 further cases of natural cycle IVF. At least four clinical pregnancies were achieved, this time within a safe luteal phase. Louise and Alistair were the first two IVF babies in the world. Another fetus was triploid, despite a virtual absence of any tripronucleate eggs in our Oldham studies. The fourth pregnancy was lost when its parents were on a walking holiday in the

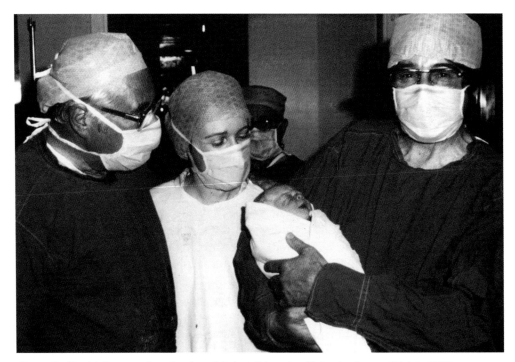

Figure 2 Patrick Steptoe, Jean Purdy and Robert Edwards with Louise Brown, 25 July 1978

hills above Skipton soon after amniocentesis for chromosomal analysis. The mother went into spontaneous labor on a hilltop, and a healthy male fetus was delivered at about 22 weeks and died after 4 days.

The birth of Louise Brown in 1978[13] (Figure 2), achieved by a small team, signified the end of these formative years, where serious competition from any other clinic had been totally lacking. I had been very surprised that virtually no competitors challenged our work or improved on it throughout 10 years. IVF clinics could have easily been established at Johns Hopkins or Chapel Hill in the 1960s, since the staff were fully trained when I had left and knew about oocyte maturation *in vitro*. For the three of us, Patrick, Jean and myself, IVF could no longer be conducted between Cambridge and Oldham. It had to be transferred to Cambridge, and a search of several suitable properties resulted in the choice and purchase of Bourn Hall in 1978 as a potential and large IVF center. It stood proudly, ancient and beautiful in its grounds. Delays in its conversion arose through fears that many abnormal babies would be born, so our first financial sponsor pulled out of the deal abruptly, overnight. Rejected financially once, we were then rejected in succession by various other venture capitalists. During this period, an IVF baby was born in

Australia. Financial problems were overcome by Alan Dexter, our new Business Director, after many months of delay, and Bourn Hall became among the first modern high-tech companies in Cambridge, linked to the University for research and teaching. It became an international symbol of assisted human conception in 1980, inheriting the mantle of the original work. Staff eager to work there included John Webtser, Patrick's assistant, who helped to develop a center capable of treating hundreds, and even thousands of patients annually. The embryology laboratories were built in temporary cabins (Figure 3), which lasted just long enough for us to build new facilities 5 years later.

Bourn Hall now became dominant in IVF for several years. Starting with natural cycles, dozens of pregnancies were established within a month or so. We were back in business! It was essential to conceive as many children as possible, and the rooms and corridors of Bourn Hall soon filled up with patients from far and wide. Over the next 12–18 months, more pregnancies were achieved at Bourn Hall than in the rest of the world combined. Many new studies were carried out, on male infertility, oocyte donation, cryopreservation, bacteriology, hormonal patterns, surrogate births, treating patients with spinal injuries, etc., far too many to discuss here. Simon Fishel and Jacques Cohen joined

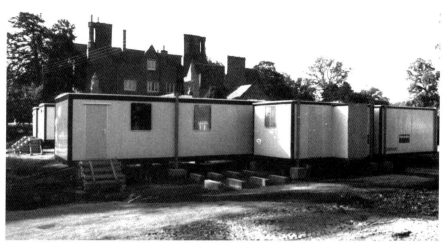

Figure 3 The temporary Portakabins housing the wards, operating theater and laboratories at Bourn Hall in the early 1980s

the embryology team, and John Webster was joined by several colleagues including Peter Brinsden for a short while. Louise received an IVF sister, and pregnancies conceived at Bourn Hall were established worldwide, including the first IVF babies in the USA, Germany, several Middle Eastern countries and others elsewhere. PhD students came from Cambridge, and occasionally elsewhere. The Hall and its grounds responded as a place for fun and fireworks. Everything was progressing wonderfully, even branching into London. Out of the blue, however, Jean developed a melanoma, and Patrick's prostatic cancer was confirmed.

Even as the lights of the Hall began to dim, it was clear that our IVF message had succeeded, perhaps beyond our wildest dreams. A thousand children had been conceived in the Hall by 1988, and IVF was now practiced worldwide. The early dream was ending, but Bourn Hall maintained its traditions. The UK Government passed liberal legislation in the late 1980s, accepting all the work we had done on human IVF. Bourn Hall may now be slimmer, but its luster remains.

1.2

The Bourn Hall story continues

Peter R. Brinsden

The team that Steptoe and Edwards set up at Bourn Hall was able to continue its pioneering work helping infertile couples to have children. After the first year, *The Times* (London) newspaper (6th October 1981) reported: 'Five New Test Tube Babies and Sixty More on the Way'. Although other *in vitro* fertilization (IVF) clinics were opening around the world, by the end of 1981, Bourn Hall had achieved more pregnancies than any other clinic. Certain highlights of the first 24 years of the life of Bourn Hall Clinic are worth recording.

1980

- Bourn Hall Clinic opened its doors to its first patients in October.

- The clinical, operating and laboratory facilities were all located in temporary Portakabins (see Figure 3, Chapter 1.1)

- Infertile couples from all over the world sought treatment, as Bourn Hall was the only clinic to offer such specialized treatments.

1981

- The First Bourn Hall Meeting on IVF was held at the Clinic (Figure 1). This was the world's first international meeting on IVF, at which many of the leading pioneers met to discuss the issues of the day.

1982

- Bourn Hall achieved its first 100 IVF pregnancies.

- Ms Gill Williams introduced the concept of ovarian follicular scanning by ultrasound at Bourn Hall.

- Parts of the old Hall became used for the first time, and the Endocrinology Laboratories were opened in the Tudor stable block.

1983

- The cryopreservation program was initiated.

- Design work began on the Clinic's new in-patient ward and operating-theater block.

- The first papers on the data of frozen embryo replacements were published.

1984

- The first babies were born at Bourn Hall from frozen–thawed human embryos.

1985

- Bourn Hall was host to the Second Bourn Hall Meeting on IVF.

- Dr Rajat Goswamy joined Bourn Hall, and introduced the new technique of transvesical ultrasound-directed oocyte recovery, and later that year, the transvaginal technique.

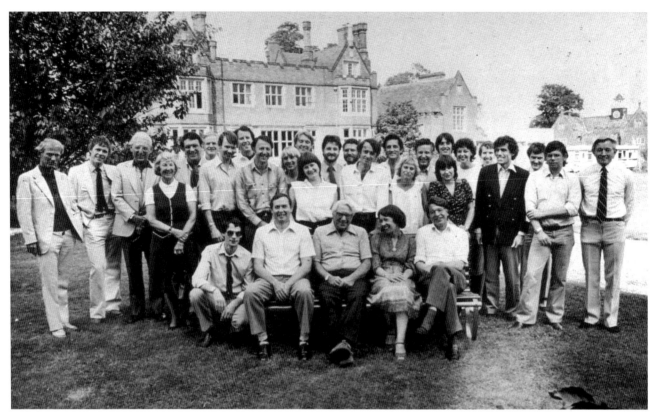

Figure 1   The First Bourn Hall and the World's First Conference on IVF in 1981

1986

- Drs Howles and Macnamee publish the first paper on tonic levels of luteinizing hormone in the follicular phase, which led to the use of gonadotropin releasing hormone (GnRH) analogs at Bourn Hall.

- A further milestone in freezing technology occurred with the birth of the second frozen embryo 'time-warp twin'.

- Building work began on the new ward block.

1987

- The Clinic helped to organize the first UK Meeting of the European Society of Human Reproduction and Embryology, held in Cambridge.

1988

- Mr Patrick Steptoe died on the 21st March 1988.

- Dr Patrick Taylor was appointed Medical Director of Bourn Hall. Professor Robert Edwards remained Scientific Director.

- The Hallam Medical Centre in London, founded by Dr Bridget Mason, merged with Bourn Hall to form Bourn–Hallam, at that time the world's largest assisted conception treatment group, performing about 2500 assisted reproductive technologies (ART) cycles a year.

- Bourn Hall converted to a fully out-patient based treatment service.

- The Bourn–Hallam Group was acquired by Ares-Serono, now Serono International SA, a multinational pharmaceutical company, based in Geneva.

- Bourn Hall celebrated the birth of its 1000th IVF baby.

1989

- Patrick Taylor returned to Canada and Peter Brinsden was appointed Medical Director.

- To commemorate the life and work of Patrick Steptoe, Bourn Hall Clinic invited their 1400 babies and parents to join in a dedication ceremony and celebration hosted by Professor Robert

Edwards and Mrs Sheena Steptoe. They opened the new ward block which is dedicated to the memory of Patrick Steptoe (Figure 2). Over 660 children and their parents attended the party in the grounds of Bourn Hall (Figure 3).

- A new training and conference center was completed at Bourn Hall, and Professor Edwards, as Scientific Director, inaugurated the first foundation course in assisted human reproduction.

- With the increasing proliferation of IVF units world-wide, Bourn–Hallam had become a place where not only childless couples came, but also clinicians and scientists wishing to gain experience of the latest techniques in assisted conception.

1990

- The Bourn–Hallam Group's 2500th IVF baby was born: Robert Patrick Peter, named after Bourn Hall's founders and the doctor who carried out the successful procedure.

- Bourn Hall launched a number of new collaborative projects, including one with Stoke Mandeville Hospital to help spinally injured men to become fathers, and another with Addenbrooke's Hospital, Cambridge, to provide infertility treatment for National Health Service patients.

- Dr Bridget Mason retired as the Medical Director of the Hallam Medical Center and John Yovich was appointed and held the post until August 1991, when he returned to Australia to continue his work in his unit in Perth.

1991

- Professor Edwards retired as Scientific Director of Bourn–Hallam, thus severing the last direct links with Bourn Hall's original founders. He was succeeded by Dr Mike Macnamee.

- Professor John Aitken, who at that time led the Medical Research Council's Research Programme in Gamete and Developmental Biology in Edinburgh, was appointed as Scientific Consultant to Bourn–Hallam's expanding research program in reproductive medicine.

1992

- Bourn Hall, as a wholly private clinic, developed contracts with the National Health Service in the

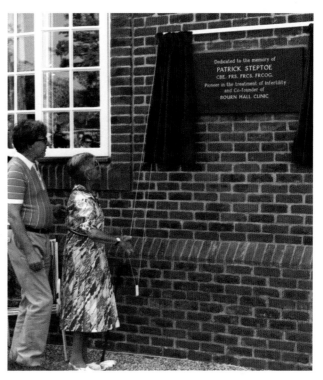

Figure 2 Sheena Steptoe and Robert Edwards opening the new wing of Bourn Hall, dedicated to the memory of Patrick Steptoe, in 1989

United Kingdom to provide treatment for patients funded by their local Health Authorities.

- The first edition of *A Textbook of In Vitro Fertilization and Assisted Reproduction* (popularly known as 'The Bourn Hall Textbook') was published, edited by Peter Brinsden and Paul Rainsbury, the then Deputy Medical Director.

1993

- Bourn Hall and the Department of Obstetrics and Gynaecology at the University of Cambridge hosted the Annual Meeting of the British Fertility Society.

- Phase 1 of the newly established Clinical Pharmacology Unit, with 36 beds, was opened.

1994

- The Hallam Clinic, the London-based sister clinic to Bourn Hall, changed management and became The London Women's Clinic.

- Phase 2 of the Clinical Pharmacology Unit opened.

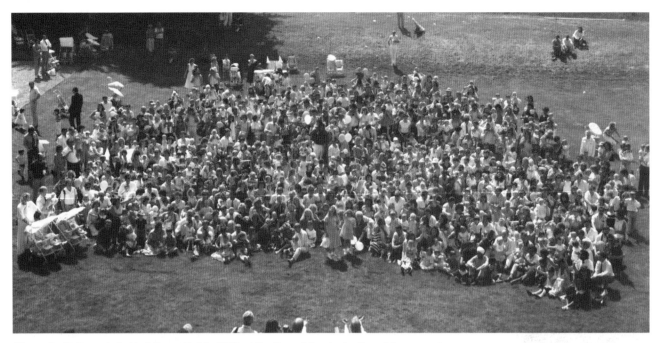

Figure 3 Baby party held at Bourn Hall in 1989, at the time of the dedication of the new wing

1995

- Bourn Hall hosted the Third Bourn Hall Conference on IVF.

1996

- The new Clinical Investigation Unit opened and conducted a large hormone replacement therapy (HRT) trial.

1997

- Bourn Hall hosted the Fourth Bourn Hall Conference on IVF, arranged by Professors Jean Cohen, Lars Hamberger and Howard Jones, with the support of Dr Colin Howles and the Ares-Serono Symposium Foundation (Figure 4).

1999

- The second edition of *A Textbook of In Vitro Fertilization and Assisted Reproduction* was published.

2003

- Bourn Hall celebrated the 25th birthday of Louise Brown, with Robert Edwards, Alastair Macdonald (the second IVF 'baby' and first boy) and 1100 Bourn Hall 'babies', varying in ages from 2 weeks to 25 years (Figure 5)!

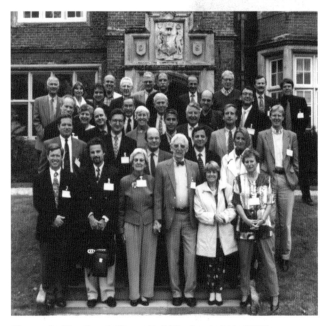

Figure 4 The Fourth Bourn Hall Meeting held in 1997

THE BOURN HALL PROGRAM

Bourn Hall provides a number of teaching courses each year, covering different areas of interest in assisted reproductive technologies (ART), from general ART,

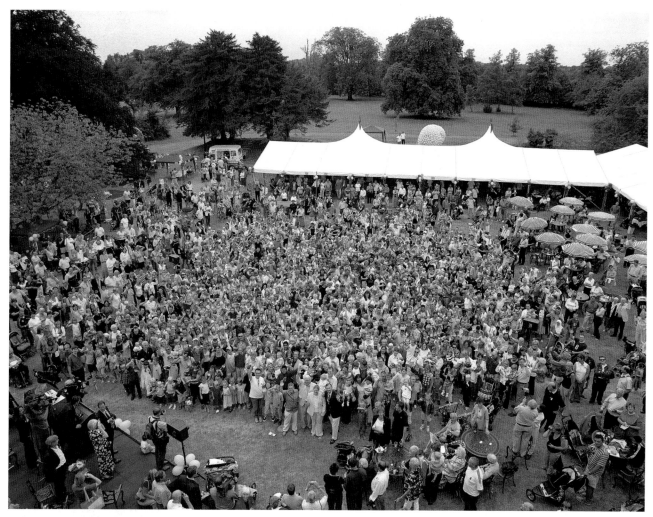

Figure 5 Robert Edwards with Louise Brown and Alastair Macdonald (front of group) at Louise's 25th birthday celebration at Bourn Hall in July 2003

to more specialized programs on cryopreservation and intracytoplasmic sperm injection. The Program Director is Dr Kay Elder, who is both a clinician and a scientist, as well as a founding member of Alpha. The aim of these courses is to increase the knowledge and skills of clinicians, scientists, nurses and others involved in the care of infertile couples. By the end of 2004, more than 3900 doctors, scientists and nurses from around the world had attended courses at Bourn Hall.

The clinical services provided for infertile couples by Bourn Hall now include:

- Diagnostic facilities for the investigation of infertility;

- Ovulation induction and monitoring of treatment cycles;

- Intrauterine insemination with monitoring of superovulation;

- Follicular and early pregnancy ultrasound scanning;

- *In vitro* fertilization (IVF);

- The investigation and treatment of male factor infertility, including:
    - Intracytoplasmic sperm injection (ICSI);
    - Percutaneous epididymal aspiration of sperm (PESA);
    - Testicular aspiration of sperm (TESA);
    - Treatment of men with ejaculatory disorders, including spinal cord injured men;
    - Cryopreservation of sperm and testicular tissue;
    - A donor insemination program;

- Embryo and oocyte cryopreservation;

- Ovum and embryo donation programs;

- An IVF surrogacy program.

In the following chapters, we describe our current approaches to all these treatment options. While we do not for one moment believe that we have the answers to all the problems and dilemmas posed by this most fascinating of specialties, as a Clinic, we have had approaching 25 years' experience in the field, and many specialists from all over the world have found it beneficial to share these experiences with us. This third edition of our textbook is therefore based on our teaching courses, describing our current clinical and scientific practices, with additional contributions from a number of distinguished friends and colleagues, many of whom have been associated with Bourn Hall through our founders since the very earliest days of IVF.

REFERENCES

1. Edwards RG. Meiosis in ovarian oocytes of adult mammals. Nature (London) 1962; 196: 446–50
2. Edwards RG, Sharpe DJ. Social values and research in human embryology. Nature (London) 1971; 231: 87–91
3. Cole RJ, Edwards RG, Paul J. Cytodifferentiation and embryogenesis in cell colonies and tissue cultures derived from ova and blastocysts of the rabbit. Dev Biol 1966; 13: 385–407
4. Edwards RG. Maturation in vitro of human ovarian oocytes. Lancet 1965; 2: 926–9
5. Gardner RL, Edwards RG. Control of the sex ratio at full term in the rabbit by transferring sexed blastocysts. Nature (London) 1968; 218: 346–8
6. Gardner RL. Mouse chimeras obtained by the injection of cells into the blastocyst. Nature (London) 1968; 220: 596–7
7. Edwards RG, Bavister BD, Steptoe PC. Early stages of fertilization in vitro of human oocytes matured in vitro. Nature (London) 1969; 221: 632–5
8. Steptoe PC, Edwards RG, Purdy JM. Human blastocysts grown in culture. Nature (London) 1971; 229: 132–3
9. Edwards RG, Surani MAH. The primate blastocyst and its environment. Uppsala J Med 1978; 22 (Suppl): 39–50
10. Steptoe PC, Edwards RG, Purdy JM. Clinical aspects of pregnancies established with cleaving embryos grown in vitro. Br J Obstet Gynaecol 1980; 87: 757–68
11. Edwards RG, Steptoe PC, Purdy JM. Establishing full-term human pregnancies using cleaving embryos grown in vitro. Br J Obstet Gynaecol 1980; 87: 737–56
12. Steptoe PC, Edwards RG. Reimplantation of a human embryo with subsequent tubal pregnancy. Lancet 1976; 1: 880–2
13. Steptoe PC, Edwards RG. Birth after reimplantation of a human embryo. Lancet 1978; 2: 366

2

Patient selection and management

Amir Lass

Normal fertility is usually defined as achieving a pregnancy within 2 years by regular coital exposure[1]. It is estimated that about 84% of couples will achieve pregnancy in the first year and 92% within 2 years[2]. There are variations in the incidence of infertility in different regions and countries[3]. Although the prevalence of infertility has probably remained constant in the past two decades, attendance of patients for fertility treatment has increased dramatically all over the world, with, in parallel, the creation of more new fertility centers. In the UK alone there are currently 78 centers performing more than 30 000 IVF cycles a year[4]. This observation is probably the result of the higher profile of infertility issues in the public arena, manifested by intensive coverage in newspapers, magazines, radio and television programs. Moreover, in the past, and in many cultures, infertility was associated with shame and guilt, and many couples tended to hide the problem. Thankfully, this phenomenon is disappearing. In addition, the abundance of treatment facilities, and easier access to fertility specialists, has increased the awareness of patients and health-care providers who seek expert assistance much sooner. In only a minority of cases is one partner completely sterile, thus eliminating the possibility of a natural pregnancy occurring (i.e. azoospermia, bilateral tubal occlusion, absence of uterus, anovulation); fertility impairment is therefore seen in both partners more frequently than expected[5].

ASSESSMENT OF COUPLES BEFORE ASSISTED CONCEPTION TREATMENT

Most patients are referred for assisted conception treatment (ACT) in a tertiary center such as Bourn Hall Clinic by their general practitioner (GP), gynecologist or andrologist after completion of basic infertility investigations. A substantial proportion of these patients have already undergone some infertility treatment, such as ovulation induction, intrauterine insemination or tubal surgery. Moreover, some couples have had treatment by *in vitro* fertilization (IVF) cycles in other centers.

In February 2004, the National Institute of Clinical Excellence (NICE) in the UK published a clinical guideline for fertility assessment and treatment for couples with fertility problems[6]. The following protocols and recommendations based on the treatment at Bourn Hall Clinic are in line with this guideline.

General condition

We encourage both partners to attend the primary consultation in the clinic together, and thoroughly investigate them as a 'unit'. We ask them to supply any relevant information and test results that are in their possession, with a cover letter from their GP or consultant. In this interview, a detailed family and medical history is obtained to rule out other health problems.

The woman's weight is an important factor in fertility potential, and probably the best measure is the body mass index (BMI). Normal acceptable BMI[7] is in the range of 18.5–30 kg/m². Being both overweight and underweight can affect normal ovulation, alter response to superovulation with gonadotropins, reduce the chance of conceiving, increase miscarriage rate[8,9], increase pregnancy complications and neonatal morbidity and increase the risks involved in anesthesia and surgical retrieval of oocytes[10,11]. Patients whose BMI is not in the recommended range are referred to a dietician in order to achieve that goal before they are allowed to continue with assisted conception treatment. In many cases, being overweight is associated with polycystic ovarian syndrome (PCOS), and further evaluation and treatment are discussed in Chapter 8.

Being overweight and obese also have an effect on the fertility of the male partner. The total number of normal-motile sperm is reduced[9,12], with more sperm DNA fragmentation[13] as well as erectile dysfunction disturbances[14].

Any potential exposure to occupational hazards, such as toxins, irradiated material, etc., should be evaluated. Habits such as alcohol consumption and smoking, as well as prescribed, over-the-counter and recreational drug use, should be determined. While there are conflicting reports on the effect of alcohol consumption on female fertility[15,16], it is clear that excessive consumption is harmful for the fetus. Heavy drinking has been shown to have a detrimental effect on semen quality[17,18]. There is a significant association between smoking and reduced fertility among female smokers[19,20], which might even include passive smoking[21].

Due attention is given to exclude conditions that can contribute to the infertility, such as diabetes mellitus, endocrinopathies or autoimmune disorders. The menstrual history is recorded and any previous investigations and pregnancies are noted. Although sometimes embarrassing, it is important to verify the frequency of intercourse and its timing related to the menstrual cycle. Coitus every 2–3 days is likely to maximize the overall chance of natural conception, as spermatozoa survive in the female genital tract for up to 7 days after insemination[22]. Any sexual problems such as impotence or premature ejaculation must be excluded. It is still surprising that inappropriate intercourse due to sexual problems or lack of knowledge contributes up to 6% of the causes of infertility. It is not rare to discover that some couples with sexual problems present themselves as suffering from infertility.

A complete physical and pelvic examination of the female and genital examination of the male (Chapter 3) are an integral part of the primary consultation.

Our policy is to assess patients promptly, without unnecessary repetition of previous examinations, and to offer the appropriate treatment to suitable patients.

The basic groups of investigations required are shown in Table 1.

Laboratory examinations

Couples are routinely required to be tested for human immunodeficiency virus (HIV) within the 6 months preceding treatment, and they are offered the option of counseling regarding the implication of this blood test. Similarly, it is essential that they have been tested for hepatitis B (HBV) and hepatitis C virus (HCV) antibodies. While a few years ago it was common practice to deny assisted reproductive technology (ART) treatment to patients who tested positive for HIV, the current trend, due to low vertical transmission of the disease (~2%) if the appropriate measures are taken, such as antiretroviral medication, elective Cesarean section (CS) and avoidance of breast-feeding, is that IVF is a reasonable option if required. It is advisable, however, that patients with positive results are referred for specialist counseling, and that the ART treatment, if required, is performed in specially designated centers that have appropriate expertise and facilities to provide safe risk-reduction investigation and treatment[23,24].

Where relevant, the woman is tested for rubella immunity; if the test is negative, she is strongly advised to be immunized before continuing with fertility treatment. However, as the vaccine is a live attenuated virus, natural conception or fertility treatment should be deferred by 1 month[25].

Cervical cytology is obtained if she has not been tested within the preceding 3 years or if clinical examination suggests the presence of a suspicious lesion. It has been reported that the incidence of abnormal cervical smears in infertile women ranges between 5 and 13%[26]. Routine high-vaginal or cervical swab cultures are not usually taken unless there are symptoms or

Table 1 Investigation of infertility

General	body mass index (BMI)* HIV antibodies* hepatitis B and C antibodies* hemoglobin* *Rubella immu* *Sickle cell*
Ovulation	basal temperature charts cycle day 2–6: serum LH, FSH, estradiol (E₂), prolactin day-21 progesterone* serial ultrasound scans of the ovaries
Ovarian reserve	cycle day 2–6: serum FSH, estradiol (E₂)* *AFC & AMH* ovarian volume by ultrasound
Sperm	semen analysis 2–3 samples*
Tubal and peritoneal factors	hysterosalpingogram laparoscopy
Uterus	hysterosalpingogram ultrasound* hysteroscopy D&C with histology of endometrium Doppler scan of uterine arteries

*Tests that are considered essential, the rest are optional depending on clinical necessity; HIV, human immunodeficiency virus; LH, luteinizing hormone; FSH, follicle stimulating hormone; D&C, dilatation and curettage

signs of infection. The hemoglobin level is estimated and should be more than 10 g before embarking upon IVF.

Ovulation assessment

Normal ovulation is defined by rupture of the follicle with release of an oocyte[27]. The only true evidence of ovulation is a subsequent pregnancy, and, regretfully, there is no established method to confirm completion of ovulation. The most common means of assessing ovulation in the menstruating woman include: basal body-temperature recordings, cervical mucus changes, luteinizing hormone (LH) surge testing and serial ultrasound scans. Fortuitous laparoscopic examination may demonstrate actual ovulation or the ovarian stigma.

Temperature recordings are still a mainstay of many infertility clinics, and something which many infertile women may use before seeking the advice of a general medical practitioner. Such charts are rarely 'textbook' in result, and are notoriously difficult for couples to interpret in helping them to decide on the best time for coitus. A biphasic temperature chart indicates that at least some progesterone is being produced, and even a luteal phase plateau suggests that the progesterone output is satisfactory, while multiple peaks may indicate 'luteal phase deficiency'. Hence, as this method is unreliable, its use is not recommended (NICE)[6].

Home-testing of morning urine samples for the LH surge with one of the easily available proprietary kits may give more definite answers and more accurate timing[28]. However, patients do not always find them easy to interpret. Furthermore, some may notice a lack of correspondence between cervical mucus changes, temperature response and the LH surge. Serum progesterone level > 16 nmol/l a week after the LH surge or mid-cycle temperature change is indicative of adequate ovulation[28], but only serial ultrasound scans or fortuitous direct inspection will confirm that the dominant follicle has ruptured. Even then, there is the possibility that the egg may still be trapped within the follicle (a not uncommon experience of gynecologists used to laparoscopic oocyte recovery).

While progesterone levels can be measured on day 21 in a 28-day cycle of regularly menstruating women, timing of the test may be performed later if the woman has a longer cycle and adjusted to the individual circumstances.

Anovulatory infertility is the most common cause of female infertility, often characterized by irregular menstruation and amenorrhea or oligomenorrhea; however, ovulatory dysfunction may occur coincidentally with apparently regular cycles. Women who suffer from primary amenorrhea have usually been evaluated previously and not in the context of infertility, the investigation and management of which are outside the scope of this chapter.

The ovulatory disorders are classified into three groups by the World Health Organization (WHO):

(1) Group 1: hypogonadotropic hypogonadism;

(2) Group 2: normogonadotropic anovulation;

(3) Group 3: hypergonadotropic hypogonadism.

We may take a blood sample between days 2 and 6 of the menstrual cycle for: prolactin, follicle stimulating hormone (FSH), luteinizing hormone (LH) and estradiol (E_2) to identify the four main causes of ovulatory failure: hypogonadotropic hypogonadism, normogonadotropic anovulation, hypergonadotropic hypogonadism and hyperlactinemia.

WHO group 1 Hypogonadotropic hypogonadism is usually idiopathic, and is a result of primary hypothalamic or pituitary failure. Other causes include excessive stress or exercise, malnutrition or underweight[29]. This group accounts for up to 10% of ovulatory disorders. This condition is best diagnosed by low LH and FSH levels (< 5 mIU/ml) and a low estradiol level (< 40 g/ml)[30], along with a negative gestagen challenge test (no withdrawal bleeding).

WHO group 2 In normogonadotropic anovulation, the majority of patients are likely to have polycystic ovaries. This condition is discussed in Chapter 8.

WHO group 3 Hypergonadotropic hypogonadism is defined by raised FSH levels (> 20 mIU/ml) and low estrogen, indicating ovarian failure, and accounts for ~5% of ovulatory disorders. It may occur at any age. While in younger women the cause is mostly genetic (i.e. Turner's syndrome), in older women near the end of their reproductive life a raised FSH level is due to aging of the ovary and therefore imminent menopause. If the woman is < 40 years old, she is classified as suffering from premature ovarian failure (POF), an entity that applies to 1% of the population[31]. Patients younger than 30 years of age should have a karyotype determination. The incidence of chromosomal abnormalities in POF patients with secondary amenorrhea is estimated to be 2–5%. The presence of a Y chromosome requires surgical removal of the gonads, as there is a 25% risk of malignant tumor formation[32,33]. The most common cause of POF in adults is probably autoimmune failure, and investigations for autoimmune disorders should take place. Other rare causes of high level gonadotropins are summarized in Table 2.

Prolactin measurement Although raised prolactin levels have been found in up to 11% of ovulatory infertile women[34], there was no significant correlation between its levels, progesterone levels and/or cumulative pregnancy rates[35,36]. Therefore the NICE guideline recommends that prolactin levels should not be routinely measured if there is no ovulatory disorder, galactorrhea or pituitary tumor.

If the prolactin level is raised to more than 800 mIU/ml[37], then a repeat estimation is made and a new sample sent also for estimation of thyroid stimulating hormone level. If there is occult hypothyroidism, then a thyroid function test, including measurement of thyroid autoantibodies, should be performed. Although stress remains the commonest cause of a rise in prolactin level, polycystic ovaries (see Chapter 5), psychotherapeutic medication and the premenopausal state must be considered, as well as the comparatively rare pituitary prolactinoma. Galactorrhea may be present.

Table 2 Causes of hypergonadotropic hypogonadism (World Health Organization group 3)
Idiopathic
Concomitant autoimmune disease thyroiditis, myasthenia gravis, idiopathic thrombocytopenic purpura (ITP), rheumatoid arthritis, adrenal insufficiency, vitiligo, autoimmune hemolytic anemia
Resistant ovary syndrome
Previous surgery
Chemotherapy and/or radiotherapy
Infection
Galactosemia
17-Hydroxylase deficiency
Tumors producing gonadotropins: lung cancer, pituitary adenoma

ASSESSMENT OF OVARIAN RESERVE

A major factor in successful IVF treatment is the ability of the ovary to respond to gonadotropin stimulation and to develop several follicles. That response reflects the ovarian function or 'ovarian reserve'. A reduction of ovarian reserve is apparently due to reduced numbers of ovarian primordial follicles, from about a million at birth, to over 250 000 at menarche, to very few at the end of reproductive life. This loss accelerates around the age of 37 and precedes the menopause by 10–12 years[38,39]. There is a wide variation in the number and rate of depletion of follicles.

Some women fail to respond to gonadotropin stimulation, and the cycles are canceled. This is common, particularly in older women. Obviously, it would be clinically and economically very helpful if we could predict a poor response before treatment.

Age of the female partner is an important factor in fertility, and as a woman becomes older her fertility diminishes[40–42]. More women in developed countries[43] are now choosing to delay starting a family for various social reasons. Therefore, one can assume that the age of those attending for infertility treatments will increase[44]. Although many women are fertile into their mid-40s, most are not, but the precise reason for this loss of fertility is not understood. There are thought to be a number of factors, including a decline in the frequency of intercourse[44], decreasing numbers of primordial follicles[45], poorer oocyte quality[46], problems in the uterus[47] and embryo loss sometimes due to chromosomal abnormalities[48]. At Bourn Hall we do not limit the upper age for treatment as long as women are not in their menopause phase. We explain to patients at the end of their reproductive lives about their very low chance of conceiving. Recently, in a large observational study in the UK comprising 1427 started cycles, around 12% of treatment cycles were performed in women of 40 years of age or older, while the average age was 36.3 years[49].

Age and regularity of menses alone are unreliable ways of predicting ovarian reserve. Biological age is more important than chronological age[50]. In the aging process, the ovaries become progressively less responsive to exogenous gonadotropins, until they are totally refractory at the time of the menopause. Oddly, the ovaries cease to respond to stimulation even though some follicles still remain in the stroma. Ovarian reserve may be evaluated by the following.

Basal serum FSH levels

Once the ovary is more or less exhausted, increased pituitary production of FSH follows. This event takes place a few years before the actual menopause. Currently, the FSH level is the best marker to assess ovarian reserve and for predicting response to superovulation, with a good correlation to pregnancy rates[51–53]. However, lack of a clear cut-off point, huge variations between different laboratories and monthly variations in FSH secretion mean that FSH measurement is of only limited value in assessing the prognosis of IVF treatment[46,54]. Increasing chronological age affects mainly implantation and pregnancy rates, whereas relatively young patients with elevated FSH levels have a higher chance of cycle cancelation due to poor response but fair to good implantation rates[55].

Age

At Bourn Hall Clinic we check the day-2 FSH level in the treatment cycle of all patients of 38 years or older and women with previously reduced response to superovulation. Our cut-off point is 12 IU/ml, and if the level is above that threshold we postpone treatment and check the FSH again in the next cycle. Once the FSH levels start to fluctuate, there is already a decreased ovarian reserve, and it is not clear whether starting stimulation in a later month with 'normal' FSH levels will give a better result[56]. We have shown that, in women whose early follicular phase FSH levels were raised to > 12 mIU/ml, there was an increased risk (> 50%) that in subsequent cycles levels would remain raised, and it was not possible to predict which individuals would have favorable FSH levels. If the cycle day-2 FSH returned to a 'normal' level of < 12 mIU/ml, women aged 40 and above had substantial cycle cancelation rates (43%), but patients who achieved the stage of embryo transfer had a good chance of conceiving, regardless of their age[57]. It is important for each fertility center to define their cut-off point, depending on their experience and results.

Basal estradiol level

Measurement of basal estradiol (E_2) in addition to FSH might improve the ability to predict fertility potential compared with basal FSH and chronological age alone[58–60]. Cycle day-3 E_2 levels of less than 80 pg/ml with normal FSH levels in women aged 38–42 give a good prognosis of successful treatment[58].

Other tests that are not widely used clinically and are performed only in special circumstances in our clinic include the following.

Ultrasonic measurements: ovarian volume, follicular count and stromal blood flow

Increased age is associated with decreased ovarian volume. Transvaginal measurement of ovarian volume is quick, accurate and cost-effective. Decreased ovarian volume is a sign of ovarian aging that may be observed earlier than a rise in FSH levels. Small ovaries are associated with a poor response to superovulation and a high cancelation rate in IVF[61–63]. Other researchers have claimed that a low antral follicular count is associated with poor outcome[64]. Since the introduction of transvaginal pulsed color Doppler ultrasound, numerous researchers have investigated the uterine artery blood flow and the implantation site, but only limited information is available on the intraovarian or extraovarian blood circulation in the context of reproductive medicine. The last two tests are not in routine practice in the clinic. The role of ultrasound in reproductive medicine is discussed in depth in Chapter 10.

Basal inhibin B level

Inhibin B is a heterodimeric glycoprotein released by the granulosa cells of the follicle. A recent study has shown that women with low day-3 inhibin B levels (< 45 pg/ml) had a poorer response to superovulation for IVF and were less likely to conceive a clinical pregnancy. It has also shown that a decrease in inhibin B probably precedes the increase in FSH levels[65]; however, the role of inhibin B in predicting pregnancy outcome is unclear[66,67].

Anti-Mullerian hormone levels

Anti-Mullerian hormone (AMH), a member of the transforming growth factor (TGF) family, was identified as a factor that causes regression of the Mullerian ducts during male fetal development. In females, AMH, also known as Mullerian inhibiting substance, is produced in the granulosa cells of ovarian follicles and is secreted into the circulation. A few early studies demonstrated that serum levels decrease with age earlier than other markers such as FSH and antral follicle count[68].

Dynamic tests

The clomiphene challenge test (CCT) was first described in 1987 by Navot and colleagues[69]. This simple test consists of measuring serum FSH on day 3 and again on cycle day 10 after administration of 100 mg of clomiphene from day 5 to day 9. An abnormal test is defined by elevated FSH levels on cycle day 10. This provocative test unmasks patients who might not be detected by basal FSH screening alone. An abnormal test is highly predictive of diminished ovarian reserve in natural cycles, during ovulation induction and in IVF[70–72]. It is superior to early follicular FSH screening, but has poor predictive value in women over 40 in terms of response to superovulation and pregnancy rate in ART cycles[70,71].

The gonadotropin releasing hormone (GnRH)-agonist challenge test has been proposed recently[73,74]. In this test, a change in E_2 levels from cycle day 2 to day 3 is measured after subcutaneous administration of leuprolide acetate[73], or an FSH increase 2 h after buserelin injection[74]. However, although the dynamic tests are strongly predictive of stimulation outcome, it is not yet clear whether they are more useful than measurement of basal FSH in predicting IVF outcome.

Ovarian biopsy

Regretfully, the predictive power of all these tests alone or in combination is quite limited. This lack of sufficient and adequate tests to predict the ovarian reserve led researchers to assess directly the non-renewable pool of primordial follicles. Obviously, the only definite way of slicing the ovary and counting all follicles in its entire cortex is out of the question. We have suggested a novel method of quantifying the number of small follicles in ovarian biopsies from infertile patients[75]. The promising results of a negative correlation between patient's age and follicular density, and fewer follicles in unexplained infertility compared with tubal infertility, led this author to suggest considering ovarian biopsy as a diagnostic tool quite early in infertility investigations[76].

However, two recent studies have demonstrated that the distribution of follicles in the ovarian cortex is erratic and without any pattern[77,78]. The presence of a sufficient number of follicles (how many is still not clear) is probably quite reassuring for adequate reserve, but an empty cortex or very few follicles might be just incidental and meaningless. However, the finding that the distribution of follicles in the ovarian cortex is random and erratic, combined with the possible risks of this procedure, suggests that on a risk–benefit balance this procedure is not justified based on the current available data, and the author does not recommend it for this indication[79].

A unique group of patients with some concern about their adequate ovarian reserve are those with only one ovary. A few studies have shown that although the response to superovulation is slightly reduced, the pregnancy rate and the chance of having a child is the same as for women with two intact ovaries, providing that they reach the stage of embryo transfer[80–84].

SEMEN ANALYSIS

While this topic is surveyed at greater length in Chapter 3, there are some points worth emphasizing here. The WHO laboratory manual for the examination of human semen and semen–cervical mucus interaction[85] contains a wealth of practical information and outlines the criteria of fertility commonly used for semen samples. These include:

(1) Volume of ejaculate 2.0 ml or more;

(2) Liquefaction time within 60 min;

(3) Sperm concentration $\geq 20 \times 10^6$ spermatozoa/ml;

(4) Total sperm count $\geq 40 \times 10^6$ spermatozoa per ejaculate;

(5) Motility $\geq 50\%$ with forward progression, or $\geq 25\%$ with rapid linear progression, within 60 min of ejaculation;

(6) Morphology $\geq 30\%$ with normal forms;

(7) Vitality 75% or more live;

(8) White blood cells $\leq 1 \times 10^6$/ml.

The grading of sperm activity on an arbitrary scale of 0–4 is useful for comparing samples from the same man; problems tend to arise with fertilization should the score be less than 2. As described in later chapters, the addition of culture medium to specimen pots before semen collection results in improved sperm motility if there has been marked viscosity of previous semen samples. Likewise, addition of 50% Albuminar®-5, (A5; Armour Pharmaceutical Co. Ltd, Eastbourne, UK) to the pots may alleviate sperm agglutination or diminish the effect of proven antibodies. The mixed antiglobulin reaction (MAR) test will distinguish immunoglobulin G (IgG) antibodies attached to the motile spermatozoa and therefore present in the seminal plasma. Should the MAR test be positive, then an indirect test with immunobeads will distinguish the presence of not only IgG, but also IgA antibodies. The MAR/immunobead test is regarded as positive when more than 10% of the motile spermatozoa have adherent particles/beads. However, there are conflicting reports regarding the reliability and usefulness of antisperm antibody tests and the lack of effective treatment[86,87].

Many non-specialized laboratories quote only a percentage of sperm motility and fail to assess the grade of sperm progression. A reported 'normal' result may thus exonerate a man who in fact has a sperm motility problem. Sperm progression and motility may appear unexpectedly poor on assessment if a long time has elapsed between production and testing of the sample. The significance of abnormal results must always be measured against the length of abstinence before production of the semen sample, and ought also to take into account tobacco and alcohol consumption, concurrent medications and a history of any recent (within the last 2–3 months) debilitating disease, such as influenza.

It is still not uncommon to find that the only previous medical contact with the male partner of an infertile couple has been indirect, via a semen sample report. If any abnormality is present in the semen analysis, a full history should be taken from the male and an examination of at least his external genitalia and prostate gland should be performed. It is not now usual clinic practice to culture the seminal fluid, unless there is excessive leukocytosis or genitourinary symptoms. A history of previous sexually transmitted disease would make it wise not only to culture the urine, but also to take a urethral swab after prostatic massage. The reader is referred to Chapter 3 for a fuller exposition of the investigation and management of the infertile male, and to Chapter 19 for details concerning the newer techniques of assisted reproduction when male infertility factors predominate.

TUBOPERITONEAL FACTOR

Tubal factor accounts for 14% of causes of infertility in women[1]. Knowledge about tubal patency and function is crucial for deciding which treatment is the best for a couple. Clearly, women with severe tubal damage need IVF and cannot be treated by other methods such as intrauterine insemination (IUI), with or without superovulation. However, couples whose only chance of conceiving using their own gametes is by IVF, for example with severe oligospermia, probably do not need investigation of the Fallopian tubes.

The first-line diagnostic tool to assess tubal status is hysterosalpingography (HSG). It is a relatively easy procedure, provides a measure of tubal diameter, locates tubal occlusion and identifies pathologies such as hydrosalpinx, salpingitis isthmica nodosa or tubal polyps. HSG cannot, however, distinguish between genuine occlusion and tubal spasm, although the administration of a non-steroidal anti-inflammatory agent prior to the procedure can reduce the occurrence of spasm. Moreover, HSG is not reliable for the evaluation of peritubal adhesions[88]. HSG has a high false-positive value. In a large metanalysis[89] it was established that when HSG suggests the presence of tubal obstruction, it will be confirmed by laparoscopy in only 38% of cases, but when HSG indicates normal patency, it is confirmed by laparoscopy in 94% of cases. Therefore, in cases with a normal HSG without any relevant medical history, laparoscopy is probably not required[90].

HSG has therapeutic value, especially in the first few months following the procedure, possibly by removing mucus plugs and debris. The effect is stronger with oil-soluble rather than water-soluble media[91,92]. Among women with patent tubes on HSG, 18% were found to have tubal obstruction or peritubal adhesions on laparoscopy[93].

Tubal patency on HSG does not necessarily indicate normal tubal function, and where there is any history of pelvic inflammation or surgery, laparoscopy is essential to confirm the normality of the tubo-ovarian relationships, especially tubal motility, and the state of the fimbriae. A rigid tube, even with free flow of dye on laparoscopy, is unlikely to be functional. Laparoscopy is the only accurate means of detecting and staging endometriosis. Periadnexal adhesive disease and tubal occlusive disease can be identified and staged.

Laparoscopy is more a patency test rather than a functional one because it does not provide information about the mucosa and the lumen of the tube. To achieve this, a new endoscope, the falloposcope, which can be introduced into the tube via a laparoscope[94,95] or transcervically[96,97], has been developed. A few studies have claimed that falloposcopy has better predictive power for natural pregnancy[98], but further studies are required. The role of salpingoscopy in tubal infertility is discussed in depth by Brosens[99].

Another option to assess the patency of the Fallopian tube, although it does not give much information about its function, is hysterosalpingo-contrast sonography (HyCoSy). A combination of air and saline or contrast medium (Echovist-200) is introduced to the tubes through the cervix. The flow of media in the tubes and the spill in the pelvis is detected by ultrasound[100,101].

Laparoscopic evaluation of the Fallopian tubes, adnexa and pelvic peritoneum in patients with radiologically damaged tubes permits decisions to be made about optimum treatment. The options which may be offered include:

(1) Transcervical tubal recanalization;

(2) Laparoscopic tubal surgery;

(3) Microtubal surgery;

(4) IVF.

The indications, effectiveness, complications and costs of these different options should be fully discussed with patients with possible referral to specialized centers.

UTERINE FACTOR

In spite of much progress in the earlier days of *in vitro* fertilization (IVF), such as ovulation induction, oocyte retrieval and culture media, the maximum conception rate, even in the best units, still does not exceed 30% per embryo transfer, and at least 90% of apparently normal embryos fail to implant[4].

Uterine anomalies, fibroids, intrauterine synechiae and endometrial polyps are commonly considered to be closely associated with spontaneous and recurrent miscarriages, although there is still controversy about their incidence, classification and role in reproductive failure[102,103] and especially in IVF treatment. While these lesions, with the exemption of intrauterine adhesions, are not a cause of infertility, they can, however, cause pregnancy loss and early deliveries. It is a tragedy to establish a pregnancy by IVF only to lose it because of a preventable miscarriage. There are few accurate methods for investigating the uterine cavity: HSG, ultrasound, hydrosonography and, recently, magnetic resonance imaging (MRI)[104,105]. However, the 'gold standard' for uterine cavity assessment is diagnostic hysteroscopy. Numerous studies have demonstrated that intrauterine pathology (mainly adhesions) occurs in up to 50% of patients before IVF treatment[106–109], with a similar frequency in women who failed to conceive in one[110] or two IVF cycles[111]. Moreover, in women with a previously normal hysteroscopy, followed by three or more consecutive failed IVF–embryo transfer (ET) cycles, 18.2% demonstrated abnormalities on repeat hysteroscopy[112].

Every woman should ideally have her uterine cavity investigated by HSG and/or hysteroscopy before starting IVF treatment. We believe that diagnostic hysteroscopy is mandatory in investigation of the subfertile woman in the following situations:

(1) An intrauterine lesion suspected on HSG or on transvaginal scan:
   (a) Fibroid;
   (b) Endometrial polyp;
   (c) Congenital uterine anomaly;

(2) Relatively high risk of intrauterine adhesions:
   (a) Instrumental interventions in the past (e.g. dilatation and curettage (D&C), termination of pregnancy, complicated forceps delivery);
   (b) History of endometritis: post-delivery, post-Cesarean section, severe pelvic inflammatory disease;
   (c) Recurrent miscarriage;

(3) Failure of implantation of reasonable embryos after three consecutive IVF cycles.

If a lesion causes significant distortion of the uterine cavity and is therefore estimated to jeopardize the chances to conceive or to carry the pregnancy to term, it can be corrected successfully by surgical hysteroscopy in the majority of cases. The abdominal approach is required for large intramural fibroids. Pregnancy rates following myomectomy in women whose fibroids were the unique cause of infertility, or after surgical correction of intrauterine anomalies, were satisfactory[110,113,114]. A recent meta-analysis of 11 studies demonstrated that women with submucous myomata have lower pregnancy rates compared to women with other causes of infertility, and myomectomy did not result in a higher delivery rate, but only a higher pregnancy rate[115].

IMMUNOLOGICAL INFERTILITY

An immunological cause of infertility accounts for up to 10% of cases of infertility.

Cervical mucus hostile to spermatozoa was usually diagnosed by the postcoital test (PCT). While some authors advocate use of this test[116,117], others have shown that the PCT has a very low predictive power for achieving a pregnancy[118–121], and the PCT has therefore become less fashionable and, with the advent

of specific new and reliable sperm antibody tests for both partners, it is now possibly outmoded. The recent NICE guideline[6] does not recommend the PCT as part of the infertility investigation. Nevertheless, the presence of a good number of motile spermatozoa 4–10h after intercourse provides direct evidence that cervical mucus hostility is not a cause of infertility. Caution must be exercised in interpreting an apparent 'shaking phenomenon' of the spermatozoa within the mucus, as this may represent preliminary coating with antibody from the male genital tract, rather than an antagonistic factor derived from the female. The sperm–mucus contact test makes it easier to ascertain that the cervical mucus itself is responsible for the 'shaking', but false-positive reactions do occur[122]. The characteristics of ovulatory cervical mucus are clearly and helpfully detailed in the WHO manual[122], to which reference should be made. Performing the test other than at the time of ovulation can produce grossly misleading results.

The association between recurrent miscarriage and antiphospholipid antibodies (APA), mainly anticardiolipin and lupus anticoagulant, have led some authors to investigate the correlation of these antibodies to infertility and repeated IVF failure[123,124]. The prevalence of APA in infertile patients is not yet clear, nor has the best treatment been established. A recent meta-analysis revealed that there was no significant association between antiphospholipid abnormalities and either clinical pregnancy or live birth in IVF patients. The authors concluded that measurement of antiphospholipid antibodies is not warranted in patients undergoing IVF[25].

Various combinations of mini-dose aspirin, heparin, steroids or immunoglobulins have been suggested for women who are APA positive[7,126–128]. The effect of treatment on improving pregnancy rates and decreasing miscarriage rates is still under evaluation.

UNEXPLAINED INFERTILITY

Following comprehensive investigation of the infertile couple, as detailed above, some 10–15% of couples will have no apparent reason for their infertility and will therefore be classified as suffering from 'unexplained infertility'.

Although couples with unexplained infertility have a 40–80% chance of conceiving spontaneously in the

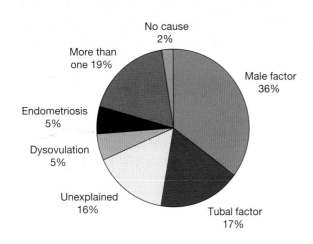

Figure 1 The causes of infertility in a large observational multicenter study in the UK, 2003[49]

3 years following investigation[1], they are usually a very anxious group of patients who find it quite difficult to come to terms with the inability of advanced scientific investigation to give them a logical explanation for their long-standing infertility. Females aged 30 or over who have an increasing duration of infertility, and who have primary infertility, decrease substantially their chances of conceiving without treatment.

Figure 1 shows the reasons for proceeding to IVF treatment in a large recent multicenter observational study conducted in the UK in 2003[49].

After completion of all investigations, the results are discussed with couples and the optimum treatment modalities decided for each couple. Today our treatment 'arsenal' is quite wide, and includes:

(1) 'Wait and see';

(2) Ovulation induction;

(3) Intrauterine insemination (IUI);

(4) IVF;

(5) IVF plus intracytoplasmic sperm injection (ICSI);

(6) Use of donated gametes or embryos;

(7) IVF surrogacy.

The final decision on the most appropriate treatment/s depends on the infertility diagnosis, the female patient's age, the estimated chance of success, cost, risks and side-effects of each method and, not least, the couple's own preferences.

Ovulation induction may be all that is required for the anovulatory woman of normal body weight[129] with normal Fallopian tubes and whose husband has normal sperm. Antiestrogens such as clomiphene citrate 50 mg daily from cycle days 2 to 6 inclusive provide a good initial starting therapy. The dose may be increased to 50 mg twice, or even three times daily. While luteal phase progesterone levels may be used to confirm ovulation (with the limitations previously described), some women react very strongly to this drug, and any pelvic pain warrants at least a pelvic examination and, more helpfully, an ultrasound scan to exclude multifollicular development and ovarian hyperstimulation syndrome (OHSS). Indeed, there are some patients for whom a dose of only 25 mg of clomiphene citrate daily is perfectly sufficient. For a small percentage of women, injection of human chorionic gonadotropin may be required to induce ovulation. At Bourn Hall, for women having timed intercourse following this sort of induction regimen, serial ultrasound scanning with hormone monitoring (estradiol, LH and progesterone) is employed, beginning on day 9 or 10 of the menstrual cycle. Another alternative, especially for women who experience some side-effects with clomiphene, is tamoxifen in an initial dose of 20 mg daily from cycle days 2 to 5 inclusive. Clomiphene is successful in inducing ovulation in 80% of women after 6 months of treatment while 40% will conceive. Rossing and colleagues[130] established an increased risk of ovarian cancer after the use of clomiphene (not tamoxifen) for more than 12 months, and the Policy and Practice Subcommittee of the British Fertility Society (BFS) has recommended limiting the use of clomiphene to 6 months[131].

Should the antiestrogens fail to induce ovulation, and hyperprolactinemia and hypergonadotropic states have been excluded, as previously described, then recourse may be made to the use of gonadotropins, and currently these are either urinary human menopausal gonadotropin (u-hMG) or the more advanced recombinant human follicle stimulating hormone (r-hFSH). At Bourn Hall we use only r-hFSH, owing to advantages in consistency, purity and safety profile. Nowadays, estrogen monitoring (urinary or blood) is regarded as insufficient by itself to exclude the possibility of hyperstimulation and multiple pregnancy, and ultrasound scan monitoring is considered essential. A few authors, including ourselves[132], have shown that in the majority of patients who are not considered to be at risk of hyperstimulation, there is probably no need to monitor blood levels of estrogen, and ultrasound alone is safe and sufficient. Alternate-day or daily doses of FSH may be employed as is most convenient to the patient and the medical attendant. At Bourn Hall, alternate-day regimens commencing with 75–150 IU of r-hFSH daily are used, especially for ovulation induction in intrauterine insemination cycles.

Table 3 Correlation between female age and pregnancy rate in 1427 *in vitro* fertilization (IVF) cycles performed in the UK in 2003[49]

Age (years)	Number of cycles (n (%))	Pregnancies (n (%))
< 35	842 (59%)	316 (37.5%)
35–40	412 (28.9%)	129 (31.3%)
> 40	173 (12.1%)	33 (19.1%)
Total	1427 (100%)	478 (33.5%)

PREGNANCY RATES IN IVF TREATMENT

Where a couple, after proper investigation and careful counseling, decide to embark on demanding and expensive IVF treatment, their main concern is usually what their real chance of success is, and whether they will become parents. Although no definite answer can be given before treatment is started, the two major factors influencing success are:

(1) The success rate of the individual clinic;

(2) The characteristics of the couple.

Pregnancy rates vary enormously in different countries and in clinics in the same country and region[4,133–135]. In the UK the national live birth rate is 21.8% per cycle started[4]. This difference may result either because clinics have different entry criteria (e.g. by limiting the upper female age, basal FSH level or the number of previous unsuccessful cycles), or because some tertiary referral centers with very good records are treating the most resistant cases. However, variations in success rates reflect genuine differences in quality of care and experience between clinics. Each clinic should therefore present couples with accurate recent pregnancy rates from their clinic, rather than quoting national or international pregnancy rates.

Numerous studies have investigated the factors that affect outcome of IVF treatment. The most comprehensive study was conducted on more than 50 000 cycles registered on the Human Fertilisation and Embryology Authority (HFEA) database[136]. Female age emerges as the single most important factor influencing the outcome of IVF[136–139]. The effect of increasing age on reduction in fertility has been discussed previously in this chapter. Our results in the

national observational study in the UK confirm this finding (Table 3). Biological age is more important than chronological age, as older women with a good response to superovulation and satisfactory cycles which result in embryos available for transfer have very reasonable chances of conceiving.

The lower pregnancy rates seen in older women seem to be due partly to a worsening response to superovulation, and, in spite of increased dosages of gonadotropins, older women generally yield fewer oocytes and have higher cycle cancelation rates. Therefore, Rest and colleagues[140] suggested recently that ovarian response was a more useful predictor of pregnancy than age alone.

The cause of infertility, even if two or more factors are involved, does not affect IVF outcome[136,139]. In the past, male infertility was associated with lower pregnancy rates in IVF[141,142], but since the introduction of intracytoplasmic sperm injection (ICSI), we now expect similar pregnancy rates in all causes of infertility (Figure 2). The HFEA database also shows a significant reduction in the success rate with increasing duration of infertility, even after adjustment for age[136] (Figure 3). Women who suffer from secondary infertility (i.e. have had a previous pregnancy) are more likely to have a live birth after IVF treatment, regardless of the pregnancy outcome[136,142].

CUMULATIVE PREGNANCY RATES

Because the chance of conception with a single IVF treatment is still relatively low, treatment cycles cannot realistically be considered in isolation. Calculations of cumulative pregnancy rates are needed, as are trends in success rates with repeated cycles. It is widely believed

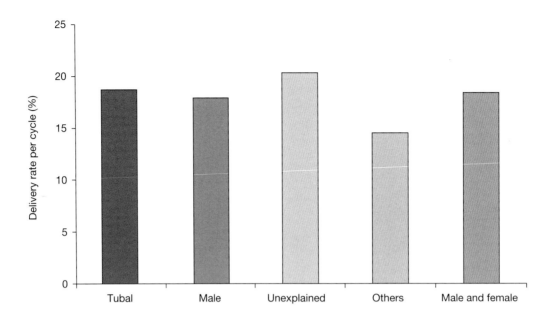

Figure 2 Delivery rate per cycle in 1943 treatment cycles during the period 1995–96 at Bourn Hall Clinic in different causes of infertility. Differences not significant

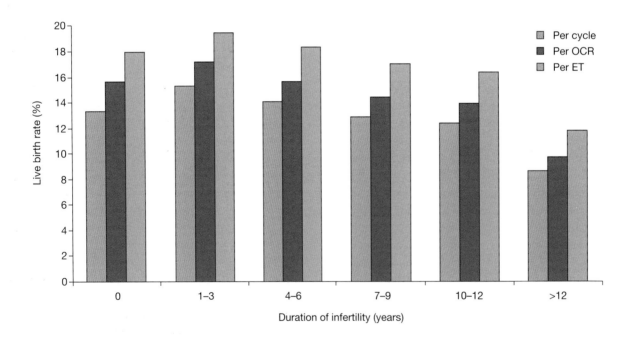

Figure 3 Live birth rates by duration of infertility (Human Fertilisation and Embryology Authority data). OCR, oocyte retrieval; ET, embryo transfer

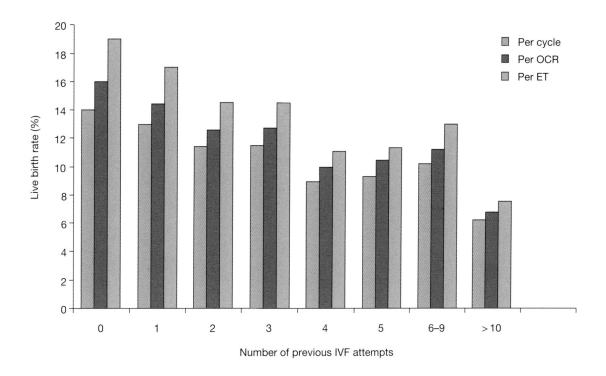

Figure 4 Live birth rates by number of previous unsuccessful *in vitro* fertilization (IVF) attempts (Human Fertilisation and Embryology Authority data). OCR, oocyte retrieval; ET, embryo transfer

that couples who discontinue IVF after a failed attempt do so because they have a poor prognosis. We have shown, in a large study of more than 9000 cycles in a single tertiary center, little evidence of this view[138]. When we compared the etiology, age, ovarian response and fertilization rates of those who returned against those who did not, we found no difference in outcome. This suggests that poorer responders were not dissuaded from returning. Rest and colleagues later confirmed these findings[143].

Women returning for a repeat IVF attempt who have delivered a live infant after an IVF cycle are reported to have a better prognosis[144]. Women who conceived an unsuccessful pregnancy in the first cycle (i.e. miscarriage, ectopic pregnancy or biochemical pregnancy) have a better chance for a live birth in the next cycle than women who did not become pregnant in the first attempt[136,139,142].

While earlier studies reported that the probability of pregnancy remains constant throughout successive IVF cycles[145], others, studying larger numbers of patients, found that there was the same chance in the first three cycles, followed by a significantly reduced chance thereafter[139], or a decreased chance with each consecutive cycle[136] (Figure 4). The overall cumulative pregnancy rates after six cycles of IVF range from 56%[146] to 72%[138], compared with a 55% cumulative probability of pregnancy after 6 months of intercourse in a normally cohabiting, fertile population.

IVF treatment should not be seen as an isolated event and biochemical and failed clinical pregnancies should be viewed with a degree of cautious optimism. All couples undergoing IVF treatment should consider that this implies a course of at least three treatments, with equal chances of pregnancy in each. Beyond three cycles, success rates per cycle fall, although cumulative pregnancy rates continue to rise, albeit at a slower rate, and the chances are still good enough to encourage those with sufficient resources and commitment to try three more attempts. While it is impossible to predict accurately those who are likely to have a child, analysis of the cumulative pregnancy rates from an IVF center provides useful information to help couples make decisions about their treatment.

CONCLUSIONS

In summary, a clinic offering IVF and associated treatment methods must pay attention at the initial consultation to past investigations of infertile couples, their previous obstetric and gynecological history and the need for further special investigations. Attention to detail throughout the whole process is necessary, and yet a flexible approach to investigation and treatment must be maintained. Failures of treatment, which sadly always exceed the successes, must be discussed with couples in the light of information drawn from both the medical and scientific records of previous treatment cycles. Only in this way can one give them soundly based advice about future therapy. In no field of medicine is there a closer relationship between clinicians, laboratory scientists, counselors and patients.

REFERENCES

1. The ESHRE Capri Workshop. Infertility revisited: the state of the art today and tomorrow. Hum Reprod 1996; 11: 1779–807
2. te Velde ER, Eijkemans R, Habbema HDF. Variation in couple fecundity and time to pregnancy, an essential concept in human reproduction. Lancet 2000; 355: 1928–9
3. Farley TM, Belsey FH. The prevalence and etiology of infertility. In Biological Components of Fertility. Proceedings of the African Population Conference, Dakar, Senegal, November 1988. Liège, Belgium: International Union for the Scientific Study of Population, 1988; 1: 2.1.15–2.1.30
4. Human Fertilisation and Embryology Authority Patients' Guide to IVF clinics. London: HFEA, 2002
5. Hargrave TB, Elton RA. Fecundability rates from an infertile male population. Br J Urol 1986; 58: 194–7
6. Fertility assessment and treatment for people with fertility problems. Clinical Guideline, February 2004. London: National Institute of Clinical Excellence, 2004 (http://www.nice.org.uk)
7. World Health Organization. Physical Status: The Use of Interpretation of Anthropometry. World Health Organization Technical Report series 854. Geneva: World Health Organization, 1995
8. Bellver J, Rossal LP, Bosch E, et al. Obesity and the risk of spontaneous abortion after oocyte donation. Fertil Steril 2003; 79: 1136–40
9. Hamilton-Fairley D, Kiddy D, Patson H, et al. Association of moderate obesity with a poor pregnancy outcome in women with polycystic ovary syndrome treated with low dose gonadotropin. Br J Obstet Gynaecol 1992; 99: 128–31
10. Pasquali R, Antenucci D, Cassimiri F, et al. Clinical and hormonal characteristics of obese amenorrheic hyperandrogenic women before and after weight loss. J Clin Endocrinol Metab 1989; 68: 173–9
11. Bray AG. Obesity and reproduction. In Basdevant A, Bringer J, Lefebvre P, eds. Weight, nutrition and hormonal events in women. Hum Reprod 1997; (Suppl 12): 26–32
12. Kort HI, Massey JB, Elsner C, et al. Men with high body mass index values present with lower numbers of normal-motile sperm cells. Fertil Steril 2003; 80 (Suppl 3): S238 (Abstr P-355)
13. Templeton A, Morris JK, Parslow W. Factors that affect outcome of in-vitro fertilization treatment. Lancet 1996; 348: 1402–6
14. Chung S, Sohn JH, Park YY. Is obesity an underlying factor in erectile dysfunction? Eur Urol 1999; 36: 68–70
15. Zaadstra B, Looman C, te Velde ER, et al. Moderate drinking: no impact on female fecundity. Fertil Steril 1994; 62: 948–54
16. Jensen TK, Hjollund NH, Henriksen TB, et al. Does moderate alcohol consumption affect fertility? Follow up study among couples planning first pregnancy. Br Med J 1998; 317: 505–10
17. Dunphy BC, Barratt CL, Cooke ID. Male alcohol consumption and fecundity in couples attending an infertility clinic. Andrologia 1991; 23: 219–21
18. Oldereid NB, Rui H, Puris K. Life styles of men in barren couples and their relationship to sperm quality. Int J Fertil 1992; 37: 343–9
19. Augood C, Duckitt K, Templeton AA. Smoking and female infertility: a systematic review and meta-analysis. Hum Reprod 1998; 13: 1539
20. Hughes EG, Brennan BG. Does cigarette smoking impair natural or assisted fecundity? Fertil Steril 1996; 66: 679–89
21. Hull MG, North K, Taylor H, et al. Delayed conception and active and passive smoking. The Avon Longitudinal Study of Pregnancy and Childhood Study Team. Fertil Steril 2000; 74: 725–33
22. Ferreira-Poblete A. The probability of conception on different days of the cycle with respect to ovulation: an overview. Adv Contracept 1997; 13: 83–95
23. Minkoff H, Santoro N. Ethical considerations in the treatment of infertility in women with human immunodeficiency virus infection. N Engl J Med 2000; 342: 1748–50
24. Gilling-Smith C, Smith JR, Semprini E. HI and infertility: time to treat. There's no justification for denying

treatment to parents who are HIV positive. Br Med J 2001; 322: 566–7

25. Leader A, Taylor PJ, Daudi F. The value of routine rubella and syphilitic serology in the infertile couple. Fertil Steril 1984; 42: 140–2

26. Fawzy M, Harrison RF. Essential pre-conceptual measures for the female partner before commencing an in vitro fertilisation programme. Ir J Med Sci 1998; 167: 14–16

27. The ESHRE Capri Workshop. Anovulatory infertility. Hum Reprod 1995; 10: 1549–53

28. Martinez AR, Voorhorst FJ, Schoemaker J. Reliability of urinary LH testing for planning of endometrial biopsies. Eur J Obstet Gynecol Reprod Biol 1992; 43: 137–42

29. Speroff L, Glass RH, Kase GN, eds. Clinical Gynecologic Endocrinology and Infertility, 4th edn. Baltimore: Williams & Wilkins, 1989: 213–32

30. Rowe PJ, Comhaire FH, Hargrave TB, Mellows HJ. WHO Manual for the Standardised Investigation of the Infertile Couple. Cambridge: Cambridge University Press, 1997

31. Coulam CB, Adamson SC, Annegers JF. Incidence of premature ovarian failure. Obstet Gynecol 1986; 67: 604–6

32. Conway GS, Kaltass G, Patel A, et al. Characterization of idiopathic premature ovarian failure. Fertil Steril 1996; 65: 337–41

33. Speroff L, Glass RH, Kase GN, eds. Clinical Gynecologic Endocrinology and Infertility, 4th edn. Baltimore: Williams & Wilkins, 1989: 173–9

34. Varkopoulou K, Dericks-Tan JS, Taubert HD. [The diagnostic value of routine prolactin determination in sterility patients]. Zentralbl Gynakol 1993; 115: 167–70

35. Glazener CM, Kelly NJ, Hull G. Prolactin measurement in the investigation of infertility in women with a normal menstrual cycle. Br J Obstet Gynaecol 1987; 94: 535–8

36. Stratford GA, Barth JH, Rutherford AJ, Balen AH. Plasma prolactin measurement is not indicated in women in the routine investigation of uncomplicated infertility. Hum Fertil (Camb) 1999; 2: 70–1

37. Lenton EA, Sulaiman R, Sobowale E, Cooke ID. The human menstrual cycle: plasma concentrations of prolactin, LH, FSH, estradiol and progesterone in conceiving and non-conceiving women. J Reprod Fertil 1982; 48: 605–7

38. Richardson, SJ, Senikas V, Nelson JF. Follicular depletion during the menopausal transition: evidence for accelerated loss and ultimate exhaustion. J Clin Endocrinol Metab 1987; 65: 1231–7

39. Faddy MJ, Gosden RG. A mathematical model of follicle dynamics in the human ovary. Hum Reprod 1995; 10: 770–5

40. Bopp BL, Alper MM, Thompson IE, Mortola J. Success rates with gamete intrafallopian transfer and in vitro fertilization in women of advanced maternal age. Fertil Steril 1995; 63: 1278–83

41. Dicker D, Goldman JA, Ashkenazi J, et al. Age and pregnancy rates in in vitro fertilization. J In Vitro Fertil Embryo Transfer 1991; 8: 141–4

42. Sharara FI, Scott RT Jr, Seifer DB. The detection of diminished ovarian reserve in infertile women. Am J Obstet Gynecol 1998; 179: 804–12

43. Speroff L. The effect of aging on fertility. Curr Opin Obstet Gynecol 1994; 6: 115–20

44. Leeton J. Patient selection for assisted reproduction. Baillière's Clin Obstet Gynaecol 1992; 6: 217–27

45. Faddy MJ, Gosden RG. A model confirming the decline in follicle numbers to the age of menopause in women. Hum Reprod 1996; 11: 1484–6

46. Wallach EE. Pitfalls in evaluating ovarian reserve. Fertil Steril 1995; 63: 12–14

47. Abdalla HI, Baber R, Kirkland A, et al. A report on 100 cycles of oocyte donation; factors affecting the outcome. Hum Reprod 1990; 5: 1018–22

48. Munne S, Alikani M, Tomkin G, et al. Embryo morphology, developmental rates, and maternal age are correlated with chromosome abnormalities. Fertil Steril 1995; 64: 382–91

49. McVeigh E, Lass A. The routine use of r-hFSH follitropin-alfa (Gonal-F®) filled-by-mass for follicular development for IVF: a large multicenter observational study in the UK. Presented at the American Society of Reproductive Medicine (ASRM), Philadelphia, USA, October 2004 (abstr)

50. Marcus SF, Brinsden PR. In-vitro fertilization and embryo transfer in women aged 40 years and over. Hum Reprod Update 1996; 2: 459–68

51. Scott RT, Toner JP, Muasher SJ, et al. Follicle-stimulating hormone levels on cycle day 3 are predictive of in vitro fertilisation outcome. Fertil Steril 1989; 51: 651–4

52. Toner JP, Philput CB, Jones GS, Mausher SJ. Basal follicle stimulating hormone level is a better predictor of in vitro fertilisation performance than age. Fertil Steril 1991; 55: 784–91

53. Levi AJ, Raynault MF, Bergh P, et al. Reproductive outcome in patients with diminished ovarian reserve. Fertil Steril 2001; 76: 666–9

54. Scott RT, Hofmann GE. Prognostic assessment of ovarian reserve. Fertil Steril 1995; 63: 1–11

55. van Rooij IA, Bancsi LF, Broekmans FJ, et al. Women older than 40 years of age and those with elevated

follicle-stimulating hormone levels differ in poor response rate and embryo quality in in vitro fertilization. Fertil Steril 2003; 79: 482–8

56. Scott RT, Hofmann GE, Oehninger S, Mausher SJ. Intercycle variability of day 3 follicle-stimulating hormone levels and its effect on stimulation quality in in vitro fertilization. Ferti Steril 1990; 54: 297–302

57. Lass A, Gerrard A, Abusheikha N, et al. IVF performance of women who have fluctuating early follicular FSH levels. J Assist Reprod Genet 2000; 17: 566–73

58. Buyalos RP, Daneshmand S, Brzechffa PR. Basal estradiol and follicle-stimulating hormone predict fecundity in women of advanced reproductive age undergoing ovulation induction therapy. Fertil Steril 1997; 68: 272–7

59. Licciardi FL, Hung-Ching L, Rosenwaks Z. Day 3 estradiol serum concentrations as prognosticators of ovarian stimulation response and pregnancy outcome in patients undergoing in vitro fertilization. Fertil Steril 1992; 64: 991–4

60. Smotrich DB, Widra EA, Gindoff PR, et al. Prognostic value of day 3 estradiol on in vitro fertilization outcome. Fertil Steril 1995; 64: 1136–40

61. Lass A, Skull J, McVeigh E, et al. Measurement of ovarian volume by transvaginal sonography before human menopausal gonadotropin superovulation for in vitro fertilisation can predict poor response. Hum Reprod 1997; 12: 294–7

62. Syrop CH, Wilhoite A, Van-Voorhis BJ. Ovarian volume: a novel outcome predictor for assisted reproduction. Fertil Steril 1995; 64: 1167–71

63. Lass A, Brinsden P. The role of ovarian volume in reproductive medicine. Hum Reprod Update 1999; 5: 256–66

64. Tomas C, Nuojua-Huttunen S, Martikainen H, et al. Pretreatment transvaginal ultrasound examination predicts ovarian responsiveness to gonadotropins in in-vitro fertilization. Hum Reprod 1997; 12: 220–3

65. Seifer DB, Lambert-Masserlian, G, Hogan JW, et al. Day 3 serum inhibin-B is predictive of assisted reproductive technologies outcome. Fertil Steril 1997; 67: 110–14

66. Corson SL, Gutmann J, Batzer FR, et al. Inhibin-B as a test of ovarian reserve for infertile women. Hum Reprod 1999; 14: 2818–21

67. Hall JE, Elt CK, Cramer D. Inhibin and inhibin B reflect ovarian function in assisted reproduction but are less useful at predicting outcome. Hum Reprod 1999; 14: 409–15

68. van Rooij IAJ, Broekmans FM, te Velde RE, et al. Serum anti-Mullerian hormone levels: a novel measure of ovarian reserve. Hum Reprod 2002; 12: 3065–71

69. Navot D, Rosenwaks Z, Margalioth E. Prognostic assessment of female fecundity. Lancet 1989; 2: 645–7

70. Scot RT, Leonardi MR, Hoffman GE, et al. A prospective evaluation of clomiphene citrate challenge test screening in the general infertility population. Obstet Gynecol 1993; 82: 539–45

71. Loumaye E, Billion JM, Mine JM, et al. Prediction of individual response to controlled ovarian hyperstimulation by means of clomiphene citrate challenge test. Fertil Steril 1990; 53: 295–301

72. Tanbo T, Dale PO, Ludne O, et al. Prediction of response to controlled ovarian hyperstimulation: a comparison of basal and clomiphene citrate stimulated follicle stimulating hormone levels. Fertil Steril 1992; 57: 819–24

73. Winslow KL, Toner JP, Brzyski RG, et al. The gonadotropin-realising hormone agonist stimulation test – a sensitive predictor of performance in the flare-up in vitro fertilization cycle. Fertil Steril 1990; 56: 711–17

74. Galtier-Dereure F, De Bouard V, Picot MC, et al. Ovarian reserve test with the gonadotropin-releasing hormone agonist buserelin: correlation with in vitro fertilization outcome. Hum Reprod 1996; 11: 1393–8

75. Lass A, Silye R, Abrams DC, et al. Follicular density in ovarian biopsy of infertile woman: a novel method to assess ovarian reserve. Hum Reprod 1997; 12: 1028–31

76. Lass A. Assessment of ovarian reserve – is there a role for ovarian biopsy? Hum Reprod 2001; 16: 1055–7

77. Schmidt KLT, Byskov AG, Nyboe Andersen A, et al. Density and distribution of primordial follicles in single pieces of cortex from 21 patients and in individual pieces of cortex from three entire human ovaries. Hum Reprod 2003; 18: 1158–64

78. Lambalk CB, de Koning CH, Flett A, et al. Assessment of ovarian reserve. Ovarian biopsy is not a valid method for the prediction of ovarian reserve. Hum Reprod 2001; 19: 1055–9

79. Lass A. Assessment of ovarian reserve – is there a role for ovarian biopsy? Debate continued. Hum Reprod 2004; 19: 467–9

80. Lass A, Silye R, Abrams DC, et al. Follicular density in ovarian biopsy of infertile woman: a novel method to assess ovarian reserve. Hum Reprod 1997; 12: 1028–31

81. Lass A, Paul M, Margara R, Winston RM. Women with one ovary have decreased response to GnRHa/HMG ovulation induction protocol in IVF programme but the same pregnancy rate as women with two ovaries. Hum Reprod 1997; 12: 298–300

82. Alper MM, Siebel MM, Oskowitz SP, et al. Comparison of follicular response in patients with one or two

ovaries in a programme of in vitro fertilization. Fertil Steril 1985; 44: 652–5

83. Bouttevile C, Mausher SJ, Acosta AA, et al. Results of in vitro fertilisation attempts in patients with one or two ovaries. Fertil Steril 1987; 47: 821–7

84. Diamond MP, Wentz AC, Herbert CM, et al. One ovary or two: differences in ovulation induction, estradiol levels, and follicular development in a programme for in vitro fertilisation. Fertil Steril 1984; 41: 524–9

85. World Health Organization. WHO Laboratory Manual for the Examination of Human Semen and Sperm-Cervical Mucus Interaction, 3rd edn. Cambridge: Cambridge University Press, 1992: 44–5

86. Helmerhorst F, Erich JJ. Antisperm antibodies: comment on the use of the MAR test using latex beads. Hum Reprod 2000; 15: 233

87. Bronson R. Detection of antisperm antibodies: an argument against therapeutic nihilism. Hum Reprod 1999; 14: 1671–3

88. Mol BW, Swart P, Bossuyt PMM, et al. Reproducibility of the interpretation of hysterosalpingiography in the diagnosis of tubal pathology. Hum Reprod 1996; 11: 1204–8

89. Swart P, Mol BW, van der Veen F, et al. The accuracy of hysterosalpingography in the diagnosis of tubal pathology: a meta-analysis. Fertil Steril 1995; 64: 486–91

90. Abdalla HI. Active management of infertility. Br J Hosp Med 1992; 48: 28–33

91. DeCherney AH, Kort H, Barney JB, DeVore GR. Increased pregnancy rate with oil-soluble hysterosalpingiography dye. Fertil Steril 1980; 33: 407–10

92. Watson A, Vandekerckhove P, Lilford R, et al. A meta-analysis of the therapeutic role of oil soluble contrast media at hysterosalpingiography: a surprising result? Fertil Steril 1994; 61: 470–7

93. Belisle S, Collins JA, Burrows EA, William AR. The value of laparoscopy among infertile women with tubal patency. J Soc Obstet Gynaecol Can 1996; 18: 326–36

94. Shapiro BS, Diamond MP, DeCherney AH. Salpingoscopy: an adjunctive technique for evaluation of the fallopian tube. Fertil Steril 1988; 49: 1076–9

95. Salpingoscopy. In Brosens IA, Gordon AG, eds. Tubal Infertility. London: Gower Medical Publishing, 1990: 4.18–4.25

96. Kerin J, Daykhovsky L, Segalowitz J, et al. Falloscopy: a microendoscopic technique for visual exploration of the human fallopian tube from the uterotubal to the fimbria using a transvaginal approach. Fertil Steril 1990; 54: 390–400

97. Scudamore IW, Dunphy BC, Cooke ID. Outpatient falloposcopy: intra-luminal imaging of the fallopian

tube by trans-uterine fibre-optic endoscopy as an outpatient procedure. Br J Obstet Gynaecol 1992; 99: 829–35

98. Dechaud H, Daures JP, Hedon B. Prospective evaluation of falloposcopy. Hum Reprod 1998; 13: 1815–18

99. Brosens IA. The value of salpingoscopy in tubal infertility. Reprod Med Rev 1996; 5: 1–11

100. Hiekkinen H, Tekay A, Volpi E, et al. Transvaginal salpingosonography for the assessment of tubal patency in infertile women: methodological and clinical experiences. Fertil Steril 1995; 64: 293–8

101. Ayida G, Kennedy S, Barlow D, Chamberline P. Contrast sonography for uterine cavity assessment: a comparison of conventional two dimensional with three-dimensional transvaginal ultrasound; a pilot study. Fertil Steril 1996; 66: 848–50

102. Bulletti C, Flamigni C, Giacommucci E. Reproductive failure due to spontaneous abortion and recurrent miscarriage. Hum Reprod Update 1996; 2: 118–36

103. Donnez J, Jadoul P. What are the implications of myomas on fertility? Need for a debate? Hum Reprod 2002; 17: 1424–30

104. de Souza NM, Brosens JJ, Schwieso JE, et al. The potential value of magnetic resonance imaging in infertility. Clin Radiol 1995; 50: 75–9

105. Turnbull LW, Lesny P, Killick SR. Assessment of uterine receptivity prior to embryo transfer: a review of currently available imaging modalities. Hum Reprod Update 1995; 1: 505–14

106. Dicker D, Goldman JA, Ashkenazi J, et al. The value of hysteroscopy in elderly women prior to in vitro fertilization–embryo transfer (IVF–ET): a comparative study. J In Vitro Fertil Embryo Transfer 1990; 7: 267–70

107. Bordt J, Belkien L, Vancaillie T, et al. Results of diagnostic hysteroscopies in an in vitro fertilization/embryo transfer program. Geburtsh Frauenheilkd 1984; 44: 813–15

108. Seinera P, Maccario S, Visentin L, DiGregorio A. Hysteroscopy in an IVF-ET program. Acta Obstet Gynecol Scand 1988; 67: 135–7

109. Shamma PN, Lee G, Gutmann JN, Lavy G. The role of hysteroscopy in in vitro fertilization. Fertil Steril 1992; 58: 1237–9

110. Golan A, Ron-El R, Herman A, et al. Diagnostic hysteroscopy: its value in an in-vitro fertilization/embryo transfer unit. Hum Reprod 1992; 7: 1433–4

111. Hamou J, Frydman R, Fernandez H. Evaluation prior to IVF by microhysteroscopy. Presented at the VIth World Congress in IVF and Alternate Assisted Reproduction, Jerusalem, Israel, 1989: abstr 40

112. Dicker D, Ashkenazi J, Feldberg D, et al. The value of repeat hysteroscopic evaluation in patients with failed

in vitro fertilization transfer cycles. Fertil Steril 1992; 58: 833–5

113. Ubaldi F, Tournaye H, Camus M, et al. Fertility after hysteroscopic myomectomy. Hum Reprod Update 1996; 1: 81–90

114. Tazuke S, Nezhat C. Management of myoma in the setting of infertility. Presented at the 10th World Congress of In Vitro Fertilization and Assisted Reproduction, Vancouver, Canada, May 1997: 1071–6

115. Pritts EA. Fibroids and infertility: a systematic review of the evidence. Obstet Gynecol Surv 2001; 56: 483–91

116. Cohlen BJ, te Velde ER, Habbema JD. Postcoital testing. Postcoital test should be performed as routine infertility test. Br Med J 1999; 318: 1008–9

117. Glazener CM, Ford C, Hull G. The prognostic power of the post-coital test for natural conception depends on duration of infertility. Hum Reprod 2000; 15: 1953–7

118. Glatstein IZ, Best CL, Palumbo A, et al. The reproducibility of the postcoital test: a prospective study. Obstet Gynecol 1995; 85: 396–400

119. Griffith CS, Grimes DA. The validity of the postcoital test. Am J Obstet Gynecol 1990; 162: 616–20

120. Oei SG, Helmerhorst F, Keirse MJ. Routine postcoital testing is unnecessary. Hum Reprod 2001; 16: 1051–3

121. Oei SG, Helmerhorst F, Bloemenkamp K, et al. Effectiveness of the postcoital test: randomised controlled trial. Br Med J 1998; 317: 502–5

122. Rowe PJ, Comhair FH, Hargreave TB, et al. WHO Manual for the Human Semen and Sperm–Cervical Mucus Interaction. Cambridge: Cambridge University Press, 2000

123. Taylor PV, Campbell JM, Scott JC. Presence of autoantibodies in women with unexplained infertility. Am J Obstet Gynecol 1989; 161: 377–9

124. Birkenfield A, Nukaida T, Minichiello L, et al. Incidence of autoimmune antibodies in failed embryo transfer cycles. Am J Reprod Immunol 1994; 31: 65–8

125. Hornstein MD, Davis OK, Massey TB, et al. Antiphospholipid antibodies and in vitro fertilization success: a meta analysis. Fertil Steril 2000; 73: 330–3

126. Kutteh WH, Yetman DI, Chantilis SJ, Crain J. Effect of antiphospholipid antibodies in women undergoing in vitro fertilization: role of heparin and aspirin. Hum Reprod 1997; 12: 1171–5

127. Kowalik A, Vichin M, Liu HC, et al. Midfollicular anticardiolipin and antiphosphatidylserine antibody titers do not correlate with in vitro fertilization outcome. Fertil Steril 1997; 68: 298–303

128. Denis AL, Guido M, Adler RD, et al. Antiphospholipid antibodies and pregnancy rates and outcome in in

vitro fertilization patients. Fertil Steril 1997; 67: 1084–90

129. Frisch RE. The right weight: body fat, menarche and ovulation. In Crosignani PG, ed. Induction of Ovulation. Clin Obstet Gynaecol 1990; 4: 419–39

130. Rossing MA, Daling JR, Weiss NS, et al. Ovarian tumors in a cohort of infertile women. N Engl J Med 1994; 331: 771–6

131. Balen A. Anovulatory infertility and ovulation induction. Hum Reprod 1997; 12 (Natl Suppl, JBFS 2): 83–7

132. Lass A, UK Timing of hCG Group. Monitoring of in vitro fertilization–embryo transfer cycles by ultrasound versus by ultrasound and hormonal levels: a prospective, multicenter, randomized study. Fertil Steril 2003; 80: 80–5

133. Anon. Assisted reproductive technology in the United States and Canada: 1995 results generated from the American Society for Reproductive Medicine/ Society for Assisted Reproductive Technology Registry. Fertil Steril 1995; 66: 697–702

134. The European IVF-monitoring programme (EIM). Assisted reproductive technology in Europe, 2000. Results generated from European registers by ESHRE. Hum Reprod 2004; 19: 490–503

135. FIVNAT. Pregnancies and births resulting from in vitro fertilization. French national registry, analysis of data 1986–1990. Fertil Steril 1995; 64: 746–55

136. Templeton A, Morris JK, Parslow W. Factors that affect outcome of in-vitro fertilisation treatment. Lancet 1996; 348: 1402–6

137. Bopp BL, Alper MM, Thompson IE, Mortola J. Success rates with gamete intrafallopian transfer and in vitro fertilization in women of advanced maternal age. Fertil Steril 1995; 63: 1278–83

138. Tan SL, Royston P, Campbell S, et al. Cumulative conception and live birth rates after in-vitro fertilisation. Lancet 1992; 339: 1390–4

139. Croucher C, Lass A, Margara R, Winston RM. Predictive value of the results of a first in vitro fertilisation cycle on the outcome of subsequent cycles. Hum Reprod 1998; 13: 403–8

140. Rest J, van Heusden AM, Mous H, et al. The ovarian response as a predictor for successful in vitro fertilization treatment after the age of 40 years. Fertil Steril 1996; 66: 969–73

141. Tournaye H, Devroey P, Camus M, et al. Comparison of in-vitro fertilization in male and tubal infertility: a 3 year survey. Hum Reprod 1992; 7: 218–22

142. Tan SL, Doyle P, Maconochie N, et al. Pregnancy and birth rates of live infants after in vitro fertilization in women with and without previous in vitro fertilization pregnancies: a study of eight thousand

cycles at one center. Am J Obstet Gynecol 1994; 170: 34–40

143. Rest J, van Heusden AM, Zeilmaker GH, Verhoeff A. Cumulative pregnancy rates and selective drop-out patients in in-vitro fertilization treatment. Hum Reprod 1998; 13: 339–41

144. Molloy D, Doody ML, Breen T. Second time around: a study of patients seeking second assisted reproduction pregnancies. Fertil Steril 1995; 64: 546–51

145. Guzick DS, Wilkes C, Jones HW. Cumulative pregnancy rates for in vitro fertilization. Fertil Steril 1986; 46: 663–71

146. Dor J, Seidman DS, Ben-Shlomo I, et al. Cumulative pregnancy rate following in-vitro fertilization: the significance of age and fertility aetiology. Hum Reprod 1996; 11: 425–8

3

The management of infertile men presenting in the assisted conception unit

Anthony V. Hirsh

INTRODUCTION

Sperm dysfunction, azoospermia or ineffective coitus is a factor in 50% of infertile couples, thus placing andrology at the core of reproductive medicine. While infertile men seek a cure, this ideal is rarely possible. However, fatherhood is usually feasible through assisted reproductive technologies (ART), and evolution of this field with the steadily reducing need for sperm has been driven substantially by male infertility. While endocrine deficiency is a rare cause of semen abnormalities, men always focus on their virility, and libidos often dissolve after the diagnosis. The best solution is to gain the ability to procreate naturally, and should be a principal resolve of specialists in clinical andrology.

The 2004 fertility guideline[1] reviews the outcome of established therapies for infertile men and confirms evidence for the increased probability of a live birth in only three uncommon conditions: hypothalamic–pituitary failure, retrograde ejaculation and obstructive azoospermia[1]. The common objective of treatment for these diverse disorders is the deposition of normal sperm during coitus. Infertile men with semen abnormalities usually eject sizeable populations of motile spermatozoa into the female tract which cannot fertilize. As there is no treatment to improve sperm function, the guideline highlights the continuing enigma

of sperm dysfunction and the need to realign the approach to the investigation of this largest-defined cause of human subfertility[2].

DIAGNOSIS, PREVALENCE AND ETIOLOGY

Infertility is defined as failure to conceive after 2 years of regular intercourse. The male partner is often seen in primary care with his spouse after 1 year, but earlier assessment is required if he has had genital surgery, treatment for cancer or previous subfertility. As a test for male fertility, the standard of seminal fluid analysis (SFA) has improved in the UK due to National External Quality Assurance Schemes (NEQAS), initiated by the British Andrology Society and allied organizations, based on World Heath Organization (WHO) reference values[3]. Thus, if the semen is normal, nothing further is needed for the man at the initial stage provided that coitus occurs frequently. If the SFA is abnormal, confirmed on repeat testing, or coitus is ineffective, he should be referred to a specialist experienced in andrology in view of the probable need for assisted reproduction.

About one in 20 men are subfertile, 80–90% with suboptimal semen quality, while azoospermia, coital dysfunction and immunological infertility each

35

Table 1 Presentation and pathogenesis of male infertility

Presentation	Explanation and examples	Incidence*
I. *Ineffective coitus* ejaculation normal retrograde ejaculation ejaculation failure	mechanical causes – normal sperm function erectile dysfunction, disability, hypospadias, phimosis bladder neck surgery, diabetes mellitus, phenothiazines anorgasmia, spinal cord or pelvic injury, multiple sclerosis	5%
II. *Azoospermia* pre-testicular non-obstructive obstructive	no spermatozoa in semen anabolic steroid abuse, Kalmann's syndrome, idiopathic HH cryptorchidism, orchitis, 47,XXY, radiotherapy, chemotherapy CBAVD, vasectomy, epididymo-orchitis, chlamydia, GC	5%
III. *Sperm autoimmunity*	antisperm antibodies impair sperm function idiopathic, genital infection, unilateral testicular obstruction	5%
IV. *Semen abnormality*	sperm dysfunction idiopathic OATS, MAGI, testis cancer, drugs, genetic, varicocele	85%
V *Sperm abnormality*	spermatozoa are structurally abnormal immotile cilia (Kartagener's) syndrome, globozoospermia	<1%

*Approximate; HH, hypogonadotropic hypogonadism; CBAVD, congenital bilateral absence of the vas deferens; 47,XXY, Klinefelter's syndrome; GC, gonorrhea; MAGI, male accessory gland infection; OATS, oligoasthenoteratozoospermia syndrome

represent about 5% of cases. Table 1 classifies the types of presentation and possible causes.

PATHOGENESIS, ENVIRONMENT AND LIFE-STYLE FACTORS

Male infertility may reflect defective spermatogenesis, sperm dysfunction, impaired sperm transport or deposition[4]. A WHO study[5] found a male factor in 51.1% of 6000 infertile couples, while sperm dysfunction was identified by Hull and colleagues[2] in 24% of couples. Surveys of the ostensible etiology are biased by referral patterns, with wide variations in the prevalence of varicocele (12.3–42.2%), testicular obstruction (0.9–14.3%), coital dysfunction (0.3–7.0%), endocrine deficiency (0.61–9%) and systemic disease (0.3–5.0%), with genetic defects hitherto unusual (0.1–0.5%)[2,5–11].

Sperm production is inefficient in man, as is reflected by high ratios of morphologically abnormal spermatozoa in normal semen that probably cannot fertilize. During fetal and later development, spermatogenesis is regarded as vulnerable to environmental or life-style factors which may cause lasting reductions in Sertoli cell numbers. Factors implicated include tobacco, alcohol, illicit and therapeutic drugs,

pesticides and chemicals at work, endocrine disruptors in food, estrogen in our water, and our sedentary lifestyle and work in modern society causing obesity and increased scrotal temperature. Falling sperm counts in some countries have not affected global fecundity, but concern arises over the associated increased incidence of testicular germ-cell cancer, cryptorchidism and hypospadias, known as the 'testicular dysgenesis syndrome'. As this is related to birth cohorts, environmental factors are implicated, with potential long-term effects on the fertility of men[12].

STRATEGIES IN CLINICAL MANAGEMENT

The high prevalence of male infertility has aroused renewed interest now that the practice of ART is standardized and professionals in the assisted conception unit (ACU) manage patients as a team.

The male partner

Infertile men should be evaluated by a reproductive medicine specialist, clinical andrologist or uroandrologist. The few disorders where natural pregnancy and birth are feasible are sought and treated, while any associated male genital or general disorders are managed or referred. Most cases require assisted reproduction. The SFA and *in vitro* fertilization (IVF) sperm preparation results, any need for surgical sperm recovery and female factors determine whether vaginal or intrauterine (IUI) insemination, IVF or intracytoplasmic sperm injection (ICSI) are indicated. Adjustments to life-style or clinical measures may marginally improve the semen quality, and can sometimes avoid surgery for the man or downgrade the complexity of ART for the woman. Lowering potential risk for both partners and any resulting child reduces stress, discomfort and the funding required.

The female partner

Female factors occur in all male diagnostic categories, with a low incidence in spouses of men with azoospermia and aspermia. The high prevalence of female factors where the SFA is subnormal means that gynecological attention may achieve the pregnancy[13]. Advancing age, or ovulatory or tubal factors, can present an overriding indication for assisted conception, while attention to any life-style issues may improve the chance of success.

Counseling

Both partners need to know about ART, the success rates, costs, side-effects and any genetic issues, when compared with male-partner therapy. After their assessments and counseling, couples should be aware of any potential for male partner therapy to initiate natural pregnancy, and whether ART is more certain. The duration of infertility, personal, economic or religious reasons[14] and need for future contraception may affect the decision, while child and family welfare issues are equally relevant.

Prognostic factors

Collins and colleagues[15] found that 14.3% of untreated infertile couples conceived naturally each year, more often if there had been a previous pregnancy, a shorter time of trying (< 3 years) or if the female partner was young (< 30 years). There was less chance of conceiving if infertility was due to endometriosis, tubal disease or a male factor.

CLINICAL ASSESSMENT OF INFERTILE MEN

The information required concerns: the duration of infertility, the frequency and effectiveness of coitus, pubertal development, any history of general disease or genitourinary infection or surgery, current medication, life-style factors and the outcome of previous ART. The examination seeks signs of hypogonadism and genital abnormality, and is carried out in private to allow the patient to volunteer anything confidential about previous fertility or sexually transmitted infections (Table 2). Table 3 lists commonly prescribed drugs and substances that impair male fertility, which is usually reversible if they are discontinued.

Full clinical assessment is valued by infertile men[16]. This engenders confidence and enables them to make decisions about their treatment. The patient seeks a diagnosis and reassurance from the andrologist that his sexual, procreative and 'macho' systems will not crash, and his hopes that this is curable. The man and his anxious spouse need to comprehend that sex and sperm production are separate processes, and that he will not become impotent. In especially severe sperm deficiencies, early referral for any further specialist advice minimizes anxiety.

Testis and prostate cancer

The association between infertility, testicular maldescent and tumors is well documented[17]. Testicular cancer may cause a semen abnormality, or can result from cryptorchidism. Most tumors are detected clinically and confirmed on ultrasound. A urological opinion is essential for any intratesticular lesion, unexplained absent testis or potentially premalignant testicular calcification found on ultrasound scan. Testicular tumors may present with gynecomastia, and scrotal ultrasound should be requested in all cases. In evaluating the prostate for urinary symptoms, any surface irregularity, asymmetry or absent median groove on rectal examination in men over 45–50 years raises the prospect of prostate cancer, the need for prostate-specific antigen (PSA) testing and referral. Semen cryobanking is undertaken if a tumor is confirmed, prior to surgery, radiotherapy or chemotherapy, but the semen quality is often poor. Protocols should be in place to inform health professionals about local sperm banking facilities for patients before they are treated for cancer.

Table 2 Common questions and various findings on assessment of infertile men

General

Infertility	duration, primary or secondary
Previous fertility	previous treatment, assisted reproduction
Coital history	frequency, erectile function, penetration, ejaculation
Family history	subfertility, cystic fibrosis, polycystic kidneys

History

Andrological	onset of puberty, libido, beard growth, loss of body hair
Recent history	pyrexia, trauma, major surgery, scrotal surgery, current medication
Endocrine	diabetes mellitus, thyroid disease, Kallman's syndrome, Klinefelter's syndrome
Neurological	spinal cord injury, pelvic surgery, multiple sclerosis, anosmia
Chronic illness	renal failure, cirrhosis, TB, schistosomiasis, sinusitis, pulmonary disease
Malignancy	testis cancer, orchidectomy, radiotherapy, chemotherapy, RPLND
Scrotal surgery	cryptorchidism, torsion, hernia, hydrocele, biopsy, varicocele, vasectomy
Genital infection	urethritis, chlamydia, gonorrhea, balanitis, orchitis, prostatitis, HIV
Micturition	LUTS, bladder-neck surgery, epispadias, hypospadias

Examination

Hypogonadism	body and pubic hair, beard growth, fat distribution, build, gynecomastia
Inguinal/scrotal scar	orchidopexy, herniorrhaphy, testicular biopsy or exploration
Penis	phimosis, balanitis, hypospadias
Testes	undescended, missing, soft or firm testes, focal lesion (?tumor)
	normal size, 4–5.5 cm (20–25 ml)
	subnormal, 3–4 cm (10–15 ml)
	atrophic, 1–2 cm (< 5 ml)
Epididymis	focal tenderness, cysts, engorgement (obstruction), absent (CBAVD)
Spermatic cord	absent vasa, vasectomy
Varicocele	grade I: cough impulse; grade II: palpable; grade III: visible
Rectal examination	prostatitis (?tender), focal lesion (?tumor)

TB, tuberculosis; HIV, human immunodeficiency virus; LUTS, lower urinary tract symptoms; CBAVD, congenital bilateral absence of the vas deferens; RPLND, retroperitoneal lymph node dissection

Table 3 Drugs that can affect male fertility

Impaired spermatogenesis	sulphasalazine, methotrexate, nitrofurantoin, colchicine, chemotherapeutic agents
Epididymal function	amiodarone
Pituitary suppression	testosterone, anabolic steroid injections
Antiandrogenic effects	cimetidine, spironolactone
Ejaculation failure	alpha-blockers, antidepressants, phenothiazines
Erectile dysfunction	beta-blockers, thiazide diuretics, metoclopramide
Drugs of abuse	anabolic steroids, cocaine

INVESTIGATIONS

Semen analysis (Tables 4 and 5)

Two abnormal SFA results are required for the diagnosis of male subfertility; these should be produced more than 3 months apart in view of the cycle of spermatogenesis, but within weeks for severe semen defects. Tests for infection include: cultures of the semen and post-prostate massage, first-catch urine samples for aerobic and anaerobic organisms and chlamydia testing. IVF preparations are discussed below.

Table 4   Normal semen parameters, World Health Organization (WHO)[3]

Volume	2.0 ml or more
Liquefaction time	within 60 min
pH	7.2 or more
Sperm concentration	20 million spermatozoa/ml or more
Total sperm number	40 million spermatozoa per ejaculate or more
Motility	50% or more motile (grades a* and b†) 25% or more with progressive motility (grade a) within 60 min
Morphology	15% (strict criteria) or 30% (WHO criteria) normal forms
Vitality	75% or more live
White blood cells	fewer than 1 million per ejaculate
Immunobead test	fewer than 50% spermatozoa with beads bound
MAR test *reaction* *Mixed antiglobulin*	fewer than 50% motile spermatozoa with adherent particles

*Grade a: rapid progressive motility (sperm moving swiftly, usually in a straight line); †grade b: slow or sluggish progressive motility (sperm may be less linear in their progression); MAR, mixed antiglobulin reaction

Table 5   Terminology of semen abnormalities

Normozoospermia	all semen parameters normal as defined by WHO values
Oligozoospermia	<20 million spermatozoa/ml
mild	>10 to <20 million spermatozoa/ml
moderate	5–10 million spermatozoa/ml
severe	<5 million spermatozoa/ml
extreme	<1 million spermatozoa/ml
Asthenozoospermia	reduced total sperm motility or reduced sperm progression
Teratozoospermia	increased proportion of abnormal forms of spermatozoa
Oligoasthenoteratozoospermia	all sperm variables are abnormal
Azoospermia	no spermatozoa in the ejaculate
Aspermia (anejaculation)	no ejaculate (ejaculation failure)
Cryptozoospermia *4 lus*	spermatozoa recovered after centrifugation *(as in retrograde ejaculation)*
Necrozoospermia	all spermatozoa are non-motile or non-viable
Leukocytospermia	increased white cells in the semen
Hypospermia	ejaculate volume <2 ml

Scrotal ultrasound

As an adjunct to the andrological examination, scrotal ultrasound is useful to distinguish varicoceles from other testicular lesions. A testicular tumor, focal calcification, rete testis or epididymal cysts may be discovered.

Transrectal ultrasound

Transrectal ultrasound (TRUS) is useful to evaluate men with low-volume ejaculates, retrograde ejaculation, pelvic pain, urinary symptoms or suspected prostate cancer. Dilated seminal vesicles may confirm ejaculatory duct obstruction, often due to a Mullerian prostatic cyst. In retrograde ejaculation there may be widening of the bladder neck, and in prostatitis evidence of calcification.

Endocrine levels   *15/3/09*

The serum follicle stimulating hormone (FSH) level rises in men with impaired spermatogenesis, and is a useful index of seminiferous tubule function[18], while inhibin B levels require further evaluation[19]. Low serum testosterone, with raised luteinizing hormone (LH) levels, indicates reduced Leydig cell mass, whereas high levels of both hormones occur in rare cases of androgen resistance. Hyperprolactinemia causes low testosterone levels, a poor libido and erectile dysfunction, but not semen abnormalities, unless a large pituitary lesion impacts on FSH and LH secretion.

Postcoital test

While there is little predictive value in terms of natural pregnancy, and sexual difficulty can arise[20], a postcoital test (PCT) can help to evaluate the effectiveness of coitus. PCTs are useful if sexual dysfunction is suspected, if a man cannot provide samples for SFA or has religious objection to masturbation, or if there is a low volume of ejaculate or male genital abnormality. Spermicide-free condoms are useful in certain situations to provide semen for analysis or assisted conception.

Genetic investigations

ICSI has led to the possibility of procreation in previously impossible situations, and raises concern about expansion of mutations in the human gene pool[21]. The principal issue is transmission of a physical defect or disease to a child, because ICSI enables sperm resulting from severely defective spermatogenesis to bypass natural selection processes to initiate pregnancies. As new genes are discovered, preimplantation genetic diagnosis (PGD) is increasingly useful to avoid genetic disease. Transmitting genes causing male infertility is of less concern, with the risk of associated somatic disease seen as small, but potential parents need to be aware. In cases involving severely defective spermatogenesis it is thus routine to offer genetic counseling and testing before treatment[22].

Chandley[23] found major chromosome changes in 2.2% of infertile men, thrice the normal incidence. There were abnormal karyotypes in 15.4% of azoospermic men, 12.9% with Klinefelter's syndrome (47,XXY). Abnormal karyotypes are less frequent if spermatogenesis is healthier: 1.76% with sperm concentration < 20 million/ml, under 1% if > 20 million/ml, 0.2% if > 100 million/ml. Microdeletions in the long arm of the Y chromosome (Yq) may cause severe oligozoospermia or non-obstructive azoospermia. These azoospermia factors (AZF) are located in three areas of Yq11, AZFa, AZFb or AZFc, with deletion of RBM1 at AZFb, DAZ (deleted in azoospermia) and SPGY1 at AZFc[24]. Yq deletions may cause future infertility in boys, while sex chromosome aneuploidy, mosaicism or an autosomal translocation could cause fetal abnormality or recurrent miscarriage[25].

In't Velt and colleagues[22] found a karyotype defect, AZF deletion or cystic fibrosis (CF) mutation in 26% of 80 severely infertile men. A risk of transmitting systemic disease arises in 66% of men with congenital bilateral absence of the vas deferens (CBAVD) due to CF mutations[26]; also in CBAVD patients without CF mutations who have renal defects such as unilateral renal agenesis[27], which may be due to autosomal dominant renal dysplasia; and bilateral vasal obstruction following renal transplantation for autosomal dominant adult polycystic kidney disease.

LIFE-STYLE ISSUES

Semen quality in men can be affected by excess alcohol intake, smoking, tight underwear, obesity, sedentary occupations (e.g. driving), heat or chemicals at work. Caffeine and foods have no effect[28]. The main issue for infertile men is alcohol intake. The safe level for fertile men is 3–4 units per day, but British males frequently binge-drink eight or more units every 1–4 weeks. If the testes are dysfunctional, one merry evening may reduce the sperm output for months due to the 3-month cycle of spermatogenesis, but this is reversible. In azoospermic alcohol abusers, Brzek reported that total abstention resulted in sperm-positive ejaculates after 3 months[29]. In the clinical situation, this can avoid the need for surgical sperm recovery in heavy drinkers with non-obstructive azoospermia. Smoking impairs semen parameters, but the relationship to infertility is uncertain, while cocaine and anabolic-steroid abuse are more likely to have an effect on fertility. In some areas (e.g. Scotland), dietary lack of selenium causes sperm defects and male subfertility (also in farm animals) with a rationale for selenium supplementation[30]. Table 6 lists a 3–6-month life-style regimen for subfertile men to try to improve their semen quality for ART, although natural conception is unlikely.

MANAGEMENT

I. Ineffective coitus

Infertility due to ineffective coitus can be categorized according to whether the patient has normal antegrade ejaculation or no ejaculate owing to retrograde ejaculation or ejaculation failure (Table 7). The diagnosis may become apparent during the inquiry into coital frequency, erectile function, penetration, orgasm and ejaculation, or explained by an existing condition or drug therapy. Any effect of sexual dysfunction on fertility would be doubtful if sperm is found on post-coital testing.

In the UK, most couples, general practitioners (GPs) and gynecologists believe that mid-cycle timing of coitus improves the chance of natural conception, but it is highest in the 6 days before ovulation[31]. Couples are advised that coitus at least every 2–3 days throughout the cycle ensures that spermatozoa, which

Table 6   Rationale for a conservative regimen for men with subnormal semen quality[28]

(1) Discontinue adverse medication or drugs of abuse: see Table 3

(2) Avoid pesticides, herbicides, X-rays, heat at work: can cause abnormal semen

(3) Stop smoking: nicotine reduces seminal plasma antioxidants and semen parameters

(4) Reduce alcohol intake or abstain: alcohol can suppress spermatogenesis

(5) Avoid scrotal heating: tight underwear and certain jobs impair semen quality

(6) Frequent coitus (alternate days): increases the output of non-senile spermatozoa

(7) Antioxidant therapy: vitamin E and selenium can improve sperm motility

Table 7   Ineffective coitus: subcategories and etiology

(1) Antegrade ejaculation: normal ejaculatory response

   (a) Asynchronous – incorrect timing

   (b) Low volume ejaculate (hypospermia) – prostatitis, unilateral ejaculatory duct obstruction

   (c) Failure of penetration – neurological, physical disability, e.g. hip disease

   (d) Abnormal semen deposition – hypospadias, phimosis

   (e) Erectile dysfunction – psychogenic or organic erectile dysfunction

   (f) Functional incompetence – retarded ejaculation

   (g) Non-consummation – vaginismus, imperforate hymen

(2) Retrograde ejaculation: cryptospermia

   (a) Neurogenic – diabetes mellitus, multiple sclerosis

   (b) Pharmacological – phenothiazines, sympathetic blocking agents

   (c) Anatomical – epispadias, congenital bladder-neck incompetence

   (d) Iatrogenic – transurethral prostatectomy, bladder-neck incision

   (e) Idiopathic

(3) Ejaculation failure: aspermia, anejaculation

   (a) Functional – primary anorgasmia

   (b) Neurogenic – spinal cord injury, multiple sclerosis

   (c) Pharmacological – antihypertensive or psychotropic medication

   (d) Iatrogenic – retroperitoneal or pelvic surgery, sympathectomy

can survive for up to 7 days inside the female tract, will always be present at ovulation. Timing coitus based on body temperature or urinary LH kits creates stress and does not improve the chance of natural conception[32], but may be useful for couples who have difficulty with frequent intercourse.

Therapeutic objectives

The effectiveness of coitus may be improved by counseling or appropriate medication. To achieve pregnancy, most cases require ART using sperm recovered from the semen or urine following stimulation of ejaculation. Vaginal or intrauterine insemination is often successful because this type of male infertility is mostly mechanical and sperm function tends to be normal, but IVF, ICSI or surgical sperm recovery is often required.

Patients with antegrade ejaculation

Initial advice on increasing coital frequency and avoiding the stress of mid-cycle timing is helpful.

Failure of consummation is mostly psychogenic in newly wed couples, often after strict religious upbringing. Reassurance, sex education and phosphodiesterase 5 (PDE5) inhibitors, e.g. sildenafil, are usually successful in initiating regular coitus. For physically disabled men a different position for coitus may assist vaginal penetration, while erectile dysfunction normally responds to PDE5 inhibitors, and studies show no adverse effect on semen quality[33]. If infertility

is an issue of timing due to long periods of travel, this is managed by semen freezing and timed IUI. Men with retarded ejaculation are unable to ejaculate intravaginally and are only occasionally helped by counseling or drugs (e.g. yohimbine), while to initiate pregnancy, semen produced by self-stimulation or clinical vibrator is utilized for artificial insemination.

Retrograde ejaculation (Figure 1)

In retrograde ejaculation, failure of bladder-neck closure during emission allows the semen to escape into the bladder. This is diagnosed from a history of orgasm without ejaculation, and is confirmed by detecting sperm and/or fructose in postorgasmic urine. Retrograde ejaculation due to sympathetic neuropathy occurs in diabetes mellitus, and may arise after sympathectomy or retroperitoneal lymph node dissection. Anatomical causes include congenital bladder-neck incompetence, bladder-neck incision or transurethral

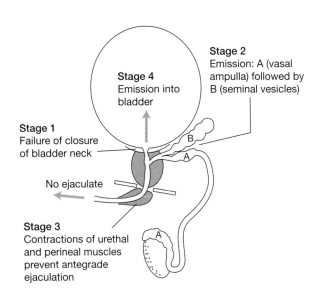

Figure 1 Mechanism of retrograde ejaculation. (Reproduced with permission form Hirsh AV. A guide to the practice of andrology in the assisted conception unit. In Rainsbury PA, Viniker DA, eds. *Practical Guide to Reproductive Medicine*. Carnforth, UK: Parthenon Publishing, 1997)

resection of the prostate, and many cases are idiopathic. Partial retrograde ejaculation is suspected if the semen volume ($<2\,ml$) or semen pH (<7.0) are reduced.

Kamischke and Nieschlag[34] found that sympathomimetic drugs (brompheniramine, ephedrine, phenylephrine, phenylpropanolamine, imipramine, midrodin, pseudoephedrine, synephrine), either alone or in combination, or prescribed with chlorpheniramine, induced antegrade ejaculation in up to 79% of patients, regardless of the etiology of the retrograde ejaculation. The side-effects of dizziness, sleep disturbance, nausea, weakness, dry mouth or sweating were tolerable. The most successful drug in inducing natural pregnancy was oral imipramine 20–150 mg daily, which resulted in 28 (39%) pregnancies in 71 couples accumulated from several reports[34].

In most cases it is necessary to proceed with timed IUI using sperm recovered from postorgasmic urine. Fluid regulation and oral sodium bicarbonate are prescribed to control urine osmolarity and pH, to minimize the toxic effects of urine on sperm. Urry and colleagues[35] reported pregnancy in 16% of cycles using IUI with washed spermatozoa. If the yield of sperm is poor, IVF and/or ICSI may be indicated. If

necessary, antegrade ejaculation can usually be induced by penile vibratory stimulation or rectal electroejaculation (see below).

Ejaculation failure (aspermia, anejaculation)

The absence of orgasm or ejaculation, with non-viscous, fructose-negative and sperm-negative post-coital urine, suggests failure of seminal emission. Cases of rare primary anorgasmia are regarded as psychogenic and usually have nocturnal emissions, but are mostly resistant to drug therapy. Sexual behavioral therapy can provide a cure, otherwise vibratory stimulation may be used to stimulate ejaculation for artificial insemination[36].

In serious neurological conditions, aspermia is incurable. Most cases seen are due to spinal cord injury (SCI), but aspermia may also be caused by pelvic injury, multiple sclerosis and retroperitoneal lymph node dissection (RPLND). Many aspermic men presenting for treatment have spinal injuries above T10, following road accidents. They are usually in wheelchairs, use a condom device for urinary drainage, or an indwelling or suprapubic catheter, and require manual evacuation of their bowels on alternate days. However, they are usually otherwise fit, both psychologically and medically, often work and marry, and want families. The lack of penetrative sex is frequently not a large problem for the couple, who are far more interested in having children. Spermatogenesis is not usually seriously impaired[37]. Erectile dysfunction may be treated by a PDE5 inhibitor or penile alprostadil injections, and ejaculation can sometimes occur during coitus. There may also be reflex ejaculation with non-penetrative sex or certain movements, when semen can be used for home vaginal insemination. Treating any urinary infection minimizes contamination of the semen.

Kamischke and Nieschlag[34] found that the most effective drugs for aspermia were intravenous or oral midrodin (α sympathomimetic agonist), subcutaneous physostigmine and intrathecal neostigmine (parasympathomimetic agonist). Retrograde or antegrade ejaculation was stimulated in up to 56% of patients, but with serious side-effects, including autonomic dysreflexia in men with SCI lesions above T6. There were only two reported cases of natural pregnancy resulting from oral drugs (two of eight couples from imipramine or brompheniramine), and three resulting from subcutaneous physostigmine. Due to side-effects and differing success, drugs are less useful for inducing ejaculation in men with aspermia (about 20%) than in cases of retrograde ejaculation (up to 80%), and the management of anejaculation is normally based on physical stimulation of ejaculation for ART[34].

Penile vibratory stimulation Most SCI men cannot ejaculate during sexual stimulation. With a lesion above T10 the reflex arcs are intact and the majority (80%) achieve antegrade ejaculation using a penile vibrator[38]. The optimum frequency of clinical vibrators is 80–100 Hz (amplitude 2.5 mm). Applying the probe to the penile frenulum is well tolerated, but there is a danger of spinal dysreflexia in men with lesions above T6, and hypertension is minimized by sublingual nifedipine. Sperm motility is usually reduced due to seminal plasma factors, but improves with repeated ejaculations. Penile vibrators used at home for vaginal insemination lead to pregnancy in 25–61% of couples, even if the semen quality is suboptimal[39].

Electroejaculation If vibratory stimulation is unsuccessful, rectal electroejaculation (REE) using a Seager probe applied to the seminal vesicles is effective in producing semen in most cases. Owing to total loss of sensation below the umbilicus in most men with SCI, the patient is often awake, but where spinal dysreflexia or discomfort are a risk, general anesthesia and sublingual nifedipine are indicated. There is normally some retrograde flow of semen, and buffering solution is first instilled into the bladder and then aspirated with sperm after REE. Poor-quality semen improves with repeated REE due to improved transit in the genital tract. The ejaculate can be used for IUI, but IVF and/or ICSI are usually required, as the semen quality tends to be inferior to that produced using penile vibratory stimulation. The average pregnancy rate is 25% per cycle[39].

Surgical sperm recovery In most assisted conception units testicular sperm aspiration (TESA) is the method of obtaining sperm for IVF–ICSI from men with aspermia if techniques to stimulate ejaculation are unsuccessful. Surgical sperm recovery under local anesthetic is also utilized as a rescue procedure for ART if the man cannot ejaculate on the day of oocyte retrieval for psychological reasons, a PDE5 inhibitor or penile vibrator have not helped, or he has eaten and cannot have a general anesthetic for REE.

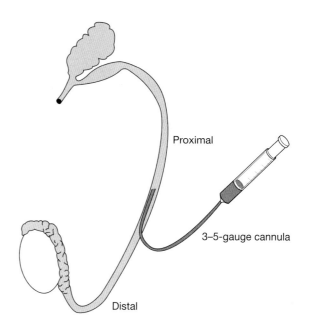

Figure 2 The technique of vas deferens aspiration (vas aspiration), which is useful in men with aspermia[40]. (Reproduced with permission from Hirsh AV. A guide to the practice of andrology in the assisted conception unit. In Rainsbury PA, Viniker DA, eds. *Practical Guide to Reproductive Medicine*. Carnforth, UK: Parthenon Publishing, 1997)

Vas aspiration (Figure 2) Vas deferens aspiration may be utilized to recover sperm from men with anejaculation[40]. The spermatozoa have traversed the epididymis and are generally of good motility and morphology, and are usually capable of fertilization. Even for spinal cord-injured men, a local anesthetic spermatic cord block is needed to avoid discomfort and possible spinal dysreflexia, because sympathetic nerve-mediated sensation of the testes is usually intact, whereas the scrotal skin is normally numb. The vas is exposed at the neck of the scrotum. A 2-French gauge (fg) umbilical cannula introduced via a microsurgical vasotomy is advanced distally to aspirate the vasal ampulla. A short intravenous cannula can be inserted proximally towards the testis while massaging the epididymis to facilitate aspiration of spermatic fluid. The vasotomy is repaired microsurgically to prevent scarring and obstruction. Vas aspiration usually harvests enough motile spermatozoa for IVF or cryostorage for several cycles, and is often adequate for IUI. Utilizing a percutaneous aspiration technique, Qiu and colleagues obtained vasal sperm and achieved 19 (56%) pregnancies in 34 cycles of IUI carried out in 26 couples[41].

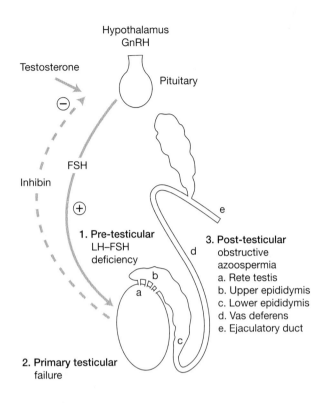

Figure 3 Pathophysiology of the three types of azoospermia, and the anatomical sites of blockages in obstructive azoospermia. GnRH, gonadotropin releasing hormone; FSH, follicle stimulating hormone; LH, luteinizing hormone. (Reproduced with permission from Hirsh AV. A guide to the practice of andrology in the assisted conception unit. In Rainsbury PA, Viniker DA, eds. *Practical Guide to Reproductive Medicine.* Carnforth, UK: Parthenon Publishing, 1997)

II. Azoospermia (Figure 3)

Azoospermia is the cause of 2% of human infertility and may be due to:

(1) Hypogonadotropic hypogonadism (hypothalamic–pituitary failure, secondary testicular failure);

(2) Non-obstructive azoospermia (NOA) (primary testicular failure, secretory azoospermia);

(3) Obstructive azoospermia (OA) (genital tract obstruction, testicular obstruction).

Hypogonadotropic hypogonadism is rare, while non-obstructive and obstructive azoospermia each cause infertility in about 1% of couples. Table 8 categorizes azoospermia according to whether the mechanism is pretesticular, testicular or post-testicular.

Diagnosis and investigations

The diagnosis of azoospermia requires two or more centrifuged semen samples, 2–4 weeks apart, to confirm that sperm are totally absent. Patients with hypogonadotropic hypogonadism have small testes (2–3 cm) and low levels of testosterone, FSH and LH. Men with non-obstructive azoospermia have small testes (2–4 cm) with high FSH levels (over twice the upper limit of normal), with usually normal virilization, but the serum testosterone level may be subnormal with a raised LH level due to a reduced Leydig cell mass. Normal-size testes (4–5 cm) and normal FSH levels support a diagnosis of obstructive azoospermia, and patients are normally virilized, as their testicular function and serum testosterone and LH levels are also normal.

Therapeutic objectives and preliminary counseling

It is important to identify hypogonadotropic hypogonadism, as gonadotropin therapy is usually effective in initiating natural pregnancy. For men with OA and palpable vasa, and men seeking vasectomy reversal, reconstructive surgery also provides an opportunity to procreate naturally. Surgical sperm recovery for ICSI is indicated if reconstruction for OA was unsuccessful and for men with congenital bilateral absence of the vas deferens (CBAVD). Many couples prefer assisted reproduction to surgery for the male partner, as the result is known sooner. Patients with NOA are offered testicular sperm recovery, as 50% have foci of spermatogenesis in the testes suitable for ICSI. All couples need advice about genetic causes of azoospermia, testing and counseling.

Hypogonadotropic hypogonadism

Hypogonadotropic hypogonadism (HH) is a rare cause of male infertility that usually presents with delayed puberty or undescended testes in adolescence. Primary HH may be idiopathic or due to Kallmann's syndrome caused by defects in gonadotropin-releasing hormone (GnRH) neurons and the olfactory bulb, with anosmia, and can be X-linked. Secondary HH results from postpubertal pituitary failure, and may be due to adenoma, head injury, hemochromatosis or metastases; hence, neurological symptoms or signs sanction imaging for a pituitary or other intracranial tumor and appropriate referral. Most men with HH

Table 8 Etiology of azoospermia

(1) Pre–testicular	gonadotropin deficiency
(a) Hypothalamic	idiopathic hypogonadotropic hypogonadism, Kallmann syndrome, craniopharyngioma, hemochromatosis
(b) Pituitary	trauma, ablation, adenoma, isolated FSH deficiency, meningitis
(c) Drugs	anabolic steroids, testosterone injections
(2) Testicular	non-obstructive azoospermia
(a) Congenital	cryptorchidism, Klinefelter's syndrome, myotonic dystrophy, sex chromosome aneuploidy, Y deletions, anorchia
(b) Acquired	mumps orchitis, torsion, castration
(c) Iatrogenic	radiotherapy, chemotherapy
(3) Post-testicular	obstructive azoospermia
(a) Congenital	CBAVD, cystic fibrosis, Mullerian prostatic cyst
(b) Acquired	gonorrhea, chlamydia, tuberculosis, schistosomiasis
(c) Iatrogenic	vasectomy, herniorrhaphy, hydrocele repair, renal transplant

FSH, follicle stimulating hormone; CBAVD, congenital bilateral absence of the vas deferens

presenting for infertility treatment are already diagnosed and maintained on testosterone injections following earlier induction of puberty, or after radiotherapy or surgery for pituitary or hypothalamic tumors. Some patients have rare congenital syndromes (e.g. cerebellar ataxia, Prader–Willi syndrome) and require genetic counseling before treatment.

HH is treated with gonadotropins, and results are best in men who did not have undescended testes[42]. Testosterone replacement can be suspended to allow the serum level to fall to a reference value. The Leydig cells are then primed to generate endogeneous testosterone with subcutaneous (SC) or intramuscular (IM) human chorionic gonadotropin (hCG) 2000–5000 units twice weekly. The serum testosterone should increase to levels above 10 nmol/l in 4–6 weeks, but the hCG dose may need to be increased. When the testosterone levels are adequate, human menopausal gonadotropin (hMG,) commencing with two ampoules (150 u FSH and 150 u LH) SC or IM three times weekly, is added to stimulate the Sertoli cells. The testes begin to grow and the semen usually reveals motile spermatozoa within 3–12 months, although the dose may also need to be increased. Natural pregnancy often occurs, even with low sperm concentrations, as the spermatozoa secreted are functionally normal. The main side-effect is painful gynecomastia, which is helped by adjusting the hCG or hMG dose. Recombinant FSH is also effective[43]. If sperm do not appear

in 12–18 months, pulsatile GnRH given by portable minipump can be tried[44], but testicular sperm recovery should be considered, as spermatogenic foci with sperm suitable for ICSI may have developed[45].

Androgen abuse

Azoospermia may be due to pituitary suppression from anabolic-steroid abuse by sportsmen. The serum testosterone level is very high, with virtually absent FSH and LH. Patients are very muscular, but may have atrophic testes, and gynecomastia can occur due to aromatization of androgens to estrogen. If the drugs are stopped, normal levels of FSH and LH are soon restored, the semen becomes normal in 3–6 months and natural pregnancy is usually soon established.

Non-obstructive azoospermia

Non-obstructive azoospermia (NOA) is due to primary seminiferous tubule (testicular) failure. There may be associated Leydig cell loss, with low serum testosterone and raised LH levels, and the libido may be affected. Most cases of NOA are idiopathic or due to late orchidopexy. Orchidopexy should be carried out before the age of 2 years to try to avoid infertility, and rarely succeeds after puberty. The most prevalent genetic causes of NOA are Klinefelter's syndrome (15–30%) and microdeletions of the Y chromosome (8–10%). Orchitis, testicular cancer, torsion, serious trauma, chemotherapy and radiotherapy are commonly encountered acquired causes of NOA.

There is little chance of restoring fertility in men with NOA. In some cases the azoospermia is a transient finding in men with severe oligozoospermia following fever, illness or excess alcohol intake. Following 3 months of alcohol abstension, motile spermatozoa may appear in the semen[29]. There are also reports of the appearance of spermatozoa after varicocele repair in NOA[46]. Cases of NOA are managed by testicular sperm recovery for IVF–ICSI. In 50% of patients, diffuse foci of spermatogenesis are present in the testes with histological appearances of the Sertoli-cell-only (del Castillo's) syndrome, or sometimes focal atrophy, maturation arrest or hypospermatogenesis.

Klinefelter's syndrome

Klinefelter's syndrome occurs in 0.2% of men, and is the most usual cause of male hypogonadism. It is due to sex chromosome aneuploidy with karyotype 47,XXY, in most cases, arising from meiotic nondisjunction of an oocyte which retains two X chromosomes and is fertilized by a Y-bearing sperm. Patients may be obese, with female body fat, scanty hair distribution and gynecomastia, but can be tall and eunuchoid. The testes are small (2 cm) and firm. The FSH and LH levels are grossly elevated, with the serum testosterone levels low due to Leydig cell dysfunction. Sexual dysfunction and other problems of androgen withdrawal are common at middle age and respond to testosterone supplementation. In rare cases there is oligozoospermia due to 46,XY/47,XXY mosaicism.

The testicular histology reveals hyalinized seminiferous tubules, absent germ cells and Leydig cell hyperplasia. Vernaeve and colleagues[47] reported recovery of testicular sperm from 48% of men with non-mosaic Klinefelter's syndrome, similar to other cases of NOA. To eliminate embryos with sex chromosome aneuploidy preimplantation genetic diagnosis is desirable, but of 36 healthy children born after ICSI using sperm from non-mosaic Klinefelter's patients only one 47,XXY fetus resulted[47].

Therapy for cancer and azoospermia

Owing to successful therapy in recent years, men cured of testicular cancer, Hodgkin's disease or other lymphoma now present for infertility treatment. Patients with these conditions should be offered semen cryopreservation before therapy, but this was not generally taken up until recently, and the semen is often azoospermic. Hansen and associates[48] reported that 53% of 41 men treated for testicular cancer by radiotherapy or chemotherapy were fertile 5 years later. Roselund and colleagues recovered sperm from 16 of 17 men (15 azoospermic) treated for testis cancer by orchidectomy and radiotherapy, chemotherapy or retroperitoneal lymph node dissection. IVF or ICSI was carried out with ejaculated sperm following masturbation in 3/3 cycles, electroejaculation in 16/17 cycles and testicular sperm extraction (TESE) in 1/2 cycles, with pregnancy in 57% of couples[49].

Obstructive azoospermia

Three categories of men with obstructive azoospermia (OA) present in the andrology clinic:

(1) Congenital bilateral absence of the vas deferens (CBAVD) – neither vas is palpable;

(2) Bilateral genital tract obstruction – both vasa are usually palpable;

(3) Men presenting for reversal of sterilization – defects in the vasa may be palpable.

Congenital bilateral absence of the vas deferens

CBAVD occurs in 0.1% of men, and 10–20% of men with OA presenting in the assisted conception unit. CBAVD is due to failure of Wolffian (mesonephric) duct development, causing bilateral aplasia of the vas deferens, seminal vesicle, ejaculatory duct, body and tail of the epididymis. The head (caput) of the epididymis engorged with sperm is usually palpable.

Azoospermia with a low volume (< 1 ml), fructose negative ejaculate is typical of CBAVD. In some men seminal vesicles develop and there is normal volume fructose-positive azoospermic semen. The diagnosis is confirmed on examination. There is normal virilization and normal-size testes, but neither vas is present. Surgical exploration is unnecessary, because spermatogenesis is invariably normal and reconstruction is impossible. Patients can be reassured in the clinic that sperm is present and can be recovered for ICSI, but the clinician must be certain that both vasa are absent.

CBAVD is a minor variant of cystic fibrosis (CF). Nearly all men affected by CF are sterile due to CBAVD. Only 4% of northern European men carry CF mutations, but 66% with CBAVD carry a major cystic fibrosis transmembrane regulator (CFTR) gene mutations, usually delta F508 combined with a 5T allele minor variant to cause the CBAVD pheno-type[26,50]. Other types of CF mutation may occur in men with CBAVD of other races. The link with CF is reflected by sinusitis or pulmonary symptoms occurring commonly. CBAVD patients without CFTR mutations may have renal anomalies, e.g. an absent, pelvic or horseshoe kidney or duplex ureters[27]. It is useful to request a renal tract ultrasound scan in case of future serious accident involving the kidneys.

Before undertaking assisted conception for CBAVD it is essential to screen both partners for CF mutations. If both partners are carriers, the 1 : 4 risk of a child affected by CF can be avoided by pre-implantation genetic diagnosis (PGD). In most cases the CBAVD patient carries one CFTR mutation and his spouse is negative, when the risk of a CF-affected child is reduced to < 1 : 300; this appears to be acceptable, as the incidence of CF in Europe is 1 : 625. Management of CBAVD is by surgical sperm recovery and ICSI. Percutaneous epididymal sperm aspiration (PESA) under local anesthesia usually recovers adequate sperm for several cycles of IVF–ICSI with cryostorage, while testicular aspiration (TESA) is an alternative.

Men with congenital unilateral absence of the vas deferens (CUAVD) are usually fertile, and this is most often discovered on examination prior to vasectomy; they have a high incidence of unilateral renal aplasia. Azoospermic men with CUAVD are often cases of CBAVD with sections of vas palpable in the scrotum, and the same precautions regarding CF screening must be carried out prior to assisted reproduction[51].

Reconstructive surgery in obstructive azoospermia (Figure 4)

The management of obstructive azoospermia and vasectomy reversal by reconstructive surgery enables natural pregnancy to be achieved. The female partner needs to be assessed in advance to ensure that she is fertile. The alternative of IVF–ICSI using surgically recovered sperm is attractive, and the comparative success rates, costs and shortcomings of both methods should be compared for both partners during their counseling, leaving adequate time for their decision.

Most cases are due to epididymal blocks from postinfective scarring (chlamydia, gonorrhea), which occur at constant sites in the genital tract. The caput epididymis is usually swollen (Bayle's sign). OA may also occur after hydrocele or hernia repair or renal transplantation, or can be due to Wolffian defects, when CF screening is indicated. OA patients with sinusitis or chest symptoms may have Young's syndrome (azoospermia with sinopulmonary disease), which is rare. Circulating sperm antibodies (immunoglobulin G, IgG) in about 50% of cases marginally affect the outcome after reconstruction.

Bilateral ejaculatory duct obstruction

If the semen volume is < 2 ml with fructose absent, the azoospermia may be due to bilateral ejaculatory duct obstruction, confirmed by transrectal ultrasound demonstrating dilatation of the seminal vesicles, often with a Mullerian duct cyst inside the prostate. Transurethral resection of the verumontanum or cyst returns sperm to the semen in 50% of cases[52].

Testicular exploration and epididymovasostomy

Having confirmed a normal semen volume, scrotal exploration under general anesthesia with a view to reconstructive microsurgery is indicated. Facilities for sperm cryopreservation should be available. Having exposed the testes, each epididymis is inspected for obstructed tubules, and there are usually symmetrical blocks in the cauda epididymis. An operative vasogram is carried out by injecting each vas with contrast to confirm patency of the ejaculatory ducts. Bilateral epididymovasostomy (EV) is undertaken by creating anastomoses between the lumen of the upper vas and an incision in a single dilated epididymal tubule swollen with sperm that is identified on microscopy.

If the vas is also blocked, this is repaired by vasovasostomy (VV)[53], but high vasal blocks seen on vasography require an inguinal approach. If there are multiple blockages the case is inoperable, while microsurgical epididymal sperm aspiration (MESA) or a testicular biopsy enables sperm to be cryopreserved.

Management if there is no epididymal obstruction

If there is no sign of epididymal obstruction, testicular biopsies are obtained and examined fresh for sperm that can be cryopreserved. Testicular tissue samples are sent for histology in Bouin's solution. If spermatogenesis is normal the block is in the rete testis, with 50% due to immune orchitis, as confirmed by raised serum sperm antibody titers (tray agglutination or

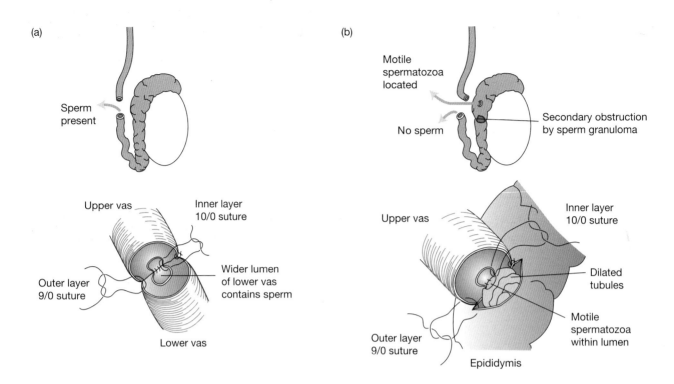

Figure 4 Microsurgical two-layer anastomoses used for vasectomy reversal and epididymal obstructions. (a) Vasovasostomy: if spermatozoa are identified in the lower (testicular) segment of the divided vas deferens, end-to-end anastomosis can be carried out. (b) Epididymovasostomy: sperm cannot enter the lower vas, owing to an obstruction in the epididymis, here caused by a secondary block from a sperm granuloma following dehiscence of an obstructed tubule. The obstruction is bypassed by anastomosing the end of the divided vas deferens to the side of an epididymal tubule where motile spermatozoa have been identified microscopically. (Reproduced with permission from Hirsh AV. A guide to the practice of andrology in the assisted conception unit. In Rainsbury PA, Viniker DA, eds. *Practical Guide to Reproductive Medicine*. Carnforth, UK: Parthenon Publishing, 1997)

immunobead tests). Therapy with oral prednisolone (5 mg three times a day after meals) may lead to sperm positive semen in 3–6 months, but natural pregnancy is unlikely. Most cases are managed by IVF–ICSI using surgically recovered testicular sperm, which avoids the potential complications of corticosteroids.

In some cases the diagnosis of OA was wrong, and the embryologist finds few or no spermatozoa in the testicular tissue. Histopathology may reveal maturation arrest or seminiferous tubule failure and the Sertoli-cell-only syndrome, with or without focal spermatogenesis. If spermatozoa are recovered and cryopreserved, appropriate genetic testing is needed before proceeding with IVF–ICSI.

Results of corrective surgery in obstructive azoospermia

Bilateral microsurgical epididymovasostomy (EV) is successful in returning sperm to the semen in over 60% of men within 6–12 months. Good results can be achieved following non-microsurgical anastomoses, especially for blocks in the tail (cauda) of the epididymis, but with poor results from anastomoses in the caput (head). Resection of ejaculatory duct obstruction returns sperm to the semen in 50% of patients. Following corrective surgery in OA, natural pregnancy results for more than 25% of couples, depending on the site of the block and operative conditions. Although early pregnancies arise following corrective surgery they usually occur after 9–12 months (Table 9)[52–56].

Vasectomy reversal

Men in second marriages often present in assisted conception units seeking details about vasectomy reversal. The couple should be counseled about the pros and cons of surgical reversal of vasectomy and ART, and the female partner requires ovulation and

Table 9 Results of epididymovasostomy (EV) in obstructive azoospermia

Technique	Author(s)	EV site	Number	Patency (%)	Pregnancy (%)
Standard	Dubin, Amelar, 1984[54]		69	20	10
	Hendry et al., 1990[53]	cauda	60	43	20
		caput	90	12	3
Microsurgical	Silber, 1989[55]	corpus	139	78	56
		caput	51	73	31
	Schlegel, Goldstein, 1993[56]		107	70	31

Table 10 Patient information: the options for reversing vasectomy

	Vasectomy reversal	Assisted reproduction
Conception	natural	medically assisted
Method	male partner surgery	assisted conception
Procedures	male partner only	both partners
Costs	male surgical procedure	sperm recovery + freezing + IVF–ICSI
Best results	reverse before 10 years	female partner under 35 years
Poor results	reverse after 10 years	female partner over 40 years
Male partner	surgical operation	sperm recovery (PESA)
Anesthetic	general	local or general
Sperm in semen	70–90% in 3 months	remains clear
Contraception	needed in the future	never required
Female partner	tests to exclude infertility	IVF–ICSI and embryo transfer
Pregnancy rates*	25% at 1 year	25% per cycle (twins 1:4)
	40–50% at 2 years	50% at 1 year[†]

*In women under 35 years (in vitro fertilization (IVF) pregnancies are less than 10% per cycle after age 40); [†]IVF cycles undertaken by infertile couples average about two per year; ICSI, intracytoplasmic sperm injection; PESA, percutaneous epididymal sperm aspiration

tubal function tests (Table 10). Production of sperm continues normally after vasectomy. The results of surgical reversal are best within 3 years, with natural pregnancy occurring in 76% of couples, whereas after 9–14 years this reduces to 30%, while the presence of sperm antibodies, which are IgG, has only slight effects on the outcome.

End-to-end vasovasostomy (VV) by a one layer standard technique results in recanalization in 80–90% of patients within 3 months, with natural pregnancy in 25–45% of couples. Results in terms of pregnancy are improved by microsurgery (Table 11). Failure to restore sperm to the semen may be due to secondary epididymal blocks arising from tubular blowouts and

sperm granuloma formation, which can be bypassed by EV if recognized. Revision (redo) of vasectomy reversal leads to sperm-positive semen in 50% of patients[57–62].

Sperm recovery techniques and ICSI in azoospermia (Figure 5)

The capacity of IVF–ICSI to enable oocyte fertilization with few immature spermatozoa has led to out-patient-oriented sperm recovery techniques to initiate pregnancies from azoospermic men, of whom 75% produce sperm. Indications for surgical sperm recovery include: obstructive (OA) and

Table 11 Results of vasectomy reversal

Technique	Author(s)	Number	Patency (%)	Pregnancy (%)
Standard	Bagshaw et al., 1980[57]	56	91	25
	Parslow et al., 1983[60]	104	93	45
	Soonawala, Lal 1984[61]	194	81	44
Microsurgery	Silber, 1977[58]	126	90	76
	Belker et al., 1991[59]	1247	86	52
	Fox, 1994[62]	103	84	48

non-obstructive (NOA) azoospermia, necrozoospermia and ejaculatory dysfunction (see above).

Sperm recovery in obstructive azoospermia

In obstructive azoospermia, sperm retrieval usually succeeds, and it is convenient to undertake this electively to accumulate frozen sperm for several ICSI cycles. Sperm recovery is indicated if:

(1) Reconstructive surgery is not feasible, e.g. CBAVD, rete testis obstruction, multiple blockages;

(2) Corrective surgery was unsuccessful, e.g. failure of vasectomy reversal or epididymovasostomy;

(3) The patient and his partner prefer assisted reproduction to surgical correction.

Couples should be advised about genetic screening as appropriate. Facilities to cryopreserve sperm should be available after routine screening for hepatitis B and C and human immunodeficiency virus (HIV) is undertaken. Sperm recovery under local anesthesia (LA) is associated with high patient satisfaction[63], but many men prefer general anesthesia (GA). The embryologist should be in the operating area to assess the recovered aspiration fluid or biopsy tissue, and inform the surgeon when sufficient viable spermatozoa are accumulated.

The procedure should be as minimally invasive as possible. Small epididymal cysts occur in 4% of men with OA, and motile spermatozoa can often be retrieved using a fine needle (23-gauge)[64]. For most cases LA is required, and is obtained by infiltrating the spermatic cord (L_1 fibers from the testis) and scrotal skin (L_{1-2} and S_{1-3} dermatomes) with 10–20 ml of 2% lignocaine mixed with 0.5% bupivacaine. This is effective for 30–60 min, with postoperative analgesia lasting 24 h.

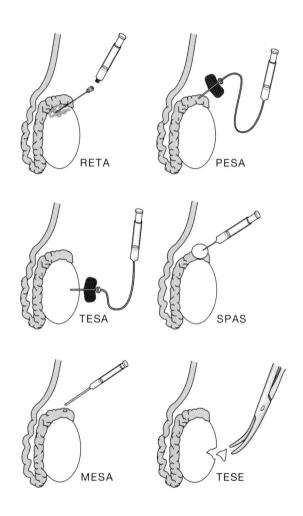

Figure 5 Methods of surgical sperm recovery for intracytoplasmic sperm injection (ICSI) utilized in men with azoospermia. RETA, rete testis aspiration; PESA, percutaneous epididymal sperm aspiration; TESA, testicular sperm aspiration; SPAS, spermatocele aspiration; MESA, microsurgical epididymal sperm aspiration; TESE, testicular sperm extraction (from a biopsy). (Reproduced with permission from Hirsh AV. A guide to the practice of andrology in the assisted conception unit. In Rainsbury PA, Viniker DA, eds. *Practical Guide to Reproductive Medicine*. Carnforth, UK: Parthenon Publishing, 1997)

Table 12 Sperm recovery techniques in 67 azoospermic men (London Women's Clinic, 1994–98)

Technique	GA (n)	Attempts (n)	Sperm (n)	Motile (n)	Suitable for ICSI (%)
Obstructive azoospermia					
SPAS	0	8	8	8	100
RETA	2	43	19	8	19
PESA	2	39	35	34	87
TESA	1	14	6	5	43
TESE	0	15	15	14	100
MESA	3	3	3	3	100
Non-obstructive azoospermia					
RETA	2	4	0	0	0
PESA	1	1	0	0	0
TESA	1	3	0	0	0
TESE	2	10 (7 nb)	6	6	60 (43% nb)
TESE	6	15 (12 sb)	15	15	100 (100% sb)

GA, procedures under general anesthesia; ICSI, intracytoplasmic sperm injection; SPAS, spermatocele aspiration; RETA, rete testis aspiration; PESA, percutaneous epididymal sperm aspiration; TESA, testicular sperm aspiration; TESE, testicular sperm extraction; MESA, microsurgical epididymal sperm aspiration; nb, patients without previous testicular biopsies; sb, patients with spermatozoa on previous testicular biopsy

Percutaneous epididymal aspiration (PESA) with a 21-gauge butterfly needle and 10-ml syringe harvests live spermatozoa, with surplus to cryopreserve in most cases[65]. Testicular sperm aspiration (TESA) with a 19-gauge butterfly needle and 20-ml syringe is undertaken if PESA fails to recover motile sperm[66]. Rete testis aspiration (RETA) with a 23-gauge needle may be useful if these procedures fail to recover any spermatozoa. Finally, a testicular biopsy for sperm extraction (TESE) may be obtained by the window technique if the yield of spermatozoa is inadequate[67]. Patients are advised to rest for 48 h and avoid alcohol. Common complications include vasovagal episodes, scrotal bruising or delayed wound healing, while hematoma and infection are unusual.

Microsurgical epididymal aspiration (MESA) is useful during corrective surgery to collect sperm for multiple cycles[68], when the incised tubules are repaired to prevent secondary blocks. However, MESA normally requires GA and is not commonly undertaken as a lone procedure, due to the advantages of LA and less invasive techniques. It is also less complicated to obtain a testicular biopsy (TESE) for sperm, saving time and effort for the microsurgical reconstruction.

Sperm recovery in non-obstructive azoospermia

Owing to the lower prevalence, patchy distribution and poor quality of spermatogenesis in NOA, sperm recovery is always uncertain. Sperm recovery should be offered in all cases, even if the testes are atrophic or the FSH levels are very high, since no test can be used to confirm or exclude sperm within the testes[69]. This should be emphasized to the patient before attempting sperm recovery.

TESA has a relatively low success rate in recovering sperm in NOA, so TESE is usually required[70]. GA is preferred because bilateral incisions and multiple biopsies may be needed to obtain sufficient spermatozoa. The biopsy should be about 5 mm in diameter. Several biopsies (1–3) may be needed, depending on how quickly sperm is recovered and on the testicular volume. A small specimen is sent for histological diagnosis, as *in situ* testicular carcinoma occurs in 1.1% of infertile men and seminoma develops in 2% of previously undescended testes[71].

Multiple TESE is useful in recovering sperm after previously failed TESE, in Klinefelter's syndrome[47] and following radiotherapy or chemotherapy. TESE suppresses spermatogenesis for 3–6 months, so that later TESE procedures in repeat ICSI cycles are undertaken only after this time interval to allow the testes to recover[72]. It is unusual for patients to develop hypogonadism following TESE, but it is good practice to assess the serum testosterone level 3–6 months later. To try to improve the yield of sperm and conserve tissue in men, microdissection TESE enables exploration of the testis between tissue planes with less trauma, and has good reported results after previously failed TESE[73].

Tournaye and colleagues[74] recovered sperm from 15 of 31 (48%) men with NOA by multiple TESE. A sperm-positive testicular biopsy was the best predictor of successful sperm recovery, but sperm was recovered from one in three men where the histology had not identified spermatozoa. AZFa and AZFb Y-chromosome deletions are poor prognostic factors for successful sperm retrieval, while men with AZFc deletions are more likely to have sperm[74]. If no sperm is recovered, spermatids used for oocyte microinjection have resulted in varying reported success[75].

Laboratory preparation of surgically recovered spermatozoa

Surgically recovered sperm may be used fresh or can be conveniently cryopreserved for future ICSI cycles. In most cases of OA, abundant viable spermatozoa are retrieved with progressive motility in epididymal (PESA and MESA) samples, and rudimentary activity in testicular aspirates (TESA) or biopsy tissue (TESE). Several ampoules of sperm can be frozen with good post-thaw motility.

Few spermatozoa are present in NOA, and identifying them in testicular tissue may require several hours and there is often no surplus to freeze. Post-thaw sperm survival is reduced in NOA, and the patient is often required for standby TESE in repeat IVF–ICSI cycles if there is doubt about the cryopreserved tissue. TESE is therefore often undertaken on the day of oocyte retrieval to obtain fresh sperm. Immotile sperm cells may become active during incubation and many units undertake TESE 24 h before oocyte collection to facilitate sperm recovery[76]. Nijs and associates observed fertilization in 52–65% of oocytes following ICSI with non-motile ejaculated, epididymal and testicular spermatozoa, but only embryos generated from testicular sperm implanted[77]. The viability of individual sperm cells can be determined by the hypo-osmotic swelling (HOS) test.

Results of sperm recovery for ICSI

Table 12 compares the effectiveness of 103 sperm recovery procedures from 67 men with OA and NOA, 92 under LA and 11 using GA, including three MESA procedures during surgery for OA. Sperm were recovered in 63 (94%) patients in 99 fresh cycles,

with failure in four of seven men with NOA. The success of the technique varied among OA and NOA cases, but with no difference in fertilization (mean 54.9%/oocyte) or pregnancy (mean 23.2%/cycle) resulting from different methods or male diagnostic categories. In OA cases, MESA enables sperm freezing for several ICSI cycles. In this series a mean of 3.6 samples (1–8) were cryobanked after 44% of PESA procedures.

As an illustration of difficulty in cases of NOA, TESA failed to recover sperm in three men with NOA, but TESE was then successful. Westlander and colleagues[78] recovered sperm by TESA in 15 of 68 (22%) men with NOA. Friedler and associates[70] retrieved sperm by TESA in four (11%) and by TESE in 16 (43%) of 37 cases of NOA. At Bourn Hall (2002–04), sperm were recovered using multiple TESE under GA from 17 (57%) of 30 men with NOA. No sperm were found on histology of two (12%) biopsies in successful cases, but there was evidence of sperm in four (30%) of 13 biopsies where no sperm were recovered (unpublished results). These converse findings reflect the patchy nature of spermatogenesis in NOA. Patients should be advised about this uncertainty beforehand.

As the intended method of sperm recovery in OA, PESA succeeded in 74 (68%) of 109 procedures carried out at four centers (Bourn Hall, London Women's Clinic, St Thomas's Hospital, Roding Hospital), 100 under LA. Spermatocele, rete testis (RETA) and testicular aspiration (TESA) improved sperm recovery to 84%. The need for TESE in 16% of men with OA reflected a learning curve for TESA, and compares to the results of Gorgy and colleagues[63] who noted the effectiveness of sperm recovery under LA and success in 90% of men when PESA and TESA results were combined.

The outcome of surgical sperm recovery and IVF–ICSI

In men with OA, successful recovery of epididymal or testicular sperm is usual in all cases, and yields similar fertilization and pregnancy results equivalent to those with ejaculated spermatozoa. In cases of NOA, sperm recovery succeeds in about 50% of cases, but although there is a similar outcome from fresh and frozen testicular sperm, the results are generally inferior when compared with OA. There is currently insufficient evidence to recommend any specific technique in favor of another, and so the least invasive method is preferable, depending on the pathology and wishes of the patient[79].

III. Sperm autoimmunity

Sperm antibodies adhere to the sperm cell membrane and impair progressive motility by causing agglutination and adherence to leukocytes in seminal plasma. Cervical mucus penetration is poor, and fertilization is marred by interference with sperm–zona binding and the acrosome reaction. The significance of sperm antibodies is unclear, but they are detectable by MAR (mixed antiglobulin reaction) or direct immunobead testing (IgG and IgA) as part of routine SFA, and confirmed in serum or seminal plasma by tray agglutination (TAT) or indirect immunobead tests. Titers of > 50% for MAR and immunobead tests, and TAT of 1/32, are considered significant. IgA antibodies are potent and may arise in genitourinary infections. IgG antibodies occurring in obstructive azoospermia, unilateral blocks and after vasectomy have low antifertility effects. Cytotoxic antibodies may also occur.

ART has replaced corticosteroid therapy for men with sperm antibodies, as their effectiveness in initiating natural pregnancy is uncertain. Side-effects of steroids are significant when considering the 1 : 3 chance of natural pregnancy after 6–9 months of therapy and a dose of 40–60 mg prednisolone daily[80]. There are risks of weight gain, insomnia, facial swelling, acne, gastric irritation, diabetes mellitis, peptic ulceration and hip necrosis. IUI gives poor results, and while sperm preparation techniques and IVF improve the fertilizing ability, this is much reduced if the immunobead titer is > 70–80%, so that ICSI is usually required[81]. Some men offer to accept the risk of steroids for the possibility of natural procreation, often where a couple cannot obtain funding for IVF–ICSI.

Unilateral testicular obstruction (Figure 6)

Obstruction of one testis may cause oligozoospermia via a cell-mediated immune orchitis, which partially obstructs the rete of the contralateral testis, reducing sperm flow into the efferent ducts. The sperm is further compromised by IgA secreted in the seminal plasma. The testes are of different sizes: the obstructed testis is usually normal with a swollen epididymis, while the opposite gland is often small due to

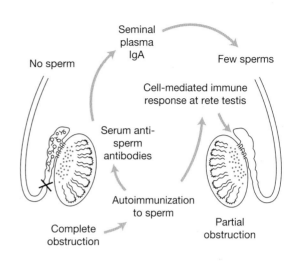

Figure 6 The etiology of immunological infertility in unilateral testicular obstruction. IgA, immunoglobulin A. (Reproduced with permission from Hirsh AV. A guide to the practice of andrology in the assisted conception unit. In Rainsbury PA, Viniker DA, eds. *Practical Guide to Reproductive Medicine*. Carnforth, UK: Parthenon Publishing, 1997)

defective spermatogenesis. The sperm antibody level may be reduced by surgical correction of the obstruction if feasible and/or corticosteroid therapy. Improved semen quality and spontaneous pregnancy were reported in 25% of couples, while removing an irreversibly obstructed testis resulted in natural pregnancy for 10% of couples[82]. IVF–ICSI has a more certain outcome with less risk.

IV. Semen abnormality

Semen abnormalities cause 25% of human infertility and 85% of male infertility. The sperm count is usually reduced (oligozoospermia), but the infertility is due to the predominance of dysfunctional spermatozoa as demonstrated by subnormal motility (asthenozoospermia) and poor morphology (teratozoospermia), which are indicators of deranged sperm maturation or production. When these primary sperm defects coexist, the abnormality is termed oligo-asthenoteratozoospermia syndrome or OATS. OATS is categorized into mild (10–20 million/ml), moderate (5–10 million/ml) or severe (< 5 million/ml) OATS, based on the count, but the problem is the quality issue of sperm dysfunction. Men with teratozoospermia or

Table 13 Etiology of semen abnormalities

Idiopathic	the majority
Developmental	cryptorchidism, late orchidopexy, varicocele
Life-style	alcohol excess, tobacco, cocaine, anabolic steroids (low dose)
Acquired	prostatitis, unilateral obstruction, torsion, orchitis, testicular cancer
Genetic	sex chromosome mosaicism, Yq deletion, translocation
Iatrogenic	salazopyrin, radiotherapy, chemotherapy, testosterone injections
Systemic disease	thyrotoxicosis, renal or liver failure, diabetes mellitus
Immunological	immune orchitis, unilateral testicular obstruction
Chemicals at work	agricultural (pesticides, herbicides), laboratory, and paint workers
Physical agents	radiotherapists (X-ray), engine drivers, diggers (vibration)
Scrotal heating	drivers, welders, bakers, tight underwear

asthenozoospermia but normal counts are considered under this category as the causes are similar, but most cases are idiopathic.

Causes of OATS and sperm dysfunction

Several factors have been implicated in the etiology of OATS. OATS patients are a heterogeneous group based on several studies of their testicular histology[83,84]. These reveal a high prevalence of about 50% with normal spermatogenesis, even with sperm counts < 1 million/ml. Subtotal testicular obstruction or 'obstructive oligozoospermia' has been reported in operative series with natural pregnancy resulting from corrective surgery[85]. In other cases, spermatogenesis is defective. These cases can be viewed as secretory or 'non-obstructive oligozoospermia', which is irreversible. There is often a history of varicocele, orchitis, orchidopexy, genitourinary infection or systemic disease. In addition, prescribed medicines, illicit drugs or alcohol intake may contribute. Environmental factors in fetal or later life, occupational influences and recessive autosomal genes are also implicated[12,86]. Many

cases of OATS appear to be multifactorial, with dysfunctional testes further suppressed by a second potentially reversible factor, e.g. varicocele, epididymitis, prostatitis, fever or illness, alcohol excess, drug abuse, smoking, obesity, tight underwear, etc. (Table 13).

The markedly reduced sperm fertilizing capacity in OATS is related to high levels of reactive oxygen species (ROS) in the seminal plasma. Low levels of ROS (free radicals) in normal semen are required for sperm capacitation and hyperactivation, regulated by seminal plasma antioxidants (e.g. vitamins C and E, selenium, zinc, catalase, superoxide dismutase, glutathione peroxidase) acting as free radical scavengers. Grossly elevated ROS levels are produced by dysfunctional spermatozoa or active leukocytes in two-thirds of men with OATS. By inducing lipid peroxidation of sperm cell membranes, ROS impair the sperm tail-powering mitochondria and acromosome enzyme mechanisms, and denature the sperm head DNA causing strand breaks. Natural antioxidants in seminal plasma may be reduced in tobacco smokers[87].

Clinical features of OATS

Most patients are normally virilized with no genital abnormality apart from reduced testis size, and have no medical or life-style infertility factors. There is rarely any problem with coitus, except for psychological reasons after the diagnosis. Serum FSH levels are often raised, with slightly reduced testosterone depending on the severity of testicular failure. In some cases epididymal swelling may indicate unilateral testicular obstruction, or focal epididymitis is associated with urinary symptoms when subclinical prostatitis is suspected. A karyotype and assessment for Y chromosome microdeletions are indicated if the sperm concentration is < 5 million/ml. As there is no effective medical or surgical treatment to improve the probability of natural pregnancy[1] it is useful to discuss ART during the initial assessment.

Therapeutic objectives in men with OATS

In couples with OATS, natural pregnancy occurs in 1–2% of cycles, commonly with a total motile sperm count of > 2 million/ml, indicating that some of the ejaculated spermatozoa are functionally normal[15,88]. Trying to improve the sperm output is a false concept. This does not address the issue of sperm dysfunction. In some men the semen may improve (possibly spontaneously) with therapy or life-style adjustment, but not the probability of natural pregnancy, because any increased sperm output is probably dysfunctional. With the high prevalence of female factors in couples with infertility attributed to OATS[8], treatment of the woman may initiate a pregnancy. However, if the semen quality improves there is potential to reduce the complexity of future ART, e.g. IUI instead of IVF.

Management of men with abnormal semen

Conservative treatment regimen (Table 6)   A 3–4-month conservative regimen may improve the semen quality if the abnormality is transient after a short illness or due to life-style factors. This aims to reduce external anti-infertility factors[28], but most effective is to curtail binge-drinking[29].

Hormone therapy   Clinical trials have shown that antiestrogens (e.g. clomiphene, tamoxifen), androgens (e.g. mesterolone) and gonadotropin injections do not improve the semen or the probability of natural pregnancy. Rarely, oligozoospermia is due to isolated FSH deficiency, which responds to gonadotropin therapy[89]. In men with reduced serum testosterone to estradiol ratios an aromatase inhibitor (e.g. anastrazole) may improve the semen quality, but not the sperm fertilizing capacity[90].

Male accessory gland infection (MAGI), antibiotics and antioxidants   Production of ROS by leukocytes in subclinical male accessory gland infection (MAGI) is often suspected in men with OATS and impaired semen liquefaction or increased viscosity, a seminal plasma pH > 8.0, leukocytospermia, prostatitis, epididymitis, previously sexually acquired infection, or testicular, perineal or ejaculatory discomfort. Semen cultures are rarely positive, as seminal plasma contains antibacterial agents, but a first catch urine sample after prostate massage may reveal red cells or increased leukocytes or chlamydia. Antibiotics are indicated only if organisms are cultured.

Antioxidants (e.g. vitamins E and C, zinc and selenium) administered to infertile men as free radical scavengers are potentially beneficial to sperm function and DNA integrity. Selenium deficiency in men (and farm animals) has been related to impaired sperm motility and infertility. Selenium supplements can improve the sperm motility in subfertile men[30].

Mast cell blocking and alpha-blocking agents   Tranilast, a mast cell blocker, improved semen quality and fertility in early studies. The alpha blocker, bunazosin, also improved the semen, but not fertility. These drugs relax smooth muscle and may enhance sperm transit in the male tract, and further studies are required[91,92].

Correction of varicocele   Varicoceles are dilatations of the pampiniform plexus due to internal spermatic vein reflux. They usually appear at puberty and are associated with atrophy of the ipsilateral testis. They occur in 15% of fertile men and in 30–40% of subfertile men. The pathogenesis of the infertility is attributed to raised testicular temperature due to disruption of scrotal heat-exchange mechanisms. Surgical correction or embolization of varicocele was traditionally recommended as treatment for male infertility, and several series demonstrated improved semen quality and fertility following surgery. However, metaanalysis of controlled studies did not confirm this[93], in contrast to proponents of varicocele correction[94]. The long-awaited final analysis of a WHO trial, and further studies, may settle the controversy, but in the mean time varicocele correction cannot be recommended for male infertility based on the available evidence, although it may prevent testicular atrophy in boys, as well as alleviating scrotal discomfort if present.

Assisted reproduction for suboptimal semen quality

The only logical treatment for OATS is ART. Fertilization and thus IUI or IVF are often feasible in mild–moderate cases, but IVF–ICSI is indicated in severe cases, especially with few ejaculated motile spermatozoa, and in men with asthenozoospermia and teratozoospermia.

Sperm preparation

The results of IVF sperm preparations and strict morphology criteria help to select the appropriate method of ART. There is no current better test of sperm function to predict the capacity of separated spermatozoa to fertilize. Washing or density gradients improve the quantity and quality of spermatozoa isolated from the semen, and the resulting 'sperm preps' have improved counts of morphologically normal progressive spermatozoa with reduced levels of ROS. Assisted conception units have different sperm selection criteria for IUI, IVF and ICSI based on their individual results.

Intrauterine insemination

If the sperm preparation harvests > 2–5 million normal spermatozoa, IUI is indicated in most units, provided that the female partner has normal tubal function. Berg and colleagues[95] determined that 0.8 million spermatozoa would suffice. The guideline recommendation of six cycles of non-stimulated IUI for mild male-factor infertility is based on meta-analyses involving several thousand IUI cycles[96]. This is low cost and avoids high-order multiple pregnancies. The conception rate of 5–10% per cycle is low, but the cumulative pregnancy rate over several cycles is likely to equate with IVF results[97].

In vitro fertilization

IVF is usually considered feasible if > 1 million normal spermatozoa are isolated, but there may be reduced fertilization in OATS[98]. Strict criteria sperm morphology assessment was originally introduced as a useful predictor of the outcome of IVF in subfertile men[99].

Intracytoplasmic sperm injection

IVF–ICSI can enable fertilization in severe cases of OATS, and is indicated if < 1 million normal spermatozoa are available, the total motility or progression (< grade 2–3/4) is reduced or there is teratozoospermia according to WHO[3] (< 30% normal) or strict[99] (< 14%) criteria. Following fertilization, the conception rate is the same as in standard IVF cycles. Scanty sperm cells in the semen need to be individually selected for ICSI, imposing demands on the skill of embryologists to recover sufficient viable spermatozoa for all retrieved oocytes. After three to five cycles the cumulative pregnancy rate reaches > 50%[100].

Necrozoospermia describes spermatozoa with no viability or motility, while the sperm count is usually normal. This may occur in chronic prostatitis, when sperm activity may be stimulated by antibiotic therapy. The sperm are probably senescent due to delayed transit in the genital tract, as sperm activity often returns with increased frequency of ejaculation. Some men with OATS also have necrozoospermia. If there is no motility in a semen sample provided for recovered oocytes, a second sample within 1 h may reveal motile spermatozoa, enabling ICSI to be carried out. As spermatogenesis is normal in most cases, testicular

sperm can usually be obtained under local anesthetic for IVF–ICSI[101].

V. Sperm abnormality

The spermatozoa are dysfunctional due to a structural defect, while the sperm concentration is normal, and the patient has normal virilization. Management involves IVF–ICSI in view of the inability of all ejaculated spermatozoa to fertilize, but genetic counseling may be required.

Immotile cilia syndrome (primary ciliary dyskinesia)

This is an autosomal recessive disorder, incidence one in 20 000, causing ultrastructural defects of all cilia in the body including the sperm flagellae. Half of these patients have Kartagener's syndrome of *situs inversus*, recurrent chest infection, bronchiectasis and sinusitis since childhood. Sperm concentration is normal, but all spermatozoa are immotile. Ultrastructural studies reveal disorganized 9 + 2 axoneme groups in the sperm tails and absence of the dynein arm muscular elements, which control flagellar activity. Before considering ART, genetic counseling is advisable owing to the clinical syndrome. ICSI is needed for fertilization[102]. The sperm cells may exhibit some activity, but the viability of cells can be assessed by the hypoosmotic swelling test prior to oocyte microinjection. As in cases of necrozoospermia (above), testicular sperm can also be utilized.

Globozoospermia

This describes the rare syndrome of 'round headed', 'marble headed' or 'acrosomeless' spermatozoa. During spermatogenesis, developing acrosomal vesicles disintegrate without fusing to the sperm heads. Patients are physically normal, with normal semen values, apart from 100% teratozoospermia due to the absence of all sperm acrosomes. Fertilization is impossible without ICSI, and several pregnancies have been reported[103].

Failed fertilization and teratozoospermia

Teratozoospermia revealed by strict morphology criteria may account for failed fertilization in IVF cycles. There is usually no clinical abnormality of the patient and such cases are resolved by ICSI. In recurrent failed embryo implantation after ICSI a recent study shows that using testicular sperm improves results, if there are high levels of sperm DNA fragmentation in the ejaculate. This novel methodology implicates a sperm factor in embryo quality[104].

Donor insemination

Owing to the success of IVF–ICSI in all types of male infertility, there is now less demand for donor insemination (DI). Men with absolutely no sperm, due to anorchia or non-obstructive azoospermia and failed testicular sperm recovery, have absolute indications for DI. DI may also be considered if there is a high risk of transmitting a genetic disorder (e.g. Huntingdon's chorea) or infectious disease (e.g. human immunodeficiency virus (HIV)) by the man, and in severe rhesus isoimmunization. In an ideal society, without economic constraint, DI would be necessary for < 1 in 200 infertile men. As DI is economic, non-invasive and very successful, this is an option for couples with infertility due to irreversible obstructive and non-obstructive azoospermia and severe semen defects, who prefer to avoid ART for various reasons, or are unable to find funding for high-technology treatment.

CONCLUSION

The issue of biological fatherhood potentially has been solved for the 99.5% of infertile men who have sperm due to developments in modern ART. Research into germ-cell and stem-cell grafting into the testes[105] may one day assist the one in 200 men with germ cell aplasia, while reproductive cloning, a potential solution for men with anorchia, has been rejected by society.

Satisfying normal desires to conceive naturally could relieve the anxiety experienced by the largest group of infertile couples, those with semen abnormalities and sperm dysfunction. Successful treatment by ART is gratifying, but not a cure. Ovarian stimulation is a risk for the female partner and fetus, ICSI may transmit genetic conditions or more infertility, while the costs limit access for many couples. Reproductive medicine needs to focus on the etiology of sperm dysfunction. We have so far directed specific treatments at a multifactorial problem, and must learn to distinguish clinically between patients with impaired or normal spermatogenesis and determine why both have sperm

dysfunction. If this can be reversed by treatment, the same goal as in therapies for the three uncommon curable causes of male infertility will be achieved, leading to natural conceptions and live births.

REFERENCES

1. National Collaborating Centre for Women and Children's Health. Fertility: Assessment and Treatment for People with Fertility Problems. London: RCOG Press, 2004: 52–6
2. Hull MGR, Glazener CMA, Kelly NJ, et al. Population study of causes, treatment, and outcome of infertility. Br Med J 1985; 291: 1693–7
3. World Health Organization. WHO Laboratory Manual for the Examination of Human Semen and Sperm–Cervical Mucus Interaction, 4th edn. London: Cambridge University Press, 1999
4. Skakkebaek NE, Giwercman A, de Kretser D. Pathogenesis and management of male infertility. Lancet 1994; 343: 1473–8
5. World Health Organization. Towards more objectivity in diagnosis and management of male infertility. Results of WHO multicenter study. Int J Androl 1987; (Suppl 7)
6. Dubin L, Amelar RD. Etiologic factors in 1294 consecutive cases of male infertility. Fertil Steril 1971; 22: 469–74
7. Greenberg SH, Lipschultz LI, Wein AJ. Experience with 425 subfertile male patients. J Urol 1978; 119: 507–10
8. Hargreave TB. Human infertility. In Hargreave TB, ed. Male Infertility, 2nd edn. London: Springer Verlag, 1994: 1–16
9. ESHRE Capri Workshop Group. Male sterility and subfertility: guidelines for management. Hum Reprod 1994; 9: 1260–4
10. Nieschlag E. Classification of andrological disorders. In Nieschlag E, Behre HM, eds. Andrology. Berlin: Springer-Verlag, 1997: 81–3
11. Sigman M, Lipschultz LI, Howards SS. Evaluation of the subfertile male. In Lipschultz LI, Howards SS, eds. Infertility in the Male, 3rd edn. St Louis, MO: Mosby, 1997: 173–93
12. Sharpe RM. Lifestyle and environmental contribution to male infertility. Br Med Bull 2000; 56: 630–42
13. Crosignani PG, Collins J, Cooke ID, et al. Unexplained infertility. Hum Reprod 1992; 8: 977–80
14. Hirsh AV. Post-coital sperm retrieval could lead to the wider approval of assisted conception by some religions. Hum Reprod 1996; 11: 245–7

15. Collins JA, Burrows EA, Wilan AR. The prognosis for live birth among untreated infertile couples. Fertil Steril 1995; 64: 22–8

16. Hirsh AV. Male subfertility. Br Med J 2003; 327: 669–72

17. Carlsen E, Giwercman A, Keiding N, Skakkebaeck NE. Evidence for decreasing quality of semen during the past 50 years. Br Med J 1992; 305: 609–13

18. Pryor JP, Hirsh AV, Fitzpatrick J, et al. The value of plasma FSH in the assessment of the infertile male. Proceedings of The 5th World Congress on Fertility and Sterility, Venice, Italy, 1978: 181–2.

19. Andersson AM, Petersen JH, Jorgensen N, et al. Serum inhibin B and FSH hormone levels as tools in the evaluation of infertile men: significance of adequate reference values from proven fertile men. J Clin Endocrinol Metab 2004; 89: 2873–9

20. Osei SG, Helmerhorst FM, Kierse MJ. When is the post-coital test normal? A critical appraisal. Hum Reprod 1995; 10: 1711–14

21. Hargreave TB. Genetic basis of male infertility. Br Med Bull 2000; 56: 650–71

22. In't Velt P, Halley DJJ, van Hemel JO, et al. Genetic counselling before ICSI. Lancet 1997; 350: 490

23. Chandley AC. Chromosomes. In Hargreave TB, ed. Male Infertility, 2nd edn. London: Springer-Verlag 1994: 149–64

24. Vogt PH, Edelmann A, Hirschmann P, et al. The Y chromosome and infertility in the male. Hum Reprod 1996; 11 (Abstr book 1): 32–3

25. Morris SM, Gleicher N. Genetic abnormality, male infertility and ICSI. Lancet 1996; 347: 1277

26. Anguiano A, Oates RD, Amos JA, et al. Congenital absence of the vas deferens: a primary genital form of cystic fibrosis. J Am Med Assoc 1992; 267: 1794–7

27. McCallum T, Milunsky J, Munarriz R, et al. Unilateral renal agenesis associated with congenital bilateral absence of the vas deferens: phenotypic findings and genetic considerations. Hum Reprod 2001; 16: 282–8

28. National Collaborating Centre for Women and Children's Health. Fertility: Assessment and Treatment for People with Fertility Problems. London: RCOG Press, 2004: 26–32

29. Brzek A. Alcohol and male fertility (preliminary report). Andrologia 1987; 19: 32–6

30. Scott R, MacPherson A, Yates RW, et al. The effect of oral selenium supplementation on human sperm motility. Br J Urol 1998; 82: 76–80

31. Wilcox AJ, Dunson D, Baird DD. The timing of the fertile window in the menstrual cycle: day specific estimates from a prospective study. Br Med J 2000; 321: 1259–62

32. Dunson DB, Baird DD, Wilcox AJ, Weinberg CR. Day-specific probabilities of clinical pregnancy based on two studies with imperfect measures of ovulation. Hum Reprod 1999; 14: 1835–9

33. Purvis K, Muirhead GJ, Harness JA. The effects of sildenafil on human sperm function in healthy volunteers. Br J Clin Pharmacol 2002; 53 (Suppl 1): 53S–60S

34. Kamischke A, Nieschlag E. Update on medical treatment of ejaculatory disorders. Int J Androl 2002; 25: 333–44

35. Urry RL, Middleton RG, McGavin S. A simple and effective technique for increasing pregnancy rates in couples with retrograde ejaculation. Fertil Steril 1986; 46: 1124–7

36. Michetti PM, Rossi R, Travaglia S, et al. Primary absolute anorgasmy in the male. Report of three clinical cases. Minerva Urol Nefrol 1999; 51: 23–6

37. Elliott SP, Orejuela F, Hirsch IH, et al. Testis biopsy findings in the spinal cord injured patient. J Urol 2000; 163: 792–5

38. Brindley GS. The fertility of men with spinal injuries. Paraplegia 1984; 22: 337–48

39. Sonksen J, Ohl DA. Penile vibratory stimulation and electroejaculation in the treatment of ejaculatory dysfunction. Int J Androl 2002; 25: 324–32

40. Hirsh AV, Mills C, Tan SL, et al. Pregnancy using sperm aspirated from the vas deferens in a patient with ejaculatory failure due to spinal injury. Hum Reprod 1993; 8: 89–90

41. Qiu Y, Wang SM, Yang DT, Wang LG. Percutaneous vasal sperm aspiration and intrauterine insemination for infertile males with anejaculation. Fertil Steril 2003; 79: 618–20

42. Ley SB, Leonard JM. Male hypogonadotrophic hypogonadism: factors influencing response to human chorionic gonadotrophin and human menopausal gonadotrophin, including prior exogenous androgens. J Clin Endocrinol Metab 1985; 61: 746–52

43. Bouloux P, Warne DW, Loumaye E. Efficacy and safety of recombinant human FSH in men with isolated hypogonadotropic hypogonadism. Fertil Steril 2002; 77: 270–3

44. Morris DV, Adeniyi Jones R, Wheeler M, et al. The treatment of hypogonadotrophic hypogonadism in men by the pulsatile infusion of luteinizing hormone-releasing hormone. Clin Endocrinol 1984; 21: 189–200

45. Fahmy I, Kamal A, Shamloul R, et al. ICSI using testicular sperm in male hypogonadotrophic hypogonadism unresponsive to gonadotropin therapy. Hum Reprod 2004; 19: 1558–61

46. Schlegel PN, Kaufmann J. Role of varicocelectomy in men with nonobstructive azoospermia. Fertil Steril 2004; 81: 1585–8

47. Vernaeve V, Staessen C, Verheyen G, et al. Can biological or clinical parameters predict sperm recovery in 47,XXY Klinefelter syndrome patients? Hum Reprod 2004; 19: 1135–9

48. Hansen PV, Glavind K, Panduro J, Pederson M. Paternity in men with testicular germ cell cancer. Pre-treatment and post-treatment findings. Eur J Cancer 1991; 27; 1385–9

49. Roselund B, Sjoblom P, Tornblom M, et al. IVF and ICSI in the treatment of infertility after testicular cancer. Hum Reprod 1998; 13: 414–18

50. Chillon M, Casals T, Mercier B, et al. Mutations in the cystic fibrosis gene in patients with congenital bilateral absence of the vas deferens. N Engl J Med 1995; 332: 1475–80

51. Mickle J, Milunsky A, Amos JA, Oates RD. Congenital unilateral absence of the vas deferens: a heterogeneous disorder with two distinct subpopulations based upon aetiology and mutational status of the cystic fibrosis gene. Hum Reprod 1995; 10: 1728–35

52. Pryor JP, Hendry WF. Ejaculatory duct obstruction in subfertile males: analysis of 87 patients. Fertil Steril 1991; 56: 725–30

53. Hendry WF, Levison D, Parkinson CM, et al. Testicular obstruction: clinico-pathological studies. Ann R Coll Surg Engl 1990; 72: 396–407

54. Dubin L, Amelar RD. Magnified surgery for epididymo-vasostomy. Urology 1984; 23: 525–8

55. Silber SJ. Results of microsurgical vaso-epididymostomy: role of epididymis in sperm maturation. Hum Reprod 1989; 4: 298–303

56. Schlegel PN, Goldstein M. Microsurgical vaso-epididymostomy: refinements and results. J Urol 1993; 150: 1165–8

57. Bagshaw HA, Masters JRW, Pryor JP. Factors influencing the outcome of vasectomy reversal. Br J Urol 1980; 52: 57–9

58. Silber SJ. Microscopic vasectomy reversal. Fertil Steril 1977; 28: 1191–202

59. Belker AM, Thomas AJ, Fuchs EF, et al. Results of 1469 microsurgical vasectomy reversals by the Vasovasostomy Study Group. J Urol 1991; 145: 505–11

60. Parslow JM, Royle MG, Kingscott MMB, et al. The effects of sperm antibodies on fertility after vasectomy reversal. Am J Reprod Immunol 1983; 3: 28–31

61. Soonawala FB, Lal SS. Microsurgery in vasovasostomy. Indian J Urol 1984; 1: 104–8

62. Fox M. Vasectomy reversal – microsurgery for best results. Br J Urol 1994; 73: 449–53

63. Gorgy A, Meniru GI, Naumann N, et al. The efficacy of local anesthesia for percutaneous epididymal sperm aspiration and testicular sperm aspiration. Hum Reprod 1998; 13: 646–50

64. Hirsh AV, Dean NL, Mohan PJ, et al. Natural spermatoceles in irreversible obstructive azoospermia – reservoirs of viable sperm for assisted conception. Hum Reprod 1996; 11: 1919–22

65. Shrivastav P, Nadkarni P, Wensvoort S, Craft I. Percutaneous epididymal sperm aspiration for obstructive azoospermia. Hum Reprod 1994; 9: 2058–61

66. Craft I, Tsirigotis M. Simplified recovery, preparation and cryopreservation of testicular spermatozoa. Hum Reprod 1995; 10: 1623–6

67. Devroey P, Liu J, Nagy Z, et al. Normal fertilization of human oocytes after testicular sperm extraction and intracytoplasmic sperm injection. Fertil Steril 1994; 62: 639–41

68. Oates RD, Lobel SM, Harris DH, et al. Efficacy of intracytoplasmic sperm injection using intentionally cryopreserved epididymal spermatozoa. Hum Reprod 1996; 11: 133–8

69. Bettocchi C, Parkinson MC, Ralph DJ, Pryor JP. Clinical aspects associated with Sertoli-cell-only histology. Br J Urol 1998; 82: 534–7

70. Friedler S, Raziel A, Strassburger D, et al. Testicular sperm retrieval by percutaneous fine needle sperm aspiration compared with testicular sperm extraction by open biopsy in men with non-obstructive azoospermia. Hum Reprod 1997; 12: 1488–93

71. Giwercman A, Berthelsen JG, Muller J, et al. Screening for carcinoma-in-situ of the testis. Int J Androl 1987; 10: 173–80

72. Schlegel PN. Physiological consequences of testicular sperm extraction. Hum Reprod 1996; 11 (Abstr book 1): 74

73. Schlegel PN. Testicular sperm extraction: microdissection improves sperm yield with minimal tissue excision. Hum Reprod 1999; 14: 131–5

74. Tournaye H, Verheyen G, Nagy P, et al. Are there any predictive factors for successful surgical sperm recovery in azoospermic patients? Hum Reprod 1997; 1: 80–6

75. Mansour RT, Fahmy IM, Taha AK, et al. Intracytoplasmic spermatid injection can result in the delivery of normal offspring. J Androl 2003; 24: 757–64

76. Zhu J, Tsirigotis M, Pelkanos M, et al. In-vitro maturation of human testicular spermatozoa [Letter]. Hum Reprod 1996; 11: 231–2

77. Nijs M, Lejeune B, Segal-Bertin G, et al. Fertilising ability of immotile sperm after ICSI. Proceedings of Andrology in the Nineties, Ghent, Belgium, October 1995: Abstr 20

78. Westlander G, Bergh C, Hanson C, et al. Recovery of epididymal and testicular sperm for ICSI in men with azoospermia. Proceedings of Treatment of Infertility: the New Frontiers. Boca Raton, FL, 1998: Abstr PO–19

79. Van Peperstraten AM, Proctor ML, Phillipson G, Johnson NP. Techniques of surgical retrieval of sperm prior to ICSI for azoospermia (Cochrane Review). In The Cochrane Library, Issue 2. Oxford: Update Software, 2003

80. Hendry WF, Hughes L, Scammel G, et al. Comparison of prednisolone and placebo in subfertile men with antibodies to spermatozoa. Lancet 1990; 335: 85–8

81. De Almeida M, Gazagne I, Jeulin C, et al. In-vitro processing of sperm with autoantibodies and IVF results. Hum Reprod 1989; 4: 49–53

82. Hendry WF, Parslow JM, Parkinson MC, et al. Unilateral testicular obstruction: orchidectomy or reconstruction? Hum Reprod 1994; 9: 463–70

83. Pryor JP, Hirsh AV, Fitzpatrick J, et al. The correlation between testicular size and histology. Proceedings of 5th World Congress on Fertility and Sterility, Venice, Italy 1978: 371–2

84. Dohle GR, van Roijen JH, Pierik FH, et al. Subtotal obstruction of the male reproductive tract. Urol Res 2003; 31: 22–4.

85. Hauser R, Temple-Smith PD, Southwick GJ, et al. Pregnancies after microsurgical correction of partial epididymal and vasal obstruction. Hum Reprod 1995; 10: 1152–5

86. Liliford R, Jones AM, Bishop DT, et al. Case control study of whether subfertility in men is familial. Br Med J 1994; 309: 570–3

87. Aitken RJ, Irvine DS. Reliability of methods for assessing the fertilizing capacity of human sperm. In Ombelet W, Bosmans E, Vandeput H, et al., eds. Modern ART in the 2000s. Studies in Profertility. 1998: Carnforth, UK: Parthenon Publishing, 1998; 8: 79–89

88. Hargreave TB, Elton RA. Is conventional sperm analysis of any use? Br J Urol 1983; 55: 780–4

89. Giltay JC, Deege M, Blankenstein RA, et al. Apparent primary FSH deficiency is a rare cause of treatable male infertility. Fertil Steril 2004; 81: 693–6

90. Pavlovich CP, King P, Goldstein M, Schlegel PN. Evidence of a treatable endocrinopathy in infertile men. J Urol 2001; 165: 837–41

91. Yamamoto M, Hibi H, Miyake K. Comparison of the effectiveness of placebo and alpha blocker therapy for the treatment of idiopathic oligozoospermia. Fertil Steril 1995; 63: 396–400

92. Yamamoto M, Hibi H, Miyake K. New treatment of idiopathic severe oligozoospermia with mast cell blocker: results of a single blind study. Fertil Steril 1995; 64: 1221–3

93. Evers JL, Collins JA. Assessment of efficacy of varicocele repair for male subfertility. Lancet 2003; 361: 1849–52

94. Sandlow J. Pathogenesis and treatment of varicoceles. Br Med J 2004; 328: 967–8

95. Berg U, Brucker C, Berg FD. Effect of motile sperm count after swim-up on outcome of intrauterine insemination. Fertil Steril 1997; 67: 747–50

96. National Collaborating Centre for Women and Children's Health. Fertility: Assessment and Treatment for People with Fertility Problems. London: RCOG Press, 2004: 75

97. Goverde AJ, McDonnell J, Vermeiden JP, et al. Intrauterine insemination or in-vitro fertilization in idiopathic subfertility and male subfertility: a randomised trial and cost-effectiveness analysis. Lancet 2000; 355: 13–18

98. Tan SL, Royston P, Campbell S, et al. Cumulative conception and live birth rates after IVF. Lancet 1992; 339: 1390–4

99. Kruger TF, Acosta AA, Simmons KF et al. Predictive value of abnormal sperm morphology in in-vitro fertilization. Fertil Steril 1998; 49: 112–17

100. Stolwijk AM, Wetzels AM, Braat DD. Cumulative probability of achieving an ongoing pregnancy after IVF and ICSI according to a woman's age, subfertility diagnosis and primary or secondary subfertility. Hum Reprod 200; 15: 203–9

101. Tournaye H, Liu J, Nagy Z, et al. The use of testicular sperm for ICSI in patients with necrozoospermia. Fertil Steril 1996; 66: 331–4

102. von Zumbusch A, Fiedler K, Mayerhofer A, et al. Birth of healthy children after intracytoplasmic sperm injection in two couples with male Kartagener's syndrome. Fertil Steril 1998; 70: 643–6

103. Stone S, O'Mahony F, Khalaf Y, et al. A normal live-birth after intracytoplasmic sperm injection for globozoospermia without assisted oocyte activation: case report. Hum Reprod 2000; 15: 139–41

104. Greco E, Scarselli F, Iacobelli M, et al. Efficiency treatment of infertility due to sperm DNA damage by ICSI with testicular spermatozoa. Hum Reprod 2005; 20: 226–30

105. Goossens E, Frederickx V, De Block G, et al. Reproductive capacity of sperm obtained after germ cell transplantation in a mouse model. Hum Reprod 2003; 18: 1874–80

4

Laboratory investigation of the infertile male

David Mortimer and Sharon T. Mortimer

INTRODUCTION

This chapter focuses on investigation of the male partner in relation to a couple's diagnostic work-up from the perspective of an assisted conception program rather than a basic infertility work-up. Space precludes detailed procedural methods for all the component laboratory techniques, which are available elsewhere. The chapter's content presumes the existence of a properly constituted diagnostic andrology laboratory, including well-trained, dedicated technical staff and a laboratory director who has both an understanding of, and a commitment to, the principles of laboratory quality control and quality assurance.

While the responsibility for interpreting test results must lie with the physician who requests them, a modern diagnostic andrology laboratory service must understand not only the diagnostic relevance and significance of the tests being performed, but also be able to discuss results with referring physicians in order to facilitate their interpretation and proper application to patient management. It is not to be inferred that a scientist can make a diagnosis, which is clearly inappropriate, but rather that the laboratory provides specific information to guide a couple's management in light of a full clinical understanding of both partners.

Structured management

Although infertility must always be considered as the couple's problem, management options will be governed by the etiologic factor(s), which may cause treatment to be focused primarily upon one or other partner. Modern comprehensive work-ups of infertile couples have revealed multifactorial infertility as more prevalent than hitherto believed. This is primarily due to the identification of previously unrecognized male factors, meaning that the prevalence of significant pathology in the male partner may be as high as 40%. However, there still remains a significant problem of idiopathic or unexplained infertility, much of which may be due to occult sperm dysfunction. It is astonishing that a semen analysis is still often the only assessment ever performed on the male partners of many infertile couples and used to ascribe a diagnosis of 'male factor' infertility, itself a classification of doubtful value[1].

The ready availability of assisted conception has led to infertile couples being referred more often straight to *in vitro* fertilization (IVF) as the most expeditious means of securing a pregnancy, and if IVF is unsuccessful then intracytoplasmic sperm injection (ICSI) is readily available as the ultimate form of treatment. The high success rates being achieved using ICSI have led to a disturbing trend in some centers for infertile couples to be referred directly for ICSI treatment after an initial infertility consultation, in the belief that this is the most cost-effective approach to achieving the desired endpoint of a pregnancy. However, ICSI treatment is the most labor-intensive, invasive and expensive form of assisted conception treatment and is unwarranted for many couples[2].

ICSI should be kept as a 'last resort' for when less invasive, lower-cost treatments have failed or are inappropriate. A more scientific approach would be to apply a management strategy using information from diagnostic testing in a progressive manner: couples who would have a good chance of pregnancy from simple insemination-based treatments would receive those treatments, while couples for whom such treatment is contraindicated (e.g. due to blocked tubes, sperm dysfunction or antisperm antibodies) would proceed directly to assisted conception procedures, and those couples in whom a severe sperm dysfunction had been identified would proceed directly to ICSI. With this approach, many couples with idiopathic infertility would begin their fertility treatment with three or four cycles of intrauterine insemination (IUI) (usually incorporating mild ovarian stimulation), only being referred on for IVF if those treatments were unsuccessful.

Such 'structured management' protocols for infertile couples determine the appropriate level of medical intervention required to achieve a reasonable chance of a pregnancy according to available diagnostic information. 'Appropriate' is judged in terms of cost (in health-care resources and to the couple), likelihood of a successful outcome, especially in consideration of the female partner's age, and associated risk factors (e.g. patient morbidity)[3,4]. However, our application and interpretation of laboratory tests needs to change: attempting to predict a positive outcome (such as fertilization *in vitro*) has poor sensitivity, being prone to a high incidence of false-positive predicted outcomes. From a patient management perspective, diagnostic tests are better used in the opposing sense, to predict the likelihood of failure of a component in the physiological processes leading to conception, and hence of particular therapeutic approaches. In other words, we need tests with good specificity, i.e. a high incidence of correctly predicted negative outcomes. Appropriate decision points will need to be based upon specific cut-offs that will certainly be very different from the traditional 'normal ranges' used to interpret semen

analyses which, it must be emphasized, were established in relation to predicting the likelihood of impaired fertility *in vivo*, not for directing assisted conception treatment. Also, because the major processes involved in gamete approximation and fertilization occur in the inaccessible domain of the female reproductive tract, assessment of sperm functional potential would be intrinsic to the development of structured management protocols.

While defective sperm–mucus interaction is often treated using IUI, this is not always the best option, because the problem may be due to sperm dysfunction, itself associated with poor fertilizing ability at IVF, which would contraindicate IUI[5]. Sperm–mucus interaction testing prior to IUI would allow patients with dysfunctional spermatozoa to be directed towards more appropriate treatment, such as ICSI. This would save time and money and, as a corollary, also increase the effective success rate of IUI. Therefore, for couples where the female partner is under 38 years and IUI is not contraindicated (e.g. due to blocked tubes, sperm dysfunction or antisperm antibodies), IUI would be the recommended first line of treatment. However, in those couples who fail to conceive after (say) three cycles, occult sperm dysfunction should be investigated to determine whether IVF or ICSI would be the better option. This is important because if all these couples went to IVF some would have an increased risk of fertilization failure, but directing everyone straight to ICSI is unnecessarily expensive for those who do not actually need it. As long as it could be provided in a cost-effective manner (see below), some sperm function testing may be justified at this point[6,7].

Couples in whom the female partner is over age 38, or where a minor 'male factor' has been identified, should proceed directly to IVF. Where the initial work-up identifies that the male partner is a significant cause in the couple's infertility, then either a first IVF attempt may be undertaken (with recognition of its possible 'diagnostic role', see below), or sperm function testing could be used to establish whether ICSI would be required to give a reasonable chance of successful fertilization. Obviously in cases where insufficient spermatozoa are available for an IVF attempt, then ICSI becomes the only viable treatment option; this would probably include all cases where spermatozoa have to be obtained from the epididymis or testis. From personal experience we have found that in routine practice, ICSI is necessary only in 35–40% of

IVF/ICSI cycles when an effective IUI program is also offered. Without the IUI option the necessary prevalence of ICSI will clearly be increased.

An example of structured management

An illustrative example of using structured management was the use of comprehensive initial sperm assessments to identify patients for whom IUI was considered to be an effective treatment option[8]. The package of assessments comprised a full semen analysis, including the sperm-morphology teratozoospermia index, testing for sperm surface antibodies using a direct immunobead test, a 'trial wash' using PureSperm® density gradients, and computer-aided sperm anaylsis (CASA)-based assessments of sperm kinematics on seminal and washed sperm populations, including an analysis of sperm hyperactivation (see below for details of these procedures).

A cohort of 69 couples for whom IUI was a recommended treatment received 128 cycles of IUI, during which 41% of them became pregnant, with a fecundity rate of 22% per cycle. Among a contemporaneous group of 56 couples who received IUI but had not been pre-screened, the success rate was only 18% pregnancy per couple with a fecundity rate of 11%. In both groups of patients only 28% of cycles involved the use of clomiphene or gonadotropins. The improved success rates in the pre-screened patients were significant ($p < 0.05$ for pregnancy rate, $p < 0.01$ for fecundity rate). Not only was IUI a cost-effective form of treatment for these couples, and a valid alternative to IVF, but its prognosis for success was significantly improved by careful work-up of the patients.

ANDROLOGY LABORATORY TESTING

When a couple has completed basic infertility investigations according to current World Health Organization (WHO) guidelines[9,10], the male partner will have had a minimum of two semen analyses (including at least a screening test for the presence of antisperm antibodies (ASABs) on the sperm surface), and participated in an assessment of the interaction between his spermatozoa and his partner's cervical mucus, either as an *in vivo* postcoital test (PCT) or an *in vitro* sperm–mucus interaction test (SMIT). In addition, his partner will have been tested for serum ASABs. If an abnormal result has been found that is considered to

decrease the man's ability to achieve a pregnancy *in vivo*, a diagnosis of a male contribution to the couple's infertility is made. A diagnosis of idiopathic infertility can only be reached when all these tests have yielded normal results, and no endocrinological or physical abnormalities are identified.

Couples proceeding to assisted conception treatment should have a sperm preparation evaluation performed (often referred to as a 'trial wash') before embarking upon active treatment, to ensure that adequate numbers and quality of spermatozoa can be obtained for the desired treatment modality.

Although many workers still consider that traditional manual/visual semen analysis methods are inaccurate and impossible to standardize, great advances have been made in establishing standard methods following the efforts of Eliasson[11–13], and since publication of the WHO's first laboratory manual in 1980[14]. Several recent monographs contain up-to-date methods for semen analysis and related sperm function tests[10,15,16].

Standardization and quality control

It is a fundamental principle of laboratory tests that they are never entirely free from error. However, understanding the source and extent of such errors is a prerequisite for correct appreciation and interpretation of test results in the diagnostic process. In order to evaluate these errors, quality control (QC) has been introduced into clinical laboratory tests and must become routine practice[15,17]. But QC is impossible without precision, and accuracy is a fundamental requirement of any laboratory measurement, and both depend on adequate staff training.

To date, the preconditions for QC in many andrology laboratories have not been met due to the belief that 'it can't be done'. Certainly there are difficulties when dealing with live gametes as analytes, and in developing standard preparations, but they are not insurmountable if commitment to the principle of QC is made. Furthermore, the lack of definitive methods for determining semen characteristics was addressed by the third and fourth editions of the *WHO Laboratory Manual*[10,18], providing a basis for QC procedures in routine semen analysis. However, most QC studies to date have only provided quantitative data to support what we already know: that different laboratories, and often different technicians within the same laboratory, produce different values. Clearly, unless everyone is trained carefully to do things in the same way, it is unreasonable to expect high levels of reproducibility[17]. Validation of this concept has been provided by the courses run by the Andrology Special Interest Group of the European Society of Human Reproduction and Embryology (ESHRE)[19].

Finally, it must be emphasized that appropriate equipment is also essential to the performance of careful assessments of semen and sperm function. Many laboratories are constrained in their ability to perform adequate examinations of sperm motility or morphology, or to establish high standards of reproducibility, by a lack of adequate microscopes (which must have phase-contrast optics, a heated stage and a good ×100 non-phase objective) or multichannel counters. Clearly, diagnostic andrology will continue to have limited value in many clinicians' eyes if laboratories are persistently denied the minimum levels of equipment necessary for reliable testing.

Specimen collection and handling

Standardization of semen analysis begins with the method of collection of the ejaculate and its delivery to the laboratory. The WHO recommends that at least two, and preferably three, semen samples be obtained over a period of at least a month to assess a man's semen quality reliably. Factors influencing specimen collection include the following.

Abstinence is a major source of variation in semen characteristics that must be controlled in order to determine true biological variation. Typically, a 3-day period of abstinence is required, as most normal ranges have been established from such data.

Specimen collection must be controlled carefully. Patients must be provided with clear, comprehensive instructions stating what should and should not be done. Also remember that giving an explanation influences people to comply more readily with instructions that might otherwise appear unimportant. Specific points to be made include:

(1) Produce the specimen by masturbation directly into a sterile plastic container provided by the laboratory. Containers whose lids have waxed cardboard, plastic or rubber liners must not be used.

(2) Do not use contraceptive condoms as the lubricant is spermicidal. Withdrawal (coitus interruptus) is also unacceptable since the first, sperm-rich, part of the ejaculate is often lost. Men objecting to masturbation on religious or moral grounds may use silastic condoms such as the seminal collection device (HDC Corp., Mountainview, CA, USA).

(3) Only remove the lid of the jar at the last moment before ejaculation to minimize microbiological contamination, and replace it immediately after completing the collection.

(4) Write the patient's full name and a second identifier on the specimen jar, along with the date and time of collection.

(5) Specimens not produced adjacent to the laboratory must be received as quickly as possible, certainly within an hour of collection, having been kept within the range of 'room' to body temperature (25–37°C).

Split ejaculates are collected in two (sometimes more) fractions so that the first fraction, which contains the majority of the spermatozoa suspended in primarily prostatic fluid, may be analyzed or used for therapeutic purposes without having been diluted by, or the spermatozoa exposed to, the later fractions of the ejaculate, consisting primarily of seminal vesicle secretions. For the laboratory this only involves numbering and taping together the required number of specimen jars, but reliable collection of split ejaculates often takes considerable practice by the patient. There is little need or justification for split ejaculates when collecting for assisted conception treatments.

Retrograde ejaculation is where spermatozoa are not ejaculated in the antegrade direction along the ureter to the exterior but, because of an incompetent bladder neck, reflux in the retrograde direction into the bladder, even though all the sensations of apparently normal ejaculation may be experienced. It can be due to a variety of reasons, including diabetes, iatrogenic surgical damage to the bladder neck innervation or pharmacological side-effects of hypertensive therapy, such as α-adrenergic blockers. The usual test to confirm retrograde ejaculation is by examining postejaculatory urine. However, exposure to urine is highly deleterious to spermatozoa, due to the combined effects of osmotic stress, low pH and urea toxicity; therefore, collection of spermatozoa from these men should employ sperm washing in conjunction with alkalinization of the urine and recovery of the spermatozoa, either by catheterization and washing of the bladder or by urination immediately after ejaculation. Alkalinization of the urine is commonly achieved by oral sodium bicarbonate[15].

Epididymal and testicular spermatozoa

Spermatozoa obtained from the epididymis (either by microsurgical epididymal sperm aspiration (MESA) or percutaneous epididymal sperm aspiration (PESA)) and the testis (testicular sperm extraction (TESE), either by microsurgical or needle-aspiration techniques) are considered elsewhere in this book.

Liquefaction and viscosity

Liquefaction of human semen occurs spontaneously after collection, typically taking less than 20 min, even at ambient temperature. Although various authorities recommend incubation of the sample at either ambient or body temperature for completion of liquefaction, because reliable visual assessment of sperm progression (as well as CASA-derived kinematics) requires analysis of the sample at 37°C, it is recommended that this temperature be used throughout.

Examination of the semen specimen begins after this incubation period. Although samples that are not fully liquefied can be incubated for a few more minutes, prolonged exposure of spermatozoa to seminal plasma can diminish their functional capacity permanently. This is very important if the sample is to be used for sperm function testing or for therapeutic purposes. All semen analyses should be commenced by 1 h post-ejaculation.

Viscosity relates to the fluid nature of the whole sample and is usually rated subjectively, e.g. according to how the semen runs out of the pipette used to measure the ejaculate volume; objective measurements are rare. It is important to distinguish between incomplete liquefaction and abnormal viscosity, the former resulting in a heterogeneous sample consisting of gelatinous material in a more fluid base with, in some cases, essentially normal overall viscosity. The clinical significance of altered semen viscosity remains uncertain, but increased viscosity can impair sperm movement and hence cervical mucus penetration. Highly viscous semen may be diluted with culture medium or even treated with chymotrypsin before preparation of sperm populations for use in function tests or for therapeutic purposes[20]. Special collection cups coated with

chymotrypsin are available from Embryotech Laboratories (Wilmington, MA, USA). However, 'needling' (passing the sample through a 19-gauge syringe needle) to reduce the viscosity of incompletely liquefied samples must be avoided as it is deleterious to motility[21].

Obviously, liquefied semen must be mixed thoroughly before commencing any analysis. Cradles or roller systems are ideal, but mixing can be achieved by swirling the sample around inside the container for 20–30 s. Avoid vortex-mixing live spermatozoa as it exposes them to excessive shearing forces that can damage the plasma membrane and even, in extreme cases, detach tails.

Semen analysis

The guidelines of the World Health Organization should be considered minimum standards for all semen analyses[10]. The clinical significance of semen characteristics has been reviewed elsewhere[15,22]. A long-term follow-up study of Danish infertility patients demonstrated that there was a better than 50% likelihood of their having had a living child over the next 5 years if the semen analysis showed more than 10×10^6 spermatozoa/ml having at least 40% motility with good progression and at least 40% normal forms[23]. However, almost 40% of patients with $< 5 \times 10^6$/ml motile spermatozoa and almost 50% of men with 60–80% morphologically abnormal spermatozoa had living children at follow-up 20 years later. Another large study revealed that the only semen characteristic predictive of *in vivo* fertility was the degree of morphological abnormality of the abnormal spermatozoa (see below)[24].

Ejaculate volume

This is measured either by collecting the specimen into a graduated container (e.g. Recisperme, Cryo Bio System, Paris, France) or using a warmed, disposable, graduated-to-contain pipette. Because some plastic syringes contain a lubricant detrimental to sperm motility, they must be checked before acceptance into routine use.

Sperm concentration

This term should be used instead of 'sperm density' to avoid confusion with the specific gravity of spermatozoa. Although sperm concentration has a positive association with the likelihood of achieving a pregnancy, there are no absolute limits to distinguish fertile from infertile except for azoospermia.

The most accurate method for determining sperm concentration suitable for routine semen analysis is volumetric dilution and hemocytometry. Because of the highly viscous nature of human semen, a positive displacement pipette must be used to ensure that an accurate aliquot is taken for dilution. There are strict rules for counting spermatozoa in the hemocytometer chamber to ensure that the result is accurate within acceptable limits of counting error. Only recognizable spermatozoa are counted; other germinal-line cells and free sperm tails are ignored; 'pinhead' spermatozoa (see below) are considered as free tails since they lack nuclear structures.

Special counting chambers for rapid semen analysis have become popular in recent years with the Makler chamber (Sefi Medical Instruments, Haifa, Israel) having gained the widest acceptance and use. Disposable chambers are also available, e.g. 2X-CEL chambers (Hamilton Thorne Biosciences, Beverly, MA, USA), Cell-VU® chambers (Millenniun Sciences Inc, www.cellvu.com) and MicroCell chambers (Conception Technologies, La Jolla, CA, USA) and the Standard Count chambers (Leja Products BV, Nieuw-Vennep, The Netherlands). Unfortunately, in routine use such chambers are prone to substantial errors, particularly those that involve loading by capillary action and especially with a liquid as viscous as human semen. Therefore, while they may simplify the work for less specialized laboratories, such chambers cannot be recommended for laboratories wishing to perform semen analyses to current WHO standards.

Recently it has been demonstrated that specialized sperm counting chambers which fill by capillary actin are subject to the Sebre–Silberberg effect, which causes a viscosity-dependent error in sperm concentration determination[25,26]. As a result of this, it has been suggested that such chambers should not be used for this purpose[27].

Sperm motility

The motility of ejaculated spermatozoa is an extremely important functional characteristic that must be evaluated as an integral part of semen analysis: the likelihood of achieving a pregnancy *in vivo* increases both with decreasing proportions of immotile spermatozoa and with increasing quality of sperm progression.

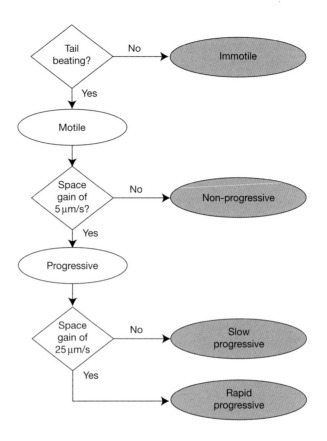

Figure 1 Principles of the World Health Organization 1992 classification scheme for human sperm motility in semen. (Redrawn from reference 17)

A wet preparation is made by placing 10 μl of thoroughly mixed, liquefied semen on a warm microscope slide and covering it with a warm 22×22 mm no. 1½ coverslip. Microscopic examination commences as soon as any 'flow' within the preparation has stopped (if not within 1 min then discard it and make another); phase-contrast optics are really essential. At least 200 spermatozoa are counted in at least four randomly selected fields, classifying each spermatozoon as described below (see Figure 1):

Class *a* = rapid progressive motility (≥25 μm/s progression velocity);

Class *b* = slow progressive motility (5–25 μm/s progression);

Class *c* = non-progressive motility (flagellar activity, but <5 μm/s 'space gain');

Class *d* = immotile (no flagellar activity).

Sperm velocity is highly temperature-dependent, showing as much as a doubling when assessed at 37°C rather than 20°C. Consequently, every effort must be made to perform such assessments as close to body temperature as possible, ideally by using a microscope fitted with a heated stage.

The motility count should be repeated on a second wet preparation, especially if the sperm concentration and/or motility is high, and the incidence of each motility class *a* to *d* expressed as an integer percentage. Where >10–15% of the spermatozoa are clumped, motility should be assessed on the free spermatozoa only.

Visual assessment of subtle features of sperm movement is not possible. For example, in the *WHO Laboratory Manual* second edition[28], the lack of a definition of 'linear' made the motility classification scheme of 'rapid and linear motility' (class *a*) versus 'slow, linear or non-linear motility' (class *b*) impossible to establish objectively. As a consequence, one laboratory that included all spermatozoa showing significant lateral head displacement as non-linear found class *b* motility to be the most significant predictor of *in vivo* fertility[29], as would be expected, since larger lateral head displacement allows more successful cervical mucus penetration (for reviews see references 15 and 30–33). This complication was resolved in the thrrd edition of the *WHO Laboratory Manual* where these two classes of progressive motility were defined simply as 'rapid' and 'slow'[18].

Although a normal semen sample has ≥ 50% motile spermatozoa, of which the majority show at least good forward progression, neither the proportion of progressively motile spermatozoa nor their concentration is the most important aspect of sperm motility; sperm kinematic information, derived from observations of individual cells, is more predictive of functional ability, and hence a man's potential fertility (see below).

Sperm vitality

Vital staining differentiates between immotile and dead spermatozoa, with the percentage of vital cells usually slightly exceeding that of motile cells. Sperm vitality assessment is particularly useful in samples where the motility is low (< 40%), allowing necrozoospermia to be distinguished from total sperm immotility (e.g. Kartagener's syndrome). Furthermore, given a similar situation, but where the vast majority of the spermatozoa are dead, further tests for the presence of spermotoxic antibodies might be more appropriate than electron microscopic investigation for absent dynein arms.

Sperm vitality is most easily assessed using the ability of live, intact cells to exclude a vital stain such as eosin, with nigrosin as a background or counterstain. The semen + stain mixture is smeared on a slide and at least 100 spermatozoa counted; those showing any pink or red coloration are considered 'dead'. Results are presented as the proportion of 'live' (unstained) cells expressed as an integer percentage. Although many authorities describe a technique where the eosin and nigrosin stains are added separately, it has recently been demonstrated that a one-step method is both faster and more reliable[34].

An alternative way of assessing sperm vitality is the *hypo-osmotic swelling test* (HOS test), whereby spermatozoa are exposed to moderate hypotonic conditions (150 mOsmol/kg).[35] Under such conditions dead spermatozoa, whose plasma membranes are no longer intact, do not show swelling. In addition, senescent spermatozoa with poor osmoregulatory ability show uncontrolled swelling that rapidly results in rupture of their overdistended plasma membranes, i.e. they do not show the swelling pattern. Therefore, the proportion of spermatozoa that show controlled swelling under test conditions is considered to reflect the potentially functional fraction. The HOS test can also be used to identify vital, but immotile, spermatozoa for ICSI. In this situation, sperm buffer is usually diluted with tissue culture-grade water to achieve the desired reduced osmolarity.

Sperm morphology

The morphology of spermatozoa is extremely important in the complete evaluation of a semen sample, but again there is no clear boundary between fertility and infertility. Normal sperm morphology is significantly related to *in vitro* tests of sperm function and *in vivo* conception (see above) and also fertilization *in vitro*[36,37].

Although the pleomorphism of human spermatozoa is a major dilemma in their morphological assessment (Figure 2), studies of sperm selection in the female reproductive tract as well as *in vitro* have helped to define the normal human spermatozoon[38,39]. However, definitions can be applied to varying levels of critical judgment, and this remains a major difficulty in establishing standardization between laboratories. The

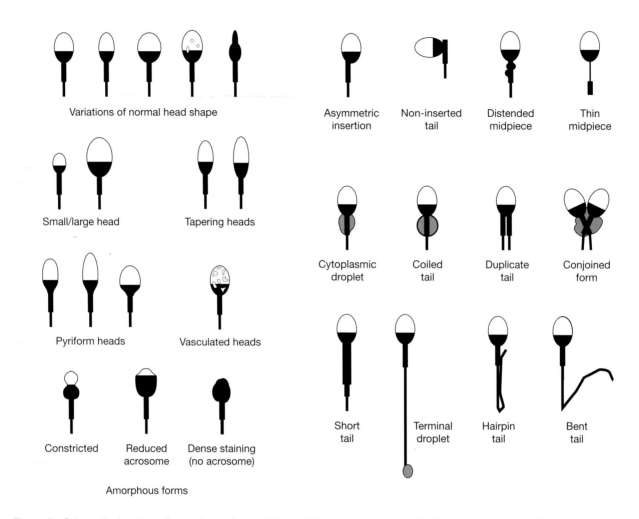

Figure 2 Schematic drawings of normal and abnormal forms of human spermatozoa. (Redrawn from reference 15)

Tygerberg 'strict' criteria (where spermatozoa showing morphological imperfection are classified as abnormal) have gained favor over older, more 'lenient' classification schemes because they are both easier to apply and have been related to endpoints of clinical interest, in this case IVF success[39,40]. The *WHO Laboratory Manual* third edition also encouraged the concept of strictness in sperm morphology assessment, but from a different perspective compared with the Tygerberg classification system[18]. This led to a perception that these two approaches would give very different results, although this was demonstrated to be false[41]. In the fourth edition of the *WHO Laboratory Manual*, the Tygerberg criteria have been accepted as the definition of 'normal' sperm morphology[10].

Because many abnormal spermatozoa possess multiple defects, careful morphology examinations need to use multiparametric rather than the older single-entry methods, which assigned priorities to the 'major' defect in the assumption that the head was more important than the midpiece, and the midpiece was more important than the tail. Determination of a 'multiple anomalies index' or MAI is clinically important[24]. In a large clinical study the MAI was the most significant seminal predictor of spontaneous *in vivo* fertility. Men with a MAI < 1.60 were almost six times more likely to achieve a pregnancy than those with a MAI > 1.90 (64% versus 11%). The 'teratozoospermia index' or TZI described in the *WHO Laboratory Manual* third edition (TZI = the average number of defects, more correctly defective regions, scored per abnormal spermatozoon) (Figure 3) is functionally equivalent to the MAI, and while the TZI has been relegated to the status of an 'optional test' in the fourth

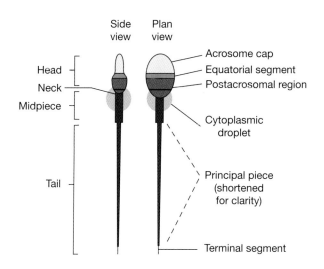

Figure 3 Diagrammatic representation of the functional regions used to assess human sperm morphology as recommended by the World Health Organization 1992. (Redrawn from reference 17)

edition, its use is considered important in the WHO clinical manual on the diagnosis and management of the infertile male[4].

Air-dried smears, prepared at the same time as the wet preparation and vital-stain smears, are later fixed, stained and mounted. The Papanicolaou method provides the best differential staining of human spermatozoa[41]. While alternative staining procedures are available, they give poorer-quality preparations that are less easy to score (especially rapid methods using prestained slides or coverslips). At least 200 spermatozoa are counted from each smear at high magnification (minimum ×1000) under oil immersion and carefully adjusted bright-field optics. Only recognizable spermatozoa are included in the count; immature germinal cells (even up to late spermatids) are not considered spermatozoa. Loose sperm heads are counted as abnormal forms, since they lack tails, but free tails are not included in the count. At the same time as the spermatozoa are being counted, the numbers of other germinal-line cells and leukocytes may be tallied so that their incidences can be expressed per 100 spermatozoa, and hence as millions/ml in the original semen.

Normal form   A normal, mature human spermatozoon has an oval-shaped head of regular outline (3–5 μm long, 2–3 μm wide), with clearly defined pale anterior

(acrosomal) and darker posterior regions in stained preparations (see Figure 3). Slightly tapering or pear-shaped heads are not necessarily abnormal since they may represent the extremes of the normal distribution for that man (or be typical of a man who is an extreme case of the population distribution), nor should the presence of a few small vacuoles (weakly stained areas) within the head be considered abnormal. Obviously tapered, pyriform or otherwise misshapen heads, large or small heads, highly vacuolated heads or more-or-less uniformly dark-staining heads are abnormal. A single tail, about 50 μm in overall length, is inserted into a symmetrically located shallow depression at the base of the head. If the head comes to a point here it is considered pyriform, indicating a weakness of the neck region. Immediately behind the head the tail is slightly thickened to form the midpiece region (7–8 μm long, maximum width 1 μm).

Head shape/size defects   These include large, small, tapering, pyriform, amorphous, vacuolated (occupying > 20% of the head area), reduced acrosome (< 40% of the head area), absent acrosome, double head or any combination of these.

Neck/midpiece defects   These include absent tail ('free head'), non-inserted or bent tail (tail forms an angle of ~ 90° to the long axis of the head), distended/irregular midpiece, abnormally thin midpiece (indicating an absent mitochondrial sheath) or any combination of these.

Tail defects   These include short, multiple, hairpin, broken (angulation of ≤ 90°), irregular width, terminal droplet, coiled or any combination of these. More than 10% coiled tails should be noted separately as it may indicate hypotonic shock (although tail coiling is also associated with sperm senescence).

Immature forms   These are defined by the presence of cytoplasmic droplets greater than the area of a normal sperm head. Cytoplasmic droplets may also be seen at other locations along the tail, or even at the tip of the tail.

Immature spermatozoa may occur in large numbers in association with frequent ejaculation (repeatedly short periods of abstinence). A high incidence of very tapered heads has been associated with 'testicular stress', such as may be experienced in cases of severe varicocele, although this remains equivocal. Scrotal heating (possibly associated with prolonged periods spent seated) may result in high proportions of morphologically abnormal spermatozoa, although not necessarily any specific type of structural defect.

It must be noted that reliable assessments of human sperm morphology cannot be made on wet preparations examined at low magnification (e.g. in a Makler chamber or on a slide), even if phase-contrast optics are used. All such assessments, regardless of the operator's self-perceived skills, will be superficial and inaccurate compared with the careful examination of properly stained smears.

Finally, similar to the 'sterilizing defects' described in domesticated species, where essentially all the spermatozoa from an individual show a specific structural defect causing sperm dysfunction, situations such as the 'round-head defect' (or 'globozoospermia') and Kartagener's syndrome have been described. Both these conditions have been circumvented using sperm microinjection, albeit with low clinical success and unknown inheritance of the man's problem[42,43]. The relationship between defective sperm morphology and pathophysiology has recently been reviewed in detail, relating structural defects to sperm fertilizing potential and/or dysfunction[44].

Leukocytes in semen

Even normal semen samples from fertile men are contaminated with substantial numbers of other cells and debris. These other cell types include germinal-line cells sloughed from the seminiferous epithelium, epithelial cells, leukocytes and, sometimes, erythrocytes, as well as occasionally bacteria and protozoa. Of these, the most important are leukocytes, whose clinical significance is two-fold: as an indication of infection within the male tract; and because of their ability to generate free radicals, and hence have a detrimental effect upon sperm function (see below). While there are some simple cytochemical methods for the estimation in semen (e.g. peroxidase staining using either benzidine–cyanosine or *o*-toluidine blue), precise identification of the classes of leukocytes present, and their exact concentrations, requires immunocytochemical methods which are only really feasible in specialized laboratories. A kit based on the benzidine–cyanosine method is available (Leuco-Screen™; FertiPro, Beernem, Belgium), and a dipstick method has been released that might be more practical for use by IVF laboratories to detect leukocytes in semen (LeukoMARQ™: Embryotech Laboratories, Wilmington, MA, USA).

For laboratories associated with assisted conception, the major importance of leukocytes is their potentially deleterious influence during sperm preparation (see below). Because this can be minimized by using appropriate sperm preparation methods, specific techniques to quantify leukocytes in semen are not described here, but are well established[10,15,45].

Semen biochemistry

While biochemical investigations of seminal plasma or spermatozoa can be of significant benefit in diagnosing some causes of male infertility, such assays have found little application in assisted conception services, with the possible exception of measuring free radicals (see below). Measurement of hormones and other esoteric compounds in semen have also found little clinical application in this area owing to limited, and often poorly reproducible, associations with clinical diagnosis and management.

Reactive oxygen species

Free radicals or reactive oxygen species (ROS) include hydrogen peroxide, the superoxide anion and the hydroxyl radical. Although the production of ROS in semen is an activity normally associated with infiltrating polymorphonuclear leukocytes, a specific subpopulation of less dense spermatozoa (when prepared on density gradients) have the capacity to generate ROS, an ability that has been implicated in the etiology of male infertility. While much work in recent years has focused upon the deleterious effects of ROS at the cellular level, it has also been recognized that ROS play key roles in the redox mechanisms that regulate normal cell physiology[46,47].

From the perspective of sperm function, the simple presence of increased numbers of spermatozoa in a semen sample with the capacity to generate ROS is indicative of impaired sperm maturation and/or morphological abnormality. The origin of this problem is that these spermatozoa have retained excessive amounts of (spermatid) cytoplasm, a defect also detectable by measuring creatine phosphokinase activity[48].

In practical terms, differential measurements of ROS production by spermatozoa and leukocytes can be made using a standardized protocol[49]. The basis of the assay is that, while both spermatozoa with retained cytoplasm and leukocytes will generate ROS in response to 12-myristate, 13-acetate phorbol ester (PMA, which bypasses surface receptors and stimulates protein kinase C directly), only polymorphs can be induced to produce ROS by the bacterial peptide mimic N-formyl-methionyl-leucyl-phenylalanine (FMLP), for which spermatozoa lack receptors.

However, while in functional terms sperm populations exhibiting high ROS-generating capacity have impaired fertilizing ability, sperm preparation procedures employed in clinical laboratory andrology will minimize this effect. A definitive role for ROS testing in the diagnostic situation remains to be established, although the detrimental impacts of ROS on male reproductive potential are now well established[50,51].

Systemic treatment of men with antioxidants has received great interest in recent years and seems to have some clinical benefit, although the story remains somewhat confused[52].

Antisperm antibodies

It has been known for almost a century that postmeiotic male germ cells, spermatozoa or sperm antigens can induce the formation of auto- and isoantibodies and so interfere with fertility. Extreme cases of such male autoimmunity can result in the destruction of all spermatogenic cells in the seminiferous epithelium, e.g. as a result of mumps orchitis. However, in clinical infertility one is usually confronted with less clear-cut problems caused by the presence of circulating antisperm antibodies (ASABs) in either or both partners, or ASABs present in the genital tract secretions as a result of either transudation from the blood or local secretory activity (e.g. in the cervix). In the male, ASABs are only clinically relevant if they are bound to the surface of the spermatozoa; hence, direct testing for sperm surface ASABs is far more useful clinically than indirect testing of blood serum. In the female, ASABs present anywhere within the genital tract may interfere with the processes of sperm transport and fertilization, particularly those secreted by the cervix, which can block sperm transport.

In spite of many doubters, and opinions based on poorly designed meta-analyses, experts still recommend that investigation for ASABs be considered imperative for all couples who undergo the various techniques of insemination and IVF[53].

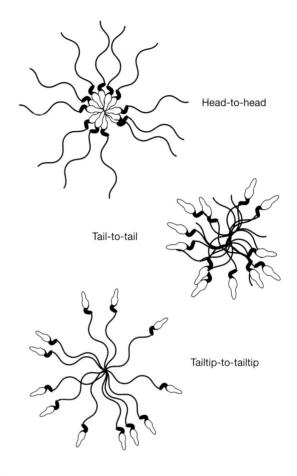

Head-to-head

Tail-to-tail

Tailtip-to-tailtip

Figure 4 Agglutination patterns of human spermatozoa. (Redrawn from reference 15)

ASABs can be classified in different ways: by immunoglobulin isotype (IgG, IgA, IgM); by their biological activity (agglutinating antibodies, cytotoxic or 'immobilizing' antibodies, or just coating antibodies); and by the region of the spermatozoon to which they bind (e.g. head, midpiece, tail, tailtip or 'all over') (Figure 4). Obviously, agglutinating and cytotoxic antibodies reduce the number of freely motile sperm and hence impair fertility, but coating ASABs cause neither effect, yet their presence on the sperm surface can interfere significantly with fertility by impairing sperm–cervical mucus interaction (causing a characteristic 'shaking' phenomenon) and sperm interaction with the oocyte via steric hindrance of sperm binding to the zona pellucida.

Immunobeads are polyacrylamide spheres with antihuman immunoglobulin antibodies covalently bound to their surface (Irvine Scientific, San Mateo,

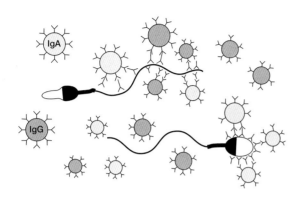

Figure 5 Diagrammatic explanation of the basis of the immunobead test. The upper spermatozoon has both immunoglobulins IgG and IgA antibodies bound to its tail, the lower spermatozoon has only IgA antibodies bound to its head. (Redrawn from reference 15)

CA, USA). The immunobead test (IBT) allows direct demonstration of human immunoglobulins bound to the sperm surface, including determination of their subcellular specificity, and their isotypes (antihuman IgG, IgA and IgM immunobeads are available) (Figure 5). There is also an immunobead which identifies all three Ig classes simultaneously, and which can be used very reliably as a screening test so that only positive samples need to be tested with separate isotype-specific immunobeads. Previously, the MAR test (mixed antiglobulin reaction, a variant of Coomb's test) was used to detect these antibodies, but, although it could be used directly upon seminal spermatozoa without the need for sperm washing, its application for isotypes other than IgG was extremely difficult. An alternative test kit is the SpermMar™ (FertiPro, Beernem, Belgium), which is essentially a MAR test that uses beads rather than sensitized sheep erythrocytes and can identify IgG and IgA antibody isotypes.

The immunobead test

The IBT can be used either directly, where washed ejaculate spermatozoa from a patient are tested for coating immunoglobulin, or as an indirect test after passive transfer of ASABs from a test sample (seminal plasma, serum or solubilized cervical mucus) to the surface of washed donor spermatozoa. After washing, these treated spermatozoa are then examined in the same way as for a direct test.

Preparation of immunobeads   Wash aliquots of the stock immunobead suspension with a ×10 volume of

phosphate-buffered saline with 3 mg/ml bovine serum albumin (PBS + 0.3% BSA w/v) and centrifuge at 600*g* for 10 min. Discard the supernatant and resuspend the pellet of immunobeads to the original aliquot volume using PBS + 5% BSA (i.e. 50 mg/ml). Store this preparation at +4°C until needed; do not leave it at ambient temperature for prolonged periods or the immunobeads will be inactivated.

Direct IBT   An appropriate aliquot of liquefied semen for the test is calculated (in μl) using the formula 500 ÷ motile sperm concentration (10^6/ml) and added to 5 ml of PBS + 0.3% BSA. After centrifugation at 600*g* for 10 min the supernatant is discarded, 5 ml of fresh PBS + 5% BSA added and the pellet resuspended. After a second centrifugation the supernatant is again discarded and the pellet resuspended in 200 μl of PBS + 5% BSA.

Indirect IBT   A washed donor sperm population in PBS + 5% BSA is prepared as for the direct IBT (although it is better to use a swim-up-from-semen or density-gradient procedure to obtain a highly motile population, see below), and its final concentration adjusted to about 25×10^6/ml. Aliquots of the sperm suspension are treated with equal volumes of a 1 + 4-diluted test sample for 30 min at 37°C before being centrifuged for 10 min at 600*g* and resuspended in PBS + 5% BSA to the original aliquot volume. Suggested volumes are 250 μl sperm suspension, 50 μl test serum or other fluid and 200 μl PBS + 5% BSA.

IBT procedure   Mix 5 μl each of the sperm suspension and the prepared immunobeads on a clean microscope slide, cover with a 22 × 22-mm no. 1½ coverslip and incubate at ambient temperature in a humid chamber for 15 min. Use separate preparations for each of the different immunobead types to identify isotype specificity. Count at least 200 motile spermatozoa under a ×40 phase-contrast objective, differentiating between those with and without immunobeads bound, and also note any localization of bead binding, i.e. head, midpiece, tail or tail-tip. The IBT result is reported according to the number of spermatozoa with beads bound, but the limits are somewhat arbitrary with 25% now suggested as the cut-off for a positive test but > 50% being required for a clinically positive result. Any sample showing ≥20% bead binding in a screening IBT should be retested using isotype-specific beads.

Testing of couples undergoing assisted conception treatment

Male partner Ideally, a direct IBT is performed. This can be undertaken in conjunction with a trial wash, although it must be established that the protein used to supplement the culture medium (either as human serum albumin (HSA) or heat-inactivated blood serum) does not contain any ASABs.

Female partner Circulating ASABs, especially if they coat the majority of spermatozoa, are directed against the sperm head, and are of both IgG and IgA isotypes simultaneously (IgA alone has a worse prognosis than IgG alone), indicate likely impairment of both sperm transport *in vivo* and fertilization. They are also a contraindication for gamete intrafallopian transfer (GIFT), and obviously preclude using that woman's serum to supplement IVF culture medium. ASABs identified in cervical mucus by abnormal sperm–mucus interaction test results (see below), or by their detection in solubilized cervical mucus, often cause a failure of sperm transport, although this may be amenable to treatment by IUI.

Although circulating ASABs have been treated by corticosteroid immunosuppression therapy, this approach is now considered rather courageous due to the high risk of undesirable sequelae, such as aseptic necrosis of the head of the femur, and is rarely attempted. Rather, the problem is bypassed using assisted conception alternatives, which can be summarized as follows:

Tail-tip IBT only: not clinically relevant;

< 50% IBT head/midpiece/tail: not clinically important;

50–80% IBT midpiece/tail: try IUI, or perhaps go straight to IVF;

50–80% IBT head: IVF (increase motile sperm numbers to compensate);

> 80% IBT midpiece/tail: try IVF, or perhaps go straight to ICSI;

> 80% IBT head: ICSI.

Semen microbiology and virology

Infections of the male tract can be contributory, or even direct causes of male infertility[54]. Because their investigation requires testing of various specimens and swabs by specialized microbiology and virology laboratories, they are outside the competence of the vast majority of diagnostic andrology and IVF laboratories and are not considered further here. In addition, such diagnoses require thorough clinical examination of the man, and perhaps seminal plasma biochemistry to evaluate accessory gland function.

Sperm washing: the 'trial wash'

Human spermatozoa need to be separated from seminal plasma to permit capacitation and expression of their intrinsic fertilizing ability. Therefore, this process is a fundamental requirement of both clinical treatments (e.g. IUI, IVF, GIFT) and *in vitro* tests of sperm fertilizing ability (see below). Performing a sperm preparation evaluation or 'trial wash' is a common feature of the work-up of many men prior to their embarking upon assisted conception treatment cycles with their partners. The ability to establish how many spermatozoa, and of what apparent functional quality, might be obtained from an ejaculate is an important factor in determining what form(s) of assisted conception treatment might be possible and/or appropriate.

Sperm washing, free radicals and iatrogenic sperm dysfunction

Apparently, a number of clinical programs still use the so-called 'classical' sperm preparation technique, involving multiple cycles of sperm washing followed by a swim-up step, to prepare a subpopulation of highly motile spermatozoa. This 'washed pellet' method was highly successful in producing sperm preparations for IVF in cases where no male factor was present, but, as the indications for IVF treatment have expanded beyond simple tubal-factor cases to couples with idiopathic infertility and, ultimately, to 'male factor' cases, the problem of fertilization failure has become more prevalent. While sperm dysfunction is generally considered a major contributory factor to IVF fertilization failures, a concept certainly borne out by many *in vitro* studies of human sperm function, there is now clear evidence for an additional component, that of iatrogenic sperm dysfunction[55].

It has been established incontrovertibly that centrifugal pelleting of unselected sperm populations from human ejaculates causes the production of ROS within the pellet, inducing irreversible damage to the spermatozoa. However, numerous clinical laboratories still argue that because there have been many IVF successes using the washed-pellet technique it cannot really be a problem. But the explanation lies in the multifactorial association between semen quality and the levels of ROS produced. Normal semen samples from fertile men contain higher proportions of morphologically normal spermatozoa and fewer leukocytes; consequently, lower ROS levels will be generated in pellets prepared from such samples than from more abnormal ones. Therefore, with increasing 'male factor' risk the level of sperm damage may become sufficient to impair, and even block, fertilization in some patients. While superficially the 'washed-pellet' technique produces populations of highly motile, morphologically normal spermatozoa, their function may have been compromised. Consequently, alternative sperm preparation methods, such as direct swim-up from liquefied semen or discontinuous density gradients, should be used to prepare spermatozoa for any purpose that will assess or require sperm fertilizing ability.

Sperm washing media

Various media can be used for sperm washing, and no one medium has been shown to be significantly better than others, although Ham's F-10 has been considered to be suboptimal because it contains iron, which can promote ROS generation. HEPES-buffered (4-(2-hydroxyethyl)-1-piperazineethanesulfonic acid) medium, often referred to as 'sperm buffer', is strongly recommended when working under an air atmosphere, but final sperm preparations for *in vitro* functional testing or clinical use should be in a bicarbonate-buffered medium ('sperm medium'), since bicarbonate ions are essential for adenylate cyclase activity, and hence capacitation. Sperm medium also needs to contain a few millimoles of calcium (commonly used media contain 2–5 mEq/l Ca^{2+}).

According to the Henderson–Hasselbach equation, to achieve a pH of 7.2–7.4 with a medium containing 25 mmol/l bicarbonate incubated at 37°C, there needs to be 5.8% CO_2 in the gas phase if working close to sea level. With only 5.0% CO_2, as is commonly used, the pH will be more alkaline and there will be a tendency to lose bicarbonate ions from the solution. Gas mixtures of 6% CO_2-in-air or 6% CO_2/5% O_2/89% N_2 should therefore be employed.

Protein, usually added as human serum albumin (HSA), is also required as a sterol acceptor for efficient capacitation. Although periovulatory oviductal fluid has been reported to contain about 3.5% (w/v) protein (equivalent to 35 mg/ml HSA), lower concentrations are often used for reasons of economy. While protein is not essential for sperm preparations to be used *in vivo*, e.g. for intrauterine insemination, at least 10 mg/ml HSA is required to reduce the sticking-to-glass phenomenon to a level that will have minimal impact upon sperm motility assessments[56].

Sperm preparation methods

Prolonged exposure to seminal plasma (> 30 min) results in marked declines in both sperm motility and vitality, and can permanently diminish the fertilizing capacity of human spermatozoa *in vitro*. Even contamination of prepared sperm populations with only traces of seminal plasma can also diminish, or even totally inhibit, their fertilizing capacity due to the presence of decapacitation factor(s). Therefore, spermatozoa for clinical procedures such as IVF or IUI, as well as for laboratory tests of sperm fertilizing ability, must be separated from the seminal environment as soon as possible after ejaculation.

Many techniques for preparing human spermatozoa have been reported, and their pros and cons have been reviewed elsewhere[15,55,57,58]. For trial wash purposes the two methods described briefly below have been found to be the most useful.

Direct swim-up from semen is the original sperm preparation method for selecting a motile subpopulation intended to replicate the migration of spermatozoa into cervical mucus *in vivo*. Aliquots of semen are taken as soon as the sample is liquefied, and placed in round-bottomed tubes (to maximize the surface area of the interface between the layers) underneath layers of culture medium. Although the tubes may be prepared by gently layering medium over the liquefied semen, the reverse procedure provides a much cleaner interface zone. For viscous semen samples, medium may be mixed with the semen prior to under-layering; 'needling' should not be used (see above). If a CO_2-enriched atmosphere is available, sperm medium may be used throughout, otherwise sperm buffer is recommended for the swim-up step.

Multiple tubes containing relatively small volumes of semen are used to increase the total interface area between semen and medium (e.g. 250 μl of semen under 600 μl of medium) and hence maximize the yield. Tubes may also be incubated at angles of 45° to the horizontal to increase the interface. After an appropriate incubation period at 37°C, most of the upper layer is removed, but great care must be taken to avoid the interface. Longer incubations give greater yields, although this should not exceed 60 min. Each migration tube should be harvested separately, and the individual preparations combined only after ascertaining that they each contain very high proportions of motile spermatozoa (typically >90–95% motile) and are not contaminated with unwanted elements from the semen fraction.

The combined preparation is then centrifuged at 600g for 5–10 min and resuspended into fresh sperm medium at the desired concentration of motile spermatozoa. Keeping a small aliquot of the preparation back while the majority is being centrifuged allows sperm concentration and motility counts to be completed during the second centrifugation.

Density gradient methods separate spermatozoa based upon their specific gravity or density; under centrifugal force the cells reach their equilibrium position on the density gradient (isopycnic point). However, routine methods typically use only two- or three-step discontinuous, rather than continuous, density gradients, with the selected spermatozoa being recovered from the lower layer or soft pellet. Percoll® (polyvinylpyrrolidone-coated colloidal silica particles) was used extensively to prepare human spermatozoa from the early 1980s until its withdrawal from clinical use, effective 1 January 1997, but several alternative products are available, all of which have the advantage of being produced specifically for clinical applications[55].

Direct Percoll replacements based on silane-coated colloidal silica particles of the same size (about 17 nm diameter) include PureSperm (Nidacon International AB, Göteborg, Sweden) and ISolate® (Irvine Scientific, San Mateo, CA, USA). Both products are sold either as 100% 'pure' material to prepare user-defined gradients or as ready-to-use gradient layers (e.g. 40 and 80% v/v dilutions). Because they are essentially isotonic there is no longer any need for a ×10 salt solution to prepare an 'isotonic' 90% stock solution for further dilution with sperm buffer or culture medium. Furthermore, these products have low endotoxin levels, unlike Percoll, which was often reported as having high endotoxin contamination. Because of the

authors' personal experience, the method given below is for PureSperm, but it should work equally well for other commercial products with the same colloid concentration.

The 100% stock PureSperm should be diluted using a sperm 'buffer', to avoid pH shifts when used under an air atmosphere, ideally containing at least 10 mg/ml HSA. Prepared PureSperm solutions can be filter-sterilized using 0.22-μm filters that do not release extractable wetting agents or other materials (e.g. Millipore Millex®-GV). Two-step discontinuous gradients of 1.5- or 2.0 ml layers of 40 and 80% are prepared in conical-bottom centrifuge tubes (e.g. Falcon 2095) and semen, either diluted or not, is layered on top (up to about 1.5 ml of semen per gradient, but this is dependent upon the sperm concentration and debris, etc. content of the specimen which can cause excessive rafting at the interfaces). Pairs of gradients are recommended, both as a precaution in case of accidental disturbance of one during recovery and to reduce problems with rafting. After a first centrifugation step at 300g for 20 min in a swing-out rotor, the seminal plasma, the upper interface, upper PureSperm layer and lower interface are removed carefully (do not remove the lower layer as this will cause substantial contamination of the pellet). Using a clean pipette the soft pellet at the bottom of the tube is then carefully aspirated, transferred to a clean tube and mixed with about 10 ml of sperm medium. This is then centrifuged at a maximum of 600g for up to 10 min, the supernatant aspirated and the pellet resuspended in fresh medium for use after determining the concentration of progressively motile spermatozoa and making any necessary adjustments.

Assessment of yields

The quality of a sperm preparation can be considered in terms of the yield of motile spermatozoa obtained. Progressive motility is used, since non-progressive spermatozoa are unlikely to be potentially functional (except perhaps for ICSI).

Relative yield is the proportion of progressively motile spermatozoa submitted to a preparative procedure that is present in the final preparation. It is calculated as:

$$Yield\ (\%) = (v \times c \times pm\%) \div (V \times C \times PM\%) \times 100$$

where v = final preparation volume, V = volume of semen used, c = concentration of spermatozoa in the final preparation, C = concentration of spermatozoa in the semen, $pm\%$ = prepared sperm population progressive motility and $PM\%$ = progressive motility in the semen.

Absolute yield is the total number of progressively motile spermatozoa that might be obtained if the whole ejaculate is used, after making an allowance for the aliquots needed to perform a standard semen analysis.

Yield quality may be important if the product is not an essentially pure preparation of motile spermatozoa, e.g. in terms of the proportions of progressively motile or morphologically normal spermatozoa.

Computer-aided sperm analysis

Since its first appearance in 1985, the development of computer-aided sperm analysis (CASA) technology has benefited enormously from the rapid evolution of microcomputers and video technology. Nevertheless, in spite of greatly improved system performance, increased clinical acceptance of CASA has not been achieved. This problem may be attributed largely to the early attempts to sell CASA systems as automated semen analyzers, an application which is only now becoming feasible. Notwithstanding such limitations, most CASA machines track moving objects reliably and derive measurements that describe their trajectories, i.e. they are functional motility analyzers. But their acceptance as such has been hampered by a perceived need for them to do something more: to replace technicians. Because this goal was unattainable, their excellent capability to analyze sperm motility has been eclipsed by inaccurate determinations of sperm concentration and percentage motility. A detailed discussion of CASA is outside the scope of this chapter, and interested readers are referred to relevant review articles[15,30,31,59–62], as well as to reports from consensus workshops held in Cairns (1994)[63], Hamburg (1995)[64] and San Miniato (1997)[65].

Much of the responsibility for the persistent misuse of CASA technology must lie with its users; instead of promulgating the measurement of traditional semen characteristics known to have only limited clinical predictive value, the advanced capabilities of CASA technology should be applied to determine values with greater clinical significance. Whether or not CASA technology is able to provide biologically

relevant information that will have clinical relevance is not in question; rather, it is the correct application of this technology to evaluate sperm functional potential which needs to be established. It is well established that it is the proportion of spermatozoa with appropriate movement characteristics (kinematics: Figure 6) which determines whether a man's spermatozoa are able to penetrate his partner's cervical mucus, or penetrate the cumulus–oocyte complex and fertilize the oocyte, either *in vivo* or *in vitro*[31,61]. Consequently, one particular application of CASA in assisted conception laboratories is in relation to assessing sperm hyperactivation (see below).

Sperm–mucus interaction and sperm migration tests

The first barrier that spermatozoa encounter *in vivo* is the mucous secretion of the cervix. Their ability to penetrate the semen–mucus interface, and also to migrate within the cervical mucus, is dependent primarily upon sperm progression. It is affected adversely by the presence of ASABs, either on the sperm surface or within the mucus itself, and concomitant with sperm penetration into mucus there is an apparent selection for morphologically normal spermatozoa. This latter process occurs as a result of the close functional relationship between sperm morphology and motility, rather than by some active selection of normal spermatozoa by the cervix.

Cervical mucus receptivity to sperm penetration is cyclic, being maximal in the immediate periovulatory period. Mucus quality is assessed by measuring its pH, using the same test strips as for semen, and using the semiquantitative Insler score (see below). Clearly, for a sperm–mucus interaction test (SMIT) to be physiologically relevant, it must be performed on the optimum day of the menstrual cycle; inappropriate scheduling may lead to false diagnoses of 'cervical hostility'. Since most variation in cycle length occurs in the follicular phase, the day of ovulation is considered equivalent to day 14 of a 'standard' 28-day cycle. Because of cycle irregularity it is better to calculate day $[14 + (x - 28)]$, where x is calculated as the average length of at least five preceding cycles. To ensure optimum mucus quality, some workers treat patients with ethinylestradiol for several days before sampling[66].

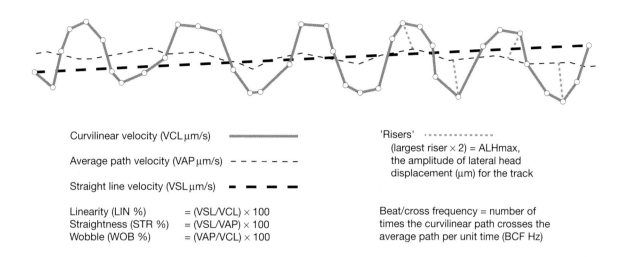

Curvilinear velocity (VCL μm/s) ————	'Risers' ·············
	(largest riser × 2) = ALHmax,
Average path velocity (VAP μm/s) − − − − − −	the amplitude of lateral head
	displacement (μm) for the track
Straight line velocity (VSL μm/s) ▬ ▬ ▬ ▬	
Linearity (LIN %) = (VSL/VCL) × 100	Beat/cross frequency = number of
Straightness (STR %) = (VSL/VAP) × 100	times the curvilinear path crosses the
Wobble (WOB %) = (VAP/VCL) × 100	average path per unit time (BCF Hz)

Figure 6 Illustrative sperm trajectory reconstructed from head-centroid positions in sequential images (white circles) to show how a computer-aided sperm analysis (CASA) instrument would derive the various 'standard' kinematic measures of sperm movement

The Insler score

This is a semiquantitative score used to assess the quantity and quality of mucus secreted by the cervix under estrogenic stimulation during the late follicular phase of the menstrual cycle. The original score has been modified to include mucus cellularity, and consequently there are now five criteria to be scored, each with a value ranging from 0 to 3. The five scores are added together to give a total out of 15: ≥ 12 indicates good ovulatory cervical mucus, and 10 or 11 indicates adequate ovulatory cervical mucus. Detailed descriptions of the method are provided elsewhere[10,15].

In vitro sperm–mucus interaction tests

These tests are derived from two basic techniques: 'slide tests' using apposed drops of semen and mucus under coverslips; and 'tube' or 'Kremer' tests where mucus-filled capillary tubes are placed with one end immersed in an aliquot of semen. Penetration in either system is assessed by counting motile spermatozoa at various distances from the semen–mucus interface at certain times after establishment of this contact. Tests must be performed using periovulatory intracervical mucus with an Insler score of ≥ 10/15 and a pH ≥ 7.0. A complete semen analysis should be performed on the ejaculate used for the test, and if the abstinence is not 3 days some tests may need to be repeated because of abnormal findings of uncertain origin.

SMITs, as with all tests of sperm function, must be commenced as quickly as possible after ejaculation. Normal semen samples are liquefied by 20 min post-ejaculation, and hence 30 min is an ideal standard starting time. If liquefaction is retarded tests may be delayed, but mucus-penetrating ability may be reduced with longer exposure of spermatozoa to seminal plasma.

Kremer tests are those based on capillary tubes, although Kremer's original cylindrical tubes have been replaced by rectangular cross-section 'flat' glass capillaries which are optically better and facilitate counting. Also, the original 'sperm penetration meter' apparatus has been superseded by disposable systems, such as a no. 00 BEEM® electron microscopy embedding capsule as the semen reservoir[15].

Due to the marked influence of temperature upon sperm progression, these tests must be run at 37°C. After a standard 60-min incubation, the capillary tube is removed from the semen reservoir and the depth and degree of sperm penetration into the mucus column assessed microscopically using a calibrated ×20 phase-contrast objective. Because some spermatozoa may have been present in the original mucus sample, at least ten fields along the length of the mucus column should be examined prior to the test to ascertain an average number of 'contaminating' spermatozoa per field. This is then subtracted from the counts at the end of the test. In addition, the furthest distance traveled by a spermatozoon within the mucus column is also determined if there are none present at 70 mm. A score is then calculated and used to derive a clinical result[18,67].

Slide tests, often called Kurzrok–Miller tests after their originators, simply involve establishing an interface between a drop of cervical mucus that has been compressed beneath a coverslip and an aliquot of liquefied semen. Because there are great problems in standardizing this test it is recommended that it be used as a qualitative assessment of sperm–mucus interaction only[18].

The *sperm–cervical mucus contact (SCMC) test* involves mixing drops of liquefied semen and mucus on a slide and can be used as a screening test for the presence of semen or cervical mucus ASABs by observing the characteristic 'shaking' pattern of sperm movement. It is especially useful in conjunction with the immunobead test in a crossed-hostility format. The difficulty of ensuring supplies of donor cervical mucus for crossed-hostility format testing can be avoided by using a control migration test in a solution of sodium hyaluronate[15].

Clinical significance of SMITs

Kremer-type SMITs have a significant prognostic value for subsequent *in vivo* fertility, much better than PCTs[66,68]. In addition, sperm-based SMIT failures have been found to predict IVF failure, indicating a general impairment of sperm function[69]. Recognition of such problems at an early stage of a couple's work-up would allow them to proceed to more aggressive IVF treatment, probably ICSI. Mucus-based problems may be amenable to treatment by IUI.

Sperm kinematics and mucus penetration

Although we have long known that spermatozoa with the 'right' kinematics are more capable of penetrating cervical mucus[28,61], and hence quantifying this sub-population would clearly be a major benefit at semen analysis, precise definitions for these spermatozoa remain to be validated. For several years we have used the following Boolean criteria for identifying spermatozoa with 'good mucus-penetrating' kinematic characteristics in a variety of situations:

VAP $\geq 25\,\mu$m/s and STR $\geq 80\%$ and ALH $\geq 2.5\,\mu$m

where VAP = average path velocity, STR = straightness and ALH = amplitude of lateral head displacement. In order to avoid including spermatozoa whose motility has been compromised by ROS induced damage, which can cause a quasi-hyperactivation pattern of movement, we have recently included a fourth term of ALH < 7.0 μm.

Hyperactivation

Hyperactivated motility is a high-energy pattern of movement characterized by the development of high-amplitude flagellar waves, with little net space gain (Figure 7). It occurs in all Eutherian spermatozoa studied, is a concomitant of capacitation *in vitro* and has been observed in free-swimming spermatozoa in the oviduct *in situ*. That hyperactivation has a physiological relevance to fertilization is now generally accepted, although whether its role is in the delivery of the spermatozoon to the proximity of the oocyte and/or to assist in penetration of the zona pellucida is still unclear (for review see references 31, 52 and 61).

The clinical significance of hyperactivation assessment is still under investigation, being confounded by a number of factors. First, in the human, inter- and intraindividual variations exist in the proportion of spermatozoa which exhibit hyperactivated motility, and spermatozoa do not remain in the hyperactivated state indefinitely[70]. Also, even though it is a flagellar phenomenon, the requirement for population-based assessments of the proportion of hyperactivated spermatozoa in a sample means that CASA analysis must be used (see above). However, commercially available CASA instruments reconstruct the trajectory of the sperm head, since it is easier to image, and the values obtained are highly machine-dependent. These shortcomings are accepted, and can be accommodated, but it must be understood that the kinematics used do not correspond directly with flagellar movement patterns for spermatozoa in capacitating medium. Alternative kinematic values which are not machine-dependent have been developed recently for use with capacitating sperm populations[71].

Validated criteria which have been established for identifying hyperactivated human spermatozoa using CASA, and work extremely well in the IVOS (integrated visual optical system for sperm analysis; Hamilton Thorne Biosciences, Beverly, MA, USA) operating at 60 Hz frame rates[61], are:

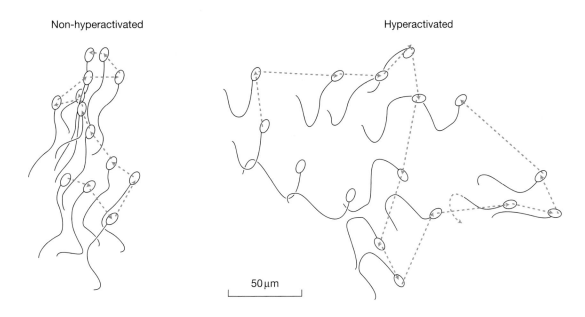

Figure 7 Illustration of the differences in sperm tail-beating and head-centroid trajectory pattern for non-hyperactivated and hyperactivated human spermatozoa. (Redrawn from reference 31)

$VCL \geq 150\,\mu m/s$ and $LIN \leq 50\%$ and $ALH \geq 7.0\,\mu m$

where VCL = curvilinear velocity, LIN = linearity and ALH = amplitude of lateral head displacement. In addition to these considerations, the need for appropriate analysis conditions is paramount, and certain fundamental requirements must be met for reliable hyperactivation studies. Many of the early studies of human sperm hyperactivation did not meet these requirements, and hence have limited value. Briefly, attention should be paid to the method used to separate spermatozoa from seminal plasma; the culture medium used should be known to support capacitation *in vitro*; analyses must be performed at 37°C; and a chamber depth of 30–50 μm is essential so as not to constrain flagellar movement[65].

Because of the variability in spontaneous sperm hyperactivation dynamics, establishing a clinical assay for hyperactivation has proven cumbersome, requiring multiple assessment time-points. Consequently, the known hyperactivation agonists progesterone and pentoxifylline were evaluated to create a similar assay to the acrosome reaction after ionophore challenge test (the ARIC test, see below). Exposure of prepared motile sperm populations to 1 μg/ml progesterone + 3.6 mmol/l pentoxifylline in sperm medium containing 30 mg/ml HSA for 60 min induced maximal levels of hyperactivation in the majority of men. Furthermore, this 'HAmax' assay has since been found, in conjunction with other sperm characteristics (many of which require CASA for their measurement), to have excellent sensitivity and specificity for predicting those cases with poor and good IVF fertilization rates (0–49% and 50–100%, respectively), even when performed weeks, or even months, prior to the actual treatment cycle (Table 1). This confirmed that a comprehensive assessment of a man's spermatozoa prior to undergoing IVF treatment can identify those patients who are at risk of poor or even failed fertilization, and may therefore allow preemptive direction of such at-risk cases towards ICSI.

Acrosome reaction testing

The finding that the fertilizing spermatozoon undergoes its acrosome reaction (AR) on the surface of the zona pellucida, in response to binding to the putative sperm receptor, the zona glycoprotein ZP3, confirmed that studies of the spontaneous AR have little positive predictive value for clinical applications. Unfortunately, the physiological inducer of the AR cannot be used in diagnostic laboratory practice because

Table 1 Results of a discriminant function analysis of the prediction of human sperm fertilizing ability using sperm kinematics, including determination of maximum level of hyperactivation (HAmax), in 29 patients (see text and Figure 6 for explanation). Overall, 88.4% of the variance in the dependent variable was accounted for, allowing good confidence in the reproducibility of the findings for a larger patient group. All tests were performed at least 1 week prior to the *in vitro* fertilization (IVF) attempt. (D. Mortimer, J. Kossakowski, S. T. Mortimer and S. Fussell, unpublished results)

Step	Variable included	R^2	ΔR^2
1	IVF oocyte quality score	0.230	0.230
2	Linearity (LIN %) of motile spermatozoa in the washed preparation	0.475	0.245
3	Straight line velocity (VSL μm/s) of motile spermatozoa in the washed preparation	0.535	0.060
4	HAmax (%) after treatment with 3.6 mmol/l pentoxifylline + 1 μg/ml progesterone for 60 min	0.627	0.092
5	Relative yield (%) of the sperm preparation	0.648	0.021
6	Hyperactivated spermatozoa (%) in the washed preparation	0.682	0.034
7	Average path velocity (VAP μm/s) of motile spermatozoa in the washed preparation	0.807	0.125
8	Proportion of rapidly progressive spermatozoa in the semen sample	0.835	0.028
9	Proportion of spermatozoa showing 'good mucus penetrating' kinematics	0.849	0.014
10	Proportion of progressive spermatozoa in the semen sample	0.861	0.012
11	Teratozoospermia index of the seminal spermatozoa	0.874	0.013
12	Straightness (STR %) of motile spermatozoa in the washed preparation	0.884	0.010

Poor fertilization (0–49%): 7/7 classified correctly = 100% specificity; good fertilization (≥50%): 22/22 classified correctly = 100% sensitivity

insufficient quantities of human zonae are available. While biologically active recombinant human ZP3 (rhuZP3) is still not yet available commercially, it remains likely that it will be the agonist for the ultimate human sperm AR test of the future.

Various current test protocols employ biological agonists or inducers of the AR[64], with human follicular fluid (hFF), calcium ionophore (most usually A23187) or progesterone being used most often. Pentoxifylline does not itself induce the human sperm AR, but rather it sensitizes the response to calcium ionophore in cases where the sperm show poor responsiveness to A23187. While hFF is a very poorly defined substance, and is impossible to standardize between centers, individual laboratories may be able to employ carefully selected pooled material. Good correlations have been found between the response of human spermatozoa to calcium ionophore and their fertilizing ability, and a modification of Cummins' original ARIC test (whose practical usefulness has been confirmed by numerous workers) is currently recommended[61]. Two types of AR pathology have

been defined from ARIC tests: AR insufficiency and AR prematurity:

AR prematurity: when >20% of spermatozoa show spontaneous ARs after 3 h incubation under capacitating conditions;

AR insufficiency: a normal result is >15% ARs inducible by ionophore treatment above the spontaneous background, <10% is abnormal and indicates a likely impairment of fertilizing ability, 10–15% is a gray area, indicating a risk of sperm dysfunction.

It has been reported that approximately 5% of infertility patients have an AR problem, about half AR insufficiency and half AR prematurity (for review see reference 64). In general, both AR prematurity and AR insufficiency are good indicators of a likely clinical problem; a poor ARIC test result is a strong indicator of poor sperm fertilizing ability at IVF (although a good ARIC result does not necessarily indicate the absence of any problem with the physiological AR). The ARIC score has been reported to be a better predictor of pregnancy during IUI treatment than conventional semen characteristics[72]. Both problems can be treated by ICSI because there is no apparent relationship between AR function and ICSI outcome, but, in the absence of other andrological indications, recourse to ICSI for treating AR insufficiency might be avoided by using spermatozoa preincubated with pentoxifylline for IVF (probably the only situation where sperm treatment with pentoxifylline is warranted). It has also been reported that AR prematurity may be alleviated by sperm pretreatment with egg yolk. However, given the overall prevalence of such problems, one cannot propose AR studies as an upfront diagnostic test like semen analysis, although automation of test scoring, and simplified protocols using rhuZP3, might make such testing more amenable to routine clinical use in the future.

Extensive studies have demonstrated that the zona-induced acrosome reaction, or ZIAR, is an interesting assessment of sperm functional potential[73–78], which has been further correlated with sperm morphology[79,80]. However, the difficulty of running this assay in routine andrology laboratories continues to hinder its wider application and acceptance into routine pretreatment evaluation.

Standardized ARIC test protocol

Because it can provide clear indications for further treatment options, the ESHRE Andrology Special Interest Group has produced a consensus protocol for reliable ARIC testing[64]:

(1) Spermatozoa must be separated from seminal plasma using a non-deleterious preparation method and suspended in a bicarbonate-based culture medium capable of supporting capacitation, supplemented with at least 10 mg/ml albumin (preferably HSA).

(2) Preincubate the prepared sperm suspension for 3 h at 37°C under 5–6% CO_2. While preincubation is not essential for responsiveness to A23187, it improves reproducibility and allows for the simultaneous assessment of spontaneous acrosome loss (i.e. AR prematurity).

(3) Assess acrosomal status before and after a rather standard ionophore treatment of 10 mmol/l A23187 (use a 2-mmol/l stock solution of A23187-free acid in dimethyl sulfoxide (DMSO)) for 15 min.

(4) Given the extensive studies validating various techniques for visualizing the human sperm acrosome, lectins (e.g. peanut, *Arachis hypogea*, or pea, *Pisum sativum*, agglutinins, i.e. PNA or PSA), monoclonal antibodies (e.g. GB24) or the triple stain may be employed. Two slides must be scored for each determination, with at least 100 spermatozoa counted per slide.

(5) A vitality assessment should be included to differentiate postmortem acrosomal degeneration or loss from a true acrosome reaction, unless the labeling technique gives an 'equatorial segment only' pattern, which is typical of a true AR and rarely seen with degenerative acrosome loss. Exclusion of the fluorescent dye Hoechst 33258 is preferred over a HOS-type test.

(6) As with any bioassay, a positive control sample is mandatory in each assay run, although a negative control is not essential. The positive control need not necessarily be from a proven fertile donor (although this is preferred), but it must be from a man proved to have a normal response in the test. Because cryopreservation alters sperm membranes, fresh semen must be used for the positive control.

Acrosin measurement

Even though a man's spermatozoa might respond to an AR agonist, this does not necessarily indicate the presence of sufficient acrosin for effective penetration of the zona pellucida. The value of biochemical assays of acrosin (either spectrophotometric or film-lysis type assays) remains inconclusive, especially in light of the perennial technical difficulties surrounding the efficient extraction of acrosin from spermatozoa, its poor solubility and the need to differentiate between acrosin's proteolytic and lectin-like activities. For the present, clinical application of such tests remains unproven[15].

Sperm–zona binding tests

Sperm binding to the zona pellucida (ZP) is an essential recognition stage in the eutherian fertilization process. After penetrating the cumulus oophorus, spermatozoa bind tightly to ZP3, which induces a signal transduction cascade within the spermatozoon leading to the acrosome reaction. Acrosome-reacted spermatozoa are then considered to bind to another zona protein (ZP2), facilitating penetration of the zona matrix and progression into the perivitelline space. Much of the species-specificity of human fertilization occurs at the level of sperm–zona pellucida interaction, including induction of the physiological acrosome reaction in the fertilizing spermatozoon, which has led to great interest in the development of tests to assess sperm binding to the human zona pellucida (for review see reference 64).

Sperm–zona binding tests (ZBTs) use non-viable, non-fertilizable human eggs from pathological specimens, or 'spare' IVF eggs which can either be cryostored using a simple freezing protocol that does not preserve oocyte function or kept in a high salt solution which denatures the ooplasm. Bisection of zonae for the hemizona assay (HZA, see below) coincidentally destroys the oocytes, although zonae for this purpose have usually been cryopreserved or salt-stored previously. ZBTs assess tight sperm binding to the zona as the primary endpoint, and have a high predictive value for *in vitro* fertilization in prospectively designed studies, as well as a high capacity to identify male-factor cases at risk for failed or poor fertilization.

The hemizona assay

The HZA involves microdissecting a zona pellucida into equal halves so that the binding of patient (or experimentally treated) and control sperm populations can be assessed on matching halves. Usual assay conditions are to prepare selected motile sperm populations over a period of about 60 min and then co-incubate them with the hemizonae for 4 h at 250 000 motile spermatozoa/ml in a droplet under oil.

The competitive zona binding test

In the competitive zona binding test (CZBT), patient and donor sperm populations are labeled with fluorochromes and mixed at equal concentrations of motile spermatozoa for simultaneous testing on the same zona(e). When using zonae that have not previously been inseminated, it is necessary only to label the donor spermatozoa (e.g. using fluorescein, FITC) to distinguish them from the patient's. If the zonae have been inseminated previously (i.e. IVF 'failed fertilization' eggs), both sperm populations must be labeled with different fluorochromes (e.g. FITC and rhodamine, TRITC) to make them distinguishable

from any spermatozoa that might be already attached to the zonae. Typically, 100 000 motile spermatozoa/ml for each of the patient and donor are mixed in 50-μl droplets under oil for co-incubation with the zonae.

Indirect ZBTs at IVF

In cases of IVF fertilization failure, all oocytes should be examined for the presence of spermatozoa bound to the zonae pellucidae as their absence might be diagnostically useful, indicating a defect of sperm–zona binding. Being a qualitative rather than quantitative assessment, this is not as reliable as a direct sperm–zona binding test, but it can provide valuable information, especially if facilities for performing a formal diagnostic ZBT do not exist.

Interpretation and application of ZBTs

Fertilization problems due to dysfunctional sperm–zona pellucida interaction are relatively common in IVF, and hence these bioassays have significant potential as diagnostic/predictive tests to identify clinical problems and in the management of individual cases, namely whether ICSI is required or not. Because the HZA and CZBT approaches employ very similar basic methodology and provide very comparable results, it has been recommended that the results of either test should be presented as an index, expressing the patient's binding results as a percentage relative to the control donor's[64]. False-positive and false-negative results do occur, but they are relatively infrequent, especially zero results. However, notwithstanding the unquestioned clinical value of ZBTs, the scarcity of suitable oocytes (especially since the advent of ICSI) makes the test impractical for most laboratories. For the future, surrogate or artificial zonae might be employed once biologically active rhuZP3 becomes readily available.

The ESHRE Andrology Special Interest Group has proposed principles for a simple, standardized protocol that can be applied with any of the ZBT formats described above[64]:

(1) Incorporation of adequate controls is essential. If separate groups of zonae are used then patient and positive control (fertile donor) sperm populations are prepared and tested in parallel on four or five zonae each. With the HZA, patient and control sperm populations are tested on identical halves of

the same zonae (requiring only one or two per test); and similarly for CZBTs.

(2) Resuspend selected motile spermatozoa at 100–250 000/ml in a protein-supplemented, bicarbonate-based, IVF culture medium. Patient and control donor preparations should be at the same motile sperm concentration.

(3) Co-incubate the spermatozoa and zonae in a droplet (e.g. 100 ml) under oil for 4 h at 37°C under a CO_2-enriched atmosphere.

(4) Remove the zonae and wash them before counting the numbers of tightly bound spermatozoa. The entire surface of the (hemi)zona needs to be scored to avoid any skewing of results due to heterogeneous distribution of spermatozoa.

Zona-free hamster egg penetration test

Although nowadays the zona-free hamster egg penetration test (HEPT) is used by only a very limited number of laboratories[64], a brief overview is given here because there is widespread clinical and patient awareness of it. Fundamentally, the HEPT assesses the ability of spermatozoa to capacitate *in vitro* and undergo the acrosome reaction, which leaves them in a fusogenic state, able to bind to and fuse with the hamster oocyte oolemma. The sperm head is then incorporated into the oocyte and its nucleus decondenses to form a swollen sperm head, whose visualization is the endpoint of the test.

There is intra- and inter-sample heterogeneity in sperm populations, both in the time needed to achieve the capacitated state and in susceptibility to undergoing spontaneous acrosome loss. Therefore, protocols that rely on spontaneous ARs will give variable results according to preincubation conditions. Attempts to eliminate this inter- and intra-sample variability gave rise to a wide range of protocols employing strategies to induce ARs artificially in more-or-less capacitated sperm populations[15,64].

Inconsistent terminology caused substantial confusion in understanding the HEPT's clinical relevance, and very few papers reported prospective studies using clinically relevant endpoints, such as the achievement of conception *in vivo* or fertilization *in vitro*. False-negative results were common in early studies based on spontaneous ARs, and false-positive results

remained a persistent problem in all but a very few studies. The ESHRE Andrology Special Interest Group consensus workshop on sperm function tests concluded that, although its value as a research tool for assessing sperm function is unquestioned, the HEPT is not a frontline clinical diagnostic test[64], a conclusion echoed by other authorities[81].

Sperm chromatin assessments

Mammalian sperm chromatin is highly condensed and inactive, with the histones being almost entirely replaced by protamines. However, the degree of condensation varies widely between spermatozoa, and several methods have been developed to investigate the degree of condensation and stability of the sperm chromatin as well as the existence of damage to the DNA itself. Detection of abnormalities in sperm DNA has been established as an important aspect of managing the infertile male, as the damaged DNA will be transmitted to embryos that are created during assisted conception treatment[82,83].

Because tests that employ optical microscopic evaluation of the spermatozoa typically analyze only 100 or 200 cells, they are inherently less robust than those which employ flow cytometry and analyze several thousand cells. Consequently, of all the sperm chromatin assessments used routinely, the sperm chromatin structure assay (SCSA) (see below) would be expected to provide the most reliable results.

Nuclear chromatin decondensation test

Human sperm chromatin has an intrinsic ability to decondense when exposed to a combination of detergent, (sodium dodecyl sulfate, SDS), to lyse the cell membranes, and a chelating agent (ethylenediaminetetra-acetic acid, EDTA), to remove zinc ions that stabilize the sulfydryl groups on the protamines not involved in disulfide bonds[84]. However, even though this decondensation ability varies between the ejaculates of fertile and infertile men, nuclear chromatin decondensation (NCD) testing has not been found to be predictive of IVF outcome.

Aniline blue staining

Staining of the sperm nucleus by aniline blue reveals disturbed chromatin condensation. Normal spermatozoa do not take up the aniline blue stain, and results are expressed as the percentage of spermatozoa with unstained heads (i.e. mature nuclei). Differentiation of degrees of aniline blue staining is of unknown value, although distinction between morphologically normal and abnormal spermatozoa may have some relevance[85].

Acridine orange fluorescence

Acridine orange (AO) staining distinguishes between spermatozoa with native DNA (green fluorescence) and single-stranded DNA (orange/red fluorescence), and can therefore be used as a marker for abnormal sperm chromatin condensation. Results of the microscopic test are expressed as the percentage incidence of cells with 'normal' or 'abnormal' DNA, perhaps incorporating a distinction between morphologically normal and abnormal spermatozoa. However, this technique has particular interest for routine application because AO fluorescence can be assessed using flow cytometry, which forms the basis of the sperm chromatin structure assay (see below).

Sperm chromatin structure assay

The sperm chromatin structure assay (SCSA®) is the flow cytometric analysis of large numbers of spermatozoa measuring a metachromatic shift from the green fluorescence of AO when intercalated into double-stranded DNA to a red fluorescence emitted when AO is associated with single-stranded DNA. The SCSA quantitates this shift when acid or heat is used to denature the sperm DNA *in situ*. It has been shown to be an objective, biologically stable and sensitive measure of semen quality in toxicology studies[86], and over recent years has become a highly informative clinical tool to study damage to human sperm DNA, and is now commercially available (www.scsadiagnostics.com). Several recent studies have confirmed the diagnostic and prognostic value of the SCSA and provide guidelines on how its results can be interpreted clinically (although, just like any other assay in infertility, the answers will never be unequivocal)[87–90]. However, similar assays run by other laboratories should not be confused with the SCSA, and must be interpreted using their own criteria established from extensive clinical trials, as for the SCSA.

DNA strand breaks

Various techniques allow the identification of breaks or 'nicks' in sperm DNA, including DNA end-labeling (transferase-mediated deoxyuridine triphosphate nick end-labeling, TUNEL assay), gel electrophoresis of DNA fragments derived from single cells (chromosomal aberration and single cell gel electrophoresis, Comet assay) and *in situ* nick translation.

Morphologically abnormal spermatozoa show an increased sensitivity of their DNA to denaturation, a feature correlated with a high presence of endogenous nicks in their DNA[91]. Furthermore, a high prevalence of spermatozoa with DNA nicks has been associated with increased likelihood of failure to initiate sperm nucleus decondensation after ICSI[92]. Only preliminary clinical application of this approach has been reported to date, but it is expected that it will become a powerful tool for investigating the deleterious effects of hazards such as smoking and free radicals upon the genome delivered to zygotes by spermatozoa from men whose reproductive health and fertility are at risk from such influences[93,94].

GENETIC TESTING

Genetic defects are associated with a variety of clinical presentations among the male partners of infertile couples, ranging from hypogonadotropic hypogonadism (e.g. Kallman's syndrome) to disturbed spermatogenesis or spermatogenic arrest to obstructive azoospermia[95–100]. Other congenital anomalies causing male sterility, sometimes referred to as 'sterilizing defects', include:

(1) Kartagener's (immotile cilia) syndrome, where all the axonemes in the body – including respiratory cilia and sperm tails – lack dynein arms and are hence immotile[101];

(2) Dyskinetic motility as a result of absent outer dynein arms or other disturbances of the axial filament complex of the sperm tail axoneme, e.g. 'sliding spermatozoa', a problem caused by the abnormal distribution and length of the outer dense fibers (these spermatozoa cannot penetrate cervical mucus)[102]; elucidation and confirmation of these defects requires transmission electron microscopy;

(3) Globozoospermia or 'round head defect', where all the spermatozoa have round nuclei surrounded by a halo of cytoplasm but no acrosome; these spermatozoa are easily recognizable under the

light microscope in stained preparations, but are distinct from more-or-less normal spermatozoa which merely have more circular-shaped heads (i.e. length : width ratio of almost 1.0).

Until recently, clinical genetic testing focused on the relationship between karyotypic anomalies (including aneuploidy and translocations) and male infertility. However, in recent years there has been a major shift away from cytogenetics to molecular genetics, employing fluorescent *in situ* hybridization (FISH), polymerase chain reaction (PCR) and the hybrid technique of primed *in situ* transcription (PRINS):

(1) FISH analysis of individual spermatozoa allows sexing (X-/Y-chromosome-bearing status) and the detection of aneuploidy;

(2) PCR analysis of DNA extracted from populations of spermatozoa enables the detection of specific defects in a gene and in particular regions of a chromosome (see below);

(3) PRINS allows PCR to be applied to individual cells with direct microscopic detection of the product.

Cytogenetics

Karyotyping allows detection of problems such as Klinefelter's syndrome (47,XXY), which accounts for a great majority of men presenting with secretory (non-obstructive) azoospermia[102]. Certain other aneuploidies are associated with disturbed spermatogenesis, presenting clinically as oligozoospermia, and in particular sex chromosome aneuploidy seems to have a higher prevalence in men presenting for ICSI, and may be transmitted to their offspring[103,104].

Fluorescent in situ hybridization

FISH analysis of sperm chromosome complements allows investigation of the transmission of chromosomal abnormalities of paternal origin, in particular aneuploidies[105]. Unfortunately, it is extremely laborious and time-consuming (and hence expensive) so that, while it can be extremely informative from a research perspective and can provide confirmation of specific diagnoses, it has little application in routine clinical practice.

Molecular genetics

A comprehensive overview of the role of molecular genetic testing in infertile men, which is becoming ever-increasingly important, is outside the scope of this chapter. However, the importance of testing for defects in cases of congenital bilateral absence of the vas deferens (CBAVD) and severe oligozoospermia, cryptozoospermia and azoospermia cannot be overemphasized and should be considered part of the basic work-up for these men[99,106–108].

Congenital bilateral absence of the vas deferens

Several hundred mutations in the cystic fibrosis (CF) transmembrane conductance regulator gene are now known. While homozygous ΔF508 deletions and some other severe mutations lead to cystic fibrosis, many other heterozygous permutations result in CBAVD. The prevalence of the various mutations is highly dependent upon the population genetic background, and hence testing strategies must consider not only the regional location, but also the ethnic origin of each patient. Testing for CF carrier status of both partners is now considered essential before treating couples by ICSI where the man has CBAVD[103,109].

Microdeletions of the Y chromosome

A wide variety of spermatogenic defects have been associated with microdeletions in an area of the long arm of the Y chromosome (Yq11.23) known as the azoospermia factor (AZF) locus[110–112]. Three AZF regions have been described (some authors describe a fourth), with AZFc being most commonly associated with severe oligozoospermia, although spermatozoa can be recovered from testicular tissue and used for ICSI. However, a deletion in the AZFa or AZFb region seems to indicate a total absence of spermatogenesis (Sertoli-cell-only phenotype) and probably contraindicates any attempt to recover spermatozoa for ICSI[113].

Molecular genetic testing of men with severe oligozoospermia or non-obstructive azoospermia is essential, not only because it can provide important information for the couple's management (i.e. whether a testicular biopsy is likely to provide spermatozoa for ICSI or not), but also because all Y-bearing spermatozoa from such men will carry the same deletion(s) and male offspring produced using ICSI will be affected in the same way as their father[114,115]. Consequently, the concept of the heritability of male sterility is now of growing concern, and the principles of informed consent require that all relevant information – and counselling[116] – is made available to the couple before embarking upon treatment.

Mitochondrial DNA

Mitochondria contain the only DNA outside the nucleus of eukaryotic cells. This extra-nuclear genome (16.6 kilobases in humans) encodes several essential components of the oxidative phosphorylation (OXPHOS) pathway. Abnormalities of mitochondrial DNA (mtDNA) underlie several neurological diseases and some forms of diabetes, and, because they accumulate in postmeiotic tissues with age, are implicated in the process of aging and the etiology of degenerative disorders[117,118]. Because mitochondria are the site of OXPHOS, they are a potent source of ROS, and hence defective mitochondria may contribute to free radical-induced problems, not only causing sperm dysfunction, but also at the testicular level. Defects in mtDNA have been implicated in sperm dysfunction by several workers[119,120] but, for the present there are no simple, readily available diagnostic tests for mitochondrial DNA defects.

CONCLUSIONS

This chapter has summarized the range of laboratory tests applicable to the male partner of infertile couples from the perspective of an assisted conception program, including tests that are expected to become more common over the next few years. Emphasis has been placed on the need to investigate the man as part of a couple, and upon using the concept of structured management to guide each couple's work-up and treatment. Patient management should be designed to provide the desired outcome for the patients as quickly – and cost-effectively – as possible, and this involves vital diagnostic laboratory input.

The summary list below is not intended to be exhaustive, merely a starting point for a unit when establishing its own management standards for best practice, a process inevitably subject to many sociological, religious, ethical, political and economic pressures, as well as personal opinions and practical constraints. However, regardless of anything else, all this must be underpinned by the provision of laboratory services that guarantee accurate and reliable results.

Basic work-up of the infertile couple

(1) *Semen analysis*: use standardized methods conforming to World Health Organization guidelines as the minimum, and include testing for sperm surface ASABs and microbiological testing of the ejaculate (perhaps also urethral swabs or expressed prostatic fluid) if there is indication of male genital tract infection.

(2) Test for circulating ASABs in the female partner, as well as microbiological testing if there is any indication of possible female genital tract infection.

(3) Evaluate sperm–cervical mucus interaction, perhaps including CASA investigation of sperm kinematics.

Prior to assisted conception treatment

(1) *Trial wash*: this is done to determine the number and quality of spermatozoa that can be recovered from the man's ejaculate.

(2) *Sperm function testing*: whether this is undertaken before commencing assisted reproductive technologies (ART) treatment, or to evaluate possible causes of failed fertilization at IVF, will depend upon many circumstances. A minimal, but very informative, package of sperm function tests would include analysis of acrosome reaction prematurity/insufficiency and sperm hyperactivation assessment. Prospective ZBTs are presently of very limited avaliability (this may change when rhuZP3-based tests are released), although an evaluation of sperm–zona interaction ia available by examining failed fertilization oocytes. For application on a prospective basis, the cost for such testing would need to be substantially less than the incremental cost for ICSI (incorporation into an 'enhanced trial wash' assessment would minimize the additional cost).

Prior to ICSI treatment

(1) CBAVD MESA cases: carry out genetic testing for CF gene mutations.

(2) Severe oligozoospermia or cryptozoospermia cases: carry out genetic testing for sex

chromosome aneuploidy and Y chromosome microdeletions.

(3) TESE cases: carry out genetic testing for sex chromosome aneuploidy and Y chromosome microdeletions prior to testicular biopsy.

Recurrent failure of embryonic development

(1) Investigate sperm DNA damage.

(2) Investigate rare cytogenetic problems, e.g. autosomal aneuploidy, translocations.

REFERENCES

1. Jequier AM, Cummins JM. Attitudes to clinical andrology: a time for change. Hum Reprod 1997; 12: 875–6

2. Mortimer D. The future of male infertility management and assisted reproduction technology. Hum Reprod 2000; 15 (Suppl 5): 98–110

3. Mortimer D. Structured management as a basis for cost-effective infertility care. In Gagnon C, ed. The Male Gamete: From Basic Science to Clinical Applications. Vienna, IL: Cache River Press, 1999: 363–70

4. Rowe PJ, Comhaire FH, Hargreave TB, Mahmoud AMA. WHO Manual for the Standardized Investigation, Diagnosis and Management of the Infertile Male. Cambridge: Cambridge University Press, 2000

5. Mortimer D. The essential partnership between diagnostic andrology and modern assisted reproductive technologies. Hum Reprod 1994; 9: 1209–13

6. Oehninger S, Franken D, Kruger T. Approaching the next millennium: how should we manage andrology diagnosis in the intracytoplasmic sperm injection era. Fertil Steril 1997; 67: 434–6

7. De Jonge CJ. The role of sperm function testing in infertility management. In Gagnon C, ed. The Male Gamete: From Basic Science to Clinical Applications. Vienna, IL: Cache River Press, 1999: 371–8

8. Mortimer ST, Hillis AJ, Fluker MR, et al. Sperm function tests in management of clinical assisted reproductive technology. Hum Reprod 2002; 17: 110–11, Abstr P-317

9. Rowe PJ, Comhaire FH, Hargreave TB, et al. WHO Manual for the Standardized Investigation and Diagnosis of the Infertile Couple. Cambridge: Cambridge University Press, 1994

10. World Health Organization. WHO Laboratory Manual for the Examination of Human Semen and Sperm–Cervical Mucus Interaction, 4th edn. Cambridge: Cambridge University Press, 1999

11. Eliasson R. Standards for investigation of human semen. Andrologie 1971; 3: 49–64

12. Eliasson R. Analysis of semen. In Behrman SJ, Kistner RW, eds. Progress in Infertility. Boston: Little, Brown & Co., 1975: 691–713

13. Eliasson R. Analysis of semen. In Burger H, de Kretser D, eds. The Testis. New York: Raven Press, 1981: 381–99

14. Belsey MA, Eliasson R, Gallegos AJ, et al. Laboratory Manual for the Examination of Human Semen and Semen–Cervical Mucus Interaction. Singapore: Press Concern, 1980

15. Mortimer D. Practical Laboratory Andrology. New York: Oxford University Press, 1994

16. Kvist U, Björndahl L. Manual on Basic Semen Analysis. Brussels: European Society of Human Reproduction and Embryology, 2002

17. Mortimer D. Laboratory standards in routine clinical andrology. Reprod Med Rev 1994; 3: 97–111

18. World Health Organization. WHO Laboratory Manual for the Examination of Human Semen and Sperm–Cervical Mucus Interaction, 3rd edn. Cambridge: Cambridge University Press, 1992

19. Björndahl L, Barratt CL, Fraser LR, et al. ESHRE basic semen analysis courses 1995–1999: immediate beneficial effects of standardized training. Hum Reprod 2002; 17: 1299–305

20. Tucker M, Wright G, Bishop F, et al. Chymotrypsin in semen preparation for ARTA. Mol Androl 1990; 2: 179

21. de Ziegler D, Cedars MI, Hamilton F, et al. Factors influencing maintenance of sperm motility during in vitro processing. Fertil Steril 1987; 48: 816–20

22. Mortimer D. Semen analysis and other standard laboratory tests. In Hargreave TB, ed. Male Infertility. London: Springer-Verlag, 1994: 37–73

23. Bostofte E, Serup J, Rebbe H. Interrelations among the characteristics of human semen, and a new system for classification of male fertility. Fertil Steril 1984; 41: 95–102

24. Jouannet P, Ducot B, Feneux D, et al. Male factors and the likelihood of pregnancy in infertile couples. I. Study of sperm characteristics. Int J Androl 1988; 11: 379–94

25. Douglas-Hamilton DH, Smith NG, Kuster CE, et al. Particle distribution in low-volume capillary-loaded chambers. J Androl 2005; 26: 107–14

26. Douglas-Hamilton DH, Smith NG, Kuster CE, et al. Capillary loaded particle fluid dynamics: effect on estimation of sperm concentration. J Androl 2005; 26: 115–22

27. Björndahl L, Barrat CLR. Semen analysis: setting standards for the measurement of sperm numbers. J Androl 2005; 26: 11

28. World Health Organization. WHO Laboratory Manual for the Examination of Human Semen and Semen–Cervical Mucus Interaction, 2nd edn. Cambridge: Cambridge University Press, 1987

29. Dunphy BC, Li T-C, Macleod IC, et al. The interaction of parameters of male and female fertility in couples with previously unexplained infertility. Fertil Steril 1990; 54: 824

30. Mortimer D. Objective analysis of sperm motility and kinematics. In Keel BA, Webster BW, eds. Handbook of the Laboratory Diagnosis and Treatment of Infertility. Boca Raton: CRC Press, 1990: 97–133

31. Mortimer ST. A critical review of the physiological importance and analysis of sperm movement in mammals. Hum Reprod Update 1997; 3: 403–39

32. Dresdner RD, Katz DF. Relationships of mammalian sperm motility and morphology to hydrodynamic aspects of cell function. Biol Reprod 1981; 25: 920–30

33. Aitken RJ. Motility parameters and fertility. In Gagnon C, ed. Controls of Sperm Motility: Biological and Clinical Aspects. Boca Raton: CRC Press, 1990: 285–302

34. Björndahl L, Soderlund I, Kvist U. Evaluation of the one-step eosin–nigrosin staining technique for human sperm vitality assessment. Hum Reprod 2003; 18: 813–16

35. Jeyendran RS, Van der Ven HH, Perez-Pelaez M, et al. Development of an assay to assess the functional integrity of the human sperm membrane and its relationship to other semen characteristics. J Reprod Fertil 1984; 70: 219–28

36. Kruger TF, Acosta AA, Simmons KF, et al. Predictive value of abnormal sperm morphology in in vitro fertilization. Fertil Steril 1988; 49: 112–17

37. Kruger TF, Menkveld R, Stander FSH, et al. Sperm morphologic features as a prognostic factor in in vitro fertilization. Fertil Steril 1986; 46: 1118–23

38. Mortimer D. Sperm form and function: beauty is in the eye of the beholder. In Van der Horst G, Franken D, Bornman R, et al. eds. Proceedings of the 9th International Symposium on Spermatology. Bologna: Monduzzi Editore S.p.A., 2002: 257–62

39. Menkveld R. Evolution of human sperm morphology assessments based on sperm functional potential. In Van der Horst G, Franken D, Bornman R, et al. eds. Proceedings of the 9th International Symposium on Spermatology. Bologna: Monduzzi Editore S.p.A., 2002: 263–8

40. Menkveld R, Stander FSH, Kotze TJVW, et al. The evaluation of morphological characteristics of human spermatozoa according to stricter criteria. Hum Reprod 1990; 5: 586–92

41. Mortimer D, Menkveld R. Sperm morphology assessment – historical perspectives and current opinions. J Androl 2001; 22: 192–205

42. Liu J, Nagy Z, Joris H, et al. Successful fertilization and establishment of pregnancies after intracytoplasmic sperm injection in patients with globozoospermia. Hum Reprod 1995; 10: 626–9

43. Nijs M, Vanderzwalmen P, Vandamme B, et al. Fertilizing ability of immotile spermatozoa after intracytoplasmic sperm injection. Hum Reprod 1996; 11: 2180–5

44. Chemes EH, Rawe YV. Sperm pathology: a step beyond descriptive morphology. Origin, characterization and fertility potential of abnormal sperm phenotypes in infertile men. Hum Reprod Update 2003; 9: 405–28

45. Wolff H, Anderson DJ. Immunohistologic characterization and quantitation of leukocyte subpopulations in human semen. Fertil Steril 1988; 49: 497–504

46. Aitken RJ, Ryan AL, Baker MA, et al. Redox activity associated with the maturation and capacitation of mammalian spermatozoa. Free Radic Biol Med 2004; 36: 994–1010

47. Baker MA, Aitken RJ. The importance of redox regulated pathways in sperm cell biology. Mol Cell Endocrinol 2004; 216: 47–54

48. Huszar G, Vigue L, Oehninger S. Creatine kinase immunocytochemistry of human sperm–hemizona complexes: selective binding of sperm with mature creatine kinase-staining pattern. Fertil Steril 1994; 61: 136–42

49. Krausz C, West K, Buckingham D, et al. Development of a technique for monitoring the contamination of human semen samples with leukocytes. Fertil Steril 1992; 57: 1317–25

50. Saleh RA, Agarwal A. Oxidative stress and male infertility: from research bench to clinical practice. J Androl 2002; 23: 737–52

51. Agarwal A, Saleh RA, Bedaiwy MA. Role of reactive oxygen species in the pathophysiology of human reproduction. Fertil Steril 2003; 79: 829–43

52. Agarwal A. Role of antioxidants in treatment of male infertility: an overview of the literature. Reprod Biomed Online 2004; 8: 616–27

53. Lombardo F, Gandini L, Dondero F, et al. Antisperm immunity in natural and assisted reproduction. Hum Reprod Update 2001; 7: 450–6

54. Fowler JE Jr. Infections of the male reproductive tract and infertility: a selected review. J Androl 1981; 3: 121–31

55. Mortimer D. Sperm preparation techniques and iatrogenic failures of in-vitro fertilization. Hum Reprod 1991; 6: 173–6

56. Chapeau C, Gagnon C. Nitrocellulose and polyvinyl coatings prevent sperm adhesion to glass without affecting the motility of intact and demembranated human spermatozoa. J Androl 1987; 8: 34–40

57. Mortimer D. Sperm recovery techniques to maximize fertilizing capacity. Reprod Fertil Dev 1994; 6: 25–31

58. Mortimer D. Sperm preparation methods. J Androl 2000; 21: 357–66

59. Boyers SP, Davis RO, Katz DF. Automated semen analysis. Curr Prob Obstet Gynecol Fertil 1989; XII: 167–200

60. Mortimer D, Mortimer ST. Value and reliability of CASA systems. In Ombelet W, Bosmans E, Vandeput H, et al., eds. Modern ART in the 2000s. Carnforth: Parthenon Publishing, 1998: 73–89

61. Mortimer ST. CASA – practical aspects. J Androl 2000; 21: 515–24

62. Mortimer ST. Practical application of computer-aided sperm analysis (CASA). In Van der Horst G, Franken D, Bornman R, et al. eds. Proceedings of the 9th International Symposium on Spermatology. Bologna: Monduzzi Editore S.p.A., 2002: 233–8

63. Mortimer D, Aitken RJ, Mortimer ST, Pacey AA. Workshop report: clinical CASA – the quest for consensus. Reprod Fertil Dev 1995; 7: 951–9

64. ESHRE Andrology Special Interest Group. Consensus workshop on advanced diagnostic andrology techniques. Hum Reprod 1996; 11: 1463–79

65. ESHRE Andrology Special Interest Group. Guidelines on the application of CASA technology in the analysis of spermatozoa. Hum Reprod 1998; 13: 142–5

66. Eggert-Kruse W, Leinhos G, Gerhard I, et al. Prognostic value of in vitro sperm penetration into hormonally standardized human cervical mucus. Fertil Steril 1989; 51: 317–23.

67. Pandya IJ, Mortimer D, Sawers RS. A standardized approach for evaluating the penetration of human spermatozoa into cervical mucus in vitro. Fertil Steril 1986; 45: 357–65

68. Eggert-Kruse W, Gerhard I, Tilgen W, et al. Clinical significance of crossed in vitro sperm–cervical mucus penetration test in infertility investigation. Fertil Steril 1989; 52: 1032–40

69. Barratt CLR, Osborn JC, Harrison PE, et al. The hypo-osmotic swelling test and the sperm mucus penetration test in determining fertilization of the human oocyte. Hum Reprod 1989; 4: 430–4

70. Mortimer ST, Swan MA. Variable kinematics of capacitating human spermatozoa. Hum Reprod 1995; 10: 3178–82

71. Mortimer ST, Swan MA, Mortimer D. Fractal analysis of capacitating human spermatozoa. Hum Reprod 1996; 11: 1049–54

72. Makkar G, Ng EH, Yeung WS, et al. The significance of the ionophore-challenged acrosome reaction in the prediction of successful outcome of controlled ovarian stimulation and intrauterine insemination. Hum Reprod 2003; 18: 534–9

73. Liu DY, Clarke GN, Baker HWG. The effect of serum on motility of human spermatozoa in culture. Int J Androl 1986; 9: 109–17

74. Liu DY, Baker HW. Frequency of defective sperm–zona pellucida interaction in severely teratozoospermic infertile men. Hum Reprod 2003; 18: 802–7

75. Liu DY, Clarke GN, Martic M, et al. Frequency of disordered zona pellucida (ZP)-induced acrosome reaction in infertile men with normal semen analysis and normal spermatozoa–ZP binding. Hum Reprod 2001; 16: 1185–90

76. Liu DY, Stewart T, Baker HW. Normal range and variation of the zona pellucida-induced acrosome reaction in fertile men. Fertil Steril 2003; 80: 384–9

77. Liu DY, Baker HW. Disordered zona pellucida-induced acrosome reaction and failure of in vitro fertilization in patients with unexplained infertility. Fertil Steril 2003; 79: 74–80

78. Liu DY, Baker HW. Defective sperm–zona pellucida interaction: a major cause of failure of fertilization in clinical in-vitro fertilization. Hum Reprod 2000; 15: 702–8

79. Bastiaan HS, Menkveld R, Oehninger S, et al. Zona pellucida induced acrosome reaction, sperm morphology, and sperm-zona binding assessments among subfertile men. J Assist Reprod Genet 2002; 19: 329–34

80. Bastiaan HS, Windt ML, Menkveld R, et al. Relationship between zona pellucida-induced acrosome reaction, sperm morphology, sperm–zona pellucida binding, and in vitro fertilization. Fertil Steril 2003; 79: 49–55

81. Oehninger S, Franken DR, Sayed E, et al. Sperm function assays and their predictive value for fertilization outcome in IVF therapy: a meta-analysis. Hum Reprod Update 2000; 6: 160–8

82. Sakkas D. The need to detect DNA damage in human spermatozoa: possible consequences on embryo development. In Gagnon C, ed. The Male Gamete: From Basic Science to Clinical Applications. Vienna, IL: Cache River Press, 1999: 379–84

83. Agarwal A, Said TM. Role of sperm chromatin abnormalities and DNA damage in male infertility. Hum Reprod Update 2003; 9: 331–45

84. Kvist U, Afzelius BA, Nilsson L. The intrinsic mechanism of chromatin decondensation and its activation in human spermatozoa. Dev Growth Differ 1980; 22: 543–54

85. Dadoune JP, Mayaux MJ, Guihard-Moscato ML. Correlation between defects in chromatin condensation of human spermatozoa stained by aniline blue and semen characteristics. Andrologia 1988; 20: 211–17

86. Sailer BL, Jost LK, Evenson DP. Mammalian sperm DNA susceptibility to in situ denaturation associated with the presence of DNA strand breaks as measured by the terminal deoxynucleotidyl transferase assay. J Androl 1995; 16: 80–7

87. Evenson DP, Larson KL, Jost LK. Sperm chromatin structure assay: its clinical use for detecting sperm DNA fragmentation in male infertility and comparisons with other techniques. J Androl 2002; 23: 25–43

88. Larson-Cook KL, Brannian JD, Hansen KA, et al. Relationship between the outcomes of assisted reproductive techniques and sperm DNA fragmentation as measured by the sperm chromatin structure assay. Fertil Steril 2003; 80: 895–902

89. Larson KL, DeJonge CJ, Barnes AM, et al. Sperm chromatin structure assay parameters as predictors of failed pregnancy following assisted reproductive techniques. Hum Reprod 2000; 15: 1717–22

90. Virro MR, Larson-Cook KL Evenson DP. Sperm chromatin structure assay parameters (SCSA®) are related to fertilization, blastocyst development, and ongoing pregnancy in in vitro fertilization and intracytoplasmic sperm injection cycles. Fertil Steril 2004; 81: 1289–95

91. Bianchi PG, Manicardi GC, Urner F, et al. Chromatin packaging and morphology in ejaculated human spermatozoa: evidence of hidden anomalies in normal spermatozoa. Mol Hum Reprod 1996; 2: 139–44

92. Sakkas D, Urner F, Bianchi PG, et al. Sperm chromatin anomalies can influence decondensation after intracytoplasmic sperm injection. Hum Reprod 1996; 11: 837–43

93. Sakkas D, Bianchi PG, Manicardi G, et al. Chromatin packaging anomalies and DNA damage in human sperm: their possible implications in the treatment of male factor infertility. In Barratt C, De Jonge C, Mortimer D, Parinaud J, eds. Genetics of Human Male Fertility. Paris: EDK, 1997: 205–21

94. Morris ID, Ilott S, Dixon L, Brison DR. The spectrum of DNA damage in human sperm assessed by single cell gel electrophoresis (Comet assay) and its relationship to fertilization and embryo development. Hum Reprod 2002; 17: 990–8

95. Mak V, Jarvi KA. The genetics of male infertility. J Urol 1996; 156: 1245–56

96. Tuerlings JHAM, Kremer JAM, Meuleman EJ. The practical application of genetics in the male infertility clinic. J Androl 1997; 18: 576–81

97. Vogt P. Molecular basis of male (in)fertility. Int J Androl 1997; 20 (Suppl 3): 2–10

98. Vogt PH. Genetic aspects of human infertility. Int J Androl 1995; 18 (Suppl 2): 3–6

99. Barratt CLR, St John JC, Afnan M. Genetic testing of the male. In Gagnon C, ed. The Male Gamete: From Basic Science to Clinical Applications. Vienna, IL: Cache River Press, 1999: 397–405

100. Maduro MR, Lo KC, Chuang WW, et al. Genes and male infertility: what can go wrong? J Androl 2003; 24: 485–93

101. Gagnon C. Genetic aspects of flagellar dyskinesia, globozoospermia. In Barratt C, De Jonge C, Mortimer D, Parinaud J, eds. Genetics of Human Male Fertility. Paris: EDK, 1997: 76–97

102. Chandley AC. Chromosomes. In Hargreave TB, ed. Male Infertility. London: Springer-Verlag, 1994: 149–64

103. Tournaye H, Lissens W, Liebaers I, et al. Heritability of sterility: clinical implications. In Barratt C, De Jonge C, Mortimer D, Parinaud J, eds. Genetics of Human Male Fertility. Paris: EDK, 1997: 123–44

104. Martin RH, Rademaker AW, Greene C, et al. A comparison of the frequency of sperm chromosome abnormalities in men with mild, moderate, and severe oligozoospermia. Biol Reprod 2003; 69: 535–9

105. Martin RH, Spriggs E, Moosani N, et al. Detection and characterization of chromosomal abnormalities in human sperm. In Barratt C, De Jonge C, Mortimer D, Parinaud J, eds. Genetics of Human Male Fertility. Paris: EDK, 1997: 164–81

106. Dohle GR, Halley DJ, Van Hemel JO, et al. Genetic risk factors in infertile men with severe oligozoospermia and azoospermia. Hum Reprod 2002; 17: 13–16

107. Griffin DK, Hyland P, Tempest HG, et al. Safety issues in assisted reproduction technology: should men undergoing ICSI be screened for chromosome abnormalities in their sperm? Hum Reprod 2003; 18: 229–35

108. Vogt PH. Molecular genetics of human male infertility: from genes to new therapeutic perspectives. Curr Pharm Des 2004; 10: 471–500

109. Schlegel P, Shin D. Urogenital anomalies and genetic defects in men with bilateral congenital absence of the vas deferens. In Barratt C, De Jonge C, Mortimer D, Parinaud J, eds. Genetics of Human Male Fertility. Paris: EDK, 1997: 98–110

110. Foresta C, Moro E, Ferlin A. Prognostic value of Y deletion analysis. The role of current methods. Hum Reprod 2001; 16: 1543–7

111. Foresta C, Moro E, Ferlin A. Y chromosome microdeletions and alterations of spermatogenesis. Endocr Rev 2001; 22: 226–39

112. Vogt PH, Fernandes S. Polymorphic DAZ gene family in polymorphic structure of AZFc locus: artwork or functional for human spermatogenesis? APMIS 2003; 111: 115–26

113. Hopps CV, Mielnik A, Goldstein M, et al. Detection of sperm in men with Y chromosome microdeletions of the AZFa, AZFb and AZFc regions. Hum Reprod 2003; 18: 1660–5

114. Rolf C, Gromoll J, Simoni M, et al. Natural transmission of a partial AZFb deletion of the Y chromosome over three generations: case report. Hum Reprod 2002; 17: 2267–71

115. Katagiri Y, Neri QV, Takeuchi T, et al. Y chromosome assessment and its implications for the development of ICSI children. Reprod Biomed Online 2004; 8: 307–18

116. Meschede D, Horst J. Genetic counselling for infertile male patients. Int J Androl 1997; 20 (Suppl 3): 20–30

117. Cummins JM. Mitochondrial DNA: implications for the genetics of human male fertility. In Barratt C, De Jonge C, Mortimer D, Parinaud J, eds. Genetics of Human Male Fertility. Paris: EDK, 1997: 287–307

118. Cummins JM, Jequier AM, Kan R. Molecular biology of human male infertility: links with aging, mitochondrial genetics, and oxidative stress. Mol Reprod Dev 1994; 37: 345–62

119. Cummins JM. Mitochondria in reproduction. Reprod Biomed Online 2004; 8: 14–15

120. Thangaraj K, Joshi MB, Reddy AG, et al. Sperm mitochondrial mutations as a cause of low sperm motility. J Androl 2003; 24: 388–92

5

Ultrasound in assisted conception

Rajat Goswamy

The use of ultrasound in the management of infertility is now routine practice, not just as an aid in the diagnosis of ovulation, but as an essential tool in the management of the infertile couple.

In the pre-ultrasound era, ovulation monitoring was based on basal body temperature charts, changes in cervical mucus and serum progesterone checks. The use of ultrasound in the management of infertility was introduced by Kratochwil and colleagues[1] in 1972, when they first described the use of static imaging to visualize the Graafian follicle. However, it was not until the development of real-time ultrasound that the report of Hackeloer and associates[2] in 1979 triggered renewed interest in this technique to track the growth of the Graafian follicle. This was followed by the widespread use of real-time ultrasound to monitor ovulation in women undergoing donor insemination and induction of ovulation with clomiphene citrate[3,4].

The historical development of ultrasound techniques is beyond the scope of this chapter. The author's aim in this chapter is to demonstrate the use of ultrasound in the management of infertility, from the initial stages of diagnosis of the cause of infertility to the eventual confirmation of pregnancy, including routine monitoring of early pregnancy.

Ultrasound research has helped in the understanding of physiological changes that occur during the ovarian cycle, especially with the widespread use of Doppler technology in assisted conception. Guidance as to the specific advantages of ultrasound techniques and their usage should help those in the field of fertility management to utilize this technology to optimize benefits to their patients and to themselves.

This chapter has been divided into four subsections, each of which is inter-related and not exclusive to the others.

ULTRASOUND IN THE DIAGNOSIS OF INFERTILITY

Ultrasound is probably the single most important test when making a diagnosis as to the cause of infertility in a particular woman. A well-performed and detailed ultrasound examination of the female pelvic organs, performed at the appropriate time of the menstrual cycle, will give more information than any other single test.

Methodology

First, it must be emphasized that ultrasound examinations should be performed with the use of transvaginal probes. The use of abdominal ultrasound probes is outdated, inaccurate and uncomfortable for patients; it lacks detail and is indicated only when a large mass in the pelvis makes it difficult to visualize the uterus, ovaries and adnexal regions adequately. Second, although many examinations are performed to monitor follicle growth, mistakes are made, and pathology is missed because a thorough systematic examination is not always carried out at each examination.

It is important that a fixed routine is practiced during each ultrasound examination so that a systematic examination of the pelvic organs is carried out. The following routine is advisable. The ultrasound probe, lubricated with jelly, is inserted slowly, pointing anteriorly so as to locate the cervix and uterus. If the uterus is not seen anteriorly, a slow movement of the probe from side to side, and then pointing posteriorly, is made. Once the uterus has been located, it is important to note its position (anteverted or retroverted) and its size. Retroversion of the uterus may be physiological, but this is also more commonly noted in the presence of endometriosis. An enlarged uterus could be as a result of pregnancy, adenomyosis or fibroids.

In vitro fertilization and assisted reproduction

The uterus should be scanned initially in the longitudinal plane, so that the 'midline' echo is located and followed from the internal os inferiorly to the fundus superiorly. The probe is then rotated so that a transverse scan of the uterus is performed. Once again, the midline echo is followed from one side of the uterine cavity to the other. After this, the probe is rocked gently from side to side, to assess the adnexal regions. Any cystic areas, appearing echo-free, can be assessed. This is especially important to distinguish hydrosalpinges from ovarian cysts (see below).

After the adnexal region is assessed, the ovaries are located on each side. By moving the probe laterally in the transverse plane, the ovaries can usually be located against the pelvic side-wall, medial or anterior to the internal iliac vessels. If the ovaries are not in the usual location, moving the probe anteriorly and posteriorly will usually help to locate them. In some cases, especially in endometriosis, the ovaries may be anchored in the pouch of Douglas. Pointing the probe towards this area may make the examination uncomfortable for the patient; hence, care should be taken that any movements are made gently and with attention to the patient's reaction. Both ovaries should be scanned sequentially, in the transverse and longitudinal planes.

Before withdrawing the probe, it is important to assess whether there are adhesions present between the genital organs, the pouch of Douglas and the ovarian fossae. This can be assessed by placing one hand on the patient's abdomen and pushing towards the pelvis, first in the midline and then downwards from each iliac fossa. If there are significant adhesions, bowel loops will not slide against the posterior or anterior wall of the uterus. Similarly, restricted mobility of the ovaries against the pelvic side-walls may be indicative of adhesions in the ovarian fossae.

To summarize, the ultrasound examination should be performed in a systematic manner. The examination is target oriented and a firm sequence should be adhered to at every examination. The simplest order of examination would be the uterus, adnexal region, ovaries and pouch of Douglas. The 'sliding organs sign' described by Timor-Tritsch and co-workers[5] should become routine practice at all gynecological ultrasound examinations.

Finally, uterine and tubal pathology can be missed, or physiological changes in the ovary may be wrongly diagnosed as pathological, if the ultrasound examination is performed at an inappropriate time of the menstrual cycle.

Frequently asked questions

(1) What information can be gained by a single ultrasound examination?

(2) When is the best time in the menstrual cycle to perform the examination?

(3) What is the benefit to the patient?

(4) What is the benefit to the clinician?

Uterine factors

The criteria for normal appearance of the endometrium and myometrium have been described previously[6,7]. Uterine size and position and the endometrial cavity are studied in detail. The endometrial cavity and contours are inspected for irregularities and echo patterns and the myometrial–endometrial interphase examined in the longitudinal and transverse planes[8,9].

The midline endometrial echo (Figure 1), where the anterior and posterior uterine walls are apposed to each other, are studied from the internal os to the fundus, and any discontinuity and distortion of this

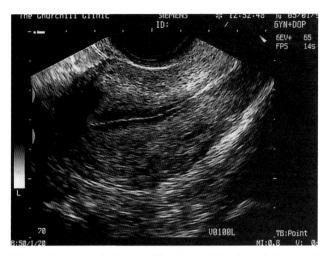

Figure 1 Longitudinal scan of the uterus. Note the uninterrupted midline echo, indicative of a normal uterine cavity

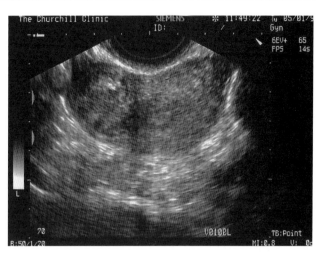

Figure 2 Cornual fibroid distorting the right tubal region

echo should be noted. Longitudinal and oblique scans are performed to study the region of the tubal ostia.

Several abnormalities in the endometrial cavity can be assessed on transvaginal sonography, and many of these would be missed by digital vaginal examination. The commonest abnormalities observed are fibroids, polyps, intrauterine adhesions, uterine septum and endometritis.

Fibroids can be diagnosed as well-defined hypoechoic areas arising from within the myometrial layer, causing attenuation of the ultrasound beam and distal shadowing. The impact of fibroids on fertility is dependent on their size and location. Large intramural and subserous fibroids can distort the uterus, resulting in difficulties in ovum pick-up because of abnormalities in the relationship between the ovary and the Fallopian tube. Intramural fibroids in the cornual region can affect tubal function (Figure 2). However, submucous fibroids are the most frequently missed pathology in women described as having unexplained infertility. Submucous fibroids distort the midline echo and are best diagnosed in the periovulatory phase (Figure 3).

Endometrial polyps (Figure 4) appear as persistent hyperechogenic areas with variable cystic spaces, and these also distort the cavity contours. They are best seen mid-cycle and are not seen clearly in the midluteal phase or in stimulated cycles. Especially in patients with polycystic ovarian disease, endometrial thickness can increase quite markedly during stimulation for *in vitro* fertilization (IVF), and polyps can be misdiagnosed or over-diagnosed.

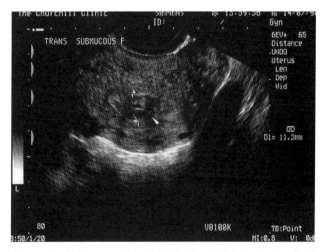

Figure 3 Submucous fibroid. Note the distal shadowing and distortion of the midline echo

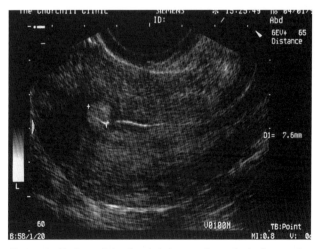

Figure 4 Endometrial polyp. It is hyperechogenic, it distorts the midline echo and there is no distal shadowing

Intrauterine adhesions cause interruptions in the midline echo (Figure 5) and are best noted in the periovulatory phase. They may result in abnormal thinning of the endometrium in response to follicle development. In cases in which endometrial thickness does not increase synchronously with follicle development, synechiae or intrauterine adhesions should be suspected, and ultrasound examination performed in a spontaneous cycle during the periovulatory phase.

Uterine septa are best diagnosed in the transverse plane when myometrial echoes divide the fundal endometrial image (Figure 6). Septa can usually be differentiated from intrauterine adhesions by the isoechoic nature of the septum compared with the surrounding myometrium. Intrauterine septa are best diagnosed in the periovulatory phase, although they can also be diagnosed in the luteal phase. This diagnosis can easily be missed if the ultrasound examination is performed when the endometrium is extremely thin in the early follicular phase.

Endometritis is diagnosed when the endometrial layers appear grainy in the periovulatory phase and the endometrium–myometrium interphase appears diffuse and ill-defined (Figure 7). The presence of such an endometrial echo is quite normal in the luteal phase, but should be considered as abnormal if there is a periovulatory follicle present in the ovary.

In a previous publication[10], in a series of 193 patients, abnormal transvaginal sonography findings as listed above were compared with hysteroscopy. The sensitivity of transvaginal sonography in detecting all abnormalities was 98.9% and the positive predictive value was 94.3%. The positive predictive value for diagnosing submucous fibroids was 91.7%, which was similar to that in the diagnosis of polyps (91.4%). Fedele and colleagues[11] reported 100% sensitivity for transvaginal sonography compared with hysteroscopic findings in patients with submucous fibroids. However, our findings indicated only 91% sensitivity for fibroids, but 98.5% sensitivity for the diagnosis of intrauterine adhesions.

Adenomyosis is probably the most difficult diagnosis to prove, although most ultrasound workers agree that high echogenicity in the myometrium, similar to endometrial findings, is indicative of adenomyosis (Figure 8). Serial ultrasound scans should be performed in at least two consecutive cycles to correlate increased echogenicity within the myometrium with endometrial echoes. Fluid-filled 'sacs' lined by

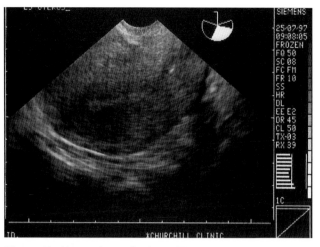

Figure 5 Intrauterine adhesions. Thin endometrium; midline echo almost invisible

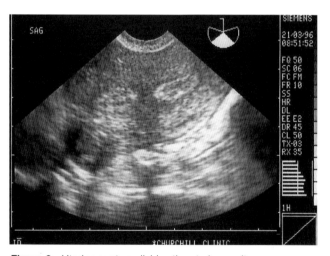

Figure 6 Uterine septum divides the uterine cavity

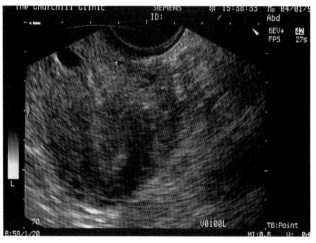

Figure 7 Endometritis. Grainy, with loss of endometrial layers

hyperechogenic thickened areas are also indicative of adenomyosis; these look like gestation sacs within the myometrium.

In reply to the 'frequently asked questions' listed above, it can be concluded that if only one examination is to be performed then this should be done in the periovulatory phase to assess and diagnose pathology in the uterine cavity accurately. The benefit to the patient is that hysteroscopic treatment can then be scheduled at the appropriate time of the cycle (day 6–10 of menses), so that diagnostic hysteroscopy can be combined with the therapeutic procedure. The benefit to the clinician is that operating list times can be adjusted accordingly and the right equipment made available for the patient, so that the other procedures can be carried out at the same time as the diagnostic procedure.

Ovarian factors

The unstimulated ovary, in premenopausal women, usually contains a small number of cystic structures. These are randomly dispersed, and, if the ultrasound examination is performed between day 6 and day 14 of the menstrual cycle, a leading follicle can be identified (Figure 9). A normal ovary usually measures $2.5 \times 2.2 \times 2.0$ cm, and ovaries with diameters in excess of 3.5 cm should be considered as abnormal. The mean volume of a normal ovary is 5.4 ml (range 4.0–7.0 ml).

In some women, the ovaries may contain ten or more cystic structures distributed peripherally around a central core of stroma (Figure 10). Such ovaries have been termed polycystic, and are usually associated with menstrual irregularity, raised luteinizing hormone (LH) levels, hirsutism, anovulation and an increased incidence of miscarriage[12–14]. Eshel and co-workers[15] have shown that the presence of polycystic ovaries is more likely to be associated with infertility if the woman has a raised body mass index.

Ovarian cysts are best diagnosed in the preovulatory phase (Figure 11). This is to avoid confusion with corpus luteum cysts, which are characteristically irregular, containing solid and semi-solid areas; in many cases corpus luteum cysts will mimic pathological cysts of the ovaries. Cysts that are sharp and smooth in their outline and unilocular are usually physiological and do not warrant surgery.

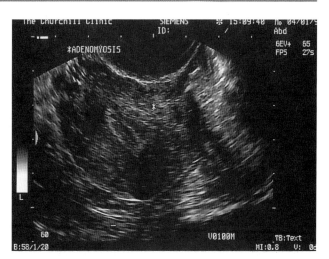

Figure 8 Adenomyosis. Echogenic areas in the posterior wall (asterisk) with thickening of posterior wall in a retroverted uterus

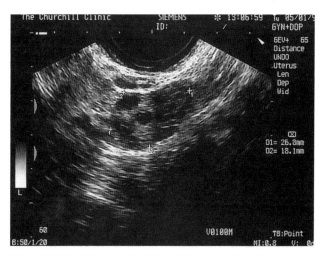

Figure 9 Normal ovary. Random distribution of follicles

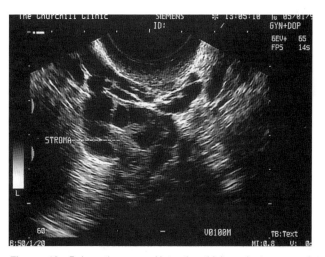

Figure 10 Polycystic ovary. Note the thickened stroma and peripheral distribution of follicles

Cysts that contain low-level echoes, which may be unilocular or multilocular, are usually indicative of ovarian endometriosis (Figure 12). Dermoid cysts can give a similar appearance to endometriosis on ultrasound examination, and the differential diagnosis can often be difficult to make. Dermoid cysts usually contain hyperechogenic areas and some of these may cause distal shadowing[16].

The presence of ovarian endometriosis[17] may have a significant bearing on the ovarian response to stimulation drugs and may become obvious only during controlled ovarian hyperstimulation, carried out for IVF therapy or intrauterine insemination[17–19].

In answer to the 'frequently asked questions' listed above, if only one ultrasound examination is to be performed, then this should be done in the periovulatory phase, in order to optimize the chances of diagnosing abnormalities accurately.

Ideally, if the diagnosis of an ovarian cyst is made, a repeat ultrasound scan should be performed approximately 8–12 weeks later, between day 6 and day 10 of the menstrual cycle. In many cases physiological cysts will subside spontaneously and do not require further surgery. The benefit to the patient is that unnecessary surgery can be avoided, and, in cases where pathological cysts are diagnosed, these cysts can be treated laparoscopically at the time of the diagnostic laparoscopy.

In cases of polycystic ovaries, where the ovaries are enlarged with diameters in excess of 3.5 cm, laparoscopic ovarian diathermy may be performed at the time of the diagnostic laparoscopy. This will avoid the risk of hyperstimulation syndrome and will increase the chances of spontaneous conception for these women.

The benefits to the patient of accurate diagnosis are that these procedures can be performed at the same time as diagnostic laparoscopy, and the risk of ovarian hyperstimulation syndrome and multiple pregnancies is decreased in cases of polycystic ovarian disease that have been treated with ovarian diathermy.

The benefit to the clinician is that the diagnosis of endometriosis or dermoid cysts can be made in advance of surgical procedures being scheduled. In cases where a dermoid cyst is suspected, ultrasound fine-needle aspiration can be performed under anesthetic, and if oily fluid is aspirated then precautions can be taken to avoid spillage intraperitoneally or laparoscopically by laparotomy. With endometriosis, if there

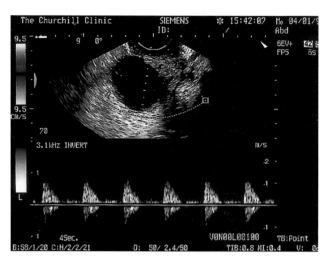

Figure 11 Simple ovarian cyst. There is poor blood flow, so it is most probably a follicular cyst

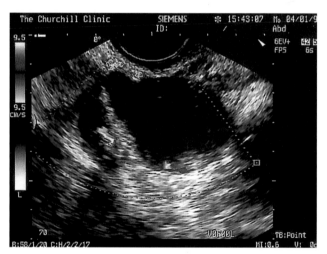

Figure 12 Intraovarian endometriosis. Note the echogenicity, with no distal shadowing

is evidence of adhesions in the pouch of Douglas or the ovarian fossae, the clinician may decide to use preoperative medical therapy for 3–6 months in order to decrease morbidity associated with laparoscopic surgery, such as bleeding and/or damage to the ureter.

Tubal factors

Normal Fallopian tubes are not seen on routine ultrasound examinations. However, the presence of hydrosalpinges is easily detected. Hydrosalpinges appear as 'cystic' and elongated, often hourglass shaped and lateral to the uterus. Sometimes, hydrosalpinges surround the ovary and can be mistaken as ovarian cysts. The presence of pseudo-septa or incomplete septa (not loculatious) can be helpful in diagnosis of hydrosalpinges. Fleming and Hull[20] and Koong and colleagues[21], showed that hydrosalpinges can decrease the chances of pregnancy in IVF treatments by up to 40%.

This makes it imperative that hydrosalpinges are either sealed at the cornual end or removed prior to IVF treatment. In the author's opinion, the former is preferable because this will not decrease uterine and/or ovarian blood flow by affecting collateral circulation to the uterus and ovaries. Decreased uterine and ovarian blood flow can decrease the chances of pregnancy, increase the risk of miscarriage and possibly affect ovarian response.

MONITORING OF TREATMENT CYCLES

Serial monitoring of follicular development is useful in both natural and stimulated ovarian cycles. In natural cycles, several small follicles may be seen in the early follicular phase. However, the dominant follicle is selected between day 5 and day 7 and other follicles will gradually decrease as this follicle develops. Follicular rupture occurs between 18 and 28 mm during natural cycles, with an average growth rate of 1.2–2.0 mm per day. It is essential that serial monitoring is carried out to determine normal growth of the Graafian follicle and to determine follicular rupture.

A baseline scan should be performed early in the menstrual cycle to avoid confusing pre-existing cystic structures with developing follicles. A luteal cyst is commonly seen, and may decrease in size during the follicular phase. In order to monitor follicular development and rupture, the first scan should be performed between day 10 and day 12 of the cycle and then, depending on the size of the leading follicle, serial scans can be performed every 2 or 3 days.

Ovulation induction and intrauterine insemination

Ovulation induction treatment may be carried out with clomiphene in combination with gonadotropins, or with gonadotropins on their own. An initial scan performed on day 2 or 3 of the cycle prior to commencing ovulation induction is again advisable; a second scan performed on day 8 or day 9 of the cycle

will help to establish the number of ovarian follicles. Ultrasound scans should be performed on alternate days, and the injection of human chorionic gonadotropin (hCG) given to induce ovulation when the mean follicular diameter of the leading follicle is between 18 and 20 mm.

In vitro fertilization

It is important that ultrasound examination is performed between day 10 and day 15 in a cycle preceding IVF, for the following reasons:

(1) The examination is used to check that the uterine cavity is normal. The presence of submucous fibroids will decrease the chances of conception with IVF.

(2) The presence of hydrosalpinges (Figure 13) should be noted because this may also decrease the chances of implantation with IVF. It is now almost routine practice in IVF centers that hydrosalpinges are removed or sealed at the cornual end in order to avoid toxic effects of hydrosalpinx fluid on embryos and implantation[20,21].

(3) The presence of ovarian cysts, especially endometriosis (Figure 14), can affect follicular development and may warrant treatment prior to IVF. In many cases, if the cyst is below 3 cm in size, aspiration of the cyst, if performed prior to stimulation, will aid the ovarian response.

(4) When ovaries are enlarged to greater than 3.5 cm, the risk of hyperstimulation syndrome is increased, and if the enlargement is due to endometriosis then the ovarian response may be compromised. However, if the ovaries are smaller than normal size, i.e. less than 2 cm in maximum diameter, this may be indicative of decreased ovarian reserve. In these cases higher than usual doses of gonadotropins may be required in order to provoke an adequate ovarian response.

(5) The examination is used to check the distribution of follicles in the ovary. Follicles should normally be randomly dispersed, with the dominant follicle being observed in one or other ovary. If the follicles are distributed around the periphery, this may indicate an increased risk of ovarian hyperstimulation. Stimulation with gonadotropins

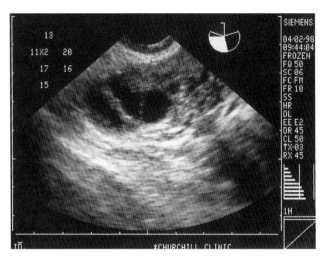

Figure 13 Hydrosalpinx. Ampullary folds of the mucosa appear as incomplete septa

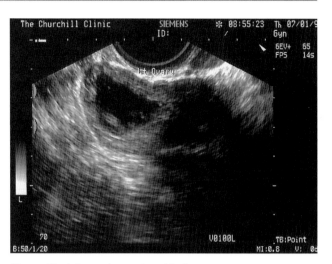

Figure 14 Intraovarian endometriosis

should be started at a lower than normal dose and can be increased after 6 or 7 days of therapy, if necessary.

Monitoring of IVF cycles is essential in order to avoid ovarian hyperstimulation syndrome (OHSS) and to assess the ovarian response during the treatment cycle. Most centers use ultrasound alone to monitor the ovarian response and to time the hCG injection, prior to oocyte recovery. The first scan should be performed prior to stimulation for the reasons given above, and the next scan should be performed approximately 6–8 days after stimulation has commenced. Subsequent ultrasound scans can be performed on a daily or alternate-day basis, depending on the ovarian response. The injection of hCG is usually given when at least two or three leading follicles are above 18 mm mean follicular diameter.

Frozen embryo replacement

Frozen–thawed embryos may be replaced in a natural cycle or in a hormone controlled cycle. In anovulatory women, clomiphene citrate or gonadotropins or a combination of both can be used to stimulate ovulation. Monitoring is performed as for a natural cycle, ovulation induction or intrauterine insemination, and embryos are usually replaced 2 or 3 days after ovulation. If urine or blood monitoring is not performed to monitor the LH surge, then ultrasound scans must be performed on a daily basis once the lead follicle reaches a mean follicular diameter of 16 mm.

DOPPLER ULTRASOUND

In previous publications I reported that the uterine response to endogenous hormonal changes in the spontaneous ovarian cycle can be demonstrated with the use of Doppler ultrasound techniques. We demonstrated that uterine perfusion increases in response to rising estrogen levels during the follicular phase, decreases with the preovulatory estrogen fall and increases in the luteal phase in response to the combined effect of estrogen and progesterone. We also reported that, in conception cycles, uterine perfusion continues to increase in the midluteal phase in contrast to non-conception cycles, and that there is a premenstrual decrease in perfusion as a result of falling progesterone levels[22].

In a second study[23], we performed Doppler examination of the uterine arteries to investigate the uterine perfusion response (Figure 15) in patients who had failed to conceive despite repeated multiple embryo replacements in IVF cycles. These patients were studied in spontaneous ovarian cycles, and, despite normal endocrine changes and basal body temperature changes, there was an inadequate uterine response in 50% of the patients recruited. The mean age of the patients was 36.9 years, and there was a significant improvement in pregnancy rate after improving uterine blood flow in those patients in whom blood flow was noted to be poor. In patients in whom the initial blood flow was noted to be normal, the pregnancy rate with subsequent IVF attempts was similar to that of the first attempt.

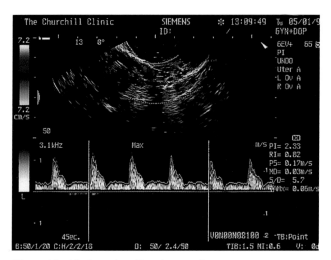

Figure 15 Uterine artery Doppler waveform

The therapy used to improve uterine blood flow was estradiol valerate 1 mg tablets taken for 21 days starting on day 5 of each cycle, for three cycles. In 10% of cases the blood flow to the uterus did not improve despite estradiol valerate. In these patients, high-dose estrogens were used, as for treatment of women receiving donated eggs, and uterine blood flow was noted to improve in all cases. The improvement in pregnancy rate was attributed to improving uterine blood flow, and hence poor uterine blood flow was considered to be a cause of previous IVF failure. Other studies found similar changes occurring in the uterine artery in the periovulatory phase[24,25]. They also confirmed indices of high resistance to flow during the luteal phase, with the peak at the midluteal phase[26,27]. This is the stage at which implantation occurs.

Continuing research in this field indicates that patients who have polycystic ovaries also have poor uterine perfusion in about 40% of cases. In our ongoing study (unpublished data), the uterine blood flow response improved in cases of polycystic ovaries after laparoscopic ovarian diathermy. This confirms a cause and effect relationship. Other reasons for poor uterine perfusion are related to previous surgery for ectopic pregnancy, and age.

Ovarian Doppler

Taylor and colleagues[28] originally obtained Doppler signals from ovarian arteries and reported this in 1985. In this paper they described technical limitations due to patient obesity, and it was not possible to obtain

signals in 27% of the women studied. They found that the resistance within the ovarian vessels decreased throughout the menstrual cycle, and blood flow peaked with the midluteal phase. Other workers confirmed this in subsequent publications when they showed that the resistance to flow decreased in the ovarian stroma and in the corpus luteum from 4 days prior to ovulation until approximately 4 days prior to the onset of menstruation. Numerous workers have studied velocities in the ovarian stroma during the periovulatory period. They found that intrafollicular blood velocity started to increase approximately 1 day before follicular rupture and that the rise continued for at least 3 days after the formation of the corpus luteum[29–32].

The practical value of these studies is still unproven. Increase in ovarian blood flow is related to angiogenesis, which starts early in the menstrual cycle when the dominant follicle or the dominant ovary has been selected. The gradual increase in ovarian blood flow is related to increasing estrogen levels, and the dramatic increase that is noted to be preovulatory is most likely to be related to a sudden increase in intrafollicular progesterone levels. It is well established that progesterone levels in the peripheral serum start to rise prior to ovulation.

More recently[33,34], attempts have been made to correlate increased blood flow with oocyte quality. There does not seem to be any practical benefit from deriving these correlations, because large follicles will yield mature oocytes and mature follicles normally produce progesterone in large quantities prior to ovulation. A simple blood test to monitor progesterone levels after the leading follicles have achieved a main follicular diameter of 16 mm is a simple way of timing the hCG injection prior to oocyte recovery, without time-consuming and inaccurate Doppler studies.

In conclusion, Doppler ultrasound scans of the ovaries have yielded information regarding angiogenesis, selection of the dominant follicle and help with the differential diagnosis of follicular cysts from corpus luteum cysts. The use of Doppler studies in the timing of oocyte recovery is of little practical value.

Doppler studies of the uterus in spontaneous ovarian cycles have helped in identifying patients who are likely to conceive, and have been shown to be a possible cause for failure of IVF treatments. However, the equipment is not sensitive enough to differentiate conception from non-conception cycles during cycles in which ovarian stimulation has been carried out using gonadotropins.

DIAGNOSIS AND MANAGEMENT OF EARLY PREGNANCY

In 1967, Kratochwil and Eisenhut[35] first reported that pregnancy could be diagnosed as early as the first week after a missed period. Their paper, first published in German, described the use of ultrasound with static techniques to diagnose an intrauterine gestation sac. In 1978, Lawson[36] reported ultrasound criteria for the diagnosis of ectopic pregnancy, but this was with the use of abdominal ultrasound and static imaging.

With the use of transvaginal ultrasound, it is possible to image a gestation sac in the uterus within 1 day of a missed period (or 4 weeks and 1 day since the last menstrual period). The uterine cavity shows a thickened endometrium with a gestation sac seen as a 2–3-mm echo-free structure surrounded by a reflective trophoblastic ring. The gestation sac is invariably located eccentrically within the uterine cavity. An echo-free space in a central position should raise suspicion of an ectopic pregnancy, requiring a careful search of the adnexal area.

In pregnancies resulting from assisted conception treatment, it is possible to diagnose multiple pregnancies at this very early stage (Figure 16). However, it is important to realise that the diagnosis of a pregnancy at this stage does not indicate viability. This can be assessed reliably only after fetal heart motion has been demonstrated. Most centers performing assisted conception techniques will conduct a blood test to check β-hCG levels approximately 15–18 days after egg recovery or insemination. By 5 weeks after insemination or ovulation, it is possible to demonstrate fetal heart motion in 99% of cases.

By 5 weeks, the yolk sac is demonstrable and measures between 3 and 4 mm. The gestation sac is double the size of the yolk sac. The need to measure these structures is discussed later, although the presence of normal-shaped structures, and their relation to each other in size, are enough to estimate gestational age to within a few days.

By 6 weeks, cystic spaces become visible on one side of the gestation sac. This is the region where the placenta will develop. In real time it is sometimes

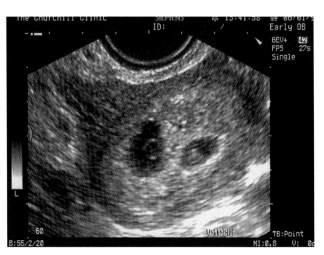

Figure 16 Twin pregnancy. Unequal sacs may indicate impending spontaneous reduction

possible to see blood flow in these spaces. The embryo is now the same size as the yolk sac, which has a diameter of 3–4 mm. By this stage, heart motion cannot always be demonstrated.

By 7 weeks, the embryo measures 7–8 mm in length and the yolk sac measures 5 mm in diameter. The head of the embryo is just distinguishable from the body. The head appears to be larger than the body, which can be recognized by the presence of heart motion within it. The heart rate, at this stage, is approximately 160 beats/min and Doppler signals can be detected.

At 8 weeks, embryonic movements, discernible limb buds and development of the central nervous system are obvious landmarks of development. The embryo measures 1 cm, twice the diameter of the yolk sac, which remains at 5 mm for the rest of the first trimester. The head contains a single cerebral ventricle, which may simulate a second yolk sac and must not be mistaken for a double-headed fetus. The finding of an equal-sized yolk sac and head is typical of this gestational age.

By the 9th week, knees and elbows have become obvious and the lower limbs are seen with their legs crossed. The coccyx is prominent and umbilical cord pulsations are easily visible. At the site of the cord insertion, in the abdomen, a physiological umbilical herniation of the gut may be seen. This appearance must be distinguished from an exomphalos. The choroid plexus becomes visible with the formation of the falx cerebri (Figure 17). The crown–rump length is approximately 2 cm.

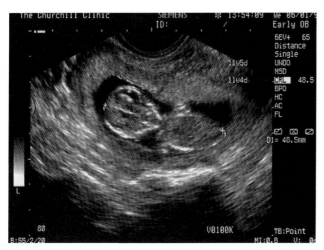

Figure 17 Ten-week pregnancy. Note the falx cerebri and choroid plexus

At 10 weeks, the yolk sac starts to disappear and the fetal heart, stomach, urinary bladder and kidneys may be seen. Organogenesis is complete, but most of the organs are difficult to distinguish until they have grown to larger than 2–3 mm in size.

By 12 weeks, the physiological umbilical hernia has started to reduce and disappear.

The incidence of spontaneous abortions varies between 20 and 50%, depending on the patient's age. It is important that anatomical landmarks are used as a way of assessing fetal growth, and that the placental site is examined at each ultrasound scan in order to diagnose bleeding at the implantation site. Color Doppler ultrasound can be used to look for increased flow patterns around the placental site. If the insertion of the cord is close to the site of placental bleeding, the prognosis of the pregnancy is extremely poor. In 50% of cases with bleeding noted near the placental site the pregnancy may still continue.

Transvaginal ultrasound is superior for imaging the implantation site. Small lacunae or cystic spaces become visible at the implantation site as early as the 6th week. Compressed by a full bladder, they may not be visualized by transabdominal ultrasound. Bleeding at the placental site may occur as a result of defective implantation in the first instance or because of decreased uterine perfusion. In most cases, however, there is no explanation for these cases of threatened abortion.

Another predictor of poor outcome that is seen by transvaginal, but not abdominal, ultrasound is the presence of large vascular spaces with increased flow waves surrounding the whole gestation sac. This is common when there is no evidence of a retroimplantation bleed and when there is no live embryo, as with missed abortions.

Ectopic pregnancy

Ectopic or extrauterine gestation is still one of the leading causes of maternal mortality and is one of the most difficult diagnoses in gynecological practice. Early detection of ectopic pregnancy is crucial to reducing mortality and morbidity, and this is even more important if future fertility is to be maintained. A combination of hormone assays and ultrasound examinations form the cornerstone for diagnosis[37]. Several studies have reported that blood levels of hCG are lower in ectopic pregnancies than those seen with viable intrauterine pregnancies[38,39].

In assisted conception, progesterone is an additional useful marker[40]. Serum progesterone levels are significantly lower on day 15 after oocyte recovery with ectopic gestation than in intrauterine pregnancies. Therefore, a low progesterone level and a low β-hCG level are indications for early transvaginal ultrasound examination.

The definitive diagnosis of ectopic gestation depends on the identification of a gestation sac outside the uterine cavity. This appears as a highly reflective ring with an echo-free area within it (Figure 18). Although ovarian ectopic pregnancy is extremely rare, it is important that this is differentiated from corpus luteum cysts, especially in superovulation cycles when rings are seen within the ovary (Figure 19). Once the gestation sac has been located, the contents must be scrutinized for the presence of a yolk sac, the embryo and heart motion. Only when embryonic structures are seen is the diagnosis of ectopic pregnancy certain. Otherwise, positive assays of β-hCG in the absence of an intrauterine pregnancy will form the basis for a presumptive diagnosis of ectopic pregnancy.

Fluid in the cul-de-sac is generally an unhelpful sign. It is not always seen with ectopic pregnancies, and its presence does not suggest an ectopic pregnancy unless there are blood clots within it. Color flow imaging and spectral Doppler to diagnose ectopic pregnancy have been proposed, but these do not improve the sensitivity.

Laparoscopic surgery is the cornerstone of treatment for ectopic pregnancy. However, in some cases

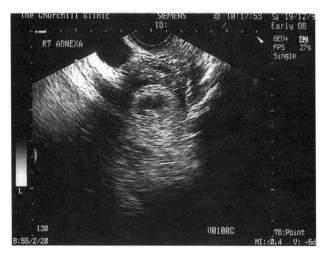

Figure 18 Ectopic pregnancy. Echogenic ring outside the uterine cavity

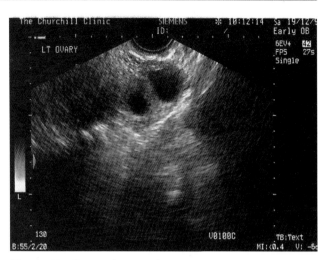

Figure 19 Corpus luteum rings, in a patient after *in vitro* fertilization therapy

when the tube is inaccessible for laparoscopic surgery, ultrasound-directed injection of methotrexate may be applied. The best agent for injection is yet to be established, results so far being similar with hyperosmolar glucose, saline, potassium chloride and methotrexate injections.

Finally, transvaginal ultrasound must replace abdominal ultrasound in early pregnancy monitoring, the diagnosis of non-viability and ectopic pregnancy. Its accuracy in diagnosis makes abdominal ultrasound examinations obsolete.

CONCLUSION

In conclusion, transvaginal ultrasound has become an essential part in the management of infertile couples. Follicle monitoring, including the timing of the post-coital test, is only the first step in its use. Its accuracy in imaging of the uterus and intrauterine abnormalities makes it imperative that the diagnosis of unexplained infertility is never made without a systematic ultrasound examination being performed at the appropriate time in the menstrual cycle.

ACKNOWLEDGMENT

The author is grateful to Juliana Cutts for her patience in preparing this manuscript.

REFERENCES

1. Kratochwil A, Urban GV, Friedrich F. Ultrasonic tomography of the ovaries. Ann Chir Gynecol 1972; 61: 211–14
2. Hackeloer BJ, Fleming R, Robinson HP. Correlation of ultrasonic and endocrinologic assessment of human follicular development. Am J Obstet Gynecol 1979; 135: 122–8
3. Siebel MM, McArdle CR, Thompson IE, et al. The role of ultrasound in ovulation induction – a critical appraisal. Fertil Steril 1981; 36: 573–6
4. Varygas JM, Marrs RP, Kletzki DA, et al. Correlation of ovarian follicle size and serum oestradiol levels on ovulatory patients following clomiphene citrate for in vitro fertilisation. Am J Obstet Gynecol 1982; 144: 569–73
5. Timor-Tritsch IE, Rottem S, Elgali S. How transvaginal sonography is done. In Timor-Tritsch IE, Rottem S, eds. Transvaginal Sonography. London: Heinemann Medical Books, 1988: 15–25
6. Fleischer AC, Gordon AN, Entman SS, et al. Transvaginal scanning of endometrium. J Clin Ultrasound 1990; 18: 337–49
7. Lewit N, Thaler I, Rottem S. The uterus: a new look with transvaginal sonography. J Clin Ultrasound 1990; 18: 331–6
8. Dodson MG, Deter RL. Definition of anatomical planes for use in transvaginal sonography. J Clin Ultrasound 1990; 18: 239–42
9. Grunfield L, Walker B, Bergh PA, et al. High-resolution endovaginal ultrasonography of the endometrium: a non-invasive test for endometrial adequacy. Obstet Gynecol 1991; 78: 200–4

10. Narayan R, Goswamy RK. Transvaginal sonography of the uterine cavity with hysteroscopic correlation in the investigation of infertility. Ultrasound Obstet Gynecol 1993; 3: 129–33

11. Fedele L, Bianchi S, Dotra M, et al. Transvaginal ultrasonography versus hysteroscopy in the diagnosis of uterine sub mucus. Obstet Gynecol 1991; 77: 745–8

12. Polson DW, Wadsworth J, Adams J, et al. Polycystic ovaries – a common finding in normal women. Lancet 1988; 1: 870–2

13. Adams J, Polson DW, Franks S. Prevalence of polycystic ovaries in women with anovulation and idiopathic ligutism. Br Med J 1986; 293: 355–9

14. Homburg R, Armar NA, Eshel A, et al. Influence of serum luteinizing hormone concentrations on ovulation, conception and early pregnancy loss in polycystic ovary syndrome. Br Med J 1988; 297: 1024–6

15. Eshel A, Abdulwahid NA, Armar N, et al. Pulsatile luteinizing hormone-releasing hormone therapy in women with polycystic ovary syndrome. Fertil Steril 1988; 49: 956–60

16. Granberg S, Wikland M. Ultrasound in the diagnosis and treatment of ovarian cystic tumours. Hum Reprod 1991; 6: 177–85

17. Dlugi AM, Coy RA, Dieterle S, et al. The effect of endometriosis on in vitro fertilization outcome. J In Vitro Fertil Embryo Transf 1989; 6: 338–41

18. Packe TD, Wladimiroff JW, DeJon, et al. Growth patterns of non-dominant ovarian follicles during the normal menstrual cycle. Fertil Steril 1990; 54: 638–42

19. Renaud RL, Macler J, Dervain I, et al. Echographic study of follicular maturation and ovulation during the normal menstrual cycle. Fertil Steril 1980; 33: 272–6

20. Fleming C, Hull MGR. Impaired implantation after in vitro fertilisation treatment associated with hydrosalpinx. Br J Obstet Gynaecol 1996; 193: 268–72

21. Koong MK, Song IO, Son IP, et al. Effect of hydrosalpinx and its surgical correction on pregnancy and implantation rates following IVF and embryo transfer. Presented at the 13th Annual Meeting of the European Society for Human Reproduction and Embryology, Edinburgh, UK. Hum Reprod 1997; 12: P-111 (abstr 1)

22. Goswamy RK, Steptoe PC. Doppler ultrasound studies of the uterine artery in spontaneous ovarian cycles. Hum Reprod 1988; 6: 721–6

23. Goswamy RK, Williams G, Steptoe PC. Decreased perfusion – a cause of infertility. Hum Reprod 1988; 8: 955–9

24. Battaglia C, Larocca E, Lanzani A, et al. Doppler ultrasound studies of the uterine arteries in spontaneous and IVF stimulated ovarian cycles. Gynecol Endocrinol 1990; 4: 245–50

25. Santolaya-Forgas J. Physiology of the menstrual cycle by ultrasonography. J Ultrasound Med 1992; 11: 139–42

26. Scholtes MCW, Wladimiroff JW, van Rijen HJM, et al. Uterine and ovarian flow velocity in the normal menstrual cycle: a transvaginal Doppler study. Fertil Steril 1989; 52: 981–5

27. Steer CV, Campbell S, Pampiglione JS, et al. Transvaginal colour flow imaging of the uterine arteries during the ovarian and menstrual cycles. Hum Reprod 1990; 5: 391–5

28. Taylor KJW, Burns PN, Wells PNT, et al. Ultrasound Doppler flow studies of the ovarian and uterine arteries. Br Obstet Gynaecol 1985; 92: 240–6

29. Merce LT, Garces D, Barco MJ, et al. Intraovarian Doppler velocimetry in ovulatory, dysovulatory and anovulatory cycles. Ultrasound Obstet Gynecol 1992; 2: 197–202

30. Kurjak A, Kupesik-Urek S, Schulman H, et al. Transvaginal colour flow Doppler in the assessment of ovarian and uterine blood flow in infertile women. Fertil Steril 1991; 56: 870–3

31. Collins W, Jurkovic D, Bourne T, et al. Ovarian morphology, endocrine function and intra-follicular blood flow during the peri-ovulatory period. Hum Reprod 1991; 6: 319–24

32. Bourne TH, Jurkovic D, Waterstone J, et al. Intrafollicular blood flow during human ovulation. Ultrasound Obstet Gynecol 1991; 1: 53–9

33. Campbell S, Bourne TH, Waterstone J, et al. Transvaginal colour blood flow imaging of the peri-ovulatory follicle. Fertil Steril 1993; 60: 433–8

34. Kupesic S, Kurjak A. Uterine and ovarian perfusion during periovulatory period assessed by transvaginal colour Doppler. Fertil Steril 1993; 60: 439–43

35. Kratochwil A, Eisenhut L. Der früheste Nachweis der fetalen Herzaktion durch Ultraschall. Geburtsh Frauenheilkd 1967; 27: 176

36. Lawson TL. Ectopic pregnancy, criteria and accuracy of ultrasonic diagnosis. Am J Roentgenol 1978; 131: 153–8

37. Pittaway D. Diagnosis of ectopic pregnancy. Obstet Gynecol 1986; 68: 440

38. Kadar N, Romero R. HCG determination in early pregnancy. Fertil Steril 1987; 47: 722

39. Kadar N, Romero R. Serial human chorionic gonadotrophin measurements in ectopic pregnancy. Am J Obstet Gynecol 1988; 158: 1239

40. Milwidsky A, Adoni A, Segal S. Chorionic gonadotrophin and progesterone levels in ectopic pregnancy. Obstet Gynecol 1977; 50: 1945

6

Diagnostic hysteroscopy in assisted conception

Karunakar Marikinti

INTRODUCTION

Depending upon their type and severity, endometrial pathologies can contribute to a less nutritive and/or to a hostile environment for the implanting blastocyst, placentation and growth of the fetus[1]. Additionally, any coexisting abnormal myometrial activity and any abnormal uterine cavity can result in premature expulsion of the products of conception[2]. Examples include: endometritis, endometrial atrophy, endometrial sclerosis, poorly developed endometrial vessels and glands, asynchronous endometrial development, endometrial polyps, submucous fibroids, intrauterine synechiae and malformations of the uterus. Intracervical pathologies account for cervical-factor infertility and are recognized causes of difficult embryo transfer during assisted conception treatments[3].

The reported incidence of uterine pathologies in infertile women varies depending on the screening or diagnostic tests used, the expertise of the technician and the clinical history of the infertile woman. Between 10 and 62% of women with infertility[1,4,5], 10 and 60% of women undergoing pretreatment assessment for *in vitro* fertilization and embryo transfer (IVF–ET)[3,6–8], 19 and 50% of women who failed to conceive following assisted reproductive technologies (ART)[9–12] and 28 and 32% of women with recurrent miscarriages following natural or assisted conception procedures[2] showed evidence of uterine pathology. A large study in 1000 women undergoing IVF–ET identified hysteroscopic abnormalities in 38% of unselected women[13] during pre-IVF assessment. It has also been reported that the presence of uterine pathologies necessitates more IVF–ET attempts per baby delivered[12].

Higher live birth rates were reported following treatment of these uterine pathologies in a number of case-controlled studies[6,8,9,14], and it has been estimated that up to 33% of women would benefit from routine screening, diagnosis and selective treatment of relevant uterine pathologies before undergoing IVF treatment[8,11,15], and up to 22% of women after repeated unsuccessful IVF treatments[9,16].

Methods to assess the uterine cavity

There are four methods of assessing the uterine cavity: transvaginal sonography (TVS), hysterosalpingography (HSG), saline contrast sonography (SCS) and hysteroscopy. Each of these techniques demands the utmost attention to detail and meticulousness: their efficacy is directly related to the experience and skill of the investigator[17]. It is common practice routinely to perform uterine cavity evaluation before commencing assisted conception treatments in the USA; HSG is the most frequently used screening test (96%), followed by pelvic ultrasound (55%) and hysteroscopy (53%)[18]. In the UK, except for a few assisted conception units, a baseline TVS is often the only screening test for uterine pathologies before starting controlled ovarian hyperstimulation (COH), and SCS or diagnostic hysteroscopy is used selectively for those found to have abnormalities on TVS or HSG. Information on the normality of the uterine cavity and endometrium is often obtained from HSG that is usually performed for assessing tubal patency.

Hysteroscopy allows direct visualization of the uterocervical canal and endometrial assessment, and is thus considered as the gold-standard reference test[4]. It has been the preferred investigation in 50–70% of all infertility evaluations in certain parts of the world[2,15], and is the second commonest investigation performed after repeated IVF treatment failures in the UK[19], but, being an invasive test, it is considered by some not to be the ideal screening test for uterine pathologies. There is now some evidence to suggest that SCS with two-dimensional (2D) or three-dimensional (3D) ultrasound can provide equally satisfactory diagnostic information in skilled hands, and can be a very useful screening test where such facilities are available.

However, with the availability of small caliber 'see and treat' hysteroscopy systems, it is now possible to diagnose and treat a range of uterine pathologies effectively and safely in one sitting on an out-patient basis, with enormous benefits to the patient and service provider[20,21].

Hysteroscopy

Traditionally, diagnostic and therapeutic hysteroscopy has been performed after cervical dilatation under general anesthesia by a few selected gynecologists. Technical expertise is now more readily available, and major improvements in the optics and light systems has led to the availability of thinner scopes with the option of performing a wide range of corrective operations under video monitoring, without the need for cervical dilatation or general anesthesia. Several studies have reported a high degree of patient compliance, safety and cost-effectiveness of out-patient operative hysteroscopy in managing women with abnormal uterine bleeding, and similar encouraging results are reported in women following reproductive surgery. Successful nurse-led diagnostic hysteroscopy services have been in use in the US for over two decades, and some centers in the UK have now begun a similar

service, making way for readily available and more user-friendly diagnostic hysteroscopy facilities[22].

Hysterosalpingography

HSG requires radiology facilities, and comparative studies of HSG versus hysteroscopy in the diagnosis of uterine pathology did not yield uniformly accurate results, with unacceptable false-positive and false negative rates[4,5,10]. Nevertheless, the World Health Organization has recommended uterine cavity assessment with an HSG in the standard evaluation of infertile women. This is still the most common method used to assess tubal patency, and many clinicians rely on it for confirmation of uterine cavity normality before commencing assisted conception treatments[23].

Transvaginal sonography

Compared with bimanual pelvic examination, TVS enables the pelvic anatomy to be identified with more accuracy and reliability. In experienced hands, a high degree of positive and negative predictive values were reported with TVS screening for uterine pathologies that subsequently underwent a diagnostic hysteroscopy[24–26]. However, a concordance rate of only 65% was shown between TVS and SCS for the diagnosis of uterine pathologies, when hysteroscopy was used as the reference test[27]. Our data, presented in the next section, suggest that when TVS is used in unselected patients seeking IVF as a screening test, without the complementary use of SCS, a wide range of uterine pathologies are underdiagnosed.

Saline contrast sonography and hysterosalpingo-contrast sonography

A few centers in Europe and the USA perform SCS and/or hysterosalpingo-contrast sonography (HyCoSy) regularly for screening infertile women prior to IVF. Reports from these centers indicate that both of these procedures are simple to perform, and effective in obtaining information on the uterine cavity, with a diagnostic accuracy of 85–100% for uterine abnormalities[6,7,28]. Targeted SCS, however, relies on the technical accuracy of TVS screening in the first place, and thus the true prevalence of uterine pathologies can be under-reported. Moreover, endometrial surface abnormalities involving epithelial glands and blood vessels cannot be reliably identified by this procedure. Other reported limitations include: a failure rate of 5.6–11.8%[27], a 19.4% incidence of severe protracted pain associated with vasovagal reactions, a 5.9% incidence of patients requiring resuscitation, and thus the availability of a qualified nurse for monitoring[27,29], and a discordance rate of 13.3%, when compared with hysteroscopy[27].

HYSTEROSCOPY AT BOURN HALL CLINIC

Set-up and service

Approximately 1200 embryo transfer cycles are performed each year at this private tertiary IVF center. Women are often referred after diagnostic work-up and/or unsuccessful IVF treatments elsewhere. A uterine cavity evaluation with HSG or contrast sonography is not a routine prerequisite before beginning IVF treatment, and diagnostic hysteroscopy is used for selected indications, which are described in the next section. An in-patient diagnostic hysteroscopy service has been available for many years, but in January 2002, a dedicated out-patient hysteroscopy service was introduced that now accounts for 80% of the procedures performed at this center.

Materials and methods

The indications for hysteroscopy are:

(1) Patients with a history of recurrent (three or more) IVF–ET or frozen embryo transfer (FET) treatment failures;

(2) New patients and those who have had less than three previous embryo transfer treatment failures, if:

(a) They have not had a hysteroscopy within a year;

(b) There is any evidence of uterine abnormalities seen on HSG or TVS;

(c) There is any history of previous instrumental intervention (such as dilatation and curettage, termination of pregnancy, evacuation of retained products);

(d) There is any history of previous uterine scarring (complicated cesarean section, myomectomy, hysterotomy, uterine perforation);

(e) There is any history of endometritis (puerperal or postabortal sepsis, chlamydia, pelvic inflammatory disease);

(f) There is any history of recurrent early pregnancy losses (two or more miscarriages).

All hysteroscopies are planned and performed close to the time of the window of implantation, avoiding conception cycles, to obtain maximum relevant information about the endometrium. Simple oral analgesia is given in the form of paracetamol 1 g, 1 h prior to the procedure. General anesthesia is reserved for medical indications and for those who request it. A history of difficult embryo transfer, suspected cervical stenosis and/or a previous cervical dilatation are not considered to be contraindications to hysteroscopy without anesthesia. Absolute contraindications are pelvic infection and uterine bleeding, and relative contraindications are a grossly distorted pelvic anatomy, suspected pelvic infection and anticipated technical difficulty. Following admission to the out-patient unit, checks are made for vital signs and the clinician responsible obtains informed consent. The option is given to the male partner to attend the procedure.

TVS is performed routinely prior to hysteroscopy to evaluate the size and direction of the uterus and any adnexal pathology. After taking measurements of endometrial thickness and length of the uterus and cervical canal, specific observations are made to ascertain the normality of the endometrium, myometrium and endometrial–myometrial interface. Any deviation in the uterine cavity shape and outline and echogenicity of the endometrium is imaged and recorded. Similar observations are made for the cervix and endocervical canal. Mock embryo transfer (MET) is then performed, in accordance with our established embryo transfer procedure guidelines. Use of a metal stylet for MET is avoided to prevent injury to the endometrium and endocervical mucosa that could interfere with hysteroscopic examination.

A Storz rigid hysteroscope with a 30°-oblique view and a single-flow-channel outer sheath (3.1 mm) is then introduced slowly through the cervix and into the uterine cavity under video monitoring, avoiding contact with the mucosa with the aid of saline distension. A nurse attends the patient constantly during hysteroscopy, and the gynecologist performing the procedure explains the progress of the investigation. Hysteroscopic diagnosis of a fibroid may be made from the presence of a firm intracavitary mass, with a broad base and acute angle with the myometrium at the uterine wall attachment. An endometrial polyp

Table 1 Indications for hysteroscopy and incidence of normal and abnormal findings in each category in a series of 170 cases

Findings	≥3ETF only	>2ETF + TVS abnormality	>2ETF + DET	>2ETF + ≥2 mis-carriages + DET	>2ETF + bleeding during treatment	>1ETF + uterine surgery	No ET before+ TVS abnormality	Bleeding during treatment	Total cases (n)
Cases (n)	72	30	37	13	2	4	11	1	170
Suspected* pathology found	—	3	0	0	1	1	0	1	6
Unsuspected* pathology found on									
hysteroscopy	24	13	25	1	1	3	6	0	73
and/or histology	19	14	12	5	0	0	3	0	53
No abnormality of cervix or uterus	29	0	0	7	0	0	2	0	38

*Transvaginal sonography (TVS) and/or clinical suspicion did not warrant diagnostic hysteroscopy at the time of suspicion in the index treatment cycle; ETF, embryo transfer failure = no pregnancy after embryo transfer; DE, difficult embryo transfer (n = 41)

may be diagnosed when a soft intracavitary mass is observed that is easily mobilized and covered by mucosa. Persistent benign-looking raised endometrial lesions are subgrouped as:

(1) Polypoid, consisting of rounded or cauliflower-shaped fleshy elevations of variable sizes, with few or no glandular openings or blood vessels;

(2) Corrugated, consisting of diffusely thick, flat elevations with intervening splits or grooves, with no visible glandular openings or blood vessels;

(3) Edematous, consisting of focal or diffuse areas of thick, pale endometrium with faintly visible glandular openings or blood vessels.

With the left-over saline acting as a contrast, SCS is performed immediately after withdrawing the hysteroscope and appropriate images are taken, so that an instant comparison may be made with the images obtained on standard TVS obtained before the hysteroscopy. At the end of the procedure, a scaled Pipelle curette is used both to measure the true uterine cavity length and to obtain a small sample of endometrium for histopathological examination. Subjective pain scores for the procedure are obtained and patients discharged shortly afterwards when the hysteroscopy is performed without anesthesia.

The true prevalence of uterine pathologies in women undergoing IVF in the UK is unknown, and studies involving SCS as a screening test have estimated it to be 10–12%[6,28], but hysteroscopy-based data are unavailable. Presented below are the findings in 170 women who underwent mid-cycle or luteal phase hysteroscopy, followed by a discussion on the post-hysteroscopy reproductive performance of 100 of these women. The relevant literature is reviewed and discussed as appropriate. Table 1 illustrates the indications for hysteroscopy and the findings in each category.

Ninety per cent of hysteroscopies in this series were performed after two or more treatment failures following the transfer of at least one good-quality embryo. A small proportion of women had the hysteroscopy performed owing to an abnormality found on TVS prior to, or during, treatment cycles (11 cases). The majority of the women were in the age group of 31–40, about 10% were below 30 and about 15% were over the age of 41 years, with a mean age of 35 years. The duration of infertility ranged from 2 to 16 years (mean ± 2SD, 6.2 ± 4.9 years) and 18 women had had at least one live birth in the past.

Eighty-two per cent of the hysteroscopies were performed in the calculated luteal phase and the rest in the calculated late proliferative phase. Unexplained and tubal factor infertility were the reasons for infertility in 46%, and ovulatory disorders, male factor, endometriosis, and psychosexual and multiple etiologies accounted for the rest.

One hundred and twenty-eight (75.3%) of the hysteroscopies were performed without any form of anesthesia, and 42 (24.7%) opted for either intravenous sedation or general anesthesia for personal reasons or if cervical dilatation or polypectomy was intended. Two cases were abandoned and rescheduled for general anesthesia due to obstructive lesions in the cervical canal or technical difficulty. Extensive endocervical synechiae required a paracervical block in one case, and the use of an os finder was required in another. Oral analgesia was routinely offered, and the majority took paracetamol 1 g an hour before the procedure. Subjective pain scores were assessed by the use of a visual analog scale following out-patient hysteroscopy of 128 women. Pain was scored as: mild in 60%, moderate in 30%, severe in 10%. Severe pain lasted for a brief period of time, and none suffered vasovagal reactions. These pain scores were similar to those reported previously in the literature[30]. One randomized controlled trial, however, reported a pain score of 4.5 when hysteroscopy was performed without any form of analgesia or anesthesia, and did not find any benefits to the use of oral and local analgesia[31]. We have adopted saline for uterine distension, as it is known to provide more detailed information on surface epithelial changes of the endometrium and is less uncomfortable for the patient[32].

Results and discussion

Concomitant TVS

The same clinician performed TVS immediately prior to hysteroscopy to assess any pathologies outside the uterine cavity, and abnormal findings were identified in 31 of the 170 cases: intramural fibroids in 19, suspected adenomyosis in seven, intramural fibroids with suspected adenomyosis in four, uterine anomaly with suspected adenomyosis in one. Table 2 summarizes the hysteroscopy findings in 170 women.

Congenital abnormalities

Major uterine malformations were present in five and mild to moderate anomalies were seen in 15 women. The true clinical relevance of these mild to moderate

Table 2 Diagnostic hysteroscopy findings in 170 women at Bourn Hall Clinic

Findings	n	%
Hysteroscopic findings: uterus		
Normal*	80	47.0
Abnormal	90	52.9
congenital abnormalities	20	
complete septum/bicornis unicollis	5	
subseptum/arcuate/mild to moderate bicornuate uterus	9	
infantile uterus/T-shaped uterus	6	
acquired abnormalities	70	
endometrial lesions		
thick, pale and polypoid	12	
thick, uneven with no glandular openings or vessels	5	
thick, pale and edematous	5	
focal elevations and ridges	7	
diffuse congestion with thin and punctate glands	4	
?? endometritis	1	
neovascularizations	2	
thin, atrophic, pale endometrium	4	
mixed lesions	1	
polyps	15	
submucous fibroids	8	
intrauterine synechiae and endometrial scarring	6	
Hysteroscopic findings: endocervix/ cervicouterine canal		
Normal	88	51.8
Abnormal	82	48.2
polyps/cysts/synechiae	52	
acute cervicouterine angle + polyps/cysts/synechiae	30	
Histology of endometrium† (n = 140)		
Normal (in-phase endometrium)	83	60
Abnormal (out-of-phase endometrium and mixed findings)	57	40

*Excluding cervical canal and histological abnormalities;
†Noyce's criteria

uterine cavity anomalies is unclear. A higher incidence of arcuate, septate and subseptate uteri was reported by Salim and colleagues in women with a history of recurrent miscarriage (RM) when compared to women without (17% vs. 3.2%)[33]. In addition, a higher incidence of mid-trimester pregnancy losses, preterm deliveries and low live-birth rates following assisted conception treatments were reported in women with uterine malformations[34–37]. Case-controlled studies[39,40] involving excision of the septum, and a recent meta-analysis[40] of studies involving hystero-scopic septoplasty or septolysis for a septate uterus, have shown increased live birth rates. Metroplasty for a T-shaped uterus and infantile or hypoplastic uterus in women with RM has also been shown to increase live birth rates[15,41,42]. Hysteroscopy forms the cornerstone of diagnosis and conservative treatment of uterine malformations, although there is growing evidence to suggest that 3D ultrasound can play a complementary role. From our data, it has emerged that TVS was able reliably to identify only four out of 20 uterine anom-alies: 1/5 with a complete septum and bicornuate uni-collis, 3/9 with a bicornuate uterus, 0/6 with infantile or T-shaped uterus, thus confirming the limitations of non-targeted TVS. It has been noticed in the past that T-shaped uteri are difficult to diagnose without hysteroscopy or 3D ultrasound[43].

Acquired and estrogen-dependent abnormalities

Polyps with abnormal vasculoepithelial changes may be detrimental to implantation, and, at times, can be a marker of a polypoid and/or a hyperplastic endo-metrium. Polyps are also associated with abnormal unscheduled bleeding and uterine irritability, which may compromise successful implantation and placen-tation. Fifteen cases in this series had endometrial polyps of varying size (at least 10 mm or more) and number (ranging from 1 to 6). The reported incidence of endometrial polyps ranged from 9 to 32% during pre-IVF work-up, and up to 35% in women during infertility work-up[8,13,25,44]. The excess risk of finding polyps in women with infertility and recurrent mis-carriages was 17 times and 3.5 times, respectively[2]. Higher live-birth rates were reported following polypectomy, irrespective of the size of the endome-trial polyp removed[8,45–47]. Hysteroscopic polypectomy is the preferred approach, as it ensures complete removal and minimizes the risk of endometrial scar-ring. A previous report from this clinic showed the limited value of blind dilatation and curettage in the successful removal of polyps[45].

Endometrial polyps can be transient and notori-ously inconspicuous at baseline scanning, and their presence can be masked by endometrial waves, which may lead to false-positive and false-negative diagnosis, and inaccurate estimation of their size (Figure 1). Therefore, pitfalls are common when TVS is used on

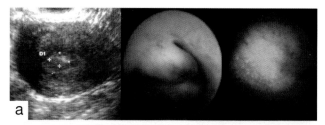
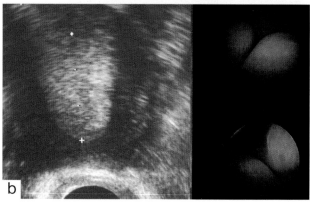

Figure 1 (a) Comparison of transvaginal sonography (TVS) and hysteroscopy. A poorly visualized and underestimated (1.0 cm) endometrial polyp on TVS. Hysteroscopy shows it to be a 2.0-cm endometrial polyp covered by out-of-phase proliferative phase endometrium. The small area of subendometrial hemorrhage evident at the 3 o'clock position resulted from mechanical injury following mock embryo transfer. (b) TVS (18 mm) thick homogeneous endometrium. Hysteroscopy shows multiple endometrial polyps

its own to diagnose and plan treatment for endo-metrial polyps.

Saline contrast sonography improves the accuracy of standard TVS, but cannot always provide inform-ation on surface changes of the polyp or associated subtle abnormalities of the endometrium, as seen in Figure 2.

Hysteroscopy, on the other hand, has the dual advantage of accurate final diagnosis and allowing simultaneous treatment, but has the drawback that it cannot normally be performed during assisted con-ception treatment cycles. In a previous study from Bourn Hall Clinic, it was reported that there was a 75% correlation between ultrasound suspicion of endometrial polyps and hysteroscopic confirmation[45]. However, in the present study, only two of 15 endometrial polyps were accurately identified and seven were missed altogether, with the rest reported as abnormal (non-homogeneous) endometrium by TVS. Careful assessment of the endometrium when no endometrial waves are present will reduce both false-positive and false-negative diagnoses of endometrial

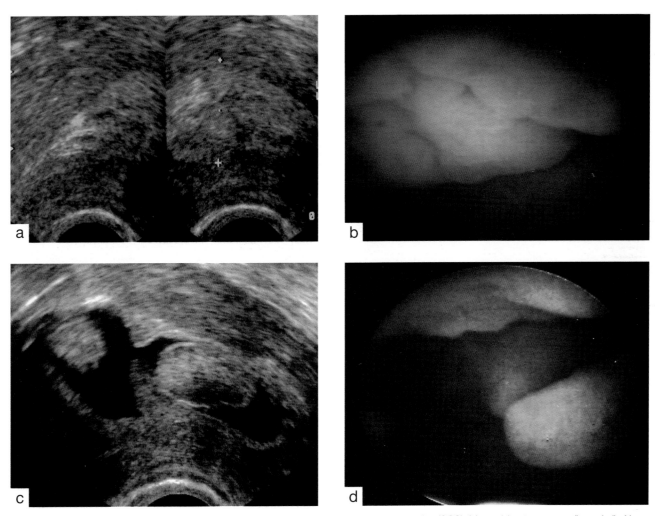

Figure 2 Comparison of transvaginal sonography (TVS) (a), saline contrast sonography (SCS) (c), and hysteroscopy (b and d). Non-homogenous endometrium on TVS (a) and intracavity lesions on SCS (c) are shown to be polypoidal endometrium and endometrial polyps on hysteroscopy (b and d)

polyps. Spontaneous expulsion of endometrial polyps is very common, and hence it is appropriate to perform a repeat scan to check for persistence of polyps before scheduling women for therapeutic hysteroscopy, particularly when there has been a time lapse from the initial diagnosis to the planned hysteroscopy.

Submucous fibroids

Eight submucous fibroids were found on hysteroscopy in the study group which were not identified by TVS, although thick endometrium was recognized in a few cases (Figure 3).

The reported incidence of submucous fibroids in women during infertility work-up, pre-IVF work-up and after repeated IVF treatment failures was: 3.9%, 9.5% and 3.3%, respectively[25,44,48]. Meta-analysis of studies in women with submucous myomas demonstrated lower pregnancy rates (relative risk 0.30) and implantation rates (relative risk 0.28) than in infertile controls[49]. Women with submucous myomas were considered separately from those with intramural and subserosal fibroids. Pregnancy was increased after myomectomy, compared with infertile controls (relative risk 1.72), and delivery rates were then equivalent to infertile women without fibroids (relative risk 0.98)[49]. Endometrial sclerosis and neovascularization can occur after resection of submucous fibroids, and it is appropriate to consider a repeat check hysteroscopy prior to commencing a new treatment cycle.

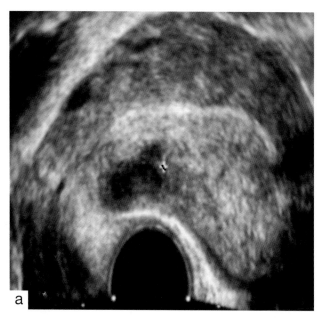
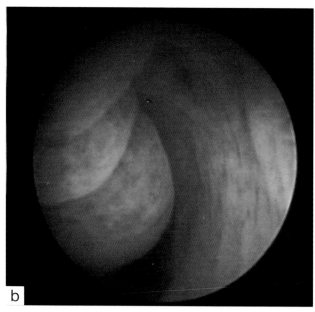

Figure 3 Comparison of transvaginal sonography (TVS) and hysteroscopy. (a) TVS showing one anterior wall intramural fibroid and non-trilaminar, ill-defined endometrium. (b) Hysteroscopy showing multiple smooth-walled submucous fibroids

Intrauterine synechiae and endometrial scarring

Six cases of intrauterine synechiae were identified on hysteroscopy out of the 170 in the present study, and none were identified on TVS in the preceding treatment cycles. However, TVS had shown thin endometrium (< 8 mm) in all cases (Figure 4).

The reported incidence of intrauterine scarring or adhesions ranged from 2.7 to 4% in women with infertility[48] and 5–39% in women with RM[50]. Improved live-birth rates were reported following hysteroscopic surgical treatment and/or 3–6 months of high-dose cyclical estrogen therapy for mild to moderate adhesions[37,50–53]. In our series, high-dose estrogen therapy was sufficient to normalize the uterine cavity of a woman who had a moderate amount of filmy adhesions, and a spontaneous conception resulted soon after completing 3 months of hormone therapy.

Mucosal elevations or ridges

Hysteroscopy identified discrete raised focal lesions of various shapes and sizes arising from apparently healthy looking endometrium in seven cases. Another study based on hysteroscopy in the follicular phase showed focal or diffuse mucosal elevations in 6.2% of infertile women[1], but the relevance of these lesions to reproductive function is unknown.

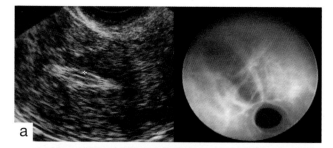
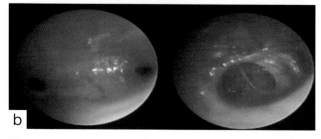

Figure 4 Comparison of transvaginal sonography (TVS) and hysteroscopy. (a) Thin (5 mm) trilaminar endometrium on TVS, moderate degree of intrauterine synechiae on hysteroscopy. (b) Hysteroscopy, obliterated uterine cavity before and after high-dose estrogen therapy

Endometritis

A significantly increased number of blood vessels in the proliferative phase of a cycle, or a reddish endometrium, in which the white openings of the glands produce a typical strawberry-like pattern, has been suggested as hysteroscopically diagnostic of endometritis (Figure 5).

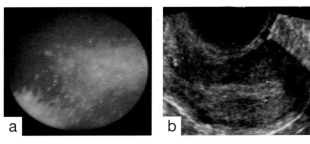

Figure 5 Comparison of transvaginal sonography (TVS) and hysteroscopy. (a) Ultrasound shows thin (6 mm) non-trilaminar endometrium. (b) Strawberry-like appearance of endometrium on hysteroscopy in an abandoned treatment cycle. The woman gave a history of repeated puerperal uterine evacuations

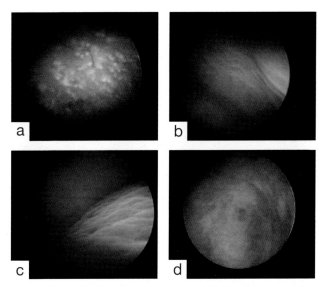

Figure 6 Comparison of endometrium at different phases of the cycle, based on histology findings: (a) late proliferative; (b) early secretory; (c) mid-secretory, and (d) late secretory endometrium

Neither microbiological examination of the cervical and uterine swabs, nor histology from Pipelle samples, seems to have any diagnostic value in such cases[1]. The endometrium appeared inflamed in five cases in our series, and the fifth case had additional features of hydrosalpinx with an abnormal uterine discharge during a frozen embryo treatment cycle. Histology of a Pipelle sample did not confirm the diagnosis in any of the five cases, and uterine swabs did not grow any pathogens in the last case. The reported incidence of endometritis in the literature based on histological examination was 17% in women during pre-IVF work-up and 12% in women with infertility, and hysteroscopy as a diagnostic test for endometritis had a very low sensitivity (16.7%) but a high specificity (93.2%)[14,54,55].

Appropriate antimicrobial and hormonal treatment for hysteroscopically suspected cases of endometritis has been shown to improve clinical pregnancy rates following natural or assisted conception[14]. In our series, there was one confirmed patient with endometritis following traumatic mock embryo transfer who successfully responded to antimicrobial and estrogen therapy and achieved a twin pregnancy after IVF.

Hysteroscopic appearance of normal endometrium

The normal appearance at various phases of the cycle is illustrated in Figure 6.

Hysteroscopic endometrial abnormalities (macroscopic): unclassified

The hysteroscopic appearance of the endometrium was abnormal in 41/170 cases (24%), examples of which were: polypoid endometrium, corrugated/ rough endometrium, pale/edematous endometrium, atrophic endometrium, inflamed endometrium, mixed distribution of blood vessels and glandular openings, neovascularization, endometrial ridges and focal elevations. Nineteen of them had out-of-phase endometrium on histological examination.

Polypoid appearance of endometrium (Figure 7) A 3% incidence of polypoid lesions of the endometrium on hysteroscopy has been reported in women undergoing pretreatment IVF work-up, and a 13.3% incidence in women who had failed to conceive, in spite of repeated IVF treatments[56]. In another study, hyperplastic appearance of the endometrium was seen on hysteroscopy in 20% of women who had undergone multiple failed IVF attempts[48], and it was also shown that the hysteroscopic description of hyperplastic endometrium may not correlate with the histological findings[45].

Thick endometrium with visible glandular openings or blood vessels This is illustrated in Figure 8.

Thick and corrugated endometrium with no visible blood vessels and glandular openings See Figure 9.

Thick endometrium with an edematous appearance See Figure 10.

Atrophic appearance with thin and faintly visible glandular openings and blood vessels See Figure 11 (hysteroscopy, Figure 11a).

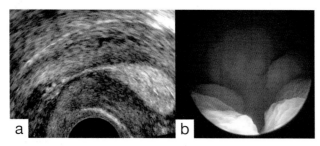

Figure 7 Comparison of transvaginal sonography (TVS) and hysteroscopy. (a) Normal (false negative) homogeneous luteal appearance of endometrium on TVS. (b) Diffuse polypoid appearance of posterior wall of endometrium on hysteroscopy

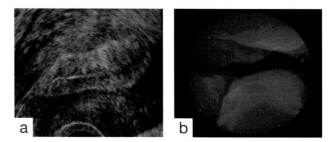

Figure 8 Comparison of transvaginal sonography (TVS) and hysteroscopy. (a) Trilaminar appearance of the endometrium on TVS. (b) Very thick and uneven growth of the endometrium

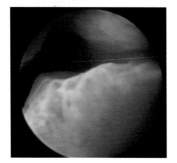

Figure 9 Hysteroscopy. Thick endometrium with no obvious glandular openings or blood vessels

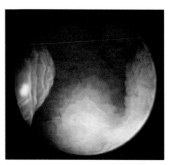

Figure 10 Hysteroscopy. Pale, edematous endometrium with focal elevations and barely visible glandular openings and blood vessels

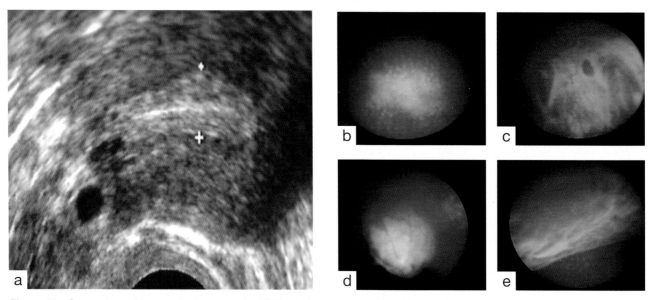

Figure 11 Comparison of transvaginal sonography (TVS) and hysteroscopy. Mixed lesions in early secretory phase. (a) Normal (false negative) trilaminar appearance of endometrium. Hysteroscopy: (b) poor-grade endometrium; (c) endometrial polyp; (d) endometrial sclerosis; (e) edematous appearance. Histology showed out-of-phase, proliferative endometrium

Poor-grade endometrium Poor grade of luteal phase endometrium (consisting of pinpoint glandular openings, instead of normal ring type openings, and thinner blood vessels, instead of varicose-type endometrial vessels) was reported in about 45–61% of women undergoing infertility investigations[57,58]. Poor-grade endometrium was noticed more often in women with a previous history of miscarriage, and resulted in fewer clinical pregnancies in their subsequent attempts to conceive[59]. There were four cases of poorly developed endometrium and one with mixed endometrial changes in the present study (Figure 11).

Endometrial dating: implications of out-of-phase endometrium

Endometrial samples were collected from 140 women in our series. Of these, 82% were in the calculated secretory phase, and 18% in the calculated proliferative phase. Histologically diagnosed out-of-phase endometrium was evident in 54.5% of cases. Seventy per cent (37/53) of those who had out-of-phase endometrium showed delayed maturation (in the secretory phase), and 16/53 (30%) showed advanced maturation, in both the proliferative and the secretory phase. Three cases showed inactive endometrium mixed with secretory or proliferative changes.

Luteal phase defect, based on out-of-phase endometrium, was reported in 3–20% of an infertile population and 23–60% of women with recurrent miscarriage[4]. However, there are very limited data on the effects of pre-existing luteal phase dysfunction on assisted conception treatments and their outcomes. A higher frequency of retarded endometrial development in women who did not become pregnant following IVF treatment was found in natural cycles preceding IVF treatment[60]. Out-of-phase endometrium was reported more often in women who had poor-grade endometrium on hysteroscopy and a previous history of miscarriage[58]. Interobserver variation between general pathologist and reproductive pathologist in the reporting of endometrial dating seems to be as high as 43%. It has also been stated that up to 48% of dys-synchronous glandular changes are underreported by standard histological examination when compared with immunohistochemistry[61]. At present, it is not standard practice to perform endometrial biopsy in the investigation of infertile women. However, pre-IVF endometrial samples are regularly collected in a few centers, to co-culture the embryos that are

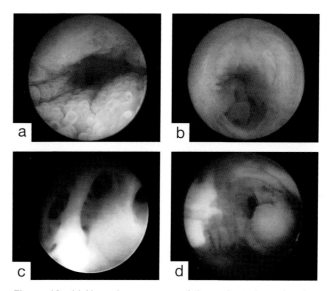

Figure 12 (a) Normal appearance of the endocervix and endocervical mucosa, with visible internal os. (b) Endocervical polyp. (c) Endocervical synechiae appearing as false/blind passages. (d) Endocervical mucosal hypertrophy and fleshy granulations after repeated attempts at cervical dilatation

produced in subsequent treatment cycles, and improved pregnancy rates are reported with this technique in women with recurrent treatment failures.

Role of hysteroscopy in ART in specific categories of patients

Abnormalities of the cervical canal: implications of findings on the embryo transfer procedure

Normal and abnormal endocervices are illustrated in Figure 12.

Eighty-two of 170 women had one or more abnormalities involving the cervical canal, endocervical mucosa and/or cervicouterine angle. These were: space-occupying lesions in 52 (30.5%) (synechiae in 17, polyps/cysts in 35), excessive cervicouterine angle and mixed lesions in 30 (17.6%). Forty-five (54.9%) of those women who had intracervical lesions gave a history of difficult embryo transfer (DET).

Mock embryo transfer (MET) was attempted in 41 (24.1%) of those women who underwent hysteroscopy with a previous history of DET. Use of a tenaculum for stabilizing the cervix and/or the use of a metal catheter to negotiate the cervical canal was considered a 'difficult embryo transfer'. In 28 (68.2%) of this group, MET was accomplished easily. Traction on the cervix with a tenaculum was sufficient to accomplish MET in a further five cases, and in the last eight cases MET could not be achieved, even with the aid of a tenaculum. No attempts were made to use a stylet to negotiate the cervix, to avoid potential damage to the endometrium.

All cases of difficult MET and failed MET showed various endocervical lesions (cysts, polyps, synechiae and Asherman's syndrome) and/or an excessive utero-cervical angle. Three from the failed MET group had blind passages evident on hysteroscopy. Figure 13 illustrates a case of undiagnosed Asherman's syndrome in which the MET catheter (highlighted in green) is shown in a false passage during ultrasound-guided MET.

Twenty of 24 women who had acute uterocervical angles, and 11 of 17 who had intracervical synechiae, gave a history of DETs in previous treatment cycles. Excessive cervicouterine angle and endocervical synechiae were the most frequent findings in women with a history of DET, but it is difficult to be certain whether synechiae are the cause or result of DET. Interestingly, in all 41 cases who gave a history of DET there was neither cervical stenosis nor was there any need for cervical dilatation to introduce the hysteroscope. In seven of 41 cases, hysteroscopy was not possible until the space-occupying lesion was removed by polypectomy or adhesiolysis. Thus, it is appropriate to consider hysteroscopic evaluation of the cervical canal and uterine cavity in women with a history of difficult embryo transfer, to identify the reason for the difficulty and so institute specific treatment. A blind cervical dilatation might break some synechiae and enable easier embryo transfers, but highly inconsistent benefits have been reported in the literature from this approach. When MET is considered, to assess the feasibility of embryo transfer, it should be performed preferably in the pretreatment cycle, so that a diagnostic hysteroscopy can be performed in cases of difficult MET to diagnose and possibly correct any obstructive lesions within the cervical canal.

Anatomical aberrations of the cervical canal, isthmus and lower uterine cavity are associated with difficult embryo transfers[62] and reduced pregnancy rates[3,63]. The reported incidence of cervicouterine abnormalities was: 15% in women during pre-IVF assessment[3], 31.2% in women who fail to conceive after repeated IVF treatments[64] and almost 100% in women who give a history of very difficult embryo transfers[65]. Hysteroscopic diagnosis and treatment of

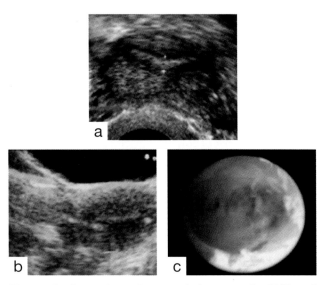

Figure 13 Comparison of transvaginal sonography (TVS) and hysteroscopy in a case of undiagnosed Asherman's syndrome. TVS (a) of thin endometrium in the luteal phase. (b) Ultrasound-guided mock embryo transfer (MET). Endometrium and uterus are highlighted in orange and the MET catheter which is in the false passage is highlighted in green. (c) Severe Asherman's syndrome

specific anatomical obstruction or distortion resulted in easier embryo transfers[3,63,66] and improved pregnancy rates[66] in their subsequent attempts to conceive.

Transvaginal ultrasound has a low sensitivity for endocervical pathologies and cervicouterine angle abnormalities, and thus has limited value in predicting a difficult embryo transfer. Interim analysis of our data on ultrasound and hysteroscopic findings in women with a history of difficult embryo transfer has shown hysteroscopic evidence of cervicouterine canal abnormalities in 21.8% of women who had normal appearance of the cervix and 60.8% of women who had abnormal findings in the cervix on TVS[62].

Hysteroscopy in women with a history of recurrent assisted conception treatment failures Seventy-two (42%) of all hysteroscopies performed in our series were in women with a history of three or more ET treatment failures. Thirty-three per cent of them had hysteroscopic abnormalities (Table 1), and an additional 26% had hysteroscopic and/or histological abnormalities in the form of out-of-phase endometrium. The occurrence of new endometrial lesions, such as hyperplasia, polyps, submucous fibroids, endometritis and synechiae in the uterus and/or cervix, has been reported in 18–50% of women undergoing a second-look hysteroscopy after repeated failures of IVF treatment[56,67]. The hyperestrogenic environment in controlled ovarian hysperstimulation cycles, and iatrogenic trauma from ET techniques, are considered to be responsible for these newly found abnormalities which may contribute to further treatment failures. Timely diagnosis and treatment enables improved outcomes[56].

Hysteroscopy in women with unexplained infertility

Forty-two of 170 (24.7%) of hysteroscopies were performed in women with a history of unexplained infertility (UEI). One or more uterine abnormalities that are recognized causes of poor reproductive outcome were found in 42.9%. Ten were found to have abnormalites of the uterus and cervix, 11 had abnormalities of the uterus only and eight had abnormalities of the cervix only. Of the 21 cases in whom uterine lesions were identified, 18 were considered significant: submucous fibroids in five, endometrial polyps (of > 1.5 cm in the longest dimension) in four, intrauterine synechiae in three, diffuse polypoid lesions in four, complete uterine septum in one and subseptum in one. Three patients underwent treatment (polypectomy, medical curettage, resection of uterine septum) and two conceived subsequently (one naturally and one after IVF).

Twelve women from this group attempted to conceive without any treatment for uterine pathologies, resulting in no clinical but one biochemical pregnancy. Two women with Asherman's syndrome chose to defer any further treatments following hysteroscopic diagnosis.

In a previous study, hysteroscopic abnormalities were reported in 15% of women with unexplained infertility associated with repeated IVF treatment failures[64]. It has also been reported that 15% of women who were scheduled for IVF for male factor infertility had uterine abnormalities, all of which required treatment and which resulted in improved pregnancy rates after treatment[68].

Meta-analysis of five randomized controlled trials on the efficacy of IVF over intrauterine insemination (IUI) treatment for women with unexplained infertility did not show any better pregnancy rates from IVF when compared with IUI[69]. This can to some extent be due to the high prevalence of undiagnosed uterine pathologies in this group of women, possibly contributing to implantation failure or miscarriage, even after replacing good-grade embryos. The estimated cost per baby through IVF in women with UEI in the UK is £9000[4]; therefore, it is worth considering these women for more thorough uterine cavity evaluation to reduce unwarranted treatment failures.

Hysteroscopy in women of advanced reproductive age Twenty-eight women who underwent hysteroscopy in this series were over the age of 40 years, and 26 of them had abnormal findings of the uterus (60%) and/or the cervix (40%). There were three miscarriages but no clinical pregnancies in the 16 women who subsequently attempted embryo transfer procedures. Such a high prevalence of uterine pathologies may to some extent explain the low (5%) take-home baby rate of women in this age group, even after the transfer of apparently good-quality embryos. The higher incidence of uterine pathologies was linked to poorer pregnancy outcome[70], and a need for an extended number of IVF attempts to acheive a pregnancy[12].

European data[71], based on IVF outcomes in women over the age of 39, reported clinical pregnancy rates of 10.7% for fresh embryo transfer and 8.9% for frozen embryo transfer, respectively. Only 34% of these women achieved a live birth, even after three cycles of the treatment, at an estimated cost of £20 056 per baby born[4]. There is therefore a genuine indication to evaluate the uteri in this group of women in order to diagnose and treat contributing uterine pathologies before beginning IVF treatments, to avoid useless IVF attempts and iatrogenic complications of such treatments, and, in addition, to reduce the costs per baby born.

Hysteroscopy in women with a history of suboptimal appearance of endometrium on TVS

The endometrium is graded as normal in the monitoring phase when there is a homogeneous appearance of a trilaminar endometrium, 8–14 mm in thickness and no additional findings of abnormal echoes. Endometrial thickness was normal but the appearance was non-homogeneous in 38 of 170 women, and 27 (71%) of these had hysteroscopic abnormalities. In the rest, the endometrium was poorly visualized and the possible reason for the non-homogeneous appearance of the endometrium was either adenomyosis and/or a fibroid uterus. In addition, hysteroscopic abnormalities were noticed in: 7/8 women with thin endometrium (Asherman's syndrome, endometrial atrophy, endometrial scarring), 7/10 women with thick endometrium (submucous fibroids, endometrial polyps, polypoid endometrium and corrugated endometrium) on TVS examination. Of 23 women who were reported to have a completely normal endometrium on TVS, hysteroscopic abnormalities were found in 14 (endometrial polyps, endometrial scarring or edematous endometrium). Our data clearly indicate the limitations of TVS in assessing the normality of the endometrium and uterus. Strict criteria should be laid down for assessing the endometrium at different stages of monitoring, and any atypical appearance should be considered for further evaluation with more accurate tools, such as SCS or hysteroscopy.

Correlation of TVS and hysteroscopy To estimate the true concordance rate and to avoid operator bias, hysteroscopic findings were correlated only with the ultrasound findings from the most recent treatment cycle. Transvaginal ultrasound was accurate only in the diagnosis of: 4/20 uterine malformations (1/5 double uterus, 3/9 bicornuate uterus, 0/6 infantile or T-shaped uterus) and 2/29 endometrial/uterine cavity abnormalities (2/15 endometrial polyps, 0/8 submucous fibroids, 0/6 intrauterine synechiae). Much better concordance rates were reported between TVS and early follicular phase hysteroscopy from those centers where contrast sonography is liberally used. Such a high discrepancy is difficult to explain, but possible

reasons include: time lag between previous treatment and hysteroscopy; higher incidence of endometrial pathologies in the mid-cycle/luteal phase in which most of the hysteroscopies were performed; iatrogenic lesions resulting from previous embryo transfer procedures; hormone-induced lesions from the hyperestrogenic environment of controlled ovarian hyperstimulation; and newly acquired gynecological pathologies unrelated to previous treatments.

Miscellaneous observations

Post-hysteroscopy saline contrast sonography TVS was performed immediately after hysteroscopy using leftover saline. This enabled better visualization of variable thicknesses of the endometrium and of the cavity outline, and better delineation of submucous fibroids. Saline contrast sonography has improved the diagnostic accuracy of TVS and appears to minimize the pitfalls of standard TVS in assessing normality of the endometrium and subtle pathologies within.

Follow-up study

Tables 3 and 4 illustrate pregnancy outcome data in relation to the pretreatment hysteroscopy findings in our series.

Table 3 Findings on hysteroscopic examination and endometrial biopsy in correlation with subsequent reproductive outcome (*n* = 100)

Findings	Clinical pregnancy (*n* = 25, 55.55%)[§]	Miscarriage (*n* = 20, 44.44%)[§]	Not pregnant (*n* = 55)
Mean age (years)	35.19	35.85	35.16
Hysteroscopy and TVS normal, no other risk factors* present	18 (72%)	1 (5%)	13 (23.63%)
Hysteroscopy and TVS normal but other risk factors* present	1 (4%)	6 (30%)	9 (16.36%)
Hysteroscopic abnormality[†] ± TVS abnormality[‡] ± other risk factors* present	6 (24%) (5/25 = 25%[†]) (were treated for pathology)	13 (65%) (8/20 = 40%[†])	33 (60%) (19/55 = 38%[†])
Histology:			
In-phase endometrium	18	6	34
Out-of-phase endometrium	7	14	18 (+3*)

*Age ≥39 years, difficult embryo transfer, recurrent miscarriages; [†]uterine malformation, submucous fibroid, small multiple or single large endometrial polyp, polypoid/atrophic endometrium and out-of-phase endometrium; [‡]multiple intramural fibroids, single large intramural fibroid, hydrosalpinx, uterine cavity fluid, severe endometriosis; [§]percentage of those who had positive day-15 pregnancy test; TVS, transvaginal sonography

Post-hysteroscopy reproductive performance

Treatment outcomes are available for 100 women who attempted further treatments within 1–16 months after their diagnostic hysteroscopies; 45 women had positive pregnancy tests (45%), 25 achieved clinical

pregnancies and 20 suffered early pregnancy losses. The mean age, etiology and duration of infertility were matched in all three groups. More women who were found to have normal uteri achieved pregnancy (72%) than those diagnosed with uterine pathologies

Table 4 Hysteroscopic endometrial abnormalities, histology correlation and subsequent assisted reproductive technologies (ART) outcomes

Findings	Number of cases	TVS findings sufficient to change management	Histology (A = in-phase B = out of phase, C = none)	Number attempted treatment	Clinical pregnancy	Biochemical pregnancy/ miscarriage
(1) Polypoid appearance	12	no	A = 6 (50%) B = 6 (50%)	9	1[†]	1[‡]
(2) Corrugated/ rough appearance (no glands/vessels)	5	no	A = 2 (40%) B = 2 (40%) C = 1 (20%)	3	1[†]	0
(3) Pale and edematous	5	no	A = 1 (20%) B = 4 (80%) C = 1	5	0	1[§]
(4) Mostly atrophic plus mixed	4	no	A = 3 (75%) B = 1 (25%) C = 0	3[††]	0	0
(5) Intense mucosal congestion– focal/diffuse (? endometritis × 1)	5	no	A = 1 (25%) B = 3 (75%) C = 1	3	0	1[‡]
(6) Neovascularization	2	no	A = 0 B = 1 (50%) C = 1 (50%)	—	—	—
(7) Patchy glandulo- vascular pattern	1	no	A = 1(100%) B = 0 C = 0	1	0	0
(8) Focal raised lesions	3	no	A = 1 (33.3%) B = 2 (66.6%) C = 0	2	0	1[‡]
(9) Endometrial ridges	4	no	A = 1 (50%) B = 1 (50%) C = 2	3	1[‡‡]	—
Total	41 (24%)[*]		A = 16 (45.71%)+ B = 19 (54.28%)++ C = 5	29	3 (10.34%)[**]	4 (57.14%)[***]
Excluding ? relevant lesions (3, 8, 9)	29 (17%)[*]		A = 12 (48%)+ B = 13 (52%)++ C = 4	19	2 (10.52%)[**]	2 (50%)[***]

[*]Percentage of total hysteroscopies performed; [**]percentage of those who attempted to conceive (n = 29); [***]percentage of those who had positive pregnancy test (n = 7); + and ++, percentage of histology reports available in A and B category, respectively; [†]had in-phase endometrium, treated with 3 months' combined pills; [‡]had out-of-phase (delayed maturation) endometrium, received no treatment; [§]had out-of-phase (advanced maturation) endometrium, received no treatment; [††]one had delayed maturation and other two had atrophic plus in-phase endometrium; [‡‡]endometrial biopsy was not performed

(24%). Sixty-five per cent of women who suffered miscarriage and 60% of those who failed to conceive following ART had uterine pathologies.

Timing of hysteroscopy in relation to IVF treatment A study evaluating the effects of performing diagnostic and therapeutic hysteroscopy in the early part of the stimulation phase of a treatment cycle found it to be safe, with no untoward effects and improved pregnancy outcome in women with hysteroscopically visible abnormalities[72].

Hysteroscopic endometrial abnormalities: implications for subsequent treatment cycles Twenty-nine of the 41 women with macroscopic endometrial abnormalities attempted further treatments resulting in seven positive pregnancy tests, successful pregnancy in three (10.3%) and early pregnancy loss in four (13.8%).

'Fertility effect' of diagnostic hysteroscopy and endometrial biopsy Improved spontaneous pregnancy rates have been reported following diagnostic HSG[73], and it has been theorized that instrumentation and distension of the uterine cavity might clear any debris, casts, mucus plugs, filmy adhesions, etc., and thus benefit women with a history of unexplained or tubal factor infertility. A similar mechanism has been postulated for improved pregnancy rates following diagnostic hysteroscopy[74]. Improved implantation rates were reported following deliberate saline irrigation of the uterus during the stimulation phase of IVF in women with a history of unexplained or tubal factor infertility who failed to conceive after repeated ART[74]. Very recently, deliberately induced local injury to the endometrium with endometrial sampling devices produced a doubling of the incidence of successful pregnancies in patients with a history of repeated IVF failures undergoing *in vitro* fertilization[75]. In our follow-up study of 100 women after hysteroscopy, 24% achieved clinical pregnancy, suggesting a trend toward a higher pregnancy rate in this category of patients.

Summary of results

A diagnostic hysteroscopy was offered at Bourn Hall Clinic to women with selected indications, and approximately 200 women in a year (20% of our annual caseload) had one or more indications. The take-up rate was about 50%, and all hysteroscopies were performed without the need for cervical dilatation, including those women with an history of difficult

embryo transfer. All hysteroscopies were performed in mid- or the later half of natural cycles, except for a few which were performed after abandoning a treatment cycle because of suboptimal endometrium identified on ultrasound. Seventy-five per cent of the hysteroscopies were carried out on an out-patient basis, with a very low conversion rate to general anesthesia or intravenous sedation (1.7%). Ten per cent of women experienced severe but transient uterine pain, but none experienced significant vasovagal reactions or postprocedural infection. A pre-hysteroscopy pelvic ultrasound scan played a complementary role in evaluating both myometrial and adnexal pathologies. A saline contrast sonograph was obtained at the end of hysteroscopy to compare data obtained from the standard 2D ultrasound scan and the diagnostic hysteroscopy. Mock embryo transfers (conventional and ultrasound-guided) provided information on the feasibility of the procedure and its effects on the endometrium. An ultrasound finding of suboptimal appearance of the endometrium (thick, thin or non-homogeneous) in the preceding treatment cycle had a 71% concordance with hysteroscopic evidence of abnormal findings, but TVS showed poor predictive value for a specific pathology: 0% for intrauterine synechiae, 0% for submucous fibroids, 7.5% for endometrial polyps and 20% for uterine malformations. Hysteroscopy revealed uterine pathologies in 60% of women who were reported to have normal appearance of the endometrium on TVS.

Acquired, estrogen-dependent pathologies of the uterus and cervix were the most frequent finding, followed by out-of-phase endometrium and congenital uterine abnormalities. Follow-up study has shown that the presence of uterine pathologies resulted in fewer pregnancies, more miscarriages and more drop-outs from pursuing further ART. In contrast, the absence of uterine pathologies was associated with a higher chance of clinical pregnancy and a reduced risk of miscarriage.

DISCUSSION AND CONCLUSIONS

The need for pretreatment evaluation and counseling

Each ART treatment cycle exposes women to the side-effects of hormonal medication, psychological and emotional stress and, at times, a small but serious risk to their lives. Repeated treatment failure is a well-recognized cause of psychological dysfunction, depression, low self-esteem and lower satisfaction with life; it is also well recognized that the longer the treatment persists the more likely women are to be depressed[76–78]. Unfortunately, 2001 European data indicate that the 'take-home-baby rate' is still only 20% for one IVF attempt, increasing to a maximum of 50% after three ART treatments in an unselected population. In addition, ART is very expensive and self-funded in most parts of the world, costing upwards of £12 000 to £20 000 per baby, when delivered between the ages of 24 and 39, respectively[4].

Karyotypically abnormal embryos have long been recognized as a leading cause of poor outcome following natural conception or assisted conception treatments[79]. Technological advances in ART now allow selection of a healthier (euploid or blastocyst) embryo, and two recent randomized controlled trials have shown that clinical pregnancy rates as high as 42% following day-3 single embryo transfer and 60% following single blastocyst transfer are achievable in good-prognosis patients[80,81]. Therefore, it is likely that the presence of structural and endometrial pathologies contribute to suboptimal conditions for the implanting embryo, resulting in treatment failure following transfer of healthy embryos in an unselected population[82].

The presence of a normal uterine environment is considered to be a good prognostic factor for success in subsequent treatment cycles, even in women with a history of recurrent IVF treatment failures, as shown in our follow-up data on 100 women. Pregnancy rates were found to be good in women with no uterine pathologies, as well as in those women who were successfully treated for any uterine pathologies found, even when they gave a history of previous assisted conception treatment failures[13–15]. Assessment of the uterus should therefore be an integral part of the pretreatment evaluation of women with or without a history of previous treatment failures, to avoid unnecessary and expensive treatment failures[83,84]. Crude cost-effective analysis indicates that hysteroscopy, as a universal screening test even before the first IVF treatment, is well justified, even in a population where there is only a 10% prevalence of uterine pathologies that are amenable to diagnosis and treatment[85].

Women who are found to have abnormal uteri before, during or after a negative ART treatment cycle should receive thorough counseling on their adjusted pregnancy chances. The treatment options available to them, depending on the pathology found, and the evidence-based treatments available for each of those pathologies should be given. Individualized treatment protocols should then be adopted with the objective of rectifying the pathology, when feasible, or to review the option of surrogacy, as appropriate. The adjusted chances of achieving a pregnancy should be emphasized for those who are either unwilling or unable to have their uterine abnormality rectified. Strong consideration should be given not to offer ART treatments to women with untreated severe uterine pathology, in order to prevent iatrogenic complications of ART and the short- and long-term negative psychosocial sequelae.

Total reliance on conventional TVS to diagnose all varieties of uterine and endometrial pathologies underestimates the true prevalence of uterine pathologies, particularly in the early luteal phase, resulting in an unacceptable false-negative rate, except in a very few skilled hands. SCS by 3D ultrasound seems to achieve very high accuracy for most, but not intraendometrial abnormalities[86], although limited availability and the need for expensive machines restricts its general use as a screening test. SCS (2D) is relatively cheap and easy to use as a screen to identify women for a confirmatory and/or therapeutic hysteroscopy[28,87].

Traditionally, diagnostic and therapeutic use of hysteroscopy is usually performed before a treatment cycle, but recent evidence suggests that it can be performed safely and effectively in the early phase of a controlled ovarian hyperstimulation cycle, with added benefits to the patient[72]. The availability of safer models of 'see-and-treat' out-patient 'Versascopy' systems, a less intensive learning curve, and a growing trend toward nurse-led out-patient hysteroscopy services[22] will perhaps lead to more liberal use of hysteroscopy in ART units.

Whether they are oocyte or embryo recipients, or using their own gametes, women of advanced reproductive age have a higher incidence of uterine pathologies than younger women. There is, therefore, a strong indication to screen them all for uterine pathologies, in order to reduce the number of useless IVF attempts and the cost per baby born[79].

Research scope

In the era of patient-centered medical care and of predominantly self-funded assisted conception treatment services, informed choices to the patient are of paramount importance. The literature is lacking on the views of patients on pretreatment evaluation, and there is a need to conduct surveys in this group to assess their awareness of the effect of uterine factors on the success of fertility treatments, their views on their willingness to undergo pretreatment assessments and the costs incurred of such an approach. Very little research has been done on hysteroscopically visible endometrial aberrations during the window of implantation (non-physiological changes) and their effects on implantation and growth of the conceptus. Comprehensive evaluation (immunocytochemistry, immunohistochemistry and implantation-marker studies) of targeted tissue samples from each of the different endometrial lesions described earlier is likely to provide much-needed information on the implications of these lesions for successful implantation.

There is also a lack of randomized, double-blind controlled trials (class A evidence) on the routine or selective use of diagnostic/therapeutic hysteroscopy in women undergoing ART and its effect on live birth rates. Adequately powered trials should address these issues and could thereby make ART a much more efficient and cost-effective medical service. A significant proportion of patients attempting new or repeated ART are found to have uterine pathologies that can compromise their live birth chances to a variable degree. Routine screening of the uterine cavity and correction of identified pathologies may therefore reduce cycle cancelation and treatment failure rates, and contribute to achieving higher success rates in selected cases. In addition, information gathered by thorough evaluation of the uterus at the outset of treatment would allow infertile women to be fully counseled on their individual progress. Moreover, this would also allow couples to make informed choices and the care provider to optimize the treatment protocols. Appropriate research is needed to explore the benefits and cost-effectiveness of hysteroscopy as a screening test for all women before commencing ART.

REFERENCES

1. Campo R, Van Bella Y, Rombauts L, et al. Office mini-hysteroscopy. Hum Reprod Update 1999; 5: 73–81
2. Valli E, Zupi E, Marconi D, et al. Hysteroscopic findings in 344 women with recurrent spontaneous abortion. J Am Assoc Gynecol Laparosc 2001; 8: 398–401
3. Frydman R, Eibschitz I, Fernandez H, et al. Uterine evaluation by microhysteroscopy in IVF candidates. Hum Reprod 1987; 2: 481–5
4. Tools to optimise the IVF–ET procedure and its cost-effectiveness. National Institute for Clinical Excellence: guidelines February 2004. London: RCOG Press, 2004
5. Valle RF. Hysteroscopy in the evaluation of female infertility. Am J Obstet Gynecol 1980; 137: 425–31
6. Wakim R, Raneiri DM, Hart R, et al. Assessment of the uterine cavity by saline hystero-contrast-sonography before IVF. Presented at the XVIIIth Annual Meeting of the ESHRE, Vienna, Austria. Program Suppl 2002; 17: 165–66
7. Ayida G, Chamberlain P, Barlow D, et al. Uterine cavity assessment prior to in vitro fertilization: comparison of transvaginal scanning, saline contrast hysterosonography and hysteroscopy. Ultrasound Obstet Gynecol 1997; 10: 59–62
8. Shokeir TA, Shalan HM, El-Shafei MM. Significance of endometrial polyps detected hysteroscopically in eumenorrheic infertile women. J Obstet Gynaecol Res 2004; 30: 84–9
9. Oliveira FG, Abdelmassih VG, Diamond MP, et al. Uterine cavity findings and hysteroscopic interventions in patients undergoing in vitro fertilization–embryo transfer who repeatedly cannot conceive. Fertil Steril 2003; 80: 1371–5
10. Golan A, Eilat E, Ron-El R, et al. Hysteroscopy is superior to hysterosalpingography in infertility investigation. Acta Obstet Gynecol Scand 1996; 75: 654–6
11. Hamou J, Frydman R, Fernandez H. Evaluation prior to IVF by microhysteroscopy. Presented at the VIth World Congress in IVF and Alternate Assisted Reproduction, Jerusalem, Israel, 1989: abstr 40
12. Kirsop R, Porter R, Torode H, et al. The role of hysteroscopy in patients having failed IVF/GIFT tranfer cycles. Aust NZ J Obstet Gynaecol 1991; 31: 263–4
13. Hinckley MD, Milki AA. 1000, office hysteroscopies for infertility: feasibility and findings. See and treat office hysteroscopy. Presented at the 58th Annual Meeting of the ASRM, San Antonio, Texas, USA. Program Suppl 2003; 80: P-215
14. Feghali J, Bakar J, Mayenga JM, et al. [Systematic hysteroscopy prior to in vitro fertilization]. Gynecol Obstet Fertil 2003; 31: 127–31
15. Seinera P, Maccario S, Visentin L, et al. Hysteroscopy in an IVF–ER program. Clinical experience with 360 infertile patients. Acta Obstet Gynecol Scand 1988; 67: 135–7
16. Demirol A, Gurgon T. Effect of treatment of intrauterine pathologies with office hysteroscopy in

patients with recurrent IVF failure. Reprod BioMed Online 2004; 5: 590–4

17. Dueholm M, Lundorf E, Sorensen JS, et al. Reproducibility of evaluation of the uterus by transvaginal sonography, hysterosonographic examination, hysteroscopy and magnetic resonance imaging. Hum Reprod 2002; 17: 195–200

18. Glatstein IZ, Harlow BL, Hornstein MD. Practice patterns among reproductive endocrinologists: the infertility evaluation. Fertil Steril 1997; 67: 443–51

19. Tan BK, Vandekerckhove F, Starr P, et al. A survey of the investigation and management of recurrent treatment failure in IVF practice in the UK. Presented at the Joint Meeting of the Association of Clinical Embryologists and the British Fertility Society Liverpool, UK. Hum Fertil 2004; 7: 45–69

20. Perez-Medina T, Bajo JM, Martinez-Cortes L, et al. Six thousand office diagnostic-operative hysteroscopies. Int J Gynaecol Obstet 2000; 71: 33–8

21. Lindheim SR, Kavic S, Shulman SV, et al. Operative hysteroscopy in the office setting. J Am Assoc Gynecol Laparosc 2000; 7: 65–9

22. Ludkin H, Quinn P. Extended training equips nurses to undertake diagnostic hysteroscopy. Nurs Times 2002; 98: 38–9

23. Rowe PJ, Comhaire FH, Hargreave TB, Mellows HJ, eds. WHO Manual for the Standardized Investigation and Diagnosis of the Infertile Couple. Cambridge: The Press Syndicate of the University of Cambridge, 1993

24. Narayan R, Goswamy RK. Transvaginal sonography of the uterine cavity with hysteroscopic correlation in the investigation of infertility. Ultrasound Obstet Gynecol 1993; 3: 129–33

25. Fabres C, Alam V, Balmaceda J, et al. Comparison of ultrasonography and hysteroscopy in the diagnosis of intrauterine lesions in infertile women. J Am Assoc Gynecol Laparosc 1998; 5: 375–8

26. Shalev J, Meizner I, Bar-Hava I, et al. Predictive value of transvaginal sonography performed before routine diagnostic hysteroscopy for evaluation of infertility. Fertil Steril 2000; 73: 412–17

27. Rogerson L, Bates J, Weston M, et al. Comparison of outpatient hysteroscopy with saline infusion hysterosonography. Br J Obstet Gynaecol 2002; 109: 800–4

28. Hamilton JA, Larson AJ, Lower AM, et al. Routine use of saline hysterosonography in 500 consecutive, unselected, infertile women. Hum Reprod 1998; 13: 2463–73

29. Stacey C, Bown C, Manhire A, et al. HyCoSy – as good as claimed? Br J Radiol 2000; 73: 133–6

30. Brown SE, Coddington CC, Schnorr J, et al. Evaluation of outpatient hysteroscopy, saline infusion hys-

terosonography, and hysterosalpingography in infertile women: a prospective, randomized study. Fertil Steril 2000; 74: 1029–34

31. De Iaco P, Marabini A, Stefanetti M, et al. Acceptability and pain of outpatient hysteroscopy. J Am Assoc Gynecol Laparosc 2000; 7: 71–5

32. Nagele F, Bournas N, O'Connor H, et al. Comparison of carbon dioxide and normal saline for uterine distension in outpatient hysteroscopy. Fertil Steril 1996; 65: 305–9

33. Salim R, Regan L, Woelfer B, et al. A comparative study of the morphology of congenital uterine anomalies in women with and without a history of recurrent first trimester miscarriage. Hum Reprod 2003; 18: 162–6

34. Marcus S, al-Shawaf T, Brinsden P. The obstetric outcome of IVF–ET in women with congenital uterine malformations. Am J Obstet Gynecol 1996; 175: 85–9

35. Raga F, Bauset C, Remohi J, et al. Reproductive impact of congenital Mullerian anomalies. Hum Reprod 1997; 12: 2277–81

36. Woelfer B, Salim R, Banerjee S, et al. Reproductive outcomes in women with congenital uterine anomalies detected by three-dimensional ultrasound screening. Obstet Gynecol 2001; 98: 1099–103

37. Lin PCJ. Reproductive outcomes in women with uterine anomalies. Women's Health 2004; 13: 33–9

38. Merviel P. Role of hysteroscopy in the diagnosis and treatment of infertility. Review. French Presse Med 2000; 29: 1302–10

39. Kupesic S, Kurjak A, Skenderovic S, et al. Screening for uterine abnormalities by three-dimensional ultrasound improves perinatal outcome. J Perinat Med 2002; 30: 9–17

40. Letterie GS. Assessing the quality of evidence in support of resection of a uterine septum. Presented at the 55th Annual Meeting of the ASRM, Toronto, Ontario, Canada. Program Suppl 1999; 72: P-165

41. Barranger E, Gervaise A, Doumerc S, et al. Reproductive performance after hysteroscopic metroplasty in the hypoplastic uterus: a study of 29 cases. Br J Obstet Gynaecol 2002; 109: 1331–4

42. Proctor JA, Haney AF. Recurrent first trimester pregnancy loss is associated with uterine septum but not with bicornuate uterus. Fertil Steril 2003; 80: 1212–15

43. Kipersztok S, Javitt M, Hill MC, et al. Comparison of magnetic resonance imaging and transvaginal ultrasonography with hysterosalpingography in the evaluation of women exposed to diethylstilbestrol. J Reprod Med 1996; 41: 347–51

44. Syrop CH, Sahakian V. Transvaginal sonographic detection of endometrial polyps with fluid contrast augmentation. Obstet Gynecol 1992; 79: 1041–3

45. Lass A, Williams G, Abusheikha N, et al. The effect of endometrial polyps on outcomes of in vitro fertilization (IVF) cycles. J Assist Reprod Genet 1999; 16: 410–15

46. Varasteh NN, Neuwirth RS, Levin B, et al. Pregnancy rates after hysteroscopic polypectomy and myomectomy in infertile women. Obstet Gynecol 1999; 94: 168–71

47. Spiewankiewicz B, Stelmachow J, Sawicki W, et al. The effectiveness of hysteroscopic polypectomy in cases of female infertility. Clin Exp Obstet Gynecol 2003; 30: 23–5

48. Borrero C, Montoya JM, Uribe JG, et al. Hysteroscopy and endometrial biopsy after failed in vitro fertilization cycles. Presented at the 54th Annual Meeting of the ASRM, San Francisco, California, USA. Program Suppl 1998; 70: P-1222

49. Pritts EA. Fibroids and infertility: a systematic review of the evidence. Obstet Gynecol Surv 2001; 56: 483–91

50. Zikopoulos KA, Kolibianakis EM, Platteau P, et al. Live delivery rates in subfertile women with Asherman's syndrome after hysteroscopic adhesiolysis using the resectoscope or the Versapoint system. Reprod BioMed Online 2004; 8: 720–5

51. Seigler AM, Valle RF. Therapeutic hysteroscopic procedures. Fertil Steril 1988; 50: 685–701

52. Pace S, Stentella P, Catania R, et al. Endoscopic treatment of intrauterine adhesions. Clin Exp Obstet Gynecol 2003; 30: 26–8

53. Kdous M, Hachicha R, Zhiou F, et al. [Fertility after hysteroscopic treatment of intrauterine adhesions]. Gynecol Obstet Fertil 2003; 31: 422–8

54. Petrozza JC, Fuarnaccia M, Haung P, et al. Prevalence of chronic endometritis in women undergoing infertility therapy. Presented at the 55th Annual Meeting of the ASRM, Totonto, Ontario, Canada. Program Suppl 1999; 72: P-356

55. Polisseni F, Bambirra EA, Camargos AF, et al. Detection of chronic endometritis by diagnostic hysteroscopy in asymptomatic infertile patients. Presented at the 57th Annual Meeting of the ASRM, Orlando, Florida, USA. Program Suppl 2001; 76: P-221

56. Schiano A, Jourdain O, Papaxanthos A, et al. [The value of hysteroscopy after repeated implantation failures with in vitro fertilization]. Contracept Fertil Sex 1999; 27: 129–32

57. Sakumoto T, Inafuku K, Miyara M, et al. Hysteroscopic assessment of midsecretory-phase endometrium, with special reference to the luteal-phase defect. Horm Res 1992; 37 (Suppl 1): 48–52

58. Masamoto H, Nakama K, Kanazawa K. Hysteroscopic appearance of the mid-secretory endometrium: relationship to early phase pregnancy outcome after implantation. Hum Reprod 2000; 15: 2112–18

59. Inafuku K. [Hysteroscopy in midluteal phase of human endometrium: evaluation of functional aspect of the endometrium]. Nippon Sanka Fujinka Gakkai Zasshi 1992; 44: 79–83

60. Bourgain CJ. [Endometrial biopsy in the evaluation of endometrial receptivity]. J Gynecol Obstet Biol Reprod (Paris) 2004; 33: S13–17

61. Dubowy RL, Feinberg R, Kliman H. Endometrial biopsy and infertility evaluation: new insights from cyclins. Presented at the 56th Annual Meeting of the ASRM, San Diego, California, USA. Program Suppl 2000; 74: P-279

62. Marikinti K, Mathews T, Ball J, et al. Ultrasound and hysteroscopic findings in women with a history of difficult embryo transfer. Presented at the 59th Annual Meeting of the ASRM, San Antonio, Texas, USA. Program Suppl 2003; 80 (Suppl 3): 14

63. Yanushpolsky EH, Ginsburg ES, Fox JH, et al. Tortuous and stenotic endocervical canal: what can be done to provide for easier access to the endometrial cavity. Presented at the 54th Annual Meeting of the ASRM, San Francisco, California, USA. Program Suppl 1998; 70: P631

64. Goldenberg M, Bider D, Ben-Rafael Z, et al. Hysteroscopy in a program of in vitro fertilization. J In Vitro Fert Embryo Transf 1991; 8: 336–8

65. Kucuk T, Pabaccu R, Atay V, et al. Hysteroscopic evaluation and treatment after difficult transcervical embryo transfer. Presented at the 54th Annual Meeting of the ASRM, San Francisco, California, USA. Program Suppl 1998; 70: P1216

66. Noyes N, Licciardi F, Grifo J, et al. In vitro fertilisation outcome relative to embryo transfer difficulty: a novel approach to the forbidding cervix. Fertil Steril 1999; 72: 261–5

67. Dicker D, Ashkenazi J, Feldberg D. The value of repeat hysteroscopic evaluation in patients with failed in vitro fertilization transfer cycles. Fertil Steril 1992; 58: 833–5

68. Alatas C, Urman B, Aksoy S, et al. Evaluation of uterine cavity by sonohysterography in women scheduled for intracytoplasmic sperm injection. Hum Reprod 1998; 13: 2461–2

69. Pandian Z, Bhattacharya S, Nikolaou D, et al. The effectiveness of IVF in unexplained infertility; a systematic Cochrane review. 2002. Hum Reprod 2003; 18: 2001–7

70. Dicker D, Goldman JA, Ashkenazi J, et al. The value of hysteroscopy in elderly women prior to in vitro fertilization-embryo transfer (IVF-ET): a comparative study. J In Vitro Fert Embryo Transfer 1990; 7: 267–70

71. Nyboe Andersen A, Gianaroli L, Nygren KG. European IVF-monitoring programme; European Society of Human Reproduction and Embryology. Assisted reproductive technology in Europe, 2000. Results generated from European registers by ESHRE. Hum Reprod 2004; 19: 490–503

72. Milki AA, Mooney SB. Does hysteroscopy immediately prior to stimulation affect IVF outcome? Presented at the 56th Annual Meeting of the ASRM, San Diego, California, USA. Program Suppl 2000; 74: P-373

73. Gillespie HW. The therapeutic aspect of hysterosalpingography. Br J Radiol 2000; 38: 301–4

74. Takahashi K, Mukaida T, Tomiyama T, et al. High pregnancy rate after hysteroscopy with irrigation in uterine cavity prior to blastocyst transfer in patients who have failed to conceive after blastocyst transfer. Presented at the 56th Annual Meeting of the ASRM, San Diego, California, USA. Program Suppl 2000; 74: P-355

75. Barash A, Dekel N, Fieldust S, et al. Local injury to the endometrium doubles the incidence of successful pregnancies in patients undergoing in vitro fertilization. Fertil Steril 2003; 79: 1317–22

76. Chiba H, Mori E, Morioka Y, et al. Stress of female infertility: relations to length of treatment. Gynecol Obstet Invest 1997; 43: 171–7

77. Olivius C, Friden B, Borg G, et al. Why do couples discontinue in vitro fertilization treatment? A cohort study. Fertil Steril 2004; 81: 258–61

78. Bryson CA, Sykes DH, Traub AI. In vitro fertilization: a long-term follow-up after treatment failure. Hum Fertil (Camb) 2000; 3: 214–20

79. Feichtinger W. Preimplantation diagnosis (PGD) – a European clinician's point of view. J Assist Reprod Genet 2004; 21: 15–17

80. Gardner DK, Surrey E, Minjarez D, et al. Single blastocyst transfer: a prospective randomised trial. Fertil Steril 2004; 81: 551–5

81. Gerris J, De Neubourg D, Mangelschots K, et al. Prevention of twin pregnancy after in-vitro fertilization or intracytoplasmic sperm injection based on strict embryo criteria: a prospective randomised clinical trial. Hum Reprod 1999; 14: 2581–7

82. Goldschlag DE, Kump LM, Schattman GL, et al. Uterine anomalies are associated with decreased delivery rates and increased embryo wastage. Presented at the 54th Annual Meeting of the ASRM, San Francisco, California, USA. Program Suppl 1998; 70: P-069

83. Shamma FN, Lee G, Gutmann JN, Lavy G. The role of office hysteroscopy in in vitro fertilization. Fertil Steril 1992; 58: 1237–9

84. Shushan A, Rojansky N. Should hysteroscopy be part of the basic infertility workup? Hum Reprod 1999; 14: 1923–4

85. La Sala GB, Montanari R, Dessanti L, et al. The role of diagnostic hysteroscopy and endometrial biopsy in assisted reproductive technologies. Fertil Steril 1998; 70: 378–80

86. Sylvestre C, Child TJ, Tulandi T, et al. A prospective study to evaluate the efficacy of two-and three-dimensional sonohysterography in women with intrauterine lesions. Fertil Steril 2003; 79: 1222–5

87. de Kroon CD, Jansen FW, Louwre LA, et al. Technology assessment of saline contrast hysterosonography. Am J Obstet Gynecol 2003; 188: 945–9

7

Historical perspectives in the management of fertility and the use of gonadotropins

Bruno Lunenfeld and Kay Elder

INTRODUCTION

So God created man in His own image, in the image of God created He him; male and female created He them. And God blessed them, and God said unto them: Be fruitful and multiply and replenish the earth and subdue it (Genesis 1:27–28).

In the Judeo-Christian tradition, the importance of procreation is inherent in man's very creation; both Old and New Testaments of the Bible refer to the tragic plight of barren women, eloquently describing the pain and agony of women experiencing difficulties with conception. Rachel's desperate plea to her husband Jacob, 'Give me children or else I will die' (Genesis 30:1), demonstrates the anguish of the childless woman, and when she did conceive, her cry that 'God hath taken away my reproach' is evidence of the stigma that childlessness carried at the time – and for many centuries thereafter. The story of Hanna (Samuel 1:2–20) is probably the first description of anorexia nervosa, successfully treated by the reduction of stress and distress; perhaps the priest Eli demonstrates the first example of psychotherapy in the management of stress-induced infertility. In the Bible, children are a joy, and their lack is a joy denied: 'Behold, children are a heritage from the Lord, the fruit of the womb is a reward' (Psalm 127:3). In the Old Testament a number

of sins are punished by infertility: If a man lies with his uncle's wife…They shall bear their sin; they shall die childless (Leviticus 20:21). There is only one mention of a woman who remained childless, and this was probably due to marital disharmony, as a result of the fact that, 'David danced naked in front of the maids': 'Therefore Michal the daughter of Saul had no children to the day of her death' (Samuel II 6: 23).

'You shall be blessed above all people; there shall not be a male or female barren among you or among your livestock' (Deuteronomy 6:14). This blessing indicates the importance given to fertility, emphasizing that fertility (of men, women and livestock) was essential for survival, and a symbol of wealth. Promotion of fertility, regulating sexual activity to optimize conception, was practiced according to the hygienic laws of the Bible (Leviticus 12), later modified by the Talmud (Niddah Tractate). Women were forbidden to have intercourse during the time of menstruation, and for 7 days thereafter. Intercourse was then to take place, after a ritual bath, at mid-cycle; it seems that the ancient Jews had observed that these were the most fertile days of the cycle.

However, records dated far earlier than the Bible confirm that fertility has been a constant fundamental priority and preoccupation, in all societies, throughout the ages of man. Fertility symbols are clearly identified in the relics of prehistoric times, of ancient civilizations in all parts of the world, a recognition of the concept that man's existence depends upon the renewal of fertility. Since the dawn of civilization, societies have developed beliefs about how to cure infertility, including prayers to deities or lucky dolls, and visits to sacred places (Figure 1). The choice of wells, springs or rivers reflects an awareness of rain and water as having power to regenerate the parched and barren earth.

The *Vedas*, ancient Sanskrit texts of Hindu wisdom that were first put into writing 5000 years ago, include an acknowledgment that men can also suffer the anguish of childlessness, as described in King Citraketu's Lamentation:

As a person aggrieved by hunger and thirst is not pleased by the external gratification of flower garlands or sandalwood pulp, I am not pleased with my empire, opulence or possessions, which are desirable even for great demigods, because I have no son.

Therefore, O great sage, please save me and my forefathers, who are descending to the darkness of hell because I have no progeny. Kindly do something so that I may have a son to deliver us from hellish conditions (Srimad Bhagavatam, Canto 6, Chapter 14 Sanskrit, original translation by Swami Prabhupâda).

Prayers for subsequent fertility are found in initiation rites and in marriage ceremonies; in India, childless women visited the Temple of Siva in order to press their naked body against the huge lingam, or phallus, of the god's statue.

EARLY RECORDS

The first systematic records that deal with fertility to be studied were Egyptian papyrus documents: the Kahun Gynecological Papyrus (1825 BC) devotes approximately 25 pages to a range of interesting cures for women's ailments[1]. Diagnosis was based on the premise that the genital organs were in continuity with the rest of the body, and in particular with the digestive tract, a concept that was subsequently embraced by Hippocrates and medieval physicians. Magic played a fundamental role in Egyptian medicine, and infertile women had their own goddess, Nephtys. Despite their preoccupation with infertility, the only remedies prescribed by their physicians relied

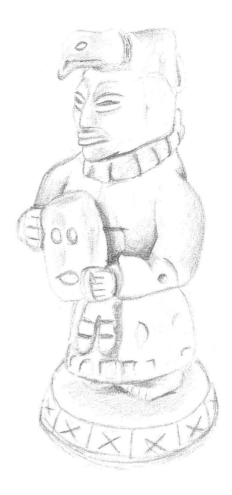

Figure 1 Ix Chel, Mother Goddess of Medicine, Fertility and the Moon, was a significant deity of the classic pre-Columbian Maya culture, one of the greatest and most extraordinary civilizations of ancient history. Ix Chel's shrine at San Gervasio on Cozumel, Mexico's 'Island of Swallows', was a site of pilgrimage, where young girls on reaching puberty traveled from the mainland to participate in ritual cleansing and prayers which would ensure their future fertility. (Image of a statue in Cozumel, sketched by Bethany Hughes)

upon faith in their gods, amulets and magic recipes, but they were able to diagnose early pregnancy (with an accuracy of 40%) by treating grains of wheat with the urine of pregnant women: 'You must put wheat and barley in a cloth bag. The woman is to urinate on it daily…. If both germinate, she will bear…' This method was adopted by Hippocrates, and was used in some parts of the world up to the 19th century[2]. The scientific basis behind this early pregnancy test was suggested by the observation that human chorionic gonadotropin (hCG) promotes adventitious root production in cuttings of *Begonia semperflorens* and *Vitis vinifera*[3].

Amongst his many treatises on medicine, Hippocrates (460–377 BC) included several books about gynecology and obstetrics, offering numerous treatments for the problem of infertility: *Diseases of Women, The Nature of Women, The Generating Seed and the Nature of the Child*[4]. Many of the diagnostic recipes he recommended were based upon those of the Egyptians, infused with magic and religion. Soranos of Ephesus (177–98 BC) practiced medicine in Rome at the time of Trajan and Hadrian, and his book *Gynaecology* defined structured principles of anatomy, physiology, obstetrics and gynecological pathologies[5].

The next recorded advance in knowledge about infertility came from the Arab school, AD 700–1200. Avicenna, or Ibn Sina (AD 980–1037) was a Persian physician, philosopher and scientist who wrote 450 books on many subjects, including *The Book of Healing* and *The Canon of Medicine (Qanun)*. His writings introduced the concept that infertility could be masculine or feminine in origin; it could be due to an abnormality of the genital tract, or to psychological troubles such as melancholy or apprehension[6]. However, the diagnostic techniques and remedies suggested were based upon those of the Greeks and Egyptians[7,8].

THE MIDDLE AGES AND RENAISSANCE

Medieval medicine was largely based upon that of the Greeks, and on the treatises of Hippocrates in particular. The perception of infertility was influenced by religious attitudes, and especially by the role of women in medieval society. In the 13th century, St Thomas Aquinas wrote that nature 'seeks the generation of children to preserve the good of the species'[9]. Infertility was considered to be a divine punishment, in particular for transgression of the laws of marriage – the consequence of sins committed, blasphemy and infidelity. Lack of children was regarded as a real threat, particularly by the aristocracy, who were concerned about preserving the family line. Fasting and prayer, appealing for divine intercession, were recommended. St Anne is the patron saint of infertile couples, and there were numerous rituals to be followed. A large variety of treatments were used, such as fumigation, purging and pessaries. Remedies included the liver or testicles of a young hare or stag, rabbit's blood, mare's

milk and sheep's urine, as well as plant remedies: mandrake and *Artemisia*, and nettle poultices applied to the womb[10].

This era was followed by a period of scientific progress during the Renaissance, particularly in Italy. Leonardo da Vinci's beautiful drawings illustrated detailed anatomy, and Vesale published his atlas *Humani Corporis Fabrica* in 1543, which included cross-sections of the female pelvis. The tubes, clitoris, vagina and placenta were described by Fallope, and the ovary and follicles by De Graaf in 1672[11]. Contributions to the field of infertility continued between the 17th and 19th centuries, with publications from Naboth[12], von Leeuwenhoek[13] and many others[8]. Marion Sims (1813–83) wrote about causes and treatments for infertility, including 'The microscope as an aid in the diagnosis and treatment of sterility'[14], an early reference to semen assessment as an infertility investigation.

THE 20TH CENTURY

Further diagnostic methods began to emerge at the beginning of the 20th century; Huhner recommended the postcoital test in 1937[15], and methods of tubal insufflation were devised to diagnose tubal obstruction[16]. Nevertheless, management of infertility remained empirical right up to the middle of the century. Knowledge about the physiological mechanisms governing reproduction was incomplete, and the therapeutic armamentarium was inadequate.

In 1905 Halberstaedter introduced the first 'site oriented therapy': X-irradiation targeting the ovarian region of the pelvis[17]. In 1926 Beclere reported that Roentgen irradiation of the pituitary had a beneficial effect[18], and X-irradiation of both the ovarian and the pituitary regions was then advocated for the relief of 'functional sterility' in the female[19]. Ovarian and pituitary irradiation was widely practiced in the USA as a treatment for infertile women, with reported success published over a 25-year period[19–21]. In 1949 Rita Finkler declared: 'Irradiation of the ovarian and pituitary regions for the relief of functional sterility in the female is a universally accepted therapeutic procedure'[22]. The benefits of radiation therapy compared with endocrine therapy (pregnant mare's serum and hCG) were demonstrated in a study of 130 patients who underwent irradiation of the ovaries and pituitary at a dose of 200 kV (a unit of electricity, not radiation). This treatment was reported as less expensive, easier to administer and requiring shorter treatment regimens than endocrine therapy[22]. The author concluded that the cumulative conception rates were independent of the treatment administered, 34.2% in patients receiving hormonal therapy and 35.2% in those receiving radiation therapy. In patients suffering from secondary amenorrhea, menstrual bleeding was re-established in 40.6% of those receiving hormonal therapy and 46.4% of those receiving radiation therapy[22]. Today we may assume that the 'positive result' was due to radiation-induced increased blood flow and hyperemia. Unfortunately, such radiation treatment remained a universally accepted procedure until 1949[20,21], and the price of this therapy was not seen until 45 years later. During the mid-1980s, an increased rate in the incidence of ovarian cancer was reported by the National Institutes of Health, with a mortality about 10% higher than that expected (based on expected rates for New York City). This observation was sadly traced back to an iatrogenic origin, X-irradiation of the ovaries[23,24], a reminder that application of the 'precautionary principle' is crucial in medical therapies.

THE INTRODUCTION OF GONADOTROPINS

As early as the second century BC, the Chinese were already anticipating modern biochemistry, isolating sex and pituitary hormones from human urine and using them for medicinal purposes. The crystals that they obtained were traditionally called 'autumn mineral', a term coined by the prince of Haua-Nan sometime before 125 BC, likening the white color and crystalline appearance to the hoar frost of the autumn[25]. Several centuries later, explicit recipes for the preparation of autumn mineral began to appear in print. To our knowledge, the first such recipe was published in 1025, in the book *Ching Yen Fang* [*Valuable tried and tested prescriptions*], written by the physician Chang Sheng-Tao[25,26]. Between AD 1025 and 1833, at least ten different methods of obtaining sex and pituitary hormones from urine were published in 39 different books. These hormones were produced on an enormous scale, using hundreds of gallons of human urine for each batch, manufacturing countless thousands of doses of the drugs for medicinal use (Figure 2). An astonishing technique was applied in hormone

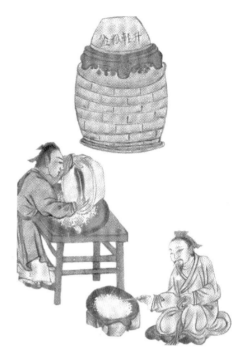

Figure 2 The process of sublimation used to collect pure crystals of human sex and pituitary hormones from human urine. The figure on the left gently brushes crystals from the sublimation lid with a feather. Two to three ounces of hormone crystals could be produced from 150 gallons of human urine. Illustration from *Essentials of the Pharmacopoeia Ranked According to Nature and Efficacy*, edited by Liu Wen T'ai in 1505. (Biblioteca Nazionale Centrale Vittorio Emanuele II, Rome)

extraction: the use of gypsum (calcium sulfate) to precipitate the hormones out of the urine. This technique was probably derived from the bean-curd industry, which uses gypsum to produce the curd. The most surprising and impressive substance used to precipitate the hormones out of solution was 'the juice of soap beans', an extract from a saponin-containing plant, *Gleditschia sinensis*. The saponins, or natural soap, as well as the proteins of the soap beans, were remarkably successful in precipitating the hormones in urine into a sediment. The earliest published method using natural soaps in this way dates from AD 1110[27].

Pituitary as well as sex hormones may have been isolated. The gonadotropins themselves would have stimulated the production of steroids by the gonads, so that by giving patients autumn mineral the ancient Chinese doctors might have felt that they were administering a 'double treatment' – the steroids themselves, and stimulants for the patient to produce more endogenous steroids. The Chinese used these hormones to treat a wide variety of ailments relating to the sex organs, including hypogonadism, impotence and sexual debility, and even to stimulate the growth of the beard. There are a number of unanswered questions about the ancient Chinese hormones, but there is no doubt whatsoever that the Chinese founded the science of endocrinology, and are entitled to the credit for that great achievement.

EARLY UNDERSTANDING OF THE HYPOTHALAMIC–PITUITARY–OVARIAN AXIS

In the Western world, however, the first experimental evidence suggesting that the pituitary had a role in regulating the gonads stemmed from the studies of Crowe and his co-workers. They showed that partial pituitary ablation resulted in atrophy of the genital organs in adult dogs, and a persistence of infantilism and sexual inadequacy in puppies[28]. Thus, by 1910 these early studies launched the idea that the reproductive organs were governed by the pituitary gland.

Two years later, Aschner confirmed these findings and also postulated that pituitary function depends upon the function of higher centers in the brain. He observed that men and women with diseases, tumors or injuries of the hypophysis, pituitary stalk and centers including and above the medulla oblongata suffered hypopituitarism and, consequently, gonadal atrophy[29]. He further demonstrated that sectioning of the pituitary stalk affected the genital organs, and therefore hypothesized that pituitary extracts may affect the gonads. He postulated that their use might have practical applications.

Another 15 years were to elapse before two different groups independently discovered the 'gonadotrophic principle'. In 1926, Smith showed that daily implants of fresh anterior pituitary gland tissue from mice, rats, cats, rabbits and guinea pigs into immature male and female mice and rats rapidly induced precocious sexual maturity, marked enlargement of the ovaries and superovulation[30,31]. In the same year, Zondek implanted anterior pituitary glands from adult cows, bulls and humans into immature animals, and this evoked the rapid development of sexual puberty[32]. These pioneering experiments revealed that ovarian function is regulated by the pituitary. In 1927 Smith demonstrated that hypophysectomized immature male or female rats and mice failed to mature sexually, and that removal of the pituitary gland from

adult animals without injury to the brain resulted in profound atrophy of genital organs, rapid regression of sexual characteristics and total loss of reproductive function in both sexes[33,34].

Only 2 years later, Zondek proposed the idea that the pituitary secretes two hormones that stimulate the gonads. He named these biological substances 'Prolan A' and 'Prolan B'[35]. The word 'Prolan' is probably derived from the Latin word 'proles', which means 'descendant'. By introducing this name, Zondek undoubtedly wished to imply that these substances were the 'spiritus movens' of sexual function, the master hormones that control all the gonadal sex hormones, and are therefore responsible for maintaining the species.

In 1930 Zondek[36] then showed that the blood and urine of postmenopausal women contained gonadotropins. He postulated that Prolan A stimulated follicular growth, that Prolan A together with Prolan B stimulated the secretion of 'foliculin', and that Prolan B induced ovulation, the formation of the corpus luteum and the secretion of lutein and foliculin. These two hormones induced glandular transformation of the endometrium, with endometrial proliferation, and also caused changes in the vaginal epithelium. Zondek realized that the dynamics of Prolan A secretion by the anterior pituitary and the correct timing of Prolan B discharge are responsible for the rhythm of ovarian function: this in turn controlled the proliferation and function of the endometrium to create optimal conditions for nidation of the fertilized egg (Figure 3). If we merely change the names of Prolan A and B to follicle stimulating hormone (FSH) and luteinizing hormone (LH), and the names of foliculin and lutein to estrogen and progesterone, we can see that by 1930 Zondek had described the pituitary–gonadal relationship as we know it today. This hypothesis was confirmed a year later with the extraction of two different hormones from the pituitary, one of which acted as a follicle stimulating factor and one as a luteinizing factor[37].

THE DISCOVERY OF HUMAN CHORIONIC GONADOTROPIN

In 1927 Ascheim and Zondek[38] demonstrated that the blood and urine of pregnant women contained a gonad-stimulating substance; injecting this substance subcutaneously into intact immature female mice

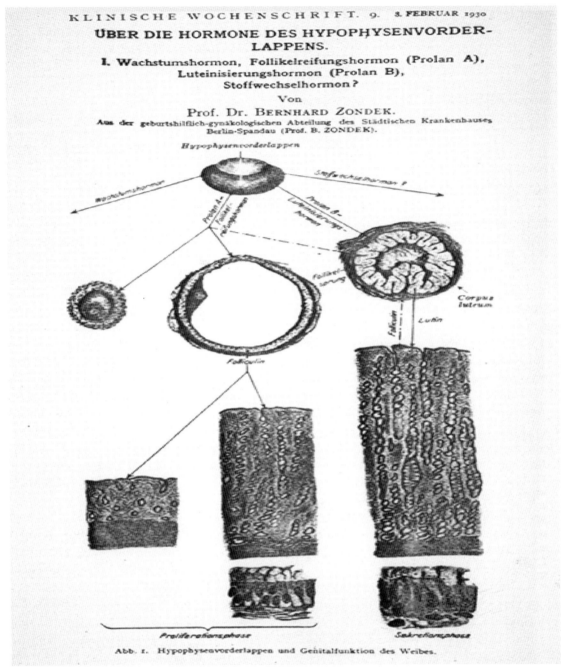

Figure 3 Zondek's illustration of the relationship between the hypothalamus, pituitary, ovaries and endometrium. Reproduced from reference 36

produced follicular maturation, luteinization and hemorrhage into the ovarian stroma. This became known as the Ascheim–Zondek pregnancy test. Ascheim and Zondek believed that this gonadotropic substance was produced by the anterior pituitary. Subsequent work by Seegar-Jones and colleagues [39] showed that this gonadotropin was produced *in vitro* in placental tissue culture, proving conclusively that the placenta and not the pituitary was responsible for the elaboration of the hormone. This gonad-stimulating property was exhibited by the chorionic villi, and was especially marked in the cytotrophoblastic Langerhans cells.

Marius Tausk's book on the history of Organon[40] describes the gonadotropic hormone hCG (extracted from human placentas) as being very similar to the pituitary hormone 'Prolan B' = LH. Organon launched this extract on the market in 1931, under the name 'Pregnon'. However, because of similarity with another trademark, the name was later changed to 'Pregnyl'. Pregnyl was released in 1932, when regulatory authorities for the evaluation and approval of medicines did not yet exist, and has survived until the present day. According to Tausk this preparation was used for 'stimulation of the ovaries' at first, and the initial hCG products were calibrated in animal units. A rat unit was defined as the smallest amount that produced vaginal opening together with estrus when injected into female immature rats. The International Standard for hCG was established in 1939, under the auspices of the League of Nations. The international unit (IU) was defined arbitrarily as the activity contained in 0.1 mg of the standard preparation. Purified urinary preparations of hCG became available in 1940[41]. Urine obtained during the first half of pregnancy (when hCG titers are highest) is chilled, filtered and acidified to pH 3.5 with glacial acetic acid. The clear filtrate is percolated through a column containing Permutit, and adsorption is complete when 10 l of urine per hour are passed through a 4-in diameter column containing 2 kg of Permutit. The active principle is eluted from the column with an alcoholic solution of ammonium acetate, and the hormone is precipitated from the eluate by increasing the concentration of alcohol. The potency of these preparations ranged from 6000 to 8500 IU/mg[42]. Clinical studies with hCG began as early as 1933[43], and were summarized by the same author 15 years later[44]; women who were scheduled for non-gynecological abdominal surgery were injected with hCG, and the ovaries were inspected during the operation. When hCG was administered in the follicular phase of the cycle, their ovaries showed no evidence of follicle stimulation, ovulation or corpus luteum formation, i.e. in the absence of FSH, no visual effect of hCG could be seen. Hamblen and Ross confirmed these results in 1937[44].

THE INTRODUCTION OF HOG AND SHEEP GONADOTROPINS FOR CLINICAL USE

These early discoveries revealing the physiological action of gonadotropins in the normal ovarian cycle

tempted many scientists to seek gonadotropic extracts with sufficient purity to allow their use in the treatment of infertile patients suffering from gonadotropin insufficiency. In 1930, gonadotropins extracted from swine pituitaries were produced by IG Farbenindustrie AG, Leverkusen, Germany, and used clinically to treat patients.

Several years later a hog preparation became available from The Armour Laboratories, and GD Searle then produced a commercially available sheep pituitary FSH preparation (Gonadophysin)[45]. Two animal pituitary gonadotropin extracts are quoted in the 1959 French drug index[46]: Gonadohormone (Laboratoires Byla) and Hormone Gonadotrope Hypophysaire Choay (Laboratoires Choay). Both were reimbursed by the French social-security system. Maddock and colleagues[45] described the increase in urinary estrogen excretion during FSH administration. Enlarged cystic ovaries measuring 7–10 cm in diameter were observed in some patients, and clear cysts as large as 2 cm in diameter were seen in other patients; microscopically these were lined with granulosa cells undergoing early lutein changes[45]. In 1959 Netter[47] also described a spectacular increase in urinary estrogen following short treatments (1–3 ampoules of 10 mouse units on alternate days for up to 9 days) with a commercially available animal pituitary gonadotropic extract (Gonadohormone, Laboratoires Byla). Gonadotropin extracts from animal pituitaries continued to be used in Europe and the USA until the early 1960s; their use began to decline after the discovery of a new phenomenon, the 'antihormones'.

Two important monographs were published independently in 1942: 'Antigonadotrophic substances' by Erling Ostergaard[48] and 'The antigonadotrophic factor with consideration of the anti-hormone problem' by Bernard Zondek and Felix Sulman[49]. Both claimed that gonadotropins from animal origin produced 'antihormones', which decreased ovarian responsiveness in humans. An exact quote from the book by Zondek and Sulman reads: 'It was noted in 1930, during chronic treatment with gonadotrophic hormone, that the effector organ, i.e. the ovary, maintains its response only in a limited period of time, at the end of which the response becomes increasingly weaker and finally disappears'. They further stated in the book: 'Chronic treatment of animals with gonadotrophic hormones evokes in them the formation of a new blood substance, called an anti-hormone. This is capable of inactivating gonadotropin hormone both *in vivo* and *in vitro*'. Thus, more than two decades before the nature of immunological phenomena was fully recognized, the authors had actually described the formation of antibodies to animal gonadotropins in women. In 1956, Maddock confirmed this previous work and described the detection of 'Antihormones' between the 44th and 76th days following prolonged treatment with animal pituitary FSH preparations[45]. The 'antihormones' prevented the action of each of the gonadotropins against which they were tested (hog FSH, human pituitary gonadotropin, human chorionic gonadotropin), and remained at detectable levels for 2–3 months after stopping gonadotropin administration. A new treatment course provoked a prompt and striking increase in antihormone titers. Following an editorial by Wilkins[50] that described 'the need for an inhibitor of gonadotropins' for certain gynecological diseases, Maddock and colleagues[45] concluded that 'the induction of antihormone formation by the administration of animal pituitary FSH may have therapeutic applications in cases in which it is desirable to inhibit pituitary gonadotropins'. The significance of this visionary statement was not to be realized for a further 25 years, when gonadotropin releasing hormone (GnRH) was isolated and synthesized[51,52]. This hormone and its analogs were found to stimulate pituitary function when administered in a precise pulsatile fashion, and to inhibit pituitary gonadotropin secretion when administered chronically. These properties led to its use as an ovulation inducer[53] (the first pregnancy was reported by Leyendecker and co-workers in 1980, see Table 1), and also as a method of 'reversible medical gonadectomy' in the treatment of diseases dependent on gonadal steroids[54].

PREGNANT MARE SERUM GONADOTROPIN

Pregnant mare serum gonadotropin (PMSG) is secreted by structures known as endometrial cups in pregnant mares, and was first described by Cole and Hart in 1930[55]. Endometrial cups, circular structures on the surface of the endometrium around the point of attachment of the fetus, secrete a highly viscous gel. PMSG first appears in this gel between days 37 and 42 of pregnancy, and reaches its highest concentration between days 50 and 70. It virtually disappears after the fourth month of gestation. The hormone

produced in the endometrial cups is also present in the blood, and PMSG was prepared by collecting blood from pregnant mares around the 65th day of pregnancy. This procedure involved fractional precipitation with acetone or alcohol, removal of impurities by proper adjustment of acidity (pH 7.0–7.5) and final precipitation of the hormone fraction in the presence of increased concentrations of acetone or alcohol. The hormone fractions were obtained as dry white, water-soluble and remarkably stable powders, and furnished a satisfactory basis for preparing sterile solutions that could be used for laboratory and clinical studies[56]. This material stimulated follicular growth, ovulation and corpus luteum formation in the ovary, and estrus changes in the uterus and vagina. Cartland and Nelson defined their rat unit as the total dose of PMSG which will produce a five-fold increase in ovarian weight.

In 1938 an International Standard for PMSG was established. One IU was defined as 0.25 mg of the standard preparation[57]. Soon afterwards commercial preparations of PMSG appeared on the market. Schering Corporation in the USA marketed 'Anteron', and Organon and Roussell in Europe marketed 'Gestyl' and 'Gonadotropine Serique'. Both preparations were reimbursed by 'social security' in France. Clinical trials in women demonstrated an ovarian response to these gonadotropins[58,59], but attempts to induce ovulation produced inconsistent results. In 1939, Hamblen showed that 'cyclic administration of PMSG during the follicular phase of the cycle, in amounts judged to be adequate, failed to result in progestational bleeding or progestational changes in the endometrium (as judged by endometrial biopsy studies) or in pregnancy'[60,61].

THE TWO-STEP PROTOCOL

The concept of the 'two-step protocol' was introduced in 1941: ovarian stimulation using gonadotropins (PMSG, or hog or sheep pituitary gonadotropins) to stimulate follicular growth and development, followed by the induction of ovulation using hCG. Mazer and Ravetz[62] used 'Synapoidin', a mixture of a human pregnancy urine extract and an extract of animal anterior pituitary lobe tissue (commercially available from Parke, Davis & Co.). The authors state: 'The combination of chorionic gonadotropin and the anterior pituitary extract evoked one or more menstrual flows in

19 of 23 severely amenorrhoeic women, some of whom had not menstruated for years'. The authors also claimed that 'the degree of the ovarian response seems to depend upon the receptivity of the ovaries, the total dosage and the duration of treatment. On the other hand the ovaries of three regularly menstruating young women were over-stimulated to a pathological degree. Each of the ovaries was 8–10 cm in diameter and studded with numerous hemorrhagic follicles which ruptured and bled at the slightest touch'. Thus, as early as 1941, the hyperstimulation syndrome was described.

In 1945 Hamblen and colleagues defined the 'ideal treatment'[63]: 'To permit effective therapy of hypofunctioning ovaries, a gonadotropin should evoke, in sequence, follicle stimulation, ovulation and corpus luteum development, and these phenomena should be in physiologic order compatible with fertility and conception.' They demonstrated that administration of PMSG during the follicular phase, followed by the application of hCG 12–18 days later, resulted in secretory endometrium and pregnancies following correctly planned coitus.

Although the antibody formation provoked by PMSG caused biological neutralization of the injected material, it did not cause anaphylactic shock or severe allergic reactions. PMSG and other gonadotropic preparations from animal pituitary sources were therefore used for many years. Despite the fact that gonadotropins of animal origin (formerly marketed as Synapoidin Steri-Vial in the USA) were shown to produce allergic reactions during the 1940s, approval of the FDA (Food and Drug Administration, USA) for Synapoidin Steri-Vial was not withdrawn until July 6, 1972 (see the Federal Register of July 6, 1972:37 FR 13284). As late as 1962, Folistiman (VEB Arneimittel-werk, Dresden), a highly purified, standardized FSH preparation from pig pituitaries, was introduced on the East German market. These preparations were used in the hope that perhaps ovulation and consequent pregnancy could be evoked within the first few months of treatment, before the immune response and its consequences had fully developed. A number of pregnancies were indeed reported[64–68]. Daume compared the results of ovulation induction by sheep gonadotropin extract with those obtained using human menopausal urinary gonadotropin[67]. The pregnancy rate per treatment cycle was 11.5% and 12.7% for the animal and human preparations, respectively. Groot-Wassink and Blawert compared the results (pregnancy rate) of an animal and a human FSH preparation[68], and found that gonadotropins derived from animal sources gave significantly better results. They explained this difference on the basis that poor results obtained with preparations derived from human sources were due to an excess of LH: the FSH/LH ratio was 11:1 in the human preparation, and 70:1 in the animal preparation. Groot-Wassink and Blawert were the first to claim that excessive LH could have adverse effects on reproductive performance[68].

PMSG eventually had to be withdrawn from the market because of the potential dangers as a consequence of provoking antibody formation. However, animal gonadotropins under the trade name Folistiman (VEB Arzneimittelwerk) were still available in some eastern European countries until 1998. Recognizing that animal gonadotropins might produce antibodies in humans which could neutralize not only the preparation applied, but also the endogenous gonadotropins, scientific and technological efforts were focused on extracting and purifying gonadotropins from human sources.

During the summer of 1953, Dr Rudi Borth and myself (Bruno Lunenfeld), with the help of Professor H. de Watteville, invited a number of scientists to Geneva to exchange information and coordinate research on gonadotropins. Egon Diczfalusy, Jim Brown, John Loraine and others were amongst those invited. The 'G Club' was founded during this meeting, and the basic and clinical goals of gonadotropic research defined. These included development of specific assay procedures, as well as bioassay standards and purification methods required to obtain gonadotropic preparations suitable for therapeutic purposes.

HUMAN PITUITARY GONADOTROPIN

In 1958 Carl Gemzell extracted gonadotropins from human pituitary glands[69]. The lyophilized glands were extracted with calcium oxide solution, and gonadotropins precipitated with ammonium sulfate, dissolved in water, dialysed and lyophilized. The clinical results achieved with the use of this preparation were published in 1958[69]. In 1961 Buxton and Hermann tested a pituitary FSH preparation prepared by Merck & Co. from lyophilized pituitaries. Gonadotropins were extracted with 40% ethanol and precipitated by increasing the alcohol concentration[70]. In 1963 Bettendorf[71,72] demonstrated that ovarian stimulation is possible in hypophysectomized individuals.

Between 1958 and 1988, human pituitary gonadotropin preparations were successfully used for ovulation induction in the treatment of ovulation disturbances in several centers throughout the world. However, it soon became clear that the reservoir of human pituitaries was too limited to cover the constantly growing demand for gonadotropin preparations. Moreover, more than 20 years after its commercial introduction, human pituitary gonadotropin (hPG) made the headlines when cases of a fatal prion disease (transmissible spongiform encephalopathy, TSE), iatrogenic Creutzfeld–Jakob disease (CJD), were discovered and linked to the use of hPG or human pituitary growth hormone; cases of CJD were identified in Australia, in France and in the UK[73,74]. The disease has a very long incubation period, presenting with dementia, ataxia and psychiatric symptoms 10 years or more later; the consequences of its transmission are therefore not recognized until long after the hormones have been administered. This very long incubation period means that individuals who are infected but do not yet display symptoms of the disease may serve as a reservoir of CJD or new variant (nv) CJD that may be transmitted to other patients iatrogenically.

It is interesting to note that none of these cases arose from the use of pituitary extracts (products) registered by pharmaceutical companies. They were traced to the use of products produced by government agencies: the Pituitary Agency in Australia, the Pituitary Agency in the UK and France-Hypophyse. hPG was subsequently withdrawn from the market, bringing another era in the history of gonadotropin use to an end.

HUMAN MENOPAUSAL GONADOTROPIN

Human menopausal gonadotropins were purified and isolated from crude extracts of large urine pools, and a number of extraction and concentration procedures were proposed. The method of Bradbury and colleagues[75], modified by Albert[76], used kaolin for adsorption and acetone for precipitation of proteins (gonadotropins), and this method was accepted by

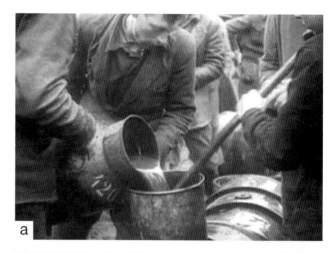

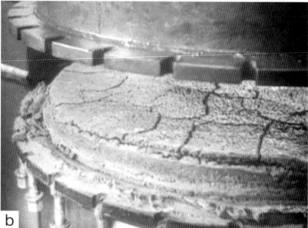

Figure 4 Extraction of gonadotropins from menopausal urine. (a) Collection of pooled urine. (b) Menopausal urine filtered through a kaolin cake

many laboratories and used successfully for many years, with minor variations (Figure 4). After numerous significant alterations, this procedure was subsequently used to produce considerable amounts of human menopausal gonadotropins for clinical use. Production of human menopausal gonadotropins (hMG) is a relatively simple procedure[77–79]. Menopausal urine is mixed with activated kaolin and shaken, and the suspension is left to settle at room temperature and then centrifuged. The supernatant is discarded, and the kaolin cake is eluted twice with $1\,mol/l\ NH_4$. The eluate containing adsorbed urinary proteins, including gonadotropins, is washed thoroughly and acidified to pH 5.5 and the proteins are then precipitated with acetone. The precipitate, after washing with acetone, ethanol and ether, is subjected to treatment with diethylaminoethyl cellulose and passed through a

Permutit chromatography column. The pH must be accurately controlled during all production stages to ensure a good yield of gonadotropins: pH must be around 4.0 at the adsorption phase and between 11.0 and 11.5 during the elution phase. Final stages of production include washing, filtering, adjustment of the FSH and LH contents and lyophilization. The first hMG preparation for clinical use 'Pergonal 25 Serono', was registered in Italy on 22 May, 1950. The definition of one unit was based upon the capacity of the product to induce estrus in 28-day-old prepubertal female rats. In 1953, hMG was successfully used for ovarian stimulation of hypophysectomized rats[80]. The second meeting of the 'G Club' took place in Birmingham during 1955, and a large batch of a menopausal urine kaolin extract (hMG 20) donated by Dr J. Dekansky from Organon Newhouse in Scotland was designated as a laboratory standard. In 1957 Borth and co-workers described the transition from animal units to the expression of results in relation to reference preparations[81,82]. The unit was initially defined in relation to the reference preparations hMG 20, hMG 20a and hMG 24[83,84]. By 1959 most of the reference preparation hMG 24 had been used, and Dr Dekansky could not make available the amount originally agreed upon. Dr Donini from Serono declared his willingness to donate 50 g of the preparation 'Pergonal 23', and this material became the 'International Reference Preparation' (IRP-hMG) for the quantitation of hMG[85]. Clinical trials using hMG preparations were then initiated. The purity of the available preparations was only 5%, containing both FSH and LH. However, in the absence of an alternative, they were accepted by both the regulatory agencies and the scientific community. In 1960 the use of this preparation in humans led to the expected and desirable changes in endometrium, vaginal epithelium and steroid excretion[86]. In 1961 we noted that amenorrheic hypogonadotropic women needed 6.8–13.6 mg of Pergonal, depending on individual sensitivity (120–240 mg equivalent of the International Reference Preparation), in order to stimulate their ovaries to produce estrogens[87]. Thereafter the first successful induction of ovulation followed by pregnancies in hypogonadotropic anovulatory women was reported, using a sequential step-up/step-down regimen. The starting dose in these women was 240 mg IRP-hMG daily, increased to 360 mg and then to 480 mg IRP-hMG, and then gradually reduced to 360 mg and finally to 240 mg IRP-hMG daily.

Ovulation was induced by administration of 10 000 IU of hCG followed by 10 000 and 5000 IU of hCG on consecutive days (Figure 5). This hCG dose was sufficient to maintain corpus luteum function until endogenous hCG appeared about 13 days later[88-90]. These results were confirmed by Palmer and Dorangeon[91] in France, and Rosenberg and colleagues[92] in the USA. In 1964 the World Health Organization (WHO) Expert Committee of Biological Standardization defined the international unit (IU) for FSH and the IU for interstitial cell stimulating hormone (ICSH) (LH) as the respective activities contained in 0.2295 mg of the IRP-hMG[93].

A retrospective conversion of IRP-hMG to IU of FSH and LH showed that the doses used were between 55 and 110 IU/daily injection. Following numerous reports of the successful induction of ovulation, Pergonal 75 was registered in Israel in 1963 and in Italy in 1965. One ampoule of this hMG preparation contained approximately 75 IU of FSH and 75 IU of LH as measured by standard bioassays.

In 1972 the WHO convened a scientific group meeting in Geneva, chaired by Professor Lunenfeld. During this meeting guidelines for the diagnosis and management of infertile couples were developed[93,94]. The effective daily dose for hypogonadotropic patients was reported to be in the range of 150–225 IU, and for anovulatory normogonadotropic patients 75–150 IU. It was also noted that the ratio of FSH to LH varies in different hMG and hPG preparations, but the available evidence indicated that preparations with ratios of 0.1–10 were acceptable therapeutic agents provided that a sufficient total dose of FSH was administered to the patient. During this time, Steptoe and Edwards had begun their pioneering in vitro fertilization (IVF) collaboration, and used hMG in their early attempts to recover oocytes by laparoscopy. In failing to achieve any pregnancies, they later reverted to natural cycles (see Chapter 1 by Edwards), until the pioneering work of Howard and Georgeanna Jones[95-97] established the use of hMG as the standard procedure for ovarian stimulation in assisted reproductive technologies (ART). The subsequent development of ovarian stimulation regimens is detailed in other chapters of this book (Chapters 9 and 10).

Two years later, in 1975, the WHO Expert Committee of Biological Standardization met (TRS 293), and noted that 'since preparations of hMG are administered to man in many countries, it is desirable

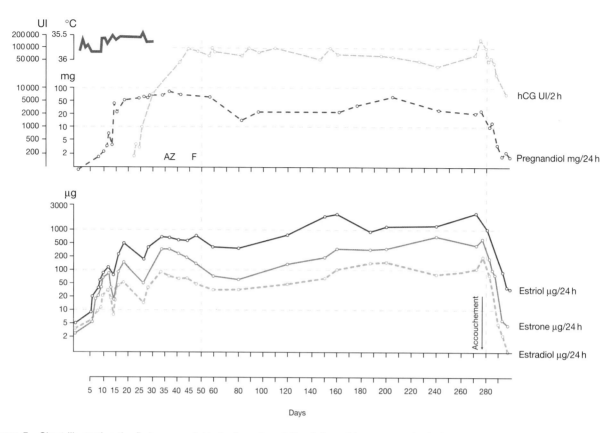

Figure 5 Chart illustrating the first successful induction of ovulation followed by pregnancies in hypogonadotropic anovulatory women, using a sequential step-up/step-down regimen. The starting dose of 240 mg (55 IU) International Reference Preparation-human menopausal gonadotropin (IRP-hMG) daily was increased to 360 mg, and then to 480 mg (110 IU) IRP-hMG, gradually reduced to 360 and finally to 240 mg IRP-hMG daily. Ovulation was induced by administration of 10 000 IU of human chorionic gonadotropin (hCG) followed by 10 000 and 5000 IU of hCG on consecutive days. Reproduced from reference 89

to have an international standard for the control of potency of such preparations'. The Committee defined the international unit for human urinary FSH for bioassay as the activity contained in 0.11388 mg and the international unit for human urinary LH (ICSH) for bioassay as the activity contained in 0.13369 mg of the International Standard. The committee also stressed that the new standard, future standards and preparations calibrated against it should have their separate activities (FSH and LH (ICSH)) individually assessed.

The Steelman and Pohley assay for FSH estimation[98] became the gold standard. In this assay, a group of immature rats are injected subcutaneously three times daily for 3 days with hCG AT different doses of the International Standard of FSH, and a second group of animals is injected with the preparation to be tested. Autopsy is performed 72 h after the first injection, at which time the ovaries are dissected and weighed

(Figure 6). The FSH content of the preparation is calculated from the curve obtained with the standard (Figure 7). When preparations with varying FSH/LH ratios were tested by this method, the LH content did not interfere[99]. However, although the assay method is specific, its precision depends on the number of animals used and is relatively low even with large numbers. A source of homogeneous FSH that could be standardized with respect to mass and bioactivity[100] would bring a significant advantage.

THE SEARCH FOR PURE PREPARATIONS

In the early 1970s, clinicians began to voice the opinion that different patient groups and individuals may need different treatment regimens, with variations in protocols and in dosages of FSH and LH. Such individually adjusted treatment regimens would

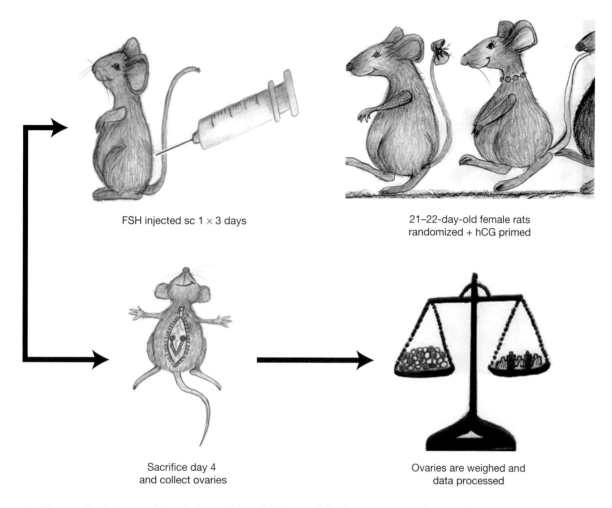

FSH injected sc 1 × 3 days

21–22-day-old female rats
randomized + hCG primed

Sacrifice day 4
and collect ovaries

Ovaries are weighed and
data processed

Figure 6 Diagramatic illustration of the Steelman–Pohley follicle stimulating hormone (FSH) bioassay. A group of immature rats is injected subcutaneously (sc) with (hCG), and then injected with the international standard of FSH once daily for 3 days; a second group of animals is injected with the same amount of hCG, and then with the preparation to be tested once daily for 3 days. Autopsy is performed 72 h after the first injection, at which time the ovaries are dissected and weighed

require therapeutic gonadotropin preparations that contained pure, or almost pure, FSH and LH. Attempts to separate FSH from LH in gonadotropin extracts were pursued via a multitude of modifications in various methods. Proteins containing FSH and LH extracted from pituitaries or from urine were subjected to digestion with trypsin[101], pancreatic enzymes[102] or urea[103]. Butt and his co-workers[104] supplemented the digestion process with removal of inert proteins by starch gel electrophoresis. Other authors proposed purifying FSH from the LH contamination by zone electrophoresis or by chromatography on diethylaminoethyl cellulose (DEAE-C)[105,106]. Gemzell's group used chromatography and Sephadex® gel filtration[107]. In 1966, Donini and associates combined

electrophoresis and chromatography with lyophilization of the eluent and its subsequent filtration on a Sephadex column. This method yielded a gonadotropin preparation containing 384.4 IU of FSH activity and 5.6 IU of LH activity per mg of protein[108]. However, none of the above efforts brought a real solution, being either too cumbersome, too complicated and expensive, or not sufficiently accurate and efficient. New developments in immunological techniques[109] opened a virtually limitless horizon for measuring and producing several hormones, including purified FSH. These new procedures were devised through the synergy of four different aspects: advances in knowledge of theoretical immunology; technical developments in macromolecular chemistry; progress in nuclear physics

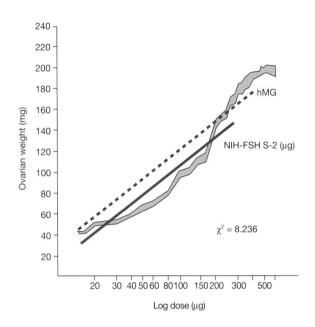

Figure 7 Standard curve used to calculate follicle stimulating hormone (FSH) content in samples tested with the Steelman–Pohley bioassay[98]. Shaded are = mean ± SD. hMG, human menopausal gonadotropin; NIH, National Institutes of Health

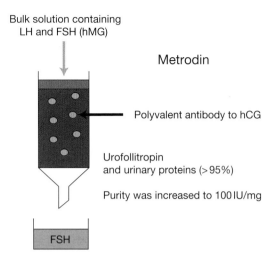

Figure 8 Metrodin was prepared by using an immunocolumn with polyclonal anti-luteinizing hormone (LH) antibodies to remove LH from a urinary human menopausal gonadotropin (hMG) preparation. All of the proteins contained in hMG, including follicle stimulating hormone (FSH), pass through the column, and LH is retained in the column, bound by the specific antibodies. The eluted FSH is then purified and lyophilized to a biologically pure FSH preparation with only minimal LH activity. hCG, human chorionic gonadotropin

which enabled *in vitro* iodination using radioactive isotopes (I^{125} and I^{131}); and availability of highly purified and potent hormone preparations. Specific hyperimmune anti-hCG serum preparation had already been attempted in the 1930s[110,111]. However, the gonadotropin preparations available at that time were crude, and contained large amounts of non-specified proteins, each of which served as a separate antigen. This resulted in the formation of a 'mixed' antiserum, which was neither sufficiently specific to recognize accurately the hCG antigen, nor sensitive enough to allow detection of small amounts of this hormone. This method was refined in the 1960s[112] by using an immunocolumn with polyclonal anti-LH antibodies. A urinary hMG preparation containing both FSH and LH was filtered through the column; all of the proteins contained in hMG, including FSH, pass through the column, and LH is retained in the column, bound by the specific antibodies. The eluted FSH is then purified and lyophilized to a biologically pure FSH preparation, with only minimal LH activity (Figure 8). The final product (Metrodin) contained 150 IU of FSH and 1 IU of LH per mg of protein.

Preparation of purified gonadotropins, coupled with the availability of macromolecules permitting the development of a whole array of efficient immunoabsorbents, enabled the pharmaceutical industry to introduce purified FSH preparations almost free from LH contamination[108].

HIGHLY PURIFIED URINARY FSH

Further technological advances made it possible to replace polyvalent antibodies with highly specific monoclonal antibodies. The production of purified urinary FSH was essentially a 'passive' process, in which LH was separated from bulk material, and FSH, together with some other urinary proteins, was collected and lyophilized for use. 'Third-generation gonadotropin', i.e. highly purified urinary FSH (FSH-HP), is produced by a more direct process. The affinity column uses highly specific monoclonal antibodies to bind selectively the FSH molecules in the hMG bulk material[113]. The unbound urinary protein and LH pass through the column and are removed, leaving pure FSH retained by the column (Figure 9). This is then extracted as a highly purified product, devoid of both LH and contaminating urinary proteins. As a result of the improved processing, this FSH preparation

(Metrodin HP) contains less than 0.1 IU of LH activity and less than 5% of unidentified urinary proteins. The specific activity of the FSH is increased from approximately 100–150 IU/mg of protein in purified urinary FSH preparations (Metrodin) to about 9000 IU/mg protein in the highly purified product (Metrodin HP). The purity is also increased from 1–2% to 95%. This enhanced purity means that the total amount of injected protein is very small, making the highly purified urinary FSH preparation suitable for subcutaneous administration. Not only is batch-to-batch variability virtually eliminated, but the product now lends itself to detailed analysis by physicochemical methods in addition to the classical *in vivo* bioassay. The technical developments that led to the production of highly purified FSH, together with a deeper understanding of the pharmacodynamics and pharmacokinetics of these preparations, has made it possible to redesign ovulation-inducing protocols (for example, low-dose regimens, low-dose increments and subcutaneous injection).

New protocols that use pure hormone preparations with complete batch-to-batch consistency offer the potential of improved efficiency by facilitating a more effective treatment plan that can be adjusted to a predictable response. Although we cannot control 'intra-patient variability', prospective management after assessing response to an initial treatment cycle can be more reliably planned, without the concern of an inconsistent response due to batch-to-batch variations in the drug preparations. This allows the design of 'tailor-made' protocols for individual patients, so that the number of developing follicles can be better controlled, reducing the risk of multiple pregnancies in ovulation-induction cycles, and of hyperstimulation in both ovulation-induction and ART cycles.

The use of highly purified FSH preparations indicated that the role of estrogen as a marker of follicular development required re-evaluation. Animal experiments[112] and studies in a patient with 17α-hydroxylase deficiency[114] indicated that follicular growth and development can take place despite extremely low levels of estrogens, and that quantitative estrogen levels do not necessarily represent an accurate assessment of follicular growth and development. When pure FSH is administered, the effect on follicular estrogen production will depend on the presence and the amount of LH produced by the patient. Since ultrasound examination can be used to assess ovarian follicular growth

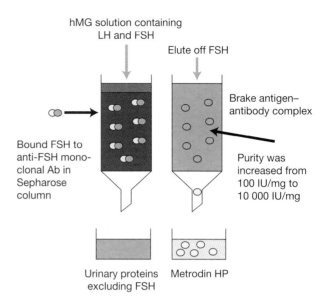

Figure 9 Highly purified urinary follicle stimulating hormone (FSH) (Metrodin HP) was produced by using an affinity column containing highly specific monoclonal antibodies (Ab) to bind selectively FSH molecules in the human menopausal gonadotropin (hMG) bulk material. Unbound urinary protein and luteinizing hormone (LH) pass through the column, leaving pure FSH retained by the column. This is then extracted as a highly purified product, devoid of both LH and contaminating urinary proteins

(a measure of FSH activity) and uterine endometrial thickness (a marker of estrogenic stimulation), ultrasound assessment of the ovaries and uterus will usually suffice to monitor the effects of FSH administration. A single estrogen determination prior to the planned ovulation induction can be used to predict hyperstimulation, and to decide on further management (e.g. withholding hCG).

In the past, human pituitary glands and menopausal urine were the sole sources for the production of human-derived pituitary gonadotropin (hPG) preparations; hPG preparations were abandoned when cases of iatrogenic Creutzfeld–Jakob disease (CJD) were recognized, and, until recently, menopausal urine represented the only primary source. It then became evident that there were serious shortcomings in the use of menopausal urine as a source. When the urinary extraction process was started, there were four urine collecting centers: one in The Netherlands, one in Spain, one in Israel and one in Italy. Altogether, 600 women participated in these collection centers, and each single woman was well known by the collectors.

If any of these women fell ill or was treated with drugs such as antibiotics, their urine samples were rejected. Over a period of 1 year, these groups of women produced 120 000 litres of urine, an amount absolutely sufficient for treating hypopituitary-hypogonadotrophic amenorrheic women (WHO grade I) worldwide at that time. At the beginning of this millennium, 120 000 000 litres of urine were necessary to satisfy the worldwide need – an increase of 100-fold, which required 600 000 donors (Figure 10). These donors were recruited from countries in Europe, Korea, China, India and South America. Since this process was no longer based upon individual collections, an increasing number of safety measures had to be included. The shortcomings of the urine extraction process can be summarized:

(1) Lack of regulatory control;

(2) Impossible to trace donor source;

(3) Quality cannot be checked during transportation;

(4) Urine sources cannot be validated;

(5) Decontamination may denature proteins;

(6) Cross-contamination cannot be avoided;

(7) Poor quality control (Figure 11);

(8) Limited source.

In addition to these drawbacks, a further cause for concern was raised when a protease-resistant form of prion protein was found in the urine of scrapie-infected hamsters, bovine spongiform encephalopathy (BSE)-infected cattle and humans suffering from CJD[115,116]. The prion protein was also identified in 29 human urine samples from 38 individuals with probable prion disease, but not in 20 patients diagnosed with Alzheimer's disease[117]. Experimental studies show that high levels of infectivity can be found in the brain and spleen of animals that do not develop clinically apparent disease during a normal life span, and it now seems that subclinical forms of prion disease exist[118]. Such asymptomatic prion 'carrier states', as well as pre-clinical/clinical prion disease, may be relevant when analyzing potential risks associated with biological products. If asymptomatic carriers of vCJD prion infection exist in the human population, they represent a potential risk to others via iatrogenic routes of

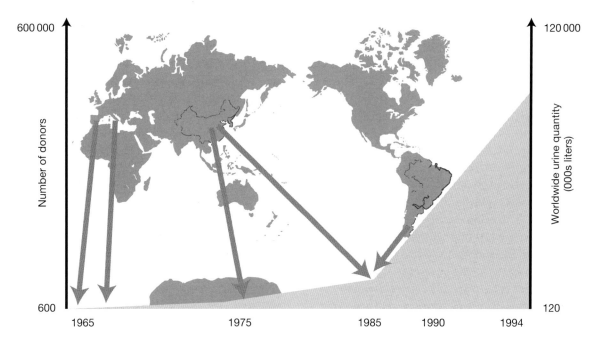

Figure 10 The potential requirement for urine as demand for gonadotropins increased between 1965 and 1995. In the 1960s, 600–1000 donors were sufficient to supply the urine necessary for the production of human menopausal gonadotropin (hMG). The development of new clinical indications and the expansion of infertility treatment on a worldwide basis resulted in an exponential increase in demand, and the number of donors required exceeded 100 000 by the early 1990s. These were recruited from Europe, Korea, China, India and South America; donor sources and urine collection could no longer be traced, controlled or regulated, leading to major concerns about safety

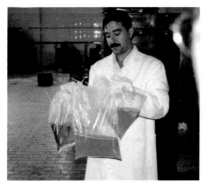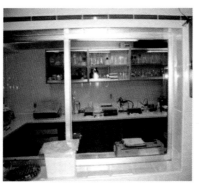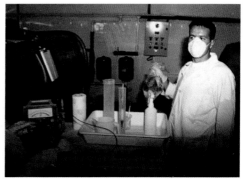

Figure 11 Quality control of urine delivered to the processing facility is limited to only four tests: color, odor, pH and density

prion transmission, although they might not develop clinical prion disease themselves.

Concerns about disease transmission led a number of countries to apply the 'precautionary principle': in 1996 the Australian Drug Evaluation Committee published its resolution on replacement of urinary with recombinant gonadotropins in view of their higher standard of purity and safety. In the same year, France introduced a class warning regarding viral safety risk on all urinary gonadotropin leaflets. In 2003, The UK Medicines Control Agency withdrew highly purified FSH (Metrodin HP) from the UK market as a precaution against the theoretical risk of CJD transmission[119]. In 2003, the Swissmedic letter[120] stated: 'Urine from countries, which belong to a GBR-class with a higher risk or in which no secured knowledge concerning status and monitoring system of Transmissible Spongiform Encephalopathy (TSE), such as China and Korea, should, as a precaution to improve safety, no longer be used. In addition, it has to be taken into account that, for certain preparations, recombinant products are now available. For those reasons, Swissmedic considers preventive measures to be reasonable and necessary.'

The future of infertility therapy clearly relies on the capacity to produce pharmaceutical-grade gonadotropins in sufficient quantities to meet the ever-increasing worldwide demand (Figure 12) and to reduce the risk of biological contamination, small as it may be. During the past 25–30 years, approximately 30 new pathogens have been identified, including the transmissible spongiform encephalopathies (prion diseases), human immunodeficiency virus (HIV), hemorrhagic viruses such as Ebola, transfusion-related hepatitis C-like viruses and, most recently, the coronavirus causing sudden acute respiratory syndrome

(SARS). These new diseases are now being defined within a context of 'emergent viruses', and it is clear that new infectious diseases may arise from a combination of different factors that prevail in modern society, including the use of biological products in medicine. Some pathogens have such lengthy incubation or latent periods before disease manifestation (e.g. prions, HIV) that the consequences of their transmission will not be detected until long after exposure. The techniques used in assisted reproduction can facilitate disease transmission by exposing pathogens to several targets (including other couples undergoing treatment and health-care personnel); breaching natural evolutionary barriers with invasive techniques such as intracytoplasmic sperm injection (ICSI) could theoretically introduce a further element of risk.

Detailed information now available regarding the physiological processes involved in the synthesis of gonadotropins by pituitary cells, along with the development of recombinant DNA technology, now allows the production of pharmacologically active pure FSH, LH and hCG preparations in unlimited quantities, minimizing the risk of disease transmission via biological contamination.

CONCLUSIONS

Throughout the history of civilization, and in many societies even now in the 21st century, a childless woman is someone to be pitied, subject to derision and perhaps condemnation. In some cultures, failure to have children may cast a heavy shadow on the physiological and social adequacy of the female, and diminish the social standing of her partner. She may be considered useless, with failure to bear children

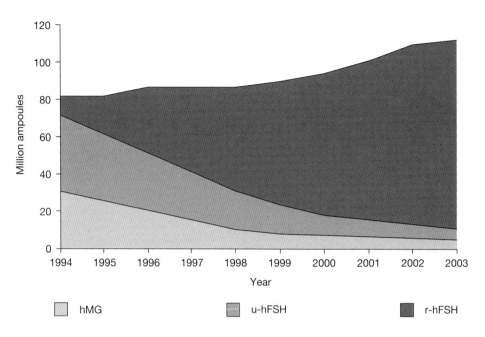

Figure 12 The change in worldwide demand for gonadotropins. Approximately 2–3 l of urine are required to prepare one vial of human menopausal gonadotropin (hMG), and one vial of purified follicle stimulating hormone (FSH) requires 6–9 l. As recombinant gonadotropins became available, the number of donors required began to decrease, and by 2003 about 40 million donors were needed to produce 20 million ampoules of urinary-gonadotropins. The benefits offered by recombinant technology, and the application of precautionary principles, are reflected in the increased use of recombinant human FSH (r-hFSH) from 1994 onwards. u-h, urinary human

accepted as a basis for annulment or divorce. Even in the absence of specific sanctions, a woman without her own children is deprived of the rewards of motherhood and suffers a loss of status, being excluded from a major part of community life. Children are regarded as an extension of self, as bearers and perpetuators of the family name and tradition, as well as an expansion of one's hopes, aims and strivings. The inability to procreate can thus be perceived as a denial of basic rights, an injustice and a disappointment, even a source of grief. This unfortunate situation was recognized and addressed in 1948 with the birth of the Universal Declaration of Human Rights. Article 16 states that 'Men and women of full age, without any limitations due to race, nationality or religion, have the right to marry and to found a family… the family is the natural and fundamental group unit of society.'

To add to the catalog of 'insult', attempts to alleviate the plight of the childless woman have sometimes resulted in iatrogenic injury. Witchcraft, the tools and rituals of magic, as well as inappropriate procedures, may sometimes do more harm than good. One can imagine that more than 2000 years ago, Hippocrates' prescription of dilating the cervix and inserting a hollow leaden probe into the uterus for the instillation of emollient substances might have led to salpingitis, permanent sterility or even death. The 20th century witnessed tragic effects of treatment that could not be recognized until decades later: irradiation of the pituitary and ovaries leading to cancer, the use of animal gonadotropins leading to antibody formation, and transmission of prion disease via pituitary hormone extracts. These lessons of the past should encourage us to apply 'the precautionary principle' and strive for the purest and safest products available, with patient-friendly medications preferred in consideration of quality of life as a further priority.

Table 1 outlines major milestones of medical treatments used in the quest to help childless women to achieve a pregnancy; Figure 13 demonstrates that major advances in technology have brought the field of gonadotropin therapy a very long way since the era of animal-, human pituitary- and urinary-derived hormones. It seems clear that new pharmaceutical products will offer the safest option for ovarian stimulation. Pure FSH preparations with approximately 13 000 IU FSH/mg protein are now accessible (see Chapter 8 by Howles), offering significant risk reduction for patients

Table 1 Significant milestones in medical treatment of infertility, indicating the first pregnancies reported after the use of increasingly refined products

First pregnancy achieved with	Author (s)
'Antophysin'	Vesell, 1938[64]
Pregnant mare serum gonadotropin/human chorionic gonadotropin (PMSG/hCG)	Hamblen et al., 1945[63]
Clomiphene	Greenblatt et al., 1961[121]
Human menopausal gonadotropin (hMG)	Lunenfeld et al., 1962[89]
Human pituitary gonadotropin (hPG)	Gemzell, 1962[122]
hPG in a hypophysectomized patient	Bettendorf, 1963[72]
Bromocriptine	Thorner et al., 1975[123]
GnRH	Leyendecker et al., 1980[53]
Recombinant human FSH in IVF (r-hFSH, Follitropin alfa)	Germond et al., 1992[124]
Recombinant hFSH (Follitropin beta) in IVF	Devroey et al., 1992[125]
Recombinant FSH in a PCOS patient	Donderwinkel et al., 2002[126]
Recombinant FSH-CTP	Beckers et al., 2003[127]

GnRH, gonadotropin releasing hormone; FSH, follicle stimulating hormone; IVF, *in vitro* fertilization; PCOS, polycystic ovarian syndrome; CTP, C-terminal peptide

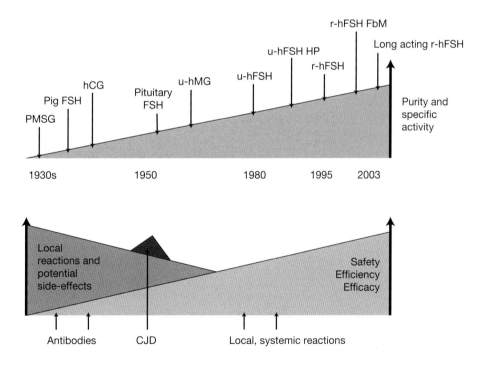

Figure 13 The continuing quest for quality and consistency. Between 1930 and 1972, gonadotropins from animal pituitaries and pregnant mare serum (PMSG) were used; due to allergic reactions and lack of efficacy, they were abandoned. Between 1958 and 1988, gonadotropins from the pituitaries of human cadavers were used; they were also abandoned, due to the threat of Creutzfeld–Jakob disease (CJD). In the early 1960s, the purity of human menopausal gonadotropin (hMG) was 5%, the remaining 95% consisted of significant amounts of known and unknown contaminating proteins. By the mid-1960s, improved purification processes were implemented that led to urinary follicle stimulating hormone (uFSH) containing less luteinizing hormone (LH), but contaminated with 95% of unwanted proteins. Improved purification processes still achieved a purity of only 40–90%. Between 1996 and 2003, precautionary principles were applied in a number of countries leading them to restrict or abandon the use of urinary gonadotropins. hCG, human chorionic gonadotropin; u-h, urinary human; HP, high purity; r-h, recombinant human; FbM, fill by mass

as well as the assurance of superior quality control over the final product. We must therefore ask ourselves if it is medically prudent and ethically admissible to use preparations derived from urine of untraceable donor source, with significant batch-to-batch variation, of different degrees of purity and contaminated with extraneous proteins. In our modern age of advanced technology and discovery, perhaps it is time to learn from the lessons of history, to take advantage of the enlightenment brought by research and increased knowledge that was denied to our predecessors.

ACKNOWLEDGMENT

The history of developments in gonadotropin therapy was adapted with permission from 'Historical perspectives in gonadotropin therapy', a review written by Bruno Lunenfeld for *Human Reproduction Update* 2004; 10: 453–67

REFERENCES

1. Dawson WR. The Egyptian medical papyri. In Brothwell DR, Sandison AT, eds. Diseases in Antiquity. London: Charles C Thomas, 1967: 98–111

2. Sanders JB. Transitions from Ancient Egyptian to Greek medicine. Lawrence: University of Kansas Press, 1963

3. Leshem Y, Lunenfeld B. Gonadotropin promotion of adventitious root production on cuttings of Begonia semperflorens and Vitis vinifera. Plant Physiol 1968; 43: 313

4. King H. Hippocrates' Woman: Reading the Female Body in Ancient Greece. New York: Routledge, 1998

5. Soranus. Gynaecology. Transl Temkin O. Baltimore, MD: The Johns Hopkins University Press, 1956

6. Ahmed M. Ibn Sina (Avicenna) – Doctor of Doctors. http://www.ummah.net/history/scholars/ibn_sina/, 1990

7. Browne EG. Arabian Medicine. Cambridge: Cambridge University Press, 1921

8. Morice P, Josset P, Chapron C, Dubuisson JB. History of infertility. Hum Reprod Update 1995; 1: 497–504

9. St Thomas of Aquinas. (1871–1873) Summa Theologica 3–3, 49, Benziger Bros edn. Transl Fathers of the English Dominican Province, 1947

10. Kennedy M. A brief history of disease, science and medicine. Cranston, RI: The Writer's Collective, 2004

11. De Graaf R. De Mullerium Organis. Paris, 1672

12. Naboth M. De Sterilitate. Lipsiae, 1707

13. von Leeuwenhoek A. Epistolae Physiologicae, 1719

14. Sims J. The Story of My Life. New York: D. Appleton & Co, 1884

15. Huhner M. The diagnosis and treatment of sexual disorders in the male and female. Philadelphia: Davis, 1937

16. Rubin IC. Non-operative determination of the patency of Fallopian tubes in sterility. J Am Med Assoc 1920; 74: 1017

17. Halberstaedter L. Berlin Klin Wochenschr 1905; 42: 64

18. Beclere A. Paris Med 1926; 13: 97

19. Rubin IC. Sterility associated with habitual amenorrhea relieved by X-ray therapy. Am J Obstet Gynecol 1926; 12: 76–82

20. Kaplan I. The use of high voltage roentgentherapy in the treatment of amenorrhea and sterility in women. Am J Roentgenol 1948; 59: 3703–79

21. Mazer C, Greenberg R. Low dosage irradiation in the treatment of amenorrhea. Am J Obstet Gynecol 1943; 46: 648–52

22. Finkler RS. Evaluation of hormonal and radiation therapy in 190 cases of functional sterility and secondary amenorrhea. Preliminary report. Am J Obstet Gynecol 1949; 58: 559–64

23. Ron E, Boice JD Jr, Hamburger S, Stovall M. Mortality following radiation treatment for infertility of hormonal origin or amenorrhoea. Int J Epidemiol 1994; 23: 1165–73

24. Radiation Epidemiology Branch, National Cancer Institute, NIH, Bethesda, MD, USA, 1985

25. Needham J. Science and Civilization in China. Cambridge: Cambridge University Press, 1983; V: 315

26. Needham J. Science and Civilization in China. Cambridge: Cambridge University Press, 2000; VI: 195

27. Temple R. The Genius of China, 3000 years of science, discovery and invention. Part 5: Medicine and Health, Chapter 53: The science of endocrinology. Cambridge, UK: Prion Books Ltd, 1999

28. Crowe SJ, Cushing H, Homans J. Experimental hypophysectomy. Bull Johns Hopkins Hosp 1910; 21: 127–67

29. Aschner B. Ueber die Beziehung zwischen Hypophysis und Genitale. Arch Gynäkol 1912; 97: 200–27

30. Smith PE. Hastening of development of female genital system by daily hemoplastic pituitary transplants. Proc Soc Exp Biol Med 1926; 24: 1311–33

31. Smith PE, Engle ET. Experimental evidence of the role of anterior pituitary in development and regulation of gonads. Am J Anat 1927; 40: 159

32. Zondek B. Ueber die Funktion des Ovariums. Zeitschr Geburtsh Gynäkol 1926; 90: 327

33. Smith PE. The disabilities caused by hypophysectomy and their repair. J Am Med Assoc 1927; 88: 158–61

34. Smith PE. Hypophysectomy and replacement therapy in the rat. Am J Anat 1930; 45: 205–74

35. Zondek B. Weitere Untersuchungen zur Darstellung, Biologie und Klinik des Hypophysenvorderlappen-hormones (Prolan). Zentralbl für Gynäkol 1929; 14: 834–48

36. Zondek B. Ueber die Hormone des Hypophysen-vorderlappens. Klin Wochenschr 1930; 9: 245–8

37. Fevold SL, Hisaw FL, Leonard SL. The gonad-stimulating and the luteinizing hormones of the anterior lobe of the hypophysis. Am J Physiol 1931; 97: 291–301

38. Ascheim S, Zondek B. Hypophysenvorderlappen-hormone und Ovarialhormone im Harn von Schwangeren. Klin Wochenschr 1927; 6: 13–21

39. Seegar-Jones GE, Gey GO, Ghisletta M. Hormone production by placental cells maintained in continuous culture. Bull Johns Hopkins Hosp 1943; 72: 26–38

40. Tausk M. Organon. De geschiedenis van een bijzon-dere Nederlandse onderneming. Nijmegen, The Netherlands: Dekker & Van de Vegt, 1978

41. Gurin S, Bachman G, Wilson DW. The gonadotropic hormone of urine of pregnancy. ii Chemical studies of preparations having high biological activity. J Biol Chem 1940; 133: 467

42. Katzman PA, Godfried M, Cain CK, Doisy EA. The preparation of chorionic gonadotropin by chromato-graphic adsorption. J Biol Chem 1943; 148: 501–7

43. Hamblen EC. Human ovarian responses to extracts of pregnancy urine – preliminary report. Virginia Med Monthly 1933; 60: 286–90

44. Hamblen EC, Ross RA. Responses of the human ovary to gonadotropic principles. Endocrinology 1947; 21: 722–6

45. Maddock WO, Leach RB, Tokuyama I, et al. Effects of hog pituitary follicle stimulating hormone in women – antihormone formation and inhibition of ovarian function. J Clin Endocrinol Metab 1956; 16: 433–48

46. Vidal L. Dictionaire des Spécialités Pharmaceutiques. Paris: Office de Vulgarisation Pharmaceutique, 1959: 696

47. Netter A. Activité en gynecologie d'un extrait gonadotrope d'origine hypophysaire. CR Soc Franc Gynecol 1959; 29: 384–90

48. Ostergaard E. Antigonadotrophic Substances. Copen-hagen: Ejnar Munksgaard, 1942

49. Zondek B, Sulman F. The antigonadotropic factor. Baltimore: Williams & Wilkins, 1942: 1–185

50. Wilkins L. The need for an inhibitor of gonadotropin. J Clin Endcrinol Metab 1953; 13: 739

51. Schally AV, Arimura A, Baba Y, et al. Isolation and properties of the FSH and LH-releasing hormone. Biochem Biophys Res Commun 1971; 43: 393–9

52. Baba Y, Matsuo H, Schally AV. Structure of porcine LH and FSH-releasing hormone. II: Conformation of the proposed structure by conventional sequential analysis. Biochem Biophys Res Commun 1971; 44: 459–63

53. Leyendecker G, Wildt L, Hansmann M. Pregnancies following chronic intermittent (pulsatile) administra-tion of Gn-RH by means of a portable pump ('Zyk-lomat') – a new approach to the treatment of infer-tility in hypothalamic amenorrhea. J Clin Endocrinol Metab 1980; 51: 1214–16

54. Haviv F, Insler V. Gonadotropin-releasing hormone analogs in perspective: a promise fulfilled. In Adashi EY, Rock AJ, Rosenwaks Z, eds. Reproductive Endo-crinology, Surgery and Technology. Philadelphia: Lip-pincott Raven, 1996: 1649–62

55. Cole HH, Hart GH. The potency of blood serum of mares in progressive stages of pregnancy in affecting the sexual maturity of the immature rat. Am J Physiol 1930; 93: 57

56. Cartland GF, Nelson JW. The preparation and purifi-cation of extracts containing the gonad-stimulating hormone of pregnant mare serum. J Biol Chem 1937; 19: 59–67

57. Burns JH, Finney DJ, Goodwin LG. Biological stan-dardization (Appendix I). London: Oxford University Press, 1950

58. Fevold HL. The gonadotropic hormones. Cold Spring Harbor Symp (Quantitative Biology) 1937; 5: 93

59. Hamblen EC. Endocrine therapy of functional ovarian failure. Am J Obstet Gynecol 1940; 40: 615–62

60. Hamblen EC. Results of preoperative administration of extract of pregnancy urine: study of ovaries and endometria in hyperplasia of endometrium following such administration. Endocrinology 1935; 19: 169–78

61. Hamblen EC. Clinical evaluation of ovarian responses to gonadotropic therapy. Endocrinology 1939; 24: 848–57

62. Mazer C, Ravetz E. The effect of combined adminis-tration of chorionic gonadotropin and the pituitary synergist on the human ovary. Am J Obstet Gynaecol 1941; 41: 474–588

63. Hamblen EC, Davis CD, Durham NC. Treatment of hypo-ovarianism by the sequential and cyclic admin-istration of equine and chorionic gonadotropins – so-called one–two cylic gonadotropic therapy. Summary of 5 years' results. Am J Obstet Gynecol 1945; 50: 137–46

64. Vesell M. Cyclic treatment of a case of secondary amenorrhea of ten years duration. Am J Obstet Gynecol 1938; 3: 1067–72

65. Rydberg E, Madsen V. The treatment of functional sterility with gonadotropic hormones. Acta Obstet Gynecol Scand 1949; 19: 222–46

66. Rydberg E, Ostergaard E. The effect of gonadotropic hormone treatment in cases of amenorrhoea. Acta Obstet Gynecol Scand 1939; 19: 222–46

67. Daume E. Comparison of HMG + HCG and sheep pituitary gonadotropin + HCG for the induction of ovulation in the human. In Clinical Application of Human Gonadotropins. Bettendorf G, Insler V, eds. Stuttgart: Georg Thieme Verlag, 1970: 103–12

68. Groot-Wassink K, Blawert H. Vergleichende untersuchungen zur Ovulationsausloesung mit Folistiman und Pergonal. Zentralbl Gynekol 1973; 9: 1019–21

69. Gemzell CA, Diczfalusy E, Tillinger G. Clinical effect of human pituitary follicle stimulating hormone (FSH). J Clin Endocrinol Metab 1958; 18: 1333

70. Buxton CL, Hermann W. Induction of ovulation in the human with human gonadotropins. Am J Obstet Gynecol 1961; 81: 584

71. Bettendorf G, Apostolakis M, Voigt KD. Darstellung hochaktiver Gonadotropin Fraktionen aus menschlichen Hypophysen und deren Anwendung beim Menschen. Proc Int Fed Gynecol Obstet 1961; 1: 76 (abstr)

72. Bettendorf G. Human hypophyseal gonadotropin in hypophysectomized women. Int J Fertil 1963; 45: 799–80

73. Dumble LD, Klein RD. Creutzfeld–Jakob disease legacy for Australian women treated with human pituitary gonadotropins. Lancet 1992; 330: 848

74. Cochius JI, Mack K, Burns RJ. Creutzfeld–Jakob disease in a recipient human pituitary derived gonadotropin. Aust NZ J Med 1990; 20: 592–6

75. Bradbury JT, Brown ES, Brown WE. Adsorption of urinary gonadotropins on kaolin. Proc Soc Exp Biol Med 1949; 71: 228–32

76. Albert A. Procedure for routine clinical gonadotropin determination in human urine. Mayo Clin Proc 1955; 30: 552–6

77. Donini P, Montezemolo R. Rassegna di Clinica, Terapia e Scienze Affini. A publication of the Biologic Laboratories of the Instituto Serono. 1949; 48: 3–28

78. Donini P, Puzzuoli D, Montezemolo R. Purification of gonadotropin from human menopausal urine. Acta Endocrinol 1964; 45: 329

79. Lunenfeld B, Donini P. Historic aspects of gonadotropins in induction of ovulation. In Greenblatt RB, ed. Ovulation. Philadelphia, PA: Lippincott Co., 1966: 105–17

80. Borth R, Lunenfeld B, de Watteville H. Activité gonadotrope d'un extrait d'urines de femmes en menopause. Experientia 1954; 10 : 266–70

81. Borth R, Diczfalusy E, Heinrichs HD. Grundlagen der statistischen Auswertung biologischer Bestimmungen. Arch Gynaecol 1957; 188: 497

82. Borth R, Lunenfeld B, de Watteville H. Le dosage des gonadotropins – méthode et intérêt clinique. Bull Soc Belge Gynecol Obstet 1957; 27: 639

83. Albert A, Borth R, Diczfalusy E, et al. Collaborative assays of two urinary preparations of human pituitary gonadotropin. J Clin Endocrinol Metab 1958; 18: 1117–23

84. Benz F, Borth R, Brown PS, et al. Collaborative assay of two gonadotropin preparations from human post-menopausal urine. J Endocrinol 1959; 19: 158–63

85. Lunenfeld B. General discussion. In Albert A, ed. Human Pituitary Gonadotropins. Springfield, IL: Charles C Thomas, 1961: 53260–9

86. Lunenfeld B, Menzi A, Volet B. Clinical effects of human post-menopausal gonadotropin. In Fuchs F, ed. Advance Abstracts of Short Communications, First International Congress of Endocrinology. Copenhagen: Excerpta Medica Foundation, 1960: 587

87. Lunenfeld B, Rabau E, Rumney G, Winkelsberg G. The responsiveness of the human ovary to gonadotropin. (Hypophysis III). Proc Third World Cong Gynecol Obstet (Vienna) 1961; 1: 220

88. Lunenfeld B, Sulimovici S, Rabau E. Les éffets des gonadotropins urinaires des femmes menopausées sur l'ovaire humain. CR Soc Franc Gynecol 1962; 32/5: 291

89. Lunenfeld B, Sulimovici S, Rabau E, Eshkol A. L'induction de l'ovulation dans les amenorrheas hypophysaires par un traitement combiné de gonadotropins urinaires menopausiques et de gonadotropins chorioniques. CR Soc Franc Gynecol 1962; 32/5: 346

90. Lunenfeld B. Treatment of anovulation by human gonadotropins. J Int Fed Gynecol Obstet 1963; 1: 153

91. Palmer R, Dorangeon P. Les gonadotropines dans les traitements de la stérilité féminine. CR Soc Franc Gynecol 1962; 32: 407–15

92. Rosenberg E, Coleman J, Damani M, Garcia CR. Clinical effect of post menopausal gonadotropin. Clin Endocrinol Metab 1962; 23: 181–9

93. WHO Expert Committee on Biological Standardization. Technical Report Series. Geneva: World Health Organization, 1972; 565: 56–57

94. WHO Expert Committee. Agents stimulating gonadal function in human. Technical Report Series. Geneva: World Health Organization, 1973: 514

95. Jones HW, Jones GS, Andrews MC, et al. The program for in vitro fertilization at Norfolk. Fertil Steril 1982; 38: 14–21

96. Garcia JE, Jones GS, Acosta A, Wright G. Human menopausal gonadotropins/human chorionic gonadotropin follicular maturation for oocyte aspiration: phase I, 1981. Fertil Steril 1983; 39: 167–73

97. Garcia JE, Jones GS, Acosta A, Wright G. Human menopausal gonadotropins/human chorionic gonadotropin follicular maturation for oocyte aspiration: phase II, 1981. Fertil Steril 1983; 39: 174–9

98. Steelman SL, Pohley FM. Assay of the follicle stimulating hormone based on the augmentation with human chorionic gonadotropin. Endocrinology 1953; 543: 604–16

99. Lunenfeld B. Methods for assay for FSH. In Bell T, Loraine JA, eds. Recent Research on Gonadotrophic Hormones. Edinburgh: E&S Livingstone Ltd, 1967: 5

100. Keene JL, Matzuk MM, Otani T, et al. Expression of biologically active human follitropin in Chinese hamster ovary cells. J Biol Chem 1989; 264: 4769–74

101. Jutisz M. General discussion. Ciba Found Study Group 1965; 22: 115–22

102. Segaloff A, Steelman SL. The human gonadotropins. Rec Prog Horm Res 1959; 14:127–42

103. Ellis S. Bioassay of luteinizing hormone. Endocrinology 1961; 68: 334–40

104. Butt WR, Cunningham FJ, Hartree A. Preparation and assay of human pituitary FSH and LH. Proc R Soc Med 1964; 57: 107–14

105. Porath J. Some recent developments in preparative electrophoresis and gel filtration. Metabolism 1964; 13: 1004–15

106. Reichert LE, Parlow AF. Partial purification and separation of human pituitary gonadotropins. Endocrinology 1964; 74: 236–43

107. Roos P. Human follicle stimulating hormone. Its isolation from pituitary glands and from post menopausal urine and a study of some chemical, physical, immunological and biological properties of the hormones from these two sources. Acta Endocrinol (Copenh) 1968; 59 (Suppl 131): 3–93

108. Donini P, Puzzuoli D, D'Alessio I, et al. Purification and separation of follicle-stimulating hormone (FSH) and luteinizing hormone (LH) from human post-menopausal gonadotropin (HMG). Acta Endocrinol 1966; 52: 169–85

109. Lunenfeld B, Givol D, Sela M. Immunologic properties of urinary preparations of human menopausal gonadotropins, with special reference to Pergonal. J Clin Endocrinol Metab 1961; 21: 478

110. Bachman C. Immunologic studies of anti-gonadotropic sera. Proc Soc Exp Biol Med 1935; 32: 851–4

111. Twombly GH. Studies on the nature of antigonadotropic substances. Endocrinology 1936; 20: 311–17

112. Eshkol A, Lunenfeld B. Purification and separation of follicle stimulating hormone (FSH) and luteinizing hormone (LH) from human menopausal gonadotropin (HMG). Part III. Acta Endocrinol 1967; 54: 919

113. Lunenfeld B, Eshkol A. Immunology of follicle stimulating hormone and luteinizing hormone. Vitam Horm 1970; 27: 131–59

114. Rabinovici J, Blankstein J, Goldman B, et al. In vitro fertilization and primary embryonic cleavage are possible in 17α-hydroxylase deficiency despite extremely low intrafollicular 17β-estradiol. J Clin Endocinol Metab 1989; 68: 693–7

115. Shaked GM, Shaked Y, Jaruv-Inbal A, et al. A protease-resistant prion protein isoform is present in urine of animals and humans affected with prion diseases. J Biol Chem 2001; 276: 1479–82

116. Gabizon R. Abnormal PrP isoforms in urine. Presented at the XVth Congress of the International Society of Neuropathology, Torino, Italy, 2003

117. Furukawa H, Shirabe S, Niwa M. Diagnostic usefulness of urine protein analysis in prion diseases. Presented at the XVth Congress of the International Society of Neuropathology, Torino, Italy, 2003

118. Hill AF, Collinge J. Subclinical prion infection in humans and animals. Br Med Bull 2003; 66: 161–70

119. SCRIP Metrodin HP withdrawn in the UK, 2003; 2824: 18

120. TSE risk of medicines manufactured from human urine, foreseen measures to ensure medical safety. Geneva, Switzerland: Swissmedic letter, 2003

121. Greenblatt RB, Barfield WE, Junck EC, Ray AW. Induction of ovulation with MRL/41. Preliminary report. J Am Med Assoc 1961; 178: 101–4

122. Gemzell CA. Induction of ovulation with human pituitary gonadotropins. Fertil Steril 1962; 13: 153–68

123. Thorner MO, Besser GM, Jones A, et al. Bromocriptine treatment of female infertility: report of 13 pregnancies. Br Med J 1975; 4: 694–7

124. Germond M, Dessole S, Senn A, et al. Successful in-vitro fertilization and embryo transfer after treatment with recombinant human FSH. Lancet 1992; 339: 1170–1

125. Devroey P, Van Steirteghem A, Mannaerts B, Coelingh Bennink H. Successful in-vitro fertilization and embryo transfer after treatment with recombinant human FSH. Lancet 1992; 339: 1170-1

126. Donderwinkel PFJ, Schoot DC, Coelingh I, et al. Pregnancy after induction of ovulation with recombinant human FSH in polycystic ovary syndrome. Lancet 2002; 340: 983–93

127. Beckers NGM, Macklon NS, Devroey PR, et al. First live birth after ovarian stimulation using a chimeric long-acting human recombinant follicle-stimulating hormone (FSH) agonist (recFSH-CTP) for in vitro fertilization. Fertil Steril 2003; 79: 621–3

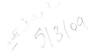

8

Superovulation for assisted conception: the new gonadotropins

Colin M. Howles

INTRODUCTION

The use of gonadotropin preparations to treat fertility problems has been known since the first half of the 20th century[1]. Initially, preparations derived from pregnant mare serum, and pig and human pituitary gland extracts, were used for ovarian stimulation. However, from the 1950s onwards, human menopausal gonadotropin (hMG) became the gonadotropin preparation of choice. hMG is extracted from the urine of postmenopausal women and contains a mixture of follicle stimulating hormone (FSH) and luteinizing hormone (LH) activity (about 5%), together with miscellaneous urinary proteins (95%). hMG was used initially to induce ovulation in women with anovulatory infertility, but from the early days of *in vitro* fertilization (IVF) in the early 1980s, it had an important role in stimulating multiple ovarian follicular development. Compared with natural cycles, ovarian stimulation with gonadotropins was associated with an increase in the number of oocytes available for collection and hence the likelihood of successful embryo replacement and pregnancy.

URINE-DERIVED GONADOTROPINS

The next step in the evolution of gonadotropins for clinical use was the application of immunoaffinity

techniques to remove LH from hMG, resulting in a product (urine-derived FSH, u-FSH) containing mainly FSH activity together with coextracted urinary proteins. Further refinement of the process in the late 1980s led to the development of highly purified u-FSH, containing approximately 9000 IU FSH activity/mg protein and < 1% urinary proteins[2]. Manufacturers have also attempted to produce purified hMG with defined levels of FSH and LH activity. They have been partially successful, resulting in preparations with a specific activity of approximately 2000 IU FSH activity/mg protein; however, in many cases, LH activity has to be added using human chorionic gonadotropin (hCG), which has a longer half-life than LH[3,4]. The presence of variable amounts of hCG in hMG preparations may further increase the variation between different batches of this product[5] and result in follicle atresia[6]. Analysis of highly purified hMG reveals the presence of at least 30% of extraneous proteins, including leukocyte elastase inhibitor, protein C inhibitor and zinc-α_2-glycoprotein[4,7].

RECOMBINANT HUMAN FSH

The isolation of the gene encoding the β subunit of FSH in 1983 made it possible to work towards the production of pure FSH using recombinant technology. The first recombinant human FSH (r-hFSH) was approved for clinical use in 1995 (follitropin alfa, GONAL-f®; Serono International SA, Geneva, Switzerland). A second r-hFSH (follitropin beta, Puregon®/Follistim®; Organon International, NJ, USA) was approved in 1996. Follitropin alfa and follitropin beta are similar in terms of immunopotency, *in vitro* biopotency and internal carbohydrate complexity, but follitropin alfa contains a higher proportion of acidic glycoforms[8]. Follitropin alfa has a specific activity of approximately 13 645 IU/mg[9], compared a mean of 9396 IU/mg (assessed from ten commercial batches of follitropin beta solution for injection)[10]. The evolution of gonadotropin preparations is illustrated in Table 1.

r-hFSH has been compared with u-FSH in many clinical trials and meta-analyses. Briefly, the results show that r-hFSH is more effective than u-FSH, as measured by the number of oocytes retrieved[11,12] and, from meta-analysis, pregnancy rates in IVF cycles[13,14]. r-hFSH is also more efficient than u-FSH, requiring a lower total dose of gonadotropin[13] and allowing treatment to be completed in a significantly shorter time[11,12]. Additionally, a very recent prospective analysis of over 24 000 ART from Germany has clearly demonstrated that treatment with r-hFSH versus hMG was associated with a significantly higher live birth rate and a reduced gonadotropin requirement per cycle[15]. While urine-derived gonadotropins are generally well tolerated, they contain protein contaminants that can affect immune function[16], and there have been reports of adverse reactions, including local and generalized skin reactions and delayed-type hypersensitivity[17-20]. Such reactions are normally resolved by switching from the urine-derived gonadotropin to a recombinant preparation[18-20]. There is also evidence of differences in tolerability between r-hFSH preparations, favoring follitropin alfa over follitropin beta[21,22].

This chapter focuses on the use of r-hFSH, particularly follitropin alfa filled-by-mass (FbM), for controlled ovarian stimulation (COS) in women undergoing assisted reproduction and ovulation induction (OI). The value of recombinant human LH (r-hLH, Luveris®; Serono International SA, Geneva, Switzerland) to supplement r-hFSH in selected patients is also discussed.

The FbM concept

The dose of gonadotropin preparations, like other peptides and proteins used pharmacologically, has traditionally been expressed in international units (IU), representing activity measured in an *in vivo* bioassay. Recent improvements in manufacturing processes, and the development of validated physicochemical techniques for determining gonadotropin structure, however, have allowed recombinant gonadotropins (r-hFSH (follitropin alfa), r-hLH and r-hCG) to be FbM. This reflects a constant relationship between mass and biological activity and guarantees consistency of dosing from batch to batch of manufactured product. The move towards products filled and released using physicochemical methods has been supported by regulatory agencies, standards agencies, such as pharmacopeial commissions[23], and joint industry-academic working parties[24], all of whom recognize the drawbacks of *in vivo* bioassays.

The bioassay used for preparations of FSH is the 50-year-old Steelman–Pohley bioassay[25]. This assay requires large numbers of laboratory animals, procedures for data generation and interpretation are cumbersome, and the coefficient of variation in a single determination can be as high as 10–20%[9]. In contrast, FbM gonadotropins are quantified by an optimized size-exclusion high-performance liquid chromatography method supported by glycan mapping, isoelectric focusing and specific activity data that demonstrate the physicochemical consistency of the product[9].

Experience with r-hFSH FbM

A number of clinical studies have compared r-hFSH (follitropin alfa) FbM with conventional r-hFSH filled by IU (FbIU). In 2002, Neuspiller and colleagues presented the results of a multinational, assessor-blind study to compare the two presentations used in a protocol for assisted reproductive technologies (ART) at a starting dose of 150 IU (11 μg r-hFSH FbM)[26]. A total of 149 women (aged 18–34 years) received r-hFSH FbM and 152 women received r-hFSH FbIU. The primary endpoint, the number of oocytes fertilized, was significantly higher in the r-hFSH FbM group (7.3 vs. 5.7, $p < 0.01$). Efficiency measures were also better in the r-hFSH FbM group, which required significantly fewer days of treatment (9.6 ± 1.6 vs. 10.2 ± 1.7 days,

Preparation	Source	FSH activity (IU/vial/ampoule)	LH activity (IU/vial/ampoule)	Co-purified non-FSH human proteins (%)
Human menopausal gonadotropin	urine	75	75	>95
Urine-derived FSH	urine	75	<0.7	>95
Highly purified, urine-derived FSH	urine	75–150	<0.001	<1
Recombinant human FSH	mammalian cells	75–150	none	none
New formulation recombinant human FSH (filled by mass)	mammalian cells	5.5 µg (75 IU)	none	none

FSH, follicle stimulating hormone; LH, luteinizing hormone

$p < 0.01$). Overall, the clinical pregnancy rate was similar, being over 30% in both groups.

A second study to compare r-hFSH FbM with the FbIU presentation was reported by Hugues and colleagues[27]. In this study, four bulk lots of r-hFSH were used to prepare four batches FbM and four batches FbIU. These eight batches were used in a double-blind clinical study in patients undergoing ART. The starting dose of r-hFSH was 150 IU or 11 µg/day. Sixty-six women were randomized to r-hFSH FbM and 65 to r-hFSH FbIU. Both preparations induced multiple follicular development and all patients underwent oocyte retrieval. In this study, outcomes related to ovarian stimulation, embryo transfer and pregnancy did not differ significantly between groups. Clinical pregnancy rates were 30.3% in the FbM group and 26.2% in the FbIU group. Variability of the response to different batches of r-hFSH was quantified and tested by comparing the highest and lowest mean value in each treatment group for the efficacy-related outcomes studied (Figure 1). Overall, the ovarian response was more consistent ($p = 0.039$) for FbM compared with FbIU.

In a recent study[28], Balasch and colleagues retrospectively compared the outcomes of 125 ART cycles using follitropin alfa FbM and 125 cycles using follitropin alfa FbIU. The duration of stimulation was significantly shorter in the FbM group, and embryo quality and implantation rates (28.6% in the FbM group vs. 18.6% in the FbIU group, $p = 0.008$) were significantly higher.

r-hFSH FbM has also been compared with r-hFSH FbIU in a sample of 180 women undergoing ovulation induction for anovulatory infertility. Both preparations were well tolerated and ovulation and pregnancy rates were similar in the two groups. The FbM group had fewer cycles requiring dose adjustment above 75 IU/day and a lower cancelation rate due to lack of response (T. Yeko, personal communication).

It should be noted that the r-hFSH FbM monodose presentation contains some constituents not present in r-hFSH FbIU (methionine and polysorbate[22]), which may affect the duration of treatment and total dose of FSH required.

Use of pen delivery devices

For successful use in clinical practice, efficacy and consistency must be combined with consistent dosing and the product must be acceptable to the patient. Pen injectors designed to improve the accuracy and compliance of self-injection have been developed for use with r-hFSH (follitropin alfa FbM and follitropin beta). The follitropin beta pen is based on an insulin pen delivery device and delivers 50–450 IU r-hFSH per injection from a separate cartridge. Injections of follitropin beta using the pen have been shown to be bioequivalent to injections given by conventional syringe[29]. The pen device appears to have advantages over conventional syringes in terms of local tolerability[30,31], and patients regard the pen as easy to use[32].

More recently, a pen injector has been developed for use with follitropin alfa FbM. This is a prefilled ready-to-use device and is available in three multidose

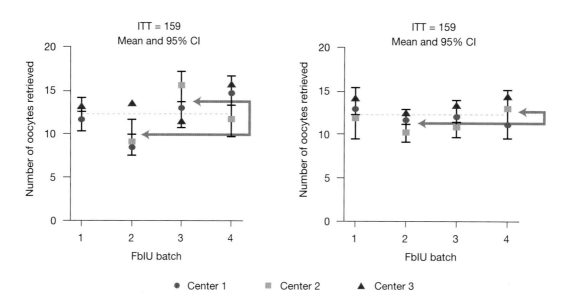

Figure 1 Consistency of ovarian response (oocytes retrieved) following treatment with four batches of recombinant human follicle stimulating hormone filled by IU (FbIU) or filled by mass (FbM). CI, confidence interval; ITT, intention to treat. Adapted from an article in *Reproductive BioMedicine Online* by Hugues *et al.*[27], reproduced with permission from Reproductive Healthcare Ltd

strengths, equivalent to 300, 450 and 900 IU. The minimum dose increment is 37.5 IU.

r-hLH and its use with r-hFSH

It has been known for some time that both FSH and LH are required for optimal estradiol (E_2) production and hence follicular maturation. The 'LH window' concept, outlined most recently by Balasch and Fabregues[33] and Shoham[34], states that in the absence of a threshold level of serum LH, E_2 production will be insufficient for follicular development and endometrial proliferation. However, exposure of the developing follicle to excessive LH results in atresia and cessation of normal development (Figure 2). Low levels of LH due to deficiency of endogenous gonadotropins are associated with anovulatory infertility (World Health Organization (WHO) type I; hypogonadotrophic hypogonadism). As noted below, LH may also fall below the threshold in some women treated with gonadotropin releasing hormone (GnRH) agonists, particularly in depot formulations.

The association of raised levels of LH with poor outcomes in assisted reproduction has been known for many years[35,36], and GnRH analogs are routinely administered to prevent a premature LH surge. It has also been suggested that raised levels of LH may be responsible for failure to conceive in some women with WHO type II anovulatory infertility treated with clomiphene citrate for OI, and in those who undergo a short protocol involving treatment with a GnRH agonist in ART[33]. Direct support for the concept of the 'LH window' comes from a study by Tesarik and Mendoza[37], in which oocyte donors were randomized to ovarian stimulation with r-hFSH alone or r-hFSH plus LH (LH activity derived from hMG). The addition of LH increased the number of developmentally competent oocytes in donors with endogenous LH suppressed below 1 IU/l at the start of stimulation. However, in donors with serum LH ≥ 1 IU/l, adding LH was associated with significantly lower embryo quality and implantation rates, compared with r-hFSH alone.

Other authors, notably Filicori and colleagues, have reported the benefits of exogenous LH activity in reducing the number of large (> 14 mm) and small (< 10 mm) follicles in women undergoing COS and OI[6,38]. The differences between groups are thought to be due to the LH activity present in hMG, and hence a reflection of the LH ceiling effect.

With the availability of pure r-hLH, it was possible to design clinical studies to validate the 'LH therapeutic window' concept. In an initial LH dose-finding study, women with hypogonadotropic hypogonadism,

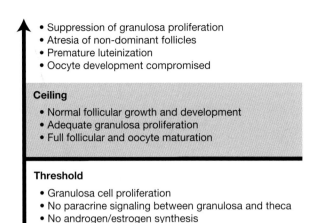

• Suppression of granulosa proliferation
• Atresia of non-dominant follicles
• Premature luteinization
• Oocyte development compromised

Ceiling
• Normal follicular growth and development
• Adequate granulosa proliferation
• Full follicular and oocyte maturation

Threshold
• Granulosa cell proliferation
• No paracrine signaling between granulosa and theca
• No androgen/estrogen synthesis
• Failure of oocyte maturation

Figure 2 The luteinizing hormone 'window' concept. Adapted from an article in *Current Opinions in Obstetrics and Gynecology* by Balasch and Fábregues[33], reproduced with permission from Lippincott Williams & Wilkins

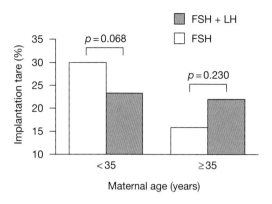

Figure 3 Implantation rates per cycle in women of different age groups following ovarian stimulation with recombinant human follicle stimulating hormone (r-hFSH) alone or r-hFSH plus recombinant human luteinizing hormone (r-hLH)[43]. Reprinted from an article in *Reproductive BioMedicine Online* by Marrs et al.[43], reproduced with permission from Reproductive Healthcare Ltd

treated with 150 IU/day r-hFSH plus 225 IU/day r-hLH, developed significantly fewer follicles compared with patients randomized to receive 75 IU LH[39]. Further testing of the LH ceiling concept was carried out in another study in women with hypogonadotropic hypogonadism[40]. Patients were randomized to receive r-hFSH, r-hLH or r-hFSH plus r-hLH during the late follicular phase following initial treatment with r-hFSH plus r-hLH. Follicular growth arrest occurred in 0/8 patients treated with r-hFSH alone, but was reported in 4/6 patients treated with r-hLH alone and in 1/6 of those who received r-hFSH plus r-hLH in the late follicular phase. In a separate study reported in the same paper, women with WHO type II infertility and known hyper-response to FSH treatment were randomized to r-hLH (225 or 450 IU/day) or placebo. In the two r-hLH groups, 5/12 patients showed follicular growth arrest, compared with none of the placebo patients. It was concluded from these two small studies that r-hLH alone can trigger follicular growth arrest in a significant number of patients, supporting the existence of an LH 'ceiling' during late follicular maturation.

Results in women with normal levels of endogenous gonadotropins were less clear-cut. However, following the introduction of down-regulation with GnRH agonists into ART protocols, a number of authors reported that a subgroup of women suffer profound pituitary and ovarian desensitization after

agonist administration[41,42]. It was suggested that such women might benefit from LH supplementation during ovarian stimulation, but these claims were not tested in large clinical studies, perhaps because of a lack of standard clinical criteria for identifying such patients[34].

In a recent study, Marrs and colleagues evaluated the effect of supplementation with 150 IU/day r-hLH from day 6 in women undergoing ovarian stimulation with r-hFSH in preparation for intracytoplasmic sperm injection (ICSI)[43]. In this large open-label study, 212 women received r-hFSH (initially 225 IU/day) plus r-hLH (150 IU/day) and 219 women received r-hFSH alone. The study included an analysis by patient age to test the hypothesis that r-hLH supplementation might be beneficial in the subgroup of women of older reproductive age (≥35 years).

The results showed no significant differences between treatment groups for most outcome measures. More embryos were transferred in the r-hFSH plus r-hLH group (2.9 ± 0.6 vs. 2.8 ± 0.7, $p = 0.037$). The results of the analysis by age showed a trend towards a higher implantation rate with r-hFSH alone in patients aged < 35 years (Figure 3). In contrast, the group aged ≥35 years had a numerically higher implantation rate in the r-hFSH plus r-hLH group (21.7 vs. 15.7%, $p = 0.230$). For clinical pregnancy rate per started cycle, differences between treatment groups were generally not significant. However, women aged

Table 2 Clinical pregnancy rates per started cycle in women of different ages undergoing ovarian stimulation with recombinant human follicle stimulating hormone (r-hFSH) alone or with r-hFSH plus recombinant human luteinizing hormone (r-hLH) from stimulation day 6[43]. Values were adjusted for the different numbers of embryos transferred in the two treatment groups using a logistic regression model. Reprinted from an article in *Reproductive BioMedicine Online* by Marrs et al.[43], reproduced with permission from Reproductive Healthcare Ltd

Age (years)	r-hFSH + r-hLH	r-hFSH alone	p Value
< 35			
ITT	63/147 (42.9%)	74/163 (45.4%)	NS
adjusted	39.8%	45.8%	NS
≥ 35			
ITT	27/65 (41.5%)	17/56 (30.4%)	NS
adjusted	35.4%	28.3%	NS
≥ 35 and undergoing first ART cycle			
ITT	22/48 (45.8%)	9/40 (22.5%)	0.027
adjusted	36.3%	19.6%	NS

ITT, intention to treat; ART, assisted reproductive technologies; NS, not significant

≥ 35 years who were undergoing their first ART cycle had significantly higher pregnancy rates in the r-hFSH plus r-hLH group (Table 2). This result was not significant after adjustment for the higher number of embryos transferred in the r-hFSH plus r-hLH group.

A similar study was reported recently by Humaidan and associates[44], who randomly assigned normogonadotropic women undergoing ART to receive r-hFSH alone ($n = 115$) or r-hFSH plus r-hLH in a 2:1 dose ratio ($n = 116$) from day 8 of stimulation. Overall, the two groups did not differ with respect to pregnancy rates. However, women aged ≥ 35 years given r-hFSH plus r-hLH had significantly higher implantation rates and lower total FSH consumption compared with those who received r-hFSH alone. In addition, the implantation rate in the subgroup with the highest endogenous LH concentration (≥ 1.99 IU/l) on day 8 was significantly increased by LH supplementation.

De Placido and colleagues[45] have recently investigated the effects of r-hLH supplementation in women with an initial poor response to r-hFSH stimulation after down-regulation. Women with serum E_2 < 180 pg/ml and with no follicles > 10 mm on stimulation day 8 were randomized to receive r-hLH at doses of 75 or 150 IU/day ($n = 23$ in each group). Normal responders ($n = 46$) continued treatment with r-hFSH alone and formed the control group. The mean number of oocytes and percentage of mature oocytes retrieved in the 150 IU r-hLH group were

significantly higher compared with the 75-IU group, and comparable to those achieved in the control group. Total r-hFSH consumption was significantly lower in the 150-IU group compared with the 75-IU group.

In summary, the results of these recent clinical studies suggest that ovarian stimulation with r-hFSH alone is appropriate for most patients in the younger age group. However, a subgroup of patients aged ≥ 35 years may benefit from supplementation with r-hLH from stimulation day 6 or 8 until hCG administration. Patients with a poor initial response to r-hFSH may also benefit from supplementation with r-hLH.

PROTOCOLS FOR ART WITH RECOMBINANT GONADOTROPINS

The most common starting dose for COS with r-hFSH is 150–225 IU/day. However, higher starting doses are used in older patients. A randomized double-blind study in women aged 30–39 years undergoing ovarian stimulation with r-hFSH (follitropin beta) for IVF or ICSI compared fixed daily r-hFSH doses of 150 and 250 IU[46]. The mean number of oocytes retrieved was 9.1 in the 150 IU group and 10.6 in the 250-IU group (not significant). The difference between the high- and the low-dose groups was 4.2 in favor of the 250-IU dose (14.8 vs. 10.6) in women aged 30–33 years, but in those aged 37–39 years slightly more oocytes were retrieved in those treated with the lower dose (8.1 vs. 7.4). This study suggests that increasing the dose of r-hFSH in women of older reproductive age does not result in increased oocyte yield.

Dosage guidelines for r-hFSH

Starting doses of r-hFSH for ART or OI tend to be decided empirically in spite of the efforts of medical societies to develop treatment guidelines. Recently, however, an attempt has been made to develop an FSH-dosing 'normogram' based on patient characteristics identified in a prospective study of 145 patients[47]. An industry-sponsored project to develop and validate dosage guidelines using data derived from statistical analysis of large databases of ART and OI clinical trials has also been initiated. The initial retrospective analysis of data from over 2000 patients demonstrated that there were four main patient characteristics that were predictive of ovarian response in an ART procedure; these were age, body mass index, baseline FSH and baseline number of small antral follicles (Howles and colleagues, manuscript in preparation). These predictive factors were fitted into a model to determine the daily dose of r-hFSH (follitropin alfa). A clinical study to validate this model is planned and a similar project for patients undergoing OI is also in progress.

GnRH analogs in cycles stimulated with r-hFSH

Most protocols involve treatment with a GnRH analog (agonist or antagonist) for prevention of a premature LH surge. Over 10 years ago, meta-analysis of clinical trials showed that the use of a GnRH agonist increases clinical pregnancy rate, decreases cycle cancelation rate and increases the number of oocytes retrieved, compared with cycles without an agonist[48]. A number of different agonists, formulations and delivery routes (subcutaneous, intranasal and depot) are available.

GnRH antagonists became available for clinical use more recently than the agonists. Antagonists have a number of potential advantages over agonists, including a rapid onset of action and lack of hormone withdrawal symptoms. GnRH antagonist treatment can be fitted into the stimulation cycle with no need

for pretreatment. Two antagonists, cetrorelix and ganirelix, are currently available for clinical use. Ganirelix is given at a daily dose of 0.25 mg, while cetrorelix can be given daily as injections of 0.25 mg or as a single 3-mg dose. A single 3-mg injection of cetrorelix offers equivalent efficacy to a long protocol involving treatment with an agonist[49].

A number of clinical studies have been carried out to compare GnRH antagonists with agonists (using a standard long protocol for the agonist cycles) in conjunction with r-hFSH[50–53] or hMG for ovarian stimulation. Following the initial clinical studies, which suggested a lower pregnancy rate per cycle following antagonist use, two meta-analyses have been published[54,55]. Both analyses demonstrated a significantly lower pregnancy rate for the antagonists, but when stratified by type of antagonist this was confirmed for ganirelix but not for cetrorelix studies. Antagonist cycles were associated with a significantly lower risk of ovarian hyperstimulation syndrome (OHSS) overall, and of severe (grade III) OHSS, which could be confirmed for cetrorelix alone. For ganirelix, the risk seems to be reduced as compared with a GnRH agonist long protocol.

Regimens involving GnRH antagonists in conjunction with r-hFSH can be refined by using programming with an oral contraceptive (OC) to reduce uncertainty in the timing of oocyte retrieval. This allows oocyte retrieval to be planned for a time convenient to both the patient and the clinic: for example, by avoiding weekends. In a randomized study by Obruca and colleagues[56], one group of patients took an OC for 18–28 days before the start of ovarian stimulation with r-hFSH. The final OC was taken on a Sunday and stimulation began the following Friday. In the control group, stimulation began on day 3 of the cycle. Both groups received cetrorelix (0.25 mg daily) from stimulation day 6 to follicular maturation. None out of 68 oocyte retrievals in the OC-treated group took place at the weekend, compared with 6/66 in the control group. Further studies using this technique are awaited.

Outcomes in cycles using cetrorelix together with r-hFSH may be further improved by using individualized starting dates for cetrorelix treatment. In a randomized study by Ludwig and colleagues[57], patients who started cetrorelix when the largest follicle was 14 mm in diameter required significantly less cetrorelix and r-hFSH and had significantly more oocytes

Table 3 Summary of results of computer modeling studies comparing cost per ongoing pregnancy with recombinant human follicle stimulating hormone (r-hFSH) vs. urine-derived FSH (u-FSH) stimulation in different health-care systems

Country	Cost per ongoing pregnancy		p Value
	r-hFSH	u-FSH	
UK[62]	£5906	£6060	<0.0001
USA[63]	$40 688 (societal perspective)	$47 096 (societal perspective)	<0.0001
	$28 481 (insurers' perspective)	$32 967 (insurers' perspective)	<0.0001
Spain: public sector[65]	€12 791	€13 007	<0.0001
Spain: private sector[66]	€19 739	€20 467	<0.0001
Germany[64]	€21 686	€22 189	<0.0001

retrieved compared with those who started cetrorelix on day 6.

r-hCG versus u-hCG

Typical criteria for the administration of hCG to induce final follicular maturation in ART would be the presence of at least one follicle of diameter ≥18 mm together with at least two other follicles ≥16 mm and E_2 concentration within the acceptable range (approximately 150 pg/ml per mature follicle). r-hCG at a dose of 250 μg is approved for this purpose, and has been compared with u-hCG (5000 and 10 000 IU) in a number of clinical trials in ART[58-60] and OI[61]. r-hCG was better tolerated than u-hCG in terms of local reactions to injection. r-hCG offers a pure and consistent product with advantages over u-hCG for the induction of final follicular maturation and ovulation.

COST-EFFECTIVENESS OF RECOMBINANT AND URINE-DERIVED GONADOTROPINS

In the current environment of constraints on health-care, it is important to demonstrate that treatments are cost-effective as well as clinically effective. This is particularly important for ART because, even when treatment is covered by the health-care system, there is often a requirement for the couple to contribute towards the cost.

A number of studies have compared the cost-effectiveness of r-hFSH (follitropin alfa) and u-FSH

for COS. These studies have used computer modeling to overcome the limitations of clinical trials for evaluating the cost-effectiveness of complex treatments such as ART in which outcomes may be affected by many different factors. Specifically, the techniques of Markov modeling and Monte-Carlo simulation have been employed to generate data on large numbers of 'virtual' patients, using assumptions based on published clinical trial data.

The results of these studies indicate that the cost per ongoing pregnancy is lower when r-hFSH is used for ovarian stimulation than when u-FSH is used (Table 3). This is true in the health-care systems of the UK[62], the USA[63], Germany[64] and Spain[65,66], and over a wide range of prices for u-FSH[67]. It appears that the greater clinical efficacy of r-hFSH compared with u-FSH[14] more than outweighs the higher acquisition cost of the recombinant product. Clinicians and policy-makers should take these data into account in making a choice between products for use in COS.

NEW DEVELOPMENTS

There are a number of new developments that are likely to affect the ways in which gonadotropin therapy is delivered in the future. One objective that might be desirable is to increase the duration of action of r-hFSH and thus reduce the number of injections required. A long-acting modified form of FSH was tested in humans in 2001[68]. This substance, designated FSH-C-terminal peptide (FSH-CTP), consists of the α subunit of hFSH together with a hybrid β subunit. The hybrid β subunit is made up of the β subunit of hFSH and the C terminus part of the β subunit of hCG, which confers an increased half-life on the molecule. A recent randomized trial in patients undergoing COS for ART showed that a single dose of FSH-CTP (120–240 μg) during the early follicular phase effectively induced multiple follicular development over a 7-day period[69]. The number of oocytes retrieved per started cycle was significantly higher in women treated with FSH-CTP, 240 μg, compared with those treated with r-hFSH, 150 IU/day (12.0 ± 7.3 vs. 7.9 ± 4.1, $p = 0.03$). However, there were no differences in the number of good-quality embryos obtained and numbers of embryos available for transfer. Further studies are required to establish the optimum dose regimen for FSH-CTP.

An alternative approach to increasing the duration of action of r-hFSH is to develop novel ways of delivering the unmodified FSH molecule. Sustained-release r-hFSH is under development. The product uses microsphere technology in which r-hFSH is encapsulated and which, when given as a single subcutaneous injection, releases FSH over a period of days, mimicking the daily dosing over the first 5–10 days of an ART or OI cycle. The quantity and duration of FSH administration depends on the loading and nature of the microsphere formulation.

In the long term, it would be desirable to replace gonadotropin injections with oral therapy if a suitable orally available gonadotropin mimetic can be found. Research to identify possible drug candidates is still at the discovery/preclinical research stage.

REFERENCES

1. Ludwig M, Felberbaum RE, Diedrich K, et al. Ovarian stimulation: from basic science to clinical application. Reprod Biomed Online 2002; 5 (Suppl. 1): 73–86

2. Loumaye E, Campbell R, Salat-Baroux J. Human follicle-stimulating hormone produced by recombinant DNA technology: a review for clinicians. Hum Reprod Update 1995; 1: 188–99

3. Stokman PG, de Leeuw R, van den Wijngaard HA, et al. Human chorionic gonadotropin in commercial human menopausal gonadotropin preparations. Fertil Steril 1993; 60: 175–8

4. Giudice E, Crisci C, Altarocca V, et al. Characterisation of a partially purified human menopausal gonadotropin preparation. J Clin Res 2001; 4: 27–33

5. Rodgers M, Mitchell R, Lambert A, et al. Human chorionic gonadotropin contributes to the bioactivity of Pergonal. Clin Endocrinol (Oxf) 1992; 37: 558–64

6. Filicori M, Cognigni GE, Taraborrelli S, et al. Luteinzing hormone activity in menotropins optimizes folliculogenesis and treatment in controlled ovarian stimulation. J Clin Endocrinol Metab 2001; 86: 337–43

7. van de Weijer BH, Mulders JW, Bos ES, et al. Compositional analyses of a human menopausal gonadotropin preparation extracted from urine (menotropin). Identification of some of its major impurities. Reprod Biomed Online 2003; 7: 547–57

8. Horsman G, Talbot JA, McLoughlin JD, et al. A biological, immunological and physico-chemical comparison of the current clinical batches of the recombinant FSH preparations Gonal-F and Puregon. Hum Reprod 2000; 15: 1898–902

9. Driebergen R, Baer G. Quantification of follicle stimulating hormone (follitropin alfa): is in vivo bioassay still relevant in the recombinant age? Curr Med Res Opin 2003; 19: 41–6

10. Bassett RM, Driebergen R. Continued improvements in the quality and consistency of follitropin alfa, recombinant human FSH. Reprod Biomed Online 2005; 10: 169–77

11. Bergh C, Howles CM, Borg K, et al. Recombinant human follicle stimulating hormone (r-hFSH; Gonal-F) versus highly purified urinary FSH (Metrodin HP): results of a randomized comparative study in women undergoing assisted reproductive techniques. Hum Reprod 1997; 12: 2133–9

12. Out HJ, Mannaerts BM, Driessen SG, et al. A prospective, randomized, assessor-blind, multicentre study comparing recombinant and urinary follicle stimulating hormone (Puregon versus Metrodin) in in-vitro fertilization. Hum Reprod 1995; 10: 2534–40

13. Daya S. Updated meta-analysis of recombinant follicle-stimulating hormone (FSH) versus urinary FSH for ovarian stimulation in assisted reproduction. Fertil Steril 2002; 77: 711–14

14. Out HJ, Driessen SG, Mannaerts BM, et al. Recombinant follicle-stimulating hormone (follitropin beta, Puregon) yields higher pregnancy rates in in vitro fertilization than urinary gonadotropins. Fertil Steril 1997; 68: 138–42

15. Ludwig M, Rabe T, Bühler K, et al. Wirksamkeit von recombinantem humanem FSH in Vergleich zu urinärem hMG nach Downregulation im langen Protokoll – eine Analyse von 24.764 ART-Zyklen in Deutschland. J Reproduktionsmed Endokrinol 1994; 4: 284–8

16. Biffoni M, Marcucci I, Ythier A, et al. Effects of urinary gonadotropin preparations on human in-vitro immune function. Hum Reprod 1998; 13: 2430–4

17. Redfearn A, Hughes EG, O'Connor M, et al. Delayed-type hypersensitivity to human gonadotropin: case report. Fertil Steril 1995; 64: 855–6

18. Whitman-Elia GF, Banks K, O'Dea LS. Recombinant follicle-stimulating hormone in a patient hypersensitive to urinary-derived gonadotropins. Gynecol Endocrinol 1998; 12: 209–12

19. Harrison S, Wolf T, Abuzeid MI. Administration of recombinant follicle stimulating hormone in a woman with allergic reaction to menotropin: a case report. Gynecol Endocrinol 2000; 14: 149–52

20. Phipps WR, Holden D, Sheehan RK. Use of recombinant human follicle-stimulating hormone for in vitro fertilization–embryo transfer after severe systemic immunoglobulin E-mediated reaction to urofollitropin. Fertil Steril 1996; 66: 148–50

21. Brinsden P, Akagbosu F, Gibbons LM, et al. A comparison of the efficacy and tolerability of two recombinant human follicle-stimulating hormone preparations in patients undergoing in vitro fertilization–embryo transfer. Fertil Steril 2000; 73: 114–16

22. Wikland M, Borg K, Decosterd G, et al. Gonal-F filled by mass is significantly better tolerated than Puregon liquid in patients undergoing ovarian stimulation for ART. Presented at the 12th World Congress on In Vitro Fertilization and Molecular Reproduction, Buenos Aires, Argentina, March 2002: Poster

23. Artiges A. Alternatives to animals in the development and control of biological products for human and veterinary use. The role of the European Pharmacopoeia. Dev Biol Stand 1999; 101: 29–35

24. Garthoff B, et al. Safety and efficacy testing of hormones and related products. Report and recommendations of the ECVAM Workshop. Altern Lab Anim 1995; 23: 699–712

25. Steelman SL, Pohley FM. Assay of the follicle stimulating hormone based on the augmentation with human chorionic gonadotropin. Endocrinology 1953; 53: 604–16

26. Neuspiller N, Kelly E, Loumaye E, et al. Technological improvements in Gonal-F manufacturing process translate into clinical benefits in ART even at 150 IU starting dose. Presented at the 12th World Congress on In Vitro Fertilization and Molecular Reproduction Buenos Aires, Argentina, March 2002: Abstr

27. Hugues JN, Barlow DH, Rosenwaks Z, et al. Improvement in consistency of response to ovarian stimulation with recombinant human follicle stimulating hormone resulting from a new method for calibrating the therapeutic preparation. Reprod Biomed Online 2003; 6: 185–90

28. Balasch J, Fabregues F, Penarrubia J, et al. Outcome from consecutive assisted reproduction cycles in patients treated with recombinant follitropin alfa filled-by-bioassay and those treated with recombinant follitropin alfa filled-by-mass. Reprod Biomed Online 2004; 8: 408–13

29. Voortman G, van de Post J, Schoemaker RC, et al. Bioequivalence of subcutaneous injections of recombinant human follicle stimulating hormone (Puregon®) by pen-injector and syringe. Hum Reprod 1999; 14: 1698–702

30. Craenmehr E, Bontje P, Hoomans E, et al. Follitropin-beta administered by pen device has superior local tolerance compared with follitropin-alpha administered by conventional syringe. Reprod Biomed Online 2001; 3: 185–9

31. Platteau P, Laurent E, Albano C, et al. An open, randomized single-centre study to compare the efficacy and convenience of follitropin beta administered by a pen device with follitropin alpha administered by a conventional syringe in women undergoing ovarian stimulation for IVF/ICSI. Hum Reprod 2003; 18: 1200–4

32. Pang S, Kaplan B, Karande V, et al. Administration of recombinant human FSH (solution in cartridge) with a pen device in women undergoing ovarian stimulation. Reprod Biomed Online 2003; 7: 319–26

33. Balasch J, Fabregues F. Is luteinizing hormone needed for optimal ovulation induction? Curr Opin Obstet Gynecol 2002; 14: 265–74

34. Shoham Z. The clinical therapeutic window for luteinizing hormone in controlled ovarian stimulation. Fertil Steril 2002; 77: 1170–7

35. Stanger JD, Yovich JL. Reduced in-vitro fertilization of human oocytes from patients with raised basal luteinizing hormone levels during the follicular phase. Br J Obstet Gynaecol 1985; 92: 385–93

36. Howles CM, Macnamee MC, Edwards RG. Follicular development and early luteal function of conception and non-conceptional cycles after human in-vitro fertilization: endocrine correlates. Hum Reprod 1987; 2: 17–21

37. Tesarik J, Mendoza C. Effects of exogenous LH administration during ovarian stimulation of pituitary down-regulated young oocyte donors on oocyte yield and developmental competence. Hum Reprod 2002; 17: 3129–37

38. Filicori M, Cognigni GE. Clinical review 126: roles and novel regimens of luteinizing hormone and follicle-stimulating hormone in ovulation induction. J Clin Endocrinol Metab 2001; 86: 1437–41

39. European Recombinant Human LH Study Group. Recombinant human luteinizing hormone (LH) to support recombinant human follicle-stimulating hormone (FSH)-induced follicular development in LH- and FSH-deficient anovulatory women: a dose-finding study. J Clin Endocrinol Metab 1998; 83: 1507–14

40. Loumaye E, Engrand P, Shoham Z, et al. Clinical evidence for an LH 'ceiling' effect induced by administration of recombinant human LH during the late follicular phase of stimulated cycles in World Health Organization type I and type II anovulation. Hum Reprod 2003; 18: 314–22

41. Fleming R, Rehka P, Deshpande N, et al. Suppression of LH during ovarian stimulation: effects differ in cycles stimulated with purified urinary FSH and recombinant FSH. Hum Reprod 2000; 15: 1440–5

42. Westergaard LG, Laursen SB, Andersen CY. Increased risk of early pregnancy loss by profound suppression of luteinizing hormone during ovarian stimulation in normogonadotrophic women undergoing assisted reproduction. Hum Reprod 2000; 15: 1003–8

43. Marrs RP, Meldrum DR, Muasher SJ, et al. Randomized trial to compare the effect of recombinant human FSH (follitropin alfa) with or without recombinant human LH in women undergoing assisted reproduction treatment. Reprod Biomed Online 2004; 8: 175–82

44. Humaidan P, Bungum M, Bungum L, et al. Effects of recombinant LH supplementation in women undergoing assisted reproduction with GnRH agonist down-regulation and stimulation with recombinant FSH: an opening study. Reprod Biomed Online 2004; 8: 635–43

45. De Placido G, Alviggi C, Mollo A, et al. Effects of recombinant LH (rLH) supplementation during controlled ovarian hyperstimulation (COH) in normogonadotrophic women with an initial inadequate response to recombinant FSH (rFSH) after pituitary downregulation. Clin Endocrinol (Oxf) 2004; 60: 637–43

46. Out HJ, Braat DD, Lintsen BM, et al. Increasing the daily dose of recombinant follicle stimulating hormone (Puregon) does not compensate for the age-related decline in retrievable oocytes after ovarian stimulation. Hum Reprod 2000; 15: 29–35

47. Popovic-Todorovic B, Loft A, Lindhard A, et al. A prospective study of predictive factors of ovarian response in 'standard' IVF/ICSI patients treated with recombinant FSH. A suggestion for a recombinant FSH dosage normogram. Hum Reprod 2003; 18: 781–7

48. Hughes EG, Fedorko DM, Daya S, et al. The routine use of gonadotropin-releasing hormone agonists prior to in vitro fertilization and gamete intrafallopian transfer: a meta-analysis of randomized controlled trials. Fertil Steril 1992; 58: 888–96

49. Olivennes F, Belaisch-Allart J, Emperaire JC, et al. Prospective, randomized, controlled study of in vitro fertilization–embryo transfer with a single dose of a luteinizing hormone-releasing hormone (LH-RH) antagonist (cetrorelix) or a depot formula of an LH-RH agonist (triptorelin). Fertil Steril 2000; 73: 314–20

50. Borm G, Mannaerts B. Treatment with the gonadotropin-releasing hormone antagonist ganirelix in women undergoing ovarian stimulation with recombinant follicle stimulating hormone is effective, safe and convenient: results of a controlled, randomized, multicentre trial. The European Orgalutran Study Group. Hum Reprod 2000; 15: 1490–8

51. European and Middle East Orgalutran Study Group. Comparable clinical outcome using the GnRH antagonist ganirelix or a long protocol of the GnRH agonist triptorelin for the prevention of premature LH surges in women undergoing ovarian stimulation. Hum Reprod 2001; 16: 644–51

52. Fluker M, Grifo J, Leader A, et al. Efficacy and safety of ganirelix acetate versus leuprolide acetate in women undergoing controlled ovarian hyperstimulation. Fertil Steril 2001; 75: 38–45

53. Roulier R, Chabert-Orsini V, Sitri MC, et al. Depot GnRH agonist versus the single dose GnRH antagonist regimen (cetrorelix, 3 mg) in patients undergoing assisted reproduction treatment. Reprod Biomed Online 2003; 7: 185–9

54. Ludwig M, Katalinic A, Diedrich K. Use of GnRH antagonists in ovarian stimulation for assisted reproductive technologies compared to the long protocol. Meta-analysis. Arch Gynecol Obstet 2001; 265: 175–82

55. Al-Inany H, Aboulghar M. GnRH antagonists in assisted reproduction: a Cochrane Review. Hum Reprod 2002; 17: 874–85

56. Obruca A, Fischl F, Huber JC. GnRH Antagonisten bei der kontrollierten ovariellen Hyperstimulation im Rahmen der IVF – Optimierung der Planbarkeit. J Reprod Fertil 2000; 4: 37

57. Ludwig M, Katalinic A, Banz C, et al. Tailoring the GnRH antagonist cetrorelix acetate to individual patients' needs in ovarian stimulation for IVF: results of a prospective, randomized study. Hum Reprod 2002; 17: 2842–5

58. Chang P, Kenley S, Burns T, et al. Recombinant human chorionic gonadotropin (rhCG) in assisted reproductive technology: results of a clinical trial comparing two doses of rhCG (Ovidrel) to urinary hCG (Profasi) for induction of final follicular

maturation in in vitro fertilization–embryo transfer. Fertil Steril 2001; 76: 67–74

59. Driscoll GL, Tyler JP, Hangan JT, et al. A prospective, randomized, controlled, double-blind, double-dummy comparison of recombinant and urinary HCG for inducing oocyte maturation and follicular luteinization in ovarian stimulation. Hum Reprod 2000; 15: 1305–10

60. European Recombinant Human Chorionic Gonadotropin Study Group. Induction of final follicular maturation and early luteinization in women undergoing ovulation induction for assisted reproduction treatment – recombinant HCG versus urinary HCG. Hum Reprod 2000; 15: 1446–51

61. International Recombinant Human Chorionic Gonadotropin Study Group. Induction of ovulation in World Health Organization group II anovulatory women undergoing follicular stimulation with recombinant human follicle-stimulating hormone: a comparison of recombinant human chorionic gonadotropin (rhCG) and urinary hCG. Fertil Steril 2001; 75: 1111–18

62. Daya S, Ledger W, Auray JP, et al. Cost-effectiveness modelling of recombinant FSH versus urinary FSH in assisted reproduction techniques in the UK. Hum Reprod 2001; 16: 2563–9

63. Silverberg K, Daya S, Auray JP, et al. Analysis of the cost effectiveness of recombinant versus urinary follicle-stimulating hormone in in vitro fertilization/intracytoplasmic sperm injection programs in the United States. Fertil Steril 2002; 77: 107–13

64. Felberbaum R, Daya S, Fischer R, et al. Kosteneffektivität von rekombinantem FSH (r-hFSH) bei assistierten Reproduktionstechnicken (ART) in Deutschland – Modellierung im Vergleich zu urinärem FSH (u-hFSH). Geburtshilfe Frauenheilkd 2002; 62: 668–76

65. Romeu A, Balasch J, Ruiz Balda JA, et al. Cost-effectiveness of recombinant versus urinary follicle-stimulating hormone in assisted reproduction techniques in the Spanish public health care system. J Assist Reprod Genet 2003; 20: 294–300

66. Barri PN, Balasch J, Romeu A, et al. Coste-efectividad de la hormona folículo-estimulante recombinante y urinaria en las técnicas de reproducción asistida en el sector sanitario privado español. Rev Iberoam Fertil 2002; 19: 195–202

67. Silverberg K, Schertz J, Falk B, et al. Impact of urinary FSH price: a cost-effectiveness analysis of recombinant and urinary FSH in assisted reproductive techniques in the USA. Reprod Biomed Online 2002; 5: 265–9

68. Bouloux PM, Handelsman DJ, Jockenhovel F, et al. First human exposure to FSH-CTP in hypogonadotrophic hypogonadal males. Hum Reprod 2001; 16: 1592–7

69. Devroey P, Fauser BC, Platteau P, et al. Induction of multiple follicular development by a single dose of long-acting recombinant follicle-stimulating hormone (FSH-CTP, corifollitropin alfa) for controlled ovarian stimulation before in vitro fertilization. J Clin Endocrinol Metab 2004; 89: 2062–70

9

The use of gonadotropin releasing hormone agonists and antagonists in infertility

Fidelis T. Akagbosu and Awoniyi O. Awonuga

See wel 158p

INTRODUCTION

In the early days of *in vitro* fertilization (IVF), natural cycles were commonly employed[1] and classic stimulation protocols involved the use of clomiphene citrate and gonadotropins. Elevated basal levels of luteinizing hormone (LH) were shown to have a poor correlation with the success of the IVF cycle[2]. Premature LH surges, which occurred due to the positive feedback of rising estradiol levels induced by the gonadotropins, led to premature luteinization and were considered reasons for cancelation of the treatment cycle. The discovery that the continued administration of gonadotropin releasing hormone (GnRH) analogs induced a state of hypophyseal desensitization and largely reduced the incidence of premature luteinization provided a welcome solution to the problems that had caused a large number of IVF cycle cancelations.

The first clinical trials of the use of GnRH analogs showed that they were effective in reducing the basal levels of LH[3,4] and in reducing the incidence of low responders[5,6]. The incidence of cycle cancelations diminished significantly, and the GnRH agonist analogs were soon in routine use. The agonists led to desensitization of the pituitary gonadotropin cells and a reduction in the number of GnRH receptors, while the antagonists produced an immediate effect by competitive blockade of the GnRH receptors.

Various protocols combining the use of agonistic analogs and gonadotropins in IVF cycles have been described. Reports in the current literature have associated the use of GnRH agonists with high pregnancy rates after IVF and embryo transfer (ET)[7]. Debatable facts include the suggestion that agonist use has a harmful effect on oocytes and embryo quality, and that agonists have direct effects on the ovary[8]. So far, there does not appear to be an increased risk of birth defects or pregnancy wastage in human pregnancies exposed to the GnRH analogs[9].

The GnRH antagonists became commercially available for use in the UK in April 1999 and in North America in May 2000. Two GnRH antagonists now commonly used in many IVF centers worldwide are cetrorelix (Serono International SA, Geneva, Switzerland) and ganirelix (Organon, Oss, The Netherlands). Antagonist use has various potential advantages, such as short-term and low medication exposure during follicular development. As there is no 'flare effect', the frequency of cyst formation should be lower, patient management should be easier and stress, cost and hyperstimulation may all be reduced. GnRH antagonists are currently used mainly to prevent premature LH surges following ovarian stimulation for IVF, in either single or multiple doses[10,11]. Promising results have been published on their use in intrauterine

---

insemination cycles and in patients with uterine myomas or endometriosis.

The use of GnRH agonists and antagonists seems safe for pregnant women and their offspring. The sex hormone-dependent disorders currently treated with GnRH agonists, including endometriosis, leiomyoma and breast cancer in women, benign prostatic hypertrophy and prostate carcinoma in men, and central precocious puberty in children, may in future be indications for a GnRH antagonist[12].

GnRH

GnRH is a decapeptide produced in the mediobasal hypothalamus by neurons located in the arcuate nucleus. Green and Harris first postulated its existence in 1947[13], and it was first isolated and characterized by Schally and colleagues in 1971[14]. In native GnRH, the amino acid sequence in positions 2 and 3 facilitates the release of gonadotropins, while the sequence in position 6 is involved in enzymatic cleavage; residues 1, 6 and 10 are important for the three-dimensional structure and thus for receptor binding. GnRH binds to specific transmembrane receptors in the gonadotropic cells in the anterior pituitary. The receptors then undergo a dimerization process and initiate a cascade of intracellular events that culminate in the synthesis and secretion of follicle stimulating hormone (FSH) and LH. Once the dimer has completed its signal transduction, it is internalized into the cell. The dimer then breaks and the receptors recycle to the surface and allow a subsequent pulse of GnRH to repeat the cycle[15]. The physiological pattern of pulsatile release also maintains GnRH receptor numbers as well as the functional intracellular transduction pathways. Knobil[16] showed that GnRH given continuously caused a decrease in LH and FSH levels.

GnRH AGONISTS

Physiology of GnRH agonists

The agonists were developed soon after the identification of the structure of native GnRH. The aim was to increase GnRH stability and binding affinity to its receptors by modifying the amino acid sequence[17,18]. The modifications were mainly at positions 6 and 10, and resulted in increased potency. For leuprolide, the

glycine in position 6 has been replaced by D-leucine and the carbonxy-terminal glycinamide has been replaced by ethylamide[19]. For buserelin, the glycine in position 6 has been replaced by (*t*-butyl) D-serine and the carboxy-terminal glycinamide replaced by ethylamide[20]. The substitutions at the number 6 position help protect against enzymatic degradation of the analogs. Unlike GnRH with a half-life of only a few minutes, the GnRH agonists have half-lives of a few hours. The agonists have a 100–200 times higher binding affinity for the GnRH receptors than does the native molecule.

The short-term effects of GnRH agonists are very similar to those of GnRH. The agonist binds to the receptors and the receptors then undergo a dimerization process and initiate a cascade of intracellular events that culminate in the synthesis and secretion of FSH and LH. Following dimerization and signal transduction, the dimer is internalized into the cell as is the case for GnRH. Over time, due to the abundance of the antagonist with a long half-life, the dimer form of the receptor is favored and the receptors are incorporated into the cell but cannot return to the cell membrane. The cell cannot therefore respond to a subsequent pulse of GnRH. This process of desensitization is achieved by down-regulation of the GnRH receptors and by an uncoupling of any remaining receptors from their intracellular machinery[21].

Agonist analog administration thus initially induces the liberation of high amounts of LH and FSH from the pituitary and an increase in the number of GnRH receptors (up-regulation). Within 12 h of administration, the so-called 'flare effect' leads to a five-fold increase of FSH, ten-fold rise in LH and four-fold elevation in estradiol[22]. Continuous (not pulsatile) GnRH analog administration causes opposite effects: internalization of the agonist-receptor complex and a decrease in the number of receptors (down-regulation). This causes paradoxical suppression of the pituitary gonadotropin synthesis and liberation (desensitization). The decreased levels of FSH and LH result in the arrest of follicular development and cause a fall in sex steroid levels to castrate levels. This is the basis for the clinical use of the agonists. GnRH agonist administration in the luteal phase causes a state of relative hypoestrogenism leading to hot flushes, insomnia, short-term memory disturbances and headaches. The pituitary blockade persists during the agonist treatment but is completely reversible after therapy. Postmenopausal estradiol levels are commonly reached after 21 days[23]. In women, a normal menstrual cycle is re-established in approximately 6 weeks.

GnRH ANTAGONISTS

Physiology of GnRH antagonists

The GnRH antagonists were developed in parallel with the agonists. Their development history was plagued mainly by the high incidence of histamine release following use of the first-generation antagonists. The first-generation antagonists were characterized by modifications in positions 2 and 3. The *in vitro* assay systems were effective, but very high doses were required. The second-generation antagonists had modifications in positions 1 and 6 and, later, the introduction of D-arginine in position 6. Allergic side-effects with the early antagonists included local erythema and induration, generalized edema and anaphylactoid reaction. The observed side-effects were caused by the induction of histamine release, due to the existence of GnRH receptors on mast cells that degranulate after binding of basic antagonist[24] and, to a much lesser extent, also of native GnRH[25].

The third- and fourth-generation antagonists are the modern antagonists. These were developed in the search for the ideal antagonist with high potency, a long duration of action and no clinically relevant side-effects. They usually have modifications in amino acid positions 1, 2, 3, 6 and 10 of GnRH. The substitutions in the first three amino acids in cetrorelix and ganirelix are identical and confer antagonist properties. The substitution in position 6 extends their half-lives relative to native. The substitutions in positions 8 and 10 have resulted in elimination of the histamine-release problem of the early antagonists[20].

Antagonists competitively bind to pituitary GnRH receptors and block the ability of GnRH to initiate dimer formation, signal transduction and FSH and LH secretion from the pituitary gonadotrope. As long as sufficient GnRH antagonist is present, suppression of FSH and LH will be sustained. Various clinical studies have confirmed that GnRH antagonists are effective at preventing the onset of a premature LH surge during controlled ovarian stimulation (COH)[26-28]. Receptor blockade is immediate and prevents the action of native GnRH. On the basis of the mechanism of competitive binding, it is possible to modulate the degree of hormone suppression by the dose of antagonist that is administered. For instance, depending upon the indication for therapy, this permits the physician to maintain defined estradiol levels, which may have the advantage of avoiding hormone withdrawal effects such as vaginal dryness or hot flushes[29].

In COH cycles, the GnRH antagonists are not initiated until the stimulation cycle is well under way and estradiol levels are elevated; consequently, no estrogen deprivation symptoms occur[30]. Since the antagonists do not cause pituitary exhaustion, these cells can respond to an adequate stimulus almost immediately. Other advantages of GnRH antagonists compared with the agonists are the substantially shorter duration of exposure to the antagonist, the reduced duration of gonadotropin treatment and the flexibility of planning treatment, knowing that the antagonist can cause rapid suppression of endogenous LH/FSH during all phases of the menstrual cycle.

There has been some concern regarding pregnancy rates (per started cycle) with antagonist versus agonist administration in the phase III studies conducted with ganirelix acetate[27,28]. The differences are not statistically significant but there is the nagging concern that, although not statistically significant, the pregnancy rates appear to be a little lower with the antagonist arms of these studies[30]. In the European study[31], it was shown that there was no difference in pregnancy rates in centers that had experience, but a larger difference in pregnancy rate when the centers lacked prior experience with the GnRH antagonists. The implication is that there is a learning curve.

CLINICAL APPLICATIONS OF GnRH ANALOGS IN ASSISTED REPRODUCTIVE TECHNOLOGIES

Raised basal levels of LH have a negative impact on the quality of oocytes and embryos and subsequently on pregnancy rate[32,33]. Pretreatment with agonists significantly reduces the occurrence of LH surges. Before the agonist era, approximately 20% of stimulated IVF cycles were canceled, owing to premature LH surges. With agonist use, this percentage has decreased to 2% and fertilization and implantation rates have increased[34].

Agonist use in assisted reproductive technologies

Different treatment schedules using GnRH analogs and gonadotropins are now in use, including the so-called 'long' protocol, which aims at complete pituitary suppression, and the 'short' and 'ultra-short' protocols, in which the 'flare-up' effect is utilized. GnRH analogs are used in IVF treatment cycles as well as in frozen embryo transfer cycles when hormone replacement is required. In the IVF cycles, the 'long' protocol is generally the most effective, and is most often used at present. However, it has the disadvantages of a long treatment period until desensitization is achieved and relatively high costs due to an increased requirement for human menopausal gonadotropin (hMG)[35]. As a result of the pituitary desensitization, and to allow recovery, luteal phase support with progesterone or human chorionic gonadotropin (hCG) is required after analog use.

Specific effects of GnRH agonist use in IVF have been documented. Hsueh and co-workers[36] noted anti-gonadotropin actions such as 83% loss of LH receptors in rat granulosa cells, decreased aromatase activity and decreased progesterone accumulation. Agonist analog use also leads to the activation of 20-OH progesterone dehydrogenase; this stimulates metabolism of progesterone to 20-OH progesterone with little progestational activity. It is usual to provide luteal support in agonist cycles.

Antagonist use in assisted reproductive technologies

The simplicity offered by antagonists in regulating the menstrual cycle and causing almost immediate suppression of LH and FSH levels has made them potentially useful in assisted reproduction cycles. Diedrich and colleagues[23] were able to stimulate patients successfully after pretreatment with cetrorelix by daily administration starting on cycle day 7 until induction of ovulation. The mean number of oocytes retrieved was 8.1 per patient and the fertilization rate was 61.5%. In 42% of the embryos, embryo quality was judged as being 'excellent' by morphological criteria. Six pregnancies were achieved in the first 42 patients treated by this regimen and three healthy babies were delivered. The mean amount of hMG required per patient was 27 ampoules, whereas 40–50 ampoules were required in the 'long' protocol of GnRH agonists at the center. The amount of hMG needed after cetrorelix treatment was comparable with the 'ultra-short' protocol, which up to then had been the least costly treatment.

Albano and colleagues[37] compared different doses of the GnRH antagonist cetrorelix during controlled ovarian hyperstimulation (COH). In 69 patients COH was carried out with hMG, starting on day 2 of the menstrual cycle; daily cetrorelix was administered from day 6 and continued up to and including the last day of hMG injection. No premature endogenous LH surge occurred in patients treated with 0.5 and 0.25 mg of cetrorelix. The minimal effective daily dose of cetrorelix able to prevent an LH surge in COH patients was 0.25 mg. Dose-finding studies[10,38] have defined 3 mg as the minimum effective dose that can prevent premature endogenous luteinizing hormone surges. The protection interval with the single 3-mg dose appears to be 4 days. If hCG is not administered within these 4 days, daily injections of 0.25 mg of antagonist can be added.

IVF results in agonist versus antagonist cycles

A nagging question has been whether the GnRH antagonists are at least as effective as the GnRH agonists when used in IVF–ET cycles. Both the North American Ganirelix Study Group[28] and The European and Middle East Study Group[27] trials showed that the duration of stimulation and the number of gonadotropin ampoules used were lower in the antagonist cycles. Fewer follicles and lower estradiol levels were observed on the day of hCG injection, with a lower number of retrieved oocytes, but no significant differences were found in the rate of metaphase II oocytes, fertilization and good-quality embryos. Lower pregnancy and implantation rates were observed with the antagonist compared with the agonist in these studies, but the finding was not statistically significant. A possible effect of GnRH antagonists on the endometrium has been suggested as an explanation for the lower pregnancy rate. Kolibianakis and colleagues[39] showed that endometrial maturation at oocyte retrieval was more advanced by around 2.5 days after the use of the GnRH antagonist, as compared with the expected chronological date.

The efficacy of GnRH antagonist versus agonist administration for COH has recently been compared in two meta-analyses. Ludwig and colleagues[40] did not show any significant difference in the pregnancy rates between the two groups. In Al-Inany and Aboulghar's Cochrane review[41], five randomized controlled trials fulfilled the inclusion criteria. In four studies, the multiple low-dose (0.25 mg) antagonist regimen was applied and, in one study, the single high-dose (3 mg) antagonist regimen was investigated. In all trials, reference treatment included a long protocol of GnRH agonist (buserelin, leuprorelin or triptorelin) starting in the mid-luteal phase of the preceding cycle. In comparison with the long protocol of GnRH agonist, the overall odds ratio (OR) for the prevention of premature LH surges was 1.76 (95% confidence interval (CI) 0.75–4.16), which was not statistically significant. There were significantly fewer clinical pregnancies in those treated with GnRH antagonists (OR 0.79, 95% CI 0.63–0.99). There was no statistically significant reduction in incidence of severe ovarian hyperstimulation syndrome between the two regimens (relative risk 0.51; OR 0.79, 95% CI 0.22–1.18). The authors concluded that the fixed GnRH antagonist protocol is a short and simple protocol with good clinical outcome. However, the lower pregnancy rate compared with the GnRH agonist long protocol and the non-significant difference between both protocols regarding prevention of premature LH surge and prevention of severe ovarian hyperstimulation syndrome necessitates counseling of subfertile couples before recommending a change from GnRH agonist to antagonist. The clinical outcome may be further improved by developing more flexible antagonist regimens, taking into account individual patient characteristics[40].

see also 178–186

GnRH antagonists in normal responders versus poor responders

In assisted reproductive technologies (ART) units with experience in their use, GnRH antagonist protocols have been shown to produce equivalent outcomes to those of the agonist protocols, with the added benefit of significantly fewer treatment/injection days. The lack of correlation between estradiol patterns on the day after initiation of a GnRH antagonist and IVF outcomes supports the concept that no intervention (such as add-back) is necessary to guard against an early decrease or plateau in estradiol during

stimulation with recombinant FSH and a GnRH antagonist[30]. Various selection criteria have been used to categorize the poor-responding patient[42,43]. Optimal stimulation of the poor responder remains a challenge. Although the use of both a GnRH agonist and a microdose flare protocol are effective at preventing an LH surge, selection of an antagonist protocol may improve cycle outcome, including a higher pregnancy rate and lower cancelation rate. The addition of the antagonist avoids ovarian suppression at the start of the cycle when it is, most likely, least beneficial for the poor-responding patient and prevents premature LH surge at mid-cycle when it is most crucial to do so. Based on accumulating data, more patients classified as poor responders who attempt IVF will achieve oocyte retrieval when an antagonist is used. The patient benefits of the antagonists, plus the determination that they provide better outcomes than leuprolide acetate down-regulation and at least as good, and potentially improved, outcomes compared with the microdose treatment, have the potential to bring changes to our existing COH protocols for the poor-responding patient[44].

To evaluate a novel protocol of ovulation induction for poor responders, D'Amato and colleagues[45] studied 145 infertile women, aged 27–39 years; 85 patients received clomiphene citrate, high-dose recombinant FSH and a delayed, multidose GnRH antagonist, whereas 60 patients underwent a standard long protocol. Patients undergoing the study protocol obtained lower cancelation rates and higher estradiol levels, oocyte retrieval and pregnancy (22.2% vs. 15.3%) and implantation rates (13.5% vs 7.6%), compared with those receiving the long protocol. Age negatively correlated with ovarian response in the latter, whereas the ovarian outcome results were comparable in younger (< 35 years) and older (> 35 years) women treated with the study protocol.

Use of the GnRH antagonist (cetrorelix) at Bourn Hall Clinic

Following earlier participation in the European Cetrorelix Study Group trial, Bourn Hall has used cetrorelix since it became commercially available in April 1999. The indications for cetrorelix use have been COH in women older than 40 years, previous poor responders to COH cycles using the luteal phase administration of agonists, FSH greater than 10 but less than 14 IU/l, previous failed 'down-regulation' or patient preference. For convenience, most treatment cycles are programmed with the oral contraceptive pill. A pelvic ultrasound scan and blood tests for FSH, LH and estradiol are performed on the second day of the menstrual cycle. If the parameters are satisfactory, then recombinant FSH (Gonal-F®; Serono International SA, Geneva, Switzerland) is administered on the same day. The ultrasound scan and blood tests for estradiol and LH are repeated on the sixth day of ovarian stimulation. Cetrorelix 0.25 mg and, if required, recombinant LH (Luveris®; Serono International SA, Geneva, Switzerland) are administered subcutaneously, with adequate follicular response (generally > 14 mm follicle). The Gonal-F and Cetrotide® are then administered daily up to the day of hCG injection. Oocyte retrieval is scheduled for 34–36 h after hCG administration. Luteal support is routinely provided following embryo transfer.

A review of IVF treatment cycles in which Cetrotide was administered between January and September 2003 showed that 69 cycles of IVF were started with an average age of 37.1 years. Fifty-two cycles were completed and 17 (24.6%) were abandoned. The average number of oocytes retrieved was 7.1 oocytes per cycle with a fertilization rate of 51%. Forty-one of the 69 patients had embryo transfer (ET) with an ET/oocyte retrieval ratio of 79%. The clinical pregnancy rate per embryo transfer was 17% and the implantation rate was 12.2% in this group that included mainly poor responders.

Luteal phase dynamics

As a result of the prolonged pituitary suppression following COH with a GnRH agonist, luteal phase deficiency is frequently observed, and luteal phase supplementation has been provided routinely[46]. Since the luteinizing hormone blockade by the GnRH antagonists is short-lasting, it is expected that the luteal phase would be less disturbed.

Felberbaum and associates[47] demonstrated pituitary responsiveness following cetrorelix use in IVF by applying a GnRH test. Patients in this study were stimulated with hMG starting on day 2 of the cycle. Cetrorelix was administered daily subcutaneously starting on cycle day 7. Three hours before ovulation induction with hCG, 25 μg of GnRH was injected. Luteinizing hormone measurements were made 30 and 80 min after the injection. As a result of the antagonist treatment, initial LH levels were very low. After 30 min, LH levels increased to about 10 mIU/ml in patients who received a dose of 3 mg and to 25 mIU/ml in those given 1 mg of cetrorelix, but fell again thereafter. Since the pituitary response is preserved following the administration of cetrorelix, ovulation may be induced with GnRH (native or agonist) instead of hCG. This could be beneficial in patients with polycystic ovarian disease (PCOD) or at risk of ovarian hyperstimulation syndrome (OHSS).

Contrary to the speculation that luteal phase supplementation is unnecessary in cycles associated with the GnRH antagonists, the serum levels of luteinizing hormone in the early and mid-luteal phases of GnRH antagonist-treated cycles have been found to be low[48], and no pregnancy was obtained in a small group of patients treated with multiple doses of cetrorelix and without luteal support[46]. In contrast, a study of intra-uterine insemination cycles showed that the use of GnRH antagonists with gonadotropins did not affect the luteal phase duration or the progesterone secretion[49]; this discrepancy could be attributed either to the non-removal of granulosa cells during follicular aspiration or to the moderately elevated steroid levels observed in these cycles. Lin and co-workers[50] reported that the granulosa cells from women regulated by the GnRH antagonist cetrorelix showed a higher degree of steroidogenesis in all cultures (testosterone, hCG and cyclic adenosine monophosphate (cAMP)) than the granulosa cells obtained from women regulated by the GnRH agonist buserelin. Until the luteal function in GnRH antagonist-treated cycles is clarified, it would be advisable to continue luteal support in all cases.

Children outcome

Follow-up of 209 children born after fresh embryo transfer and 18 children born after frozen embryo transfer in cetrorelix cycles[51], 73 infants[52] and 432 children born after ganirelix[53] has shown no adverse effects of the antagonists. Ludwig and colleagues[51] also showed that the children born from IVF cycles using cetrorelix had no increased risk of malformations. The rate of major malformation (3%) was in the range of that in the general population and among children born after intracytoplasmic sperm injection (ICSI) (2–5%). Normal physical and mental development of the children was observed in that study up to 2 years of age[51]. Long-term follow-up will be required to confirm the safety of the antagonists.

'Soft' and minimal ovarian stimulation protocols

There is renewed interest in the use of the GnRH antagonists with clomiphene citrate and gonadotropins in order to prevent LH surges, as well as reduce side-effects and the risks and costs of IVF treatment. While Engel and colleagues[54] using a multiple-dose antagonist protocol with clomiphene citrate and gonadotropins found a higher incidence of premature luteinizing hormone surges, Williams and co-workers[55] found no premature LH rises in patients using a similar protocol. The combination of clomiphene citrate–hMG or recombinant FSH–antagonist is associated with encouraging IVF results, but in some studies a high incidence of LH rises was observed[12]. In the 'soft' ovarian stimulation for IVF proposed by De Jong and colleagues[56], gonadotropins were administered on cycle day 5 and 0.25 mg GnRH antagonist co-treatment began on day 8 or later. Not only was the FSH required with this protocol substantially reduced, but a satisfactory pregnancy rate was obtained without luteal support.

Rongieres-Bertrand and colleagues[57] studied 44 natural cycles in 33 patients for IVF. When serum estradiol reached 100–150 pg/ml and a leading follicle of 12–14 mm was found, a single injection of GnRH antagonist was administered at the same time as the daily injection of 150 IU of hMG until the day of hCG. Four cycles (9%) were canceled and in ten cycles (25%) no oocyte was obtained. A total of seven clinical pregnancies were obtained (17.5% per retrieval). These preliminary data show that this treatment regimen offers an acceptable success rate. However, due to the high incidence of cycles with no oocyte retrieval, it should be applied mostly to good-prognosis patients[12].

Premenstrual GnRH antagonist administration has been shown to reduce diameters and size disparities of early antral follicles on cycle day 2, most likely through the prevention of luteal FSH elevation and early follicular development[58]. This simple approach may be used to coordinate multifollicular development in controlled ovarian stimulation. Further studies are needed to investigate whether this coordination is maintained during later stages of follicular growth and

whether it could improve the results of short GnRH agonist or antagonist COH protocols and IVF–ET outcome[59].

Polycystic ovarian disease

The treatment of polycystic ovarian disease (PCOD) patients with GnRH agonists is well established. Long-term treatment with agonists has been shown to result in the suppression of estradiol and ovarian androgen levels, owing to the inhibition of gonadotropins. The beneficial effect results from interference with the pathological LH/FSH ratio commonly found in these women. After full suppression of the endogenous gonadotropins is reached, normal follicular development and synchronization can be established by administration of exogenous LH and FSH or even FSH alone.

Pretreatment with an agonist cannot prevent the occurrence of OHSS. This complication is frequent in PCOD patients and necessitates careful monitoring in the treatment cycle. It appears that the incidence of severe OHSS is higher in hMG-stimulated cycles of 'down-regulated' patients than in those treated with hMG alone. This observation might be explained by the rapid increase in estradiol levels in the combined treatment schedule, which results from the fast and synchronized development of multiple follicles[23].

The type of luteal support recommended is important in the presence of OHSS. With the use of progesterone, the frequency of complications seems to be much lower than after multiple injections of hCG.

In comparison with the agonists, GnRH antagonist use would have the advantages of immediate suppression of gonadotropins and a greater suppression of LH compared with FSH secretion. This difference is clear during short-term treatment, and might be advantageous with regard to the higher LH/FSH ratio found in PCOD patients[23]. PCOD patients may benefit from the use of GnRH antagonists because of the reduced use of gonadotropins and the possibility of using a GnRH agonist or recombinant luteinizing hormone instead of hCG for final oocyte maturation, thereby reducing the risk of OHSS.

Ovarian hyperstimulation syndrome

Ovarian hyperstimulation is a well-known and potentially life-threatening iatrogenic complication of ovulation induction[60]. Women less than 35 years of age, suffering from PCOD with high estradiol values (> 5000 pg/ml) and multiple early-stage follicles, seem to be at particularly high risk for the development of OHSS.

In general during hMG-stimulated cycles, ovulation is induced by the administration of hCG, which has a high degree of homology and synergistic effects with LH[61], and thus can mimic the normally occurring mid-cycle LH peak. However, in spite of its high similarity to LH, hCG does not cause identical physiological reactions; it has a prolonged half-life and does not induce the typical mid-cycle increase in FSH[62]. These features may be responsible for the occurrence of the complication of OHSS after ovarian stimulation and ovulation induction with hCG. If hCG is not used for ovulation induction, OHSS may be avoided.

Successful attempts have been made to induce ovulation by the single administration of an agonist, using the flare-up effect, in cases in which an antagonist had been used in the preceding stimulatory phase. In none of the patients treated in this way was severe OHSS observed[63]. Several prospective randomized studies have shown that both cetrorelix[21] and ganirelix[28] cause less OHSS than the long GnRH agonist protocol. The trend toward lower estradiol concentrations and fewer follicles on the day of hCG in the antagonist group may be of importance.

Endometriosis and uterine myoma

Although the overall results with IVF are good in endometriosis, the optimal protocol of treatment has not yet been determined. Nakamura and colleagues[64] reported two protocols combining GnRH analogs and gonadotropins for IVF–ET in patients with various stages of endometriosis who were resistant to conventional therapies. In the ultra-long-protocol group (21 patients), GnRH analog was administered for at least 60 days prior to ovarian stimulation along with menotropin. In the long-protocol group (11 patients), the GnRH analog was started at the midluteal phase and exogenous gonadotropin was commenced between the third and the seventh day of the menstrual cycle after pituitary suppression. The clinical pregnancy rate per transfer was found to be superior with the ultra-long protocol (67 vs. 27%). Prolonged GnRH analog suppression of ovarian function before

superovulation may thus overcome some causes of infertility in patients with endometriosis.

GnRH analogs are efficient at reducing uterine fibroid volume and reversing the related symptomatology. The fibroids tend to return to their pretreatment size about 6 months after treatment is discontinued. The beneficial effects of presurgical GnRH analog use are well established. Romer[65] reported the safety of hysteroscopic myoma resection of submucous myomas with largely intramural components following pretreatment with two or three monthly injections of GnRH analogs. At Bourn Hall Clinic, GnRH agonists have been used for 2–3 months before IVF treatment in women with moderate-sized uterine fibroids. Beneficial effects of such use include some reduction in fibroid volume and thus easier access to the ovaries at transvaginal oocyte retrieval. It is important to increase the dose of gonadotropins in the stimulatory phase of the IVF cycle to achieve adequate ovarian follicular development.

In both endometriosis and uterine fibroids, the therapeutic use of GnRH agonists is well established, but again the initial 'flare effects' are undesirable. The immediate suppression produced by the administration of a GnRH antagonist would offer advantages in reducing the duration of treatment and leading to a faster improvement of subjective symptoms.

Kupker and colleagues[66] showed that following the administration of 3 mg of the antagonist weekly in women with endometriosis, basic estrogen production was preserved and regression from stage III to stage II of the disease occurred in 60% of the cases. Treatment of myomas with GnRH antagonists by daily or depot injections has been shown to result in shrinkage of the myomas by 30–50% within 1–2 months[67,68]. Future clinical trials would address the place of antagonists in suppressing endometriosis or moderate-sized uterine fibroids before IVF treatment; expectations would include a shorter period of stimulation, fewer side-effects, reduced requirements for gonadotropins and reduced cost.

GnRH antagonists and cancer treatment

GnRH analogs may be useful in steroid hormone-dependent cancers in the female such as endometrial, ovarian and breast malignancies[69]. Postulated mechanisms by which the analogs could interfere with the growth of these tumors are by inhibition of the pituitary–gonadal axis and a consequent decrease of estrogen levels and a direct effect on the proliferation of the cancer cells. Whereas an antiproliferative effect of the GnRH agonist and antagonists on cancer cells has been detected in some studies[69], others did not observe the finding[70]. Ligand heterogeneity or differences between GnRH receptors among various tumors have been postulated as the cause of the different effects of antagonists on the growth of these tumors[71]. LH-releasing hormone receptors and epidermal growth factor receptors are present in a high percentage of ovarian and prostate tumors[72,73]. *In vitro* studies[72] have reported a decrease in epidermal growth factor receptor messenger RNA to non-detectable values in the presence of GnRH agonists and antagonists. A better understanding of the mechanism of action is necessary to facilitate the development of more efficacious therapeutic approaches in the future[74].

CONCLUSIONS

It is still too early to speculate about the possible end of the 'agonist era'. GnRH agonists are well-tested and easily available pharmaceutical agents for use in sex steroid-dependent diseases and in the management of IVF cycles. Agonists are still preferred in clinical situations where the use of a single monthly injection is required. The use of antagonists has become increasingly widespread since they first became commercially available in 1999. The antagonists seem to offer many advantages compared with the agonists, but their efficacy and safety have to be proved in long-term studies.

There has been much progress, and several new clinical regimens for GnRH antagonists in infertility are now being evaluated, with promising results. Randomized controlled studies have shown that treatment with the GnRH antagonists in selected groups of women undergoing COH is an acceptable, safe, effective and convenient alternative to the use of the agonists in IVF cycles. What is clear is that there is a learning curve in using the antagonists. As with GnRH agonists, it has to be expected that GnRH antagonists, when applied for complete hormone suppression, would exert side-effects during long-term treatment based on the pharmacological action of these compounds, such as a decrease in libido or loss of bone density. Suitable sustained delivery systems

and the development of GnRH antagonists with sufficient oral bioavailability still represent present and future challenges[75].

REFERENCES

1. Edwards RG, Steptoe PC, Purdy JM. Establishing full term human pregnancies using cleaving embryos grown in vitro. Br J Obstet Gynaecol 1980; 87: 737–56
2. Howles CM, Macnamee MC, Edwards RG, et al. Effects of high tonic levels of luteinising hormone on outcome of in vitro fertilisation. Lancet 1986; 2: 521
3. Porter RN, Smith W, Craft IL. Induction of ovulation for in vitro fertilisation using buserelin and gonadotrophins. Lancet 1984; 2: 1284
4. Macnamee M, Howles CM, Edwards RG. Pregnancy after IVF when high tonic LH is reduced by long-term treatment with GnRH agonists. Hum Reprod 1987; 2: 569–71
5. Neveu S, Hedon B, Bringer J, et al. Ovarian stimulation by a combination of gonadotropin releasing hormone agonist and gonadotropins for in vitro fertilisation. Fertil Steril 1987; 47: 639–43
6. Smitz J, Devroey P, Braeckmans P, et al. Management of failed cycles in an IVF/GIFT programme with the combination of a GnRH analogue and HMG. Hum Reprod 1987; 2: 309
7. Assisted Reproductive Technology in the United States: 2000 results generated from the American Society for Reproductive Medicine/Society for Assisted Reproductive Technology Register. Fertil Steril 2004; 81: 1207–20
8. Remohi J, Pellicer A. Use of GnRH analogs in IVF. In Asch RH, Studd JWW, eds. Annual Progress in Reproductive Medicine. Carnforth, UK: Parthenon Publishing, 1993: 107–25
9. Janssens RMJ, Brus L, Cahill DJ, et al. Direct ovarian effects and safety aspects of GnRH agonists and antagonists. Hum Reprod Update 2000; 6: 505–18
10. Olivennes F, Fanehein R, Bouchard P, et al. Scheduled administration of GnRH antagonist (Cetrorelix) on day 8 of in vitro fertilization cycles; a pilot study. Hum Reprod 1995; 10: 1382–6
11. The Ganirelix Dose-finding Group. A double-blind, randomized, dose-finding study to assess the efficacy of the gonadotrophin-releasing hormone antagonist ganirelix (Org 37462) to prevent premature luteinizing hormone surges in women undergoing ovarian stimulation with recombinant follicle stimulating hormone (Puregon). Hum Reprod 1998; 13: 3023–31

12. Tarlatzis BC, Bili HN. Gonadotropin-releasing hormone antagonists: impact of IVF practice and potential non-assisted reproductive technology applications. Curr Opin Obstet Gynecol 2003; 15: 250–64

13. Green JD, Harris GW. The neurovascular link between the neurohypophysis and adenohypophysis. J Endocrinol 1947; 5: 136–46

14. Schally AV, Arimura A, Baba Y. Isolation and properties of the FSH and LH-releasing hormone. Biochem Biophys Res Commun 1971; 43: 393–9

15. Cornea A, Janovich JA, Lin X, et al. Simultaneous and independent visualization of gonadotropin-releasing hormone receptor and its ligand: evidence for independent processing and recycling in living cells. Endocrinology 1999; 140: 4272–80

16. Knobil E. The neuroendocrine control of the menstrual cycle. Recent Prog Horm Res 1980; 36: 53–88

17. Koch Y, Baram T, Hazum E, et al. Resistance to enzymatic degradation of LH-RH analogs possessing increased biological activity. Biochem Biophys Res Commun 1997; 74: 488–92

18. Schally AV, Comaru-Schally AM, Hollander V. Hypothalamic and other peptide hormones. In Hollander JR, Frei E, Bast RC, eds. Cancer Medicine, 3rd edn. Philadelphia: Lea & Febiger, 1993: 827

19. Coy DH, Labrie F, Savary, M, et al. LH-releasing activity of potent LH-RH analogues in vitro. Biochem Biophys Res Commun 1975; 67: 576–82

20. Brogden RN, Buckley M-T, Ward A, et al. Buserelin. A review of the pharmacodynamic and pharmacokinetic properties, and clinical profile. Drugs 1990; 39: 399–437

21. Gordon K, Hodgen GD. GnRH agonists and antagonists in assisted reproduction. Baillière's Clin Obstet Gynecol 1992; 6: 247–65

22. Lemay A, Maheux R, Faure N, et al. Reversible hypogonadism induced by a luteinizing hormone-releasing hormone (LH-RH) agonist (buserelin) as a new therapeutic approach for endometriosis. Fertil Steril 1984; 41: 863–71

23. Reissmann T, Felberbaum R, Diedrich K, et al. Development and applications of luteinising hormone-releasing hormone antagonists in the treatment of infertility: an overview. Hum Reprod 1995; 10: 1974–81

24. Kiesel L, Runnebaum B. Gonadotrophin-releasing-Hormone und Analoga – Physiologic and Pharmakologie. Gynakol Geburtsh Rundsch 1992; 32: 22–30

25. Weinbauer GF, Behre HM, Nieschlag E. Gonadotrophin releasing hormone analogue-induced regulation of testicular function in monkeys and men. In Bouchard P, Caraty A, Coelingh-Bennink HJT, Palou SN, eds. GnRH, GnRH- Analogs, Gonadotrophins and Gonadal Peptides. Carnforth, UK: Parthenon Publishing, 1993: 211

26. Felberbaum RE, Albano C, Ludwig M, et al. European Cetrorelix Study Group. Ovarian stimulation for assisted reproduction with hMG and concomitant midcycle administration of the GnRH antagonist cetrorelix according to the multiple dose protocol: a prospective uncontrolled phase III study. Hum Reprod 2000; 15: 1015–20

27. The European and Middle East Orgalutran Study Group. Comparable clinical outcomes using the GnRH antagonist ganirelix or a long protocol of the GnRH agonist triptorelin for the prevention of premature LH surges in women undergoing ovarian stimulation. Hum Reprod 2001; 16: 644–51

28. The North American Ganirelix Study Group. Efficacy and safety of ganirelix acetate versus leuprolide acetate in women undergoing controlled ovarian hyperstimulation. Fertil Steril 2001; 75: 38–45

29. Bouchard P, Caraty A, Medalie D. Mechanism of action and clinical uses of GnRH-antagonists in women. In Bouchard P, Haour F, Franchimont P, Schatz B, eds. Recent Progress on GnRH and Gonadal Peptides. Paris: Elsevier, 1990: 209

30. Shapiro DB. GnRH Antagonists Symposium – Introduction. Fertil Steril 2003; 80: S1–7

31. Albano C, Felbernaum RE, Smitz J, et al. Controlled ovarian stimulation with HMG: results of a prospective randomised phase III European study comparing the LHRH-antagonist cetrorelix (Cetrotide) and the LHRH agonist buserelin. Hum Reprod 2000; 15: 526–31

32. Stanger JD, Yovich JL. Reduced in vitro fertilization of human oocytes from patients with raised basal luteinizing hormone levels during the follicular phase. Br J Obstet Gynaecol 1985; 92: 385–93

33. Loumaye E. The control of endogenous secretion of LH by gonadotrophin-releasing hormone agonists during ovarian hyperstimulation for in-vitro fertilization and embryo transfer. Hum Reprod 1990; 5: 357–76

34. Diedrich K, Diedrich C, Santos E, et al. Suppression of the endogenous luteinizing hormone surge by the gonadotrophin-releasing hormone antagonist Cetrorelix during ovarian stimulation. Hum Reprod 1994; 9: 788–91

35. Smitz J, Ron-El R, Tarlatzis BC. The use of gonadotrophin releasing hormone agonists for in vitro fertilization and other assisted procreation techniques: experience from three centers. Hum Reprod 1992; 7 (Suppl 1): 49–66

36. Hsueh AJW, Wang C, Erickson GF. Direct inhibitory effect of gonadotropin-releasing hormone upon follicle-stimulating hormone induction of luteinizing hormone receptor and aromatase activity in rat granulosa cells. Endocrinology 1980; 106: 1697–705

37. Albano C, Smitz J, Camus M, et al. Comparison of different doses of gonadotropin-releasing hormone antagonist Cetrorelix during controlled ovarian hyperstimulation. Fertil Steril 1997; 67: 917–22

38. Olivennes F, Alvarez S, Bouchard P, et al. The use of new GnRH antagonist (Cetrorelix) in IVF-ET with a single dose protocol: a dose finding study of 3 versus 2 mg. Hum Reprod 1998; 13: 2411–14

39. Kolibianakis E, Bourgain C, Albano C, et al. Effect of ovarian stimulation with recombinant follicle-stimulating hormone, gonadotropin releasing hormone antagonists, and human chorionic gonadotropin on endometrial maturation on the day of oocyte pick-up. Fertil Steril 2002; 78: 1025–9

40. Ludwig M, Katalinic A, Diedrich K. Use of GnRH antagonists in ovarian stimulation for assisted reproduction technologies compared to the long protocol. Arch Gynecol Obstet 2001; 265: 175–81

41. Al-Inany H, Aboulghar M. Gonadotropin-releasing hormone antagonists for assisted conception [Cochrane review]. The Cochrane Library 2002; 1: 1–2

42. Surrey ER, Schoolcraft WB. Evaluating strategies for improving ovarian response of the poor responder undergoing assisted reproductive techniques. Fertil Steril 2000; 73: 667–76

43. Kligman I, Rosenwaks Z. Differentiating clinical profiles: predicting good responders, poor responders and hyporesponders. Fertil Steril 2001; 76: 1185–90

44. Copperman AB. Antagonists in poor-responder patients. Fertil Steril 2003; 80: S16–24

45. D'Amato G, Caroppo E, Pasquadibisceglie A, et al. A novel protocol of ovulation induction with delayed gonadotropin-releasing hormone antagonist administration combined with high-dose recombinant follicle stimulating hormone and clomiphene citrate for poor responders and women over 35 years. Fertil Steril 2004; 81: 1572–7

46. Albano C, Grimbizis G, Smitz J, et al. The luteal phase of non-supplemented cycles after ovarian superovulation with human menopausal gonadotropin and the gonadotropin-releasing hormone antagonist cetrorelix. Fertil Steril 1998; 70: 357–9

47. Felberbaum R, Bauer O, Kupker W, et al. Hormone profiles and pituitary response under ovarian stimulation with HMG and GnRH-antagonist (cetrorelix). Hum Reprod 1994; 9 (Suppl 4): 13

48. Tavaniotou A, Albano C, Smitz T, et al. Comparison of LH concentrations in the early and mid-luteal phase in IVF cycles after treatment with HMG alone or in association with the GnRH antagonist cetrorelix. Hum Reprod 2001; 16: 663–7

49. Ragni G, Vegetti W, Baroni E, et al. Comparison of luteal phase profile in gonadotrophin stimulated cycles with or without a gonadotrophin-releasing hormone antagonist. Hum Reprod 2001; 16: 2258–62

50. Lin Y, Kahn JA, Hillensjo T. Is there a difference in the function of granulosa cells in patients undergoing IVF with either GnRH agonist or GnRH antagonist? Hum Reprod 1999; 14: 885–8

51. Ludwig M, Reithmuller-Winzen H, Felberbaum RE, et al. Health of 227 children born after controlled ovarian stimulation for in vitro fertilization using the luteinizing hormone-releasing hormone antagonist cetrorelix. Fertil Steril 2001; 75: 18–22

52. Olivennes F, Mannaerts B, Struijs M, et al. Perinatal outcome of pregnancy after GnRH antagonist (ganirelix) treatment during ovarian stimulation for conventional IVF or ICSI: a preliminary report. Hum Reprod 2001; 16: 1588–91

53. Boerrigter PJ, de Bie JJ, Mannaerts B, et al. Obstetrical and neonatal outcome after controlled ovarian stimulation for IVF using the GnRH antagonist ganirelix. Human Reprod 2002; 17: 2027–34

54. Engel JB, Ludwig M, Felberbaum R, et al. Use of cetrorelix in combination with clomiphene citrate and gonadotrophins: a suitable approach to 'friendly IVF'? Hum Reprod 2002; 17: 2022–6

55. Williams S, Gibbons W, Muasher S, et al. Minimal ovarian hyperstimulation for in vitro fertilization using sequential clomiphene citrate and gonadotropin with or without the addition of a gonadotropin-releasing hormone antagonist. Fertil Steril 2002; 78: 1068–72

56. De Jong D, Nicholas S, Fauser BCJM, et al. A pilot study involving minimal ovarian stimulation for in vitro fertilization: extending the 'follicle-stimulating hormone window' combined with the gonadotropin-releasing hormone antagonist cetrorelix. Fertil Steril 2000; 73: 1051–4

57. Rongieres-Bertrand C, Olivennes F, Righini C, et al. Revival of the natural cycles in in-vitro fertilization with the use of a new gonadotrophin-releasing hormone antagonist (Cetrorelix): a pilot study with minimal stimulation. Hum Reprod 1999; 14: 683–8

58. Fanchin R, Branco AC, Kadoch IJ, et al. Premenstrual administration of gonadotropin-releasing hormone antagonist coordinates early antral follicle sizes and sets up the basis for an innovative concept of controlled ovarian hyperstimulation. Fertil Steril 2004; 81: 1554–9

59. Pelinck MJ, Hoek A, Simons AHM, et al. Efficacy of natural cycle IVF: a review of the literature. Hum Reprod Update 2002; 8: 129–39

60. Brinsden PR, Wada I, Tan SL, et al. Diagnosis, prevention and management of ovarian hyperstimulation syndrome. Br J Obstet Gynaecol 1995; 102: 767–72

61. Dufau HL, Catt RJ, Tsuruhara T. Retention of in vitro biological activities by desialylated human luteinizing hormone and chorionic gonadotrophin. Biochem Biophys Res Commun 1971; 44: 1022–9

62. Hoff YD, Quigley MB, Yen SCC. Hormonal dynamics at midcycle: a reevaluation. J Clin Endocrinol Metab 1983; 57: 892–6

63. Shalev E, Geslevich Y, Ben-Ami M. Induction of pre-ovulatory luteinizing hormone surge by gonadotrophin-releasing hormone agonist for women at risk for developing the ovarian hyperstimulation syndrome. Hum Reprod 1994; 9: 417–19

64. Nakamura K, Oosawa M, Kondou I, et al. Menotropin stimulation after prolonged gonadotropin releasing hormone agonist pretreatment for in vitro fertilization in patients with endometriosis. J Assist Reprod Genet 1992; 9: 113–17

65. Romer T. Hysteroscopic myoma resection of submucous myomas with largely intramural components. Zentralbl Gynakol 1997; 119: 374–7

66. Kupker W, Felberbaum Re, Krapp M, et al. Use of GnRH antagonists in the treatment of endometriosis. Reprod Biomed Online 2002; 5: 12–16

67. Gonzalez-Barcena D, Alvarez RB, Ochoa ER, et al. Treatment of uterine leiomyomas with luteinizing hormone-releasing hormone antagonist cetrorelix. Hum Reprod 1997; 12: 2028–35

68. Felberbaum RE, Ludwig M, Diedrich K. Medical treatment of uterine fibroids with the LHRH antagonist: cetrorelix. Contracept Fertil Sex 1999; 27: 701–9

69. Emons G, Schally V. The use of luteinizing hormone releasing hormone agonists and antagonists in gynaecological cancers. Hum Reprod Update 1994; 9: 1364–79

70. Chatzaki E, Bax CMR, Eidine KA, et al. The expression of gonadotrophin-releasing hormone and its receptors in endometrial cancer, and its relevance as an autocrine growth factor. Cancer Res 1996; 56: 2059–65

71. Srkalovic G, Bokser L, Radulovic S, et al. Receptors for luteinizing hormone-releasing hormone (LHRH) in Dunning R3327 prostate cancer and rat anterior pituitaries after treatment with a sustained delivery system of LHRH antagonist SB-75. Endocrinology 1990; 127: 3052–60

72. Moretti RM, Montagnani-Marelli M, Dondi D, et al. Luteinising hormone-releasing hormone agonists interfere with the stimulatory actions of epidermal growth factor in human prostatic cancer cell lines, LNCaP and DU 145. J Clin Endocrinol Metab 1996; 81: 3930–7

73. Lamharzi N, Halmos G, Jungwirth A, et al. Expression of mRNA for luteinizing hormone-releasing hormone receptors and epidermal growth factor receptors in human cancer cell lines. Int J Oncol 1996; 12: 671–5

74. Albano C, Platteau P, Devroey P. Gonadotropin-releasing hormone antagonist: how good is the new hope? Curr Opin Obstet Gynecol 2001; 13: 257–62

75. Reissmann T, Felberbaum R, Diedrich K, et al. Development and applications of luteinising hormone-releasing hormone antagonists in the treatment of infertility: an overview. Hum Reprod 1995; 10: 1974–81

10

Superovulation strategies in assisted conception

Peter R. Brinsden

INTRODUCTION

The first *in vitro* fertilization (IVF) pregnancy was ectopic, and the first child, Louise Brown, was conceived in a 'natural' IVF cycle[1]. This birth in 1978 not only heralded an upsurge of interest in the treatment of human infertility, but ushered in a period of particular interest in ovulation induction. The aim of superovulation for assisted conception treatment techniques is to induce women to produce a larger number of oocytes than the one or two that are required for normal ovulation-induction programs.

Many changes have occurred in the development of gonadotropins and in IVF superovulation protocols since 1978 (Table 1). These changes range from the use of clomiphene alone, through clomiphene and human menopausal gonadotropin (hMG, luteinizing hormone (LH), 75 IU and follicle stimulating hormone (FSH), 75 IU), to the use of highly purified urine-derived FSH (HP-FSH). Since 1995 we have been using the latest and most sophisticated of the gonadotropins so far developed: recombinant human FSH (r-hFSH) (Table 2).

The treatment options available to infertile couples have also expanded during this time to include simple ovulation induction and intrauterine insemination (IUI) as well as IVF and intracytoplasmic sperm injection (ICSI), the last two of which remain the principal

Table 1 Changes in superovulation protocols for *in vitro* fertilization: the historical perspective

1970s
Natural cycle
Clomiphene

1980s
Clomiphene + u-hMG
Analogs + u-hMG
  'flare'
  ultrashort and short
  long, luteal or follicular

1990s
Analogs + u-FSH (im)
Analogs + HP-FSH (sc)
Analogs + r-hFSH (sc)

Late 1990s–2000+
Antagonists + r-hFSH
  ± r-hLH
  ± r-hCG

u-hMG, urinary human menopausal gonadotropin; u-FSH, urinary follicle stimulating hormone; im, intramuscular; HP-FSH, high-purity FSH; r-hFSH, recombinant human FSH; sc, subcutaneous; r-hLH, recombinant human luteinizing hormone; r-hCG, recombinant human chorionic gonadotropin

Table 2   Changes in the use of gonadotropins at Bourn Hall: 1980–2005

1980–89	hMG
1989–93	u-FSH ± hMG
1993–94	u-FSH → HP-FSH
1994–95	HP-FSH
1995–96	HP-FSH → r-hFSH
1996–2002	r-hFSH
2002–present	r-hFSH ± r-hLH ± r-hCG

treatments for the most severe infertility problems. Many units are also now able to offer treatment by ovum, sperm and embryo donation and IVF surrogacy.

The most important factors governing the chances of successful IVF treatment are still:

(1) Female age;

(2) Response to superovulation;

(3) Number and quality of oocytes collected;

(4) Quality of semen;

(5) Number and quality of embryos transferred.

Our aim with superovulation for IVF has always been to produce a sufficient number of high-quality embryos so as to enable two to be transferred to the uterus, and to leave those that remain to be frozen for possible later use. In this way, the need for further stimulation cycles is reduced and the chance of success for each stimulation cycle is maximized. Clearly, if patients respond well to superovulation and produce high-quality oocytes, the chances of success are much greater than if they do not.

In the late 1960s, oocytes maturing in the human ovary were identified by the presence of chromosomes in diakinesis of the first meiotic division, and the first demonstration that human eggs could be fertilized *in vitro* was made[2]. Subsequently it was shown that oocyte maturation and ovulation could be timed precisely after an injection of human chorionic gonadotropin (hCG) or by observing the onset of the endogenous LH surge in both gonadotropin-stimulated and 'natural' menstrual cycles[3]. Although far in advance of work in animal species, it was a full decade before this knowledge was successfully applied clinically, and the first live birth[1] following *in vitro* fertilization and embryo transfer (IVF–ET) was achieved.

Louise Brown was the product of an embryo created following fertilization of a mature oocyte collected by timing the endogenous LH surge in a natural menstrual cycle. Her birth heralded the genesis of a new treatment for infertility and brought hope to countless thousands of couples. Following the founding of Bourn Hall Clinic in 1980, Steptoe and Edwards continued to develop the techniques of IVF, which included using gonadotropins to stimulate follicular development[4]. This required the rigorous application of endocrine monitoring and the adoption of the then newly developed techniques of ultrasound ovarian imaging, which have since led to major advances in the clinical management of superovulation cycles.

The early use of superovulation cycles for IVF established that success was principally determined by the number of embryos replaced. This key finding, backed by mathematical models, demonstrated that the replacement of three or more healthy embryos optimized the likelihood of achieving an ongoing pregnancy[5–8]. It was also found that replacement of more than three embryos increased the likelihood of higher-order multiple pregnancies, while not increasing the pregnancy rate[5,8]. Given a reasonable sperm preparation, four or five good-quality oocytes must be recovered to be reasonably sure of the replacement of two, or, very occasionally three, morphologically normal embryos. Thus, natural-cycle IVF has largely been abandoned in favor of superovulated cycles for assisted conception, although there was a resurgence of interest in natural cycle IVF[9] in the early 1990s, and it may still be of value in a limited number of patients[10].

In this chapter, the history, theoretical background and rationale for the follicular stimulation protocols currently in use at Bourn Hall are explained. The information in this chapter may be enhanced by reading the chapters on luteinizing hormone-releasing hormone (LHRH) agonists and antagonists (Chapter 9) and the new gonadotropins (Chapter 8) elsewhere in this book.

CLOMIPHENE CITRATE AND GONADOTROPINS IN SUPEROVULATION

Until the late 1980s, the most common ovarian stimulation regimen used in assisted conception was the combination of clomiphene citrate (CC), a partial agonist of estrogen, and exogenous gonadotropin preparations in the form of human menopausal gonadotropin (hMG). The rationale of this regimen is that the estrogen-driven negative feedback on endogenous gonadotropin secretion is defeated. Acting at the hypothalamic and pituitary levels, CC provokes a mild hypersecretion of pituitary gonadotropins. If administered shortly after menstruation begins, CC will stimulate the growth of a number of small follicles. The administration of exogenous gonadotropins will then sustain the growth of this cohort of recruited follicles. Thus, synchronous multiple follicle development can be induced in an otherwise mono-ovular species.

The best success rates using this combination were achieved when extensive monitoring of endogenous LH secretion in the late follicular phase was employed. If undetected, the endogenous LH surge, although severely attenuated[11], can lead to ovulation prior to surgical oocyte recovery, or to the collection of postmature oocytes, with a reduced capacity to fertilize. The onset of the LH surge is not predictable by observation of follicle size alone, or the absolute level of estrogen, or the rate of estrogen rise[11]. However, if detected and supported by the administration of human chorionic gonadotropin (hCG), and if the onset of the surge is used to time oocyte recovery, the patient's clinical performance through an assisted conception cycle is not compromised. An increasing proportion of patients will surge if ovulation is induced in the later stages of follicular growth[11].

The early results with CC/hMG stimulation demonstrated its efficacy, achieving a clinical pregnancy rate of 25–35% following the transfer of three or more embryos[6-8]. These figures equate with a 'take-home-baby rate' of around 15%. Up to the time of publication of the first edition of this book in 1992, the majority of the then estimated 10 000 babies born worldwide following IVF were the result of CC/hMG treatment; more than 1200 of these babies were from Bourn Hall alone.

Extensive endocrine and ultrasound monitoring of IVF patients stimulated with CC/hMG has allowed detailed analysis of the endocrine indicators of reproductive success that occur in the late follicular phase[11]. No difference was found between those patients who became pregnant after embryo transfer and those whose embryos failed to implant in terms of the final estrogen level, the diameter of the four largest follicles at the time of hCG administration, the number of oocytes collected, their fertilization and cleavage rates or the average number of embryos transferred per patient. However, patients who established a clinical pregnancy had a significantly lower urinary LH output in the 2 days prior to the induction of ovulation (Figure 1). A similar pattern was demonstrated for plasma levels of LH in the late follicular phase. More detailed analysis has shown that a link exists between oocyte quality and the mean tonic urinary LH output in the late follicular phase. Failure of fertilization solely attributable to poor oocyte quality (assessed by light microscopy) correlates with higher late follicular phase LH levels. Further evidence of a detrimental effect of high LH on ovarian function comes from the finding that patients discharged prior to oocyte recovery because of inadequate follicular development had high tonic levels of LH production. Principal among these findings is the fact that high follicular phase levels of LH are incompatible with implantation and are predictive of early pregnancy loss following ovulation induction, IVF[12,13] and natural conception[14]. Our data on urinary LH output and success following IVF–ET are summarized in Figure 2. Only in cases where mean late follicular phase urinary LH levels were above 0.3 IU/l per hour was a decrease in oocyte quality obvious by routine light microscopy.

USE OF THE GONADOTROPIN RELEASING HORMOME ANALOGS IN SUPEROVULATION FOR IVF

Being aware of the detrimental effects of elevated LH levels on oocyte quality, it seemed logical to reduce LH levels and to prevent premature LH surges by use of the gonadotropin releasing hormone (GnRH) analogs. The first report of their successful use was by Porter and colleagues in 1984[15]. Our own experience with their use was reported in 1987[16]. In common with others[17], we have shown improvements in follicular recruitment and growth, fertilization rates and pregnancy rates when endogenous LH secretion is reduced in stimulation cycles using GnRH analogs[18-20]. Initially, these reductions were achieved by the use of the GnRH agonist buserelin, and more recently we have also used nafarelin by nasal spray. A detailed review of the use of the GnRH agonists and

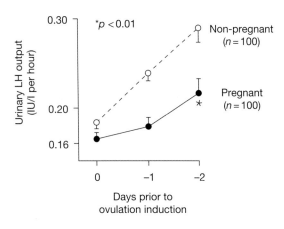

Figure 1 Profiles of urinary luteinizing hormone (LH) output in pregnant and non-pregnant *in vitro* fertilization (IVF) patients

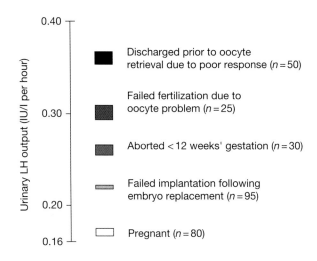

Figure 2 Outcome of *in vitro* fertilization (IVF) treatment in relation to late follicular phase output of luteinizing hormone (LH). The blocks represent mean ± SEM

antagonists is given elsewhere in this book (Chapter 9).

Superovulation strategies combining the use of GnRH agonists and hMG originally, but now recombinant human FSH (r-hFSH), fall into three categories: the so-called 'ultrashort', the 'short' and the 'long' protocols. The rationale of the long protocol is to induce a temporary state of hypogonadotropic hypogonadism. Follicular recruitment and growth are then stimulated by the administration of exogenous FSH. Both the short and the ultrashort protocols make use of the initial stimulatory phase of GnRH analogs to encourage the recruitment of follicles and to maintain a degree of hyposecretion of endogenous gonadotropins in the later part of the follicular phase. Exogenous FSH is concurrently administered to stimulate follicular growth.

Loumaye[21] has summarized the data concerning the advantages of GnRH analog therapy when compared with CC/hMG or gonadotropins alone. The major studies which he cites all claim a higher clinical pregnancy rate with the GnRH analog and gonadotropin treatments, but the magnitude of the difference is questioned when overall statistics are considered. The problem lies with the quality of the data, since many of the studies are only retrospective analyses. However, two large, well-controlled studies show a doubling of the 'take-home-baby rate' on both the long and the ultrashort protocols, when compared with CC/hMG-stimulated cycles[17,18]. This increase in

success is due to improved oocyte quality, achieved by the reduction of LH levels, and greater consistency of oocyte quality.

In conclusion, the use of GnRH analogs, in combination with exogenous gonadotropins, significantly increases the chance of pregnancy after embryo replacement when compared with treatment with CC/hMG. The physiological basis for this incremental success is attributable to the suppression of endogenous LH in the late follicular phase. The result is improved oocyte quality and the generation of 'fitter' embryos. However, endometrial factors are as important in implantation as embryo quality. To this end, a case can be made that the estrogen-sparing effect of GnRH analog treatment may also be important.

THE USE OF GnRH ANTAGONISTS

Although the 'long agonist' protocols are still preferred by the majority of centers for superovulation for IVF, an increasing number are turning to the use of the GnRH antagonists. The primary aim of both the agonists and antagonists is to prevent a premature LH surge, but 'patient friendliness' – comfort, convenience and cost – are also major considerations in addition to effectiveness. The antagonists are now being seen by many practitioners to be the preferred of the two options. This is mainly because of the much shorter treatment time: often only 4 or 5 days for the antagonist, compared with at least 21 days or more for the agonist.

Our early experience was with cetrorelix in a large multicenter trial, comparing it with long down-regulated cycles using buserelin; the results of the study were published in 2000[22]. Similar results were achieved between the two groups in fertilization, cleavage and pregnancy rates.

Two GnRH antagonists are currently available: cetrorelix (Cetrotide®; Serono International SA, Geneva, Switzerland) and ganirelix (Orgalutron® or Antagon®; Organon, Oss, The Netherlands). Our own experience is with cetrorelix, but in the majority of cycles at Bourn Hall, the long agonist protocol is still used. We have tended to use cetrorelix for 'poor responders', and for women undertaking a second or third cycle of treatment for whom we wish to try a different approach to stimulation. Most published series comparing agonist and antagonist cycles have shown equivalent results, or slightly worse with the antagonist. We believe that, with increasing experience of use of the antagonists, as good or better results are being achieved with the antagonists. A meta-analysis by Ludwig and colleagues[23] showed no difference in pregnancy rates between cetrorelix and agonists, but ganirelix showed a significantly lower pregnancy rate per embryo transfer.

In our own protocol, cetrorelix 0.25 mg is given subcutaneously from stimulation day 6 or when the leading follicle reaches 14 mm in diameter. In older women (> 30–40), previous 'poor responders' and women responding poorly in the current cycle, we

have added r-hLH at the start of the cetrorelix in order to achieve an improved response, although, thus far, good evidence of its real need or effectiveness, from our own unit or from others, is still lacking.

THE INTRODUCTION AND USE OF RECOMBINANT GONADOTROPINS

The development of the recombinant gonadotropins is reviewed by Colin Howles in Chapter 8. The changes that have occurred in the use of gonadotropins in our own superovulation protocols for assisted reproductive technologies (ART) at Bourn Hall over the past 25 years are shown in Table 2.

As r-hFSH became available to us in 1994/1995, so clinical trials were conducted elsewhere using this new preparation. Bergh and colleagues[24] and Frydman and associates[25] were the first to publish large series of patients comparing the use of r-hFSH (Gonal-F®) with HP-FSH (Metrodin-HP®). In both of these series it was found that significantly fewer numbers of ampoules of r-hFSH were used, compared with HP-FSH; significantly more oocytes were recovered and significantly more embryos were available to transfer to the uterus or cryopreserve (Table 3).

Between the years 1993 and 1999, a large number of papers were published comparing the use of r-hFSH with urinary FSH (u-FSH). Daya and Gunby[26] reviewed 12 reports that were suitable for inclusion in a meta-analysis. All of the trials, except one, showed a trend in favor of the use of r-hFSH, but were not individually significant. However, the common odds ratio showed a significant benefit to the use of r-hFSH over u-FSH in terms of clinical

Table 3 Comparison of the use of urinary high-purity follicle stimulating hormone (HP-FSH), Metrodin®-HP with recombinant human FSH (Gonal-F®). Results are expressed as mean ± SD

Study	Treatment	Ampoules (75 IU)	Oocytes	Embryos
Bergh et al.[24] 1997	Gonal-F (n = 119)	21.9 ± 5.1	12.2 ± 5.5	8.1 ± 4.2
	Metrodin-HP (n = 102)	31.9 ± 13.4	7.6 ± 4.4	4.7 ± 3.5
Frydman et al.[25] 1998	Gonal-F (n = 130)	27.6 ± 10.2	11.0 ± 5.9	5.0 ± 3.7
	Metrodin-HP (n = 116)	40.7 ± 13.6	8.8 ± 4.8	3.5 ± 2.9

$p < 0.0001$, significant difference between Gonal-F and Metrodin-HP in numbers of ampoules used, numbers of oocytes recovered and numbers of embryos for transfer or cryopreservation

pregnancy (Figure 3). This meta-analysis also showed benefit of follitropin alpha over follitropin beta (Puregon®), and was the first to point out that there may be a difference in follicular response and clinical outcome between the two recombinant hFSH preparations. Brinsden and co-workers[27] also compared the efficacy and tolerability of the α and β preparations of r-hFSH. There was no significant difference in any of the clinical outcomes; however, when the local tolerance of the two preparations was compared, the proportion of injections that led to at least one report of a symptom (itching, swelling, redness, bruising or pain) differed significantly between the α and the β preparations ($p = 0.014$). Similar differences between the two preparations are reported in two other studies[28,29].

Manassiev and colleagues[30] compared the effectiveness of r-hFSH against u-FSH or HP-FSH in five clinical trials and produced similar results to those of Daya and Gunby[26]. All five studies showed improved pregnancy rates with recombinant FSH. As in the Daya study, however, all confidence intervals included 1, but the combined meta-analysis showed significantly improved pregnancy rates, with a common odds ratio of 1.35 and confidence intervals of 1.08–1.74 in favor of r-hFSH.

A number of more recent studies have confirmed that follicular stimulation with r-hFSH alone achievesa more satisfactory follicular response than HP-FSH or u-FSH. Raga and colleagues[31] looked at the effect of r-hFSH use in 30 young infertile women with previous poor responses to stimulation, but who had normal basal concentrations of FSH and estradiol. They prospectively randomized these women to receive either r-hFSH or HP-FSH. They concluded that r-hFSH was more effective than HP-FSH in young previously poor responders with normal serum FSH levels. Similarly, De Placido and associates[32] looked at the outcome of 'poor responders' to previous stimulation with HP-FSH. There were fewer, but not significant, numbers of days of stimulation and numbers of ampoules of gonadotropin used in the r-hFSH group. However, the estradiol levels at three different stages in the cycle were significantly better with r-hFSH, and there were significantly more mature oocytes recovered, better fertilization rates and highly significantly more ($p = 0.007$) pre-embryos available for transfer.

An unpublished study by Gearon and Abdalla (personal communication) of the Lister Hospital in

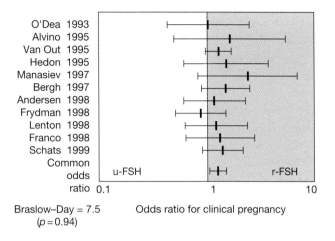

Art trials of urinary-FSH versus recombinant h-FSH
Clinical pregnancy per cycle start

Figure 3 Meta-analysis by Daya and Gunby[26] of trials comparing urinary follicle stimulating hormone (u-FSH) and recombinant human FSH (r-hFSH): clinical pregnancy per cycle started.

London showed significantly improved pregnancy rates with r-hFSH in a large series (r-hFSH, $n = 297$ vs. HP-FSH, $n = 306$) However, the most significant finding in this study is that, although the women under 38 years of age achieved better pregnancy rates in the r-hFSH group, but not significantly so, the older women (≥ 38 years of age) showed a significantly improved pregnancy rate of 32.7% vs. 13.6% ($p = 0.011$) of the r-hFSH group versus the HP-FSH group. They attribute this finding to improved oocyte and embryo quality achieved with r-hFSH over HP-FSH. This is the first study that has shown such a significant improvement in the quality of oocytes in older women treated with r-hFSH.

The issue of the consistency of batches of the recombinant gonadotropins has been addressed by Serono International SA, by changing from the old system of quantifying r-hFSH by the *in vivo* Steelman–Pohley bioassay technique to a liquid chromatography method, which is very accurate and allows vials to be filled by mass[33]. Batches of Gonal-F are now very much more consistent in the amount of FSH in each vial and from batch to batch. Hughes and colleagues[34] reported the results of a multicenter, double-blind, randomized, parallel-group study to compare the safety and efficacy of r-hFSH (Gonal-F) filled and released by mass (FbM) and r-hFSH (Gonal-F) filled by the traditional IU (FbIU) method for stimulating follicular development for IVF. There were 66 and 65 subjects in each arm of the study, respectively. Their conclusions were that the consistency of patients' responses to stimulation were significantly superior ($p = 0.039$) and clinical pregnancy rates significantly higher ($p = 0.001$) with the FbM r-hFSH. Their final conclusion was that this new method of quantifying r-hFSH produces an improved consistency in clinical outcome.

Balasch and co-workers[35] compared 125 patients undergoing IVF with the traditional r-hFSH with 125 patients receiving r-hFSH with ampoules filled by mass. They concluded that women treated with the new r-hFSH filled by mass achieved significant improvements in terms of embryo quality, implantation rates and a reduced number of days of stimulation. Another recent advance has been the introduction of multidose vials and 'pens', with which the daily dose of r-hFSH can be dialed up on the pen and the exact dose injected. No longer is it necessary to mix one or more ampoules of powder with diluent – a real benefit to our patients.

One further advance that is still undergoing trials is production of a sustained-release r-hFSH which would last for several days, thereby reducing the number of injections patients must receive. These advances have all made for more reliable, consistent and 'user-friendly' care of our patients.

THE NEED FOR LH IN STIMULATION PROTOCOLS

As practitioners have continued to gain experience with the use of r-hFSH alone, which is effective for the majority of patients, so the question has again arisen as to whether some groups of patients might benefit by receiving some added LH, as either hMG or r-hLH, to supplement their stimulation protocols. There is good evidence that profound suppression of serum LH in analog long down-regulated cycles has a negative effect on the outcome of IVF cycles. Fleming and colleagues[36] showed significantly reduced numbers of oocytes, embryos, spare embryos available for cryopreservation and an increase in the number of days' stimulation required when serum LH levels were < 0.5 IU/l in long analog cycles. There is no doubt that the addition of exogenous LH is necessary in stimulation protocols for anovulatory hypogonadotropic

hypogonadal women (World Health Organization (WHO) Group 1)[37,38]. Women who are 'heavily down-regulated' in long analog cycles, with consequently low endogenous LH levels, may also benefit by the addition of LH to their cycles[39], since they are, in effect, in an induced hypogonadal hypogonadotropic state. However, it has also been shown that the addition of LH, either as r-hLH or as hMG, does not improve the outcomes in all down-regulated IVF cycles[40–42]. Nevertheless, in the management of 'poor responders' to FSH stimulation in down-regulated cycles, there is evidence that the addition of LH may improve the outcome[43,44], and the results of adding LH to the cycles of women more than 35 years of age may also show an improvement[41,44,45].

Humaidan and colleagues[46], in a large prospective randomized trial, compared women receiving treatment in GnRH-agonist down-regulated IVF cycles. Half the patients received r-hFSH only and half received r-hFSH with r-hLH added in a ratio of 2:1 Supplementation with r-hLH significantly improved implantation rates in women ≥ 36 years, and significantly reduced the total dose of r-hFSH required for stimulation.

In another study in which r-hFSH-only cycles were supplemented with 75 or 150 IU of r-hLH, De Placido and associates[47] found that women with poor initial responses to r-hFSH alone benefited by the addition of 150 IU r-hLH from stimulation day 8.

As r-hLH (Luveris®) has become more available to practitioners, so its usefulness instead of hCG to induce final follicular maturation has been investigated. A multicenter, double-blind, comparative, parallel-group, dose-finding, phase II clinical study comparing the safety and efficacy of r-hLH with u-hCG for inducing final follicular maturation and early luteinization in women undergoing superovulation with r-hFSH prior to IVF was published by Loumaye and colleagues[48]. They concluded that a single injection of r-LH (Luveris) is effective in inducing final follicular maturation and early luteinization in IVF patients achieving embryo transfer. A dose of 5000 IU of r-hLH appeared to be as effective as 5000 IU of u-hCG, and was well tolerated in doses up to 30 000 IU administered subcutaneously. Significantly, they found that a single administration of r-hLH was associated with a reduction in moderate ovarian hyperstimulation syndrome (OHSS), especially in patients with estradiol levels in excess of

3000 pg/ml and/or > 20 follicles on the day of administration of hCG or LH.

STIMULATION PROTOCOLS FOR IVF AS USED AT BOURN HALL

The evolution of ovarian follicular stimulation protocols for ART over the past 25 years is mentioned earlier in this chapter. For the past 9 years at Bourn Hall, all follicular stimulation protocols have involved the use of r-hFSH (Gonal-F) only. More recently, r-hLH (Luveris) has been added, as and when we consider it to be appropriate, in a limited number of cycles (see below). Our policy is always to check the serum FSH, LH, estradiol and prolactin levels of all women over 35–36 years of age before a treatment cycle, and also, if they have had previous treatment, we carefully review their previous responses to stimulation.

'Down-regulation' is achieved with buserelin (Suprecur®) 500 µg subcutaneously (sc) daily, or nafarelin (Synarel®) 400 µg intranasally, both from menstrual cycle day 21 onwards, until the 'baseline' evaluation, which takes place in the first few days of menstruation. If baseline levels of estradiol (< 50 pg/ml), LH (< 5 IU/l) and progesterone (< 2 pg/ml) have been achieved, then the dose of buserelin or nafarelin is reduced to 200 µg intranasally daily. The start of follicular stimulation with r-hFSH is timed so that the collection of oocytes is programmed for the convenience of the patient and the clinic.

The starting doses of r-hFSH in first IVF cycles are:

Age < 35: start 150 IU r-hFSH sc daily;

Age 35–39: start 225 IU r-hFSH sc daily;

Age 40+: start 300 IU r-hFSH sc daily.

After 5–7 days of stimulation the dosages may be adjusted upwards or downwards depending on the follicular response. If women have had poor responses or exaggerated responses to treatment using this protocol in previous cycles, the starting dosage will be increased or decreased accordingly, depending on that experience.

Recombinant-hLH, in a dose of 75 or 150 IU, may be added to stimulation regimens, particularly for the following groups:

(1) 'Older women' – usually those over 38 years of age;

(2) Women whose serum LH levels at the 'baseline' assessment are < 1.5 IU;

(3) Women with a history of a previous poor response to stimulation;

(4) Women responding poorly to a standard stimulation protocol in the current treatment cycle;

(5) When serum estradiol levels in the current treatment cycle are low;

(6) Cycles in which the GnRH antagonist are being used.

Recombinant-hCG has been shown to have significant advantages over u-hCG in terms of luteal phase progesterone levels and local tolerance[49,50], and is increasingly becoming available in many countries. At Bourn Hall, r-hCG (Ovitrelle®) is usually administered when two or more follicles have achieved 18 mm or more in diameter. However, flexibility is exercised with the timing of hCG, with particular attention being paid to the quality of the endometrium and to achieving estradiol levels of approximately 100 pg/ml per follicle > 12–14 mm in diameter, both of which are evidence of a satisfactory follicular response. A dose of 250 µg r-hCG (equivalent to 6500 IU of u-hCG; or, before r-hCG was available, 10 000 IU of u-HCG (Profasi®)), is given 34–36 h before the planned time of oocyte recovery.

Luteal phase support is provided with progesterone only. No luteal phase hCG has been used for the past 15 years at Bourn Hall, even in patients at low risk of OHSS. Progesterone in the form of Cyclogest® (Shire Pharmaceuticals Ltd, Andover, UK) 400 mg vaginally or rectally is given 12-hourly, starting on the evening of oocyte collection. More recently, progesterone gel (Crinone®; Serono UK Ltd) 8% vaginally has been used. The use of Crinone with its plastic vaginal applicator and ease of use is popular with patients. The serum hCG level on day 15 post-oocyte recovery is tested, and, if pregnancy is achieved, a vaginal ultrasound scan is carried out on day 35 following oocyte recovery to confirm a clinical pregnancy. The progesterone is continued for up to 11 weeks. We see no indication to use painful intramuscular injections of progesterone, as the vaginal route has been shown to be as or more effective and is certainly more 'patient-friendly'[51–53].

THE COST–BENEFIT OF RECOMBINANT GONADOTROPINS

The American Society for Reproductive Medicine (ASRM) in their Practice Committee Report of June 1998[54] states: 'Recombinant FSH was more effective for IVF than urinary FSH in stimulating multiple follicular development and, when results from cryopreserved embryos were included, was associated with higher pregnancy rates'. Similarly, the Royal College of Obstetricians and Gynaecologists in the UK, in a report: 'Management of infertility in tertiary care', Evidence based clinical guideline no. 6, published in January 2000[55], reported that 'Recombinant FSH produces significantly more oocytes in an IVF cycle compared to urinary derived high-purity gonadotropin preparations, however pregnancy rates in fresh and embryo replacement cycles are similar' (grade A evidence), but, 'If fresh and frozen embryo replacements are considered, the use of recombinant FSH produces a higher pregnancy rate when compared to urinary derived high-purity gonadotrophin preparations' (grade A evidence). The report goes on to state that: 'Because of the small differences in outcome, additional factors should be considered when choosing a gonadotrophin regimen, including patient acceptability, costs and drug availability' (grade C evidence).

There is now no doubt about the clinical benefits of recombinant gonadotropins, which are listed in Table 4[56]. The only disadvantage that could be attributed to the use of r-hFSH is the apparent increased cost of treatment. With the increasing awareness of cost–benefit analysis, which is being conducted for all treatments in medicine today, it is important to establish any cost–benefit to the use of r-hFSH. This has been reviewed by Ledger[57], who looked at the effectiveness of treatment – i.e. 'success' – as judged by an ongoing pregnancy beyond 12 weeks' gestation, the cost of an ongoing pregnancy and the mean number of cycles that it takes to achieve an ongoing pregnancy. Using the Markov model with 100 000 'virtual patients', 37 358 successes could be expected with u-FSH and 40 575 successes with r-hFSH. The cost per u-FSH successful pregnancy was £6060 ($US9696) and per r-hFSH success was £5906 ($US9449) (standard deviation £232; $p < 0.0001$). When assessing the mean number of cycles that it took to achieve a successful pregnancy, with u-FSH it was 5.25 cycles and with r-hFSH 4.59 cycles. This

Table 4 List of the clinical benefits of recombinant gonadotropins. Abstracted from reference 53

Advantages
Improved logistics of the pharmaceutical process
Controlled manufacture
More homogeneous product
Reduced batch-to-batch variability
Potentially unlimited supply
Should never be shortages
Not reliant on a supply of urine
No risk of infection
No risk of contamination with drugs or metabolites
No seroconversion to antigonadotropin antibodies
Effective, safe and less traumatic subcutaneous
  administration
Greater purity and specificity
? Smaller doses needed
? More predictable responses

Disadvantages
Cost (?)

highly sophisticated but well-validated statistical analysis, when applied to model the cost-effectiveness of recombinant versus urinary gonadotropins, demonstrated that the use of recombinant gonadotropins is associated with a lower cost per pregnancy and a lower number of treatment cycles per success. This finding was further validated by a study of Sykes and colleagues[58], which again used the Markov model, but with data taken from a paper by van Out and co-workers[59], together with data from 20 UK IVF clinics and the experience of an expert panel. The authors of this study confirm the conclusions of Ledger[57], that recombinant FSH is the most cost effective therapy for follicular stimulation for ART.

CONCLUSIONS

There have been major changes in the approach to follicular stimulation for IVF over the past 25 years, from no stimulation at all in natural cycles, to sophisticated protocols using GnRH antagonists and recombinant gonadotropins, the development of which has been one of the most significant advances in assisted reproduction. The purity and consistency of the recombinant products and ease of administration are two of the most important factors from the point of view of patients, and the evidence from most studies over the past 10 years is that r-hFSH is superior or at least equivalent in effectiveness to HP-FSH, u-FSH and hMG; however, the controversy between proponents of the different preparations will continue for some years yet. It is this author's firm belief that the urinary-derived products are bound eventually to be withdrawn from markets worldwide, as indeed they have been in certain countries already. The single factor that has delayed the more widespread acceptance of the recombinant preparations has been the apparent increased cost of using them in treatment cycles. The recent evidence that has become available from analysis of the large body of data now available, and from the use of Markov models, has shown that r-hFSH is the most cost-effective preparation for follicular stimulation in ART today.

One of our aims has always been to simplify a patient's treatment as much as possible: to make it easier, cheaper and more convenient for them. The development of the most highly purified subcutaneous preparation possible, in the form of r-hFSH, is one major step in achieving this aim. It has enabled patients to self-administer their drugs, and ensures that they do not receive the extraneous proteins contained in the older hMG preparations. Increasing use of the shorter GnRH antagonist cycles, and less painful, more consistent drugs self-administered by a 'dial pen' system, have all greatly contributed to making treatment easier, and in the future, long-acting and even oral preparations of the gonadotropins may be possible.

Another simplification of treatment cycles would be to rely on ultrasound monitoring of cycles only and to discontinue all endocrine monitoring. At Bourn Hall, however, we have continued to monitor serum estradiol levels, as we believe the information is still useful in assisting the decision-making process. Also, when we are looking back at any failed treatment cycles, it is of help in deciding how to modify future treatment cycles. It also provides useful research data. However, in an attempt to reduce patient stress further, we are developing new protocols to decrease the number of blood tests and ultrasound examinations.

REFERENCES

1. Steptoe PC, Edwards RG. Birth after the reimplantation of human embryo. Lancet 1978; 2: 366

2. Edwards RG, Bavister BI, Steptoe PC. Early stages of fertilization in vitro of human oocytes matured in vitro. Nature (London) 1969; 221: 632–5

3. Steptoe PC, Edwards RG. Laparoscopic recovery of preovulatory human oocytes after priming of ovaries with gonadotrophins. Lancet 1970; 1: 6831

4. Edwards RG. In vitro fertilization and embryo replacement. Ann NY Acad Sci 1985; 442: 1–22

5. Edwards RG, Steptoe PC. Current status of human in vitro fertilization and implantation of human embryos. Lancet 1983; 2: 1265–9

6. Trounson AO, Wood C. IVF results 1979–1982 at Monash University–Queen Victoria–Epworth Medical Centre. J In Vitro Fertil Embryo Transf 1984; 1: 42–7

7. Steptoe PC, Edwards RG, Walters DE. Observations on 767 clinical pregnancies and 500 births after human in vitro fertilization. Hum Reprod 1986; 1: 89–94

8. Jones H. Embryo transfer. Ann NY Acad Sci 1985; 442: 375–80

9. Lenton EA, Hooper M, King H, et al. Normal and abnormal implantation in spontaneous and in vitro human pregnancies. J Reprod Fertil 1991; 92: 555–65

10. Nargund G, Waterstone J, Bland J, et al. Cumulative conception and live birth rates in natural (unstimulated) IVF cycles. Hum Reprod 2001; 16: 259–62

11. Macnamee MC, Edwards RG, Howles CM. The influence of stimulation regimes and luteal phase support on the outcome of IVF. Hum Reprod 1988; 3 (Suppl 2): 43–52

12. Stanger JD, Yovich JL. Reduced in vitro fertilization of human oocytes from patients with raised basal luteinizing hormone levels during the follicular phase. Br J Obstet Gynaecol 1985; 92: 385–93

13. Homburg R, Armar NA, Eshel A, et al. Influence of serum luteinising hormone concentrations on ovulation, conception, and early pregnancy loss in polycystic ovary syndrome. Br Med J 1988; 297: 1024–6

14. Regan L, Owen EJ, Jacobs HS. Hypersecretion of luteinising hormone, infertility and miscarriage. Lancet 1990; 336: 1141–4

15. Porter RN, Smith W, Craft IL. Induction of ovulation for in vitro fertilisation using buserelin and gonadotrophins. Lancet 1984; 2: 1284

16. Macnamee MC, Howles CM, Edwards RG. Pregnancies after IVF when high tonic LH is reduced by long-term treatment with GnRH agonists. Hum Reprod 1987; 2: 569–71

17. Rutherford AS, Suback-Sharpe RJ, Dawsib KJ, et al. Improvement of in vitro fertilization after treatment with buserelin, an agonist of luteinizing hormone releasing hormone. Br Med J 1988; 296: 1765

18. Macnamee MC, Howles CM, Edwards RG, et al. Short-term luteinising hormone-releasing hormone agonist treatment, prospective trial of a novel ovarian stimulation regimen for in vitro fertilization. Fertil Steril 1989; 52: 264–9

19. Marcus SF, Brinsden PR, Macnamee MC, et al. A comparative trial between an ultrashort and long stimulation protocol of LH-RH analogue with gonadotrophin for in vitro fertilization. Hum Reprod 1993; 8: 238–43

20. Howles CM, Macnamee MC, Edwards RG. Follicular development and early luteal function of conception and non-conceptual cycles after human in vitro fertilization. Hum Reprod 1987; 2: 17–21

21. Loumaye E. The control of endogenous secretion of LH by gonadotrophin-releasing hormone agonists during ovarian hyperstimulation for in vitro fertilization and embryo transfer. Hum Reprod 1990; 5: 357–76

22. Albano C, Felberbaum RE, Smitz J, et al. Controlled ovarian stimulation with HMG: results of a prospective randomized phase III European study comparing the LHRH-antagonist cetrorelix (cetrotide) and the LHRH-agonist buserelin. Hum Reprod 2000; 15: 526–31

23. Ludwig M, Katalinic A, Diedrich K. Use of GnRH antagonists in ovarian stimulation for assisted reproductive technologies compared to the long protocol. Arch Gynecol Obstet 2001; 265: 175–82

24. Bergh C, Howles CM, Borg K, et al. Recombinant human follicle stimulating hormone (r-hFSH; Gonal F) versus highly purified urinary FSH (Metrodin HP): results of a randomized comparative study in women undergoing assisted reproductive techniques. Hum Reprod 1997; 12: 2133–9

25. Frydman R, Haverell C, Camier B. A double blind randomized study comparing the efficacy of recombinant human (FSH: Gonal-F®) versus highly purified urinary FSH (Metrodin-HP) in inducing superovulation in women undergoing assisted reproductive techniques. Hum Reprod 1998; 13: 180–5

26. Daya S, Gunby J. Recombinant versus urinary follicle stimulating hormone for ovarian stimulation in assisted reproduction. Hum Reprod 1999; 14: 2207–15

27. Brinsden P, Akagbosu F, Gibbons L, et al. A comparison of the efficacy and tolerability of two recombinant human follicle-stimulating hormone preparations in patients undergoing in vitro fertilisation–embryo transfer. Hum Reprod 2000; 73: 114–16

28. Sargent S. A study to evaluate the ease of use and tolerability by patients of gonadotrophins old and new. Presented at the 16th Annual Meeting of the ESHRE, Bologna, Italy, June 2000

29. Afnan MA, Kennefick A. Recombinant gonadotrophins: is there a difference in the tolerability of these products? BFS Abstr Book 1999; 75: 1

30. Manasiev NS, Tenekedjier KI, Collins J. Does the use of recombinant follicle stimulating hormone instead of urinary follicle stimulating hormone lead to higher pregnancy rates in in vitro fertilisation–embryo transfer cycles? Assist Reprod 1999; 9: 7–12

31. Raga F, Bonilla-Musoles F, Casan E, et al. Recombinant follicle stimulating hormone stimulation in poor responders with normal basal concentrations of follicle stimulating hormone and oestradiol: improved reproductive outcome. Hum Reprod 1999; 14: 1431–4

32. De Placido G, Alviggi C, Mollo A, et al. Recombinant follicle stimulating hormone is effective in poor responders to highly purified follicle stimulating hormone. Hum Reprod 2000; 15: 17–20

33. Driebergen R, Baer G. Quantification of follicle stimulating hormone (follitropin alfa): is in vivo bioassay still relevant in the recombinant age? Curr Med Res Opin 2003; 19: 41–6

34. Hughes J-N, Barlow D, Rosenwaks Z, et al. Improvement in consistency of response to ovarian stimulation with recombinant human follicle stimulating hormone from a new method of calibrating the therapeutic preparation. Reprod Biomed Online 2004; 6: 185–90

35. Balasch J, Fabregues F, Penarrubia J, et al. Outcome from consecutive assisted reproduction cycles in patients treated with recombinant follitropin alfa filled-by-bioassay and those treated with recombinant follitropin alfa filled-by-mass. Reprod Biomed Online 2004; 8: 408–13

36. Fleming R, Rehka P, Deshpande N, et al. Suppression of LH during ovarian stimulation: effects differ in cycles stimulation with purified urinary FSH and recombinant FSH. Hum Reprod 2000; 15: 1440–5

37. European Recombinant Human LH Study Group. Recombinant human luteinizing hormone (LH) to support recombinant human follicular stimulating hormone (FSH) induced follicular development in LH and FSH deficiency anovulatory women: a dose finding study. J Clin Endocrinol Metab 1998; 83: 1507–14

38. Filicori M. The role of luteinizing hormone in folliculogenesis and ovulation induction. Fertil Steril 1999; 71: 404–14

39. Levy DP, Navarro JM, Schattman GL, et al. The role of LH in ovarian stimulation: exogenous LH: let's design the future. Hum Reprod 2000; 15: 2258–65

40. Ben Amor A-F. The effect of luteinising hormone administered during luteal follicular phase in normo-ovulatory women undergoing in vitro fertilisation. Hum Reprod 2000; 15 (Suppl 1): 46 (abstr 0–116)

41. Balasch J, Vidal E, Penarrubia J, et al. Suppression of LH during ovarian stimulation: analysing threshold values and effects on ovarian response and the outcome of assisted reproduction in down-regulated women stimulated with recombinant FSH. Hum Reprod 2001; 16: 1636–43

42. Lisi F, Rinaldi L, Fishel S, et al. Use of recombinant follicle-stimulating hormone (Gonal F) and recombinant luteinizing hormone (Luveris) for multiple follicular stimulation in patients with suboptimal response to in vitro fertilisation. Fertil Steril 2003; 79: 1037–8

43. Surrey ES, Schoolcraft WB. Evaluating strategies for improving ovarian response of poor responders undergoing assisted reproductive techniques. Fertil Steril 2000; 73: 667–76

44. Phelps JY, Figueira-Armada L, Levine AS, et al. Exogenous luteinizing hormone (LH) increases estradiol response patterns of poor responders with low serum LH concentrations. J Assist Reprod Genet 1999; 16: 363–8

45. Marrs R, Meldrum D, Muasher S, et al. Randomized trial to compare the effect of recombinant human FSH (follitropin alfa) with or without recombinant human LH in women undergoing assisted reproduction treatment. Reprod Biomed Online 2004; 8: 175–82

46. Humaidan P, Bungum M, Bungum L, et al. Effects of recombinant LH supplementation in women undergoing assisted reproduction with GnRH agonist down-regulation and stimulation with recombinant FSH: an opening study. Reprod Biomed Online 2004; 6: 635–43

47. De Placido G, Alviggi C, Mollo A, et al. Effects of recombinant LH (rLH) supplementation during controlled ovarian hyperstimulation (COH) in normogonadotrophic women with an initial inadequate response to recombinant FSH (rFSH) alter pituitary downregulation. Clin Endocrinol 2004; 60: 637–43

48. Loumaye E, Piazzi A, Engrand P. Results of a phase II, dose finding clinical study comparing recombinant human luteinising hormone (r-hLH) with human chorionic gonadotrophin (HCG) to induce final follicular maturation prior to in vitro fertilisation. Fertil Steril 1998; (Suppl) 0–236–S–88

49. The European Recombinant Human Chorionic Gonadotrophin Study Group. Induction of final follicular maturation and early luteinization in women undergoing ovulation induction for assisted reproduction treatment – recombinant HCG versus urinary HCG. Hum Reprod 2000; 15: 1446–51

50. The International Recombinant Human Chorionic Gonadotropin Study Group. Induction of ovulation in World Health Organization group II anovulatory women undergoing follicular stimulation with recombinant human follicle-stimulating hormone: a comparison of recombinant human chorionic gonadotropin (rhCG) and urinary hCG. Fertil Steril 2001; 75: 1111–18

51. Schoolcraft WB, Hesla JS, Gee MJ. Experience with progesterone gel for luteal support in a highly successful IVF programme. Hum Reprod 2000; 15: 1284–8

52. Penzias AS. Luteal phase support. Fertil Steril 2002; 77: 318–23

53. Ludwig M, Diedrich K. Evaluation of an optimal luteal phase support protocol in IVF. Acta Obstet Gynecol Scand 2001; 80: 452–66

54. American Society for Reproductive Medicine. Practice Committee Report. Fertil Steril 1998; June (Suppl)

55. Guideline development group, Royal College of Obstetricians and Gynaecologists. Management of infertility in tertiary care. Evidence based clinical guideline no. 6. London: RCOG, 2000: 46

56. Balen AH, Hayden CJ, Rutherford AJ. What are the clinical benefits of recombinant gonadotrophins? Clinical efficacy of recombinant gonadotrophins. Hum Reprod 1999; 14: 1411–17

57. Ledger W. A cost-effective analysis of Gonal-F® (follitropin alpha) compared to urinary FSH-HP in ART: results from the UK. Presented at the European Society of Human Reproduction and Embryology (Serono Symposium), Bologna, Italy, June 2000

58. Sykes D, Out HJ, van Loon J. Economic evaluation of recombinant follicle-stimulating hormone (Puregon) in infertile women undergoing IVF in the UK. J Reprod Fertil 2000; 48: 24 (Fertil abstr series 25 for BFS meeting)

59. van Out H, Mannaerts B, Driessen S, et al. A prospective, randomized, assessor blind, multi-centre study comparing recombinant urinary follicle-stimulating hormone (Puregon vs Metrodin) in in vitro fertilisation. Hum Reprod 1995; 10: 2534–40

11

Polycystic ovaries and their relevance to assisted conception

Adam H. Balen

INTRODUCTION

In vitro fertilization (IVF) is not the first-line treatment for polycystic ovarian syndrome (PCOS), but many patients with the syndrome may be referred for IVF, either because there is another reason for their infertility or because they fail to conceive despite ovulating for more than 6 months (i.e. their infertility remains unexplained). Furthermore, approximately 30% of women have polycystic ovaries as detected by ultrasound scan. Many will have little in the way of symptoms and may present for assisted conception treatment because of other reasons (for example tubal factor or male factor). When stimulated, these women with asymptomatic polycystic ovaries have a tendency to respond sensitively and are at increased risk of developing the ovarian hyperstimulation syndrome (OHSS). An understanding of the management of such patients is therefore important to specialists involved in IVF.

Four issues need to be considered. First, what are polycystic ovaries and how are they diagnosed? Second, how large is the problem within the context of IVF? Third, does a diagnosis of polycystic ovaries matter and do patients with polycystic ovaries respond differently at any of the stages of IVF? Finally, should such patients be managed differently, and if so, how?

The association of enlarged, sclerocystic ovaries with amenorrhea, infertility and hirsutism, as described by Stein and Leventhal in 1935[1], is now described as the polycystic ovarian syndrome (PCOS). In recent years it has become apparent that polycystic ovaries may be present in women who are not hirsute and who have a regular menstrual cycle. Thus, a clinical spectrum exists between the typical Stein– Leventhal picture (PCOS) and symptomless women with polycystic ovaries. Even the clinical picture of patients with PCOS exhibits considerable heterogeneity[2]. This heterogeneous disorder may present, at one end of the spectrum, with the single finding of polycystic ovarian morphology as detected by pelvic ultrasound. At the other end of the spectrum symptoms such as obesity, hyperandrogenism, menstrual cycle disturbance and infertility may occur either singly or in combination (Table 1). Metabolic disturbances (elevated serum concentrations of luteinizing hormone (LH), testosterone, insulin and prolactin) are common, and may have profound implications for the long-term health of women with PCOS. PCOS is a familial condition and a number of candidate genes have been implicated[3]. PCOS appears to have its origins during adolescence, although it may present at any time and is particularly associated with an increase in weight[4].

PCOS is a heterogeneous collection of signs and symptoms that, gathered together, form a spectrum of

189

Table 1   The spectrum of clinical manifestations of heterogeneous polycystic ovarian syndrome

Symptoms (% patients affected)	Associated endocrine manifestations	Possible late sequelae
Obesity (38%)	↑ androgens (testosterone and androstenedione)	diabetes mellitus (11%) cardiovascular disease
Menstrual disturbance (66%)		
Hyperandrogenism (48%)	↑ luteinizing hormone	hyperinsulinemia
Infertility (73% of anovulatory infertility)	↑ LH : FSH ratio ↑ free estradiol	low LDL endometrial carcinoma
Asymptomatic (20%)	↑ fasting insulin ↑ prolactin ↑ sex hormone-binding globulin	hypertension

LH, luteinizing hormone; FSH, follicle stimulating hormone; LDL, low-density lipoprotein

a disorder with a mild presentation in some, whilst in others, there is a severe disturbance of reproductive, endocrine and metabolic function. The pathophysiology of PCOS appears to be multifactorial and polygenic. The definition of the syndrome has been much debated. Key features include menstrual cycle disturbance, hyperandrogenism and obesity. There are many extraovarian aspects to the pathophysiology of PCOS, yet ovarian dysfunction is central. At a recent joint European Society of Human Reproduction and Embryology/ American Society for Reproductive Medicine (ESHRE/ASRM) consensus meeting a refined definition of PCOS was agreed: namely, the presence of two out of the following three criteria:

(1) Oligo- and/or anovulation;

(2) Hyperandrogenism (clinical and/or biochemical);

(3) Polycystic ovaries, with the exclusion of other etiologies[5].

DIAGNOSIS

The diagnosis of polycystic ovaries is best made not on the clinical presentation, but rather on the ovarian morphology. With the advent of high-resolution ultrasound, identification of polycystic ovaries has been simplified, and ovarian biopsy, which is invasive and possibly damaging to future fertility because it can cause adhesions, is now unnecessary. Ovaries are described as polycystic if there are ten or more cysts,

2–8 mm in diameter, arranged around a dense stroma or scattered throughout an increased amount of stroma[6] (Figure 1b). They should be distinguished from multicystic ovaries (Figure 1c), which occur normally during puberty and are associated with recovering weight loss-related amenorrhea. These ovaries do not contain increased stroma and the size of the cysts is usually larger than in polycystic ovaries[6].

At the recent joint ESHRE/ASRM consensus meeting a refined definition of PCOS was agreed, encompassing a description of the morphology of the polycystic ovary. According to the available literature, the criteria fulfilling sufficient specificity and sensitivity to define the polycystic ovary should have at least one of the following: either 12 or more follicles measuring 2–9 mm in diameter or increased ovarian volume (> 10 cm^3). If there is a follicle greater than 10 mm in diameter, the scan should be repeated at a time of ovarian quiescence in order to calculate volume and area. The presence of a single polycystic ovary is sufficient to provide the diagnosis. The distribution of the follicles and the description of the stroma are not required in the diagnosis. Increased stromal echogenicity and/or stromal volume are specific to polycystic ovaries, but it has been shown that measurement of the ovarian volume (or area) is a good surrogate for quantification of the stroma in clinical practice[7].

High-resolution ultrasound scanning has made it possible for an accurate estimate to be made of the prevalence of polycystic ovaries in the general population. Several studies have estimated the prevalence of

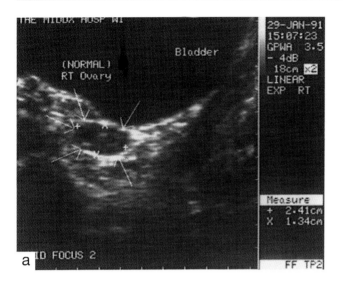

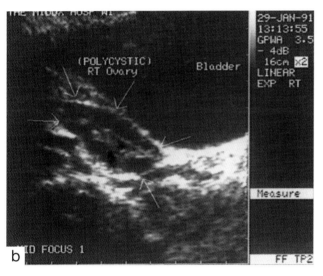

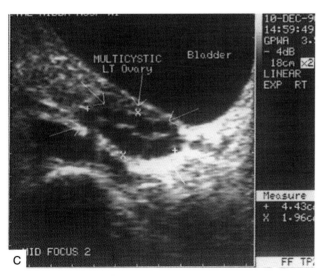

Figure 1 (a) Transabdominal scan of a normal ovary, (b) a polycystic ovary and (c) a multicystic ovary

polycystic ovaries in 'normal' adult women and have found rates of approximately 20–33%[8–12], but it is not known at what age they first appear. Bridges and colleagues[13] found that polycystic ovaries could be detected as early as the age of 6 years. The proportion of children in whom polycystic ovaries could be identified rose throughout childhood to the figure of 20–25% in young adults. It is important to differentiate between polycystic ovaries and PCOS. The former term describes the morphological appearance of the ovary, whereas the latter term is only appropriate when polycystic ovaries are found in association with a menstrual disturbance, most commonly oligomenorrhea, the complications of hyperandrogenization (seborrhea, acne and hirsutism) and obesity.

PCOS is often associated with endocrinological abnormalities, and in particular with alterations in the serum concentrations of LH, prolactin, estrogens and androgens (especially testosterone and androstenedione). In about 40% of cases, plasma concentrations of LH are raised[2]. In a proportion of patients with PCOS, moderate hyperprolactinemia (usually 600–2000 mU/l) is present. Futterweit[14] reported a 27% prevalence of raised prolactin level in 394 women. Hyperprolactinemia may be caused by the stimulation of pituitary lactotrophs by acyclical estrogen production[15] rather than by a primary pituitary defect. Estrogen levels may be altered in PCOS patients who are anovulatory. Estradiol levels are similar to those found in normal women during the early follicular phase of the cycle. Estrone levels are raised, mostly because of extraovarian conversion of androstenedione[16,17], which largely takes place in adipose tissue. Finally, the polycystic ovary tends to produce an excess of androgens. As with the clinical picture, these endocrine changes are variable, and patients with PCOS may have normal hormone concentrations. Therefore, the measurement of these hormones is not as helpful as ultrasound in making the diagnosis.

The polycystic ovary is usually detected by ultrasound, the images correlating well with histopathological studies[18,19]. The original ultrasound definition was provided by transabdominal ultrasonography[6,20], which is still used in current publications[2,21,22]. While Swanson and colleagues[20] described a characteristic appearance without the need for reporting the particular number of cysts, Adams and co-workers[6] proposed a quantifiable definition, with a prerequisite number of at least ten cysts in a single plane. It is now accepted that transvaginal sonography provides greater resolution and that there is a need to redefine the ultrasound criteria for the polycystic ovary[23]. Indeed, Fox and associates[23] suggested the requirement of at least 15 cysts per ovary in their study. Apart from the number of cysts, it is necessary to consider the stromal thickness or density – the latter usually being a subjective assessment – and the ovarian volume, neither of which is clearly defined[24–26]. van Santbrink and co-workers[27] characterized PCOS by taking values for the diagnostic criteria of the syndrome (increased follicle number and ovarian volume, elevated serum concentrations of testosterone, androstenedione and LH) as the 95th centile of a control population. They found considerable overlap between the sonographic and endocrine criteria for the diagnosis of PCOS in women with normogonadotropic oligomenorrhea or infertile women with amenorrhea. The predictive value of polycystic ovaries detected by ultrasound for endocrine parameters, however, was limited[27] – a finding supported by others[28].

Jonard and colleagues[29] studied 214 women with PCOS (oligo-/amenorrhea, elevated serum LH and/or testosterone and/or ovarian area $>5.5\,cm^2$) and 112 with normal ovaries to determine the importance of follicle number per ovary (FNPO). A 7-MHz transvaginal ultrasound scan was performed and three different categories of follicle size analyzed separately (2–5, 6–9 and 2–9 mm). Size range of the follicles has been considered important by some, with polycystic ovaries tending to have smaller follicles than normal or multicystic ovaries. The mean FNPO was similar between normal and polycystic ovaries in the 6–9-mm range, but significantly higher in the polycystic ovaries in both the 2–5- and 2–9-mm ranges. A FNPO of ≥ 12 follicles 2–9 mm gave the best threshold for the diagnosis of PCOS (sensitivity 75%, specificity 99%)[29]. The authors suggest that intraovarian hyperandrogenism promotes excessive early follicular growth up to 2–5 mm, with more follicles able to enter the growing cohort, which then become arrested at the 6–9-mm size. Thus, the consensus definition for a polycystic ovary is one that contains 12 or more follicles of 2–9 mm diameter. This should help to discriminate polycystic ovaries from the other causes of multifollicular ovaries.

A large study of 80 oligo-/amenorrheic women with PCOS was compared with a control group of 30 using a 6.5-MHz transvaginal probe[30]. Based on mean

± 2 standard deviation (SD) data from the control group, the cut-off values were calculated for ovarian volume ($13.21\,cm^3$), ovarian total area ($7.00\,cm^2$), ovarian stromal total area ($1.95\,cm^2$) and stromal/total area ratio (0.34). The sensitivity of these parameters for the diagnosis of PCOS was 21%, 4%, 62% and 100%, respectively, suggesting that a stromal/total area ratio >0.34 is diagnostic of PCOS[30]. Whilst these data may be useful in a research setting, the measurement of ovarian stromal area is not easily achieved in routine daily practice. Thus, the consensus definition for a polycystic ovary includes an ovarian volume of greater than $10\,cm^3$. It is recognized that not all polycystic ovaries will be enlarged to this size or greater, and that the consensus is based on the synthesis of evidence from many studies that have reported a greater mean ovarian volume for polycystic ovaries combined with a consistent finding of a smaller mean volume than $10\,cm^3$ for normal ovaries.

Transabdominal ultrasound has been largely superseded by transvaginal scanning because of greater resolution and, in many cases, patient preference, as the need for a full bladder is avoided, which saves time and may be more comfortable. Whilst this may be the case in the context of infertility clinics, where women are used to having repeated scans, it was found that 20% of women who were undergoing routine screening declined a transvaginal scan after having first had a transabdominal scan[31].

The transvaginal approach gives a more accurate view of the internal structure of the ovaries, avoiding apparently homogeneous ovaries as described with transabdominal scans, particularly in obese patients. With the transvaginal route, high-frequency probes ($>6\,MHz$) having a better spatial resolution, but less examination depth, can be used because the ovaries are close to the vagina and/or the uterus and because the presence of fatty tissue is usually less disruptive (except when very abundant).

Recent studies with computerized three-dimensional reconstructions of ultrasound images of the polycystic ovary have shown that the major factor responsible for the increase in ovarian volume is an increase in the stroma, with little contribution from the cysts themselves[32]. Zaidi and co-workers[33], using color and pulsed Doppler ultrasound, have shown that the stroma of the polycystic ovary has a very high rate of blood flow, consistent with histological studies showing increased stromal vascularity[34], and the recent finding of large amounts of vascular endothelial growth factor (VEGF) in the theca cells of the polycystic ovary[35].

There have been many reviews over the years which have attempted to piece together the complexities of the syndrome[17,36–44], but that is beyond the scope of this chapter. It is fascinating to follow the evolving ideas on the spectrum and pathogenesis of PCOS, yet at the same time frustrating that a consensual definition has not, until recently, been accepted, and this has meant that, when we turn to the literature on the treatment of the condition, it proves impossible to compare studies from different centers that use differing starting points.

Hypersecretion of LH is particularly associated with menstrual disturbances and infertility. Indeed, it is this endocrine feature that appears to result in reduced conception rates and increased rates of miscarriage in both natural and assisted conception[45]. The finding of a persistently elevated early to mid-follicular phase LH concentration in a woman who is trying to conceive suggests the need to suppress LH levels, either by pituitary desensitization with a gonadotropin releasing hormone agonist (GnRH-a), or by laparoscopic ovarian diathermy. There are, however, no large, prospective randomized trials that demonstrate a therapeutic benefit from a reduction in serum LH concentrations during ovulation induction protocols.

We, and others, have found that the patient's body mass index (BMI) correlates with an increased rate of hirsutism, cycle disturbance and infertility[2,46]. Obese women with PCOS hypersecrete insulin, which stimulates ovarian secretion of androgens, and is associated with hirsutism, menstrual disturbance and infertility. It is seldom necessary to measure the serum insulin concentration, as this will not overtly affect the management of the patient, but the prevalence of diabetes in obese women with PCOS is 11%[47], so a measurement of impaired glucose tolerance is important in these women. Obese women (BMI $> 30\,kg/m^2$) should therefore be encouraged to lose weight. Weight loss improves the symptoms of PCOS and improves the patient's endocrine profile[46,48].

Heterogeneity of PCOS

An initial report of 556 patients who attended the Endocrine Clinic at The Middlesex Hospital, London, described the heterogeneity of PCOS and clarified the significance of three endocrine patterns (raised concentrations of LH, testosterone and prolactin) and identified five clinical subgroups (hirsutism, infertility, obesity, alopecia and acanthosis nigricans)[49]. We subsequently extended that study and described the features of what at present is the largest series of patients with ultrasound-detected polycystic ovaries, to produce a reference for the spectrum of this disorder and to highlight the features of ultrasound morphology with endocrine parameters[2]. A total of 1871 women who attended the clinic were identified as having polycystic ovaries, and 130 patients (6.9%) were excluded from the analysis because they were additionally found to be menopausal ($n = 13$) or also had weight-related amenorrhea ($n = 46$), pituitary disease ($n = 27$), a prolactinoma ($n = 25$) or congenital adrenal hyperplasia ($n = 19$). There were no patients with abnormal thyroid function tests or androgen-secreting tumors. The findings for the remaining 1741 patients are recorded in Table 2.

The clinical data included age, BMI and the presence of acne and hirsutism, which were defined using the Ferriman and Gallwey score. Acanthosis nigricans was diagnosed by clinical appearance. The menstrual cycle was described as being regular, oligomenorrheic (a cycle interval longer than 35 days but less than 6 months) or amenorrheic (no menstruation for more than 6 months). The fertility status was classified as 'proven fertile' (those with a previous pregnancy and no subsequent infertility), 'fertility untested' (those who had never tried to conceive) or 'primary/secondary' infertility of at least 1 year's duration.

Serum was collected for measurement of LH, follicle stimulating hormone (FSH), testosterone, prolactin and thyroid function. The assays that were used are described in detail in the paper of Conway and colleagues[49]. In particular, the Chelsea radioimmunoassay (RIA) kit for measurement of LH (which employs polyclonal antiserum F87 and NIBSC 68/40 International Reference Preparation) was used, and a value of 10 IU/l was 2 SD above the mean for normal women in the follicular phase. The hormone measurements were usually performed in the follicular phase of the menstrual cycle and were excluded from the analysis if measurements of FSH were elevated ($> 10\,IU/l$), which suggested the presence of either a mid-cycle surge or a perimenopausal state.

The variables BMI, serum LH and prolactin concentrations and ovarian volume were log-transformed

Table 2 Characteristics of 1741 women with ultrasound-detected polycystic ovaries. Values are expressed as mean and 5–95 centiles[2]

	Mean	Normal range	5–95th centiles
Age (years)	31.5		14–50
Ovarian volume (cm³)	11.7	< 10	4.6–22.3
Uterine cross-sectional area (cm²)	27.5		15.2–46.3
Endometrium (mm)	7.5		4.0–13.0
BMI (kg/m²)	25.4	19–25*	19.0–38.6
FSH (IU/l)	4.5	1–10*	1.4–7.5
LH (IU/l)	10.9	1–10*	2.0–27.0
Testosterone (nmol/l)	2.6	0.5–2.5*	1.1–4.8
Prolactin (mU/l)	342	<350	87–917

BMI, body mass index; FSH, follicle stimulating hormone; LH, luteinizing hormone

before parametric analysis, and geometric means are presented for these variables. Group means were compared by analysis of variance with Duncan's procedure for multiple comparisons. Grouped variables (BMI and LH) and discrete data were tested with the χ^2 test, and associations between continuous variables were sought with Pearson's correlation coefficients. Multiple regression analysis was performed using the stepwise method with a threshold of $p < 0.05$ for inclusion.

Of the study population, 38.4% of patients were overweight (BMI $> 25\,\mathrm{kg/m^2}$), 39.8% had an elevated serum concentration of LH ($> 10\,\mathrm{IU/l}$) and 28.9% had an elevated serum testosterone concentration ($> 2.5\,\mathrm{nmol/l}$). With respect to menstrual history, 47.0% had oligomenorrhea, 29.7% had a normal menstrual cycle, 19.2% had amenorrhea, 2.7% had polymenorrhea and 1.4% had menorrhagia. Of the patients, 66.2% had hirsutism: mild (20.6%), moderate (40.7%) or severe (4.9%). Furthermore, 34.7% of patients had acne and 2.5% had acanthosis nigricans.

By Pearson's correlation coefficient, the patients' BMI was found to correlate significantly with ovarian volume ($r = 0.11$; $p < 0.0005$) and uterine cross-sectional area ($r = 0.15$; $p < 0.0005$). Despite the effect of obesity on reducing the synthesis by the liver of sex hormone-binding globulin (SHBG), BMI was positively associated with a rise in serum testosterone concentration ($r = 0.254$; $p < 0.0005$) and the prevalence of hirsutism ($p = 0.0002$) (Figure 2). Obesity was

also associated with an increased rate of infertility and cycle disturbances. The rates of primary (15%) and secondary (8%) infertility were fairly constant with a BMI of 20–30 kg/m², but rose to 26% and 14%, respectively, when the BMI was $> 30\,\mathrm{kg/m^2}$ ($p < 0.00005$). Similarly, the percentage of women with a regular menstrual cycle fell from approximately 32 to 22% when the BMI rose above $30\,\mathrm{kg/m^2}$ ($p = 0.032$).

With respect to fertility, 804 of a total of 1269 women (63.4%) had not yet tested their fertility by the end of the study. Of the remaining 465 women, 228 (49%) had primary infertility, 121 (26%) had secondary infertility and 116 (25%) had proven fertility. The LH concentrations in relation to fertility are recorded in Table 3. The mean serum LH concentration of those with primary infertility was significantly higher than that of women with secondary infertility and both were higher than the LH concentration of those with proven infertility ($p < 0.00001$). The rate of infertility increased if the serum LH concentration was $> 10\,\mathrm{IU/l}$ (Figure 3; χ^2 58.72; degrees of freedom (df) 12; $p < 0.00001$). There was also a significant increase in the rate of cycle disturbance with LH concentrations of $> 10\,\mathrm{IU/l}$ (χ^2 68.96; df 24; $p < 0.00001$).

The ovarian volume correlated with serum concentrations of LH ($r = 0.24$; $p < 0.0005$), testosterone ($r = 0.16$; $p < 0.0005$) and the BMI ($r = 0.11$; $p < 0.0005$). These variables were independent of each other when tested with multiple regression analysis. A

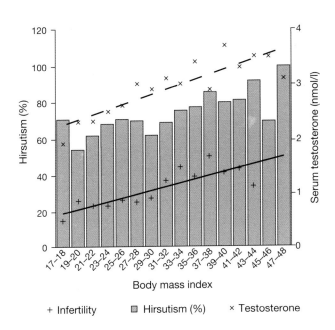

+ Infertility   ■ Hirsutism (%)   × Testosterone

Figure 2 The relationship between body mass index and the rates of hirsutism and serum testosterone concentration

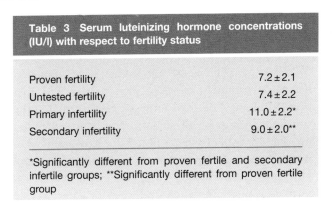

Table 3 Serum luteinizing hormone concentrations (IU/l) with respect to fertility status	
Proven fertility	7.2±2.1
Untested fertility	7.4±2.2
Primary infertility	11.0±2.2*
Secondary infertility	9.0±2.0**

*Significantly different from proven fertile and secondary infertile groups; **Significantly different from proven fertile group

rising serum concentration of testosterone was associated with an increased risk of hirsutism ($p < 0.0005$), infertility ($p = 0.0225$) and cycle disturbance ($p = 0.0007$). Ovarian morphology appears to be the most sensitive marker of PCOS, compared with the classical endocrine features of raised serum LH and testosterone, which were found in only 39.8% and 28.9% of patients, respectively, in our study.

PREVALENCE

The prevalence of polycystic ovaries in women with ovulatory disorders has been well documented. With the use of high-resolution ultrasound, it is now apparent that as high a proportion as 87% of patients with oligomenorrhea and 26% with amenorrhea have polycystic ovaries[50]. Polson and colleagues[8] found a prevalence of 22% in a volunteer 'normal' population, and a number of other studies have found a similar prevalence (see above). We studied 224 normal female volunteers between the ages of 18 and 25 years and identified polycystic ovaries using ultrasound in 33% of participants[12]. Fifty per cent of the participants were using some form of hormonal contraception, but the prevalence of polycystic ovaries in users and non-users

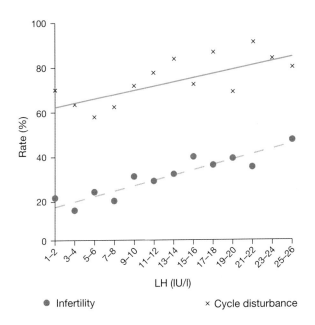

● Infertility   × Cycle disturbance

Figure 3 The relationship between serum luteinizing hormone (LH) concentration and the rates of infertility and cycle disturbance

of hormonal contraception was identical. Polycystic ovaries in the non-users of hormonal contraception were associated with irregular menstrual cycles and significantly higher serum testosterone concentrations when compared with women with normal ovaries; however, only a small proportion of women with polycystic ovaries (15%) had 'elevated' serum testosterone concentrations outside the normal range. Interestingly there were no significant differences in acne, hirsutism, body mass index (BMI) or body fat percentage between women with polycystic and with normal ovaries, and hyperinsulinism and reduced insulin sensitivity were not associated with polycystic ovaries in this group.

The prevalence in patients referred for IVF is not so well known. Three of our studies have suggested that many patients have polycystic ovaries. The first involved a review of ultrasound scans performed in the early follicular phase of an IVF treatment cycle, and 50% of 42 patients were noted to have polycystic ovaries[51]. A more recent study identified 58 (33%) with polycystic ovaries compared with 117 with normal ovaries[52]. In patients referred for natural-cycle IVF, all with regular ovulatory menstrual cycles, 43.5% had polycystic ovaries[52].

Polycystic ovaries, with or without clinical symptoms, are therefore a common finding in patients referred for IVF. It must be stressed that the first-line treatment for PCOS is not IVF. Occasionally, the IVF specialist will be presented with a patient with PCOS, referred for IVF, who either has never had induction of ovulation or has been inadequately stimulated. Provided there is no other cause for their infertility, for example tubal damage, it then behoves the clinician to try induction of ovulation first.

Infertility in patients with polycystic ovaries is caused either by PCOS (i.e. failure to ovulate at a normal rate, and/or hypersecretion of LH), or by all the other causes of infertility, or a combination of the two. Ovulation induction is appropriate for the first group (PCOS). IVF may be necessary in the second group (other causes), and in patients with PCOS who have failed to conceive despite at least six ovulatory cycles (i.e. those who have coexisting 'unexplained' infertility).

THE RESPONSE OF THE POLYCYSTIC OVARY TO STIMULATION FOR IVF

The response of the polycystic ovary to stimulation in the context of ovulation induction aimed at the development of unifollicular ovulation is well documented, and differs significantly from that of normal ovaries. The response tends to be slow, with a significant risk of ovarian hyperstimulation and/or cyst formation[53-57]. Conventional IVF currently depends on inducing multifollicular recruitment[54]. It is thus to be expected that the response of the polycystic ovary within the context of an IVF program should also differ from the normal, but this has previously been

assumed rather than documented. Jacobs and co-workers[51] described an increase in follicle production in patients with polycystic ovaries, and others[55] have referred to the 'explosive' nature of the ovarian response. Dor and co-workers[56] compared 16 patients with PCOS with a control group with normal ovaries, who were all undergoing IVF, and noted an increase in number of follicles and oocytes and in estrogen levels, associated with a decrease in fertilization rates.

There are several possible explanations for this 'explosive' response. There are many partially developed follicles present in the polycystic ovary, and these are readily stimulated to give rise to the typical multifollicular response. Thecal hyperplasia (in some cases with raised levels of LH and/or insulin) provides large amounts of androstenedione and testosterone, which act as substrates for estrogen production. Granulosa cell aromatase, although deficient in the 'resting' polycystic ovary, is readily stimulated by FSH. Therefore, normal quantities of FSH act on large amounts of substrate (testosterone and androstenedione) to produce large amounts of intraovarian estrogen. Ovarian follicles, of which there are too many in polycystic ovaries, are increasingly sensitive to FSH (receptors for which are stimulated by high local concentrations of estrogen), and as a result there is multiple follicular development associated with very high levels of circulating estrogen. In some cases, this may result in the ovarian hyperstimulation syndrome (OHSS), to which patients with polycystic ovaries are particularly prone.

There are two additional factors to be considered. The first is that many women with PCOS, particularly those who are obese, have compensatory hypersecretion of insulin in response to the insulin resistance specifically related to PCOS[58] and that caused by obesity. Since the ovary is spared the insulin resistance, it is stimulated by insulin, acting, as it were, as a co-gonadotropin. Insulin augments theca cell production of androgens in response to stimulation by LH[59] and granulosa cell production of estrogen in response to stimulation by FSH[60].

The second factor to be considered relates to the already mentioned widespread expression of VEGF in polycystic ovaries. VEGF is an endothelial cell mitogen that stimulates vascular permeability, and hence its involvement in the pathophysiology of OHSS. VEGF is normally confined in the ovary to the blood vessels and is responsible there for invasion of the relatively avascular Graafian follicle by blood vessels after ovulation. The increase of LH at mid-cycle leads to the expression of VEGF, which has recently been shown to be an obligatory intermediate in the formation of the corpus luteum[61]. In polycystic ovaries, however, Kamat and colleagues[35] have shown widespread expression of VEGF in theca cells in the increased stroma. More recent studies[62] have shown that, compared with women with normal ovaries, women with polycystic ovaries or PCOS have increased serum VEGF, both before and during LH-releasing hormone (LHRH) analog therapy and gonadotropin treatment.

The above data serve to remind us of the close relationship of polycystic ovaries with OHSS, and also provide a possible explanation for the multifollicular response of the polycystic ovary to gonadotropin stimulation. One of the mechanisms that underpins the unifollicular response of the normal ovary is diversion of blood flow within the ovaries, first from the non-dominant to the dominant ovary, and second from cohort follicles to the dominant follicle. This results in diversion of FSH away from the cohort follicles and permits them to undergo atresia. We postulate that the widespread distribution of VEGF in polycystic ovaries prevents this diversion of blood flow, leaving a substantial number of small- and intermediate-sized follicles in 'suspended animation' and ready to respond to gonadotropin stimulation. The distribution of VEGF in the polycystic ovary therefore helps to explain one of the fundamental features of the polycystic ovary, namely loss of the intraovarian autoregulatory mechanism that permits unifollicular ovulation to occur.

We examined the outcome of IVF in 76 patients diagnosed as having polycystic ovaries on pretreatment ultrasound scan and compared it with 76 control patients who had normal ovaries. The subjects were matched for age, cause of infertility and stimulation regimen[57]. Despite receiving significantly less human menopausal gonadotropin (hMG), patients with ultrasound-diagnosed polycystic ovaries had significantly higher serum estradiol concentrations on the day of human chorionic gonadotropin (hCG) administration (5940 vs. 4370 pmol/l; $p < 0.001$), developed more follicles (14.9 vs. 9.8; $p < 0.001$) and produced more oocytes (9.3 vs. 6.8; $p < 0.003$). Fertilization rates, however, were reduced in patients with polycystic ovaries (52.8% vs. 66.1%; $p < 0.007$). There was no significant difference in cleavage rates. The pregnancy rate per embryo transfer was 25.4% in the polycystic

ovary group and 23.0% in the group with normal ovaries. There were three high-order multiple pregnancies in the polycystic ovary group but none in the group with normal ovaries. Of the patients with polycystic ovaries, 10.5% developed moderate/severe OHSS compared with none in the controls ($p = 0.006$). Patients with and without polycystic ovaries undergoing IVF had similar pregnancy and live birth rates, as each had similar numbers of good-quality embryos for transfer. The study indicated the importance of the diagnosis of polycystic ovarian morphology prior to 'controlled' ovarian stimulation, because it is less likely to be controlled in women with polycystic ovaries and these patients are more likely to develop OHSS and multiple pregnancy. Similar observations in women with polycystic ovaries undergoing IVF have been reported by others[63].

It should be noted that there are a small number of patients with polycystic ovaries who are poor responders, rather than over-responders. Such patients are often very resistant to gonadotropin stimulation and may benefit from the addition of growth hormone[64].

PRECONCEPTION COUNSELING

Women with polycystic ovaries encounter specific problems during assisted conception treatment cycles. By our diagnostic criteria, many women are unaware that their ovaries are polycystic and may have presented with another cause of subfertility. When polycystic ovaries have been diagnosed by ultrasound, it is helpful to discuss this finding with the patient, as a preliminary knowledge of the behavior of the polycystic ovary in response to superovulation regimens acts as a foundation for both an explanation of the drugs chosen and advice about potential problems – specifically OHSS and multiple pregnancy[54].

Some women will already have been diagnosed as having either polycystic ovaries or PCOS, and may be aware of the sequelae. The latter group will usually have had endocrinological and metabolic problems, and for them, preconception counseling should involve more than an outline of the consequences of treatment. There are additional problems that may occur during pregnancy, and there may be a chance to reduce their risk by appropriate measures, such as weight loss, even before embarking upon assisted conception regimens.

There are thus two aspects to the counseling and subsequent management of women with polycystic ovaries: first, the general behavior of the polycystic ovary itself; and second, the additional features of PCOS. Ovaries that are morphologically polycystic contain multiple antral follicles and are extremely sensitive to stimulation. It is the woman with PCOS who will benefit most from preconception counseling. She has not only an endocrine disorder but also a metabolic one. She may therefore have hyperandrogenism and insulin resistance; it is the consequences of the latter that have a particular bearing on pregnancy. Hyperinsulinemia may lead to obesity, which in turn is associated with hypertension, pre-eclampsia and gestational diabetes[65,66]. Although hypertension and pre-eclampsia have been directly associated with PCOS[67], it appears that it is the resultant obesity that is the prime factor[68]. Dietary restriction and reduction of weight gain during pregnancy do not reduce the incidence of pre-eclampsia[65], yet if an ideal weight can be attained before conception, pre-eclampsia may be avoided[66]. The role of insulin-lowering drugs in the context of IVF are still being evaluated.

It is established that women with polycystic ovaries exhibit insulin resistance, particularly if they are obese[47], and it has been postulated that hyperinsulinemia may have an etiological role in PCOS, possibly through effects on ovarian insulin-like growth factor I (IGF-I) receptors[58]. Even if exposure to high insulin or IGF-I levels is not etiological, it is thought to result in increased ovarian androgen secretion[47]. Fasting insulin levels are raised in two-thirds of obese and one-third of lean women with PCOS; those women with hyperinsulinemia are more likely to present with menstrual disturbances and hyperandrogenism than those with normal insulin levels[41]. The most effective management is advice on diet and weight loss. One should also be aware that type 2 diabetes mellitus may be precipitated by some treatments, such as synthetic sex steroids[69]. Screening women with PCOS for glucose intolerance should now be standard practice, with a 75-g oral glucose tolerance test being performed in all women with a BMI of greater than $30 \, \text{kg/m}^2$. Gestational diabetes is also more prevalent amongst women with PCOS, our study quoted a prevalence of 8.1%, as compared with a population prevalence of 0.25%[68]. Of the 89 pregnancies studied, the rate was greatest (19%) in the obese women; none of those with a normal weight became diabetic in pregnancy.

Although dietary restriction is employed in the management of obesity, active steps towards weight loss during pregnancy itself are not advised[66].

Obesity in pregnancy also leads to an increased incidence of urinary tract infections, fetal malpresentations and dystocia, postpartum hemorrhage and thromboembolism. The perinatal mortality rate in the infants of obese women (> 110th centile, Metropolitan Life Insurance tables) is also double that of the normal population[66]. Current research suggests that in later life women with PCOS may be at risk from hypertension, type 2 diabetes mellitus and cardiovascular disease, because insulin resistance is also associated with a reduction of the cardioprotective high-density lipoprotein 2 (HDL_2). Women with endometrial hyperplasia and carcinoma are traditionally obese, with hypertension and diabetes, and they are likely to have polycystic ovaries. Therefore, preconception counseling is important not only to advise short-term weight loss, in order to reduce maternal and neonatal morbidity, but also to prevent later morbidity by encouraging obese women to become slim, and non-obese women to stay slim[54].

There has been disagreement in the past about the association of PCOS with congenital abnormalities, especially as treatment regimens may have an influence[70]. The miscarriage rate is increased in women with polycystic ovaries[71]. This is thought to be secondary to an abnormal endocrine environment, specifically hypersecretion of LH, affecting either oocyte maturation or endometrial receptivity[71,72]. There is, however, no evidence of an increased incidence of congenital abnormalities either in women with PCOS[68] or in women undergoing ovulation induction[73,74] and IVF[75,76]. That PCOS does not cause congenital anomalies is also supported by the high prevalence of the syndrome in our clinic, whose statistics are included in the reports of the Medical Research Council[75] and Beral and colleagues[76]. Couples can thus be given appropriate reassurance at the time of their first consultation.

IMPLICATIONS OF PCOS IN RELATION TO FERTILITY

Anovulation is the main cause of infertility in women with PCOS. Many regimens have been evolved to induce ovulation, and the interested reader is referred to the review by Balen[77]. In recent years there has been increasing evidence that hypersecretion of LH is deleterious both to fertility and to pregnancy outcome[78–82]. LH has several functions in the control of the developing follicle. In the early follicular phase, low levels of LH induce a change in function of the theca interstitial cells from progesterone to androgen production[83]. FSH then promotes the conversion of androgen to estradiol by the granulosa cells. Not only does LH initiate theca cell androgen production, but it is also involved in the reversal to progesterone secretion at the time of the preovulatory surge. LH is also involved in the supression of oocyte maturation inhibitor (OMI). The action of OMI is to maintain the meiotic arrest of the oocyte at the diplotene stage of prophase I. The precise nature of OMI is uncertain, but it is known that cyclic adenosine monophosphate (cAMP) activates OMI or is itself OMI[84]. By reducing cAMP in the oocyte, LH enables the reactivation of meiosis and hence the attainment of oocyte maturity prior to ovulation[85]. Inappropriate release of LH may profoundly affect this process such that the released egg either is unable to be fertilized[82], or, if fertilized, miscarries[72].

There has been debate about the predictive value of an elevated follicular phase level of LH for either conception or pregnancy outcome. It was first demonstrated in 1985 that oocytes obtained from women undergoing IVF who had a serum LH value greater than 1 SD above the mean on the day of hCG administration had a significantly reduced rate of fertilization and cleavage[79]. This relationship was subsequently confirmed with urinary LH measurements in the Bourn Hall IVF program[81] and in our ovulation induction clinic[82]. It has also been shown not only that ovulation and fertilization are affected by high tonic LH levels, but also that miscarriage is more likely[82]. A study of women attending a recurrent miscarriage clinic demonstrated that 82% had polycystic ovaries[71], and women attending this clinic were also found to have abnormalities in follicular phase LH secretion[86]. A field study of 193 women planning to become pregnant showed that mid-follicular phase LH levels of > 10 IU/l were associated with both a significant drop in conception rate (67%) and a major increase in miscarriage rate (65%), compared with those women with normal LH levels (88% and 12%, respectively)[72]. There has been some disagreement over the significance of an elevated LH, with one group suggesting no

deleterious effect in IVF cycles[87]. In this study it was considered that only cycles that result in a pregnancy should be used to provide the normal range of LH concentrations, and that by taking LH levels above the 75th centile, no adverse effect on fertilization or cleavage was detected. An effect on miscarriage was not addressed.

The occurrence of a 'premature' endogenous LH surge in exogenously stimulated cycles is not related to basal hypersecretion of LH, but is a reflection of endocrine feedback from the leading follicle(s). The 'prematurity' is not an indication of abnormality, but rather of a surge that has occurred before the planned intervention by egg collection. If an LH surge is identified at its initiation, the treatment cycle is sometimes abandoned, but it may instead be augmented with hCG (as the LH surge is usually markedly attenuated[88]) and therapy continued. If, however, the surge is established – also demonstrated by a rising serum progesterone level – the patient may have ovulated by the time that oocyte retrieval is attempted[89]. Others have had similar experiences, with women who do not conceive having significantly higher LH values in the 24–48 h prior to hCG administration[90–92]. This has led to the practice of canceling cycles in which a spontaneous surge is observed, unless it is 'caught' within 12 h of its onset. This approach requires intense endocrine monitoring, with serum or urine LH measurements at least 4-hourly.

Basal hypersecretion of LH is a defect found only in PCOS. There is increasing evidence that both high follicular phase LH levels and an endogenous LH surge are deleterious to conception and pregnancy outcome[78]. Although the precise mechanism resulting in hypersecretion of LH in PCOS is unclear[93], the therapeutic approach to ovulation induction in women with polycystic ovaries should be aimed at preventing inappropriate gonadotropin levels.

To assess the risk of miscarriage after IVF with respect to age, cause of infertility, ovarian morphology and treatment regimen, we performed an analysis of the first 1060 pregnancies conceived between July 1984 and July 1990 as a result of 7623 IVF cycles[45]. Ovarian stimulation had been achieved either by the administration of clomiphene citrate (100 mg/day, days 2–6 of the menstrual cycle) and hMG (Pergonal; Serone Ltd, Welwyn Garden City, UK) and/or FSH (Metrodin; Serono, UK); or by the combined use of the GnRH-a buserelin (Suprefact; Hoechst,

Table 4 The outcome of 1060 *in vitro* fertilization (IVF) pregnancies in relation to patient age

	Number	Mean age (SD) (years)	Age range (years)
Successful pregnancy	724 (68.3%)	32.18 (3.86)	22–44
Spontaneous miscarriage	282 (26.6%)	33.17 (4.09)	22–44
Ectopic pregnancy	54 (5.1%)	32.19 (3.15)	24–38
Heterotopic pregnancy	4 (0.4%)	29.50 (2.08)	27–32
Total pregnancies	1060		

Hounslow, UK) and hMG or FSH. Three regimens of administration of buserelin (500 µg per day given subcutaneously) and hMG/FSH were used. In the 'long' protocol, buserelin was administered from day 1 of the menstrual cycle, and treatment with hMG or FSH commenced after pituitary desensitization had been achieved at least 14 days later[94]. In the 'short' protocol, buserelin was administered from day 2 and hMG or FSH from day 3 of the menstrual cycle, and both continued until the day of hCG administration[95]. In the 'ultrashort' protocol, buserelin was administered on days 1–3 and hMG or FSH were given from day 2 of the cycle until the day of hCG administration[96].

Of the 1060 pregnancies, 724 (68.3%) were ongoing, 282 (26.6%) ended in a spontaneous miscarriage and 54 (5.1%) were ectopic. There were four heterotopic pregnancies (0.4%). The mean age of women who had ongoing pregnancies (32.2, SD 3.9 years) was significantly lower ($p < 0.008$) than that of the women who miscarried (33.2, SD 4.1 years) (Table 4). There was no difference in miscarriage rates in the 20–24-, 25–29- and 30–34-year age groups (17.4%, 22.7% and 28.7%, respectively), but this increased significantly to 31.9% in the 35–39-year age group ($p < 0.01$) and even further to 53.3% in those aged 40–44 years ($p < 0.04$).

There was no relationship between the miscarriage rate and the indication for IVF (Table 5). On the other hand, of the 538 patients who had a pretreatment baseline ultrasound scan, those with normal ovaries had a 23.6% miscarriage rate compared with a rate of 35.8% in those with polycystic ovaries ($p = 0.0038$, 95% confidence interval (CI) of the difference 4.7–23.1%) (Table 6). The mean age of women who had successful pregnancies and those who miscarried was similar, whether they had normal or polycystic ovaries (Table 7).

Table 5 Cause of infertility and pregnancy outcome

Diagnosis	Successful (n)	Miscarriage (n)
Tubal damage	417	158 (27.5%)
Male factor	178	61 (25.5%)
Unexplained	120	59 (33.0%)
Endometriosis	106	27 (20.3%)
Anovulation	29	18 (38.3%)
Total	680	282

$\chi 2 = 9.344$, degrees of freedom (df) = 4, not significant

Of the 689 women who received a clomiphene citrate regimen, 31.1% miscarried. There was no difference in the miscarriage rate in patients who received either hMG (30.2%) or FSH (36.8%) with clomiphene. The proportion who miscarried after receiving treatment with a buserelin regimen was 21.5%, and this was significantly less than the miscarriage rate with clomiphene citrate ($p = 0.0018$, 95% CI 3.9–15.3%) (Table 8).

We found a highly significant difference ($p = 0.001$, 95% CI 5.4–18.3%) between the miscarriage rates in patients who received the 'long' buserelin regimen (19.1%) compared with those who received clomiphene citrate, but no difference between those who received 'short' (28.0%) or 'ultrashort' (24.7%) buserelin regimens and clomiphene citrate. There was no significant difference in the miscarriage rate in patients who received hMG (21%) or FSH (16.5%) and a long buserelin regimen (Table 8). In women who were scanned pretreatment, the prevalence of polycystic ovaries in those who received clomiphene citrate (41.4%, 108/261) was comparable to that in those on the 'long' buserelin regimen (44.1%, 74/168).

Table 6 Prevalence of polycystic ovaries in 538 women with baseline ultrasound scans

	Successful pregnancy (n)	Miscarriage (n)	Total (n)
Normal ovaries	266 (76.4%)	82 (23.6%)	348
Polycystic ovaries	122 (64.2%)	68 (35.8%)	190

Fisher's exact probability = 0.0038 (95% confidence interval 4.7–23.1%)

Table 7 Mean age (years) of women with normal and polycystic ovaries

	Successful pregnancy	Miscarriage	Total (n)
Normal ovaries	32.26 ± 3.92	33.19 ± 3.64	348
Polycystic ovaries	32.14 ± 4.29 (NS)	33.04 ± 3.98 (NS)	190

NS, not significant

Table 8 Treatment regimen and pregnancy outcome in 1006 *in vitro* fertilization (IVF) pregnancies (54 ectopic pregnancies excluded from this analysis)

	Successful (n)	Miscarriage (n)	Total (n)
Clomiphene regimens			
Clomiphene + hMG	420 (69.8%)	182 (30.2%)	602
Clomiphene + FSH	55 (63.2%)	32 (36.8%)	87
Total clomiphene	475 (68.9%)	214 (31.1%)	689
Buserelin regimens			
Long buserelin (all)	164 (80.8%)	39 (19.2%)	203
long buserelin + hMG	98 (79.0%)	26 (21.0%)	124
long buserelin + FSH	66 (83.5%)	13 (16.5%)	79
Short buserelin	18 (72.0%)	7 (28.0%)	25
Ultra-short buserelin	67 (75.3%)	22 (24.7%)	89
Total buserelin	249 (78.5%)	68 (21.5%)	317
Overall total	724 (72.0%)	282 (28.0%)	1006

hMG, human menopausal gonadotropin; FSH, follicle stimulating hormone

The number of patients with polycystic ovaries on the 'short' buserelin regimen (4.2%, 1/24) and the 'ultra-short' buserelin regimen (8.2%, 7/85) was significantly lower ($p = 0.004$ and $p < 0.00005$, respectively, compared with the long buserelin regimen). These figures reflect the fact that the short regimens of buserelin were generally avoided in patients with polycystic ovaries.

The rate of miscarriage in patients who received clomiphene citrate was 47.2% in those with polycystic ovaries and 20.3% in those with normal ovaries ($p < 0.00005$, 95% CI 15.6–38.3%). In patients who received the 'long' buserelin regimen, there was no significant difference in miscarriage rates between those with polycystic ovaries (20.3%) and those with normal ovaries (25.5%). There was also no difference in the

Table 9 Miscarriage rate by ovarian morphology and treatment with either clomiphene citrate (CC) or long buserelin (LTB)

	Successful (n)	Miscarriage (n)	Total (n)
(a) Normal ovaries + CC	122	31 (20.3%)	153
(b) Normal ovaries + LTB	70	24 (25.5%)	94
(c) Polycystic ovaries + CC	57	51 (47.2%)	108
(d) Polycystic ovaries + LTB	59	15 (20.3%)	74

(a) vs. (b) not significant (NS), (a) vs. (c) $p < 0.00005$, (b) vs. (d) NS, (c) vs. (d) $p = 0.0003$

Table 10 Miscarriage rate by ovarian morphology and treatment with clomiphene citrate and long buserelin with either human menopausal gonadotropin (hMG) or follicle stimulating hormone (FSH)

	hMG		FSH	
	Successful (n)	Miscarriage (n)	Successful (n)	Miscarriage (n)
Normal ovaries				
Clomiphene	96	23 (19.3%)	26	8 (23.5%)
Long buserelin	52	17 (24.6%)	18	7 (28.0%)
Polycystic ovaries				
Clomiphene	43	39 (47.6%)	14	12 (46.2%)
Long buserelin	41	9 (18.0%)	18	6 (25.0%)

miscarriage rates in women with normal ovaries who received clomiphene citrate (20.3%) or the 'long' buserelin regimen (25.5%). There was, however, a highly significant difference ($p = 0.0003$, 95% CI 13.8–40.1%) in miscarriage rates between women with polycystic ovaries who received clomiphene (47.2%) and those who received the 'long' buserelin regimen (20.3%) (Table 9). Miscarriage rates were not affected by treatment with hMG versus FSH in patients with normal (24.6% vs. 28%) or polycystic ovaries (18% vs. 25%) who were treated with the 'long' buserelin regimen, and similarly between hMG versus FSH in patients with normal (19.3% vs. 23.5%) or polycystic ovaries (47.6% vs. 46.2%) who were treated with a clomiphene citrate regimen (Table 10).

In this series of 1060 consecutive IVF pregnancies the rate of miscarriage was 26.6%, which is similar to the miscarriage rates of other large IVF series (reviewed by Balen and Yovich[97]). It is difficult to compare figures obtained after assisted conception procedures with miscarriage rates after spontaneous conceptions because of the more intensive early-pregnancy monitoring and earlier diagnosis of pregnancy after IVF treatment. If one takes the timing of the miscarriage into account, the abortion rates that follow natural and assisted conception are similar[98].

As expected, there was an increased risk of miscarriage with increasing maternal age. Women attending infertility clinics tend to be older than the average couple attending an antenatal clinic. The mean age of women giving birth in England and Wales is 28.8 years[99], whilst the mean age of patients in our series was 32.2 years. In addition to the difficulty in becoming pregnant, older women have a greater risk of miscarriage[100]. There are extensive data that confirm a rising incidence of chromosomal anomalies with increasing maternal age[101,102], and this accounts, in a large part, for the increasing miscarriage rate. With respect to chromosomal abnormalities following assisted conception, a recent study compared miscarriage following spontaneous and assisted conception and found no significant increase in the rate of chromosomal abnormalities after gamete manipulation[103]. Thus, the miscarriage rate is a reflection of maternal characteristics rather than the gamete handling procedures. Over the time period of the present study there was a considerable increase in the experience of IVF practitioners (both medical and scientific), together with an improvement in the pregnancy rate. Analyzing the data year by year, we found no significant difference in the miscarriage rates by cause of infertility or treatment regimen.

Abdalla and co-workers[104], in an IVF/gamete intrafallopian transfer (GIFT) program, compared the outcome of 14 pregnancies following treatment with clomiphene and hMG with 33 pregnancies in which ovarian stimulation had been performed with buserelin and hMG. They found a significantly higher rate of early pregnancy loss, defined as a loss of pregnancy within 6 weeks of oocyte retrieval, in the group that received clomiphene compared with the group that received buserelin (5/14 vs. 3/33). There was, however, no significant difference in the rate of miscarriage that occurred after 6 weeks of gestation. The outcome of pregnancy from 25 units in Australia and New Zealand following IVF and GIFT in 1988–89 has been reported[105]. In 2646 pregnancies following stimulation with a clomiphene citrate regimen the spontaneous miscarriage rate was 23.8%, compared with a 19.5% miscarriage rate in 731 pregnancies which resulted after a buserelin regimen ($p < 0.05$). The type of buserelin regimen was not known to the authors. There was no correlation with the cause of infertility, and ovarian morphology was not studied.

The high rate of miscarriage in those who received clomiphene may be related to the deleterious effects of elevated serum LH levels. Clomiphene citrate causes an exaggerated early follicular phase release of both gonadotropins, and the resultant elevated level of LH may reduce the chance of conception and increase the risk of miscarriage[106]. The protective effect of GnRH-a, such as buserelin, is presumably mediated by the functional hypogonadotropic hypogonadism and suppressed LH levels that they induce. This notion is consistent with the observation that the 'long' protocol of treatment with buserelin, but not the 'short' or 'ultra-short' protocol, was associated with the reduction in miscarriage rates. It is well documented that use of the 'short' or 'ultra-short' protocol of GnRH-a is associated with a rise of LH concentrations to pre-ovulatory surge levels[95], so the developing ovarian follicle may be exposed to inappropriately high LH levels, especially in patients with polycystic ovaries, in whom return to baseline levels of LH takes longer than average. In this respect, use of the 'short' or

'ultra-short' protocol of GnRH-a exposes the patient to the same adverse effects as when clomiphene citrate is used.

Our study cannot distinguish between the proposed beneficial effect of pituitary desensitization and the detrimental effect of clomiphene citrate. This issue, however, has been clarified by Homburg and colleagues[107], who studied the outcome of 97 pregnancies in women with the polycystic ovary syndrome. The patients were treated by either ovulation induction or IVF with either hMG alone or hMG after pituitary desensitization with the GnRH-a Decapeptyl®. The miscarriage rate in the agonist-treated patients (17.6%) was significantly lower than the miscarriage rate in the women treated with hMG alone (39.1%; $p = 0.03$). The study demonstrates that pituitary desensitization is the important factor in reducing miscarriage rates in women with polycystic ovaries, rather than clomiphene citrate being the adverse factor, as clomiphene was not given to the patients in that study.

The use of a GnRH-a to achieve pituitary desensitization has become popular in IVF clinics because of the flexibility in programming oocyte recovery[108]. There is debate whether the improved pregnancy rate observed by some clinics[109,110] is seen consistently[111]. We have found, however, that in women with an ultrasound diagnosis of polycystic ovaries, the use of the GnRH-a buserelin is associated with a significant reduction in the rate of miscarriage in the particular group of women at greatest risk. There appears to be no beneficial effect on the rate of miscarriage, however, for women with normal ovaries. Pretreatment pelvic ultrasonography is therefore important in order to select the treatment regimen that will optimize outcome.

SUPEROVULATION STRATEGIES FOR WOMEN WITH POLYCYSTIC OVARIES AND/OR PCOS

When ovarian stimulation is required for IVF, a different approach to therapy is required, because the objective is to achieve multifollicular development, resulting in the collection of several appropriately mature eggs, but without causing OHSS. The latter is a particular problem in women with PCOS as they usually exhibit greater sensitivity than women with normal ovaries to exogenous stimulation[112]. Women with PCOS may require IVF for reasons other than their ovarian dysfunction (for example tubal damage, male factors, etc.). In addition, there is a group who do not conceive with either oral antiestrogens or gonadotropin therapy[113], and for these women assisted conception is a reasonable option[56,114]. Such a patient, who is still not pregnant following at least six ovulatory cycles, becomes a case of 'unexplained' infertility. There have been no specific studies examining whether IVF confers any advantage over other treatments, such as GIFT, for women with polycystic ovaries, and so treatment should be individualized to the other needs of the patient. It is important to be able to assess fertilization, and this can be examined either by IVF or with spare oocytes collected during GIFT. We consider the various regimens used with specific reference to PCOS.

The initial experience in ovulation induction for IVF was with a combination of clomiphene citrate with either or both hMG and FSH, or sometimes with a high-dose gonadotropin alone[115]. Irrespective of ovarian morphology, these treatment regimens do not suppress pituitary responsiveness to the secretory products of the developing follicle. Premature luteinization and a premature LH surge may both occur, with a deleterious effect on the developing oocytes[79,116] or ovulation prior to oocyte recovery. These problems are more often encountered in women with PCOS[116,117]. As already mentioned, the mechanism resulting in inappropriate LH release in PCOS is not yet understood.

Many strategies have evolved to achieve superovulation for IVF, and several were evaluated at the Hallam Medical Centre[118,119]. It is interesting to note that, contrary to earlier beliefs, ovarian stimulation resulting in the collection of large numbers of oocytes (more than ten) results in a poor outcome, the optimum number being between seven and nine[120]. This is of particular relevance to women with polycystic ovaries in whom there is often a high number of oocytes, yet poor rates of fertilization and implantation[56], the overall effect being to achieve an equivalent pregnancy rate to that of a control group[56] but a higher miscarriage rate.

The above experience relates to the use of clomiphene with exogenous gonadotropins. The move towards pituitary desensitization with a GnRH-a[121] has become almost universal in assisted conception

clinics. The reversible hypogonadotropic hypogonadism so produced permits unimpeded control over follicular development[122] and improved pregnancy rates in IVF programs[109,123]. As already mentioned, the suppression of endogenous LH by GnRH-a is of particular relevance and advantage to the woman with PCOS[51,117]. Thus, many oocyte-containing follicles may develop in the sensitive polycystic ovary free from the adverse environment of high tonic LH levels. These oocytes appear to fertilize better than those obtained in cycles without pituitary desensitization[104,124], suggesting that it is indeed the abnormal hormonal milieu, rather than the polycystic ovary itself, that is the problem for women with PCOS.

SHORT AND LONG PROTOCOLS

There are few studies that have specifically compared different treatment regimens for women with and without polycystic ovaries, and those that have vary in their definition and diagnosis of the syndrome[51,125,126]. The two particular aims of therapy in this group of women are correction of the abnormal hormone milieu, by suppressing elevated LH and androgens, and avoidance of ovarian hyperstimulation. Pituitary desensitization avoids the initial surge of gonadotropins with the resultant ovarian steroid release that occurs in the short GnRH protocol. Although the long protocol theoretically provides controlled stimulation, the polycystic ovary is still more likely than the normal ovary to become hyperstimulated[112]. With both long and short protocols, significantly more eggs are collected from women with polycystic than normal ovaries[51], and, interestingly, the total dose of exogenous gonadotropins is the same for either regimen. It has also been proposed that a longer period of desensitization (30 instead of 15 days) is of benefit by reducing androgen levels[125]; in the latter study, the longer duration of treatment did not improve pregnancy rates but did apparently decrease the incidence of hyperstimulation.

The other debate in ovulation induction for women with PCOS is whether the use of FSH alone has any benefit over hMG: is the hypersecretion of LH responsible for the exaggerated response to stimulation of the polycystic ovary? Does minimizing circulating LH levels by giving FSH alone improve outcome? Preparations of purified urinary FSH contain some

LH activity, usually less than 1%, and preliminary work has suggested that ovulation induction can be achieved without exogenous LH[127]. In patients with hypogonadotropic hypogonadism, however, follicular maturation is often incomplete and inconsistent[128,129], as LH, by its action on the thecal cells, is required for full ovarian steroidogenesis. Thus, the presence of some LH facilitates normal follicular development. Most studies have found no benefit over hMG from the use of urinary FSH alone in ovulation induction for either *in vivo*[51,130,131] or *in vitro* fertilization[51,126,132–135]. The most probable reason is that there are only 75 units of LH activity in each ampoule, and, when hMG is given in standard doses to patients who are receiving treatment with buserelin, the serum LH levels barely rise to above 5 IU/l. In patients with PCOS the serum LH concentration is usually 2–4 times that level: that is, the serum level represents a higher 'secretion rate' than that mimicked by injections of hMG.

As far as IVF is concerned Agrawal and colleagues. have reported the results of a meta-analysis of randomized controlled comparisons of urinary derived FSH and hMG[136]. Our analysis showed that, in studies in which the long protocol of GnRH desensitization was used, we could detect no difference in outcome between ovarian stimulation with urinary derived FSH or with hMG preparations.

In recent years, recombinant follicle stimulating hormone (rFSH) has increasingly been used in ovulation induction and IVF treatments. Although there is pituitary suppression by GnRH agonists during IVF treatment, a low endogenous LH level is sufficient to permit adequate steroidogenesis in mature follicles. rFSH is synthesized by transfecting Chinese hamster ovary cell lines with both FSH subunit genes. It has a higher bioactivity than urinary FSH[137], and results in a higher number of oocytes retrieved in IVF treatment, and a shorter duration of treatment in clomiphene-resistant anovulatory patients[138]. The same group also reported that the initial dose of rFSH can be reduced to 100 U, achieving a similar response to that with the usual starting dose of 150–225 U[139]. Marci and colleagues, in 2001, demonstrated that a low-dose stimulation protocol with rFSH can lead to high pregnancy rates in IVF patients with polycystic ovaries who are at risk of a high ovarian response to gonadotropins. This protocol may potentially reduce the risk of OHSS[140]. Teissier and associates, in 1999, demonstrated that women with PCOS undergoing

IVF cycles using hMG had higher testosterone and estradiol levels compared with those using rFSH, due to higher serum LH levels[141]. A recent meta-analysis of 18 randomized trials on the effectiveness and the outcomes of IVF cycles with a long protocol using GnRH agonist, comparing ovarian stimulation with rFSH and with urinary FSH, was published in the Cochrane Database of Systematic Reviews[142]. This review concluded that rFSH is more effective, and has greater batch-to-batch consistency and higher bioactivity than urinary FSH. The total amount of gonadotropins required in IVF treatment was significantly lower with rFSH than with urinary FSH. Additionally, the clinical pregnancy rates per cycle started were also higher with rFSH, although the magnitude of the observed difference was small, 3.7%. No significant differences were detected in the rates of miscarriage, multiple pregnancy and OHSS. It seems then that rFSH may have some additional benefit over hMG in IVF treatment. However, these results will of course need to be updated when data become available from randomized controlled trials using recombinant gonadotropin preparations and GnRH antagonists rather than superactive agonists, and from trials that are focused specifically on patients with polycystic ovaries and PCOS rather than the usual mélange of clinic patients. On the other hand, as described above, polycystic ovaries occur so commonly in patients presenting for IVF that the results from general clinic populations are likely to be sufficiently generalizable for them to be valid for patients with polycystic ovaries.

We recommend the long protocol of pituitary desensitization for women identified as having polycystic ovaries and a dose of 75–100 U of FSH or hMG, which is intentionally lower than our usual starting dose of 150 U. The dose may, of course, be modified if the patient has exhibited either an exuberant or a poor response in a previous cycle. Follicular development is then monitored principally by daily ultrasonography from day 8 of stimulation, with additional measurements of serum estradiol being helpful in some cases.

The recent introduction of schedules of gonadotropin stimulation that incorporate treatment with GnRH antagonists holds promise for patients with polycystic ovaries and PCOS, although the results of specific trials in this condition are not yet available. GnRH antagonists do not activate the

GnRH receptors, and produce a rapid suppression of gonadotropin secretion within hours. The new IVF protocol using GnRH antagonists can offer a shorter and simpler treatment in comparison with the long protocol using GnRH agonists[143–145]. A recent Cochrane review showed that there was a trend of reduction of ovarian hyperstimulation syndrome in the GnRH antagonist-treatment groups with the combined odds ratio of 0.47 (95% CI 0.18–1.25)[146].

Another advantage of using GnRH antagonists is that the native GnRH or GnRH agonist can displace the antagonist from the GnRH receptors at the pituitary level. Therefore, in a GnRH antagonist IVF cycle, GnRH agonist can be administered to induce an LH surge and to trigger the final oocyte maturation and ovulation. Itslovitz-Eldor and colleagues[147] demonstrated a rapid rise of LH concentrations after administration of GnRH agonist, and a peak in LH levels at 4 h after the injection. The pattern of the induced LH surge was similar to that observed in the natural cycle. Fauser and associates[148] showed that the outcomes of IVF treatment in terms of the number of oocytes retrieved, the proportion of metaphase II oocytes, the fertilization rates, the number of good-quality embryos and the implantation rates were comparable to those using hCG to trigger ovulation. Triggering of ovulation with GnRH agonist is potentially more physiological and can reduce the risk of OHSS compared with using hCG, due to a shorter half-life of LH (60 min versus 32–34 h). Exogenous hCG has been known to be associated with OHSS, and in fact hCG activity can still be detected 8 days after administration. Further studies are needed to evaluate this potential advantage, especially among higher responders, and women with polycystic ovaries and PCOS.

A recent multicenter, double-blind study revealed that new recombinant human luteinizing hormone can be as effective as hCG in inducing final follicular maturation in IVF treatment[149], with a lower incidence of OHSS. This clinical effect can be beneficial for women with polycystic ovaries undergoing either GnRH antagonist or GnRH agonist IVF cycles.

OBESITY AND INSULIN RESISTANCE

Patients with PCOS undergoing IVF appear to have an increased risk of cycle cancellation[150]. Patients with android obesity, which is a common feature of PCOS, and a high BMI ($> 25\,kg/m^2$) were found to have low pregnancy rates after IVF[151,152]. These observations were consistent with the early studies on pregnancy outcomes after ovulation induction with gonadotropin in obese PCOS women[153]. Fedorcsak and colleagues[151] concluded that obesity ($> 25\,kg/m^2$), independent of insulin resistance, is associated with the gonadotropin resistance. Fewer oocytes were also retrieved from obese women. The number of oocytes collected and the quality of transferred embryos were positively correlated. In other words, embryo quality declined along with the number of oocytes recovered. Therefore, obese patients should be advised to lose weight before IVF treatment.

Insulin resistance and compensatory hyperinsulinemia contribute to the pathogenesis of PCOS. A number of studies have investigated the effects of using insulin-lowering agents, mainly metformin, in women with PCOS. The initial studies were small and non-randomized. A recent meta-analysis of appropriately conducted randomized studies has confirmed a beneficial effect of metformin in improving rates of ovulation when compared with placebo, and also improving rates of both ovulation and pregnancy when used with clomiphene citrate when compared with clomiphene citrate alone[154,155]. The data indicate that serum concentrations of insulin and androgens improve, although, contrary to popular belief, body weight does not fall.

There are no guidelines for the use of metformin in women with anovulatory PCOS. It is the author's practice to consider metformin therapy for overweight PCOS women wishing to conceive, initially alone for 3 months, in order to acclimatize to side-effects, and then combined with clomiphene citrate, although it is preferable to prescribe the latter once the patient's BMI has fallen to 30–$32\,kg/m^2$. Metformin therapy may be commenced after appropriate screening and advice about diet, life-style and exercise for anovulatory women with PCOS who wish to conceive. The usual dose is either 850 mg twice daily or 500 mg three times daily. Baseline investigations should include an oral glucose tolerance test, full blood count, urea and electrolytes and liver function tests. Side-effects are predominantly gastrointestinal (anorexia, nausea, flatulence and diarrhea), and may be reduced by taking metformin just before food and gradually increasing the dose from 850 mg at night to 850 mg twice a day. after 1 week. Metformin therapy is not thought to cause lactic acidosis in non-diabetic women with PCOS and normal renal and liver function. Metformin should be discontinued for 3 days after iodine-containing contrast medium has been given. Metformin is usually discontinued in pregnancy, although there is no evidence of teratogenicity, and preliminary reports from retrospective studies suggest a reduced rate of gestational diabetes.

There is also some evidence suggesting that metformin can improve response to clomiphene and gonadotropin ovulation induction therapy[156–158]. Hyperinsulinemia is often associated with hyperandrogenism. Teissier and colleagues[159] suggested that the follicular endocrine microenvironment is related to oocyte quality in women undergoing IVF. The study showed that testosterone levels in the follicular fluid were significantly elevated in PCOS follicles, compared with normal patients. They also demonstrated significantly higher levels of follicular testosterone concentrations in those follicles with meiotically incompetent oocytes, compared with follicles with meiotically competent oocytes. It was concluded that the excess follicular androgen concentration could affect oocyte maturation and quality. Hence, high androgen levels may contribute to a lower fertilization rate among oocytes retrieved from women with PCOS compared with those without. Therefore, co-treatment with metformin in IVF treatment may also improve the response to exogenous gonadotropins. A recent publication by Stadtmauer and co-workers[160] demonstrated that the use of metformin in patients with PCOS undergoing IVF treatment improved the number of mature oocytes retrieved, and the overall fertilization and pregnancy rates. However, caution is required to interpret the retrospective observational data. We are currently performing a randomized controlled trial to evaluate the extent of the potential benefit of using metformin in women with polycystic ovaries and PCOS undergoing IVF treatment.

IN VITRO MATURATION OF OOCYTES

In recent years, *in vitro* maturation (IVM) has attracted a lot of interest as a new assisted reproductive technique[161,162]. The immature oocytes are retrieved from antral follicles of unstimulated (or minimally stimulated) ovaries via the transvaginal approach. The oocytes are subsequently matured *in vitro* in a special

formulated culture medium for 24–48 h. The mature oocytes are fertilized, usually by intracytoplasmic sperm injection (ICSI), and the selected embryos are transferred to the uterus 2–3 days later.

Although IVM is labor-intensive compared with conventional IVF treatment, there are a number of clinical advantages with the avoidance of exogenous gonadotropins, most importantly by avoiding the risk of OHSS. Since patients with PCOS have more antral follicles and a higher risk of developing OHSS compared with those without, IVM may be a promising alternative to conventional IVF.

Some studies have reported that the maturation rate of immature oocytes recovered from patients with PCOS is lower than of those from women with normal regular menstrual cycles[163]. However, Chan and Chian[164] demonstrated that priming with hCG before the retrieval of immature oocytes from unstimulated women with PCOS improved the maturation rate. In a prospective observational study of 180 cycles carried out by Child and colleagues[162], it was demonstrated that significantly more immature oocytes were retrieved from polycystic ovary (10 ± 5.1) and PCOS (11.3 ± 9.0) groups than from women with normal ovaries (5.1 ± 3.7), $p < 0.05$. The overall oocyte maturation and fertilization rates were similar among the three groups. The subsequent pregnancy and live birth rates per transfer were significantly higher in the polycystic ovary and PCOS groups. This could be partially explained by the fact that there was a greater choice in the embryos selected for transfer in these two groups. However, women with polycystic ovaries and PCOS were significantly younger and had more embryos transferred than women with normal ovaries.

Furthermore, Child's group[163] also reported a case–control study comparing 170 IVM and 107 IVF cycles for women with PCOS. IVM yielded significantly fewer mature oocytes than did IVF cycles (7.8 vs. 12, $p < 0.01$) and fewer embryos per retrieval (6.1 vs. 9.3, $p < 0.01$). The pregnancy rates per retrieval were similar between the groups. However, the implantation rate in the IVM group was significantly lower than in the IVF group (9.5% vs. 17.1%, $p < 0.01$), with the fact that patients in IVM cycles received more embryos than those in IVF cycles (3.2 ± 0.7 vs. 2.7 ± 0.8, $p < 0.01$). The lower implantation rate may be due to reduced oocyte potential or reduced endometrial receptivity. Interestingly, these authors also reported that the incidence of OHSS in the IVF group was 11.2%. Continuous improvements in the culture medium and synchrony between endometrial and embryonic development will hopefully result in a better IVM success rates in the future. It is also important that infants born after IVM treatment should have long-term follow-up to ensure the safety of this new technology.

LUTEAL SUPPORT AND OVARIAN HYPERSTIMULATION SYNDROME

The OHSS is a well-recognized complication of ovulation induction. In its severe form, it is characterized by ascites, ovarian enlargement with cyst formation, pleural effusion and electrolyte disturbances[166]. Oliguria and vascular complications may ensue, and there have been fatalities. OHSS is believed to be relatively rare in patients undergoing ovarian stimulation for IVF, despite the multiple follicular development and high estrogen levels that commonly occur, and it has been suggested that the protective mechanism is mediated through aspiration of ovarian follicular fluid at the time of oocyte collection[167]. However, OHSS does occur in IVF[55,168,169], and, when severe, is the only life-threatening condition associated with ovarian stimulation in IVF.

It has been apparent for some time that patients with polycystic ovaries undergoing straightforward ovulation induction are particularly at risk of developing OHSS[166,170]. This has been confirmed in IVF as well[55,169]. In a total population of 1302 patients we identified 15 patients who underwent ovarian stimulation for IVF or other assisted conception techniques at the Hallam Medical Centre, between July 1989 and July 1990, and who developed OHSS of sufficient severity to merit hospital admission (prevalence of 1.2%, with 0.6% having severe OHSS). Of these patients, 53% had ultrasonically diagnosed polycystic ovaries and 87% were undergoing their first attempt at IVF. All had received luteal support in the form of hCG. Although the pregnancy rate in this group was very high (93.3%), the multiple pregnancy rate was 57%, with a miscarriage rate of 14.3%[169]. As a result of this analysis, we recommend that all patients undergoing IVF have a pelvic ultrasound scan performed either prior to or early in the treatment cycle. If polycystic ovaries are identified, the dose of gonadotropins should be minimized (see above).

It has been observed that OHSS is rare in patients with hypopituitary hypogonadism[170]. The use of luteinizing hormone-releasing hormone (LHRH) agonists has been recommended in patients with polycystic ovaries[133], in the hope that, by converting the patient to a hypogonadal state, OHSS might be prevented. Unfortunately, this does not seem to be the case[55], and, in fact, a number of recent reports suggest that OHSS is actually more common when LHRH agonists are used, especially if patients have polycystic ovaries[171]. Incidentally, this observation provides further evidence to suggest that the primary lesion in PCOS is in the ovary itself, since its response to gonadotropin stimulation is abnormal even after suppression of abnormal gonadotropin secretion.

Recent studies have suggested that the increased propensity of polycystic ovaries to become overstimulated is due to increased expression of VEGF in the stroma of the polycystic ovary, which itself has increased blood flow, as assessed by color Doppler[33]. A recent study explored this association further by performing pulsed and color Doppler studies together with measurements of serum VEGF concentrations in 36 women with normal ovaries and 24 women with polycystic ovaries (ten of whom had the syndrome) undergoing IVF. Serum VEGF concentrations and blood flow were significantly higher in the women with polycystic ovaries/PCOS than in those with normal ovaries, and this might explain the greater risk of OHSS in these patients[62,169].

Careful monitoring of estrogen levels and numbers of follicles by ultrasound scanning during stimulation for IVF can also help to identify those at risk. In patients thought to be at risk of OHSS (age less than 30 years, and/or polycystic ovaries, and/or estrogen levels greater than 8000 pmol/l, and/or more than 20 follicles at oocyte collection), luteal support in the form of hCG should be withheld. It is now our practice to use progesterone pessaries instead of hCG as luteal support in all patients.

Transfer of a maximum of two embryos in this group reduces the multiple pregnancy rate with its attendant obstetric and neonatal problems. Alternatively, embryos may be frozen for transfer at a later date, and, in the case of patients on LHRH analogs, the analog is continued until the onset of menstruation (by giving a long-acting depot), and hormone replacement therapy for the frozen embryo replacement cycle is commenced at that stage.

CONCLUSION

Women with PCOS may have presented with symptoms of endocrine or metabolic disturbance prior to seeking assisted conception or they may be diagnosed at their first attendance at the infertility clinic, a proportion of them having polycystic ovaries on ultrasound scan, but no symptoms. We have demonstrated that women with polycystic ovaries require careful management to achieve follicular maturation in an environment free from elevated luteinizing hormone levels in order to enhance fertilization and pregnancy outcome. The sensitivity of the polycystic ovary to exogenous stimulation and the risk of ovarian hyperstimulation syndrome have been emphasized. The association between insulin resistance and the pathogenesis of PCOS has resulted in interest in the potential for insulin-lowering drugs, such as metformin, which appear to benefit anovulatory women with PCOS and may also enhance ovarian response to stimulation. More research is required in this area. In addition to offering assisted conception, we feel that the infertility clinic is an ideal place to offer preconceptional counseling and advice as to how to minimize the metabolic sequelae of PCOS that may occur later in life.

REFERENCES

1. Stein IF, Leventhal ML. Amenorrhea associated with bilateral polycystic ovaries. Am J Obstet Gynecol 1935; 29: 181–91

2. Balen AH, Conway GS, Kaltsas G, et al. Polycystic ovary syndrome: the spectrum of the disorder in 1741 patients. Hum Reprod 1995; 8: 2107–11

3. Franks S, Ghasani N, Waterworth D, et al. The genetic basis of polycystic ovary syndrome. Hum Reprod 1997; 12: 2641–8

4. Balen AH, Dunger D. Pubertal maturation of the internal genitalia [Commentary]. Ultrasound Obstet Gynecol 1995; 6: 164–5

5. Fauser B, Tarlatzis B, Chang J, et al. The Rotterdam ESHRE/ASRM-sponsored PCOS consensus workshop group. Revised 2003 consensus on diagnostic criteria and long-term health risks related to polycystic ovary syndrome (PCOS). Hum Reprod 2004; 19: 41–7

6. Adams J, Polson DW, Abdulwahid N, et al. Multifollicular ovaries: clinical and endocrine features and response to pulsatile gonadotrophin releasing hormone. Lancet 1985; 2: 1375–8

7. Balen AH, Laven JSE, Tan SL, Dewailly D. Ultrasound assessment of the polycystic ovary: international consensus definitions. Hum Reprod Update 2003; 9: 505–14

8. Polson DW, Wadsworth J, Adams J, Franks S. Polycystic ovaries: a common finding in normal women. Lancet 1988; 2: 870–2

9. Tayob Y, Robinson G, Adams J, et al. Ultrasound appearance of the ovaries during the pill-free interval. Br J Fam Plann 1990; 16: 94–6

10. Clayton RN, Ogden V, Hodgekinson J, et al. How common are polycystic ovaries in normal women and what is their significance for the fertility of the population? Clin Endocrinol 1992; 37: 127–34

11. Farquhar CM, Birdsall M, Manning P, Mitchell JM. Transabdominal versus transvaginal ultrasound in the diagnosis of polycystic ovaries on ultrasound scanning in a population of randomly selected women. Ultrasound Obstet Gynecol 1994; 4: 54–9

12. Michelmore KF, Balen AH, Dunger DB, Vessey MP. Polycystic ovaries and associated clinical and biochemical features in young women. Clin Endocrinol (Oxf) 1999; 51: 779–86

13. Bridges NA, Cooke A, Healy MJR, et al. Standards for ovarian volume in childhood and puberty. Fertil Steril 1993; 60: 456–60

14. Futterweit W. Pathologic anatomy of polycystic ovarian disease. In Futterweit W, ed. Polycystic Ovarian Disease. New York: Springer-Verlag, 1984: 41–6

15. Franks S, Adams J, Mason H, Polson D. Ovulatory disorders in women with polycystic ovary syndrome. Clin Obstet Gynaecol 1985; 12: 605–32

16. Baird DT, Corker CS, Davidson DW. Pituitary–ovarian relationships in polycystic ovary syndrome. J Clin Endocrinol Metab 1977; 45: 798–809

17. Yen SSC. The polycystic ovary. Clin Endocrinol 1980; 12: 177–207

18. Saxton DW, Farquhar CM, Rae T, et al. Accuracy of ultrasound measurements of female pelvic organs. Br J Obstet Gynaecol 1990; 97: 695–9

19. Takahashi K, Eda Y, Okada S, et al. Morphological assessment of polycystic ovaries using transvaginal ultrasound. Hum Reprod 1993; 6: 844–9

20. Swanson M, Sauerbrei EE, Cooperberg PL. Medical implications of ultrasonically detected polycystic ovaries. J Clin Ultrasound 1981; 9: 219–22

21. Obhrai M, Lynch SS, Holder G, et al. Hormonal studies on women with polycystic ovaries diagnosed by ultrasound. Clin Endocrinol (Oxf) 1990; 32: 467–74

22. Robinson S, Rodin DA, Deacon A, et al. Which hormone tests for the diagnosis of polycystic ovary disease? Br J Obstet Gynaecol 1992; 99: 232–8

23. Fox R, Corrigan E, Thomas PA, Hull MGR. The diagnosis of polycystic ovaries in women with oligo-amenorrhoea: predictive power of endocrine tests. Clin Endocrinol 1991; 34: 127–31

24. Puzigaca Z, Prelevic GM, Stretenovic Z, Balint-Peric L. Ovarian enlargement as a possible marker of androgen activity in polycystic ovary syndrome. Gynecol Endocrinol 1991; 5: 167–74

25. Pache TD, de Jong FH, Hop WC, Fauser BCJM. Association between ovarian changes assessed by trans-vaginal sonography and clinical and endocrine signs of the polycystic ovary syndrome. Fertil Steril 1993; 59: 544–9

26. Dewailly D, Robert Y, Helin I, et al. Ovarian stromal hypertrophy in hyperandrogenic women. Clin Endocrinol (Oxf) 1994; 41: 557–62

27. van Santbrink EJP, Hop WC, Fauser BCJM. Classification of normogonadotrophic infertility: polycystic ovaries diagnosed by ultrasound versus endocrine characteristics of polycystic ovary syndrome. Fertil Steril 1997; 67: 452–8

28. Abdel Gadir A, Khatim MS, Mowafi RS, et al. Implications of ultrasonically diagnosed polycystic ovaries. I. Correlations with basal hormonal profiles. Hum Reprod 1992; 4: 453–7

29. Jonard S, Robert Y, Cortet-Rudelli C, et al. Ultrasound examination of polycystic ovaries: is it worth counting the follicles? Hum Reprod 2003; 18: 598–603

30. Farquhar CM, Birdsall M, Manning P, Mitchell JM. Transabdominal versus transvaginal ultrasound in the diagnosis of polycystic ovaries in a population of randomly selected women. Ultrasound Obstet Gynecol 1994; 4: 54–9

31. Fulghesu AM, Ciampelli M, Belosi C, et al. A new ultrasound criterion for the diagnosis of polycystic ovary syndrome: the ovarian stroma/total area ratio. Fertil Steril 2001; 76: 326–31

32. Kyei-Mensah AA, LinTan S, Zaidi J, Jacobs HS. Relationship of ovarian stromal volume to serum androgen concentrations in patients with polycystic ovary syndrome. Hum Reprod 1998; 13: 1437–41

33. Zaidi J, Campbell S, Pittrof R, et al. Ovarian stromal blood flow in women with polycystic ovaries: a possible new marker for diagnosis. Hum Reprod 1995; 10: 1992–6

34. Goldzieher JW, Green JA. The polycystic ovary. I. Clinical and histological features. J Clin Endocrinol Metab 1962; 22: 325–38

35. Kamat BR, Brown LF, Manseau EJ. Expression of vascular endothelial growth factor vascular permeability factor by human granulosa and theca lutein cells. Role in corpus luteum development. Am J Pathol 1995; 146: 157–65

36. Goldzieher JW, Axelrod LR. Clinical and biochemical features of polycystic ovarian disease. Fertil Steril 1963; 14: 631–53

37. Leventhal ML. The Stein–Leventhal syndrome. Am J Obstet Gynecol 1958; 76: 825–38

38. Vaitukaitis JL. Polycystic ovary syndrome – what is it? N Engl J Med 1983; 309: 1245–6

39. Hull MGR. Epidemiology of infertility and polycystic ovarian disease: endocrinological and demographic studies. Gynecol Endocrinol 1987; 1: 235–45

40. Jacobs HS. Review: polycystic ovary syndrome. Gynecol Endocrinol 1987; 1: 113–31

41. Barnes R, Rosenfield RL. The polycystic ovary syndrome: pathogenesis and treatment. Ann Intern Med 1989; 110: 386–99

42. Franks S. Polycystic ovary syndrome: a changing perspective. Clin Endocrinol 1989; 31: 87–120

43. Insler V, Lunenfeld B. Pathophysiology of polycystic ovarian disease: new insights. Hum Reprod 1991; 6: 1025–9

44. Homburg R. Polycystic ovary syndrome – from gynecological curiosity to multisystem endocrinopathy. Hum Reprod 1996; 11: 29–39

45. Balen AH, Tan SL, MacDougall J, Jacobs HS. Miscarriage rates following in-vitro fertilization are increased in women with polycystic ovaries and reduced by pituitary desensitization with buserelin. Hum Reprod 1993; 8: 959–64

46. Kiddy DS, Hamilton-Fairley D, Bush A, et al. Improvement in endocrine and ovarian function during dietary treatment of obese women with polycystic ovary syndrome. Clin Endocrinol 1992; 36: 105–11

47. Conway GS. Insulin resistance and the polycystic ovary syndrome. Contemp Rev Obstet Gynaecol 1990; 2: 34–9

48. Clark AM, Ledger W, Galletly C, et al. Weight loss results in significant improvement in pregnancy and ovulation rates in an ovulatory obese women. Hum Reprod 1995; 10: 2705–12

49. Conway GS, Honour JW, Jacobs HS. Heterogeneity of the polycystic ovary syndrome: clinical, endocrine and ultrasound features in 556 patients. Clin Endocrinol 1989; 30: 459–70

50. Adams J, Polson DW, Franks S. Prevalence of polycystic ovaries in women with anovulation and idiopathic hirsutism. Br Med J 1986; 293: 355–8

51. Jacobs HS, Porter R, Eshel A, Craft I. Profertility uses of luteinising hormone releasing hormone agonist analogues. In Vickery BH, Nestor JJ, eds. LHRH and its Analogs. Lancaster: MTP Press, 1987: 303–22

52. MacDougall JM, Tan SL, Hall V, et al. Comparison of natural with clomiphene citrate-stimulated cycles in IVF: a prospective randomized trial. Fertil Steril 1994; 61: 1052–7

53. Balen AH, Braat DDM, West C, et al. Cumulative conception and live birth rates after the treatment of anovulatory infertility. An analysis of the safety and efficacy of ovulation induction in 200 patients. Hum Reprod 1994; 9: 1563–70

54. Balen AH, Jacobs HS. Ovulation induction. In Balen AH, Jacobs HS, eds. Infertility In Practice. Edinburgh: Churchill Livingstone, 1997: 131–80

55. Smitz J, Camus M, Devroey P, et al. Incidence of severe ovarian hyperstimulation syndrome after gonadotropin releasing hormone agonist/HMG superovulation for in-vitro fertilization. Hum Reprod 1991; 6: 933–7

56. Dor J, Shulman A, Levran D, et al. The treatment of patients with polycystic ovary syndrome by in-vitro fertilization: a comparison of results with those patients with tubal infertility. Hum Reprod 1990; 5: 816–18

57. MacDougall JM, Tan SL, Balen AH, Jacobs HS. A controlled study comparing patients with and without polycystic ovaries undergoing in-vitro fertilization and the ovarian hyperstimulation syndrome. Hum Reprod 1993; 8: 233–7

58. Dunaif A, Graf M. Insulin administration alters gonadal steroid metabolism independent of changes in gonadotropin secretion in insulin-resistant women with the polycystic ovary syndrome. J Clin Invest 1989; 83: 23–9

59. Franks S. Polycystic ovary syndrome. N Engl J Med 1995; 333: 853–61

60. Adashi EY, Resnick CE, D'Ercole AJ, et al. Insulin-like growth factors as intraovarian regulators of granulosa cell growth and function. Endocr Rev 1985; 6: 400–20

61. Ferrara N, Chen H, Davis-Smyth T, et al. Vascular endothelial growth factor is essential for corpus luteum angiogenesis. Nature Med 1998; 4: 336–40

62. Agrawal R, Sladkevicius P, Engman L, et al. Serum vascular endothelial growth factor concentrations and ovarian stromal blood flow are increased in women with polycystic ovaries. Hum Reprod 1998; 13: 651–5

63. Homburg R, Berkowitz D, Levy T, et al. In-vitro fertilization and embryo transfer for the treatment of infertility associated with polycystic ovary syndrome. Fertil Steril 1993; 60: 858–63

64. Owen EJ, Shoham Z, Mason BA, et al. Cotreatment with growth hormone after pituitary suppression for ovarian stimulation in IVF: a randomized double-blind placebo-control trial. Fertil Steril 1991; 56: 1104–10

65. MacGillivray I. Pre-Eclampsia – The Hypertensive Disease of Pregnancy. London: WB Saunders, 1983: 44–5, 227–8

66. Treharne I. Obesity in pregnancy. In Studd J, ed. Progress in Obstetrics and Gynaecology. Edinburgh: Churchill Livingstone, 1984; 4: 127–38

67. Diamant YZ, Rimon E, Evron S. High incidence of pre-eclamptic toxemia in patients with polycystic disease. Eur J Obstet Gynecol Reprod Biol 1982; 14: 199–204

68. Gjonnaess H. The course and outcome of pregnancy after ovarian electrocautery in women with polycystic ovarian syndrome: the influence of body weight. Br J Obstet Gynaecol 1989; 96: 714–19

69. Fox R, Wardle PG. Maturity onset diabetes mellitus in association with polycystic ovarian disease. J Obstet Gynaecol 1990; 10: 555–6

70. Ahlgren M, Kallen B, Rannevik G. Outcome of pregnancy after clomiphene therapy. Acta Obstet Gynecol Scand 1976; 55: 371–5

71. Sagle M, Bishop K, Alexander FM, et al. Recurrent early miscarriage and polycystic ovaries. Br Med J 1988; 297: 1027–8

72. Regan L, Owen EJ, Jacobs HS. Hypersecretion of luteinising hormone, infertility and miscarriage. Lancet 1990; 336: 1141–4

73. Harlap S. Ovulation induction and congenital malformation. Lancet 1976; 2: 961

74. Kurachi K, Aono T, Minagawa J, Miyake A. Congenital malformations of newborn infants after clomiphene-induced ovulation. Fertil Steril 1983; 40: 187–9

75. Medical Research Council. Births in Great Britain resulting from assisted conception, 1978–87. Br Med J 1990; 330: 1229–33

76. Beral V, Doyle P, Tan SL, et al. Outcome of pregnancies resulting from assisted conception. Br Med Bull 1990; 46: 753–68

77. Balen AH. PCOS: mode of treatment. In Shoham Z, Howles CM, Jacobs HS, eds. Female Infertility Therapy. London: Martin Dunitz, 1999: 45–68

78. Balen AH, Tan SL, Jacobs HS. Hypersecretion of luteinising hormone – a significant cause of infertility and miscarriage. Br J Obstet Gynaecol 1993; 100: 1082–9

79. Stanger JD, Yovich JL. Reduced in-vitro fertilisation of human oocyte from patients with raised basal

luteinising hormone levels during the follicular phase. Br J Obstet Gynaecol 1985; 92: 385–93

80. Abdulwahid NA, Adams J, Van der Spuy ZM, Jacobs HS. Gonadotrophin control of follicular development. Clin Endocrinol 1985; 23: 613–26

81. Howles CM, Macnamee MC, Edwards RG, et al. Effect of high tonic levels of luteinising hormone on outcome of in-vitro fertilisation. Lancet 1986; 1: 521–2

82. Homburg R, Armar NA, Eshel A, et al. Influence of serum luteinising hormone concentrations on ovulation, conception and early pregnancy loss in polycystic ovary syndrome. Br Med J 1988; 297: 1024–6

83. Erickson GF, Magoffin DA, Dyer CA, Hofeditz C. The ovarian androgen producing cells: a review of structure/function relationships. Endocrinol Rev 1985; 6: 371–99

84. Downs SM. Maintenance of meiotic arrest in mammalian oocytes. In Bavister BD, Cummins J, Roldan ERS, eds. Fertilization in Mammals. Norwell, MA: Serono Symposia, 1990: 5–16

85. Dekel N, Galiani D, Aberdam E. Regulation of rat oocyte maturation: involvement of protein kinases. In Bavister BD, Cummins J, Roldan ERS, eds. Fertilization in Mammals. Norwell, MA: Serono Symposia, 1990: 17–24

86. Watson H, Hamilton-Fairley D, Kiddy D, et al. Abnormalities of follicular phase luteinizing hormone secretion in women with recurrent early miscarriage. J Endocrinol 1989; 123 (Suppl): Abstr 25

87. Thomas A, Okamoto S, O'Shea F, et al. Do raised serum luteinising hormone levels during stimulation for in-vitro fertilisation predict outcome? Br J Obstet Gynaecol 1989; 96: 1328–32

88. Messinis IE, Templeton A, Baird DT. Relationships between the characteristics of endogenous luteinizing hormone surge and the degree of ovarian hyperstimulation during superovulation induction in women. Clin Endocrinol 1986; 25: 393–400

89. Van Uem JFHM, Garcia JE, Liu HC, Rosenwaks Z. Clinical aspects with regard to the occurrence of an endogenous luteinizing hormone surge in gonadotropin-induced normal menstrual cycles. J In-vitro Fertilization Embryo Transf 1986; 3: 345–9

90. Lejeune B, Degueldre M, Camus M, et al. In vitro fertilization and embryo transfer as related to endogenous luteinizing hormone rise or human chorionic gonadotropin administration. Fertil Steril 1986; 45: 377–83

91. Howles CM, Macnamee MC, Edwards RG. Follicular development and early luteal function of conception and non-conception cycles after human in-vitro

fertilization: endocrine correlates. Hum Reprod 1987; 2: 17–21

92. Punnonen R, Ashorn R, Vilja P, et al. Spontaneous luteinizing hormone surge and cleavage of in vitro fertilized embryos. Fertil Steril 1988; 49: 479–82

93. Balen AH, Rose M. The control of luteinising hormone secretion in the polycystic ovary syndrome. Contemp Rev Obstet Gynaecol 1994; 6: 201–7

94. Kingsland C, Tan SL, Bickerton N, et al. The routine use of gonadotropin releasing hormone agonists for all patients undergoing in vitro fertilization. Is there any medical advantage? A prospective randomized study. Fertil Steril 1992; 57: 804–9

95. Tan SL, Kingsland C, Campbell S, et al. The long protocol of administration of gonadotropin releasing hormone agonist is superior to the short protocol for ovarian stimulation for in vitro fertilization. Fertil Steril 1992; 57: 810–14

96. Macnamee MC, Howles CM, Edwards RG, et al. Short-term luteinizing hormone releasing hormone agonist treatment: prospective trial of a novel ovarian stimulation regimen for in-vitro fertilization. Fertil Steril 1989; 52: 264–9

97. Balen AH, Yovich JL. Miscarriage following assisted conception. In Stabile I, Grudzinskas JG, Chard T, eds. Spontaneous Abortion, Diagnosis and Treatment. London: Springer-Verlag, 1992: 133–48

98. Steer C, Campbell S, Davies M, et al. Spontaneous abortion rates after natural and assisted conception. Br Med J 1989; 299: 1317–18

99. Office of Population and Censuses and Surveys (OPCS). Series FM1. London: HMSO, 1988

100. Brambati B. Fate of human pregnancies. In Edwards RG, ed. Establishing a Successful Human Pregnancy, Serono Symposia. New York: Raven Press, 1980; 6: 269–81

101. Hook EB, Woodbury DF, Albright SG. Rates of Trisomy 18 in Livebirths, Stillbirths and at Amniocentesis. Birth defects: Original Article Series. New York: AR Liss, 1979: 81–9

102. Hassold T, Jacobs P, Kline J, et al. Effect of maternal age on autosomal trisomies. Ann Hum Genet 1980; 44: 29–36

103. Lower AM, Mulcahy MT, Yovich JL. Chromosome abnormalities detected in chorionic villus biopsies of failing pregnancies in a subfertile population. Br J Obstet Gynaecol 1991; 98: 1228–33

104. Abdalla HI, Ahuja KK, Leonard T, et al. Comparative trial of luteinizing hormone releasing hormone analogue/HMG and clomiphene citrate/HMG in an assisted conception program. Fertil Steril 1990; 53: 473–8

105. Saunders DM, Lancaster PAL, Pedisich EL. Increased pregnancy failure rates after clomiphene following assisted reproductive technology. Hum Reprod 1992; 7: 1154–8

106. Shoham Z, Borenstein R, Lunenfeld B, Pariente C. Hormonal profiles following clomiphene citrate therapy in conception and nonconception cycles. Clin Endocrinol 1990; 33: 271–8

107. Homburg R, Levy T, Berkovitz D, et al. Gonadotropin releasing hormone agonist reduces the miscarriage rate for pregnancies achieved in women with polycystic ovaries. Fertil Steril 1993; 59: 527–31

108. Tan SL, Balen AH, Hussein EH, et al. A prospective randomized study of the optimum timing of human chorionic gonadotropin administration after pituitary desensitization in in vitro fertilization. Fertil Steril 1992; 157: 1259–64

109. Rutherford AJ, Subak-Sharpe RJ, Dawson KJ, et al. Improvement of in-vitro fertilisation after treatment with buserelin, an agonist of luteinising hormone releasing hormone. Br Med J 1988; 296: 1765–8

110. Frydman R, Fries N, Testart J, et al. Luteinizing hormone releasing hormone agonists in in-vitro fertilization: different methods of utilization and comparison with previous ovulation stimulation treatments. Hum Reprod 1988; 3: 559–61

111. Polson DW, MacLachlan V, Krapez JA, et al. A controlled study of gonadotropin-releasing hormone agonist (buserelin acetate) for folliculogenesis in routine in vitro fertilization patients. Fertil Steril 1991; 56: 509–14

112. Salat-Baroux J, Antoine JM. Accidental hyperstimulation during ovulation induction. Baillière's Clin Obstet Gynaecol 1990; 4: 627–37

113. Wang CF, Gemzell C. The use of human gonadotropins for the induction of ovulation in women with polycystic ovary syndrome. Clin Endocrinol 1980; 12: 479–86

114. Ashkenazi J, Feldberg D, Dicker D, et al. In-vitro fertilization–embryo transfer in women with refractory polycystic ovary disease. Eur J Obstet Gynecol Reprod Biol 1989; 30: 157–61

115. Fleming R, Coutts JRT. Induction of multiple follicular development for in-vitro fertilisation. Br Med Bull 1990; 46: 596–615

116. Gemzell CA, Kemman E, Jones JR. Premature ovulation during administration of human menopausal gonadotrophins in non-ovulatory women. Infertility 1978; 1: 1–10

117. Fleming R, Coutts JRT. Luteinising hormone releasing hormone analogues for ovulation induction, with particular reference to polycystic ovary syndrome. Baillière's Clin Obstet Gynaecol 1988; 2: 677–88

118. Riddle A, Sharma V, Mason B, et al. Two years experience of ultrasound directed oocyte recovery. Fertil Steril 1987; 48: 454

119. Sharma V, Riddle A, Mason B, et al. Studies on folliculogenesis and in-vitro fertilization outcome after the administration of follicle stimulating hormone at different times during the menstrual cycle. Fertil Steril 1989; 51: 298–303

120. Sharma V, Riddle A, Mason BA, et al. An analysis of factors influencing the establishment of a clinical pregnancy in an ultrasound-based ambulatory in-vitro fertilization program. Fertil Steril 1988; 49: 468–78

121. Porter RN, Smith W, Craft IL, et al. Induction of ovulation for in-vitro fertilisation using buserelin and gonadotrophins. Lancet 1984; 2: 1284–5

122. Fleming R, Haxton MJ, Hamilton MPR, et al. Successful treatment of infertile women with oligomenorrhoea using a combination of a luteinising hormone releasing hormone agonist and exogenous gonadotrophins. Br J Obstet Gynaecol 1985; 92: 369–74

123. Frydman R, Belaisch-Allart J, Parneix I, et al. Comparison between flare up and down regulation of luteinizing hormone releasing hormone agonists in an in-vitro fertilization program. Fertil Steril 1988; 50: 471–5

124. Fleming R, Jamieson ME, Hamilton MPR, et al. The use of GnRH analogues in combination with exogenous gonadotropins in infertile women. Acta Endocrinol 1988; 119 (Suppl 288): 77–84

125. Salat-Baroux J, Alvarez S, Antoine JM, et al. Comparison between long and short protocols of luteinising hormone releasing hormone agonist in the treatment of PCOD by in-vitro fertilization. Hum Reprod 1988; 3: 535–9

126. Tanbo T, Dale PO, Kjekshus E, et al. Stimulation with HMG versus follicle stimulating hormone after pituitary suppression in polycystic ovary syndrome. Fertil Steril 1990; 53: 798–803

127. Jones GS, Garcia JE, Rosenwaks Z. The role of pituitary gonadotropins in follicular stimulation and oocyte maturation in the human. J Clin Endocrinol Metab 1984; 59: 178–83

128. Couzinet B, Lestrat N, Brailly S, et al. Stimulation of ovarian follicular maturation with pure follicle stimulating hormone in women with gonadotropin deficiency. J Clin Endocrinol Metab 1988; 66: 552–6

129. Shoham Z, Balen AH, Patel A, Jacobs HS. Results of ovulation induction using hMG or purified FSH in hypogonadotropic hypogonadism patients. Fertil Steril 1991; 56: 1048–53

130. Homburg R, Eshel A, Kilborn J, et al. Combined luteinizing hormone releasing hormone analogue and exogenous gonadotropins for the treatment of infertility associated with polycystic ovaries. Hum Reprod 1990; 5: 32–5

131. Sagle MA, Hamilton-Fairley D, Kiddy DS, Franks S. A comparative, randomised study of low dose human menopausal gonadotrophin and follicle stimulating hormone in women with polycystic ovary syndrome. Fertil Steril 1991; 55: 56–60

132. Messinis IE, Templeton AA, Baird DT. Comparison between clomiphene plus human menopausal gonadotropin and clomiphene plus pulsatile follicle stimulating hormone in induction of multiple follicular development in women. Hum Reprod 1986; 4: 223–6

133. Salat-Baroux J, Alvarez S, Antoine JM, et al. Results of in-vitro fertilization in the treatment of polycystic ovary disease. Hum Reprod 1988; 3: 331–5

134. Bentick B, Shaw RW, Iffland CA, et al. A randomized comparative study of purified follicle stimulating hormone and human menopausal gonadotropin after pituitary desensitisation with buserelin for superovulation and in-vitro fertilization. Fertil Steril 1988; 50: 79–84

135. Larsen T. Comparison of urinary human follicle stimulating hormone and HMG for ovarian stimulation in polycystic ovary syndrome. Fertil Steril 1990; 53: 426

136. Agrawal R, Holmes J, Jacobs HS. Follicle-stimulating hormone or human menopausal gonadotropin for ovarian stimulation in in vitro fertilization cycles: a meta-analysis. Fertil Steril 2000; 73: 338–43

137. Out H, Mannaerts B, Driessen S, Bennink H. A prospective, assessor-blinded, multicentre study comparing recombinant and urinary follicle stimulating hormone (Puregon vs Metrodin) in in-vitro fertilisation. Hum Reprod 1995; 10: 2534–40

138. Coelingh Bennink H, Fauser B, Out H. The European Puregon Collaborative Anovulation Study Group. Recombinant FSH (Puregon) is more efficient than urinary FSH (Metrodin) in clomiphene-resistant normogonadotropic chronic anovulatory women. A prospective multicentre, assessor-blend, randomised, clinical trial. Fertil Steril 1998; 69: 19–25

139. Devroey P, Tournaye H, Hendrix P, Out H. The use of a 100 IU starting dose of recombinant follicle stimulating hormone (Puregon) in in-vitro fertilisation. Hum Reprod 1998; 13: 565–6

140. Marci R, Senn A, Dessole S, et al. A low-dose stimulation protocol using highly purified follicle-stimulating hormone can lead to high pregnancy rates in in vitro fertilization patients with polycystic ovaries who are at risk of a high ovarian response to gonadotrophins. Fertil Steril 2001; 75: 1131

141. Teissier M, Chable H, Paulhac S, et al. Recombinant human follicle stimulating hormone versus human menopausal gonadotrophin induction: effects in mature follicle endocrinology. Hum Reprod 1999; 14: 2236–41

142. European and Middle East Orgalutran Study Group. Comparable clinical outcome using the GnRH antagonist ganirelix or a long protocol of the GnRH agonist triptorelin for the prevention of premature LH surges in women undergoing ovarian stimulation. Hum Reprod 2001; 16: 644–51

143. North American Ganirelix Study Group. Efficacy and safety of ganirelix acetate versus leuprolide acetate in women undergoing controlled ovarian hyperstimulation. Fertil Steril 2001; 75: 35–45

144. European Orgalutran Study Group, Borm G, Mannaerts B. Treatment with the gonadotrophin-releasing hormone antagonist ganirelix in women undergoing controlled ovarian hyperstimulation with recombinant follicle stimulating hormone is effective, safe and convenient: results of a controlled, randomized, multicentre trial. Hum Reprod 2000; 15: 1490–8

145. Olivennes F, Taieb J, Frydman R, Bouchard P. Triggering of ovulation by a gonadotrophin releasing hormone agonist in patients pretreated with a GnRH antagonist. Fertil Steril 1996; 66: 151–3

146. Al-Inany H, Aboulghar M. Gonadotrophin releasing hormone antagonist for assisted conception (Cochrane Review). In The Cochrane Library, Issue I Oxford: Update Software, 2002

147. Itslovitz-Eldor J, Kol S, Mannaerts B, Use of a single bolus of GnRH agonist triptorelin to trigger ovulation after GnRH antagonist ganirelix treatment in women undergoing ovarian stimulation for assisted reproduction, with special reference to the prevention of OHSS: preliminary report. Hum Reprod 2000; 15: 1965–8

148. Fauser B, Jong D, Olivennes F, et al. Endocrine profile after triggering of final oocytes maturation with GnRH agonist after co-treatment with the GnRH antagonist ganirelix during ovarian hyperstimulation for IVF. J Clin Endocrinol Metab 2002; 87: 709–15

149. The European Recombinant LH Study Group. Recombinant human LH is as effective as, but safer than, urinary human chorionic gonadotrophin in inducing final follicular maturation and ovulation in in vitro fertilisation. Results of a multicentre double blind study. J Clin Endocrinol Metab 2001; 86: 2607

150. Kodama H, Fakuda J, Karube H, et al. High incidence of embryo transfer cancellations in patients with

polycystic ovarian syndrome. Hum Reprod 1995; 10: 1962–7

151. Fedorcsak P, Dale P, Storeng R, et al. The impact of obesity and insulin resistance on the outcome of IVF or ICSI in women with polycystic ovarian syndrome. Hum Reprod 2001; 16: 1086–91

152. Wass P, Rossner S. An android body fat distribution in women impairs the pregnancy rates of in vitro fertilisation and embryo transfer. Hum Reprod 1997; 12: 2057–60

153. Dale P, Tanbo T, Haug E, Abyholm T. The impact of insulin resistance on the outcome of ovulation induction with low-dose follicle stimulating hormone in women with polycystic ovary syndrome. Hum Reprod 1998; 13: 567–70

154. Fleming R, Hopkinson Z, Wallace A, et al. Ovarian function and metabolic factors in women with oligomenorrhoea treated with metformin in a randomized double blind placebo-controlled trial. J Clin Endocrinol Metab 2002; 87: 569–74

155. Lord JM, Flight IHK, Norman RJ. Metformin in polycystic ovary syndrome: systematic review and meta-analysis. Br Med J 2003; 327: 951–5

156. Nestler J, Jakubowicz D, Evans W, Pasquali R. Effects of metformin on spontaneous and clomiphene-induced ovulation in the polycystic ovary syndrome. N Engl J Med 1998; 338: 1876–80

157. Kocak M, Caliskan E, Simsir C, Haberal A. Metformin therapy improves ovulatory rates, cervical scores, and pregnancy rates in clomiphene citrate-resistant women with polycystic ovary syndrome. Fertil Steril 2002; 77: 101

158. Vandermolen D, Ratts V, Evans W, et al. Metformin increases the ovulatory rate and pregnancy rate from clomiphene citrate in patients with polycystic ovary syndrome who are resistant to clomiphene citrate alone. Fertil Steril 2001; 75: 310

159. Teissier M, Chable H, Paulhac S, Aubard Y. Comparison of follicle steroidogenesis from normal and polycystic ovaries in women undergoing IVF: relationship between steroid concentrations, follicle size, oocyte quality and fecundability. Hum Reprod 2000; 15: 2471–7

160. Stadtmauer L, Toma S, Riehl R, Talbert L. Metformin treatment of patients with polycystic ovary syndrome undergoing in vitro fertilization improves outcomes and is associated with modulation of the insulin-like growth factors. Fertil Steril 2001; 75: 505

161. Trounson A, Wood C, Kausche A. In vitro maturation and the fertilisation and development competence of oocytes recovered from untreated polycystic ovarian patients. Fertil Steril 1994; 62: 353–61

162. Child T, Abdul-Jalil A, Gulekli B, Tan S. In vitro maturation and fertilization of oocytes from unstimulated normal ovaries, polycystic ovaries, and women with polycystic ovary syndrome. Fertil Steril 2001; 76: 936

163. Child T, Phillips S, Abdul-Jalil A, et al. A comparison of in vitro maturation and in vitro fertilization for women with polycystic ovaries. Am J Obstet Gynecol 2002; 100: 665

164. Chan K, Chian R. Maturation in vitro of immature human oocytes for clinical use. Hum Reprod Update 1998; 4: 103–20

165. Chian RC, Buckett WM, Tulandi T, Tan SL. Prospective randomized study of human chorionic gonadotrophin priming before immature oocyte retrieval from unstimulated women with PCOS. Hum Reprod 2000; 15: 165–70

166. Schenker JG, Weinstein D. Ovarian hyperstimulation syndrome: a current survey. Fertil Steril 1978; 30: 255

167. Friedman CI, Schmidt GE, Chang FE, Kim MH. Severe ovarian hyperstimulation following follicular aspiration. Am J Obstet Gynecol 1984; 150: 436–7

168. Golan A, Ron-el R, Herman A, et al. Ovarian hyperstimulation syndrome: an update review. Obstet Gynaecol Surv 1989; 44: 430–40

169. MacDougall MJ, Tan SL, Jacobs HS. In-vitro fertilization and the ovarian hyperstimulation syndrome. Hum Reprod 1992; 7: 597–600

170. Lunenfeld B, Insler V. Classification of amenorrhoeic states and their treatment by ovulation induction. Clin Endocrinol 1974; 3: 223–37

171. Charbonnel B, Krempf M, Blanchard P, et al. Induction of ovulation in polycystic ovary syndrome with a combination of a luteinizing hormone-releasing hormone analog and exogenous gonadotropins. Fertil Steril 1987; 47: 920–4

12

Classification, pathophysiology and management of ovarian hyperstimulation syndrome

Botros Rizk and Mohamed Aboulghar

INTRODUCTION

Whilst mild ovarian hyperstimulation syndrome (OHSS) is of no clinical relevance, severe OHSS, characterized by massive ovarian enlargement, ascites, pleural effusion, oliguria, hemoconcentration and thromboembolic phenomena, is a life-threatening complication[1,2].

Significant advances have been made in the understanding of the pathophysiology of OHSS over the past decade. Rizk and colleagues[3] have extensively investigated the role of vascular endothelial growth factor (VEGF) nd other interleukins in the pathogenesis of this syndrome. More recent publications have made our review on the pathophysiology obsolete only 5 years after its publication[4]. Rizk and Smitz[5] have shown that the use of gonadotropin releasing hormone agonist (GnRH-a) does not make an impact on the occurrence of OHSS in *in vitro* fertilization (IVF) cycles. On the other hand, Rizk and Thorneycroft[6] have shown that even the use of a low-dose protocol of gonadotropins does not abolish the risk of OHSS. Rizk and colleagues[7] have shown that patients with polycystic ovarian syndrome (PCOS) are at high risk for OHSS regardless of other factors. This could probably be related to VEGF and interleukin production in patients with PCOS. In this chapter, we propose a new classification for OHSS. The role of VEGF and interleukins pertinent to the pathogenesis of OHSS is presented.

It is important for all clinicians, especially gynecologists, to be aware of the current principles of prevention and management of OHSS[8]. Rizk and Nawar[9] critically evaluated the classic as well as novel methods for the prevention of OHSS. It is natural that, as there has been an increase in the variety of ovarian stimulation protocols, so there are newer options for prevention. This is specifically evident with the use of GnRH-a and recombinant luteinizing hormone (r-hH) for triggering ovulation. Our protocol for the treatment of OHSS is summarized. Rizk and Aboulghar[10] established the basic principles for the treatment of OHSS. In comparison with our protocol published almost 15 years ago, there has been steady progress, but much less compared with options for prevention. This is a healthy sign, implying that most researchers focus on prevention rather than treatment. The most significant advance in treatment relies on our understanding of the role of VEGF as a key component of this syndrome.

CLASSIFICATION

There has been no unanimity in classifying OHSS, and divergent classifications have made comparisons between studies difficult[4]. Aboulghar and Mansour[11] reviewed the classifications used for OHSS over the past four decades. Rabau and colleagues[12] proposed the first classification of OHSS. This was later reorganized by Schenker and Weinstein[13] into three main clinical categories and six grades according to the severity of symptoms and signs and laboratory findings:

(1) *Mild hyperstimulation*:

Grade 1 is defined by laboratory findings of estrogen levels above 150 µg/24 h and pregnanediol excretion above 10 mg/24 h;

Grade 2 in addition includes enlargement of the ovaries; sometimes small cysts are present;

(2) *Moderate hyperstimulation*:

Grade 3 in addition to elevated urinary steroid levels and ovarian cysts includes the presence of abdominal distension;

Grade 4 includes also nausea, vomiting and/or diarrhea;

(3) *Severe hyperstimulation*:

Grade 5 in addition to the above includes large ovarian cysts as well as ascites and/or hydrothorax;

Grade 6 includes marked hemoconcentration with increased blood viscosity which may result in coagulation abnormalities.

More recently, Golan and colleagues[14] proposed the following classification:

(1) *Mild OHSS*:

Grade 1 with abdominal distension and discomfort;

Grade 2 with features of grade 1 plus nausea, vomiting and/or diarrhea; ovaries are enlarged from 5 to 12 cm;

(2) *Moderate OHSS*:

Grade 3 with features of mild OHSS plus ultrasonic evidence of ascites;

(3) *Severe OHSS*:

Grade 4 with features of moderate OHSS plus evidence of ascites and/or hydrothorax and breathing difficulties;

Grade 5 with all of the above plus a change in the blood volume, increased blood viscosity due to hemoconcentration, coagulation abnormality and diminished renal perfusion and function.

Yet more recently, Rizk and Aboulghar[15] classified the syndrome into only two categories:

(1) *Moderate OHSS*:

Discomfort, pain, nausea, abdominal distension, no clinical evidence of ascites, but ultrasonic evidence of ascites and enlarged ovaries, normal hematological and biological profiles;

(2) *Severe OHSS*:

Grade A
dyspnea, oliguria, nausea, vomiting, diarrhea, abdominal pain;
clinical evidence of ascites plus marked distension of abdomen or hydrothorax;
ultrasound scan showing large ovaries and marked ascites;
normal biochemical profiles;

Grade B
all symptoms of grade A, plus:
massive tension ascites, markedly enlarged ovaries, severe dyspnea and marked oliguria;
biochemical changes in the form of increased hematocrit, elevated serum creatinine and liver dysfunction;

Grade C
OHSS complicated by respiratory distress syndrome, renal shut-down or venous thrombosis.

The mild degree of OHSS, as in previous classifications by Rabau and co-workers[12], Golan and co-workers[14] and Schenker and Weinstein[13], was omitted from our new classification, as this degree occurs in the majority of cases of ovarian stimulation, and mild OHSS has no complications and does not require special treatment. The great majority of cases of OHSS presenting with symptoms belong to the moderate degree of OHSS. Our new classification can be correlated with the treatment protocol and prognosis more clearly. Moderate OHSS requires observation at home and regular phone calls or visits to the clinic for monitoring progress. Severe OHSS grade A is treated on an out-patient basis by transvaginal aspiration of ascitic fluid and regular follow-up. Severe OHSS grade B

Table 1	Classification of ovarian hyperstimulation syndrome (OHSS)			
Study	*Mild*	*Moderate*	*Severe*	
Rabau et al.[12] (1967)	**grade 1**: estrogen > 150 μg and pregnanediol > 10 mg/24 h **grade 2**: + enlarged ovaries and possibly palpable cysts grades 1 and 2 were not included under the title of mild OHSS	**grade 3**: grade 2 + confirmed palpable cysts and distended abdomen **grade 4**: grade 3 + vomiting and possibly diarrhea	**grade 5**: grade 4 + ascites and possibly hydrothorax	**grade 6**: grade 5 + changes in blood volume, viscosity and coagulation time
Schenker and Weinstein[13] (1978)	**grade 1**: estrogen > 150 μg/24 h and pregnanediol > 10 mg/24 h **grade 2**: + enlarged ovaries, sometimes small cysts	**grade 3**: grade 2 + abdominal distension **grade 4**: grade 3 + nausea, vomiting and/or diarrhea	**grade 5**: grade 4 + large ovarian cysts, ascites and/or hydrothorax	**grade 6**: marked hemoconcentration + increased blood viscosity and possibly coagulation abnormalities
Golan et al.[14] (1989)	**grade 1**: abdominal distension and discomfort **grade 2**: grade 1 + nausea, vomiting and/or diarrhea, enlarged ovaries 5–12 cm	**grade 3**: grade 2 + ultrasound evidence of ascites	**grade 4**: grade 3 + clinical evidence of ascites and/or hydrothorax and breathing difficulties	**grade 5**: grade 4 + hemoconcentration, increased blood viscosity, coagulation abnormality and diminished renal perfusion
Navot et al.[16] (1992)			severe OHSS: variable enlarged ovary; massive ascites ±hydrothorax; Hct > 45%; WBC > 15 000; oliguria; creatinine 1.0–1.5, creatinine clearance ≥ 50 ml/min; liver dysfunction; edema	critical OHSS: variable enlarged ovary; tense ascites ± hydrothorax; Hct > 55%; WBC ≥ 25 000; oliguria; creatinine ≥ 1.6, creatinine clearance < 50 ml/min; renal failure; thromboembolic phenomena; ARDS
Rizk and Aboulghar[15] (1999)	discomfort, pain, nausea, distension, ultrasonic evidence of ascites and enlarged ovaries, normal hematological and biological profiles	**grade A**: dyspnea, oliguria, nausea, vomiting, diarrhea, abdominal pain, clinical evidence of ascites, marked distension or hydrothorax, US showing large ovaries and marked ascites, normal biochemical profile	**grade B**: grade A plus massive tension ascites, markedly enlarged ovaries, severe dyspnea and marked oliguria, increased hematocrit, elevated serum creatinine and liver dysfunction	**grade C**: complications as respiratory distress syndrome, renal shut-down or venous thrombosis

Hct, hematocrit; WBC, white blood cell count; ARDS, adult respiratory distress syndrome; US, ultrasound requires admission to hospital with aspiration of the ascitic fluid and correction of the hemoconcentration and electrolyte imbalance. Severe OHSS grade C requires appropriate treatment according to the type of complication.

This simple classification is practical and may be used very easily to compare the incidence and the outcome of different treatment protocols worldwide (Table 1).

Distinction between early and late ovarian hyperstimulation syndrome was studied by Mathur and colleagues[17]. They concluded that early OHSS relates to 'excessive' preovulatory response to stimulation, whereas late OHSS depends on the occurrence of pregnancy, is likelier to be severe and is only poorly related to preovulatory events.

COMPLICATIONS OF OHSS

Rizk[4] reviewed the myriad of complications following the development of OHSS. While vascular complications are the most dreaded, pulmonary, gastrointestinal and renal complications commonly follow in severe cases. Delvigne[18] investigated, in a series of multicenter studies, the complications of OHSS as well as epidemiology and pathophysiology.

Vascular complications

Cerebrovascular complications are by far the most serious in OHSS[2]. Mozes and associates[1] reported two severe cases of thromboembolic phenomena following human menopausal gonadotropin (hMG) and human chorionic gonadotropin (hCG) treatment, which caused the death of one patient (carotid artery embolism) and required amputation of a limb in the other. Rizk and colleagues encountered a case of hemiplegia as a result of severe OHSS after gamete intrafallopian transfer; the hemiplegia resolved gradually and the pregnancy continued successfully, ending in the vaginal delivery of a healthy girl[2].

Three large series of OHSS cases reported from Belgium, Israel and Egypt noted thromboembolic complications. In Belgium during a period of 4 years, one case of cerebral thrombosis (0.8%) was documented among 128 cases of OHSS (87% moderate and severe)[19]. In Israel, over a period of 10 years, an incidence of 2.4% of thromboembolic complications was observed among 209 cases of severe forms of OHSS[20]. Serour and colleagues[21] reported 10% of thromboembolic phenomena among patients with severe OHSS. The authors studied in detail the complications of assisted reproductive technology in 3500 IVF cycles. Ovarian hyperstimulation occurred in its moderate form in 206 cycles (5.9%) and in its severe form in 60 cycles (1.7%). Deep vein thrombosis occurred in four patients (0.12%) and hemiparesis in two patients (0.06%). All cases in this series were associated with severe OHSS.

Delvigne[18] found 68 cases of thrombosis reported in the literature. Among these, 34.3% of the cases were arterial and 65.7% were venous. The upper and lower body distribution was interesting: 83% were localized in the upper part of the body and 17% in the lower part. Of the upper body thromboses, 60% were venous and 40% were arterial. Of the lower body, 81% were venous and 19% were arterial. There were as many patients with early and late OHSS complicated by thrombosis and also as many singleton as multiple pregnancies complicated by thrombosis.

Aboulghar and colleagues[22] described two patients who developed moderate OHSS without evidence of hemoconcentration; both developed serious cerebrovascular thromboses resulting in hemiparesis, were treated with anticoagulants and recovered. This report emphasizes the role of other factors that can result in vascular thrombosis and illustrates that cerebrovascular accidents may complicate moderate OHSS. Delvigne[18] advised caution in all cases of OHSS since thrombosis complicated about 12% of moderate OHSS cases as well as about 12% of mild OHSS. Furthermore, thromboses could appear at as late as 20 weeks' gestation, even in the absence of hemoconcentration, and in severe cases the event occurred several weeks after OHSS[18].

Stewart and co-workers[23] reported three cases of upper-limb deep venous thrombosis in association with assisted conception, the cause of which was largely unexplained. The authors stressed that not only did these thromboses occur in unusual sites, but they also occurred well after the assumed peak period of risk.

Loret de Mola and colleagues[24] reported two cases of subclavian deep vein thrombosis associated with the use of recombinant follicle stimulating hormone, complicating mild OHSS. A case of cortical vein thrombosis presenting as intracranial hemorrhage was described in a patient with OHSS after IVF and embryo transfer (ET). Veno-occlusive disease of the brain could appear as a hemorrhagic lesion on magnetic resonance imaging (MRI), and this made the initial diagnosis of cortical vein thrombosis difficult. The patient developed deep vein thrombosis 2 weeks after the intracranial event, and the diagnosis of cortical vein thrombosis was made at the time of MRI study after resolution of the hemorrhage. The patient actually developed generalized thrombosis as a complication to OHSS. Although the initial MRI picture may be misleading, the diagnosis of thrombosis should always be kept in mind, as it is the commonest cause of intracranial lesions after OHSS[25]. Belaen and colleagues[26] reported a case of internal jugular vein thrombosis after ovarian stimulation with gonadotropins. Screening for hereditary hypercoagulability for this patient was negative. The patient was successfully treated with low-molecular-weight heparin, and a twin pregnancy was diagnosed. Mancini and colleagues[27] reported a case of forearm amputation after ovarian stimulation for IVF–ET. The patient underwent many cycles of IVF–ET. She had a coagulation disorder as a result of OHSS, with thrombosis of the axillary vein, recurring after thromboarterectomy and leading to the paradoxical result of the amputation of an arm. Turkistani and colleagues[28] reported a case of severe OHSS presenting with central retinal artery occlusion, a combination not reported previously. Foong and associates[29] performed measurement and quantification of the cutaneous arteriolar vasoconstrictor response using laser Doppler fluximetry. They found that women with OHSS have impaired vascular reactivity when compared with normal women.

Hemoconcentration and OHSS

Hemoconcentration and increased hematocrit values, in the presence of normal coagulation parameters, were found in nine of 25 patients by Schenker and Weinstein[13]. Increased levels of factor V, platelets, fibrinogen, profibrinolysin, fibrinolytic inhibitors and thromboplastin generation were observed by Phillips and colleagues[30]. Kaaja and co-workers[31] described deep venous thrombosis in a case of severe OHSS.

Etiopathology of thromboembolic complications

Dulitzky and co-workers[32] found an increased prevalence of thrombophilia among women with severe OHSS. These findings suggested that prophylactic

screening for this disorder and possible use of heparin prophylaxis for thromboembolic phenomena should be considered in these patients. Kodama and associates[33] studied the plasma hemostatic markers in OHSS. They found that the levels of thrombin–antithrombin III and plasma α_2–antiplasmin complexes in the plasma began to rise within a few days after hCG administration, with significantly higher levels during the midluteal phase. In OHSS patients who became pregnant, elevation of these markers continued for 3 weeks after the onset of the disease. There were also some characteristic changes in OHSS cycles in other hemostatic markers, such as a decrease in the levels of antithrombin III and prekallikrein and shortened activated partial thromboplastin time. The practice in that unit was to provide preoperative subcutaneous heparin (5000 IU, single dose) in women undergoing oocyte retrieval and during hospitalization with symptomatic OHSS (subcutaneous 5000 IU twice daily). Balasch and colleagues[34] found an increased expression of induced monocyte tissue factor in plasma from patients with severe OHSS. This increase in the procoagulant activity of blood monocytes, which is mediated principally by tissue factor expression, may be important in thrombotic events associated with the syndrome. Venous compression due to enlarged ovaries and ascites, together with immobility and a transient change in coagulation factors, were thought to be the main etiological factors[35]. Ong and co-workers[36] reported internal jugular vein thrombosis occurring >6 weeks after ovulation, and Mills and associates[37] reported subclavian vein thrombosis 7 weeks after egg collection for IVF. These two late complications suggest a generalized effect on the coagulation system which may persist for several weeks.

Kodama and co-workers[38] studied the status of the plasma kinin system in patients with OHSS, in order to investigate whether activation of the plasma kinin system correlates with increased blood coagulability. They concluded that activation of the plasma kinin system occurs specifically and occasionally in OHSS patients, and is associated with increased blood coagulability, and that, when an OHSS patient demonstrates a low value of plasma kinin, more careful management is required to prevent thromboembolic complications.

Stewart and associates[39] reviewed the world literature for reports of venous and arterial thrombosis as a complication of OHSS. The authors stressed the fact that little was known about the pathogenesis and suggested that, if possible, those women at greater risk should be identified so that prophylactic measures can be taken.

Aune and colleagues[10] reported that ovarian stimulation for IVF induced a hypercoagulable state. They followed up 12 IVF cycles, measuring whole blood clotting time (WBCT), whole blood clot lysis time (CLT), antithrombin III, plasma fibrinogen and factor VII, both before stimulation and after hCG administration, at the peak of estradiol concentration. Their findings showed a significant increase in fibrinogen and a reduction in antithrombin III concentration, and a significant increase in CLT over this time, implying a disruption of the balance of coagulation and thrombolysis leading to a relative increase in coagulability.

Todros and colleagues[41] reported a case of spontaneous OHSS occurring in a pregnant woman carrying the factor V Leiden mutation. Even though prophylactic treatment for thromboembolism was adopted by administering low-molecular-weight heparin, the pregnancy was complicated by thromboses of the left subclavian, axillary, humeral and internal jugular veins during the second trimester of gestation. The pregnancy was managed conservatively and a healthy newborn was delivered at term. To avoid unnecessary laparotomy, the authors emphasized the importance of careful diagnosis in order to differentiate spontaneous OHSS from ovarian carcinoma, as well as the necessity to look for the presence of coagulation disorders in women affected by OHSS.

A 33-year-old female with OHSS with thrombosis of the right internal jugular vein, subclavian vein and superior vena cava underwent IVF. A pregnancy progressed, and edema, pain and a tingling sensation developed. A computed tomography (CT) scan confirmed thrombus in the right internal jugular and subclavian veins and a free-floating tip in the superior vena cava. Following treatment with intravenous heparin therapy and subcutaneous low-molecular-weight heparin until delivery, the symptoms improved[42].

Andrejevic and co-workers[43] reported a 28-year-old patient with polycystic ovary syndrome who presented with fever and laboratory markers of inflammation. Intracardiac thrombosis was diagnosed in the presence of antiphospholipid antibodies. The authors suggested that primary antiphospholipid syndrome was possibly triggered by ovulation induction.

Elford and colleagues[44] presented a case of a previously healthy woman who underwent IVF and experienced a middle cerebral artery thrombosis that was subsequently lysed with intra-arterial recombinant tissue plasminogen activator (rt-PA). To the authors' knowledge, this was the first reported case of successful use of rt-PA to lyse a cerebral arterial thrombus resulting from severe OHSS. The patient made a near complete neurologic recovery and delivered a healthy infant at term, illustrating that intra-arterial thrombolysis can be used with relative safety even in very early pregnancy.

Ulug and colleagues[45] reported a case of bilateral internal jugular venous thrombosis following successful assisted conception in the absence of OHSS.

McGowan and colleagues[46] reported a case of deep vein thrombosis followed by internal jugular vein thrombosis as a complication of IVF in a woman heterozygous for the prothrombin 3′ untranslated region (UTR) and factor V Leiden mutations. They suggested that neck pain and swelling in a pregnant woman, especially one who has undergone IVF, should be taken seriously and investigated. Women with a personal or family history of thrombosis undergoing IVF should be made fully aware of the potential thrombotic risks and should be considered for a thrombophilia screen.

Fabregues and associates[47] conducted a case–control study of the prevalence of thrombophilia in women with severe OHSS, and cost-effectiveness of screening. The cost of preventing one thrombotic event in a patient developing severe OHSS after IVF and having factor V Leiden or prothrombin G20210A mutation was calculated. None of the OHSS patients or controls had antithrombin, protein C or free protein S deficiencies. All of them tested negative for antiphospholipid antibodies.

Ou and co-workers[48] reported a case of thromboembolism after ovarian stimulation and successful management of a woman with superior sagittal sinus thrombosis after IVF–ET. The authors recommended dose-adjusted heparinization as the first-line treatment of choice, while intravascular thrombolysis or operative thrombectomy is an aggressive but effective treatment. Continuation of pregnancy is considered safe, without any increased risk of fetal congenital anomalies.

Nakauchi-Tanaka and colleagues[49] reported a 31-year-old nulligravida woman who developed an acquired factor VIII inhibitor associated with severe OHSS. She developed hematuria, ecchymosis and intramuscular bleeding following the severe OHSS. Laboratory examinations showed a markedly prolonged activated partial thromboplastin time and a low level of factor VIII activity. Treatment with prothrombin concentrate and factor VIII inhibitor bypassing agent was successful in reducing the inhibitor so that she delivered a healthy baby via spontaneous vaginal delivery. Acquired hemophilia is a life-threatening disorder. This was the first case report of acquired hemophilia in OHSS.

Myocardial infarction

Akdemir and colleagues[50] reported a case of a patient with myocardial infarction associated with OHSS.

Liver dysfunction

Abnormal liver function tests occur in 25–40% of cases[18]. Sueldo and co-workers[51] and Younis and co-workers[52] were the first to report liver dysfunction in severe OHSS. Since then, abnormal hepatic function has been increasingly recognized as a complication of severe OHSS that may persist for > 2 months[53]. It was interesting to note that, although the liver function tests were markedly abnormal, liver biopsy showed significant morphological abnormalities only at the ultrastructural level[51].

The relationship of serum proinflammatory cytokines and VEGF with liver dysfunction in severe OHSS was studied by Chen and colleagues[54]. Concentrations of interleukin-6 (IL-6) in the active phase of OHSS were significantly higher in the abnormal liver function test group than in the normal liver function test group. These results suggest that the IL-6 cytokine system may play a role in the pathogenesis of liver dysfunction in severe OHSS. Abnormal liver function tests were associated with lower clinical pregnancy rates.

Elter and associates[55] reported a case of hepatic dysfunction associated with moderate OHSS, suggesting that hepatic dysfunction is not limited to severe forms of OHSS. Liver function should be analyzed even in moderate cases.

Davis and associates[56] reported a severe case of OHSS with liver dysfunction and malnutrition in which the patient's albumin dropped to 9 g/l, with

liver function abnormalities peaking at: alanine aminotransferase, 46 IU/l; alkaline phosphatase, 706 IU/l; bilirubin, 26 μmol/l; and prothrombin time, 19 s. The judicious use of paracentesis and commencement of total parenteral nutrition coincided with rapid clinical improvement. One month after discharge, the patient was asymptomatic with normal liver function.

Respiratory complications

Pulmonary manifestations were observed in 7.2% of severe OHSS cases. Dyspnea and tachypnea were the commonest symptoms appearing in 92% of these cases. A small proportion of patients who had pulmonary manifestations presented with complications such as local pneumonia (4%), adult respiratory distress syndrome (2%) and pulmonary embolism (2%)[20]. Respiratory distress, secondary to ascitic fluid accumulation, is common in severe OHSS and is usually relieved by aspiration of ascitic fluid. Adult respiratory distress syndrome was reported in a patient with severe OHSS[57].

Jewelewicz and Van de Wiele[58] reported a rare case of pleural effusion as the sole presentation of OHSS following superovulation. Kingsland and colleagues[59] reported the first case where a patient after IVF developed OHSS manifested only by pleural effusion. Rabinerson and co-workers[60] reported severe unilateral hydrothorax as the only manifestation of OHSS. A 35-year-old woman presented with mild dyspnea 2 weeks after ovarian stimulation with hMG and hCG and IVF–ET. Chest X-ray revealed a large pleural effusion on the right side. Three consecutive thoracocenteses were needed to drain a total of 6800 ml of fluid. Following drainage, the respiratory symptoms disappeared. An uneventful pregnancy progressed.

Cordani and colleagues[61] discussed a case of massive unilateral hydrothorax as the only clinical manifestation of OHSS. The published literature on OHSS presenting with pleural effusion is shown in Table 2.

Semba and colleagues[63] reported an autopsy case of severe OHSS in a 28-year-old Japanese female. The patient developed bilateral chest pain and progressive dyspnea during the course of administration of human gonadotropins. Pleural effusion and hypouresis clinically disappeared 4 days after the onset of the symptoms, but the patient died suddenly of rapid respiratory insufficiency. Autopsy examination revealed

Table 2 Isolated pleural effusion as the only manifestation of ovarian hyperstimulation syndrome (OHSS). Adapted from reference 62

Author (year)	Age (years)	Peak follicular estradiol level	Number of oocytes retrieved	Luteal support	Onset of OHSS	Hydrothorax	Fluid drained (l)	Presence of ascites	Conception
Jewelewicz et al. (1975)	24	180 μg/24 h	none	none	13 days after hCG	right side	none (resolved spontaneously)	none	in vivo
Kingsland et al. (1995)	35	1221 nmol/24 h	7	none	10 days after oocyte retrieval	right side	3.5	none	IVF–ET followed by miscarriage
Daniel et al. (1995)	27	1900 ng/ml	none	none	10 days after hCG	right side	2	none	in vivo
Bassil et al. (1996)	39	2650 pg/ml	11	progesterone	12 days after oocyte retrieval	left side	2.5	none	IVF–ET (twins)
Wood et al. (1998)	29	3479 pg/ml	18	hCG	12 days after oocyte retrieval	right side	4	none	none (after IVF–ET)
Friedler et al. (1998) (case 1)	29	>3000 pg/ml	22	progesterone	12 days after oocyte retrieval	right side (recurrent)	1.7	minimal	IVF–ET (twins)
Friedler et al. (1998) (case 2)	33	>3000 pg/ml	19	progesterone	5 days after oocyte retrieval	right side	4.5	none	none
Man et al. 1997 (4 cases)	24–29	NM	NM	NM	NM	right side (one left-sided)	1.2–2	none	IVF–ET in one case (NM for other cases)
Arikan et al. (1997)	29	NM	NM	NM	12 days after oocyte retrieval	left side	4	minimal	IVF–ET (twins)
Gore et al. (2002)	27	1840 pg/ml	none (IUI)	hCG, progesterone	10 days after hCG	right side (recurrent)	10.4	none	in vivo

NM, not mentioned; IUI, intrauterine insemination; hCG, human chorionic gonadotropin; IVF–ET, *in vitro* fertilization–embryo transfer massive pulmonary edema, intra-alveolar hemorrhage and pleural effusion, without any evidence of pulmonary thromboembolism. Histopathological examination of the ovary demonstrated multiple well-developed follicle formations, consistent with OHSS. This is the first autopsy report of a patient with severe OHSS.

Renal complications

Prerenal failure is a complication of hypovolemia secondary to fluid transudation in the peritoneal cavity. Balasch and colleagues[64] reported a case of prerenal failure after treatment with indomethacin, and advised against the use of prostaglandin synthetase inhibitors. Ovarian hyperstimulation syndrome in a renal transplant patient undergoing assisted conception treatment was reported. Ovarian enlargement secondary to OHSS resulted in obstruction in the transplanted kidney and deterioration of renal function. Conservative management was successful and a twin live birth was later achieved by replacement of two frozen–thawed embryos[65].

Gastrointestinal complications

With the widespread use of ovulation induction for assisted conception, it is mandatory that general practitioners become aware that gastrointestinal symptoms may be the initial presentation of ovarian hyperstimulation. One such case presented to us with a cerebrovascular accident because such symptoms were ignored[2].

Benign intracranial tension

In an IVF patient and shortly after embryo transfer, a patient developed clinical signs of moderate OHSS with symptoms which were later diagnosed as benign intracranial hypertension (BIH). This was treated effectively using repeated lumbar puncture and diuretics. Spontaneous labor and delivery occurred at 40 weeks' gestation. There was no neurological sequela and no recurrence of the BIH, 2 years after the pregnancy. The possible link between OHSS and BIH as well as the risks of further pregnancy should be considered[66].

Obstetric complications

Schenker[67] reported that among IVF patients with severe and critical OHSS, pregnancy, multiple gestation, miscarriage, preterm premature rupture of the membranes, prematurity and low birth weight rates are significantly higher than those reported previously for pregnancies after assisted conception. Raziel and colleagues[68] reported increased early pregnancy loss in IVF patients with severe OHSS, 38% as compared with 15% in the control group.

INCIDENCE OF OHSS

Rizk and Smitz[5] studied the factors that influence the incidence of OHSS. They found a wide variation among different centers. This is partly because of different definitions for the grades of severity and partly because of the adoption of different criteria for prevention. The incidence of mild OHSS is approximately 20–33% of IVF cycles[17], and the incidence of moderate OHSS is 3–6%. The severe form is reported at between 0.1 and 2% of IVF cycles[21].

Table 3 Incidence of ovarian hyperstimulation syndrome (OHSS) in human menopausal gonadotropin/human chorionic gonadotropin (hMG/hCG) cycles. Modified from reference 4

Author	Year	Mild (%)	Moderate (%)	Severe (%)
Rabau	1967	–	–	3.5
Tyler	1968	23	–	1.5
Taymor	1968	20	–	2
Thompson and Hansen	1970	–	–	1.2
Godfarb and Rakoff	1973	10	0.005	0.008
Jewelewicz et al.	1973	20	7	1.8
Hammond and Marshall	1973	21	–	10
Caspi et al.	1974	–	6	1.17
Lunenfeld and Insler	1974	8.4	–	0.8
Schwartz	1980	–	6.3	1.4

Table 4 Literature data concerning frequencies of ovarian hyperstimulation syndrome (OHSS; moderate and severe), the nature of the gonadotropin releasing hormone (GnRH) agonist used, the protocol for human menopausal gonadotropin (hMG) therapy, the type of luteal support and the occurrence of pregnancies in these women. Modified from reference 5

Reference	Study group	Incidence of OHSS (%)	GnRH agonist used	Dose	% OHSS pregnant	hMG regimen	Luteal support
Golan et al. (1988)	143 cycles, 117 patients	8.4	D-Trp 6	3.2 mg, long-acting	83	started with 3 ampoules	2500 IU hCG every 72 h and adjusted to estradiol
Belaisch-Allar and De Niyzib (1989)	304 embryo transfers	5.9	D-Trp 6 or D-Ser (TBU) 6	NM	NM	NM	2500 IU hCG (151 patients), or placebo (153 patients) randomized
Buvat et al. (1989)	171 embryo transfers	1.8 (moderate)	D-Trp 6	short-acting	NM	NM	3×1500 IU hCG or 400 mg progesterone p.o. daily
Herman et al. (1990)	36 embryo transfers	14	D-Trp 6	3.2 mg, long-acting	80	started with 3 ampoules and adjusted to estradiol	2500 IU every 3rd day or placebo (18 patients)
Fornan et al. (1990)	413 cycles	1.9 (severe)	D-Trp 6 or D-Ser (TBU) 6	3.75 mg long-acting injection 100 ng/day or nasal spray 500 ng/day	88	started with 2 ampoules and adjusted to estradiol	didrogesterone 30 mg/day p.o. or 2500 IU hCG every 72 h
Smitz et al. (1990)	1673 cycles	0.6 (severe)	D-Ser (TBU) 6	600 ng daily nasal spray	70	started with 2 ampoules hCG and adjusted to estradiol	1500 IU every 72 h or progesterone vaginal or i.m.
Rizk et al. (1993)	1562 cycles	1.3 (severe)	D-Ser (TBU) 6	subcutaneous injection 200 µg/day or nasal spray 500 µg/day	57	started with 2 ampoules hCG and adjusted to estradiol	2000 IU on days 2 and 5 or progesterone 200 mg/day vaginal suppository

NM, not mentioned; hCG, human chorionic gonadotropin; p.o., orally; i.m., intramuscularly

It is interesting to note that the incidence of moderate and severe OHSS before the introduction of transvaginal sonography and estradiol assays in the 1970s (Table 3) appears to be comparable with results of more recent series of OHSS in IVF programs (Table 4). This possibly represents an increase in aggressiveness in stimulation during the 1980s. Delvigne and Rozenberg[69] and Delvigne[18] recently evaluated the epidemiology of OHSS and studied the factors that influence its incidence. In a retrospective study from 13 Belgian IVF centers, 128 cases of OHSS and 256 selected controls were identified from January 1988 to December 1991. Clinical and biological parameters were significantly different between the OHSS cases and the controls, although a considerable overlap of their distributions was observed. Therefore, discriminant analysis was performed in a separate study in order to derive a formula that could be predictive of the risk of OHSS.

Factors that influence the incidence of OHSS

Age

It is commonly observed that women suffering from ovarian hyperstimulation are significantly younger. This does not mean that older women are not at risk for OHSS, but it means that younger women are at higher risk. Delvigne and colleagues[70] in a large Belgian study including 128 cases of OHSS and 256 controls observed that the mean age for OHSS patients was 30.2 ± 3.5 vs. 32.0 ± 4.5 years for controls.

Body mass index

Most clinicians have the impression that OHSS is more common in patients with a lower body mass index (BMI). Navot and colleagues[71] described a positive correlation between lean body mass and OHSS, whereas Delvigne and colleagues[70] did not find such a correlation.

Etiology of infertility

OHSS has been observed equally in primary and secondary infertility[18]. The duration of infertility does not influence the occurrence of OHSS[71]. Most certainly, women who have previously developed OHSS are at increased risk[70]. A significantly higher incidence of OHSS is reported in group II patients (World Health Organization (WHO) classification, 1973). Lunenfeld and Insler[72] found the incidence of mild and severe OHSS in 621 cycles of patients belonging to group I to be 5.5% and 0.6%, respectively, compared with 10.8% and 1.2% in 784 cycles in group II. Thompson and Hansen[73] analyzed 3002 hMG/hCG cycles in 1280 patients and found no cases of hyperstimulation

syndrome in patients with primary amenorrhea (group I). Similar observations have been made by Caspi and colleagues[74], Schenker and Weinstein[13] and Tulandi and co-workers[75].

Polycystic ovarian syndrome

Rizk and Smitz[5] found polycystic ovarian syndrome (PCOS) to be the major predisposing factor for OHSS. Schenker and Weinstein[13] found that 12 of 25 patients who developed severe OHSS had PCOS as determined by endoscopy. Charbonnel and colleagues[76] encountered ovarian hyperstimulation in all 33 cycles in PCOS patients. Bider and associates[77] found a higher proportion of severe OHSS, 38% in PCOS patients. Smitz and colleagues[78] found a hormone profile suggestive of hyperandrogenism in eight of ten patients who developed severe OHSS. Aboulghar and colleagues[79] reported that 15 of 18 patients with severe OHSS had PCOS. Rizk and colleagues[7] found that 13 of 21 patients with severe OHSS had PCOS confirmed by ultrasound and endocrine criteria.

Ovarian stimulation protocol

Gonadotropin releasing hormone agonist

It had been hoped that the use of GnRH-a/hMG protocols would decrease the incidence of OHSS. With the use of GnRH-a, the practice of IVF has been simplified, the blocking of the LH surge permitting further stimulation of the ovaries, increasing the number of oocytes. Golan and colleagues[80] observed a high incidence of OHSS, 8.4% after combined GnRH-a and hMG for superovulation. The French

Table 5 Comparison of the stimulation characteristics of ovarian hyperstimulation syndrome (OHSS) cycles with those of normo-ovulatory women who became pregnant after treatment with the same gonadotropin releasing hormone agonist/human menopausal gonadotropin (GnRH-a/hMG) protocol. Modified from reference 78

	OHSS (n = 10)	Normal cycles (n = 40)	Significance
Number of days before desensitization	30.2 ± 6.0	21.0 ± 7.0	$p < 0.01$
Days of hMG stimulation	9.6 ± 1.7	12.3 ± 2.5	$p < 0.01$
Number of ampoules of hMG used	21.9 ± 6.9	39.2 ± 14.2	$p < 0.001$
Preovulatory estradiol concentration (ng/l)	3735.0 ± 1603	1634 ± 492	$p < 0.001$
Number of oocytes retrieved	19.1 ± 10.3	7.5 ± 4.2	$p < 0.001$

report of FIVNAT results for 1989[81] showed that the use of GnRH-a led to significantly higher preovulatory estradiol concentrations, and to more frequent severe hyperstimulation (4.6% vs. 0.6% for non-GnRH-a/hMG cycles). Rizk and Smitz[5] summarized the major reports of OHSS after the use of GnRH and gonadotropins for IVF (Table 4).

Human menopausal gonadotropin

Rabau and co-workers[12] found no relationship between the incidence of OHSS and the dose of gonadotropin administered. In animal studies, Schenker and Weinstein[13] found a direct relationship between the dose of hMG administered and the production of OHSS. In humans, however, they found no correlation between the dose of hMG and the occurrence of OHSS. OHSS occurred in 0.008–23% of hMG/hCG cycles (Table 3), compared with 0.6–14% in GnRH-a/hMG/hCG cycles (Table 4). Comparison of the endocrine patterns (Table 5) in patients who developed OHSS, and normo-ovulatory patients who became pregnant after treatment with the same ovarian stimulation protocol, showed that the former required less hMG to achieve a higher preovulatory serum estradiol concentration and a higher number of mature oocytes[78].

Rizk and Smitz[5] found that, in the groups reporting the lowest frequency of severe OHSS, ovarian stimulation was started with 2×75 IU hMG, whereas most other groups used 3×75 IU hMG[5]. The amount of follicle stimulating hormone (FSH) injected at the start could possibly induce the growth of a larger number of follicles, which could develop sufficiently to acquire receptors for LH, and, as a result, luteinize massively. Interestingly, Rizk and Vere found that a fixed-regimen protocol, with a predetermined date of retrieval, has a similar incidence of OHSS[82].

Follicle stimulating hormone

It has been suggested by Raj and colleagues[83] that the use of FSH in anovulatory patients with PCOS offers a safe treatment compared with hMG, resulting in higher pregnancy rates and lower hyperstimulation rates. These authors suggested that endogenous LH levels in patients with polycystic ovaries are quite adequate for follicular development, and that the administration of exogenous LH is therefore unwarranted. However, Check and co-workers[84] found an incidence of 23.7% of OHSS in 18 women treated

with 38 FSH cycles. Severe OHSS occurred in 5.3%, indicating that FSH is no safer than hMG. In a more recent prospective randomized study, Rizk and Thorneycroft[6] found that the use of recombinant FSH did not abolish the risk of OHSS; the incidence was comparable to that of purified urinary FSH in a similar low-dose protocol.

Clomiphene citrate

Severe OHSS with clomiphene citrate (CC) is rare[4]. Southan and Janovsky[85] reported a patient with polycystic ovaries who developed massive ovarian enlargement, ascites and hydrothorax after the administration of 100 mg of CC for 14 days. Scommegna and Lash[86] reported a case of ovarian hyperstimulation associated with conception after treatment with CC.

OHSS in a spontaneous cycle

Rizk[4] found rare reports of OHSS in spontaneous cycles. In the world literature, only a few cases have been reported. The condition was reported in a hypothyroid patient with Down's syndrome[87]. Zalel and co-workers[88] reported a case of OHSS in a spontaneous cycle in a patient with PCOS, and Zalel and colleagues[89] reported recurrence of OHSS in a spontaneous pregnancy in the same patient with PCOS. More recently, Ayhan and co-workers[90], Lipitz and co-workers[91] and Regi and co-workers[92] reported one case each in a normal female. The clinical presentation with ascites and pleural effusion, which is typical of advanced ovarian cancer, resulted in an exploratory laparotomy in the Ayhan case. Surgery is generally not advised in the treatment of OHSS, and yet, in these extremely rare cases, surgery is often performed, based on an incorrect diagnosis.

Chae and colleagues[93] reported a case of severe OHSS in a spontaneously pregnant woman with no underlying disease. Di Carlo and colleagues[94] reported a case of spontaneous recurrent familial OHSS, associated with high concentrations of renin and aldosterone. Both the patient and her only sister had suffered from a similar condition in their previous pregnancies. The authors suggested that similar cases of spontaneous OHSS, when admitted to a surgical emergency department, may undergo unnecessary surgical treatment by medical staff with no experience in reproductive medicine. With the increasing awareness of these conditions, more and more cases should be detected and reported.

Montanelli and associates[95,96] described a new familial case of recurrent OHSS. The affected women were heterozygous for a different mutation involving codon 449, where an alanine was substituted for threonine. Similar to D567N, the T449 A FSHr mutant shows an increase of its sensitivity to both hCG and thyroid stimulating hormone (TSH), together with an increase in basal activity.

Jung and Kim[97] described a case of severe spontaneous OHSS with magnetic resonance (MR) findings. MR scans showed bilateral symmetric enlargement of ovaries with multiple cystic changes, giving the classic 'wheel-spoke' appearance. There was no definite abnormally thickened or enhanced wall, but there was internal hemorrhage in some chambers. The authors emphasized the importance of careful diagnosis to differentiate spontaneous OHSS from ovarian cystic neoplasms.

Luteal phase support and the role of luteal hCG in the genesis of OHSS

The World Collaborative Report on IVF compiled by Seppala[98] pointed out the non-uniform approach to luteal phase support. Many centers used progesterone and its derivatives, others used hCG and some avoided any luteal support. The introduction of GnRH-a offers advantages in terms of pituitary desensitization and prevention of a premature LH surge, thereby resulting in lower cancellation rates and an increased number of preovulatory follicles. However, its effect on corpus luteum function requires careful treatment if a satisfactory luteal phase endometrium is to be maintained. Smitz and colleagues[99] were the first to document luteal phase insufficiency, in 23 IVF cycles treated with GnRH-a when luteal phase support with progesterone was omitted. Golan and colleagues[80] observed a high incidence of OHSS (8.4%) after the use of hCG for luteal support. Herman and co-workers[100], in a prospective randomized trial, compared the pregnancy rate and incidence of OHSS after luteal hCG in IVF cycles stimulated with GnRH-a and hMG. Nine of the 18 patients who received hCG conceived, compared with three of 18 patients in the placebo group. OHSS occurred in five out of 18 patients treated with hCG. None of the 18 patients without luteal hCG support developed OHSS, including those patients who became pregnant. Because the number of patients who conceived in the placebo group was small (three of 18), the authors

Table 6 Incidence of pregnancy in patients with ovarian hyperstimulation syndrome (OHSS). Modified from reference 4

Author	Year	Incidence (%)	Number of patients	Multiple pregnancies
Rabau	1967	42	6/14	2/6
Schenker and Weinstein	1978	40	10/25	5/10
Tulandi	1984	34.6	10/29	4/10
Golan	1988	91	10/11	1/10
Borenstein	1989	35	14/39	3/14
Herman	1990	80	4/5	1/4
Forman	1990	88	7/8	2/7
Smitz	1990	70	7/10	3/7
Rizk	1991	57	12/21	5/12

concluded that the question of whether repeated early luteal hCG injections are more important in the pathogenesis of OHSS than endogenous hCG secreted later by the developing conceptus remains unresolved. Imoedemhe and co-workers[101] found no cases of OHSS, even amongst pregnant patients, when GnRH-a was used instead of hCG to trigger ovulation. They suggested that the preovulatory hCG dose may play a more important role in initiating the syndrome. The role of hCG generated by the presence of a pregnancy may therefore essentially augment the prevailing condition, initiated by preovulatory hCG administration. Luteal phase support is an essential prerequisite to achieve satisfactory pregnancy rates in IVF after GnRH-a/hMG. Progesterone, intramuscular or vaginal, should be given to patients at risk of OHSS, otherwise hCG may be used.

Conception cycles

Rizk[4] found OHSS to be much more frequent in conception cycles (Table 6). Haning and co-workers[102] found that OHSS was four times more frequent in pregnancy than in non-pregnancy cycles and to be three times that in non-hyperstimulated cycles. The pregnancy rate in the reported series of hyperstimulation varied from 34.6 to 91%. A high incidence of multiple pregnancy (10–42%) was also observed. However, OHSS is very rarely reported in association with heterotopic pregnancy[103,104]. The duration of

OHSS is longer and its expression is more severe when pregnancy ensues. Bider and colleagues[77] found the average hospitalization stay in pregnant patients with OHSS to be longer, compared with non-pregnant patients. Koike and colleagues[105] observed that severity of OHSS is related to the number of conceptuses, which is reflected in the number of days of hospital stay.

Oocyte quality in OHSS

Aboulghar and co-workers[106] studied oocyte quality in patients with severe OHSS. They reported that the inferior quality and maturity of oocytes in OHSS reduced the fertilization rate but did not affect the quality or the number of embryos transferred, or the pregnancy rate. The effect on oocyte quality could be due to the prevalence of polycystic ovaries in this group of patients.

PATHOPHYSIOLOGY OF OHSS

Rizk and colleagues[3] have extensively reviewed the pathophysiology of OHSS. OHSS is marked by massive bilateral cystic ovarian enlargement. The ovaries are noted to have a significant degree of stromal edema, interspersed with multiple hemorrhagic follicular and theca-lutein cysts, areas of cortical necrosis and neovascularization. The second pathological phenomenon is that of acute body fluid shifts, resulting in ascites and pleural effusion. Most investigators believe that these fluid shifts are the result of enhanced capillary permeability[107]. Three decades ago, Schenker and Weinstein demonstrated this increased permeability in the rabbit model[13]. More recently, Tollan and co-workers[108] showed that during ovarian stimulation for IVF there is infiltration of fluid from the vascular space to the interstitial compartment, 1 day before oocyte aspiration. Significant advances have been made in our understanding of the nature of the vasoactive agents involved (Figure 1).

Delbaere and colleagues[109] reported the recent identification of mutations in the FSH receptor gene which display an increased sensitivity to hCG and are responsible for the development of spontaneous OHSS; this provides, for the first time, the molecular basis for the pathophysiology of spontaneous OHSS.

Based on these recent findings, the authors underlined the differences between spontaneous and iatrogenic OHSS and proposed a model to account for the different chronology between the two forms of the syndrome. In the iatrogenic form, follicular recruitment and enlargement occur during ovarian stimulation with exogenous FSH, while in the spontaneous form, follicular recruitment occurs later through stimulation of the FSH receptor by pregnancy-derived hCG. In both forms, massive luteinization of enlarged stimulated ovaries ensues, inducing the release of vasoactive mediators, leading to development of the symptoms of OHSS.

Enskog and colleagues[110] found that peripheral blood concentrations of inhibin B are elevated during gonadotropin stimulation in patients who later develop ovarian OHSS, and inhibin A concentrations are elevated after OHSS onset.

The selectins, a group of cell adhesion molecules, are major mediators of inflammatory, immunologic and angiogenic reactions. Ascitic fluid of women with OHSS contains appreciable amounts of soluble selectins, suggesting their ovarian origin and possible involvement in the syndrome[111].

Abramov and colleagues[112] studied the potential involvement of the soluble endothelial cell-leukocyte adhesion molecules E-selectin and intercellular adhesion molecule (ICAM-1) in the pathophysiology of capillary hyperpermeability in OHSS. They found that soluble ICAM-1 and soluble E-selectin seem to be involved in the pathophysiology of capillary hyperpermeability in severe OHSS. In a retrospective study, Ogawa and associates[113] noted that a rise of the serum level of von Willebrand factor occurs before clinical manifestation of the severe form of OHSS but not in patients with mild OHSS. Evbuomwan and colleagues[114] studied the hypothesis that decreases in and maintenance of a new steady state in plasma osmolality and sodium level in OHSS are due to altered osmoregulation of arginine vasopressin secretion and thirst. They found that the osmotic thresholds for arginine vasopressin secretion and thirst are reset to lower plasma osmolality during superovulation for IVF–ET. This new lower body tonicity is maintained until at least day 10 after hCG in OHSS. Decreases in plasma osmolality and plasma sodium levels in OHSS are due to altered osmoregulation rather than electrolyte losses; correction of apparent 'electrolyte imbalance' in OHSS is therefore inappropriate.

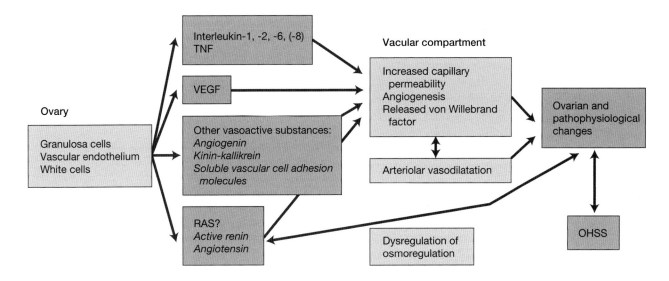

Figure 1 Pathophysiology of ovarian hyperstimulation syndrome (OHSS). TNF, tumor necrosis factor; VEGF, vascular endothelial growth factor; RAS, renin–angiotensin system. From reference 18, with permission

In contrast to our classic concept[4] of increased capillary permeability, Balasch and co-workers[115] adopted a very different and interesting view. They studied the hemodynamic changes in severe OHSS and suggested that the circulatory disturbances are not secondary to reduction in circulating blood volume, but are a consequence of an intense peripheral arteriolar vasodilatation that leads to underfilling of the arterial vascular component, arterial hypotension and a compensatory increase in heart rate and cardiac output. However, it must be mentioned that none of their patients had hemoconcentration – a common finding among patients with severe OHSS[115].

The hemodynamic relationship between hematocrit and plasma volume was nicely illustrated by Van Beaumont[116]. It is accepted that, in the face of a constant red cell volume, a rising hematocrit signifies a fall in plasma volume. It appears that, when the red cell volume remains constant, the change in hematocrit can never be numerically commensurate with the change in plasma volume. The change in plasma volume must always be larger than the change reflected by the hematocrit. Thus, a change of 2 points in the hematocrit from 45 to 47% is four times smaller than the actual 8% drop in plasma volume. This is extremely important to keep in mind when treating patients with OHSS. Any increase in the hematocrit as it approaches 45% does not accurately reflect the

magnitude of plasma volume depletion, and thus the seriousness of the patient's condition. Likewise, in the face of hemoconcentration, small drops in the hematocrit may represent significant improvements in plasma volume.

Alteration of osmoregulation of OHSS

Evbuomwan and colleagues[117] observed an alteration of osmoregulation during OHSS with an osmotic threshold for arginine vasopressin secretion that is reset to lower plasma osmolality during superovulation. This is maintained for at least 10 days after hCG administration in patients with OHSS. The decreasing plasma osmolality and sodium levels in these patients is attributed to altered osmoregulation rather than electrolyte losses.

Immunoglobulins and metabolic changes in OHSS

Significantly lower levels of gamma-globulins, specifically IgG and IgA, were detected in the plasma of patients with severe OHSS, whereas alpha- and beta-globulin levels as well as IgM levels were not significantly different from those in controls[118]. Metabolic characteristics of women who developed ovarian hyperstimulation syndrome showed that there is no evidence for an increased prevalence of hyperinsulinism among women who developed OHSS[119].

Source of the peritoneal fluid

In the absence of ovarian stimulation, the volume of normally present peritoneal fluid was found to be directly related to cyclical ovarian activity; it was consistently low in normal males[120], postmenopausal women and women on oral contraceptives[121]. Abdalla and Rizk[122] found that, in normal, ovulatory women, the volume of peritoneal fluid was diminished in the early proliferative phase and increased until the time of ovulation. Following ovulation, there was a sudden increase in the volume of peritoneal fluid, which lingered throughout the luteal phase and diminished at the commencement of menses[121]. Since this peritoneal fluid production was not dependent on the patency or presence of the Fallopian tubes or uterus, its origin was felt to be ovarian or peritoneal.

Yarali and co-workers[123] assessed the direct ovarian contribution to ascites formation in OHSS in the rabbit by the microsurgical isolation of the ovaries from the peritoneal cavity. Despite extraperitonealization of both ovaries, ascites occurred in all animals. This was considered to be evidence against a direct ovarian contribution to ascites formation. They postulated that the development of ascites was caused by a substance that increased capillary permeability of the peritoneum and the omentum, and possibly the pleura.

Mediators of increased capillary permeability

Estrogens

Asch and co-workers[124] reported an overall incidence of 1% for severe OHSS, but when the estradiol concentration on the day of hCG administration was more than 22 000 pmol/l, the incidence of severe OHSS rose to 38%. Estrogens were shown to induce increased capillary permeability of the uterine and ovarian circulation. Because levels of estrogen are greatly increased in OHSS patients, it was postulated that the increase in its production and levels causes the increase in capillary permeability. However, large doses of estrogens could not reproduce OHSS in the rabbit model[125]. Furthermore, Pellicer and colleagues[126] reported moderate to severe OHSS during pregnancy in a woman with partial 17,20-desmolase deficiency and very low serum estradiol concentrations, therefore questioning the role of estradiol in the pathogenesis of OHSS.

Levy and colleagues[127] presented a case report of a woman with hypogonadotropic hypogonadism who developed severe OHSS during ovulation induction with urinary FSH and hCG in the presence of low circulating estradiol concentrations. The authors emphasized that the serum estradiol concentration is not a completely reliable predictor of OHSS.

The ovarian renin–angiotensin system

Fernandez and co-workers[128] demonstrated preovulatory follicular fluid levels of prorenin up to 12 times higher than those of plasma prorenin after gonadotropin stimulation. The magnitude of the mid-cycle rise of prorenin in response to hCG is related to the number of ovarian follicles.

Navot and colleagues[129] found a direct correlation between plasma renin activity and the severity of OHSS. A report by Ong and colleagues[36] of patients with OHSS found pronounced elevations in plasma renin activity and plasma aldosterone concentrations despite significant therapeutic plasma volume expansion.

Delbaere and co-workers[130] measured total renin, active renin, prorenin, renin activity and aldosterone in the plasma and ascites of nine patients who developed severe OHSS. Total renin and prorenin concentrations were significantly higher in the ascites than in the plasma.

Sahin and colleagues[131] investigated the possible effects of the angiotensin-converting enzyme (ACE) inhibitor cilazapril and angiotensin II antagonist saralasin on ovulation, ovarian steroiodogenesis and ascites formation in OHSS in the rabbit model. They concluded that the ACE inhibitor cilazapril and the angiotensin II antagonist saralasin did not prevent ascites formation in OHSS. The ovarian renin–angiotensin system may not be the only factor acting in ascites formation in OHSS. Teruel and associates[132] studied the hemodynamic state and the role of angiotensin II in OHSS in the rabbit. ACE inhibition decreases the incidence of OHSS in the rabbit model by 30%, suggesting that angiotensin II may play a role in the formation of ascites.

Teruel and associates[133] studied the effect of ACE inhibitor on renal function in OHSS in the rabbit. They found that angiotensin II may play a significant role in this phenomenon, since ACE inhibition normalized the pressure–natriuresis relationship.

Morris and colleagues[134] conducted an experiment to determine whether the use of the ACE inhibitor enalapril would prevent the occurrence of OHSS in the rabbit model. ACE inhibition resulted in a 40% decrease in the occurrence of OHSS in the rabbit model. It is tempting to speculate that ACE inhibitors may be useful in the treatment of OHSS in humans. Since severe OHSS usually occurs with pregnancy, possible fetal effects are important. However, ACE inhibitors may alter steroid synthesis within the ovary[135] and may inhibit ovulation[136], resulting in retention of oocytes and follicular fluid, leading to larger ovaries.

Prostaglandins

Prostaglandins were proposed as possible mediators by Schenker and Polishuk[137] and prostaglandin synthetase inhibitors were used to prevent the fluid shift responsible for the manifestations of OHSS[13,138]. However, Pride and colleagues[139] found that indomethacin, in pharmacological doses, did not influence the clinical features of OHSS (ovarian weight and ascites formation). Therefore, the rationale of treatment of OHSS with non-steroidal anti-inflammatory drugs should be seriously questioned[3,122].

Balasch and co-workers[115] suggested that renal prostaglandin (PG) E_2, and PGI_2, by antagonizing the renal vasoconstrictor effect of angiotensin II and norepinephrine (noradrenaline), play a major role in the maintenance of renal function in severe OHSS.

Vascular endothelial growth factor

Rizk and colleagues[3] extensively reviewed the role of vascular endothelial growth factor (VEGF) in the pathogenesis of OHSS. VEGF is a member of a family of heparin-binding proteins that act directly on endothelial cells to induce proliferation and angiogenesis[140]. In vivo, VEGF is a powerful mediator of vessel permeability[141]. It is also strongly implicated in the initiation and development of angiogenesis in the developing embryo[142] and in adult tissue undergoing profound angiogenesis such as cycling endometrium[143] and the luteinizing follicle[144]. In addition to its physiological role, VEGF is implicated as a critical angiogenic factor in the development of tumor vascularization[145] and the excessive neovascularization seen in conditions such as rheumatoid arthritis[146]. Its levels are also increased in the peritoneal fluid of women with endometriosis compared with normal controls[147,148].

Kamat and colleagues[149] used immunohistochemistry to demonstrate the increased activity of VEGF with Graafian follicle development, which showed strong cytoplasmic staining for VEGF with the formation of the corpus luteum.

VEGF may also play a role in the regulation of cyclic ovarian angiogenesis, and its ability to increase vascular permeability may be an important factor in the production of Fallopian tube effluent and fluid formation in ovarian cysts. Gordon and co-workers[150] showed that, in normal ovaries, VEGF within healthy follicles was localized to the theca cell layer with minimal VEGF peptide detected in the granulosa cell layer. VEGF was not expressed in atretic follicles or degenerating corpus luteum. However, intense VEGF immunostaining was observed within the highly vascularized corpora lutea. In normal ovaries from postmenopausal women, VEGF was detected only in epithelial inclusion cysts and sera cystadenoma. The authors concluded that, during reproductive life, VEGF plays an important role in growth and maintenance of ovarian follicles and corpus luteum by mediating angiogenesis. In addition, VEGF within the Fallopian tube luminal epithelium increased the vascular permeability and modulated the tubal luminal secretions. Similarly, VEGF in the epithelial lining of benign ovarian neoplasms may contribute to fluid formation in ovarian cysts.

Yan and associates[151] were the first to demonstrate the presence of VEGF mRNA in human luteinized granulosa cells. Neulen and colleagues[152], from the same group, later showed that the expression of VEGF mRNA is enhanced by hCG in a dose- and time-dependent fashion. VEGF mRNA expression in granulosa cells was enhanced by increasing amounts of hCG with maximum enhancement at 1 IU of hCG/ml of medium. Further dosage increments revealed no additional augmentation of VEGF expression. VEGF mRNA expression also reached maximum values at 3 h.

McClure and colleagues[153] investigated the role of VEGF in OHSS. They found strong evidence of the role of VEGF in OHSS. Hybridization studies have demonstrated VEGF mRNA expression in the rat ovary[145], but predominantly after the LH surge. This surge is also essential for OHSS. Luteal phase treatment with GnRH-a to suppress LH secretion decreased VEGF mRNA expression, implying that such expression is dependent on LH[153]. Similarly, luteal phase supplementation with progesterone rather than hCG decreased the likelihood of OHSS. Also, ovarian angiogenesis is normally restricted to a single follicle. Therefore, the agent responsible for ovarian follicular capillary permeability may not be contained within the individual follicles but may spill over into the peritoneal cavity. Moreover, it has been demonstrated that VEGF is the major capillary permeability factor in OHSS ascites. These results led the authors to conclude that the major capillary permeability agent in OHSS ascitic fluid is VEGF.

Gomez and colleagues[154] found that administration of moderate and high doses of gonadotropins to female rats increases ovarian VEGF and VEGF receptor-2 expression that is associated with vascular hyperpermeability.

McElhinney and co-workers[155] studied the variations in serum VEGF binding profiles and the development of OHSS, and found that patients who do not develop OHSS appear to have a high-molecular-weight protein that binds VEGF to a greater degree than occurs in patients who develop OHSS.

Gomez and colleagues[156] reported that VEGF receptor-2 activation induces vascular permeability in hyperstimulated rats, and this effect is prevented by receptor blockade.

Mathur and associates[157] investigated whether serum VEGF levels can distinguish highly responsive women who subsequently develop OHSS from women with a similar ovarian response who do not. They found that serum VEGF levels are poorly predictive of subsequent OHSS in highly responsive women undergoing assisted conception.

Artini and colleagues[158] studied VEGF, interleukin-6 (IL-6) and IL-2 in serum and follicular fluid of patients with OHSS. These patients presented follicular fluid IL-6 levels higher than in both patients at risk and controls ($p < 0.05$). On the day of the oocyte retrieval, patients developing OHSS showed serum and follicular VEGF values higher than those of patients at risk ($p < 0.05$). Serum and follicular fluid IL-2 levels showed no differences between the examined groups. IL-2, IL-6 and VEGF values were not correlated with each other. The authors concluded that angiogenesis and inflammation processes are both present in severe OHSS.

Krasnow and colleagues[159] measured VEGF in serum, peritoneal fluid and follicular fluid of eight patients considered at risk for OHSS. Serum VEGF was significantly higher in the group who developed severe OHSS compared with those who did not. The detection of high serum VEGF levels in the circulation of patients with OHSS suggests that this factor may play a role in the pathogenesis of OHSS. The large amount of VEGF in follicular fluid relative to serum or peritoneal fluid suggests that the ovary is a significant source of VEGF. In an unstimulated menstrual cycle, the development of a single corpus luteum does not result in OHSS. In patients with severe OHSS in whom VEGF was significantly higher in the serum, a mean of 21 follicles were present before hCG administration. It is possible that the hCG that rescues the corpus luteum results in an increase in ovarian VEGF secretion, which in turn causes an exacerbation of OHSS, confirming the work of Neulen and colleagues[152]. The effect of follicular aspiration on the incidence of OHSS has been debated in clinical studies[79].

Abramov and co-workers[160] followed the kinetics of VEGF in the plasma of seven patients with severe OHSS from the time of admission to hospital until clinical resolution. High levels of VEGF were detected in the plasma of all patients admitted for severe OHSS compared with controls, who received similar ovulation-induction regimens but did not develop OHSS after IVF and embryo transfer. Levels dropped significantly, along with clinical improvement, reaching minimum values after complete resolution. A statistically significant correlation was found between plasma VEGF levels and certain biological characteristics of OHSS and of capillary leakage such as leukocytosis with increasing VEGF levels. Ascitic fluid obtained from the study patients also confirmed high VEGF levels. These findings suggest the involvement of VEGF in the pathogenesis of capillary leakage in OHSS.

In a prospective cohort study, Enskog and colleagues[161] evaluated whether differences in plasma VEGF(165) concentrations exist during gonadotropin stimulation in IVF patients developing severe OHSS, compared with matched controls. They found that patients developing OHSS do not have raised plasma VEGF(165) levels during gonadotropin stimulation. The lack of positive correlation between VEGF(165) levels and follicle numbers/progesterone levels in the OHSS group suggests a disruption in OHSS of normal, controlled, follicular VEGF expression.

Lee and associates[162] studied the relationship between serum and follicular fluid levels of VEGF, estradiol and progesterone in patients undergoing IVF, to quantify the effects of hCG on serum levels of VEGF during early pregnancy and to report serial measurements of serum and ascitic fluid levels of VEGF in a patient with severe OHSS. They found a significant ovarian contribution to the circulating VEGF levels in early pregnancy. They concluded that elevated serum VEGF levels may be a factor in the etiology of OHSS symptoms.

Agarwal and co-workers[163] suggest that serum VEGF concentrations in IVF cycles predict the risk of OHSS, and that VEGF rise may have an advantage over estradiol concentration, the number of follicles and the number of oocytes, which individually predict only 15–25% of cases.

Kitajima and colleagues[164] found that GnRH-a administration reduced VEGF, VEGF receptors and vascular permeability of the ovaries of hyperstimulated rats. They speculated that GnRH-a treatment may prevent early OHSS by reducing vascular permeability through the decrease in VEGF and its receptors.

The prognostic importance of serial cytokine changes in ascites and pleural effusion in women with severe OHSS was evaluated and compared with ascitic fluid in IVF cycles before oocyte retrieval[165]. The results suggest that local cytokines might be involved in the evolution of severe OHSS and possibly serve as a prognostic marker for this syndrome. Geva and colleagues[166] concluded that preovulatory follicular fluid levels should not serve as a possible predictive factor for development of OHSS. The increased capillary permeability found in OHSS may be due to its systemic effect.

A soluble receptor for VEGF has been detected that antagonizes the activity of VEGF[167]. This receptor is produced by endothelial cells, allowing them to modify their response to circulating VEGF. Administration of the soluble receptor is able to bind circulating VEGF, thus preventing it from interacting with the endothelial cell receptor[167]. Its clinical applicability in OHSS is awaited with interest.

Interleukins

Recent investigations in ovarian physiology have established the role of cytokines in the process of ovulation[168]. Rizk and colleagues[3] have reviewed the role of interleukins in the pathogenesis of OHSS. D'Ambrogio and associates[169] found that serum VEGF levels before starting gonadotropin treatment in women

who developed moderate forms of OHSS showed no significant difference from those in the control group. Chen and co-workers[170] suggest that follicular fluid IL-6 concentrations at the time of oocyte retrieval and serum IL-8 concentrations on the day of embryo transfer may serve as early predictors for this syndrome.

Interleukin-2 Interleukin-2 does not appear to be at the center of the cascade of events leading to OHSS. Barak and associates[171] addressed the correlation between IL-2 and estradiol, progesterone and testosterone levels in periovulatory follicles of IVF patients. They found no correlation between follicular fluid IL-2 concentration and follicular fluid estradiol and progesterone concentrations. In addition, they found no correlation between follicular fluid IL-2 and serum estradiol concentrations. Orvieto and colleagues[172] elected to use pooled aspirated follicular fluid from each patient rather than to evaluate each follicle separately. They demonstrated a significantly higher IL-2 concentration in follicular fluid obtained at the time of oocyte recovery from patients who developed OHSS, compared with the control group. The authors suggested a possible role for follicular fluid IL-2 concentrations in the prediction of OHSS.

In a multicenter study, Revel and co-workers[173] found IL-2 levels to be undetectable in all samples of peritoneal fluid from patients with severe OHSS. It therefore appears that intraperitoneal leakage of IL-2 in OHSS is mediated, if indeed IL-2 is central in the cascade of pathogenic events.

Interleukin-6 Circulating levels of IL-6 increase in a variety of acute illnesses, including septic shock[176]. IL-6 mediates the acute phase response to injury, a systemic reaction characterized by leukocytosis, increased vascular permeability and increased levels of acute phase proteins synthesized by the liver. IL-6 has been described in the follicular fluid in women undergoing stimulation[177]. A role for IL-6 in normal ovarian function has been suggested by the observation that IL-6 RNA is produced during the neovascularization or angiogenesis that occurs in the development of ovarian follicles[178]. The rapid growth and luteinization of the stimulated ovary require extensive angiogenesis.

Friedlander and co-workers[179] examined the role of IL-6 and other cytokines in four patients with OHSS. Five healthy women at the time of elective laparoscopic tubal ligation served as controls. Control serum was also obtained from healthy volunteers, and control peritoneal fluid was obtained from patients on peritoneal dialysis. Both serum and ascitic fluid from women with OHSS contained significantly greater levels of IL-6 than control serum and peritoneal fluid. No significant differences in tumor necrosis factor (TNF) levels in serum, ascitic fluid or peritoneal fluid could be found by enzyme-linked immunosorbent assay (ELISA) or bioassay. The mechanism by which IL-6 might mediate the pathogenesis of this syndrome is not clear. However, elevated levels of plasma IL-6 have been recorded in both acute pancreatitis and acute alcoholic hepatitis, conditions in which ascites and hypotension are common complications of severe disease[180]. It was also found that the albumin level was markedly lower than would be expected in two of the patients with severe OHSS[179]. This observation provides further clinical support for the hypothesis that IL-6 plays a key pathophysiological role in OHSS, because IL-6 is a potent inhibitor of hepatic albumin production, switching the liver to synthesis of acute phase reactants[181].

More recently, Loret de Mola and co-workers[182] examined the production and immunolocalization of IL-6 in patients with OHSS. Significantly higher serum and ascites IL-6 levels were found in OHSS compared with postovulatory serum and peritoneal fluid from normal controls, or serum after menotropin stimulation. The same authors, having found a significant increase in cytokines in OHSS, addressed the possibility of whether preovulatory cytokine levels could predict the occurrence of OHSS[183]. Cytokine preovulatory values were similar in OHSS compared with controlled ovarian hyperstimulation. They therefore concluded that cytokine measurement cannot be used to predict the occurrence of OHSS prior to the administration of hCG.

Abramov and colleagues[160] studied the kinetics of four inflammatory cytokines in the plasma of patients who developed severe OHSS after IVF. Higher concentrations of IL-1, IL-6 and TNF were detected in all individuals upon admission for severe OHSS. Concentrations dropped significantly with clinical improvements, with normal values recorded after complete resolution. A statistically significant correlation was found between plasma cytokine concentration and certain biological characteristics of the syndrome, such as leukocytosis, increased hematocrit and elevated plasma estradiol concentrations.

Interleukin-8 IL-8 is a chemoattractant and an activating cytokine to neutrophils, and a potent angiogenic agent. IL-8 is produced by a number of cell types including monocytes, endothelial cells, fibroblasts, mesothelial cells and endometrial stromal cells. Significantly higher peritoneal fluid levels of IL-8 were found in 12 patients with severe OHSS compared with 20 controls[173]. However, no statistical significance was observed in the serum levels of patients and controls. This might imply a direct spill of IL-8 from the ovaries to the peritoneal fluid. Abdalla and Rizk[122] suggested that IL-8 may mediate the intraperitoneal acute phase response seen in OHSS.

Interleukin-10 Manolopoulos and colleagues[174] found high concentrations of IL-10 in peritoneal fluid and suggested a role of this anti-inflammatory cytokine during OHSS. 17β-Estradiol and progesterone were elevated in peritoneal fluid and serum during OHSS, but no correlation with IL-10 concentrations was found. Therefore, they assumed that IL-10 has a role in OHSS as a local mediator of inflammation; however, it presents different aspects of OHSS compared with the sex steroids 17β-estradiol and progesterone.

The role of endothelial cells in the pathogenesis of OHSS was studied by Albert and colleagues[175]. They showed that the endothelium may be a primary target of hCG, causing an acute release of VEGF and a significant increase in IL-6, and resulting in an autocrine–paracrine action that may increase vascular permeability

Angiogenin

Aboulghar and associates[184] investigated the possible role of angiogenin in the pathogenesis of OHSS. The study group consisted of ten healthy women who developed severe OHSS, following ovarian stimulation by the long GnRH-a/hMG protocols for IVF. A control group of ten patients underwent stimulation with the same protocol and did not develop OHSS. Blood samples were taken from the OHSS group on the day of admission to hospital for treatment, and in the control group 1 week after oocyte retrieval. Ascitic fluid samples were aspirated during the routine aspiration of ascitic fluid as treatment for severe OHSS, and peritoneal fluid samples were aspirated transvaginally before oocyte retrieval in the control group.

In the OHSS group, the mean serum level of angiogenin, mean ascitic fluid level of hCG administration and the mean hematocrit were 8390 ± 6836 ng/ml, 2794 ± 1024 ng/ml, 6300 ± 2450 pg/ml and 46.6 ± 4.4, as compared with 234 ± 91 ng/ml, 254 ± 105 ng/ml, 1850 ± 1100 pg/ml and 36.8 ± 4.6 in the control group, respectively. The difference was highly significant between all parameters. Angiogenin seems to play an important role in the formation of neovascularization responsible for the development of OHSS.

Increased erythrocyte aggregation

Levin and colleagues[185] conducted a study to evaluate the erythrocyte aggregation in OHSS. The degree of erythrocyte aggregation is enhanced in the peripheral venous blood of patients with both controlled ovarian hyperstimulation and OHSS. This finding, which is known to cause capillary leak, may contribute to the pathophysiology of OHSS.

MANAGEMENT OF OHSS

Rizk and Aboulghar[10] established that the first priority in the management of OHSS should be given to prediction and prevention. The basis for the clinical treatment and management is reviewed below.

Prediction

Rizk[4,186] stated that the most effective treatment of OHSS is its precise prediction and active prevention. Abdalla and Rizk[122] advised the combined use of ultrasound and endocrine monitoring of follicular development for the precise prediction of OHSS during ovarian stimulation (Figure 2).

Endocrine monitoring

Haning and colleagues[102] compared plasma 17β-estradiol, 24-h urinary estriol glucuronide and ultrasound as predictors of ovulation in 70 ovulation induction cycles. Plasma estradiol was the best predictor of the hyperstimulation score. No case of OHSS occurred when the plasma estradiol level was < 1000 pg/ml, and the authors considered 4000 pg/ml to be the level above which hCG should be withheld, because OHSS occurred in all pregnancies when the estradiol level was > 4000 pg/ml. Several authors have reported severe OHSS with peak follicular plasma estradiol levels well below 1500 pg/ml. On the other

hand, only a small fraction of patients with excessive estrogen levels will develop severe OHSS[187].

Two studies from California highlight how the prevalence of OHSS could vary among patients with similar estradiol levels. Asch and colleagues[124] observed severe OHSS in 38% of patients with serum levels of estradiol > 6000 pg/ml. No OHSS was observed in patients with serum estradiol levels < 3500 pg/ml. On the other hand, Morris and colleagues[188] from the University of Southern California observed only 17% of OHSS cases in 34 patients with serum estradiol levels > 6000 pg/ml.

Follicular monitoring by ultrasound

Ultrasound is widely used for monitoring follicular development in assisted conception. The number, size and pattern of distribution of the follicles are important in the prediction of OHSS. Tal and co-workers[189] found a positive correlation between the mean number of immature follicles and OHSS. The diagnosis of polycystic ovaries at ultrasound examination (the necklace sign) improved the prediction of OHSS to 79% in the Belgian multicenter study[70]. Blankstein and colleagues[190] stated that a decrease in the fraction of mature follicles and an increase in the fraction of very small follicles correlated with an augmented risk for the development of severe OHSS.

Danninger and associates[191] studied the baseline ovarian volume prior to stimulation, to investigate whether it would be a suitable predictor for the risk of OHSS. They performed three-dimensional volumetric ultrasound assessment of the ovaries prior to ovarian stimulation and on the day of hCG injection. There was a significant correlation between the baseline ovarian volume and the subsequent occurrence of OHSS. The authors suggested that volumetry of the ovaries could help to detect patients at risk.

Research into the use of transvaginal color flow Doppler for prediction of OHSS is currently being undertaken[122]. Moohan and co-workers[192] assessed the intraovarian blood flow in relation to the severity of OHSS by using transabdominal ultrasonography with color flow and pulsed Doppler imaging. The authors suggested that measurements of intraovarian vascular resistance in patients undergoing controlled ovarian hyperstimulation may help in predicting those patients at particular risk of developing OHSS. The authors agreed with Golan and colleagues[14] that the combination of estradiol and ultrasonography offers

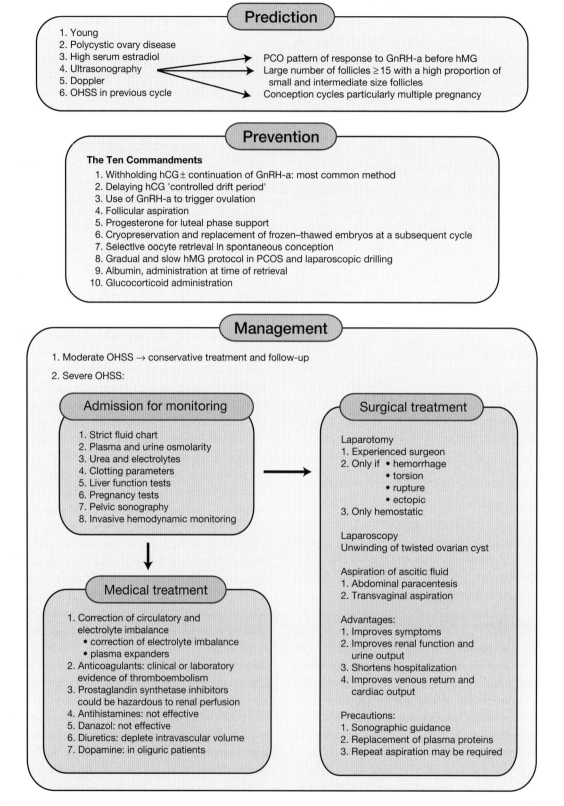

Figure 2 Prediction, prevention and management of ovarian hyperstimulation syndrome (OHSS). PCO, polycystic ovary; GnRH-a, gonadotropin releasing hormone agonist; hMG, human menopausal gonadotropin; hCG, human chorionic gonadotropin; PCOS, polycystic ovarian syndrome

the best chance for the prediction of OHSS. Ultrasonographic follow-up of the leading follicles should be used for the determination of hCG administration and serum estradiol measurement, and sonographic visualization of small and intermediate follicles should be used to determine the likelihood of OHSS.

Prevention

Rizk[186] suggested the use of 'ten commandments' for the prevention of OHSS (Figure 2).

Withholding hCG

Rizk and Aboulgar[10] found that withholding hCG is the most commonly used method of preventing OHSS in patients predicted to be at high risk of developing the syndrome. Strict criteria for withholding hCG will lower and possibly abolish the incidence of OHSS, but at the expense of canceling the cycle. Rizk and Nawar[9] highlighted that cancellation of the IVF cycle creates a frustrating situation for both the physician and the patient. The serum estradiol levels above which hCG should be withheld vary widely among different centers[10]. Schenker and Weinstein[13] withheld hCG when serum estradiol levels exceeded 800 pg/ml. Blankstein and colleagues[190] suggested 1700 pg/ml, and Haning and associates[102] accepted 4000 pg/ml as the upper limit.

Delaying hCG administration (coasting)

Serum estradiol levels at the time of ovulation triggering have been considered as a predictor of the risk of developing OHSS. It has therefore been proposed to postpone hCG administration to allow the serum estradiol levels to drop below a certain threshold. This has been termed 'coasting' or 'controlled drift period'. This method has the great attraction of the cycle not being canceled, fresh embryos still being transferred and no additional gonadotropins or medications being used. Although coasting is a very effective method to reduce the incidence of severe OHSS it does not abolish the syndrome completely, as some patients (2.5%) in this group of hyper-responders still present with the severe form of the syndrome[193].

Coasting acts through down-regulation of VEGF gene expression and protein secretion[194]. The fact that medium and small size follicles are more sensitive to undergoing atretic changes is of crucial relevance in both steroid and vasoactive mediator secretion.

Garcia-Velasco and co-workers[194] observed that a significantly higher percentage of granulosa lutein cells become apoptotic after coasting. This difference is even greater for immature follicles.

Currently, this is the most popular method among physicians to prevent OHSS[195]. More than 15 studies have been published, and several reviews have analyzed the impact of coasting on OHSS (Table 7). These studies are very heterogeneous, and only one trial had a randomized control design comparing a coasting approach with early unilateral follicular aspiration.

Several authors have reported successful reduction in severe OHSS by delaying hCG or 'coasting'[197–199]. Rabinovici and colleagues[197] were the first to report their experience with the rescue of 12 gonadotropin-induced cycles that were liable to develop hyperstimulation. Treatment with hMG was stopped in 12 patients who either had overt biochemical overstimulation or were at an increased risk of hyperstimulation. The duration of the pause in treatment ranged from 2 to 10 days. In nine patients, including six who were overstimulated, the plasma estradiol levels declined despite the continuing growth of most follicles. None of these patients conceived following hCG. Pregnancies occurred in three patients whose estradiol levels continued to rise until the day of hCG. They therefore concluded that, although rescue of the overstimulated cycles is sometimes possible, the resulting conceptions seem to be associated with a continuing rise of estradiol during the period of treatment pause.

Urman and colleagues[198] studied 40 cycles in 32 patients with PCOS. The authors used a controlled drift period to avoid cancellation. The clinical pregnancy rate per cycle was 25% (10/40). OHSS occurred in 2.5% (1/40). The authors did not share the same conclusion about the relationship between pregnancy and the rise of estradiol suggested by Rabinovici and colleagues[197].

Sher and co-workers[199] suggested that prolonged coasting in GnRH-a/hMG/FSH cycles could prevent life-endangering complications of OHSS. They withheld menotropins in 17 patients whose serum estradiol exceeded 6000 pg/ml and continued daily GnRH-a until estradiol levels had fallen below 3000 pg/ml, and then 10 000 IU of hCG was administered to trigger ovulation. The estradiol levels continued to rise rapidly in the 48 h following initiation of the coasting period, then plateaued and began to fall 96–168 h after the menotropins were stopped. The coasting period lasted

Table 7   The 'coasting' approach: studies between 1995 and 2002. Modified from reference 196

Authors	Year	Design	n	Coasting duration (days)	Result: moderate/ severe OHSS*
Shet *et al.*	1995	descriptive	51	6.1	12/0 (0)
Benadiva *et al.*	1997	retrospective	22	1.9 ± 0.9	1/0 (0)
Tortoriello *et al.*	1998	retrospective	44	2.6 ± 0.3	6/3 (6.8)
Dhont *et al.*	1998	retrospective	120	1.94 ± 0.8	7/1 (0.8)
Lee *et al.*	1998	retrospective	20	2.8 ± 1.3	—/4 (20)
Fluker *et al.*	1999	descriptive	63	5.3 ± 0.2	11/1 (1.6)
Waldenstrom *et al.*	1999	descriptive	65	4.3	11/2 (3.1)
Egbase *et al.*	1999	prospective	15	4.9 ± 1.6	3/0 (0)
Dechaud *et al.*	2000	descriptive	14	1.6	—/0 (0)
Ohata *et al.*	2000	descriptive	5	4	5/0 (0)
Aboulghar *et al.*	2000	retrospective	24	2.92 ± 0.92	4/0 (0)
Al-Shawaf *et al.*	2001	retrospective	50	3.4 ± 1.6	2/0 (0)
Egbase *et al.*	2002	descriptive	102	3 (fixed)	0 (0)

*Number in parentheses is percentage with severe ovarian hyperstimulation syndrome (OHSS)

between 4 and 9 days and the day of hCG administration fell on cycle days 12–16. Six of the 17 cycles (35%) produced viable pregnancies. All 17 patients developed signs of grade 2 or 3 OHSS but none developed severe OHSS.

Benadiva and co-workers[200] reported that withholding gonadotropin administration was an effective alternative to prevent the development of severe OHSS in a high-risk population. Although the risk of cancellation cannot be completely eliminated, this strategy can provide a high pregnancy rate without the need to repeat multiple frozen-thawed cycles.

Decrease in hCG dosage

Abdalla and colleagues[201] reported a significantly lower successful oocyte recovery in patients who received 2000 IU of hCG (77.3%) compared with patients who received either 5000 IU of hCG (95.5%) or 10 000 IU of hCG (98.1%; $p < 0.001$). Abdalla and Rizk highlighted the limitations of using a small dose of hCG to prevent OHSS, as shown in this study[122].

GnRH antagonist as an alternative to the long agonist protocol

In a recent Cochrane review[202], the efficacy of GnRH antagonist was compared with the long agonist

protocol in assisted conception. The overall odds ratio (OR) for the prevention of premature LH surge was 1.76 (95% confidence interval (CI) 0.75–4.16), which was not statistically significant. There were significantly fewer pregnancies in the GnRH antagonist group (OR 0.79, 95% CI 0.63–0.99). There was no statistically significant reduction in the occurrence of severe OHSS (relative risk 0.50; OR 0.79, 95% CI 0.22–1.18)

The use of GnRH-a to trigger ovulation

In gonadotropin cycles   Revel and Casper[203] carefully analyzed the use of GnRH-a instead of hCG to trigger ovulation in cycles where gonadotropins and clomiphene citrate had been used for ovulation induction. They evaluated the efficacy of GnRH-a and pursued the concept of whether GnRH-a would prevent OHSS. They analyzed the data from uncontrolled clinical trials as well as controlled studies comparing GnRH-a with hCG in terms of its ability to trigger the LH surge or to prevent OHSS. In uncontrolled studies, when GnRH-a was used to trigger ovulation, the incidence of OHSS was 0.9% (3/334). In controlled studies, the incidence of OHSS was 1.5% in the hCG group compared with 0.7% in the GnRH-a group. It appears therefore that

GnRH-a is as effective as hCG in triggering ovulation in gonadotropin-only cycles, with only half the incidence of OHSS.

Gonen and colleagues[204] and Itskovitz and colleagues[205] used the initial flare-up effect of the agonist to achieve ovulation and subsequent pregnancies. In patients at risk of OHSS, intranasal buserelin (200 mg three times at 8-h intervals) was used to trigger ovulation and a 22% pregnancy rate resulted, without any cases of OHSS[206]. Imoedemhe and co-workers[101] used GnRH-a in 38 women considered at risk of OHSS, having serum estradiol levels > 4000 pg/ml, with 11 pregnancies and no cases of OHSS. The major limitation to the use of GnRH-a is that it could not be used in cycles where ovarian stimulation with hMG was performed after pituitary desensitization using GnRH-a[122].

In GnRH-antagonist/gonadotropin cycles Rizk[207] reviewed the approaches that have been successfully used to induce the final stages of oocyte meiosis maturation in GnRH antagonist and gonadotropin cycles. These include hCG, GnRH-a, native GnRH, recombinant LH and withdrawal of GnRH antagonist. GnRH-a has been successfully shown to induce these final stages of oocyte maturation in monkeys and humans[208]. Felberbaum and colleagues[209] and Olivennes and associates[210] elegantly demonstrated ovulation triggering by GnRH-a after GnRH antagonist treatment.

From the point of view of OHSS stimulation, at least two studies suggested the safe use of GnRH-a to trigger ovulation in women who underwent ovulation induction with recombinant FSH and GnRH antagonist. Itskovitz-Eldor and colleagues[211] reported the use of a single bolus of GnRH-a (decapeptyl) 0.2 mg to trigger ovulation in women at risk for OHSS after treatment with recombinant FSH and ganirelix. All women had serum estradiol levels greater than 3000 pg/ml and more than 20 follicles, and none developed signs or symptoms of OHSS, and four conceived.

Bracero and associates[212] who studied 19 women who underwent controlled ovarian hyperstimulation for IVF using gonadotropins and ganirelix 0.5 mg. They concluded that leuprolide acetate instead of hCG should be used for triggering ovulation to prevent OHSS in cycles where gonadotropins and GnRH antagonist have been used.

Recombinant human LH to trigger ovulation

hCG is a promoter of OHSS, whereas an endogenous LH surge rarely causes OHSS. A prospective randomized, double-blind, multicenter study evaluated the safety of recombinant LH in patients undergoing IVF compared with 5000 IU of hCG. The European recombinant LH study group concluded that a dose of between 5000 and 15 000 IU of r-hLH induced significantly fewer moderate and severe cases of OHSS[213].

Follicular aspiration

The incidence of OHSS is not increased in IVF cycles, despite very high serum estradiol levels and multiple follicular developments prior to hCG administration[186]. The first case of severe OHSS in an IVF program was reported by Friedman and associates[214]. The incidence of moderate and severe OHSS in the major IVF series varied from 0.6% to 6.0%. Rabinowitz and colleagues[197] postulated that multiple follicular aspirations, which empty most of the follicles of follicular fluid granulosa cells, may have a protective effect against OHSS. Four of the 81 patients in the series who developed OHSS during a cycle where egg retrieval was canceled did not develop the syndrome in cycles when multiple follicular punctures and aspiration were performed.

Follicular aspiration at the time of oocyte retrieval In a retrospective study, Aboulghar and co-workers[79] found that follicular aspiration had no protective effect on the occurrence of OHSS. They studied the incidence of moderate and severe OHSS following the same superovulation protocol in 182 patients who underwent follicular aspiration, compared with 137 patients who did not. Anovulatory infertility, particularly PCOS, was the main predisposing factor in OHSS, and follicular aspiration had no protective effect.

Follicular aspiration prior to hCG In a prospective randomized study, Egbase and associates[215] performed unilateral follicular aspiration prior to administration of hCG for the prevention of severe OHSS. They concluded that unilateral follicular aspiration does not reduce the incidence of severe OHSS in women at risk.

Intravenous albumin administration

Asch and co-workers were the first to suggest that intravenous albumin during follicular aspiration could potentially be useful to prevent OHSS[216]. Following the publication of their trial, two groups of investigators conducted prospective trials and agreed with their conclusion[217,218]. Other authors have disagreed with the conclusion[219–222].

The effectiveness of human albumin administration in prevention of severe OHSS was reviewed[223] using the Cochrane 'menstrual disorders and subfertility group' literature search strategy. Only randomized controlled trials comparing the effect of human albumin compared with placebo or no treatment were included. Seven randomized controlled trials were identified, five of which met the inclusion criteria and enrolled 378 women: 193 in the albumin group and 185 in the control group. There was a significant reduction in the occurrence of OHSS in the albumin group (OR 0.28, 95% CI 0.11–0.73); the relative risk was 0.35 (95% CI 0.14–0.87) and the absolute risk reduction was 5.5. For every 18 women at risk for severe OHSS, albumin infusion may save one more case of OHSS. Based on this review, there is a clear benefit from the administration of intravenous albumin at the time of oocyte retrieval[223]. However, this delicate topic remains controversial.

Experience in subjects with different forms of third-space fluid accumulation have shown that albumin is efficacious in preventing and correcting hemodynamic instability. Using a similar approach in an effort to increase the oncotic pressure and to reverse the leakage of fluids from the intravascular space, high-risk subjects for severe OHSS were treated with albumin[216,217]. The authors proposed that the role of albumin in prevention of OHSS is multifactorial. First, it acts to sequester vasoactive substances released from the corpora lutea. Albumin has a half-life of 10–15 days. Patients generally develop OHSS symptoms 3–10 days after hCG injection, regardless of the embryo transfer. Timely administration of albumin, during oocyte retrieval and immediately following, may serve to bind and inactivate this factor. It also serves to sequester any additional substances which may have been synthesized as a result of OHSS. The oncotic properties of albumin also serve to maintain intravascular volume and prevent the ensuing effects of hypovolemia, ascites and hemoconcentration.

Hydroxyethyl starch solution administration

Rizk[207] reviewed the role of synthetic macromolecules used to prevent OHSS and avoid the potential risks from using human products such as albumin.

Hydroxyethyl starch (HES) is a synthetic colloid, glycogen-like polysacharride which is derived from amylopectin. It has been used as an effective volume expander and is available in several types of molecular weight with different chemical properties. Graf and colleagues[224] used 1000 ml of 6% HES at the time of oocyte retrieval and an additional 500 ml 48 h later in 100 patients considered at high risk of OHSS, with estradiol > 11 000 pmole/l and 20 follicles or more. They compared the outcome with that of a historical control group of 82 patients without any prophylactic measure. Seven cases of severe OHSS and 32 cases of moderate OHSS occurred in the control group, compared with two cases of severe and ten cases of moderate OHSS in the HES group ($p < 0.05$ and $p < 0.001$, respectively). Konig and colleagues[225] in a prospective, randomized trial evaluated HES and placebo in patients with estradiol levels > 1500 pg/ml and ten follicles on the day of hCG. The dose of HES was 1000 ml after oocyte retrieval. In the HES group, there was one case of moderate OHSS and no severe cases, compared with six cases of moderate OHSS and one case of severe OHSS in the control group.

Glucocorticoid administration

The pathophysiology of OHSS suggests involvement of an inflammatory mechanism during development of the fluid leakage associated with the syndrome. Therefore, investigators hypothesized that glucocorticoids could possibly prevent OHSS in patients at high risk. Tan and colleagues[226], in a prospective randomized study of 17 patients, failed to demonstrate any efficacy of steroid administration. Intravenous hydrocortisone was immediately administered after the retrieval of oocytes, and this was followed by oral treatment with decreasing doses for 10 days. At the present time, we do not recommend administering steroids for prevention of OHSS.

Intramuscular progesterone

Costabile and colleagues[227] compared the use of intramuscular progesterone versus intravenous albumin for the prevention of OHSS. Progesterone was administered at the time of oocyte retrieval and continued throughout the luteal phase. The OHSS rates in this interesting study do not permit a conclusion to be drawn. The authors suggested that progesterone appears likely to be safer than albumin, with a possible benefit to pregnancy rates.

Luteal phase support with progesterone

Rizk and Smitz[5] demonstrated that the use of hCG for luteal phase support increases the incidence of OHSS. Progesterone, intravaginally or intramuscularly, should be used for luteal phase support in patients at risk of OHSS.

Cryopreservation of embryos and subsequent replacement

The availability of cryopreservation has made it possible not to lose the cycle and to achieve pregnancy by replacement of the frozen–thawed embryos at a later cycle. In one of the first reports, Amso and co-workers[228] presented four cases in which cryopreservation and later replacements resulted in pregnancies and avoided hyperstimulation. In Bourn Hall Clinic there were no cases admitted with severe OHSS in 1989 and 1990[186]. Cryopreservation of embryos was performed for all patients at risk. Replacement at a subsequent cycle resulted in a 37% clinical pregnancy rate[229]. Wada and colleagues[230] electively cryopreserved all the embryos from women with serum estradiol levels > 3500 pg/ml on the day of hCG. They demonstrated a reduction in the severity, but not the incidence of OHSS.

Queenan and co-workers[231] reported that cryopreservation of all prezygotes in patients at risk of severe hyperstimulation did not eliminate the syndrome, but the chances of pregnancy were excellent with subsequent frozen–thawed transfers. In their series of 15 patients, two patients (13%) developed severe OHSS and two others developed moderate OHSS. Subsequent transfer of the cryopreserved embryos resulted in a 58% pregnancy rate.

In a Cochrane review, D'Angelo and Amso[232] identified 17 studies, two of which met the inclusion criteria. When elective cryopreservation was compared with fresh embryo transfer, no difference was found between the two groups in the incidence of OHSS. This Cochrane review at present suggests that there is insufficient evidence to support routine cryopreservation, and also insufficient evidence to be able to determine the relative merits of intravenous albumin versus cryopreservation.

Prevention of OHSS in PCOS patients

Rizk and Smitz[5] highlighted that ovarian stimulation for patients with PCOS carries the highest risk for development of the severe form of OHSS. Today, this is one of the major challenges in PCOS patients. Several approaches have been used, which include: low-dose gonadotropins, which are widely used in non-IVF stimulations, and laparoscopic ovarian drilling, which is popular in Europe and Australia, but less popular in the United States as a method to prevent OHSS.

Low-dose gonadotropins in PCOS patients Prevention of OHSS in this group of patients is rather difficult because of the narrow margin between the dose required to induce reasonable stimulation and the dose which may result in the development of OHSS. The low-dose hMG or FSH step-up protocol is safe for non-IVF stimulation[233].

Aboulghar and colleagues[234] compared low-dose recombinant FSH and hMG protocols in the treatment of patients with a history of severe OHSS. The recombinant FSH low-dose protocol proved to be as effective as the low-dose hMG protocol in producing reasonable ovulation and pregnancies in PCOS patients with a history of severe OHSS; the protocol was safe with regard to the risk of developing OHSS. Rosenwaks[235] highly recommended a very gentle stimulation approach as the key component in preventing OHSS. This involves both lower gonadotropin and hCG dosages.

If ovarian hyperstimulation is performed for IVF, it is recommended to start with lower doses of hMG or FSH. In our experience, we believe that coasting, by stopping hMG injection and monitoring estradiol with assays until it drops to 4000 pg/ml, is an excellent and safe treatment if the patient is found to be at risk for developing OHSS. The other option is to withhold the hCG injection, as discussed earlier.

Metformin in PCOS patients Metformin is widely used for the treatment of insulin resistance in women with PCOS. De Leo and colleagues[236] performed a prospective randomized trial in 21 women with clomiphene-resistant PCOS which demonstrated that metformin use results in a reduction of intraovarian androgens by reducing hyperinsulinism. This leads to a reduction in estradiol and favors orderly follicular growth in response to exogenous gonadotropins.

Laparoscopic ovarian drilling in PCOS patients Laparoscopic ovarian drilling has been used successfully for prevention of OHSS in patients with polycystic ovaries. Rizk and Nawar[237] reviewed the treatment of PCOS by ovarian drilling using electrosurgery and laser therapy. Similar ovulation and pregnancy rates were observed. The pregnancy rates varied from 20 to 60%. Both ovarian diathermy and laser vaporization have been used immediately prior to the commencement of ovarian stimulation in patients at risk of OHSS[238–241]. Ovarian diathermy has been performed in either one or both ovaries. The results of these trials have been encouraging.

Is there an ideal protocol for prevention of OHSS?

Rizk[207] proposed the following protocol as an ideal protocol for the prevention of OHSS (Table 8). We suggest that to minimize the risk of OHSS, pretreatment with oral contraceptive and low-dose gonadotropin is initiated, GnRH antagonist is used to prevent the LH surge, GnRH agonist is used to trigger ovulation and progesterone given for luteal phase support. We emphasize that no comparison of pregnancy rates has been performed between this protocol and more conventional protocols, and there may be a drop in pregnancy rates if any or all of the above are adopted; however, it can be estimated that the incidence of severe OHSS would decrease from 1–2 to 0.5–0.8%. It has to be mentioned that with any protocol there will still be a 0.5% chance of OHSS, unless a more liberal policy for cancelation is adopted.

TREATMENT OF OHSS

Based on our proposed classification, moderate OHSS will be followed up by regular telephone calls and office visits. The patient should be instructed to report to the hospital if she develops dyspnea, if the volume of urine is diminished or upon development of any unusual symptoms.

Severe OHSS grade A is treated in hospital by aspiration of ascitic fluid, administration of intravenous fluids and evaluating all biochemical parameters on an out-patient basis. Patients with severe OHSS grade B are admitted to hospital for treatment (Figure 2). Great caution is required in all grades because complications can occur suddenly.

Delvigne and Rozenberg[193] reviewed the clinical course and treatment of OHSS. They stated that the clinical course of OHSS may involve, according to its severity and the occurrence of pregnancy, electrolytic

Table 8 Ideal protocol for the prevention of ovarian hyperstimulation syndrome (OHSS). Modified from reference 207

Pretreatment with oral contraceptives

Low-dose gonadotropins

GnRH antagonist to prevent LH surge

GnRH agonist to trigger ovulation

Progesterone for luteal phase support

GnRH, gonadotropin releasing hormone; LH, luteinizing hormone

imbalance, neurohormonal and hemodynamic changes, pulmonary manifestations, liver dysfunction, hypoglobulinemia, febrile morbidity, thromboembolic phenomena, neurological manifestations and adnexal torsion. Treatment of the acute phase relies only on an empirical and symptomatic approach. The general approach will be adapted to the levels of severity. Specific approaches, such as paracentesis or pleural puncture, can be carried out.

Clinical and biochemical monitoring in hospital

The patient's general condition requires regular assessment, with documentation of vital signs, together with daily weight and girth measurement. Strict fluid balance recording is needed, particularly of urine output[122].

Biochemical monitoring should include serum and electrolytes, renal and liver function tests, a coagulation profile and blood count. Serum and urinary osmolarity and urinary electrolyte estimation may be required as the severity of the disease process increases. Respiratory compromise and/or significant deterioration of renal function require evaluation of blood gases and acid–base balance. The frequency of these investigations will depend on the severity of the condition.

Ultrasonographic examination provides accurate assessment of ovarian size and the presence or absence of ascites, as well as pleural or pericardial effusion. Also, it will help in the diagnosis of intra- or extrauterine pregnancy as well as multiple or heterotopic pregnancy. Chest X-ray will also provide information on the presence of hydrothorax. Assay of β-hCG will help to diagnose pregnancy as early as possible.

Invasive hemodynamic monitoring (central venous pressure and pulmonary artery pressure) may be needed under certain circumstances when volume expanders are being employed.

Medical treatment

Circulation and electrolytes

The main line of treatment is correction of the circulatory volume and the electrolyte imbalance. Efforts should be directed towards restoring a normal intravascular volume and preserving adequate renal function. This may be achieved by using colloid plasma expanders or human albumin. One concern with using plasma expanders is that the beneficial effect is transitory before their redistribution into the extravascular space, further exacerbating ascites formation[242]. Appropriate solutions will correct electrolyte imbalances; if hypokalemia is significant, a cation exchange resin may be needed. Sodium and water restriction were advocated by Shapiro and colleagues[242] and Haning and colleagues[243], but Thaler and colleagues[244] found no change in the patient's weight, abdominal circumference or peripheral edema when sodium and water were restricted. Therefore, salt and water restriction are not widely advocated[14].

Anticoagulant therapy

Anticoagulant therapy is indicated if there is clinical evidence of thromboembolic complications or laboratory evidence of hypercoagulability[1,2,122]. As has been shown in the recent literature, reviewed earlier, venous thrombosis is the most common serious complication of OHSS; it is believed that prophylactic heparin should be given for a long period in all cases with severe OHSS.

Diuretics

Diuretic therapy without prior volume expansion may prove detrimental, by further contracting the intravascular volume, thereby worsening hypotension and its sequelae. Diuretics will increase blood viscosity and increase the risk of venous thrombosis. Diuretics may be used in the management of pulmonary congestion or edema.

Dopamine

Dopamine has been used recently in oliguric patients with severe OHSS, resulting in significant improvement in renal funcion[245]. Dopamine produces its renal effect by increasing renal blood flow and glomerular filtration. This is accomplished via stimulation of the dopaminergic receptors present in the vascular kidney. The rationale for treating oliguric patients with dopamine is to avoid fluid and salt retention and to prevent acute renal failure. However, dopamine therapy should be given cautiously and under strict observation.

Tsunoda and colleagues[246] reported 27 patients, hospitalized because of OHSS and refractory to the initial therapy with intravenous albumin, who were treated by docarpamine. A 750-mg tablet of docarpamine was taken every 8 h. In 19 (86.4%) of 22 patients treated, clinical symptoms associated with ascites gradually improved after administration of docarpamine. Moreover, there were no major adverse effects of docarpamine in this study. These findings indicate that oral docarpamine administration could be one of the options in the management of patients with OHSS using dopamine therapy.

Aspiration of ascitic fluid and pleural effusion in severe OHSS

Abdominal paracentesis

Thaler and associates[244], in a case report, showed that paracentesis was followed by increased urinary output shortly after the procedure, with a concomitant decrease in the patient's weight, leg edema and abdominal circumference. They also showed that there was an increased creatinine clearance rate of 50% following the procedure.

Levin and colleagues[247] studied the effect of paracentesis of ascitic fluids on urinary output and blood indices in patients with severe OHSS. Paracentesis of ascitic fluids in women with severe OHSS had an isolated effect in improving renal function, as was evidenced by the increased urinary output and reduced blood urea nitrogen.

Bider and co-workers[77] treated 12 patients with severe OHSS, accompanied by pleural effusion or ascites causing respiratory discomfort and dyspnea, using abdominal puncture. Drainage of abdominal or pleural effusion improved the symptoms in all patients. The amount of fluid aspirated ranged between 200 and 1400 ml. The risk of injury to an ovarian cyst was minimized by ultrasonographic guidance. Paracentesis offered temporary relief of respiratory distress, but, since the fluid tended to recur, some patients needed repeated paracentesis and drainage of effusions before spontaneous improvement ensued. The experience with this group of patients indicates that the actual risk of paracentesis is negligible. However, a possible drawback is the loss of fluid that is rich in proteins.

Padilla and colleagues[248] demonstrated that abdominal paracentesis is a well-tolerated treatment to relieve severe pulmonary compromise caused by severe ascites and pleural effusion in OHSS. The improvement in renal function may be another benefit that deserves further investigation. Al-Ramahi and co-workers[249] reported three cases in which an indwelling peritoneal catheter was used to decrease the need for repeated paracentesis. Under ultrasound guidance, a closed-system Dawson–Mueller catheter with 'simp-loc' locking design was inserted to allow continuous drainage of the ascitic fluid. A total of 23, 20 and 28 l was subsequently aspirated from the three patients. There was a significant decrease in abdominal discomfort and improvement of the urine output, with no complications. The only possible drawback to this technique would be depletion of a huge amount of plasma protein. We believe that monitoring of plasma proteins is essential if this treatment is applied, and human albumin should be infused whenever necessary[122]. Koike and associates[250] investigated prospectively the clinical efficacy of a newly developed continuous autotransfusion system of ascites (CATSA) without protein supplement in patients with severe OHSS. The CATSA was performed for 5 h at a rate of 100–200 ml/h once a day. Eighteen patients were treated with the CATSA (CATSA group) and 36 were treated with an intravenous 37.5 g/day of albumin supplement (albumin group). Hospital stay was significantly shorter in the CATSA group than in the albumin group (10.0 ± 5.7 versus 13.9 ± 6.2 days, $p < 0.01$). Using a single procedure, hemoconcentration, urinary output and pulse pressure were markedly improved in the CATSA group compared with the albumin group. Discomfort due to massive ascites diminished promptly and did not recur in nine of 18 CATSA group patients, whereas it persisted in all 36 patients in the albumin group. The serum concentration of protein was maintained in the CATSA group, whereas it did not

increase in the albumin group despite daily supplementation with 37.5 g of albumin. The mean values of several parameters in the serum pertinent to the coagulation–fibrinolysis system did not change significantly in either group after the procedure. It was concluded that the CATSA procedure expanded circulating plasma volume without exogenous albumin and appeared to lead to a prompt recovery from severe conditions of OHSS.

Abuzeid and co-workers[251] studied the efficacy and safety of percutaneous pigtail catheter drainage for the management of ascites complicating severe OHSS. A pigtail catheter was inserted under transabdominal ultrasound guidance and kept in place until drainage ceased. Percutaneous placement of a pigtail catheter is a safe and effective treatment modality for severe OHSS. It may represent an attractive alternative to multiple vaginal or abdominal paracentesis.

Transvaginal ultrasound-guided aspiration

Aboulghar and associates[252], in a prospective randomized clinical trial, investigated the effects of transvaginal aspiration of ascitic fluid under sonographic guidance in patients with severe OHSS. The average hospital stay and the period with severe symptoms and disturbed electrolyte balance were much shorter in the group in which aspiration of ascitic fluid was performed, when compared with the group who underwent conservative treatment. Rizk and Aboulghar[10] found that aspiration of ascitic fluid immediately relieved the symptoms of the patients, improved the general condition and increased urinary output. A marked improvement in symptoms was noted after drainage of as little as 900 ml of ascitic fluid. There were no adverse hemodynamic effects as a result of the aspiration of large volumes of ascitic fluid. Replacement of the plasma proteins was mandatory because of the high protein content of ascitic fluid. This was essential, as repeated aspiration was required in 30% of patients. The rate of accumulation of ascitic fluid varied significantly. However, recollection of a large volume of ascitic fluid sufficient to cause discomfort would require, on average, 3–5 days.

Aboulghar and colleagues[253] reported three cases of severe OHSS treated by transvaginal aspiration of ascitic fluid and autotransfusion of the aspirated fluid. Marked improvement of the symptoms, general condition and urine output followed shortly after the aspiration. No reactions were noted during or after autotransfusion. The blood parameters were corrected, and the general condition and urine output continued to improve. The procedure is simple, safe and straightforward, and shows a striking physiological success in correcting the maldistribution of fluid and proteins without the use of heterogeneous biological material. However, we do not recommend autotransfusion of ascitic fluid because of the possible reinjection of cytokines into the circulation. Cytokine levels in a patient with severe OHSS before and after ultrafiltration and reinfusion of ascitic fluid showed that cytokine concentrations decline in parallel with the improvement of clinical conditions and resolution of OHSS[254].

Abdalla and Rizk[122] urged early and prompt management of ascitic fluid. Aboulghar and co-workers[255] assessed the value of intravenous fluid therapy and ascitic fluid aspiration in the management of severe OHSS. Forty-two women with severe OHSS were treated by ultrasonically guided transvaginal aspiration of ascitic fluid and intravenous fluid infusion. Ten women with the same condition treated conservatively constituted a comparison group. The main outcome measures included percentage change in hematocrit, creatinine clearance and urine output before and after aspiration. The duration of hospital stay was compared between the groups. Marked improvement of symptoms and general condition followed soon after aspiration. Hematocrit readings decreased by 22%, creatinine clearance increased by 79.3% and urine output increased by 220.7%. The average volume of aspirated fluid was 3900 ml. The average duration of hospital stay was 3.8 days for the treated women. In the comparison group, severe symptoms and electrolyte imbalance continued for an average of 9 days, and the average hospital stay was 11 days. Intensive intravenous fluid therapy and transvaginal aspiration of ascitic fluid are safe and effective in improving symptoms, preventing complications and shortening the hospital stay in severe OHSS.

Transvaginal ultrasound-guided aspiration is an effective and safe procedure[122,252]. Injury to the ovary is easily avoided by puncture under ultrasonic visualization. No anesthesia is required for the procedure, and better drainage of the ascitic fluid is accomplished because the pouch of Douglas is the most dependent part.

Surgical treatment

Management of ovarian torsion

Hurwitz and colleagues[256] reported the first case of unwinding of a cystic ovary which had undergone torsion in a patient with OHSS. The pregnancy continued to term, resulting in a normal twin delivery. Mashiach and co-workers[257] reported 12 pregnant women who presented with torsion of hyperstimulated ovaries. They suggested that torsion of ovaries in patients who conceived after gonadotropin therapy should be considered a special entity, which requires more attention to achieve early diagnosis. Although the adnexa appeared dark, hemorrhagic and ischemic, they suggested that it could be saved by simply unwinding it.

Laparotomy

Rizk stated that laparotomy, in general, should be avoided in OHSS[4]. If deemed necessary, it should be performed by an experienced gynecologist and only hemostatic measures undertaken to preserve the ovaries. Bider and co-workers[77] reported operative procedures in 16 patients with severe OHSS because of torsion, rupture and bleeding in the ovarian cysts.

Aboulghar and associates[258] treated surgically a case of severe OHSS complicated by ectopic pregnancy. The diagnosis of ectopic pregnancy in this case was very difficult because internal bleeding occurred when the patient was already complaining of severe OHSS and the amount of blood loss was not severe enough to be reflected in her general condition. Diagnosis of tubal pregnancy by vaginal ultrasound examination at this stage is not always possible. The presence of large ovaries filling the pelvis makes ultrasound scanning of other structures difficult. Fluid in the pouch of Douglas is suspicious of the presence of ascites. Shiau and colleagues[259] described a case of severe OHSS coexisting with a bilateral ectopic pregnancy.

SUMMARY

Ovarian hyperstimulation syndrome is an iatrogenic complication of ovulation induction by gonadotropins. The syndrome can result in serious life-threatening complications, which include cerebrovascular accidents due to venous thrombosis, liver dysfunction, acute renal failure, respiratory complications and adnexal torsion. It is known that the most important predisposing factor for the development of severe forms of OHSS is polycystic ovarian disease.

The syndrome is characterized by leakage of fluid from the intravascular compartment, with accumulation of fluid in the peritoneal and pleural cavities, resulting in hypotension and a decrease in renal blood flow and volume of urine. Increased capillary permeability is the most accepted hypothesis for the initial pathophysiological event.

Vascular endothelial growth factor and other cytokines are pivotal in the pathogenesis of OHSS. A new classification of the syndrome has been proposed, with mild OHSS omitted. Moderate OHSS is treated conservatively, by observation on an out-patient basis. Severe OHSS, without an abnormal biochemical profile, is treated by ascitic fluid aspiration and intravenous fluid therapy on the basis of day–care treatment. Cases of severe OHSS with electrolyte imbalance or other complications must be admitted to hospital for appropriate treatment. Surgical treatment is reserved for torsion or rupture of adnexal cysts or an ectopic pregnancy. Novel medical treatments might open new horizons in the treatment of OHSS.

REFERENCES

1. Mozes M, Bogowsky H, Anteby E, et al. Thromboembolic phenomena after ovarian stimulation with human menopausal gonadotropin. Lancet 1965; 2: 1213–15

2. Rizk B, Meagher S, Fisher AM. Ovarian hyperstimulation syndrome and cerebrovascular accidents. Hum Reprod 1990; 5: 697–8

3. Rizk B, Aboulghar MA, Smitz J, Ron-El R. The role of vascular endothelial growth factor and interleukins in the pathogenesis of severe ovarian hyperstimulation syndrome. Hum Reprod Update 1997; 3: 255–66

4. Rizk B. Ovarian hyperstimulation syndrome. In Studd J, ed. Progress in Obstetrics and Gynecology. Edinburgh: Churchill Livingstone, 1993; 11: 311–49

5. Rizk B, Smitz J. Ovarian hyperstimulation syndrome after superovulation for IVF and related procedures. Hum Reprod 1992; 7: 320–7

6. Rizk B, Thorneycroft IH. Does recombinant follicle stimulating hormone abolish the risk of severe ovarian hyperstimulation syndrome? Presented at the 52nd Annual Meeting of the American Society for Reproductive Medicine, Boston, MA, 1996: S151–2 (abstr)

7. Rizk B, Aboulghar MA, Mansour RT, et al. Severe ovarian hyperstimulation syndrome: analytical study of twenty-one cases. Proceedings of the VII World Congress on In Vitro Fertilization and Assisted Procreations, Paris. Hum Reprod 1991; 6 (Suppl): 368–9

8. Brinsden PR, Wada I, Tan SL, et al. Diagnosis, prevention and management of ovarian hyperstimulation syndrome. Br J Obstet Gynaecol 1995; 102: 767–72

9. Rizk B, Nawar MG. Ovarian hyperstimulation syndrome. In Serhal P, Overton C, eds. Good Clinical Practice in Assisted Reproduction. Cambridge: Cambridge University Press, 2004: 164–6

10. Rizk B, Aboulghar M. Modern management of ovarian hyperstimulation syndrome. Hum Reprod 1991; 6: 1082–7

11. Aboulghar MA, Mansour RT. Ovarian hyperstimulation syndrome: classifications and critical analysis of preventive measures. Hum Reprod Update 2003; 9: 275–89

12. Rabau E, Serr DM, David A, et al. Human menopausal gonadotrophin for anovulation and sterility. Am J Obstet Gynecol 1967; 98: 92–8

13. Schenker JG, Weinstein D. Ovarian hyperstimulation syndrome: a current survey. Fertil Steril 1978; 30: 255–68

14. Golan A, Ron-El R, Herman A, et al. Ovarian hyperstimulation syndrome: an update review. Obstet Gynecol Surv 1989; 44: 430–40

15. Rizk B, Aboulghar MA. Classification, pathophysiology and management of ovarian hyperstimulation syndrome. In Brinsden P, et al. A Textbook of In Vitro Fertilization and Assisted Reproduction, 2nd edn. Lancaster, UK: Parthenon Publishing, 1999: 131–55

16. Navot D, Bergh PA, Laufer N. Ovarian hyperstimulation syndrome in novel reproductive technologies: prevention and treatment. Fertil Steril 1992; 58: 246–61

17. Mathur RS, Akande AV, Keay SD, et al. Distinction between early and late ovarian hyperstimulation syndromes. Fertil Steril 2000; 73: 901–7

18. Delvigne A. Epidemiology and pathophysiology of ovarian hyperstimulation syndrome. In Gerris J, Olivennes F, de Sutter P, eds. Assisted Reproductive Technologies: Quality and Safety. New York: Parthenon Publishing, 2004: 149–62

19. Delvigne A, Demoulin A, Smitz J, et al. The ovarian hyperstimulation syndrome in in-vitro fertilization: a Belgian multicentric study. I. Clinical and biological features. Hum Reprod 1993; 8: 1353–60

20. Abramov Y, Elchalal U, Schenker JG. Pulmonary manifestations of severe ovarian hyperstimulation syndrome: a multicenter study. Fertil Steril 1999; 71: 645–51

21. Serour GI, Aboulghar M, Mansour R, et al. Complications of medically assisted conception in 3500 cycles. Fertil Steril 1998; 70: 638–42

22. Aboulghar MA, Mansour RT, Serour GI, et al. Moderate ovarian hyperstimulation syndrome complicated by deep cerebrovascular thrombosis. Hum Reprod 1998; 13: 2088–91

23. Stewart JA, Hamilton PJ, Murdoch AP. Upper limb thrombosis associated with assisted conception treatment. Hum Reprod 1997; 12: 2174–5

24. Loret de Mola JR, Kiwi R, Austin C, Goldfarb JM. Subclavian deep vein thrombosis associated with the use of recombinant follicle-stimulating hormone (Gonal-F) complicating mild ovarian hyperstimulation syndrome. Fertil Steril 2000; 73: 1253–6

25. Tang OS, Ng EH, Wai Cheng P, Chung Ho P. Cortical vein thrombosis misinterpreted as intracranial haemorrhage in severe ovarian hyperstimulation syndrome: case report. Hum Reprod 2000; 15: 1913–16

26. Belaen B, Geerinckx K, Vergauwe P, Thys J. Internal jugular vein thrombosis after ovarian stimulation. Hum Reprod 2001; 16: 510–12

27. Mancini A, Milardi D, Di Pietro ML, et al. A case of forearm amputation after ovarian stimulation for in vitro fertilization–embryo transfer. Fertil Steril 2001; 76: 198–200

28. Turkistani IM, Ghourab SA, Al-Sheikh OH, et al. Central retinal artery occlusion associated with severe ovarian hyperstimulation syndrome. Eur J Ophthalmol 2001; 11: 313–15

29. Foong LC, Bhagavath B, Kumar J, Ng SC. Ovarian hyperstimulation syndrome is associated with reversible impairment of vascular reactivity. Fertil Steril 2002; 78: 1159–63

30. Phillips LL, Glanstone W, Van de Wiele R. Studies of the coagulation and fibrinolytic systems in hyperstimulation syndrome after administration of human gonadotrophin. J Reprod Med 1975; 14: 138

31. Kaaja R, Sieberg R, Titinen A, et al. Severe ovarian hyperstimulation syndrome and deep venous thrombosis. Lancet 1989; 2: 1043

32. Dulitzky M, Cohen SB, Inbal A, et al. Increased prevalence of thrombophilia among women with severe ovarian hyperstimulation syndrome. Fertil Steril 2002; 77: 463–7

33. Kodama H, Fukuda J, Karube H, et al. Status of the coagulation and fibrinolytic systems in ovarian hyperstimulation syndrome. Fertil Steril 1996; 66: 417–24

34. Balasch J, Reverter JC, Fabregues F, et al. Increased induced monocyte tissue factor expression by plasma from patients with severe ovarian hyperstimulation syndrome. Fertil Steril 1996; 66: 608–13

35. Smith BH, Cooke ID. Ovarian hyperstimulation: actual and theoretical risks. Br Med J 1991; 298: 127–8

36. Ong ACM, Eisen V, Rennie DP, et al. The pathogenesis of the ovarian hyperstimulation syndrome (OHS): a possible role of ovarian renin. Clin Endocrinol 1991; 34: 43–9

37. Mills MS, Eddowes HA, Fox R, et al. Subclavian vein thrombosis; a late complication of ovarian hyperstimulation syndrome. Hum Reprod 1992; 7: 370–1

38. Kodama H, Takeda S, Fukuda J, et al. Activation of plasma kinin system correlated with severe coagulation disorders in patients with ovarian hyperstimulation syndrome. Hum Reprod 1997; 12: 891–5

39. Stewart JA, Hamilton PJ, Murdoch AP. Thromboembolic disease associated with ovarian hyperstimulation syndrome and assisted conception techniques. Hum Reprod 1997; 12: 2167–73

40. Aune B, Hoie KE, Oian P, et al. Does ovarian stimulation for in vitro fertilization induce a hypercoagulable state? Hum Reprod 1991; 6: 925–7

41. Todros T, Carmazzi CM, Bontempo S, et al. Spontaneous ovarian hyperstimulation syndrome and deep vein thrombosis in pregnancy: case report. Hum Reprod 1999; 14: 2245–8

42. Lamon D, Chang CK, Hruska L, et al. Superior vena cava thrombosis after in vitro fertilization: case report and review of the literature. Ann Vasc Surg 2000; 14: 283–5

43. Andrejevic S, Bonaci-Nikolic B, Bukilica M, et al. Intracardiac thrombosis and fever possibly triggered by ovulation induction in a patient with antiphospholipid antibodies. Scand J Rheumatol 2002; 31: 249–51

44. Elford K, Leader A, Wee R, Stys PK. Stroke in ovarian hyperstimulation syndrome in early pregnancy treated with intra-arterial rt-PA. Neurology 2002; 59: 1270–2

45. Ulug U, Aksoy E, Erden H. Bilateral internal jugular venous thrombosis following successful assisted conception in the absence of ovarian hyperstimulation syndrome. Eur J Obstet Gynecol Reprod Biol 2003; 109: 231–3

46. McGowan BM, Kay LA, Perry DJ. Deep vein thrombosis followed by internal jugular vein thrombosis as a complication of in vitro fertilization in a woman heterozygous for the prothrombin 3′ UTR and factor V Leiden mutations. Am J Hematol 2003; 73: 276–8

47. Fabregues F, Tassies D, Reverter JC, et al. Prevalence of thrombophilia in women with severe ovarian hyperstimulation syndrome and cost-effectiveness of screening. Fertil Steril 2004; 81: 989–95

48. Ou YC, Kao YL, Lai SL, et al. Thromboembolism after ovarian stimulation: successful management of a woman with superior sagittal sinus thrombosis after

IVF and embryo transfer: case report. Hum Reprod 2003; 18: 2375–81

49. Nakauchi-Tanaka T, Sohda S, Someya K, et al. Acquired haemophilia due to factor VIII inhibitors in ovarian hyperstimulation syndrome: case report. Hum Reprod 2003; 18: 506–8

50. Akdemir R, Uyan C, Emiroglu Y. Acute myocardial infarction secondary thrombosis associated with ovarial hyperstimulation syndrome. Int J Cardiol 2002; 83: 187–9

51. Sueldo CE, Price HM, Bachenberg K, et al. Transient liver function test abnormalities of ovarian hyperstimulation syndrome: a case report. J Reprod Med 1988; 33: 387–90

52. Younis JS, Zeevi D, Rabinowitz R, et al. Transient liver function test abnormalities of ovarian hyperstimulation syndrome. Fertil Steril 1988; 50: 176–8

53. Ryley NG, Froman R, Barlow D, et al. Liver abnormality in ovarian hyperstimulation syndrome. Hum Reprod 1990; 5: 938–43

54. Chen CD, Wu MY, Chen HF, et al. Relationships of serum pro-inflammatory cytokines and vascular endothelial growth factor with liver dysfunction in severe ovarian hyperstimulation syndrome. Hum Reprod 2000; 15: 66–71

55. Elter K, Scoccia B, Nelson LR. Hepatic dysfunction associated with moderate ovarian hyperstimulation syndrome: a case report. J Reprod Med 2001; 46: 765–8

56. Davis AJ, Pandher GK, Masson GM, et al. A severe case of ovarian hyperstimulation syndrome with liver dysfunction and malnutrition. Eur J Gastroenterol Hepatol 2002; 14: 779–82

57. Zosmer A, Katz Z, Lancet M, et al. Adult respiratory distress syndrome complicating ovarian hyperstimulation syndrome. Fertil Steril 1987; 47: 524–6

58. Jewelewicz R, Van de Wiele RL. Acute hydrothorax as the only symptom of ovarian hyperstimulation syndrome. Am J Obstet Gynecol 1975; 121: 1121

59. Kingsland C, Collins JV, Rizk B, et al. Ovarian hyperstimulation presenting as acute hydrothorax after in vitro fertilization. Am J Obstet Gynecol 1989; 161: 381–2

60. Rabinerson D, Shalev J, Royburt M, et al. Severe unilateral hydrothorax as the only manifestation of the ovarian hyperstimulation syndrome. Gynecol Obstet Invest 2000; 49: 140–2

61. Cordani S, Bancalari L, Maggiani R, et al. Massive unilateral hydrothorax as the only clinical manifestation of ovarian hyperstimulation syndrome. Monaldi Arch Chest Dis 2002; 57: 314–17

62. Gore et al. Middle East Fertil Soc J 2002; 7: 211–13

63. Semba S, Moriya T, Youssef EM, et al. An autopsy case of ovarian hyperstimulation syndrome with massive

pulmonary edema and pleural effusion. Pathol Int 2000; 50: 549–52

64. Balasch J, Carmona F, Llach J, et al. Acute prerenal failure and liver dysfunction in a patient with severe ovarian hyperstimulation syndrome. Hum Reprod 1990; 5: 3448–51

65. Khalaf Y, Elkington N, Anderson H, et al. Ovarian hyperstimulation syndrome and its effect on renal function in a renal transplant patient undergoing IVF treatment: case report. Hum Reprod 2000; 15: 1275–7

66. Lesny P, Maguiness SD, Hay DM, et al. Ovarian hyperstimulation syndrome and benign intracranial hypertension in pregnancy after in-vitro fertilization and embryo transfer: case report. Hum Reprod 1999; 14: 1953–5

67. Schenker JG. Clinical aspects of ovarian hyperstimulation syndrome. Eur J Obstet Gynecol Reprod Biol 1999; 85: 13–20

68. Raziel A, Friedler S, Schachter M, et al. Increased early pregnancy loss in IVF patients with severe ovarian hyperstimulation syndrome. Hum Reprod 2002; 17: 107–10

69. Delvigne A, Rozenberg S. Epidemiology and prevention of ovarian hyperstimulation syndrome (OHSS): a review. Hum Reprod 2002; 8: 559–77

70. Delvigne A, Dubois M, Battheu B, et al. The ovarian hyperstimulation syndrome in in-vitro fertilization: a Belgian multicenter study. II. Multiple discriminant analysis for risk prediction. Hum Reprod 1993; 8: 1361–6

71. Navot D, Relou A, Birkenfeld A, et al. Risk factors and prognostic variables in the ovarian hyperstimulation syndrome. Am J Obstet Gynecol 1988; 159: 210–15

72. Lunenfeld B, Insler V. Classification of amenorrheic states and their treatment by ovulation induction. Clin Endocrinol (Oxf) 1974; 3: 223–37

73. Thompson C, Hansen M. Pergonal: summary of clinical experience in induction of ovulation and pregnancy. Fertil Steril 1970; 21: 844

74. Caspi E, Levom S, Bukovsky I, et al. Induction of pregnancy with human gonadotrophin after clomiphene failure in menstruating ovulatory infertility patients. Isr J Med Sci 1974; 10: 249

75. Tulandi T, McInnes RA, Arronet GH. Ovarian hyperstimulation syndrome following ovulation induction with hMG. Int J Fertil 1984; 29: 113–17

76. Charbonnel B, Krempf M, Blanchard P, et al. Induction of ovulation in polycystic ovary syndrome with a combination of luteinizing hormone releasing hormone analogue and exogenous gonadotrophin. Fertil Steril 1987; 47: 920–4

77. Bider D, Menashe Y, Oelsner G, et al. Ovarian hyperstimulation due to exogenous gonadotrophin admin-

istration. Acta Obstet Gynecol Scand 1989; 69: 511–14

78. Smitz J, Camus M, Devroey P, et al. Incidence of severe ovarian hyperstimulation syndrome after GnRH-agonist/HMG superovulation for in vitro fertilization. Hum Reprod 1990; 5: 933–7

79. Aboulghar MA, Mansour RT, Serour GI, et al. Follicular aspiration does not protect against the development of ovarian hyperstimulation syndrome after GNRH-agonist/HMG superovulation for in vitro fertilization. J Assist Reprod Genet 1992; 9: 238–43

80. Golan A, Ron-El R, Herman A, et al. Ovarian hyperstimulation syndrome following D-Trp-6 luteinizing hormone-releasing hormone microcapsules and menotrophin for in vitro fertilization. Fertil Steril 1988; 50: 912–16

81. Bilan FIVNAT. Résponses aux stimulations de l'ovulation dans les procréations médicalement assistes (pMA). Contracept Fertil Sex 1989; 18: 592–4

82. Rizk B, Lenton W, Vere M. The use of gonadotropin releasing hormone agnoist in programmed oocyte retrievel for GIFT. Hum Reprod 1991: S368

83. Raj SG, Berger MJ, Grimes EM, Taymor ML. The use of gonadotrophin for the induction of ovulation in women with polycystic ovarian disease. Fertil Steril 1977; 28: 1280–4

84. Check JH, Wu CH, Gocial B, et al. Severe ovarian hyper-stimulation syndrome from treatment with urinary follicle stimulating hormone: two cases. Fertil Steril 1985; 43: 317–20

85. Southan AL, Janovsky NA. Massive ovarian hyperstimulation with clomiphene citrate. J Am Med Assoc 1962: 200

86. Scommegna A, Lash SR. Ovarian overstimulation with massive ascites and singleton pregnancy after clomiphene. J Am Med Assoc 1969; 207: 753

87. Rotmensch S, Scommegna A. Spontaneous ovarian hyperstimulation syndrome associated with hypothyroidism. Am J Obstet Gynecol 1989; 160: 1220–2

88. Zalel Y, Katz Z, Caspi B, et al. Spontaneous ovarian hyperstimulation syndrome concomitant with spontaneous pregnancy in a woman with polycystic ovary disease. Am J Obstet Gynecol 1992; 167: 122–4

89. Zalel Y, Oriveto R, Ben-Rafael Z, et al. Recurrent spontaneous ovarian hyperstimulation syndrome associated with polycystic ovary syndrome. Gynecol Endocrinol 1995; 9: 313–15

90. Ayhan A, Tuncer ZS, Aksu AT. Ovarian hyperstimulation syndrome associated with spontaneous pregnancy. Hum Reprod 1996; 11: 1600–1

91. Lipitz S, Grisaru D, Achiron R, et al. Spontaneous ovarian hyperstimulation mimicking ovarian tumor. Hum Reprod 1996; 11: 720–1

92. Regi A, Mathai M, Jasper P, et al. Ovarian hyperstimulation syndrome (OHSS) in pregnancy not associated with ovulation induction. Acta Obstet Gynecol Scand 1996; 75: 599–600

93. Chae HD, Park EJ, Kim SH, et al. Ovarian hyperstimulation syndrome complicating a spontaneous singleton pregnancy: a case report. J Assist Reprod Genet 2001; 18: 120–3

94. Di Carlo C, Bruno PA, Cirillo D, et al. Increased concentrations of renin, aldosterone and Ca125 in a case of spontaneous, recurrent, familial, severe ovarian hyper-stimulation syndrome. Hum Reprod 1997; 12: 2115–17

95. Montanelli L, Delbaere A, Di Carlo C, et al. A mutation in the follicle-stimulating hormone receptor as a cause of familial spontaneous ovarian hyperstimulation syndrome. J Clin Endocrinol Metab 2004; 89: 1255–8

96. Montanelli L, Van Durme JJ, Smits G, et al. Modulation of ligand selectivity associated with activation of the transmembrane region of the human follitropin receptor. Mol Endocrinol 2004; 18: 2061–73

97. Jung BG, Kim H. Severe spontaneous ovarian hyperstimulation syndrome with MR findings. J Comput Assist Tomogr 2001; 25: 215–17

98. Seppala M. The World Collaborative Report on in-vitro fertilization and embryos replacement: current state of art in January 1984. Ann NY Acad Sci 1985; 442: 558–63

99. Smitz J, Devroey P, Camus M, et al. The luteal phase and early pregnancy after combined GnRH-agonist/HG treatment for superovulation in IVF and GIFT. Hum Reprod 1988; 3: 585–90

100. Herman A, Ron-El R, Golan A, et al. Pregnancy rate and ovarian hyperstimulation after luteal human chorionic gonadotropin in vitro fertilization stimulated with gonadotropin-releasing hormone analog and menotropins. Fertil Steril 1990; 53: 92–6

101. Imoedemhe DAG, Chan RCW, Signe AB, et al. A new approach to the management of patients at risk of ovarian hyperstimulation in an in vitro fertilization program. Hum Reprod 1991; 6: 1088–91

102. Haning RV Jr, Austin CW, Carlson IH, et al. Plasma estradiol is superior to ultrasound and urinary estriol glucuronide as a predictor of ovarian hyperstimulation during induction of ovulation with menotropins. Fertil Steril 1983; 40: 31–6

103. Rizk B, Tan SL, Morcos S, et al. Heterotopic pregnancies after in vitro fertilizations and embryo transfer. Am J Obstet Gynecol 1991; 164: 161–4

104. Reyad RM, Aboulghar MA, Serour GI, et al. Bilateral ectopic pregnancy with an intact intrauterine preg-

nancy following an ICSI procedure. Middle East Fertil Soc J 1988; 3: 91

105. Koike T, Minakami H, Araki S, et al. Severity of ovarian hyperstimulation syndrome: its relation to the number of conceptuses. Int J Fertil Women's Med 2004; 49: 36–42

106. Aboulghar MA, Mansour RT, Serour GI, et al. Oocyte quality in patients with severe ovarian hyperstimulation syndrome. Fertil Steril 1997; 68: 1017–21

107. Aboulghar MA, Mansour RT, Serour GI, et al. Ovarian hyperstimulation syndrome: modern concepts in patho-physiology and management. Middle East Fertil Soc J 1996; 1: 3–16

108. Tollan A, Holst N, Forsdahl F, et al. Transcapillary fluid dynamics during ovarian stimulation for in vitro fertrilization. Am J Obstet Gynecol 1990; 162: 554

109. Delbaere A, Smits G, Olatunbosun O, et al. New insights into the pathophysiology of ovarian hyperstimulation syndrome. What makes the difference between spontaneous and iatrogenic syndrome? Hum Reprod 2004; 19: 486–9

110. Enskog A, Nilsson L, Brannstrom M. Peripheral blood concentrations of inhibin B are elevated during gonadotrophin stimulation in patients who later develop ovarian OHSS and inhibin A concentrations are elevated after OHSS onset. Hum Reprod 2000; 15: 532–8

111. Daniel Y, Geva E, Amit A, et al. Soluble endothelial and platelet selectins in serum and ascitic fluid of women with ovarian hyperstimulation syndrome. Am J Reprod Immunol 2001; 45: 154–60

112. Abramov Y, Schenker JG, Lewin A, et al. Soluble ICAM-1 and E-selection levels correlate with clinical and biological aspects of severe ovarian hyperstimulation syndrome. Fertil Steril 2001; 76: 51–7

113. Ogawa S, Minakami H, Araki S, et al. A rise of the serum level of von Willebrand factor occurs before clinical manifestation of the severe form of ovarian hyperstimulation syndrome. J Assist Reprod Genet 2001; 18: 114–19

114. Evbuomwan IO, Davison JM, Murdoch AP. Coexistent hemoconcentration and hypoosmolality during superovulation and in severe ovarian hyperstimulation syndrome: volume homeostasis paradox. Fertil Steril 2000; 74: 67–72

115. Balasch J, Arroyo V, Carmona F, et al. Severe ovarian hyperstimulation syndrome: role of peripheral vasodilation. Fertil Steril 1991; 56: 1077–83

116. Van Beaumont W. Evaluation of hemoconcentration from hematocrit measurements. J Appl Physiol 1872; 5: 712–13

117. Evbuomwan IO, Davison JM, Baylis PM, et al. Altered osmotic thresholds for arginine vasopressin secretion and thirst during superovulation and in the ovarian hyperstimulation syndrome (OHSS): relevance to the pathophysiology of OHSS. Fertil Steril 2001; 75: 933–41

118. Abramov Y, Naparstek Y, Elchalal U, et al. Plasma immunoglobulins in patients with severe ovarian hyperstimulation syndrome. Fertil Steril 1999; 71: 102–5

119. Delvigne A, Kostyla K, De Leener A et al. Metabolic characteristics of women who developed ovarian hyperstimulation syndrome. Hum Reprod 2002; 17: 1994–6

120. Maathuis JB, Van Look PF, Michie EA. Changes in volume, total protein and ovarian steroid concentrations of peritoneal fluid through the human menstrual cycle. J Endocrinol 1978; 76: 123–4

121. Donnez J, Langerock S, Thomas K. Peritoneal fluid volume and 17β-estradiol and progesterone concentrations in ovulatory, anovulatory, and postmenopausal women. Obstet Gynecol 1982; 59: 687–92

122. Abdalla HI, Rizk B, eds. Assisted Reproductive Technology. Abingdon, Oxford: Health Press, 2004: 37–9

123. Yarali H, Fleige-Zahradka BG, Yuen BH, et al. The ascites in the ovarian hyperstimulation syndrome does not originate from the ovary. Fertil Steril 1993; 59: 657–61

124. Asch RH, Li HP, Balmeceda JP, et al. Severe ovarian hyperstimulation syndrome in assisted reproductive technology; definition of high risk groups. Hum Reprod 1991; 6: 1395–9

125. Pride SM, James C, Ho Yuen B. The ovarian hyperstimulation syndrome. Semin Reprod Endocrinol 1990; 8: 247–60

126. Pellicer A, Miru F, Sampaia M, et al. In vitro fertilization as a diagnostic and therapeutic tool in a patient with partial 17,20 desmolase deficiency. Fertil Steril 1991; 55: 970–5

127. Levy T, Oriveto R, Homburg R, et al. Severe ovarian hyperstimulation syndrome despite low plasma oestrogen concentrations in a hypogonadotrophic, hypogonadal patient. Hum Reprod 1996; 11: 1177–9

128. Fernandez LA, Twickler J, Mead A. Neovascularization produced by angiotensin II. J Lab Clin Med 1985; 105: 141

129. Navot D, Margalioth E, Laufer N. Direct correlation between plasma renin activity and severity of the ovarian hyperstimulation syndrome. Fertil Steril 1987; 48: 57–61

130. Delbaere A, Bergmann PJM, Gervy-Decoster C, et al. Prorenin and active renin concentrations in plasma and ascites during severe ovarian hyperstimulation syndrome. Hum Reprod 1997; 12: 236–40

131. Sahin Y, Kontas O, Muderris I, et al. Effects of angiotensin converting enzyme inhibitor cilasaprin and angiotensin II antagonist saralasin in ovarian hyperstimulation syndrome in the rabbit. Gynecol Endocrinol 1997; 11: 231–6

132. Teruel MJ, Carbonell LF, Llanos MC, et al. Hemodynamic state and the role of angiotensin II in ovarian hyperstimulation syndrome in the rabbit. Fertil Steril 2002; 77: 1256–60

133. Teruel MJ, Carbonell LF, Teruel MG, et al. Effect of angtiotensin-converting enzyme inhibitor on renal function in ovarian hyperstimulation syndrome in the rabbit. Fertil Steril 2001; 76: 1232–7

134. Morris RS, Wong IL, Kirkham E, et al. Inhibition of ovarian-derived prorenin to angiotensin cascade in the treatment of ovarian hyperstimulation syndrome. Hum Reprod 1995; 10: 1355–8

135. Pepperell JR, Nemeth G, Plaumbo A, et al. The intraovarian rennin–angiotensin system. In Adashi EY, Leung PCK, eds. The Ovary. New York: Raven Press, 1993: 363–80

136. Pellicer A, Palumbo A, DeCherney AH, et al. Blockage of ovulation by an angiotensin antagonist. Science 1988; 240: 1660–1

137. Schenker JG, Polishuk WZ. The role of prostaglandins in ovarian hyperstimulation syndrome. Obstet Gynecol Surv 1976; 31: 742

138. Katz Z, Lancet M, Borenstein R, et al. Absence of teratogenicity of indomethacin in ovarian hyperstimulation syndrome. Int J Fertil 1984; 29: 186

139. Pride SM, Ho Yuen B, Moon YS, et al. Relationship of gonadotropin-releasing hormone, danazol and prostaglandin blockage to ovarian enlargement and ascites formation of the ovarian hyperstimulation syndrome. Am J Obstet Gynecol 1986; 154: 1155–60

140. Ferrara N, Houck K, Jakeman L, et al. Molecular and biological properties of the vascular endothelial growth factor family of proteins. Endocr Rev 1992; 13: 18–32

141. Keck PJ, Hauser SD, Krivi G, et al. Vascular permeability factor, an endothelial cell mitogen related to PDGF. Science 1989; 246: 1309–12

142. Millauer B, Wizigmann-Voos S, Schnurch H, et al. High affinity VEGF binding and developmental expression suggest FLK-1 as a major regulator of vasculogenesis and angiogenesis. Cell 1993; 72: 835–46

143. Charnock-Jones DS, Sharkey AM, Rajput-Williams J, et al. Identification and localization of alternately spliced mRNAs for vascular endothelial growth factor in human uterus and estrogen regulation in endometrial carcinoma cell line. Biol Reprod 1993; 48: 1120–60

144. Ravindranath N, Little-Ihrig LL, Phillios HS, et al. Vascular endothelial growth factor messenger ribonucleic acid expression in the primate ovary. Endocrinol 1992; 131: 254–60

145. Kim KJ, Li B, Winer J, et al. Inhibition of vascular endothelial growth factor induced angiogenesis suppresses tumor growth in vivo. Nature (London) 1993; 362: 841–4

146. Koch AE, Harlow LA, Haines GK, et al. Vascular endothelial growth factor: a cytokine modulating endothelial function in rheumatoid arthritis. J Immunol 1994; 152: 4149–56

147. McLaren J, Prentice A, Charnock-Jones DS, et al. Vascular endothelial growth factor (VEGF) concentrations are elevated in peritoneal fluid of women with endometriosis. Hum Reprod 1996; 11: 220–3

148. Abdalla HI, Rizk B. Pathogenesis of endometriosis. In Abdalla HI, Rizk B, eds. Endometriosis 1998. Abingdon, Oxford: Health Press, 1998: 42–4

149. Kamat BR, Brown LF, Manseau EJ, et al. Expression of vascular permeability factor/vascular endothelial growth factor by human granulosa and theca lutein cells. Am J Pathol 1995; 146: 157–65

150. Gordon JD, Mesiano S, Zaloudek CJ, et al. Vascular endothelial growth factor localization in human ovary and fallopian tubes: possible role in reproductive function and ovarian cyst formation. J Clin Endocrinol Metab 1996; 81: 353–9

151. Yan Z, Weich HA, Bernart W, et al. Vascular endothelial growth factor (VEGF) messenger ribonucleic acid (mRNA) expression in luteinized human granulosa cells in vitro. J Clin Endocrinol Metab 1993; 77: 1723–5

152. Neulen J, Yan Z, Raczek S, et al. Ovarian hyperstimulation syndrome: vascular endothelial growth factor/ vascular permeability factor from luteinized granulosa cells is the patho-physiological principle. Presented at the 11th Annual Meeting of the ESHRE, Hamburg, 1995: abstr

153. McClure N, Healy DL, Rogers PA, et al. Vascular endothelial growth factor as capillary permeability agent in ovarian hyperstimulation syndrome. Lancet 1994; 344: 235–6

154. Gomez R, Simon C, Remohi J, et al. Administration of moderate and high doses of gonadotropins to female rats increases ovarian vascular endothelial growth factor (VEGF) and VEGF receptor-2 expression that is associated to vascular hyperpermeability. Biol Reprod 2003; 68: 2164–71

155. McElhinney B, Ardill J, Caldwell C, et al. Variations in serum vascular endothelial growth factor binding profiles and the development of ovarian hyperstimulation syndrome. Fertil Steril 2002; 78: 286–90

TEXTBOOK OF *IN VITRO* FERTILIZATION AND ASSISTED REPRODUCTION

156. Gomez R, Simon C, Remohi J, et al. Vascular endothelial growth factor receptor-2 activation induces vascular permeability in hyperstimulated rats, and this effect is prevented by receptor blockade. Endocrinology 2002; 143: 4339–48

157. Mathur R, Hayman G, Bansal A, et al. Serum vascular endothelial growth factor levels are poorly predictive of subsequent ovarian hyperstimulation syndrome in highly responsive women undergoing assisted conception. Fertil Steril 2002; 78: 1154–8

158. Artini PG, Monti M, Fasciani A, et al. Vascular endothelial growth factor, interleukin-6 and interleukin-2 in serum and follicular fluid of patients with ovarian hyperstimulation syndrome. Eur J Obstet Gynecol Reprod Biol 2002; 101: 169–74

159. Krasnow JJ, Berga SL, Guzick DS, et al. Vascular permeability factor and vascular endothelial growth factor in ovarian hyperstimulation syndrome. Fertil Steril 1996; 65: 552–5

160. Abramov Y, Schenker JG, Lewin A, et al. Plasma inflammatory cytokines correlate to the ovarian hyperstimulation syndrome. Hum Reprod 1996; 11: 1381–6

161. Enskog A, Nilsson L, Brannstrom M. Plasma levels of free vascular endothelial growth factor (165) (VEGF(165)) are not elevated during gonadotropin stimulation in in vitro fertilization (IVF) patients developing ovarian hyperstimulation syndrome (OHSS): results of a prospective cohort study with matched controls. Eur J Obstet Gynecol Reprod Biol 2001; 96: 196–201

162. Lee A, Christenson LK, Stouffer RL, et al. Vascular endothelial growth factor levels in serum and follicular fluid of patients undergoing in vitro fertilization. Fertil Steril 1997; 68: 305–11

163. Agarwal R, Tan SL, Wild S, et al. Serum vascular endothelial growth factor concentrations in in vitro fertilization cycles predict the risk of ovarian hyperstimulation syndrome. Fertil Steril 1999; 71: 278–93

164. Kitajima Y, Endo T, Manase K, et al. Gonadotropin-releasing hormone agonist administration reduced vascular endothelial growth factor (VEGF), VEGF receptors, and vascular permeability of the ovaries of hyperstimulated rats. Fertil Steril 2004; 81 (Suppl 2): 842–9

165. Chen CD, Wu MY, Chen HF, et al. Prognostic importance of serial cytokine changes in ascites and pleural effusion in women with severe ovarian hyperstimulation syndrome. Fertil Steril 1999; 72: 286–92

166. Geva E, Amit A, Lessing JB, et al. Follicular fluid levels of vascular endothelial growth factor. Are they predictive markers for ovarian hyperstimulation syndrome? J Reprod Med 1999; 44: 91–6

167. Kendall RL, Rhomas KA. Inhibition of vascular endothelial cell growth factor activity by an endogenously encoded soluble receptor. Proc Natl Acad Sci USA 1993; 90: 10705–9

168. Adashi EY. The potential relevance of cytokines to ovarian physiology: the emerging role of resident ovarian cells of the white blood cell series. Endocr Rev 1990; 11: 454–64

169. D'Ambrogio G, Fasciani A, Monti M, et al. Serum vascular endothelial growth factor levels before starting gonadotropin treatment in women who have developed moderate forms of ovarian hyperstimulation syndrome. Gynecol Endocrinol 1999; 13: 311–15

170. Chen CD, Chen HF, Lu HF, et al. Value of serum and follicular fluid cytokine profile in the prediction of moderate to severe ovarian hyperstimulation syndrome. Hum Reprod 2000; 15: 1037–42

171. Barak V, Mordel N, Zakicek G, et al. The correlation between interleukin 2 and interleukin 2 receptors to oestradiol, progesterone and testosterone levels in pre-ovulatory follicles of in vitro fertilization patients. Hum Reprod 1992; 7: 926–9

172. Orvieto R, Voliovitch I, Fishman P, et al. Interleukin-2 and ovarian hyperstimulation syndrome: a pilot study. Hum Reprod 1995; 10: 24–7

173. Revel A, Barak V, Lavy Y, et al. Characterization of intraperitoneal cytokines and nitrites in women with severe ovarian hyperstimulation syndrome. Fertil Steril 1996; 66: 66–71

174. Manolopoulos K, Lang U, Gips H, et al. Elevated interleukin-10 and sex steroid levels in peritoneal fluid of patients with ovarian hyperstimulation syndrome. Eur J Obstet Gynecol Reprod Biol 2001; 99: 226–31

175. Albert C, Garrido N, Mercader A, et al. The role of endothelial cells in the pathogenesis of ovarian hyperstimulation syndrome. Mol Hum Reprod 2002; 8: 409–18

176. Damas P, Ledoux D, Nys M, et al. Cytokine serum level during severe sepsis in humans IL-6 as a marker of severity. Ann Surg 1992; 215: 356–62

177. Buyalos RP, Watson JM, Martinez Maza O, et al. Detection of IL-6 in human follicular fluid. Fertil Steril 1992; 57: 1230–40

178. Motro B, Itin A, Sacjs L, et al. Pattern of IL-6 gene expression in vivo suggests a role for this cytokine in angiogenesis. J Cell Biol 1990; 87: 3092–6

179. Friedlander MA, de Mola JR, Goldfarb JM. Elevated levels of interleukin-6 in ascites and serum from women with ovarian hyperstimulation syndrome. Fertil Steril 1993; 60: 826–32

180. Finkel MS, Oddis CV, Jacob TD, et al. Negative isotropic effects of cytokines on the heart mediated by nitric oxide. Science 1992; 257: 387–9

181. Kishimoto T. The biology of IL-6. Blood 1989; 74: 1–10

182. Loret de Mola JR, Flores JP, Baumgardner GP, et al. Elevated interleukin-6 levels in the ovarian hyperstimulation syndrome: ovarian imunohistochemical localization of interleukin-6 signal. Obstet Gynecol 1996; 87: 581–7

183. Loret de Mola JR, Baumgardner GP, Goldfarb JM, et al. Ovarian hyperstimulation syndrome: pre-ovulatory serum concentrations of interleukin-6, interleukin-1 receptor antagonist and tumor necrosis factor cannot predict its occurrence. Hum Reprod 1996; 11: 1377–80

184. Aboulghar MA, Mansour RT, Serour GI, et al. Elevated levels of angiogenin in serum and ascitic fluid from patients with severe ovarian hyperstimulation syndrome. Hum Reprod 1998; 13: 2068–71

185. Levin I, Gamzu R, Hasson Y, et al. Increased erythrocyte aggregation in ovarian hyperstimulation syndrome: a possible contributing factor in the pathophysiology of this disease. Hum Reprod 2004; 19: 1076–80

186. Rizk B. Prevention of ovarian hyperstimulation syndrome: the Ten Commandments. Presented at the 1993 European Society of Human Reproduction and Embryology Symposium, Tel Aviv, Israel, 1993: 1–2

187. Schwartz M, Jewelewicz R, Dyrenfurth I. The use of the human menopausal and chorionic gonadotropins for induction of ovulation. Sixteen years experience at Sloane Hospital for women. Am J Obstet Gynecol 1980; 138: 801

188. Morris RS, Paulson RJ, Sauer MV, et al. Predictive value of serum oestradiol concentrations and oocyte number in severe ovarian hyperstimulation syndrome. Hum Reprod 1995; 10: 811–14

189. Tal J, Faz B, Samberg I, et al. Ultrasonographic and clinical correlates of menotrophin versus sequential clomiphene citrate: menotrophin therapy for induction of ovulation. Fertil Steril 1985; 4: 342–9

190. Blankstein J, Shalev J, Saadon T, et al. Ovarian hyperstimulation syndrome prediction by number and size of preovulatory ovarian follicles. Fertil Steril 1987; 47: 597–602

191. Danninger B, Brunner M, Obruca A, et al. Prediction of ovarian hyperstimulation syndrome of baseline ovarian volume prior to stimulation. Hum Reprod 1996; 11: 1597–9

192. Moohan JM, Curcio K, Leoni M, et al. Low intraovarian vascular resistance: a marker for severe ovarian hyperstimulation syndrome. Fertil Steril 1997; 57: 728–32

193. Delvigne A, Rozenberg S. Review of clinical course and treatment of ovarian hyperstimulation syndrome (OHSS). Hum Reprod Update 2003; 9: 77–96

194. Garcia-Velasco JA, Zuniga A, Pacheco A. Coasting acts through downregulation of VEGF gene expression and protein secretion. Hum Reprod 2004; 19: 1530–8

195. Delvigne A, Rozenberg S. A qualitative systematic review of coasting, a procedure to avoid ovarian hyperstimulation in IVF patients. Hum Reprod Update 2002; 8: 291–6

196. Guibert J, Olivennes F. Ovarian hyperstimulation syndrome: prevention in IVF and non-IVF treatment. In Gerris J, Olivennes F, de Sutter P, eds. Assisted Reproductive Technologies: Quality and Safety. New York: Parthenon Publishing, 2004: 169–80

197. Rabinowitz J, Kushnir O, Shalev J, et al. Rescue of menotropin cycles prone to develop ovarian hyperstimulation. Br J Obstet Gynaecol 1987; 94: 1098–102

198. Urman B, Pride SM, Ho Yuen B. Management of over-stimulated gonadotrophin cycles with a controlled drift period. Hum Reprod 1992; 7: 213–17

199. Sher G, Salem R, Fernman M, et al. Eliminating the risks of life-endangering complications following over-stimulation with menotropin fertility agents: a report on women undergoing in vitro fertilization and embryo transfer. Obstet Gynecol 1993; 81: 1009–11

200. Benadiva CA, Davis O, Kilgman I, et al. Withholding gonadotropin administration is an effective alternative for the prevention of ovarian hyperstimulation syndrome. Fertil Steril 1997; 67: 724–7

201. Abdalla HI, Ahmoye N, Brinsden P, et al. The effect of the dose of human chorionic gonadotropin and the type of gonadotropin stimulation on oocyte recovery rates in an in vitro fertilization program. Fertil Steril 1987; 48: 958–63

202. Al-Inany H, Aboulghar M. GnRH antagonist in assisted reproduction: a Cochrane review. Hum Reprod 2002; 17: 874–85

203. Revel A, Casper RF. The use of LHRH agonists to induce ovulation. In Devroey P, ed. Infertility and Reproductive Medicine Clinics of North America: GnRH analogues. Philadelphia: WB Saunders, 2001: 105–18

204. Gonen Y, Balakier H, Powell W, et al. Use of gonadotrophin-releasing hormone agonist to trigger follicular maturation for in vitro fertilization. J Clin Endocrinol Metab 1990; 71: 918–22

205. Itskovitz J, Boldes R, Levron J, et al. Induction of preovulatory luteinizing hormone surge and prevention of hyperstimulation syndrome by gonadotrophin-

releasing hormone agonist. Fertil Steril 1991; 56: 213–20

206. Emperaire JC, Ruffie A. Triggering ovulation with endogenous luteinizing hormone may prevent ovarian hyperstimulation syndrome. Fertil Steril 1991; 56: 506–10

207. Rizk B. Can OHSS in ART be eliminated? In Rizk B, Meldrum D, Schoolcraft W, eds. A Clinical Step-by-step Course for Assisted Reproductive Technologies. 35th Annual Postgraduate Program, Middle East Fertility Society. Presented at the ASRM 58th Annual Meeting, Seattle, WA, 2002: 65–102

208. Rizk B, ed. Ovarian Hyperstimulation syndrome: Pathophysiology, Prevention and Management. Cambrige: Cambridge University Press, 2005: 254–49

209. Felberbaum RE, Reissmann T, Kupker W, et al. Preserved pituitary response under ovarian stimulation with hMG and GnRH antagonist (cetrorelix) in women with tubal infertility. Eur J Obstet Gynecol Reprod Biol 1995; 61: 151–5

210. Olivennes F, Fanchin R, Bouchard P, et al. Triggering of ovulation by a gonadotropin-releasing hormone (GnRH) agonist in patients pretreated with GnRH antagonist. Fertil Steril 1996; 66: 151–3

211. Itskovitz-Eldor J, Kol S, Mannaerts B. Use of a single bolus of GnRH agonist triptorelin to trigger ovulation after GnRH antagonist ganirelix treatment in women undergoing ovarian stimulation for assisted reproduction, with special reference to the prevention of ovarian hyperstimulation syndrome: preliminary report: short communication. Hum Reprod 2000; 15: 1965–8

212. Bracero MW, Jurema MN, Posada JG, et al. Triggering ovulation with leuprorelide acetate (LA) instead of human chorionic gonadotropin (hCG) after the use of ganirelix for in vitro fertilization-embryo transfer (IVF–ET) does not compromise cycle outcome and may prevent ovarian hyperstimulation syndrome. Presented at the American Society for Reproductive Medicine 57th Annual Meeting, Orlando, FL, 2001: General Program Prize, Abstracts of the scientific oral and poster sessions program supplement, abstr 0–245, S–93

213. The European Recombinant LH Study Group. Recombinant human leuteinizing hormone is as effective as, but safer than, urinary human chorionic gonadotrophin in inducing final follicular maturation and ovulation in in vitro fertilization procedures: results of a multi-center double blind study. J Clin Endocrinol 2001; 86: 2607–16

214. Friedman CI, Schmidt GE, Chang FE, et al. Severe ovarian hyperstimulation syndrome following follicular aspiration. Am J Obstet Gynecol 1984; 150: 436–7

215. Egbase PE, Makhseed M, Al Sharhan M, et al. Timed unilateral ovarian follicular aspiration prior to administration of human chorionic gonadotrophin for the prevention of severe ovarian hyperstimulation syndrome in in-vitro fertilization: a prospective randomized study. Hum Reprod 1997; 12: 2603–6

216. Asch RH, Ivery G, Goldsman M, et al. The use of intravenous albumin in patients at high risk for severe ovarian hyperstimulation syndrome. Hum Reprod 1993; 8: 1015–20

217. Shoham Z, Weissman A, Barash A, et al. Intravenous albumin for the prevention of severe ovarian hyperstimulation syndrome in an in vitro fertilization program: a prospective, randomized, placebo controlled study. Fertil Steril 1994; 62: 137–42

218. Shalev E, Giladi Y, Matilsky M, et al. Decreased incidence of severe ovarian hyperstimulation syndrome in high risk in-vitro fertilization patients receiving intravenous albumin: a prospective study. Fertil Steril 1994; 62: 137–42

219. Ng E, Leader A, Claman P, et al. Intravenous albumin does not prevent the development of severe ovarian hyperstimulation syndrome in an in-vitro fertilization programme. Hum Reprod 1995; 10: 107–10

220. Mukherjee T, Copperman AB, Sandler B, et al. Severe ovarian hyperstimulation despite prophylactic albumin at the time of oocyte retrieval for in vitro fertilization and embryo transfer. Fertil Steril 1995; 64: 641–3

221. Shaker AG, Zosmer A, Dean N, et al. Comparison of intravenous albumin and transfer of fresh embryos with cryopreservation of all embryos for subsequent transfer in prevention of ovarian hyperstimulation syndrome. Fertil Steril 1996; 65: 992–6

222. Lewit N, Kol S, Ronene N, et al. Does intravenous administration of human albumin prevent severe ovarian hyperstimulation syndrome? Fertil Steril 1996; 66: 656

223. Aboulghar M, Evers JH, Al-Inany H. Intravenous albumin for preventing severe ovarian hyperstimulation syndrome. Cochrane Database Syst Rev 2000; 2: CD001302

224. Graf MA, Fischer R, Naether OG, et al. Reduced incidence of ovarian hyperstimulation syndrome by prophylactic infusion of hydroxyaethyl starch solution in an in-vitro fertilization programme. Hum Reprod 1997; 12: 2599–602

225. Konig E, Bussen S, Sitterlin M, Steck T. Prophylactic intravenous hydroxyethyl starch solution prevents moderate–severe ovarian hyperstimulation in in-vitro fertilization patients: a prospective, randomized, double-blind and placebo-controlled study. Hum Reprod 1998; 13: 2421–4

226. Tan SL, Balen A, el Hussein E, et al. The administration of glucocorticoids for the prevention of ovarian hyperstimulation syndrome in in-vitro fertilization: a prospective randomized study. Fertil Steril 1992; 58: 378–83

227. Costabile L, Unfer V, Manna C, et al. Use of intramuscular progesterone versus intravenous albumin for the prevention of ovarian hyperstimulation syndrome. Gynecol Obstet Invest 2000; 50: 182–5

228. Amso NN, Ahuga KK, Morris N, et al. The management of predicted OHS involving gonadotrophin-releasing analogue with elective cryopreservation of all pre-embryos. Fertil Steril 1990; 53: 1087–90

229. Rizk B, Manners CV, Davies MC, et al. Immunohistochemical expression of endometrial proteins and pregnancy outcomes in frozen embryo replacement cycles. Hum Reprod 1992; 7: 413–17

230. Wada I, Matson PL, Trooup SA, et al. Does elective cryopreservation of all embryos from women at risk of ovarian hyperstimulation syndrome reduce the incidence of the condition? Br J Obstet Gynaecol 1993; 10: 265–9

231. Queenan JT Jr, Veeck LL, Toner JP, et al. Cryopreservation of all prezygotes in patients at risk of severe hyperstimulation does not eliminate the syndrome, but chances of pregnancy are excellent with subsequent frozen–thaw transfers. Hum Reprod 1997; 12: 1573–6

232. D'Angelo A, Amso NN. Embryo freezing for preventing ovarian hyperstimulation syndrome: a Cochrane review. Hum Reprod 2002; 17: 2787–94

233. Homburg R, Armar NA, Eshel J, et al. Influence of serum luteinizing hormone concentrations on ovulation, conception and early pregnancy loss in polycystic ovary syndrome. Br Med J 1988; 297: 1024–6

234. Aboulghar MA, Mansour RT, Serour GI, et al. Recombinant follicle-stimulating hormone in the treatment of patients with history of severe ovarian hyperstimulation syndrome. Fertil Steril 1996; 66: 757–60

235. Rosenwaks Z. Ovarian hyperstimulation syndrome (OHSS): strategies for prevention. In Muasher SJ, Rizk B, eds. American Society for Reproductive Medicine 59th Annual Meeting. 36th Postgraduate Program. Birmingham, AL: American Society for Reproductive Medicine, 2003: 153–73

236. De Leo V, la Marca A, Ditto A, et al. Effects of metformin on gonadotropin-induced ovulation in women with polycystic ovary syndrome. Fertil Steril 1999; 72: 282–5

237. Rizk B, Nawar MG. Laparoscopic ovarian drilling for surgical induction of ovulation in polycystic ovarian syndrome. In Allahbadia G, ed. Manual of Ovulation Induction. Mumbai, India: Rotunda Medical Technologies, 2001: 140–4

238. Fukaya T, Murakami T, Tamura M, et al. Laser vaporization of the ovarian surface in polycystic ovary disease results in reduced ovarian hyperstimulation and improved pregnancy rates. Am J Obstet Gynecol 1995; 173: 119–25

239. Egbase P, Al-Awadi S, Al-Sharhan M, Grudzinskas JG. Unilateral ovarian diathermy prior to successful in vitro fertilisation: a strategy to prevent ovarian hyperstimulation syndrome? J Obstet Gynaecol 1998; 18: 171–3

240. Rimington MR, Walker SM, Shaw RW. The use of laparoscopic ovarian electrocautery in preventing cancellation of in vitro fertilization treatment cycles due to risk of ovarian hyperstimulation syndrome in women with polycystic ovaries. Hum Reprod 1997; 12: 1443–7

241. Almeida OD Jr, Rizk B. Microlaparoscopic ovarian drilling under local anesthesia. Middle East Fertil Soc J 1998; 3: 189–91

242. Shapiro AG, Thomas T, Epstein M. Management of hyperstimulation syndrome. Fertil Steril 1977; 28: 237–9

243. Haning RV, Stawn EY, Nolten WE. Pathophysiology of the ovarian hyperstimulation syndrome. Obstet Gynecol 1985; 66: 220–4

244. Thaler I, Yoffe N, Kaftory J, et al. Treatment of ovarian hyperstimulation syndrome: the physiologic basis for a modified approach. Fertil Steril 1981; 36: 110–13

245. Ferraretti AP, Gianaroli L, Diotallevi L, et al. Dopamine treatment for severe hyperstimulation syndrome. Hum Reprod 1992; 7: 180–3

246. Tsunoda T, Shibahara H, Hirano Y, et al. Treatment of ovarian hyperstimulation syndrome using an oral dopamine prodrug, docarpamine. Gynecol Endocrinol 2003; 17: 281–6

247. Levin I, Almog B, Avni A et al. Effect of paracentesis of ascitic fluids on urinary output and blood indices in patients with severe ovarian hyperstimulation syndrome. Fertil Steril 2002; 77: 986–8

248. Padilla SL, Zamaria S, Baramki TA, et al. Abdominal paracentesis for the ovarian hyperstimulation syndrome with severe pulmonary compromise. Fertil Steril 1990; 53: 365–7

249. Al-Ramahi M, Leader A, Claman P, et al. A novel approach to the treatment of ascites associated with ovarian hyperstimulation syndrome. Hum Reprod 1997; 12: 2614–16

250. Koike T, Araki S, Minakami H, et al. Clinical efficacy of peritoneovenous shunting for the treatment of severe ovarian hyperstimulation syndrome. Hum Reprod 2000; 15: 113–17

251. Abuzeid MI, Nassar Z, Massaad Z, et al. Pigtail catheter for the treatment of ascites associated with ovarian hyperstimulation syndrome. Hum Reprod 2003; 18: 370–3

252. Aboulghar MA, Mansour RT, Serour GI, et al. Ultrasonically guided vaginal aspiration of ascites in the treatment of ovarian hyperstimulation syndrome. Fertil Steril 1990; 53: 933–5

253. Aboulghar MA, Mansour RT, Serour GI, et al. Autotransfusion of the ascitic fluid in the treatment of severe ovarian hyperstimulation syndrome (OHSS). Fertil Steril 1992; 58: 1056–9

254. Ito M, Harada T, Iwabe T, et al. Cytokine levels in a patient with severe ovarian hyperstimulation syndrome before and after the ultrafiltration and reinfusion of ascitic fluid. J Assist Reprod Genet 2000; 17: 118–20

255. Aboulghar MA, Mansour RT, Serour GI, et al. Management of severe ovarian hyperstimulation syndrome by ascitic fluid aspiration and intensive intravenous fluid therapy. Obstet Gynecol 1993; 81: 108–11

256. Hurwitz A, Milwidsky A, Yagel S, et al. Early unwinding of torsion of an ovarian cyst as a result of hyperstimulation syndrome. Fertil Steril 1983; 40: 393

257. Mashiach S, Bider D, Moran O, et al. Adnexal torsion of hyperstimulated ovaries in pregnancies after gonadotrophin therapy. Fertil Steril 1990; 53: 76–80

258. Aboulghar MA, Mansour RT, Serour GI, et al. Severe ovarian hyperstimulation syndrome complicated by ectopic pregnancy. Acta Obstet Gynecol Scand 1992; 70: 371–2

259. Shiau CS, Chang MY, Chiang CH, et al. Severe ovarian hyperstimulation syndrome coexisting with a bilateral ectopic pregnancy. Chang Gung Med J 2004; 27: 143–7

13

Intrauterine insemination

Samuel F. Marcus

INTRODUCTION

Intrauterine insemination (IUI) has been performed for many years. It is almost 200 years since John Hunter advised a man with hypospadias to inject his seminal fluid into his wife's vagina with a syringe, which resulted in a normal pregnancy[1]. In the 19th century, Sims artificially inseminated six women with negative postcoital tests. He used their husband's semen obtained from the vagina after intercourse; one pregnancy was achieved[2]. The first reported case of human donor insemination was by William Pancoast in 1884 in Philadelphia, USA[3]. Bunge and Sherman[4] first reported the successful use of frozen semen in 1953, but widespread use did not begin until the mid-1970s. The use of cryopreserved semen in donor insemination programs is now mandatory in most countries to minimize the possibility of transmission of human immunodeficiency virus (HIV) to the recipients. The term 'artificial insemination' (AI) covers a range of techniques for insemination, which can be done intravaginally, intracervically, by intrauterine, intrafallopian or intrafollicular methods[5,6], or intraperitoneally. AI has been used for a number of different indications, and either the husband/partner's sperm (AIH) or donor sperm (AID) may be used.

The rationale for the use of IUI is to reduce the effect of factors that may impede the progress of spermatozoa, such as vaginal acidity and cervical mucus hostility, and to benefit from the deposition a bolus of concentrated, motile, morphologically normal sperm as close as possible to the oocytes. Sperm preparation methods developed for *in vitro* fertilization and embryo transfer[7–9] have led to a resurgence of interest in IUI, making this a frequent first choice of the assisted conception techniques (ACT) that may be used for the treatment of infertile women with patent Fallopian tubes. The employment of washed prepared sperm for IUI has resulted in a significant reduction in the side-effects associated with the use of neat semen for IUI, such as painful uterine cramps, collapse and infection[9,10]. Couples seeking artificial insemination should be fully evaluated, including a complete medical history, a clinical examination and investigation of the presence of any abnormality such as tubal damage or ovulatory disorder.

COUNSELING

Couples seeking intrauterine insemination should receive adequate counseling prior to starting their treatment, especially when donor sperm is to be used. Couples should also be assured of complete confidentiality, and informed of the means by which donors are selected, screened and matched, the cost of treatment, the probability of success, complications and, in the United Kingdom when using donor sperm, the regulations imposed by the Human Fertilisation and Embryology Authority (HFEA), such as: 'any child born to a married woman following donor insemination is legally the child of her husband, unless he did not consent to his wife's treatment. For unmarried couples, any child born to a woman following donor insemination is legally the child of her male partner. Furthermore, the male partner may not have parental responsibility for that child under The Children Act 1989'[11]. Furthermore, in 2005 the UK government is to change the law which safeguards the anonymity of men who have donated sperm to childless couples, giving children born as a result of their donation the right to know their identity. There are several psychological issues surrounding insemination. Men may feel a loss of esteem and the fear of losing a wife or a partner because of infertility, and women may feel guilt or anger directed toward the male partner for having infertility problems; furthermore, the couple may feel that someone has intruded into their sexual life and this may affect their intimacy. These issues should be discussed and resolved before undergoing insemination.

INDICATIONS

Indications for donor insemination

The main indications for donor insemination are listed in Table 1. Many couples experiencing gross male subfertility may choose to undergo donor insemination in order to achieve pregnancy and childbirth. The introduction of oocyte–sperm micromanipulation procedures, such as intracytoplasmic sperm injection (ICSI), into *in vitro* fertilization and embryo transfer (IVF-ET) programs[12] has made it possible to achieve fertilization and pregnancies when only very few spermatozoa are available. Prior to the development of techniques such as percutaneous epididymal sperm aspiration (PESA)[13] and more recently testicular sperm extraction (TESE)[14], men with bilateral congenital absence of the vas, surgically unreconstructable vasa or other causes of vasal obstruction had very little chance of fathering their own children. Now, however, if these techniques are combined with ICSI, these men can be offered a real chance of achieving paternity with their own sperm[15,16]. Also, recent advances in preimplantation

Table 1 Main indications for insemination with donor semen

(1) Gross male subfertility
   obstructive azoospermia, e.g. congenital bilateral absence of the vasa deferentia
   non-obstructive azoospermia, e.g. Klinefelter's syndrome
   severe oligozoospermia
   severe asthenozoospermia
   severe teratozoospermia
   oligoasthenoteratozoospermia
   failed fertilization with ICSI
(2) Infectious disease in the male partner such as HIV
(3) Familial/genetic diseases e.g. hemophilia, Huntington's disease
(4) Severe rhesus incompatibility
(5) Lesbian couples or single women

ICSI, intracytoplasmic sperm injection; HIV, human immunodeficiency virus

diagnosis have enabled couples with hereditary or genetic diseases such as hemophilia and cystic fibrosis to have IVF, preimplantation embryo biopsy and transfer of normal embryos[17]. These methods have reduced the demand for donor insemination, but the cost of these procedures puts them beyond the means of many couples.

Increasing numbers of single women and lesbian couples are requesting artificial insemination with donor sperm. The practice of inseminating lesbian and single women remains a controversial issue. Some clinics, as a matter of policy, do not offer treatment to single women or lesbian couples. The reasons for refusing such treatment include: the absence of a father figure and the impact of his absence on the child's psychological development; an assumption that the daughters of lesbian mothers will themselves grow up to be homosexual. To date, there is no evidence to support an adverse effect of lesbian motherhood on childhood development[18]. Many single women would have liked to have a child within a partner relationship, but their age often forces them to decide between single motherhood or unwanted childlessness.

Indications for husband/partner insemination

There are a number of indications for IUI using husband's or partner's semen; these are summarized in

Table 2 Main indications for insemination with husband's/partner's semen

(1) Ejaculatory failure   *ANPR*
   Anatomical (e.g. hypospadias)
   Neurological (e.g. spinal-cord injury)
   Retrograde ejaculation (e g. multiple sclerosis)
   Psychological (e.g. impotence)

(2) Cervical factor
   Cervical mucus hostility
   Poor cervical mucus

(3) Mild male subfertility
   Hypospermia
   Oligospermia
   Asthenozoospermia
   Teratozoospermia
   Oligoasthenoteratozoospermia

(4) Immunological
   Male antisperm antibodies
   Female antisperm antibodies (cervical, serum)

(5) Unexplained infertility

(6) Endometriosis
   minimal
   mild

(7) Ovulatory dysfunction

(8) Human immunodeficiency virus (HIV)-positive male partner and HIV-negative female partner

(9) Combined infertility factors

Table 2. Ejaculatory failure is the classical indication, because of the inability of the partner to ejaculate into the vagina, and cervical mucus hostility is another logical indication for IUI, as it bypasses the cervical canal. The most common indications for IUI are some of the less severe forms of male-factor infertility and unexplained infertility, and yet these are the most controversial. Other indications for IUI include immunological causes of infertility and minimal to mild endometriosis. Ovulatory dysfunction, in the author's view, should be treated initially by ovulation induction and timed sexual intercourse, and if these measures fail, then IUI with controlled ovarian stimulation would be indicated. Other rare indications for IUI using husband/partner sperm include allergy to sperm[19,20] and poor response to superovulation in an IVF program, provided that no tubal pathology exists. Recently, insemination of HIV-negative women with the processed semen of HIV-positive partners has been carried out to reduce the risk of male to female sexual transfer of HIV[21–23]. Recent advances in cancer treatment and the better chance of survival have also led some centers, such as Bourn Hall, to offer cryopreservation of semen for men prior to them receiving cancer chemotherapy, radiotherapy or orchidectomy for testicular cancer[24]. Recently, cytometrically separated sperm cells (MicroSort®) has been used for preconception gender selection[25]. Preconception sex selection for non-medical reasons raises many legal, social and ethical issues[26].

METHODS OF INTRAUTERINE INSEMINATION

Step

The steps involved in intrauterine insemination are:

(1) Ovarian stimulation;

(2) Monitoring of follicular growth and endometrial development;

(3) Timing of insemination;

(4) Semen preparation;

(5) IUI with prepared sperm.

Ovarian stimulation

Intrauterine insemination may be carried out in either a natural or a stimulated cycle.

Several studies have reported an increase in pregnancy rates when superovulation was combined with intrauterine insemination[27–29]. Many ovarian stimulation protocols have been devised for use with IUI, including clomiphene citrate alone or in combination with gonadotropins and human chorionic gonadotropin (hCG); gonadotropins alone, or combined with the use of a gonadotropin releasing hormone (GnRH) agonist or antagonists and hCG. Table 3 summarizes the main drugs which are commonly used for superovulation. The protocol most used at Bourn Hall for IUI is follicle stimulating hormone (FSH) only, in a dose of 75 IU of recombinant human FSH (r-hFSH) from day 3 of menstruation. When the mean diameter of the leading follicle is ≥ 18 mm, hCG 5000–10 000 IU is administered. The rationale of hCG administration is to achieve final follicular maturation and rupture. Manzi and co-workers[30] reported

Table 3 Commonly used superovulation drugs for intrauterine insemination

Agent	Trade name	Company	Route of administration	Reported side-effects
Antiestrogens				
Clomiphene citrate	Clomid	Aventis	oral	hot flushes, headaches, blurred vision,
	Serophene	Serono	oral	hair loss, abdominal distension, rash, nausea
Tamoxifen	Nolvadex	AstraZeneca	oral	
Gonadotropins				
Follicle stimulating hormone	Menogon	Ferring	IM	headaches, breast tenderness, ovarian
and luteinizing hormone	Menopur	Ferring	SC/IM	hyperstimulation, multiple pregnancy,
				allergic reaction
Recombinant follicle	Gonal-F	Serono	SC/IM	
stimulating hormone	Puregon/	Organon	SC/IM	
	Follistim			
Human chorionic	Choragon	Ferring	IM	edema, ovarian hyperstimulation,
gonadotropin	Pregnyl	Organon	SC/IM	allergic reaction and mood changes
Recombinant human	Ovidrel/	Serono	SC	
chorionic gonadotropin	ovitrelle			
Gonadotropin releasing hormone agonists				
Buserelin	Suprefact	Aventis	nasal/ SC	headaches, local irritation, hot flushes,
	Suprecur	Aventis	nasal/ SC	vaginal dryness, loss of libido, blurred vision,
				ovarian cysts, allergic reaction
Naferelin	Synarel	Pharmacia	nasal	
Goserelin	Zoladex	AstraZeneca	SC implant	
Leuprorelin	Prostap SR	Wyeth	IM implant	
Gonadotropin releasing	Cetrotide	Serono	SC	local irritation, nausea, headache,
hormone antagonists	Orgalutron/	Organon	SC	hypersensitivity reaction
	Antagon			

SC, subcutaneous; IM, intramuscular

significant improvement of pregnancy outcome when they selectively used GnRH agonist and human menopausal gonadotropin (hMG) in women who had previously shown evidence of premature luteinization on hMG alone. The rationale for the use of superovulation with IUI is to increase the number of oocytes available for insemination, and thus the chance of implantation occurring. Stimulation also increases steroid production, which may also improve the chance of fertilization and embryo implantation[28,31]. When considering whether or not to use ovarian stimulation for IUI, the benefit of increased success rates achieved compared with natural cycles must be balanced against the increased cost of medication and monitoring, as well as the potential side-effects of these medications. These include ovarian hyperstimu-

lation syndrome (OHSS), which is the most serious complication, and the increased incidence of maternal and neonatal complications associated with high-order multiple pregnancies[32–34]. The patients should also be informed that a possible association between superovulation drugs and later development of ovarian cancer remains uncertain, but none has yet been proven[35,36]. Specialists should confine the use of ovulation induction drugs to the lowest effective dose and duration of use. The National Institute of Clinical Excellence (NICE) in the UK[37] advocates that ovarian stimulation should not be offered where IUI is used to manage a male-factor fertility problem and unexplained infertility because of the risk of multiple pregnancy. At Bourn Hall, patients are offered the choice of stimulated- or natural-cycle IUI.

Monitoring of follicular growth and endometrial development

It is essential that ovarian stimulation be carefully monitored in order to see whether an excessive number of follicles develop, indicating the possibility of developing OHSS and high-order multiple pregnancies. Monitoring of follicular growth is achieved by serial pelvic ultrasound scanning and measurement of plasma estradiol (E_2), luteinizing hormone (LH) and progesterone. Ideally, a baseline ultrasound scan should be performed as well as plasma FSH, LH and E_2, measurement on day 2 or 3 of menstruation, in order to exclude the presence of ovarian cysts or endometrial pathology, such as endometrial polyps. Elevated LH and FSH levels may predict poor follicular response, while a raised LH/FSH ratio may provide the first indication of polycystic ovaries and hence an excessive follicular response. From day 7 or 8 of stimulation, serial ultrasound scanning and plasma levels of LH, E_2 and progesterone are performed and the results charted. Plasma E_2 is an index of follicular maturity, while LH will detect a possible premature LH surge and progesterone will detect premature luteinization of the follicles.

Timing of insemination

The rationale behind the timing of insemination is that viable spermatozoa should be present in the female genital system at the time of ovulation. There are several methods for timing ovulation in natural or stimulated cycles, including simple methods such as the measurement of basal body temperature (BBT), found to be the least accurate, and assessment of cyclical changes in the cervical mucus, which is also unreliable. Templeton and colleagues[38] showed that in 35% of cycles the optimum mucus score was observed the day before the LH surge, in 44% of cycles it was optimum on the day of the LH surge and in 18% of cycles on the day after the LH surge, and in 3% it occurred 2 days after the LH surge. More recently, detection of the serum or urinary LH surge and ultrasound assessment of follicular growth and rupture have proved to be the most accurate methods of monitoring cycles. Vermesh and co-workers[39] showed that the use of a 'dipstick' LH test kit predicted ovulation in 84% of cycles in their series. In a stimulated cycle, if hCG is administered when the average diameter of the leading follicle is 20 mm, rupture of the follicle may be expected 34–46 h later, with a mean time interval of 38 h[40,41]. If the number of mature follicles exceeds four or the total number of follicles over 12 mm in diameter exceeds eight, hCG administration should be withheld and the couple advised to abstain from intercourse. The couple should be offered IVF/gamete intrafallopian transfer (GIFT) as an alternative if appropriate[31]. Many clinicians will perform two inseminations at 24 and 48 h from the timing of hCG administration. The efficacy of two versus one insemination has not yet been resolved[42–44]. The NICE fertility guidelines in the UK[37] advocate single rather than double intrauterine insemination. At Bourn Hall, approximately 38 h after hCG administration, the patient will have a pelvic ultrasound scan, and if she has ovulated by then, IUI will be performed; however, if the scan result indicates that the patient has not yet ovulated then she will have two inseminations, one on the same day and another 24 h later.

Sperm preparation and insemination procedure

Fresh semen is usually produced by masturbation and collected into one or two pots (split ejaculate). The highest sperm concentration is commonly present in the first part of the ejaculate. The addition of culture medium to the specimen pots before semen collection results in improved motility if there has been previous marked viscosity of the semen; likewise, addition of 50% albuminar 5 (A5; Armur Pharmaceutical Ltd, Eastbourne, UK) to the pot will reduce sperm agglutination if there are antisperm antibodies in the ejaculate. The ideal sperm preparation technique is the one which will achieve the largest number of morphologically normal motile spermatozoa in a small volume of physiological culture medium free from seminal plasma, leukocytes and bacteria[45]. Although there is no threshold of sperm concentration below which pregnancy is impossible, most conceptions occur when the concentration of inseminated motile sperm is more than 1 million/ml. The degree of motility and percentage of morphologically normal spermatozoa are the most important variables in fertility prognosis[46]. There are several different sperm preparation techniques for IUI, and each has its own advantages and disadvantages[47]. The most simple and cheapest is the conventional swim-up procedure. Sperm preparation using a density gradient technique yields the highest number of motile spermatozoa when compared with simple washing or swim-up methods, and the sperm density gradient technique significantly reduces bacterial contamination[47,48]. For many years, Percoll™ (LKB Biotechnology, Sweden) was the most commonly used density gradient. Percoll gradient is no longer available in the UK for human assisted reproduction; various other density gradients are available such as SilSelect (Microm, Fam, UK). The different methods used for sperm preparation are described in a later chapter.

Not only should insemination be carried out using aseptic techniques to avoid the risk of infection, but the procedure should also be carried out gently to avoid traumatizing the endometrium, as this could induce cramping and bleeding that may adversely affect survival of the spermatozoa. The procedure is performed in the dorsal position; the cervix is exposed with a bivalve speculum and cleaned. The preparation of spermatozoa is then withdrawn using a tuberculin syringe attached to an IUI catheter, the catheter is then threaded into the uterine cavity and semen is injected gently. There are several IUI catheters available such as the Wallace™ artificial insemination catheter (H G Wallace Ltd, Colchester, UK).

RESULTS OF INTRAUTERINE INSEMINATION

The results of IUI in terms of pregnancy rates per treatment cycle vary considerably between clinics. Evaluation of results is difficult because of the heterogeneity of patient populations and the different ovarian stimulation protocols used in the studies. Although there are a large number of published studies of IUI, most of these are retrospective and/or in small numbers; only a few are prospective and randomized trials. There is an undoubted need for a large prospective randomized study to evaluate the effectiveness of IUI, to elicit which group of patients will benefit most from this treatment and to assess the value of controlled ovarian hyperstimulation.

Table 4 summarizes the results of some published series on IUI treatment. During the period from 1989 to 1993, 237 patients underwent IUI at Bourn Hall; a total of 452 IUI treatment cycles were performed using husband/donor sperm, and 103 pregnancies were achieved, including: 11 biochemical (10.7%), ten abortions (9.7%), two ectopic pregnancies (1.9%), one

Table 4 Pregnancy rates for IUI related to the cause of infertility[49,50,52]. Values are expressed in percentage (range)

Indication for IUI	Martinez et al. (1993)	Crosignani et al. (1991), Crosignani and Walters (1994)
Idiopathic infertility (%)	18 (0–40)	27 (0–67)
Cervical mucus hostility (%)	14 (5–29)	—
Immunological infertility (%)	10 (3–18)	—
Endometriosis (%)	11 (0–18)	—
Male subfertility (%)	10 (0–20)	12.8 (0–40)
Ejaculatory failure (%)	11 (0–18)	—

heterotopic pregnancy with the intrauterine pregnancy resulting in a live birth (1%) and 79 deliveries (76.7%). The clinical pregnancy rates per treatment cycle were 12.3% for unexplained infertility, 16.4% for cervical mucus hostility, 10% for immunological infertility, 21% for mild male subfertility, 13.3% for ejaculatory failure, 0% for moderate/severe endometriosis and 15.8% for combined factors. The European Society of Human Reproduction and Embryology (ESHRE) multicenter prospective study[49] compared ovulation induction alone with ovulation induction in conjunction with IUI, intraperitoneal insemination (IPI), GIFT and IVF in the treatment of unexplained infertility. The pregnancy rate achieved from superovulation alone was less than when combined with IUI, IPI, GIFT or IVF. The ESHRE multicenter trial[50], which compared ovulation induction alone and ovulation induction combined with IUI, IPI, GIFT and IVF in the treatment of male subfertility, showed that ovulation induction with IUI, GIFT and IVF gave better results than IPI and ovulation induction alone. Recently, Cohlen and colleagues[51] systematically reviewed the literature for the Cochrane database and reported that IUI offers couples with male subfertility benefit over timed intercourse.

Martinez and colleagues[52], in an extensive review of the English literature from 1980 to 1991, showed that there was marked variation in the results of IUI between different clinics. An overall live birth rate of 11.0% per donor insemination cycle was reported in the latest Annual Report of the Human Fertilisation and Embryology Authority in the UK[53]. Again, there was a wide variation of results between clinics (0–25.0%). The multiple pregnancy rates also varied between clinics. In relation to maternal age, the live birth rate was 12.1% per treatment cycle in women aged < 38 years compared with 7.6% in women aged ≥ 38 years. Bourn Hall Clinic IUI (donor) results during the same time period gave a live birth rate of 13.6%, with an 11% multiple pregnancy rate (all twins).

FACTORS AFFECTING SUCCESS RATES

The success of IUI depends upon several factors, which include:

(1) Cause of infertility;

(2) Age of both partners;

(3) Duration of infertility;

(4) Treatment cycle rank;

(5) Sperm parameters.

Increasing female age is associated with a deterioration of natural fertility, mainly because of decreasing oocyte quality and, to a lesser extent, endometrial receptivity[54–56]; the decline is irrespective of previous childbirth[31]. Plosker and co-workers[56] reported cycle fecundity of 0.11–0.14 in women aged 25–39, compared with 0.04 in women aged >40 years. Corsan and colleagues[57] retrospectively analyzed the results of IUI in women 40 years or older, and found no viable pregnancies in 136 cycles in women aged ≥ 43 years. In their series, the fecundity rates for women aged 40, 41 and 42 were 9.6, 5.2 and 2.4 per cycle, respectively. They concluded that women aged 43 or more should consider other alternatives such as adoption or egg donation. At Bourn Hall, the pregnancy rate in women aged < 25 was 28.7%, compared with 10% in women aged 40 and more, and there were no pregnancies in the three women aged 45 years or more. Furthermore, increasing age of the male partner negatively influences the pregnancy rate[58,59]. This is possibly through an increased incidence of non–disjunction in the spermatozoa[60]. Most clinics have upper age limits for women they are prepared to treat. The chance of conception also declines with the duration of infertility[58,61].

Remohi and associates[62] reported a series of 489 cycles of controlled ovarian stimulation and IUI. The cycle fecundity rate was 0.07 for the first four cycles and 0.03 for the fifth through tenth cycle. In this series, 94% of the pregnancies occurred in the first four attempts. Other retrospective analyses of IUI data[28,63,64], using life-table analysis, showed a relatively constant probability of becoming pregnant after each IUI treatment through six cycles, which thereafter was hardly increased by continuing for longer. Agarwal and Buyalos[65] reported that the vast majority of the pregnancies in their series occurred in the first four treatment cycles. Most clinicians agree that further evaluation and discussion of the other treatment options available to couples, such as IVF or GIFT, should be carried out with them after four to six cycles of IUI. The NICE fertility guidelines[37] in the UK advocate up to six cycles of IUI for couples with mild male-factor fertility problems, unexplained fertility problems or minimal or mild endometriosis. The value of GIFT for women who fail to conceive through IUI has not yet been resolved, mainly because GIFT does not provide any information on fertilization and embryo cleavage[31].

The degree of motility and percentage of morphologically normal spermatozoa are the most important sperm parameters which affect fertility[46,61,66,67].

COMPLICATIONS OF TREATMENT

There are few complications to treatment by IUI; failure of the treatment could be said to be the most frequent. The complication that causes couples the most concern is the possibility of using the wrong semen sample. It is the duty of all staff involved to take all necessary measures to prevent this from happening. Other complications include the possibility of transmission of venereal disease. However, there have been no reported cases of HIV seroconversion, in either partner or child born after sperm washing, in over 3000 cycles of treatment where the male partner was HIV-positive and his female partner was HIV-negative[68]. Nevertheless, couples should be counseled that semen wash is a risk-reduction and not a risk-elimination technique for this group of patients.

Other complications include the remote possibility of consanguineous insemination when using donor sperm. Uterine contractions, intrauterine infection and anaphylaxis may also occur, especially if neat semen is used, which it should never be. Finally, there is a chance of ovarian hyperstimulation occurring from the drugs used for ovulation induction[69]. This is the most serious complication. Younger women and those with polycystic ovaries are at high risk; also, the risk is increased in cycles employing GnRH. Multiple pregnancy with its associated risks should also be considered as a possible complication of treatment. The main group at risk for multiple pregnancy after ovarian stimulation with gonadotropins and IUI is that of younger women < 30 years of age, who develop more than six mature follicles, with E_2 > 1000 pg/ml[70]. The risk of multiple pregnancy can be minimized by careful monitoring of treatment cycles.

CONCLUSIONS

Intrauterine insemination is a relatively simple and effective method of treatment for certain groups of subfertile couples. IUI is less invasive and cheaper than IVF or GIFT. With insemination, many couples can experience pregnancy, childbirth and the joy of raising children. However, careful selection of patients is important. Those who will benefit most are young women with patent Fallopian tubes, no ovulatory disorder, no endometriosis of moderate or severe degree and no severe degree of male-factor infertility in their partner. All couples require in-depth advice and counseling about the method, the effectiveness and the complications of treatment. The increased pregnancy rates achieved with superovulation as compared with natural cycles must be balanced against the cost of drugs and monitoring, as well as the complications such as multiple pregnancy and ovarian hyperstimulation syndrome. It is generally accepted that re-evaluation and discussion about other treatment options such as IVF should be carried out with couples after 4–6 cycles. IUI can be provided more easily to more infertile couples in District General Hospitals than can the more specialized techniques such as IVF, provided that there are adequate facilities for semen preparation and cycle monitoring. Although the main advantage of IUI over IVF is its simplicity, there are many advantages of IVF over IUI: principally, a higher pregnancy rate, the knowledge obtained about fertilization of oocytes and the ability to cryopreserve any spare embryos that may result from a treatment cycle.

While ICSI is the only realistic treatment for couples with severe male-factor infertility, IVF remains the realistic option for women with severe endometriosis and infertility due to severe tubal damage. Although IUI can be performed outside specialist units, a clinic with IVF facilities offers the best setting in case complications such as ovarian hyperstimulation occur, as patients can be offered the chance to convert to IVF and the possibility of freezing any surplus embryos.

REFERENCES

1. Shields FE. Artificial insemination as related to females. Fertil Steril 1950; 1: 271
2. Sims JM. Clinical notes on uterine surgery with special reference to the management of the sterile condition. London: Harolwiche, 1866
3. Hard AD. Artificial impregnation. Med World 1909; 27: 253
4. Bunge RG, Sherman JK. Fertilizing capacity of frozen human spermatozoa. Nature (London) 1953; 173: 767–9
5. Nuojua-Huttunen S, Tumivaara L, Tuntunen K, et al. Intrafollicular insemination for the treatment of infertility. Hum Reprod 1995; 10: 91–3
6. Nuojua-Huttunen S, Tumivaara L, Tuntunen K, et al. Comparison of fallopian sperm perfusion with intrauterine insemination in the treatment of infertility. Fertil Steril 1997; 5: 939–42
7. Sher G, Knutzen VK, Stratton CJ, et al. In vitro sperm capacitation and transcervical intrauterine insemination for the treatment of refractory infertility. Fertil Steril 1984; 41: 260–4
8. Sun SL, Gastaldi C, Paterson E, et al. Comparison of techniques for selection of bacteria-free sperm preparations. Fertil Steril 1987; 48: 659–63
9. Yovich JL, Matsen PL. The treatment of infertility by the high intrauterine insemination of the husband's washed spermatozoa. Hum Reprod 1988; 3: 939–43
10. Allen MC, Herbert I, Maxson WS, et al. Intrauterine insemination: a critical review. Fertil Steril 1985; 44: 569–80
11. Human Fertilisation and Embryology Act 1990. London: HMSO, 1990
12. Palermo G, Joris H, Devroey P, Van Steirtegheim AC. Pregnancies after intracytoplasmic injection of single spermatozoa into an oocyte. Lancet 1992; 340: 17–18
13. Craft IL, Khalifa Y, Boulos A, et al. Factors influencing the outcome of in-vitro fertilization with percutaneous aspirated epididymal spermatozoa and intracytoplasmic sperm injection in azoospermic men. Hum Reprod 1995; 10: 1791–4

14. Silber SJ, Van Steirtegheim AC, Liu J, et al. High fertilization and pregnancy rates after intracytoplasmic sperm injection with spermatozoa obtained from testicle biopsy. Hum Reprod 1995; 10: 148–52

15. Devroey P, Nagy Z, Goossens A, et al. Pregnancies after testicular sperm extraction and intracytoplasmic sperm injection in non-obstructive azoospermia. Hum Reprod 1995; 6: 1457–60

16. Sherman J, Silber SJ, Nagy Z, et al. The use of epididymal and testicular spermatozoa for intracytoplasmic sperm injection: the genetic implication for male infertility. Hum Reprod 1995; 10: 2031–43

17. Liu J, Lissens W, Silber SJ, et al. Birth after preimplantation diagnosis of cystic fibrosis delta F508 mutation by polymerase chain reaction in human embryos resulting from intracytoplasmic sperm injection with epididymal sperm. J Am Med Assoc 1994; 23: 1858–60

18. Golombok S, Tasker F. Donor insemination for single heterosexual and lesbian women: issues concerning the welfare of the child. Hum Reprod 1994; 9: 1972–6

19. Shapiro SS, Kooistra B, Schwartz D, et al. Induction of pregnancy in a woman with seminal plasma allergy. Fertil Steril 1981; 36: 405–7

20. Wuthrich B, Stern A, Johansson SG. Severe anaphylactic reaction to bovine serum albumin at the first attempt of artificial insemination. Allergy 1995; 50 179–83

21. Semprini AE. Insemination of HIV-negative women with processed semen of HIV-positive partner [Letter, comment]. Lancet 1993; 341: 1343–4

22. Semprini AE, Fiore S, Savasi V, et al. Assisted conception to reduce risk of male to female sexual transfer of HIV in sero discordant couples: an update. Presented at the Annual Meeting of the American Society for Reproductive Medicine, Boston, 1996: Abstr

23. Semprini AE, Fiore S, Pardi G. Reproductive counseling for HIV discordant couples [Letter; comment]. Lancet 1997; 349: 1401–2

24. Lass A, Akagbosu F, Abusheikha N, et al. A programme of semen cryopreservation for patients with malignant disease in a tertiary infertility centre: lessons from 8 years' experience. Hum Reprod 1998; 13: 3256–61

25. Fugger E, Black S, Keyvanfar K, Schulman J. Births of normal daughters after MicroSort sperm separation and intrauterine insemination, in-vitro fertilization, or intracytoplasmic sperm injection. Hum Reprod 1998; 13: 2367–70

26. Dahl E, Beutel M, Brosig B, Hinsch K. Preconception sex selection for non-medical reasons: a retrospective survey from Germany. Hum Reprod 2003; 18: 2231–4

27. Dodson WC, Whitesides DB, Hughes CL, et al. Superovulation with intrauterine insemination in the treatment of infertility: a possible alternative to gamete intrafallopian transfer and in vitro fertilization. Fertil Steril 1987; 48: 441–3

28. Wallach EE. Gonadotrophin treatment of the ovulatory patient: the pros and cons of empiric therapy for infertility. Fertil Steril 1991; 55: 478–80

29. Hughes EE. The effectiveness of ovulation induction and intrauterine insemination in the treatment of persistent infertility: a meta-analysis. Hum Reprod 1997; 12: 1865–72

30. Manzi DL, Dumez S, Scott LB, Nulsen JC. Selective use of leuprolide acetate in women undergoing superovulation with intrauterine insemination results in significant improvement in pregnancy outcome. Fertil Steril 1995; 63: 866–73

31. Edwards RG, Brody SA. Natural cycle and ovarian stimulation in assisted conception. In Edwards RG, Brody SA, eds. Principles and Practice of Assisted Human Reproduction. Philadelphia: WB Saunders, 1995: 233–84

32. Sheldon R, Kemmann E, Bohrer M, Pasquale S. Multiple gestation is associated with the use of high sperm numbers in the intrauterine insemination specimen in women undergoing gonadotrophin stimulation. Fertil Steril 1988; 49: 607–10

33. Levene MI, Wild J, Steer P. Higher multiple births and the modern management of infertility in Britain. Br J Obstet Gynaecol 1989; 99: 607–13

34. Lipitz S, Fishel S, Watts C, et al. High order multifetal gestation – management and outcome. Obstet Gynecol 1990; 76: 215–18

35. Cohen J, Forman R, Harlaps S, et al. IFFS expert group report on the Whittemore study related to the risk of ovarian cancer associated with the use of infertility agents. Hum Reprod 1993; 8: 996–9

36. Whittemore AS. Fertility drugs and the risk of ovarian cancer. Hum Reprod 1993; 8: 999–1000

37. National Institute of Clinical Excellence. Fertility: assessment and treatment for people with fertility problems, Clinical Guidelines No 11. London: Abba Litho Ltd UK, 2004

38. Templeton AA, Penney GC, Lees MM. Relation between the luteinizing hormone peak, the nadir of basal body temperature and the cervical mucus score. Br J Obstet Gynaecol 1982; 89: 985–8

39. Vermesh M, Kletzky OA, Davajam V, Israel R. Monitoring techniques to predict and detect ovulation. Fertil Steril 1987; 47: 259–64

40. O'Herlihy C, Pepperell RJ, Robinson HP. Ultrasound timing of human chorionic gonadotrophin

administration in clomiphene stimulated cycles. Obstet Gynecol 1982; 59: 40–5

41. Anderson AG, Als-Nielson B, Hornness PJ, French Anderson L. Time interval from human chorionic gonadotrophin (HCG) injection to follicular rupture. Hum Reprod 1995; 10: 3202–5

42. Ransom MX, Blotner MB, Bohrer M, et al. Does increasing frequency of intrauterine insemination improve pregnancy rates significantly during superovulation cycles. Fertil Steril 1994; 61: 303–7

43. Khalifa Y, Redgment CJ, Tsirigotis M, et al. The value of single versus repeated insemination in intrauterine donor insemination cycles. Hum Reprod 1995; 10: 153–4

44. Cantineau AE, Heineman MJ, Cohlen BJ. Single versus double intrauterine insemination (IUI) in stimulated cycles for subfertile couples. Cochrane Database Syst Rev 2003; 1: CD003854

45. Pardo M, Bancells N. Artificial insemination with husband's sperm (AIH). Techniques for sperm selection. Arch Androl 1989; 22: 15–27

46. Ombelet W, Deblaere K, Bosmans E, et al. Semen quality and intrauterine insemination. Reprod Biomed Online 2003; 7: 485–92

47. Berger T, Marrs RP, Moyer DL. Comparison of techniques for selection of motile spermatozoa. Fertil Steril 1985; 43: 268–73

48. Punjabi V, Gerris J, Van Bijilen J, et al. Comparison between different pre-treatment techniques for sperm recovery prior to intrauterine insemination, GIFT or IVF. Hum Reprod 1990; 5: 75–8

49. Crosignani PG, Walters DE, Soliani A. The ESHRE multicentre trial on the treatment of unexplained infertility: a preliminary report. Hum Reprod 1991; 6: 953–8

50. Crosignani PG, Walters DE. Clinical pregnancy and male subfertility, the ESHRE multicentre trial on the treatment of male subfertility. Hum Reprod 1994; 9: 1112–18

51. Cohlen BJ, Vandekerckhove P, te Velde ER, Habbema JD. Timed intercourse versus intrauterine insemination with or without ovarian hyperstimulation for subfertility in men. Cochrane Database Syst Rev 2000; 2: CD000360

52. Martinez AR, Bernardus RE, Vermeiden JPW, Schoemaker J. Basic questions on intrauterine insemination: an update. Obstet Gynecol Surv 1993; 48: 811–28

53. Human Fertilisation and Embryology Authority. The Patient's Guide to Donor Insemination. London: HFEA, 2002

54. Marcus SF, Edwards RG. High rates of pregnancy after long-term down-regulation of women with severe endometriosis. Am J Obstet Gynecol 1994; 171: 812–17

55. Marcus SF, Brinsden PR. In vitro fertilization and embryo transfer in women aged 40 years and more. Hum Reprod Update 1996; 2: 459–648

56. Plosker SM, Jacobson W, Amao P. Predicting and optimizing success in an intrauterine insemination program. Hum Reprod 1994; 9: 2014–21

57. Corsan G, Trias A, Trout S, Kemmann E. Ovulation induction combined with intrauterine insemination in women 40 years and older: is it worthwhile. Hum Reprod 1996; 11: 1109–12

58. Mathieu C, Ecochard R, Bied V, et al. Cumulative conception rate following intrauterine artificial insemination with husband spermatozoa: influence of husband age. Hum Reprod 1995; 10: 1090–7

59. Brzechffa PR, Buyalos RP. Female and male partners' age and menotrophin requirement influence pregnancy rates with human menopausal gonadotrophin therapy in combination with intrauterine insemination. Hum Reprod 1997; 12: 29–32

60. Griffin DK, Abruzzo MA, Millie EA, et al. Nondisjunction in human sperm: evidence of an effect of increasing paternal age. Hum Mol Genet 1995; 4: 2227–32

61. Tomlinson MJ, Amissah Arthur JB, Thompson KA, et al. Prognostic indicators for intrauterine insemination (IUI): statistical mode for IUI success. Hum Reprod 1996; 11: 1892–6

62. Remohi J, Gastaldi C, Patrizio P, et al. Intrauterine insemination and controlled ovarian hyperstimulation in cycles before GIFT. Hum Reprod 1989; 4: 918–20

63. Martinez AR, Bernardus RE, Vermeiden JPW. Factors affecting pregnancy results after intrauterine insemination. Presented at the 4th Meeting of the European Society of Human Reproduction and Embryology, Barcelona, Spain July 1988: Abstr 35

64. Roger A, Lalich DO, Edward L, et al. Life table analyses of intrauterine insemination pregnancy rates. Am J Obstet Gynecol 1988; 158: 980–4

65. Agarwal SK, Buyalos RP. Clomiphene citrate with intrauterine insemination: is it effective therapy in women above the age of 35 years? Fertil Steril 1996; 65: 759–63

66. Toner JP, Mossad H, Grow DR, et al. Value of sperm morphology assessed by strict criteria for prediction of the outcome of artificial intrauterine insemination. Andrologia 1995; 27: 143–8

67. Berg U, Brucker C, Berg FD. Effect of motile sperm count after swim-up on the outcome of intrauterine insemination. Fertil Steril 1997; 67: 747–50

68. Gilling-Smith C, Almeida P. HIV, hepatitis B and hepatitis C and infertility: reducing risk. Hum Fertil 2003; 6: 106–12

69. Brinsden PR, Wada I, Tan SL, et al. Diagnosis, prevention and management of ovarian hyperstimulation syndrome. Br J Obstet Gynaecol 1995; 102: 767–72

70. Valbuena D, Simon C, Remero JL, et al. Factors responsible for multiple pregnancies after ovarian stimulation and intrauterine insemination with gonadotrophins. J Assist Reprod Genet 1996; 13: 663–9

14

Oocyte recovery and embryo transfer techniques for *in vitro* fertilization

Peter R. Brinsden

INTRODUCTION

The first culture of human oocytes *in vitro* from ovarian tissue removed at laparotomy is ascribed to Gregory Pincus some 25 years before the same experiments were repeated by Robert Edwards[1]. The need to retrieve individual human oocytes by a less invasive procedure, initially for research and later for the treatment of infertility, was recognized early on by Edwards. He came to hear of Patrick Steptoe, a consultant gynecologist in Oldham, Lancashire, who in 1968 was the only man in England operating with the laparoscope. He was therefore able to see the female pelvis in a minimally invasive way and to see ovarian follicles, with the potential of aspirating oocytes from them[2]. It was for this reason that Edwards, the scientist, and Steptoe, the gynecologist, came together to collaborate and ultimately to create the first child born as a result of *in vitro* fertilization and embryo transfer (IVF–ET)[3].

Oocytes were collected for IVF exclusively by laparoscopy from then until the great technological advances made in ultrasound imaging allowed ovarian follicles to be clearly seen[4]. Systems were continuously improved, particularly with regard to real-time scanning, until by 1981 it was shown to be possible consistently to retrieve oocytes by needling follicles with transabdominal ultrasound guidance[5]. From then, as

the technology further improved and with further miniaturization of transducers, oocyte recovery via the vagina using vaginal scanners became possible[6]. Thus, methods of oocyte recovery became increasingly simple, less traumatic to patients and simpler for their surgeon. Ultrasound-guided retrieval also meant that all patients could be treated as day-cases, since the retrievals could be performed with sedation only or light general anesthesia.

Unlike oocyte recovery, the technique for embryo transfer (ET) has hardly changed since the first successful transfer in 1978[3]. Embryos are still transferred at Bourn Hall in exactly the same way as was taught by Steptoe. The only other recent developments that have occurred are those involving the transfer of embryos, either laparoscopically or transcervically, to the Fallopian tube; these are described in Chapter 19.

This chapter describes the methods of oocyte recovery and embryo transfer that have evolved over the past 26 years, and how they are now practiced at Bourn Hall.

PRELIMINARY ASSESSMENT

It goes without saying that a complete infertility assessment should always have been carried out in all couples who are about to embark upon assisted conception treatment; nevertheless, there are many couples who receive assisted conception treatment who have been inadequately investigated.

The proper assessment of couples prior to IVF, gamete intrafallopian transfer (GIFT), intrauterine insemination (IUI) and other techniques is described in detail elsewhere in this volume (Chapter 2). However, it is appropriate to discuss briefly the place of assessment or preliminary laparoscopy in the management of patients.

The need for preliminary laparoscopy

Prior to the advent of ultrasound-guided oocyte recovery, laparoscopy was the only technique available. Then, it was essential that the current state of the pelvic organs was known, particularly with regard to the accessibility of the ovaries for oocyte recovery. It was, therefore, normal practice to carry out a laparoscopic assessment in every patient who had not had one in the previous 6–12 months[7,8].

This preliminary laparoscopy allowed one:

(1) To plan the route of entry of the collecting needles, laparoscope and trochar: this was especially important when there was extensive adhesion formation;

(2) To divide adhesions in the pelvis, particularly around the ovaries, to allow future access;

(3) To decide whether in fact a laparotomy was required to separate adhesions and to bring the ovaries into full view;

(4) To occlude Fallopian tubes that were patent but abnormal, so as to prevent the occurrence of ectopic pregnancies following embryo transfer;

(5) To record in exact detail any abnormal findings.

We do not now consider that a preliminary laparoscopy is necessary for all patients prior to IVF, unless there are clear indications to perform one. If standard IVF with ultrasound-directed oocyte recovery is the selected treatment, then the presence of pelvic adhesions is of little consequence, especially if the tubes are known to be blocked. However, if either GIFT or zygote intrafallopian transfer (ZIFT) are proposed, then it is essential that a recent assessment of the tubes should have been made. These treatment options are not now practiced at Bourn Hall.

OOCYTE RECOVERY TECHNIQUES

The change from laparoscopic oocyte recovery to ultrasound-directed oocyte recovery (UDOR) is now almost universal. UDOR has revolutionized the way that IVF is carried out, as it can be practiced without anesthesia and as an out-patient procedure. There are, however, still three remaining indications for laparoscopic oocyte recovery:

(1) When suitable ultrasound facilities and experience with ultrasound-directed oocyte recovery are not available: this should seldom be the case in reputable units;

(2) When it is considered desirable to assess the state of the pelvis at the same time as the oocytes are collected in order to save a second procedure: if this is done, it will not be possible to assess the Fallopian tubes, unless all the embryos are frozen in that cycle for future transfer;

(3) If it is intended to make an attempt at GIFT: however, on the increasingly rare occasions that GIFT is carried out, the oocytes may be collected by transvaginal ultrasound-directed recovery, then proceeding to laparoscopy for GIFT.

Each of the major oocyte recovery techniques is now described.

Laparoscopic oocyte recovery

As early as 1968, Patrick Steptoe devised a method of aspirating oocytes laparoscopically from human pre-ovulatory follicles (Figure 1). In 1976, a pregnancy was achieved following IVF of oocytes from laparoscopic oocyte recovery, the first ever IVF pregnancy, but this was subsequently found to be an ectopic pregnancy[9]. It was a further 2 years before a live birth was achieved. Laparoscopic oocyte recovery has not been practiced at Bourn Hall since 1988; however, the technique is described. There have been no developments since then that would improve upon the method originally described by Steptoe and Webster[8], except for the introduction of video monitoring of the operation, rather than by direct vision through the laparoscope. The selection of patients, their investigation, ovulation induction and monitoring are described elsewhere in this book.

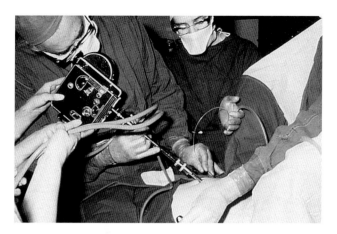

Figure 1 Mr Steptoe performing a laparoscopic oocyte recovery procedure (with teaching camera)

Full general anesthesia is induced. Patients are prepared, draped and placed in the Trendelenberg and lithotomy position as for any laparoscopy, and the urinary bladder is emptied. A 1-cm transverse subumbilical incision is made and a Verre's needle is inserted through the abdominal wall and directed towards the concavity of the pelvis. The needle is connected to a gas insufflator, which delivers a steady flow of CO_2 at a pressure of less than 100 mmHg. When an adequate pneumoperitoneum has been achieved, the CO_2 is changed to a gas mixture of 5% O_2, 5% CO_2 and 90% N_2; this has always been the practice at Bourn Hall, as 100% CO_2 causes acidification of follicular fluid[8,10], which has subsequently been confirmed[11,12].

Semms or Palmer grasping forceps are inserted in the midline, or laterally about 2.5 cm above the symphysis pubis or inguinal ligament (Figure 2). A fine trochar and cannula are passed into the peritoneal cavity from a lateral position and a double-lumen follicular aspiration needle is passed down it, having been attached by fine plastic tubing to the collection tube or pot and to a vacuum pump, the suction pressure of which can be controlled by a foot switch. We used the Craft pump (Rocket of London, UK) originally, and more recently we have used the Cook pump (Cook (UK) Ltd, Letchworth, UK) (Figure 3).

A good view of the pelvic organs is essential, particularly of the ovaries, which can be maneuvered into a suitable position for oocyte recovery by grasping and manipulating the ovarian ligament or the infundibulopelvic ligament (Figure 4). If minor adhesions obscure access to the ovaries, these may be gently divided by blunt dissection or by the use of laparoscopic scissors.

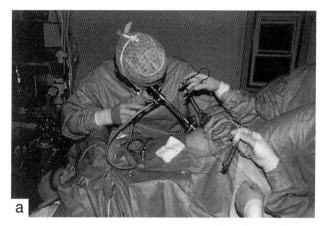

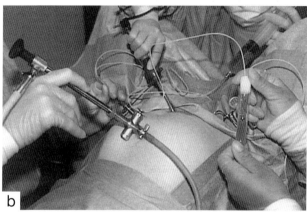

Figure 2 Laparoscopic oocyte recovery (before the use of video monitors). (a) General view showing the position of the operator and assistants. (b) Close-up view to show the position of the instruments. (Reproduced with the kind permission of Professor Ian Craft)

When the ovary is in a suitable position and the follicles are clearly seen, collection may begin. The follicle to be aspirated is best maintained uppermost and punctured from the side through an avascular area (Figure 4b), rather than through its thin dome, since this may cause rupture of the follicle and loss of the contents. Puncture from the side, where the tissue is thicker, allows a better seal around the needle to be obtained.

Before aspiration, the needle and tubing are flushed through with flushing medium (Earle's medium with heparin). The needle is inserted into the follicle and a vacuum is applied up to a pressure of 100–110 mmHg. The clear follicular fluid is seen to enter the collecting tube. The first clear aspirate is then passed through to the embryologist to detect the oocyte. If it is not found, the follicle is flushed with an equal volume of flushing medium and aspirated until it is identified.

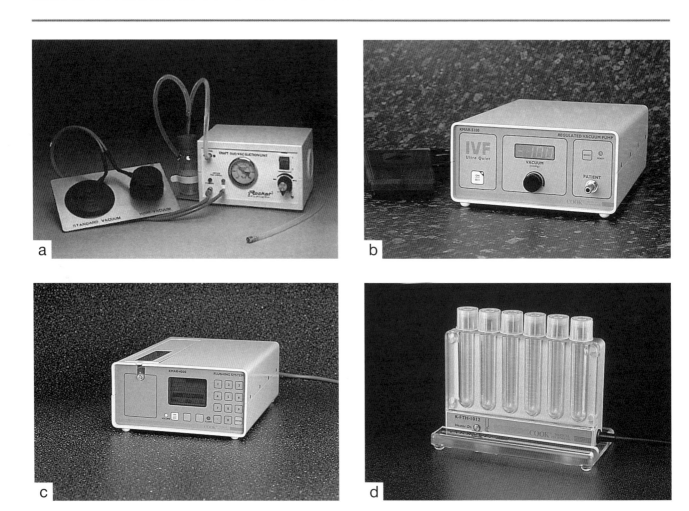

Figure 3 (a) Craft Vacuum Pump (Rocket of London, UK); (b) Cook K-MAR-5100 vacuum pump with foot control (Cook (UK) Ltd, Letchworth, UK); (c) Cook-K-MAR-4000 follicle flushing system (Cook (UK) Ltd; d) Cook K-FTH-1012 test-tube heater (Cook (UK) Ltd

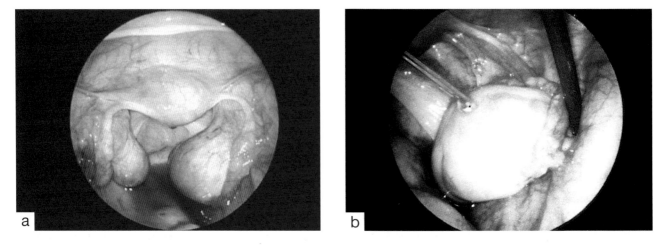

Figure 4 (a) Laparoscopic view of the female pelvis, showing normal uterus, Fallopian tubes and stimulated ovaries. (b) Right infundibulopelvic ligament grasped by forceps to steady the ovary, with the aspiration needle entering the follicle at an angle

Often the oocyte is found in the second or third flush. The embryologist will be able to determine the maturity of the follicle by the appearance of the granulosa and cumulus cells. The laboratory methods for oocyte recovery and IVF are described in detail in Chapter 15.

All visible follicles, even small ones, are aspirated. If difficulty is experienced in obtaining the oocyte, the follicle may be gently curetted as the vacuum is applied. At completion of the recovery, the pouch of Douglas should be aspirated clear of all blood and flushing fluid; occasionally an oocyte may be found which has dropped into the pouch.

On completion of the procedure, the laparoscope, grasping forceps and needle are withdrawn and the gas mixture is released. The peritoneal cavity may be flushed through with 100% CO_2, which is then also released. Every effort should be made to remove all remaining gas, in order to prevent postoperative chest and shoulder pains.

Laparoscopic oocyte recovery is a straightforward procedure for an experienced laparoscopist, but a number of problems can arise which can turn it into a frustrating and prolonged procedure. The major problems are the unexpected finding of adhesions obscuring the ovary, endometriosis, bleeding and difficulty in recovering oocytes. Proper selection and preparation of patients, with increasing experience and expertise, can make laparoscopic oocyte recovery a most rewarding procedure, but for most of us, a procedure of the past.

Ultrasound-guided follicular aspiration techniques

Apart from laparoscopy, ultrasound imaging of the pelvis has been the greatest advance in the diagnosis and management of gynecological conditions. From the earliest pioneering days of Ian Donald in Glasgow and crude A-scan and B-scan static images of fetuses *in utero*, we have progressed to real-time images on vaginal scanning which can even detect the minute cumulus– oocyte complexes in mature ovarian follicles, and we also have the ability to measure blood flow to the uterus and ovaries with color Doppler imaging.

Following the pioneering work of Kratochwil and colleagues[4], who developed techniques for ultrasonically guided transcutaneous needle biopsy of

abdominal organs, observations on ovarian follicular development were made[13]. This was followed by the first recorded aspiration of oocytes from follicles under ultrasound guidance by Lenz and colleagues in 1981[5]. Soon, other units were practicing ultrasound-directed oocyte recovery (UDOR) successfully[14], and it was found that recovery rates were as good as those by laparoscopy, with fewer complications and easier ovarian access[15]. Shortly thereafter, oocytes were successfully collected by the transvaginal route, but with abdominal ultrasound to guide the aspiration of follicles[16,17] (Figure 5).

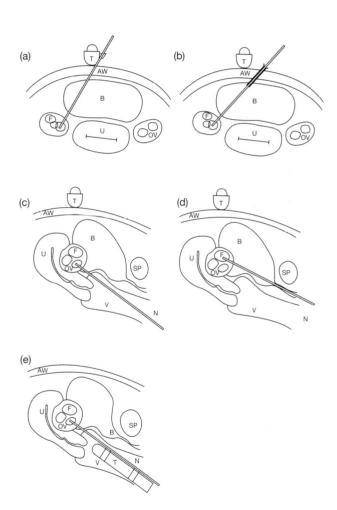

Figure 5 Diagrammatic representations of different ultrasound-guided oocyte recovery techniques: (a) transabdominal– transvesical oocyte recovery (fixed technique); (b) transabdominal– transvesical oocyte recovery (freehand technique); (c) transabdominal-transvaginal oocyte recovery technique; (d) transabdominal-perurethral oocyte recovery technique; (e) transvaginal oocyte recovery using a transvaginal ultrasound probe with needle guide attached. T, transducer; AW, abdominal wall; B, full bladder; SP, symphysis pubis; OV, ovary; F, follicle; U, uterus; V, vagina; N, needle

At present, the very large majority of IVF units collect oocytes by the transvaginal ultrasound-directed oocyte recovery (TV-UDOR) technique. This approach has very significant advantages: simplicity of use, ease of learning, proximity of the transducer to the ovaries, patient acceptance without the need for general anesthesia and relatively few complications. Briefly described below are the early UDOR techniques, followed by a detailed description of the transvaginal recovery technique, as practiced at Bourn Hall.

Transabdominal–transvesical ultrasound-directed oocyte recovery

This was the original method described by Lenz and colleagues[5] for the recovery of oocytes from ovarian follicles. It was used by most IVF units until it was superseded by the vaginal ultrasound technique as the method of choice, and gave oocyte recovery rates and fertilization rates as good as those with laparoscopic retrieval[15,18]. The technique was originally described as using a fixed needle guide attached to the abdominal transducer, but others found that this limited the flexibility of approach, and that a 'freehand' method, without the guide, was preferable[19] (Figure 5a and b).

Methods

Transabdominal–transvesical ultrasound-directed oocyte recovery may be performed under general anesthesia, but its great advantage over laparoscopy is that sedation alone can be used. This can be achieved with premedication 1 h before the procedure: intravenous diazepam 5–10 mg and pethidine 25–100 mg are then given, intraoperatively, as required. Alternatively, we have found that midazolam (Hypnovel®; Roche Products Ltd, Welwyn Garden City, UK) 10 mg intravenously provides excellent sedation, with almost complete amnesia following the experience. The operation may be carried out in a 'clean' procedure room, but we prefer to use the operating theater, with full aseptic technique.

The bladder is catheterized and emptied of urine, and an indwelling self-retaining catheter is inserted and connected to a 500-ml bag of normal saline or Hartman's solution attached to a drip stand. The bladder is then filled. The abdomen is prepared with chlorhexidine (Savlodil®; ICI Pharmaceuticals UK, Wilmslow, UK) and washed off with sterile water, and sterile abdominal drapes are applied. We have used a

number of different ultrasound machines and abdominal probes and found that they all perform adequately. The abdominal probe is placed in a sterile polythene sleeve containing contact gel, and the pelvis is scanned to define the uterus and ovaries.

When the follicles have been identified, a small bleb of 1% lignocaine is raised in the skin, followed by a small nick with a scalpel close to the transducer, to ease the passage of the needle through the skin. A double-lumen needle is passed down along the track of the ultrasound beam 'freehand' (Figure 6) through the abdominal wall and the distended bladder towards the selected ovary. The tip of the needle, which becomes visible as a point of increased echogenicity if one is in the right plane, is thrust firmly into the most accessible follicle, which is then aspirated (Figure 7). The collecting needle is attached by tubing to a sterile plastic collecting tube, and on to a suction pump. Pressures of 100–120 mmHg may be applied, controlled with a foot pedal. Most pumps have a 'red button' or second foot control for higher vacuum pressures, to clear the needle and tubing of blood clot or tissue. If the oocyte is not in the first aspirate, the follicle is flushed with a volume of flushing medium (Earle's solution with heparin) equal to that aspirated, and flushed and aspirated until the oocyte is obtained or until the embryologist indicates that there is little prospect of recovering one. The same procedure is repeated for all follicles on each side. At the end of the procedure the flushing medium and blood that have accumulated in the pouch of Douglas are aspirated.

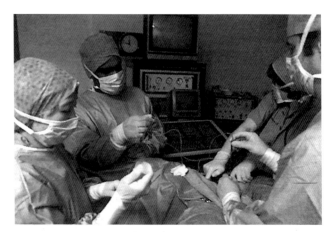

Figure 6 Transabdominal–transvaginal 'freehand' technique, with transducer held by an ultrasonographer. (Reproduced with the kind permission of Professor Ian Craft)

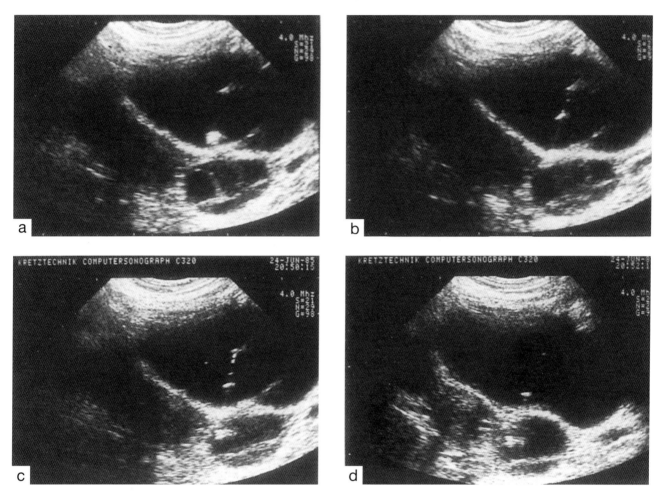

Figure 7 Ultrasound picture of a transabdominal–transvesical oocyte recovery: (a) the needle tip entering the full bladder; (b) the needle tip entering the far wall of the bladder; (c, d) the needle in the follicle

Discussion

Transabdominal–transvesical ultrasound-directed oocyte recovery was a very considerable advance technically over laparoscopy for the recovery of oocytes. Its disadvantage is that it is quite painful for a number of patients, particularly because the needle passes through the sensitive bladder wall. Quite severe hematuria is not infrequent, with occasional clot retention of urine postoperatively. The other major problem is the relative distance of the ovaries from the ultrasound probe, making accurate needling of the follicles more difficult. This technique is now very seldom used, and has been entirely superseded by the vaginal approach. Very occasionally, ovaries are situated high in the pelvis and are difficult to access with a vaginal probe; the direct abdominal approach will often solve the problem in these cases.

Transabdominal–transvaginal ultrasound-directed oocyte recovery

This method, which involves the use of a transabdominal ultrasound probe with needle aspiration of the ovarian follicles through the vagina (Figure 5c), was first described by Gleicher and colleagues[16], followed by Dellenbach and co-workers[17], who also later presented the results from a large series of patients[20].

The method is seldom used today because of the advent of vaginal ultrasound probes, which have made the vaginal approach very much more accurate, as the ovaries are much closer to the end of the probe. The only indication now for the use of this method is if a unit does not have a vaginal probe, or if a probe malfunctions during a procedure.

Transabdominal–perurethral ultrasound-directed oocyte recovery

Parsons and colleagues[21] first described the method of collection of oocytes via the urethra and bladder using transabdominal ultrasound probes (Figure 5d). They presented data on a series of 242 cases[22] with no serious complications.

If vaginal transducer technology had not advanced so rapidly, then this technique would have been much more widely used. It will continue to be used in units that do not have vaginal probes, or if a vaginal probe is out of order. It may also be used if the ovaries are inaccessible vaginally, or in the presence of vaginal infection.

Transvaginal ultrasound-directed oocyte recovery

It was not until 1985 that vaginal ultrasound probes became commercially available, when their usefulness for oocyte recovery immediately became apparent. Wikland and colleagues[6] first suggested the potential of vaginal ultrasound for oocyte recovery in 1985, at which time they also described the method of guiding the collecting needle alongside the transducer to achieve very accurate puncture of follicles (Figure 5e). Now, almost every IVF unit collects oocytes by the TV-UDOR method, since it is the easiest, the most accurate and the most acceptable to patients of all the collection methods.

Methods

At Bourn Hall, TV-UDOR is performed in the operating theater under full aseptic technique. The patient is placed in the lithotomy position, the vulva and vagina are prepared with Savlodil and rinsed thoroughly with normal saline, and the area is covered with a sterile drape. Patients are offered either a light general anesthetic or analgesia with local anesthesia. If the latter is requested, then it is administered as described above for transabdominal–transvesical ultrasound-directed oocyte recovery, together with a local anesthetic for a paracervical block and infiltration of the vaginal vault. The vaginal transducer is covered with a sterile polythene sleeve or special 'condom', with a small amount of coupling gel to cover the end of the probe. The needle guide (Casmed, Cheam, UK) is attached to the ultrasound probe. A Cook (Cook (UK) Ltd) single- or double-lumen needle is attached to the plastic tubing, which, in turn, is connected to a collecting tube for the follicular fluid and on to the Cook K-MAR-4000 vacuum pump and follicle flushing systems (Cook UK Ltd) (Figure 3b–d). The system is flushed through with flushing fluid – warm normal saline is now used at Bourn Hall – and the needle is then inserted part-way into the needle guide. The transducer, with the needle guide attached and needle within, is then introduced into the vagina, and the pelvis is scanned thoroughly to confirm the position of the uterus, the quality of the endometrium, the position and accessibility of the ovaries and the number of follicles to be aspirated. The ultrasound probe is then manipulated and rotated until the follicles appear in close proximity to the needle guide lines. One of the follicles nearest to the probe is selected, its maximum diameter is found and the needle is then thrust gently but purposefully into it (Figure 8). The echo from the tip of the needle, which is scored to increase its echogenicity, can be seen in the follicle, which is then aspirated until empty. The follicular fluid passes into the plastic tubes which are located in a 'hot block' or test-tube heater (Cook (UK) Ltd) (Figure 3d). The full tubes are passed to the embryologist in the adjacent laboratory, and the oocytes are identified (Chapter 15). If an oocyte is not found in the first aspirate, the follicle is flushed with an equal volume of warmed flushing medium, previously Earle's medium with heparin, but we now use warmed normal saline. The follicle is then aspirated again and this is repeated until the oocyte is recovered. Gentle manipulation of the needle tip within the follicle, in effect curetting the follicle wall, may assist release of oocytes that are reluctant to separate.

Ovaries are often mobile and tend to 'run away' from the tip of the needle. This effect can be reduced by ensuring that the needle tips are kept very sharp; this is assured by using single-use disposable needles, whereas in the early days, needles were reused many times. By using a short stabbing movement and by applying pressure suprapubically, either by hand or by means of an abdominal pressure cuff[23], the mobility of the ovaries can be reduced and entry into the follicles made easier. Although some recommend that the needle be withdrawn and flushed after each oocyte has been recovered[24], we believe that the number of stabs through the vaginal vault and ovaries should be kept to an absolute minimum, in order to reduce trauma

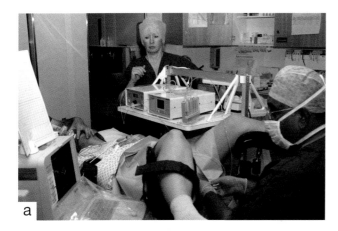

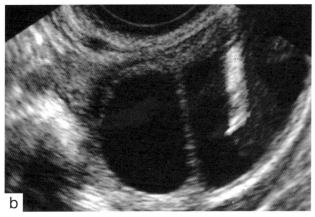

Figure 8 (a) Set-up for transvaginal oocyte recovery at Bourn Hall. (The procedure may be done under light general anesthesia or sedation. (b) Ultrasound picture of a transvaginal oocyte recovery, with the echogenic tip of the needle visible in a follicle

and the possibility of bleeding. It is usually possible to keep the needle tip within the ovary and aspirate several follicles, one after the other, by careful manipulation and by choosing the order in which they are aspirated. In this way it is often possible to aspirate all the follicles from both ovaries with a single puncture on each side. We aspirate all follicles that are visible, even those of less than 10 mm in diameter, as mature oocytes, which can be fertilized, may be obtained from smaller follicles. When all follicles are seen to have been emptied, the pouch of Douglas is aspirated of any visible pool of flushing fluid and blood. The transducer is then withdrawn and the vaginal vault is checked with a speculum for signs of bleeding. If bleeding does occur, it will invariably stop with firm pressure for a minute or two using a sponge in a sponge forceps; occasionally it may be necessary to insert an absorbable suture at the site of bleeding.

At Bourn Hall, we give prophylactic antibiotics during the procedure in the form of Augmentin® (SmithKline Beecham, Brentford, UK) 1.2 g intravenously, and Flagyl® (RPR Ltd, Eastbourne, UK) 1 g rectally at the end of the procedure.

Complications

The incidence of complications for TV-UDOR is variously reported. Brinsmead and colleagues[25] reported relatively high complication rates, with venous puncture 2–7%, bladder bleeding 40%, vaginal bleeding 24%, bowel perforation 14%, postoperative pain 10% and pelvic infection 3%. There are no other recent reports with as much detail as this, but it is our experience that complications are now very much less frequent than in this report from 1989. Wikland and colleagues[24] reported no serious complications in 50 cases.

In the past 5 years at Bourn Hall there have been no admissions to hospital for bleeding following oocyte recovery. There is an average of one or two pelvic infections each year, an incidence of about 0.5–1%, a similar incidence to that reported by Bennett and associates[26] of 0.6%. These infections have frequently been associated with aspiration of endometriotic cysts. In spite of the administration of prophylactic antibiotics intraoperatively, the aspiration of cysts, particularly endometriotic cysts, unless indicated for therapeutic reasons, appears to be better avoided. We also recommend that hydrosalpinges, if detected for the first time at oocyte collection, should not be aspirated, because the risk of pelvic infection, as with endometriomata, may be increased[27]. Among other, but much more rare, complications that have been reported are: massive retroperitoneal bleeding following TV-UDOR[28]; vertebral osteomyelitis[29]; and acute ureteral obstruction[30]. When compared with the incidence and severity of complications that can occur at laparoscopic oocyte recovery, we believe that TV-UDOR is a very much safer procedure and will remain the method of choice for oocyte recovery long into the future.

Discussion

Vaginal ultrasound has undoubtedly been the greatest advance in our ability to visualize the pelvic organs since laparoscopy. As the use of laparoscopy was extended to oocyte recovery, so was vaginal ultrasonography, and very effectively. How the 'fashion' changed in the use of different methods of oocyte recovery, as described in this chapter, is demonstrated in Figure 9. This shows the Scandinavian experience during the change from laparoscopic to transvaginal ultrasound-directed oocyte recovery, which occurred between 1981 and 1989[31]. The same very major changes in our own practice occurred at the same time. The majority of IVF units throughout the world now perform their oocyte recoveries by transvaginal ultrasound guidance.

The major advantages of transvaginal over transabdominal–transvesical ultrasound-directed oocyte recovery are:

(1) The better image obtained with the vaginal probe, because of its closer proximity to the ovaries;

(2) Greater ease of use and shorter learning phase;

(3) Less pain, because the bladder wall is not pierced, thus necessitating less analgesia and sedation, with a consequently quicker return to normal activity;

(4) The fact that, because of better visualization of the ovaries and of smaller follicles, more oocytes are recovered, more embryos are available to transfer and freeze and therefore higher pregnancy rates have, in general, been reported;

(5) The fact that, because there is no need to catheterize the bladder or pass the aspirating needle through it, there is much less chance of dysuria, infection or hematuria than after transabdominal–transvesical ultrasound-directed oocyte recovery;

(6) Less risk of perforation of a viscus because of the proximity of the ovaries to the vaginal vault;

(7) Much better patient acceptance, because it is less painful than ultrasound-directed or laparoscopic oocyte recovery, both intraoperatively and postoperatively.

There are a number of measures that can be taken to ensure that the transvaginal method is made easier and safer:

(1) Pressure applied with a pad to the lower abdomen may help to stabilize a mobile ovary.

(2) A double-lumen needle with flushing and aspirating channels may achieve more efficient and

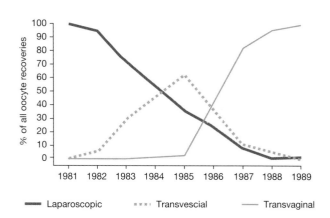

Figure 9 The Scandanavian experience of the changes in 'fashion' of oocyte recovery techniques between 1980 and 1989. (Courtesy of Oxford University Press, the publishers of *Human Reproduction* (reference 31), and updated to 1989 (A. Sunde, personal communication)

rapid retrieval of oocytes, although many surgeons prefer single-channel needles because of their smaller diameter, thus causing less pain[32].

(3) Sharpness of the needles is essential. A firm and rapid thrusting motion of the needle should be used to penetrate the follicle; a gentle approach will tend just to push the ovary away from the needle.

(4) The number of entries of the needle through the vault of the vagina, as well as the ovary, should be minimized. It will often be possible to aspirate all follicles from one ovary with one stab only.

(5) When scanning follicles, it is always wise to look at them in two planes, by rotating the transducer, before entering them. There are occasions when an apparently 'good-looking follicle' turns out to be the internal iliac vein in cross-section! Rotation of the probe will show it to be a long tubular structure.

(6) We advocate the routine administration of antibiotics in the form of clavulanic acid (Augmentin; SmithKline Beecham) intraoperatively and metronidazole (Flagyl; RPR) rectally, immediately postoperatively.

(7) Whether or not flushing of the follicles is necessary or useful is really a matter of personal choice. We favor having the ability to flush, but advocate

minimal flushing. Tan and colleagues[33] found that there was no significant difference in the oocyte recovery or pregnancy rates between patients who had follicles flushed or not, but there was a halving of the time taken for the procedure (15 min vs. 30 min), and a significant reduction in the amount of analgesia required for patients without flushing.

EMBRYO TRANSFER

'Meticulous embryo transfer technique is essential to IVF success'[34].

The basic technique of transferring embryos to the uterus following IVF has changed very little at Bourn Hall over the past 15 years. We no longer place patients in the knee–chest position when transferring to an anteverted uterus, as was originally recommended by Steptoe (personal communication), nor do we keep patients lying down for 12 h after transfer; otherwise, the procedure is practiced much as it always has been.

Generally, embryo transfer (ET) is carried out about 48–50 h after oocyte collection, which is about 44–48 h after insemination of the oocytes. The embryos are usually at the 2–4-cell stage of cleavage by then. In the UK, the Human Fertilisation and Embryology Authority restricts the number of embryos that can be transferred (see Chapter 39.1 for more detail). The rule, as from 2003, is for a maximum of two embryos, with very occasional exceptions being permitted for women over 40 years of age for three embryos to be transferred.

Methods

Embryo transfer is carried out in the operating theater under sterile conditions with scrubbing up and gloving, but not gowning up. Husbands are encouraged to attend, suitably gowned and with overshoes.

On arrival in the theater, the identity of the patient is checked by the accompanying nurse, the surgeon and the embryologist attending the case, and all then sign the case records to confirm that they have checked the identity of the patient and her embryos using at least three separate identifiers: their name, date of birth and unique clinic number. The embryologist explains to the couple what has occurred with regard to fertilization and cleavage of their embryos, their

quality, the number to be transferred and the number being cryopreserved for future use.

The patient is placed in the lithotomy position, a perineal drape is placed over her and, after having the process explained to her, a Cuscoe speculum, lubricated with warm saline solution only, is inserted into the vagina. The cervix is exposed gently and any vaginal and cervical secretions are gently removed with small pledgets of cotton wool, moistened with warm normal saline. If there is a plug of mucus in the cervical canal, this is wiped away or aspirated.

In the laboratory, the embryos are identified by the embryologist and scored, and their details are entered into the log. Those embryos that are to be transferred are placed into a drop of Earle's medium. A Wallace (Bourn) embryo transfer catheter (Smiths Industries Medical Systems (SIMS), Lancing, UK) is used for the majority of transfers (Figure 10). The catheter is fitted with a 1-ml tuberculin-type syringe and flushed through with medium. The embryo(s) are drawn up

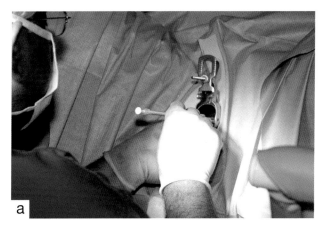

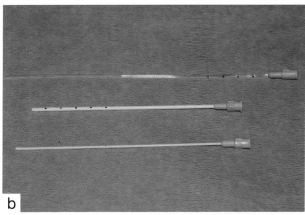

Figure 10 (a) Embryo transfer using a Wallace (Bourn) catheter. (b) The Wallace catheter, as used at Bourn Hall Clinic

into the already charged catheter, so that a volume of 15–25 μl is transferred; Chapter 15 gives more detail on the laboratory aspects of the transfer procedure. The catheter is taken through to the theater and passed to the surgeon. At this stage the lights in the theater are kept dimmed, but are switched up when the surgeon is ready to do the transfer. The catheter is gently maneuvered through the cervical canal and into the uterus. The length of the uterine cavity will usually have been measured at the time of the 'baseline' ultrasound scan, so that the tip of the catheter can be placed in the mid- or low–mid-uterine cavity, usually about 5–5.5 cm from the external cervical os. If difficulty is experienced in passing the catheter through the cervical canal, then the stiffer outer sheath can be introduced into the cervical canal and the inner catheter 'persuaded' through. If this fails, an Aliss single-tooth forceps may be applied to the anterior or posterior lip of the cervix and gentle traction applied to straighten the cervical canal. If it is still found to be impossible to pass the catheter after every reasonable means has been tried, and after a maximum of 2 min (because of the cooling effect on the embryos), then the embryos are returned to the laboratory and replaced in the culture dish.

The Wallace catheter is now available with an optional stiffener for the outer sheath. The embryo transfer catheter is removed from the outer sheath and replaced by the stiffener, which, because it has a 'memory', can be molded to a shape that may facilitate navigation of the cervical canal. If the internal os is negotiated successfully, the outer sheath is held in position and the stiffener withdrawn. The embryologist then returns with the embryo transfer catheter, which is then threaded up the sheath and will usually enter the uterine cavity. If it still proves impossible to transfer the embryos because the catheter cannot be passed into the uterus, then the procedure is abandoned and arrangements are made for the transfer to take place the following day under general anesthesia.

When the operator is confident that the catheter is properly placed, the embryologist or the surgeon can slowly and gently inject the embryos into the uterus; the catheter is left in position for a few moments and then gently and slowly removed. The catheter is returned to the laboratory and checked to ensure that the embryos have not been retained. If they have, the embryologist will draw up the embryo(s) again into

the catheter and a further attempt will be made to transfer them to the uterus.

On completion of the transfer, the speculum is withdrawn and the patient is made comfortable. The surgeon then explains to the patient about what medication, usually vaginal progesterone, she should take and when a pregnancy test will be performed. She is encouraged to return to her normal daily activities, including work, but to avoid violent exercise and sexual relations.

In earlier days the patient remained resting with a slight head-down tilt to her bed for 2 h before being allowed home. There is no evidence that this is necessary, and currently at Bourn Hall, patients walk back to the ward after the transfer, where they relax in a comfortable chair for 15–30 min, before being allowed home.

Luteal phase support is given to all patients who have been on luteinizing hormone releasing hormone (LHRH) agonist or antagonist protocols. We use either Cyclogest® (Shire Pharmaceuticals Ltd, Andover, UK) vaginal pessaries, 400 mg twice or three times a day, or, more recently, Crinone® 8% (Serono UK Ltd). Rarely, if the vaginal preparations are not well tolerated, intramuscular progesterone in the form of Gestone® (Ferring Pharmaceuticals Ltd, Langley, UK) 50–100 mg daily is used. Human chorionic gonadotropin is never used for luteal phase support.

Discussion

Between 1978 and 2001, there were more than 40 500 publications on the topic of IVF, of which only 45 concerned one of the most critical stages in the whole process – embryo transfer, even though it is well known that good embryo transfer technique is essential to the success of IVF[34]. It has been shown that there may be significant differences in success between different operators, even in the same unit[35], and that up to 30% of all IVF failures are due to poor transfer technique[36].

In our own practice, we have standardized the ET procedure to what we believe is a reasonable and evidence-based protocol, a summary of which is given in Table 1 (see also the the CD that accompanies this book for the full Bourn Hall Embryo Transfer Protocol). We require all operators to adhere to the protocol, in order to achieve uniformity of care.

One of the several contentious issues that provoke discussion about ET is whether or not it should be

Table 1 Summary of embryo transfer (ET) protocol at Bourn Hall

(1) Check identity of patient with embryos

(2) Relaxed atmosphere, reassurance

(3) Lithotomy position

(4) Sterile technique

(5) Clean cervix (saline) and remove cervical mucus

(6) Check cavity length in notes and any indication of difficulty (e.g. uterocervical angle)

(7) Load Wallace catheter

(8) Operator receives Wallace catheter and attempts transfer – gentle technique

(9) Place embryos mid- to low–mid-cavity (±2 cm from fundus). Do *not* touch fundus

(10) Expel embryos gently. Short delay before withdrawal of catheter

(11) Return catheter to embryologist – check for retained embryos and presence of blood and mucus on catheter

If difficult ET:

(1) Try passing outer sheath of catheter just through internal cervical os

(2) If not successful, return catheter to embryologist and gently pass stylet and outer sheath just through internal os

(3) As a last resort use a tenaculum on the cervix to straighten uterocervical angle

(4) Very last resort: refer for ET under general anesthetic

Table 2 Factors affecting the success of embryo transfer (ET). From references 45 and 46

Rank	Factor	Score/10
1	removal of hydrosalpinges	6.8
2	absence of blood/mucus	6.6
3	type of catheter	6.1
4	no touch of fundus	5.8
5	avoid tenaculum	5.7
6	remove cervical mucus	5.2
7	prior ultrasound of cavity	4.3
8	leave catheter 1 min	4.2
9	bed rest 30 min	3.8
10	trial ET	3.1
11	ultrasound monitoring of ET	2.6
12	antiprostaglandin treatment	1.9

done under ultrasound guidance. Earlier research showed no evidence of a difference[37,38], whereas Coroleu and colleagues[39] showed a pregnancy rate of 38% and 25%, with and without ultrasound, respectively; similarly, Wood and associates[40] showed rates of 50% and 33%. More recently, Mirkin and co-workers[41], in a large series of 823 patients, compared the 'clinical touch' technique with transabdominal ultrasound-guided transfers. They showed that there was no significant difference between the two techniques (44% vs. 48%, respectively). Our own experience and belief is that fully trained and experienced operators do not need ultrasound guidance routinely for ET, but that if difficulty is expected or experienced, it is beneficial to use ultrasound guidance to be certain of the correct placement of the embryos.

We are certain that soft catheters, such as the Wallace and Cook catheters, are more effective than harder catheters, and the findings of Wood and associates[40], which showed a pregnancy rate of 36% with a soft catheter and 17% with a hard catheter, confirm this. Similarly, Mirkin and co-workers[41] found that the use of a soft catheter was the only significant variable associated with pregnancy success (odds ratio 2.74).

We are firm believers that gentleness at all stages of the procedure is essential, not only for the comfort of the patient, but because it is well known that any manipulation of the cervix or uterus, particularly touching the uterine fundus with the tip of the transfer catheter, provokes uterine contractions, which cannot be good; other authors have confirmed this[42–44].

The most important factors which govern successful ET, and their relative importance, are shown in Table 2, which has been drawn up from data abstracted from references 45 and 46.

CONCLUSIONS

Since the earliest reports of oocyte recovery from human ovaries by laparoscopy[9], several major changes in technique and technology have simplified the procedure and made it much more acceptable to patients. Laparoscopic oocyte recovery techniques have changed little in the past 28 years, except for refinements in instrumentation such as laparoscopes, fiberoptic light sources and video imaging. The dramatic improvements that have occurred in ultra-sound equipment in these same nearly three decades have enabled us to monitor closely even small changes in follicular size and endometrial texture. The development of ultrasound-guided intra-abdominal biopsy techniques in the early 1980s enabled fertility specialists to 'biopsy' ovarian follicles and aspirate oocytes from them[5]. From there, attempts were made to move closer to the ovaries by perurethral and transvaginal routes. With the development of smaller and smaller ultrasound transducers, vaginal probes have given us the ability to view the pelvic organs in great detail. It was then only a short step to using guides mounted upon these probes to enable very accurate localization and aspiration of ovarian follicles to be carried out.

Vaginal ultrasound has brought a new dimension to the diagnosis and management of gynecological disorders, and has certainly revolutionized the practice of oocyte recovery. The simplicity of the procedure is its great merit, as it is easier for surgeons to learn, is safer, requires no anesthesia and has much greater patient acceptance than laparoscopic and transvesical ultrasound-guided oocyte recovery.

Embryo transfer has always been, and will always be, a critical part of the whole IVF process. Done badly and by poorly trained operators, pregnancy rates may be severely reduced. There are many factors that contribute to a successful transfer, and each must be addressed with meticulous attention to detail in order to achieve the optimum chance of success.

REFERENCES

1. Edwards R, Steptoe P. A Matter of Life. The Story of a Medical Breakthrough, 1st edn. London: Hutchinson, 1980: 40
2. Steptoe PC. Laparoscopy and ovulation. Lancet 1968; 2: 913
3. Steptoe PC, Edwards RG. Birth after reimplantation of a human embryo. Lancet 1978; 2: 366
4. Kratochwil A, Urban G, Freidrich F. Ultrasonic tomography of the ovaries. Ann Chir Gynaecol Fenn 1972; 61: 211–14
5. Lenz S, Lauritsen JG, Kjellow M. Collection of human oocytes for in vitro fertilization by ultrasonically guided follicular puncture. Lancet 1981; 1: 1163–4
6. Wikland M, Enk L, Hamberger L. Transvesical and transvaginal approaches for the aspiration of follicles by the use of ultrasound. Ann NY Acad Sci 1985; 442: 683–9
7. Edwards RG, Steptoe PC, Purdy JM. Establishing full term pregnancies using cleaving human embryos in vitro. Br J Obstet Gynaecol 1980; 87: 737
8. Steptoe PC, Webster J. Laparoscopy for oocyte recovery. Ann NY Acad Sci 1985; 442: 178–81
9. Steptoe PC, Edwards RG. Reimplantation of a human embryo with subsequent tubal pregnancy. Lancet 1976; 1: 880–2
10. Edwards RG, Steptoe PC. Current status of in vitro fertilization and implantation of human embryos. Lancet 1983; 2: 1265–9
11. Daya S. Follicular fluid pH changes following intraperitoneal exposure of Graafian follicles to carbon dioxide: a comparative study with follicles exposed to ultrasound. Hum Reprod 1988; 3: 727–30
12. Verbessem D, Camu F, Devroey P, Van Steirteghem A. Pneumoperitoneum induced pH changes in follicular and Douglas fluids during laparoscopic oocyte recovery in humans. Hum Reprod 1988; 3: 751–4
13. Hackeloer BJ, Hansmann M. Ultrasound diagnosis of follicular growth and ovulation. In Beier HM, Lindner HR, eds. Fertilization of the Human Egg In Vitro. Biological Basis and Clinical Application. Berlin: Springer-Verlag, 1983: 83–94
14. Wikland MD, Nilsson L, Hansson R, et al. Collection of human oocytes by the use of sonography. Fertil Steril 1983; 39: 603–8
15. Feitchinger W, Kemeter P. Laparoscopic or ultrasonically guided follicular aspiration for in vitro fertilization? J In Vitro Fertil Embryo Transf 1984; 1: 244–9
16. Gleicher M, Friberg J, Fullan N, et al. Egg retrieval for in vitro fertilization by sonographically controlled culdocentesis. Lancet 1983; 2: 508–9
17. Dellenbach P, Nisand I, Moreau L, et al. Transvaginal sonographically controlled ovarian follicle puncture for egg retrieval. Lancet 1984; 1: 1467
18. Wikland M, Hamberger L. Ultrasound as a diagnostic and operative tool for in vitro fertilization and embryo replacement (IVF/ER) programs. J In Vitro Fertil Embryo Transf 1984; 1: 213–16
19. Riddle AF, Sharma V, Mason BA, et al. Two years' experience of ultrasound-directed oocyte retrieval. Fertil Steril 1987; 48: 454–8
20. Dellenbach P, Nisand I, Moreau L, et al. Transvaginal sonographically controlled follicle puncture for oocyte retrieval. Fertil Steril 1985; 44: 656–62
21. Parsons J, Riddle A, Booker M, et al. Oocyte retrieval for in-vitro fertilization by ultrasonically guided needle aspiration via the urethra. Lancet 1985; 1: 1076
22. Parsons J, Pampiglione JS, Campbell S. Ultrasound directed follicle aspiration for oocyte collection using the perurethral technique. Fertil Steril 1990; 53: 97–102

23. Yovich J, Grudzinskas G. The Management of Infertility. A Manual of Gamete Handling Procedures, 1st edn. London: Heinemann, 1990: 127

24. Wikland M, Enk L, Hammarberg K, Nilsson L. Use of a vaginal transducer for oocyte retrieval in an IVF/ET program. J Clin Ultrasound 1987; 15: 245–51

25. Brinsmead M, Stanger J, Oliver M, et al. A randomised trial of laparoscopy and transvaginal ultrasound-directed oocyte pickup for in vitro fertilization. J In Vitro Fertil Embryo Transf 1989; 6: 149–54

26. Bennett SJ, Waterstone JJ, Cheng WC, et al. Complications of transvaginal ultrasound-directed follicle aspiration: a review of 2670 consecutive procedures. J Assist Reprod Genet 1993; 10: 72–7

27. Varras M, Polyzos D, Tsikini A, et al. Ruptured tubo-ovarian abcess as a complication of IVF treatment: clinical, ultrasonographic and histopathologic findings. A case report. Clin Exp Obstet Gynecol 2003; 30: 164–8

28. Azem F, Wolf Y, Botchan A, et al. Massive retroperitoneal bleeding: a complication of transvaginal ultrasonography-guided oocyte retrieval for in vitro fertilisation–embryo transfer. Fertil Steril 2000; 74: 405–6

29. Almog B, Rimon E, Yovel I, et al. Vertebral osteomyelitis: a rare complication of transvaginal ultrasound guided oocyte retrieval. Fertil Steril 2000; 73: 1250–2

30 Miller PB, Price T, Nichols JE, et al. Acute ureteral obstruction following transvaginal oocyte retrieval for IVF. Hum Reprod 2002; 17: 137–8

31. Sunde A, von During V, Kahn JA, Molne K. IVF in the Nordic Countries 1981–1987: a collaborative survey. Hum Reprod 1990; 5: 959–64

32. Aziz N, Bilijan MM, Taylor CT, et al. Effect of aspirating needle calibre on outcome of in-vitro fertilization. Hum Reprod 1993; 8: 1098–100

33. Tan SL, Waterstone J, Wren M, et al. A prospective randomised study comparing aspiration only vs aspiration and flushing for transvaginal ultrasound-directed oocyte recovery. Fertil Steril 1992; 58: 356–60

34. Meldrum DR, Chetkowski R, Steingold KA, et al. Evolution of a highly successful in vitro fertilization program. Fertil Steril 1987; 48: 86–93

35. Hearns-Stokes RM, Miller BT, Scott L, et al. Pregnancy rates after embryo transfer depend on the provider at embryo transfer. Fertil Steril 2001; 75: 449–50

36. Cohen J. How to avoid multiple pregnancies in assisted reproduction. Hum Reprod 1998; (Suppl 13): 197–214

37. Kan AK, Abdalla HI, Gafar AH, et al. Embryo transfer: ultrasound-guided versus clinical touch. Hum Reprod 1999; 14: 1259–61

38. Al-Shawaf T, Dave R, Harper J, et al. Transfer of embryos into the uterus: how much do technical factors affect pregnancy rates? J Assist Reprod Genet 1993; 10: 31–6

39. Coroleu B, Carreras O, Veiga A, et al. Embryo transfer under ultrasound guidance improves pregnancy rates after in vitro fertilisation. Hum Reprod 2000; 15: 616–20

40. Wood EG, Batzer FR, Go KJ, et al. Ultrasound-guided soft catheter embryo transfers will improve pregnancy rates in in-vitro fertilization. Hum Reprod 2000; 15: 107–12

41. Mirkin S, Jone EL, Mayer JF, et al. Impact of transabdominal ultrasound guidance on performance and outcome of transcervical uterine embryo transfer. J Assist Reprod Genet 2003; 20: 318–22

42. Knutzen V, Stratton CJ, Sher G, et al. Mock embryo transfer in early luteal phase, the cyclebefore in vitro fertilization and embryo transfer: a descriptive study. Fertil Steril 1992; 57: 156–62

43. Dorn C, Reisenberg J, Schlebusch H, et al. Serum oxytocin concentration during embryo transfer procedure. Eur J Obstet Gynecol Reprod Biol 1999; 87: 77–80

44. Mansour RT, Aboulghar MA. Optimizing the embryo transfer technique. Hum Reprod 2002; 17: 1149–53

45. Kovaks GT. What factors are important for successful embryo transfer after in-vitro fertilization? Hum Reprod 1999; 14: 590–2

46. Schoolcraft WB, Surrey ES, Gardner DK. Embryo transfer: techniques and variables affecting success. Fertil Steril 2001; 76: 863–70

15

Routine gamete handling: oocyte collection and embryo culture

Kay Elder

INTRODUCTION

Successful assisted reproduction involves the careful co-ordination of both a medical and a scientific approach toward each couple who undertake a treatment cycle, with close collaboration between doctors, scientists, nurses and counselors. Only meticulous attention to detail at every step of each patient's treatment can optimize their chance of delivering a healthy baby as a result. Appropriate patient selection, ovarian stimulation, monitoring and timing of oocyte retrieval should provide the *in vitro* fertilization (IVF) laboratory with viable gametes capable of producing healthy embryos. It is the responsibility of the IVF laboratory to ensure a stable, non-toxic, pathogen-free environment, with optimum parameters for oocyte fertilization and embryo development. The clinical biologist must always be aware that control mechanisms exist that are exquisitely sensitive to even apparently minor changes in the environment of gametes and embryos: in particular, temperature, pH and any other factors which potentially affect cells at the molecular level. Because so many multiple variables are involved[1], the basic science of each step must be carefully controlled, whilst allowing for individual variation between patients and between treatment cycles.

Full sterile precautions and techniques must be adopted in the IVF laboratory, with restricted access and change of clothing into clean operating-room dress, including shoes, hats and masks. In order to ensure a pathogen-free environment, a strict discipline of sterile procedures should be enforced in all daily routines[2], with manipulations carried out in biological safety cabinets and gloves worn when handling gametes and embryos[3]. A class I biological safety cabinet (BSC) has an open front with negative-pressure ventilation; this provides personnel and environmental protection, but no protection for the material being handled. Class II BSCs provide product, personnel and environment protection, using a stream of unidirectional air moving at a steady velocity along parallel lines ('laminar flow'). The laminar flow, together with high-efficiency particulate air (HEPA) filtration, captures and removes airborne contaminants and provides a particulate-free work environment. A class II BSC is recommended in order to provide a microbe-free IVF cell culture environment, and should be used during any manipulations that may cause aerosols, such as sperm preparation procedures (Figure 1). A horizontal laminar flow 'clean bench', in which HEPA-filtered air is discharged across the work surface towards the user, provides only product protection, and is not a BSC. These can be used for clean activities, but should never be used when handling cell cultures or infectious materials.

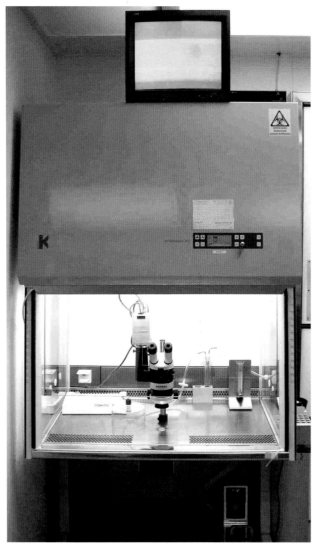

Figure 1 Class II biological safety cabinet. Air flows in sheets (laminar flow), acting as a barrier to particles outside the cabinet area and directing the flow of contaminated air into the high-efficiency particulate air (HEPA) filters. Air that enters the cabinet and flows over the infectious material, as well as the air to be exhausted, is sterilized. A class IIA cabinet is self-contained with ~70% of the air recirculated. The exhaust air in class IIB cabinets is discharged outside the building

DAILY CLEANING ROUTINE

During the course of procedures, any spillage should be immediately cleaned with dry tissue. No detergent or alcohol should be used whilst oocytes/embryos are being handled. Should it be necessary to use either of the above, allow residual traces to evaporate for a period of at least 20 min before removing oocytes/embryos from incubators.

At the end of each day:

(1) Clean flow hoods, work benches and all equipment by washing with a solution of distilled water and 7× laboratory detergent (Flow Laboratories), followed by wiping with 70% methylated spirit;

(2) Prepare each work station for the following day's work.

QUALITY CONTROL PROCEDURES

The ultimate test of quality control must rest with pregnancy and live birth rates per IVF treatment cycle. An ongoing record of the results of fertilization, cleavage and embryo development provide the best short-term evidence of good quality control. Therefore, daily records in the form of a laboratory log book are essential, summarizing details of patients and the outcome of laboratory procedures: age, cause of infertility, stimulation protocol, number of oocytes retrieved, semen analysis, sperm preparation details, insemination time, fertilization, cleavage, embryo transfer, cryopreservation. It is also essential to record details of media and oil batches for reference, along with the introduction of any new methods or materials used. Chapter 30 describes the details of Bourn Hall's IVF laboratory quality management systems.

TISSUE CULTURE SYSTEMS

Tissue culture media

A great deal of scientific research and analysis has been applied to the development of media that will successfully support the growth and development of human embryos, and many controlled studies have shown fertilization and cleavage to be satisfactory in a variety of simple and complex media. Rigorous quality control is essential in media preparation, including the source of all ingredients – especially the water, which must be endotoxin-free, low in ion content and guaranteed free of organic molecules and micro-organisms[4,5]. Each batch of culture media prepared must be subjected to rigorous quality control procedures, with results documented[6,7]. Commercially prepared, pre-tested high-quality culture media are now available for purchase from a number of suppliers worldwide;

media preparation in the laboratory is no longer necessary, and may not be a cost-effective exercise when time and quality control are taken into account. There is no scientific evidence that any commercially prepared medium is superior to another in routine IVF. The choice should depend upon considerations such as quality control and testing procedures applied in its manufacture, cost and, in particular, a guaranteed efficient supply in relation to shelf-life. After delivery, the medium may be aliquoted in suitable smaller volumes, such that one aliquot can be used for a single patient's gamete preparation and culture (including sperm preparation). Media containing HEPES (4-(2-hydroxyethyl)-1-piperazineethanesulfonic acid), which maintains a stable pH in the bicarbonate-buffered system, can be used for sperm preparation and oocyte harvesting and washing. However, HEPES is known to alter ion channel activity in the plasma membrane[8] and may well be embryotoxic. The gametes must therefore subsequently be washed in HEPES-free culture medium before insemination and overnight culture. Media specially designated for 'sperm washing' are also commercially available. In 2001, Biggers[9] published a comprehensive overview of culture media development that describes the evolution of the current approach to early human embryo culture *in vitro*, from early biological and balanced salt solution systems, to modern stage–specific chemically defined media. *In vitro* culture systems used during the 1980s and early 1990s sustained embryo development through extended culture to the blastocyst stage, but implantation rates resulting from transfer of these blastocysts were disappointingly low[10]. Further research in embryo development and metabolism, with the help of co-culture systems, led to the formulation of stage-specific culture media; this can now be used for extended culture, so that embryos can be cultured to a viable blastocyst stage, with implantation rates in the order of 50% per blastocyst[11,12].

Serum supplements

Commercially prepared media are supplied complete, and do not require the addition of any supplements – most contain a serum substitute such as Albuminar™, human serum albumin. No significant differences were found in fertilization, cleavage or pregnancy rates when maternal serum was compared with human serum albumin supplemented culture media[13,14].

Although development to the blastocyst stage may be enhanced when maternal serum is used, the availability of stage-specific media for blastocyst culture now allows the use of maternal serum to be discontinued in human IVF.

Follicular flushing

Ideally, if a patient has responded well to follicular phase stimulation with appropriate monitoring and timing of ovulation induction by human chorionic gonadotropin (hCG) injection, the oocyte retrieval may proceed smoothly with efficient recovery of oocytes without flushing follicles. However, if the number of follicles is low or the procedure is difficult for technical reasons, follicles may be flushed with a physiological solution to assist recovery of all the oocytes present. Balanced salt solutions such as Earle's (EBSS) or physiological saline may be used for follicular flushing, and heparin may be added at a concentration of 2 u/ml to prevent coagulation in blood-stained aspirates. HEPES-buffered media can also be used for flushing. Temperature and pH of flushing media must be carefully controlled, and the oocytes recovered from flushing media subsequently washed in culture media before transfer to their final culture droplet or well.

Tissue culture systems

Vessels successfully used for *in vitro* fertilization include test-tubes, four-well culture dishes, organ culture dishes and Petri dishes containing microdroplets of culture medium under a layer of paraffin or mineral oil. Whatever the system employed, it must be capable of rigidly maintaining fixed stable parameters of temperature, pH and osmolarity. Human oocytes are extremely sensitive to transient cooling *in vitro*, and modest reductions in temperature can cause irreversible disruption of the meiotic spindle, with possible chromosome dispersal[15,16]. Analyses of embryos produced by IVF have shown that a high proportion are chromosomally abnormal[17–20], and it is possible that temperature-induced chromosome disruption may contribute to the high rates of preclinical and spontaneous abortion that follow IVF. Therefore, it is essential to control temperature fluctuation from the moment of follicle aspiration and during all oocyte and embryo manipulations, by using heated microscope stages and heating blocks or platforms.

The choice of culture system used is a matter of individual preference and previous experience; two systems which are both widely and successfully used by different IVF groups are described here.

Microdroplets under oil

Pour previously equilibrated mineral oil into 60-mm Petri dishes that are clearly marked with each patient's surname. Using either a Pasteur pipette or adjustable pipettor and sterile tips, carefully place eight or nine droplets of medium around the edge of the dish. One or two drops may be placed centrally, to be used as wash drops. Examination of the follicular growth records will indicate approximately how many drops/dishes should be prepared – each drop may contain one or two oocytes. Droplet size can range from 50 to 250 μl per drop (Figure 2).

Four-well plates

Prepare labeled and numbered plates containing 0.5–1.0 ml of tissue culture medium and equilibrate overnight in a humidified incubator. Each well is normally used to incubate three oocytes. Small Petri dishes with approximately 2 ml of HEPES-containing medium may also be prepared, to be used for washing oocytes immediately after identification in the follicular aspirates. This system may also be used in combination with an overlay of equilibrated mineral oil, allowing the use of non-humidified incubators.

An overlay of equilibrated oil as part of the tissue culture system confers specific advantages[21]:

(1) The oil acts as a physical barrier, separating droplets of medium from the atmosphere and airborne particles or pathogens;

(2) Oil prevents evaporation and delays gas diffusion, thereby keeping pH, temperature, and osmolality of the medium stable during gamete manipulations, protecting the embryos from significant fluctuations in their microenvironment;

(3) Oil prevents evaporation: humidified and preequilibrated oil allows the use of non-humidified incubators, which are easier to clean and maintain.

(It has also been suggested that oil could enhance embryo development by removing lipid-soluble toxins from the medium.)

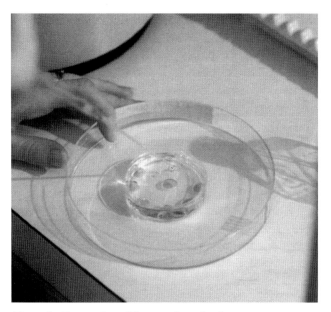

Figure 2 Preparation of tissue culture droplets

Because the physical properties of oil result in very slow diffusion of gas through the overlay, it must be prepared and equilibrated in advance: unequilibrated oil could absorb gas from the media, producing an alkaline pH with adverse effects upon the gametes or embryos. Culture dishes with an oil overlay should be equilibrated in the incubator for at least 1 h before gametes or embryos are added to the medium.

OOCYTE RETRIEVAL AND EMBRYO CULTURE

Preparation for each case

The laboratory management of an assisted reproduction cycle has become increasingly complex with the addition of new techniques and *in vitro* technologies, including intracytoplasmic sperm injection (ICSI), extended culture to blastocyst stage, assisted hatching and cryopreservation. An effective system of communication is essential to ensure that the laboratory staff are fully informed about all details of each treatment cycle, and written confirmation regarding the patients' wishes and consents regarding the handling, transfer, storage and disposal of their gametes and embryos. The laboratory staff have a responsibility to ensure that all appropriate consent forms have been signed by both partners, including consent for special procedures and storage of cryopreserved embryos. It is helpful to review details of any previous assisted conception treatment, including response to stimulation, number and quality of oocytes, timing of insemination, fertilization rate, embryo quality and embryo transfer procedure, in order to judge whether any parameters at any stage could be altered or improved in the present cycle. A repeat semen assessment may be required at the beginning of the treatment cycle, especially if the male partner has suffered recent illness, stress or trauma that could affect spermatogenesis. If necessary, a back-up semen sample may also be cryopreserved after this assessment.

The risk of introducing any infection into the laboratory via gametes and samples must be absolutely minimized; as of December 2004, the legislating authority in the UK, the Human Fertilisation and Embryology Authority (HFEA), requires that both partners should be screened for human immunodeficiency virus (HIV) and hepatitis B and C viruses at the beginning of the treatment cycle.

After administration of hCG to induce ovulation, the embryologist should again examine the case notes and prepare the laboratory records for the following day's oocyte retrievals, with attention to the following details:

(1) Previous history, with attention to laboratory procedures: any modifications required?

(2) Semen assessment: any special preparations or precautions required for sample collection or preparation?

(3) Current cycle history: number of follicles, endocrine parameters, any suggestion of ovarian hyperstimulation syndrome?

(4) Special procedures, such as assisted hatching or extended culture to blastocyst stage?

(5) Patient wishes regarding number of embryos for transfer, cryopreservation and storage of gametes and embryos.

Laboratory case notes, media, culture vessels and tubes for sperm preparation are prepared during the afternoon prior to each case, with clear and adequate labeling throughout, using printed labels when possible. Culture dishes must be clearly identified with the patient's name, and if samples are being handled from patients with similar names, an additional means of

identification must also be used. Tissue culture dishes or plates are equilibrated in the CO_2 incubator overnight.

see also 278p

Oocyte retrieval and identification

Before beginning each oocyte retrieval (OCR) procedure, the following details must be checked by the nurse and by the embryologist:

(1) Surname and first name;

(2) Date of birth;

(3) Medical number;

(4) Any allergies (e.g. penicillin);

(5) HIV + hepatitis B and C results;

(6) Ensure that consent forms have been signed; indicate number of years' storage for cryopreserved embryos on OCR record sheet;

(7) Record the cycle number on the medical records.

Immediately prior to OCR:

(1) Ensure that heating blocks, stages and trays are warmed to 37°C;

(2) Pre-warm collection test-tubes and 60-mm Petri dishes for scanning aspirates;

(3) Prepare a fire-polished Pasteur pipette and holder and a fine-drawn blunt Pasteur pipette as a probe for manipulations;

(4) Check the names on dishes and laboratory case notes with medical notes; this procedure should be witnessed by an independent witness if possible.

Examine follicular aspirates under a stereo dissecting microscope with transmitted illumination base and heated stage (Figure 3). Aliquot the contents of each test-tube into two or three Petri dishes, forming a thin layer of fluid which can be quickly, carefully and easily scanned for the presence of an oocyte in the follicular tissue. Low-power magnification (6–12×) can be used for scanning the fluid, and oocyte identification verified using higher magnification (25–50×).

The oocyte usually appears within varying quantities of cumulus cells and, if very mature, may be pale and difficult to see (immature oocytes are dark and also difficult to see). Granulosa cells are clearer and

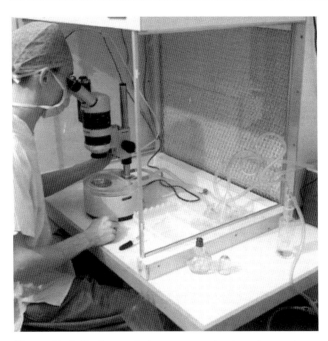

Figure 3 Follicular aspirates are examined under a stereo dissecting microscope with heated stage. Culture droplets are maintained on another heated stage in the corner of the hood, in an atmosphere of 5% CO_2 in air

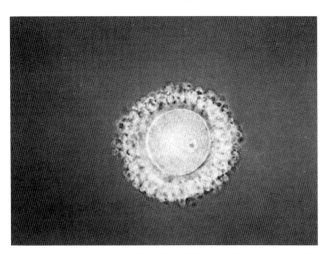

Figure 4 Germinal vesicle with tightly packed cumulus (by permission of Lucinda L. Veeck)

more 'fluffy', and appear in amorphous, often iridescent clumps. Blood clots, especially from the collection needle, should be carefully dissected with 23-gauge needles to check for the presence of cumulus cells.

When an oocyte/cumulus complex (OCC) is found, its stage of maturity is assessed by noting the volume, density and condition of the surrounding coronal and cumulus cells. If the oocyte can be seen, the presence of a single polar body indicates that it is a metaphase II oocyte, ready for insemination. OCC assessment may include the following six categories:

(1) *Germinal vesicle stage* (Figure 4) The oocyte is very immature; there is no expansion of the surrounding cells, which are tightly packed around the egg. A large nucleus (the germinal vesicle) is still present, and may be seen with the help of an inverted microscope.

(2) *Immature* (Figure 5) The oocyte is surrounded by a tightly apposed layer of corona cells, with tightly packed cumulus cells around this. The oocyte will no longer show a germinal vesicle, and the absence of a polar body indicates that it has reached the metaphase I stage.

(3) *Pre-ovulatory* (Figure 6) This is the optimal level of maturity, appropriate for successful fertilization. The oocyte is surrounded by a radiating 'crown' of corona cells (corona radiata), and the cumulus has expanded into a fluffy mass that can be easily stretched with a Pasteur pipette. The presence of an extruded polar body indicates that it has reached the stage of metaphase II.

(4) *Very mature* (Figure 7) The oocyte can often be seen clearly as a pale orb; very little coronal material is present, and may be dissociated from the oocyte. The cumulus is very profuse, but is still cellular.

(5) *Post-mature or luteinized* (Figure 8) The oocyte is very pale and is often difficult to find. The cumulus has broken down and becomes a gelatinous mass around the oocyte. These oocytes have a very low probability of fertilization.

(6) *Damaged or non-viable* (Figure 9) Granulosa cells are fragmented, and have a lace-like appearance. The oocyte is very dark, and can be difficult to identify.

Morphological assessment of oocyte maturity is highly subjective, and prone to inaccuracies[22–24]. Since 1990, micromanipulation procedures have been widely introduced into routine IVF; because the procedure involves completely denuding oocytes from surrounding cells using hyaluronidase, this allows accurate assessment of the cytoplasm and nuclear maturity. It is now apparent that gross OCC morphology does not

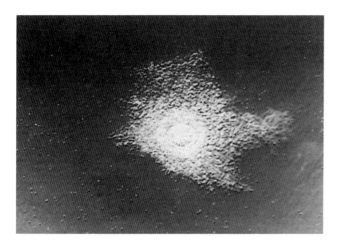

Figure 5 Immature oocyte (by permission of Lucinda L. Veeck)

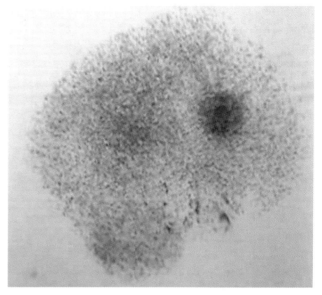

Figure 6 Pre-ovulatory oocyte, with expanded corona and cumulus cells

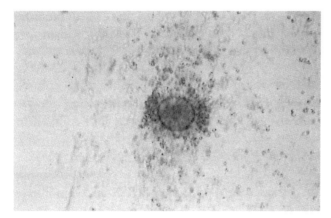

Figure 7 Very mature oocyte

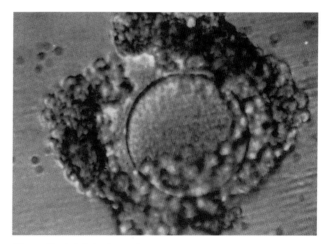

Figure 8 Luteinized oocyte

necessarily correlate with nuclear maturity. Alikani and colleagues[25] used ICSI to analyze its developmental consequences in dysmorphic human oocytes. Of 2968 injected oocytes, 806 (27.2%) were classified as dysmorphic, on the basis of cytoplasmic granularity, areas of necrosis, organelle clustering, vacuolization, or accumulating saccules of smooth endoplasmic reticulum. Anomalies of the zona pellucida and non-spherical oocytes were also noted. No single abnormality was found to be associated with a reduction in fertilization rate, and fertilization was not compromised in oocytes with multiple abnormalities. Overall pregnancy and implantation rates were not altered in patients in whom at least one oocyte was dysmorphic; however, exclusive replacement of embryos which originated from dysmorphic oocytes led to a lower implantation rate, and a higher incidence of biochemical pregnancies. They suggest that aberrations in the

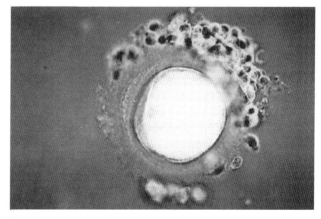

Figure 9 Atretic oocyte (by permission of Lucinda L. Veeck)

morphology of oocytes – possibly a result of ovarian hyperstimulation – are of no consequence to fertilization or early cleavage after ICSI. It is possible that embryos generated from dysmorphic oocytes have a reduced potential for implantation and further development. A later study by Meriano and colleagues[26] suggests that tracking of oocyte dysmorphisms for ICSI patients may prove relevant to the outcome in subsequent patient cycles.

Homburg and Shelef[27] reviewed the factors affecting oocyte quality, including morphology, chromosome anomalies, age, follicular microenvironment (in relation to ovulation-induction protocol) and endocrine factors. They concluded that nuclear maturity is an important factor in the assessment of oocyte quality, and that the environment of the oocyte has a significant effect upon its quality. Luteinizing hormone (LH) plays a central role in the maturation process of the oocyte, and an imbalance in the secretion of LH may upset the mechanisms involved. LH is required for completion of the first meiotic division, and inappropriate secretion of LH impairs oocyte quality. A working hypothesis has been proposed which suggests that inappropriately high levels of LH cause a premature maturation of the oocyte, causing it to become physiologically aged, less readily fertilized and, if embryo implantation occurs, possibly more prone to early abortion[28]. High follicular phase LH levels result in a poor prognosis for IVF and pregnancy, and patients with a poor previous history of IVF, including poor oocyte and embryo quality, may benefit from management with long-term gonadotropin releasing hormone (GnRH) down-regulation and LH monitoring during the follicular phase[29,30].

In summary, the procedure for oocyte collection is as follows:

(1) Scan follicular aspirates immediately, on a heated microscope stage;

(2) Wash oocytes; if necessary dissect free of blood clots or granulosa cells;

(3) Transfer immediately to culture system; maintain at 37°C in an atmosphere of 5% CO_2;

(4) At the end of the procedure, assess and record the optimum time for insemination;

(5) For microdroplet/oil systems, prepare oil dish(es) for insemination, and equilibrate in the incubator;

(6) Maintain a stable pH and temperature throughout.

INSEMINATION AND INTRACYTOPLASMIC INJECTION

If the oocytes are to be prepared for ICSI, they must first be denuded of all cells using enzymatic digestion with hyaluronidase, followed by mechanical dissection[25,31]:

(1) Prepare a culture dish containing one drop of prepared hyaluronidase solution and five wash drops of culture medium, covered with an overlay of equilibrated mineral oil (denudation can also be carried out in Nunc four-well dishes). Incubate at 37°C in the CO_2 incubator for a minimum of 60 min.

(2) Prepare a thin glass probe and denudation pipettes of suitable diameter (these are commercially available).

(3) Remove the oocyte and hyalase dishes from the incubator; group the oocytes together in small batches (4–8 oocytes per drop) and then wash the groups of oocytes through the hyalase drop, agitating gently until the cells start to dissociate (usually in less than 1 min). Carefully aspirate the oocytes, leaving as much cumulus as possible behind. Wash by transferring them through at least five drops of culture medium, and change to a fine-bore pipette for aspiration in order to remove finally all of the corona cells. These cells must be removed, as they will hinder the injection process by blocking the needle or obscuring clear observation of the cytoplasm and sperm.

(4) Assess the quality and maturity of each oocyte under an inverted microscope. Use the glass probe to roll the oocytes around gently in order to identify the polar body, and examine the ooplasm for vacuoles or other abnormalities. Separate metaphase I or germinal vesicle oocytes (no polar body, Figure 10) from metaphase II oocytes (polar body extruded, Figure 11), and label them.

(5) Set up the ICSI dish with 3–5-μl drops under oil, one drop per oocyte and one central drop for sperm.

(6) Culture the dissected oocytes for a minimum of 1 h before beginning micromanipulation.

(7) Examine the oocytes again before starting the injection procedure to see if any more have extruded the first polar body. ICSI is carried out

on all morphologically intact oocytes that have extruded the first polar body.

Important: Before adding sperm and oocytes to the ICSI dish, the embryologist and an independent witness should ensure that the identifying information on the dishes and the sperm correspond, and they should then sign the worksheet to confirm that this check has been performed.

INSEMINATION FOR IVF

For routine IVF without ICSI, oocytes are routinely inseminated with a concentration of 100,000 normal motile sperm per ml.

Microdroplets under oil

At the end of the oocyte retrieval procedure, prepare insemination dishes by pouring mineral oil into the appropriate number of 60-mm Petri dishes, and equilibrate these in the incubator along with the collected oocytes in their collection dishes. Pre-ovulatory oocytes are inseminated after 3 h pre-incubation *in vitro*. Each oocyte is transferred into a drop containing motile sperm at a concentration of approximately 100 000 per ml.

(1) Assess the volume of sperm suspension required according to the number of oocytes, and make an appropriate dilution of prepared sperm in a test-tube. Check the dilution by examining a drop of suspension on a plain glass slide under the microscope: it should contain ten normal motile sperm per high power field (100×). Adjust the dilution accordingly until the number of progressively motile normal sperm appears adequate. Incubate the diluted sperm suspension at 37°C in the CO_2 incubator for at least 30 min, leaving the cap of the tube loose in order to allow equilibration with CO_2.

(2) When removing the sample from the incubator, the embryologist and an independent witness should ensure that the identifying information on the dish and on the sample correspond, and sign the worksheet accordingly.

(3) Using a Pasteur pipette, place droplets of the sperm suspension into the paraffin dishes prepared at the end of the oocyte collection.

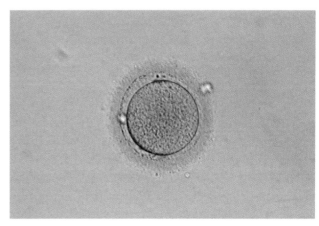

Figure 10 Metaphase I oocyte after denudation prior to intracytoplasmic sperm injection (ICSI); the first polar body has not been extruded

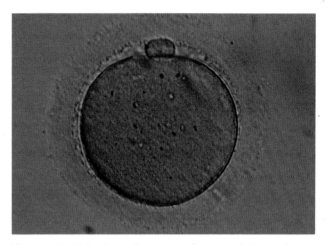

Figure 11 Metaphase II oocyte after denudation prior to intracytoplasmic sperm injection (ICSI), with first polar body clearly visible

(4) Examine each oocyte before transfer to the insemination drop; it may be necessary to dissect the cumulus in order to remove bubbles, large clumps of granulosa cells or blood clots.

(5) Prepare labeled 35-mm Petri dishes containing equilibrated paraffin at this time – these will be used for culture of the zygotes after scoring for fertilization the following day.

If the oocyte culture droplets have been created to a measured (e.g. 240 μl) volume, the oocytes can be inseminated by adding 10 μl of prepared sperm suspension whose concentration has been adjusted to 2.5 million/ml (final concentration approximately 100 000 sperm per ml, or 25 000 per oocyte).

Four-well dishes

Add a measured volume of prepared sperm suspension to each well, to a total concentration of approximately 100 000 progressively motile sperm per well.

see also 347-8

SCORING OF FERTILIZATION ON DAY 1

Oocytes that have been denuded prior to an ICSI procedure can be readily assessed for signs of fertilization, since prior removal of cells renders their cytoplasm clearly visible. Inseminated oocytes must be dissected the day following insemination in order to assess fertilization. Oocytes at this time are normally covered with a layer of corona and cumulus cells (Figure 12). These are carefully dissected away in order to visualize clearly the cell cytoplasm and examine for the presence of two pronuclei indicating normal fertilization. Pronuclear scoring should be carried out between 17 and 20 h after insemination, before the pronuclei merge during syngamy.

Zygote dissection

When removing the insemination dish from the incubator, there should be again a witnessing procedure to confirm that identity of dish and worksheet correspond. Place the microscope on 25× magnification, and choose a narrow-gauge pipette tip (e.g. 'stripper' tip) with a diameter slightly larger than the oocyte, approximately 125 μm. Aspirate 2 cm of clean culture medium into it, providing a protective buffer. This allows easy flushing of the oocyte, and prevents it from sticking to the inside surface of the pipette. Place the pipette over the oocyte and gently aspirate it into the shaft. If the oocyte does not easily enter, change to a larger diameter pipette (however, if the diameter is too large, it will be ineffective for cumulus removal). Gently aspirate and expel the oocyte through the pipette, retaining the initial buffer volume, until sufficient cumulus and corona is removed, allowing clear visualization of the cell cytoplasm and pronuclei.

An OCC that has been collected in a bloody aspirate may be lodged in a blood clot, and require additional dissection techniques.

Needle dissection Use two 26-gauge needles attached to 1-ml syringes, with the microscope on 25× magnification. Use one needle as a guide, anchoring a piece

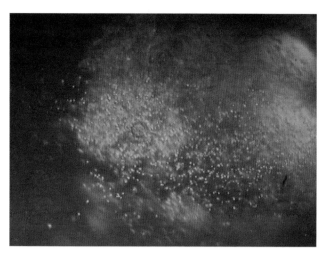

Figure 12 Oocyte after insemination for *in vitro* fertilization (IVF)

of cellular debris if possible; slide the other needle down the first one, 'shaving' cells from around the zona pellucida with a scissor-like action.

'Rolling' Use one 23-gauge needle attached to a syringe, and a fine glass probe. With the microscope on 12× magnification, use the needle to score lines in each droplet on the base of the plastic dish. Adjust the magnification to 25×, and push the oocyte gently over the scratches with a fire polished glass probe until the adhering cells are teased away from the oocyte.

Great care must be taken with either technique to avoid damaging the zona pellucida or the oocyte either by puncture or over-distortion. Breaks or cracks in the zona can sometimes be seen, and a small portion of the oocyte may extrude through the crack (this may have occurred during dissection or during the aspiration process). Occasionally, the zona is very fragile, fracturing or distorting at the slightest touch. In cases such as this, it is probably best not to continue the dissection.

Pronuclear scoring

An inverted microscope is recommended for accurate scoring of fertilization; although the pronuclei can be seen with dissecting microscopes, it can often be difficult to distinguish normal pronuclei from vacuoles or other irregularities in the cytoplasm. Normally fertilized oocytes should have two pronuclei, two polar bodies, a regular shape with an intact zona pellucida and a clear healthy cytoplasm (Figure 13). However, a variety of different features may be observed. The cytoplasm of normally fertilized oocytes is usually slightly granular, whereas the cytoplasm of unfertilized oocytes tends to be completely clear and featureless. The cytoplasm can vary from slightly granular and healthy-looking, to brown or dark and degenerate. The shape of the oocyte may also vary, from perfectly spherical to irregular. A clear halo of peripheral cytoplasm 5–10 μm thick is an indication of good activation and reinitiation of meiosis.

Single pronucleate (PN) zygotes obtained after conventional IVF were analyzed by fluorescence *in situ* hybridization (FISH) to determine their ploidy[32]: of 16 zygotes, ten were haploid and six were diploid (four XY and two XX). Therefore, it seems that during the course of their interaction, it is possible for human gamete nuclei to associate together and form diploid, single PN zygotes. These findings confirm a newly recognized variation of human pronuclear interaction during syngamy, and the authors suggest that single pronucleate zygotes which develop with normal cleavage may be safely replaced[32,33].

Details of morphology and fertilization should be recorded for each zygote, for reference when choosing embryos for transfer on day 2. Remove zygotes with normal fertilization at the time of scoring from the insemination drops or wells, transfer them into new dishes or plates containing pre-equilibrated culture medium, and return them to the incubator for a further 24 h of culture. Those with abnormal fertilization such as multipronucleate zygotes must be cultured separately, so that there is no possibility of their being selected for embryo transfer; after cleavage these are indistinguishable from normally fertilized oocytes.

Although the presence of two pronuclei confirms fertilization, their absence does not necessarily indicate fertilization failure, and may instead represent either parthenogenetic activation, or a delay in timing of one or more of the events involved in fertilization. A study showed that in 40% of oocytes with no sign of fertilization 17–27 h after insemination, 41% had the appearance of morphologically normal embryos on the following day, with morphology and cleavage rate similar to that of oocytes with obvious pronuclei on day 1. However, 30% of these zygotes arrested on day 2, compared with only 7% of 'normally' fertilized oocytes, and they showed a reduced implantation rate of 6% compared with 11.1%. Cytogenetic analysis of these embryos revealed a higher incidence of chromosomal anomalies (55% vs. 29%), and a high rate of

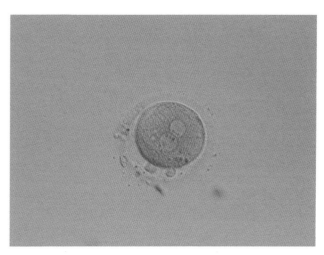

Figure 13 Fertilized oocyte (zygote) on day 1, showing two polar bodies and pronuclei, with nucleolar precursor bodies aligned within the nuclei

haploidy (20%), confirming parthenogenetic activation. Nine per cent were triploid, and 26% mosaic[32,33].

Delayed fertilization, with the appearance of pronuclei on day 2, may also be observed, and these embryos tend to have an impaired developmental potential. Oehninger and colleagues[34] suggest that delayed fertilization could be attributed to morphological or endocrine oocyte defects in 37% of their cases, and sperm defects in 14.8%. Thirty-three per cent of the cases studied had no obvious association with either oocyte or sperm defects.

Re-insemination

Although oocytes which fail to demonstrate clear pronuclei at the time of scoring for fertilization can be re-inseminated or injected by the ICSI procedure, this practice has been widely questioned scientifically[35]. Fertilization or cleavage may then be seen on day 2, but this may be as a consequence of the initial insemination, and the delay in fertilization may be attributed to either functional disorders of the sperm, or maturation delay of the oocyte.

Selection of surplus zygotes for cryopreservation

If a large number of oocytes have two clearly visible pronuclei on day 1, a selected number can be kept in culture for transfer on day 2, and the remainder considered for pronucleate stage cryopreservation. The decision as to the number of embryos to be frozen at pronucleate stage should take into consideration the patient's previous history regarding cleavage and quality of embryos; zygotes to be frozen should have a regular outline, distinct zona and clearly visible pronuclei. The microtubular apparatus that supports the spindle apparatus is more stable and able to withstand the cryopreservation procedure when it is enclosed within the pronuclear membrane; therefore the process must be initiated whilst the pronuclei are still clearly visible, before the onset of pronuclear membrane breakdown and initiation of syngamy. At this point the spindle will be 'free' in the cytoplasm, and is more likely to dissociate under the stress of the procedure (Table 1).

EMBRYO QUALITY AND SELECTION FOR TRANSFER

In current IVF practice, the selection procedure for choosing the right embryos for transfer must be safe, non-invasive and easy to perform within the routine of a busy IVF laboratory. Both objective and subjective strategies have been applied to the problem, and the application of different strategies to measure human embryo viability objectively have yielded a vast body of scientific literature:

(1) Blastomere or polar body biopsy for cytogenetic analysis[36–38];

(2) Metabolic assessment of culture media[39,40];

(3) High-resolution videocinematography[41];

(4) Delayed embryo transfer[42];

(5) Culture of cumulus cells, apoptosis in granulosa cells[43–45];

(6) Oxygen levels in follicular fluid and perifollicular vascularization[46–48];

(7) Distribution of mitochondria and adenosine triphosphate (ATP) levels in blastomeres[49];

(8) Gene expression profiles[50].

Although each of these strategies has its problems, and many are not suitable for routine daily assessment of embryos, they have all helped to contribute a great deal of information about embryo development,

which has led to an overall improvement in our understanding of culture conditions. We have also gained an increasing number of clues to help in the evaluation of embryo morphology, which continues to be the selection procedure used in routine IVF practice.

Historically, cleaved embryos have been graded on the basis of their cleavage rate and blastomere appearance, and the presence of anucleate fragments. However, we now know that correlations between gross morphology and implantation potential are weak and inaccurate, except when embryos are clearly degenerating. We also know that embryo morphology changes with time, and that embryos with apparently the 'worst' morphology and many fragments do sometimes implant: time-lapse photographic studies clearly demonstrate that fragments can sometimes be absorbed[51]. Further studies by Alikani and colleagues[52] indicate that the pattern and distribution of fragments within the embryo may be significant, and that surgical fragment removal may be beneficial. High-resolution videocinematography of embryos prior to transfer, followed by retrospective correlation with their implantation[41], suggested two further features of embryo morphology which relate to implantation potential: thickness of the zona pellucida, and cell–cell contact between the blastomeres on day 3. Although 'bad' morphology may indicate 'bad quality', good morphology does not always mean high developmental capacity – even the 'ugliest' embryo can sometimes produce a beautiful baby! The problems inherent in adequately assessing embryo competence have therefore led to a more detailed and combined approach that not only judges the embryo on its esthetic appearance at the time of transfer, but follows its evolution and development from the time of oocyte retrieval. It seems 'intuitively' correct to assume that cytoplasmic defects in oocytes such as granular cytoplasm, necrotic regions, vacuoles, refractile bodies, organelle clustering or an abnormally large perivitelline space may reflect inherent abnormalities that will compromise further development. Abnormally 'large' or 'giant' oocytes have been associated with digynic embryos[53,54]. Although there are conflicting reports about the significance of cytoplasmic defects with respect to embryo implantation, nonetheless these features are worth noting on day 0[25,26]. The first polar body starts to appear at 36–44 h post-hCG, and it begins to disintegrate approximately 20 h later. Ebner and

Table 1 *In vitro* fertilization scoring chart

Day 1	Options	Day 2	Day 3	Rationale
2PN	maintain in culture or freeze as pronucleate	(a) transfer or freeze if cleaved (b) if not cleaved, may be transferred if insufficient cleaved embryos are available (c) if no cleaved embryos are available, continue culture	(a) transfer or freeze if cleaved (b) transfer if cleaved (day-3 transfer)	normal fertilization
3PN	discard	—	—	abnormal fertilization
Single PN or pale central area ('light spot')	discard	—	—	abnormal fertilization
0PN +1 polar body	culture	(a) if 2PN, may be transferred if insufficient cleaved embryos are available for transfer (b) if no cleaved embryos are available for transfer, continue culture if 2PN visible	(b) transfer if cleaved	late fertilization
0PN + 0 polar body	culture	if 2PN visible, culture, freeze or add to cleaved embryos for transfer	transfer or freeze if cleaved	late maturation

PN, pronucleate

colleagues[55] suggest that features of the polar body such as abnormal size or early fragmentation may also be associated with a poor prognosis for that oocyte.

Attention has also been focused on evaluating the development and appearance of pronuclei on day 1 after fertilization. Payne and associates[56] observed the formation of pronuclei and extrusion of polar body by time-lapse videocinematography, and witnessed circular periodic waves of granulation in the ooplasm. Garello and colleagues[57] measured the angle between the two polar bodies, and also the angle between the polar axis (the line passing through the two pronuclei) and each polar body. They propose that pronuclear orientation may reflect cytoplasmic or pronucelar rotation relative to the polar bodies, and the angles might reflect the degree of cytoplasmic pronuclear rotation that has occurred since oocyte maturation: this feature might be related to oocyte maturity and/or competence. However, other studies have been unable to confirm these observations[58,59].

In 1998, Scott and Smith[60] suggested a system of zygote evaluation that noted alignment of pronuclei and nucleoli, in conjunction with the appearance of a 'halo' in the cytoplasm. Sadowy and colleagues[61] studied pronuclear dysmorphism, and observed that zygotes with pronuclei of uneven or unequal size more frequently had arrested development, and an increased incidence of mosaicism. Tesarik and co-workers[62,63] also studied the association of pronuclear structure and architecture with development, and suggest that assessment of the number and distribution of nucleolar precursor bodies within pronuclei can help to predict implantation potential. However, since these early stages are largely dependent on maternal reserves, which become depleted after approximately 60 h in culture and the new zygote genome does not become activated and translated until the 4–8-cell stage, any factors that influence this maternal–embryonic transition stage can cause even the most apparently 'perfect' zygote to fail at a later stage.

Cleavage rate has also been used as a prognostic indicator: it appears that 'faster growing' embryos may have greater implantation potential[64-67]. However, accelerated growth may also be associated with increased mosaicism[68], and cleavage rates are clearly influenced by culture conditions: judgment of this parameter should also be made with caution. Evidence suggests that, in an optimized culture system, optimal implantation rates are obtained by selecting embryos that have reached the two-cell stage by the end of day 1, have 4–6 cells on day 2, 7–9 cells on day 3, and show signs of early compaction on day 3.

The presence of multinucleated blastomeres has also been correlated with implantation potential. These can only be clearly seen on day 2, and embryos displaying this feature apparently have severely impaired implantation potential[69-71].

In summary, it seems that no single parameter or morphological feature is paramount when choosing the right embryo by non-invasive detailed observation. A strategy towards choosing a single embryo for transfer could include an assessment of as many parameters as possible following the time sequence of events after fertilization, but this must also be balanced by consideration of the potential damage caused by subjecting the embryo to physiological stresses as a result of excessive exposure and manipulation.

Applying this strategy also requires, first of all, that each oocyte and embryo should be cultured and tracked individually in single microdroplets. Second, there must be an excellent microscope available, with heated stage, high-power magnification and optimal resolution/optics. Finally, this strategy requires dedicated attention, time, patience and perseverance. Ultimately, a final ingredient will be the application of background scientific knowledge, common sense and a balance of judgment that includes appreciation of the intricacies and delicate choreography of mechanisms involved in the creation of a competent embryo, and a new life.

Blastocyst transfer

The development of stage-specific sequential culture media systems which support embryo development to the blastocyst stage has made it possible to delay embryo transfer until day 5/6 (Figure 18). The aim of extended culture is to produce blastocysts with better implantation potential than cleavage-stage embryos, by identifying those embryos with little developmental competence. Transfer of only one or two blastocysts may thus result in successful pregnancy, reducing the number of multiple gestations and increasing the overall efficiency of IVF. Transfer on day 5 can eliminate those embryos that are unable to develop after activation of the zygote genome due to genetic or metabolic defects, and may also have the advantage of allowing better synchrony between the embryo and endometrium. Current data suggest that blastocyst transfer has a place in the treatment of selected groups of patients, in particular those with a high risk of multiple gestation or for whom a multiple pregnancy represents an obstetric disaster. An important prerequisite for blastocyst culture is an optimal IVF laboratory environment; extended culture yields no advantage unless satisfactory implantation rates are already being achieved with embryos cultured to day 2 or 3. In patients who develop three or more good-quality eight-cell embryos on day 3, extended culture to the blastocyst stage has achieved implantation rates in the order of 40% per embryo, with pregnancy rates of at least 65% per transfer[11,12].

The ability to identify healthy viable blastocysts is an important factor in the success of blastocyst transfer, and a grading system has been devised that takes into consideration the degree of expansion, hatching status, the development of the inner cell mass and the development of the trophectoderm[11]. Satisfactory implantation rates after blastocyst transfer are only achieved with selection after careful assessment of all morphological parameters available. If embryos are to be cultured beyond day 2 for potential blastocyst development, the culture medium should be changed on day 2 or 3 to a stage-specific formulation, according to the manufacturer's instructions.

Selection of embryos for transfer

As outlined above, many studies have researched more objective criteria for judging embryo viability and implantation potential, but the method most commonly used still relies upon subjective morphological assessment of the rate of division judged by the number of blastomeres, the size, shape, symmetry and cytoplasmic appearance of the blastomeres, and the presence of anucleate cytoplasmic fragments[72-74].

Based upon these criteria, embryos may be arbitrarily classified.

See also 347, 348

Grade 1

Embryos have even, regular, spherical blastomeres with moderate refractility (i.e. not very dark) and with intact zonae. Allowance must be made for the appearance of blastomeres that are in division or that have divided asynchronously with their sisters, i.e. three-, five-, six- or seven-cell embryos. These may be uneven but are perfectly normal. As always, individual judgment is important, and this is a highly subjective assessment. Grade 1 embryos have no, or very few fragments (less than 10%) (Figure 14).

Grade 2

Embryos have uneven or irregularly shaped blastomeres, with mild variation in refractility and no more than 10% fragmentation of blastomeres (Figure 15).

Grade 3

Embryos show fragmentation of no more than 50% of blastomeres. The remaining blastomeres must be at least in reasonable (grade 2) condition and with refractility associated with cell viability; the zona pellucida must be intact (Figure 16).

Grade 4

More than 50% of the blastomeres are fragmented, and there may be gross variation in refractility. The remaining blastomeres should appear viable (Figure 17).

Grade 5

Zygotes have two pronuclei on day 2, either as a result of delayed fertilization or re-insemination on day 1.

Grade 6

Embryos are non-viable, with lysed, contracted or dark blastomeres.

Fragments

Most IVF embryologists would agree that fragmentation is the norm in routine IVF, but it is not clear whether this is an effect of culture conditions and follicular stimulation, or a characteristic of human embryo development. The degree of fragmentation varies from 5 or 10% to 100%, and the fragments may be either localized or scattered. Alikani and colleagues[52] used an analysis of patterns of cell fragmentation in the human

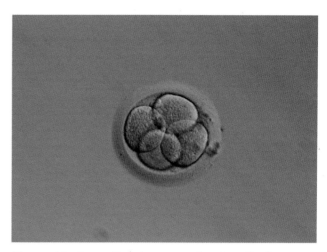

Figure 14 Four-cell embryo, on day 2, with four even blastomeres and no fragments, grade 1

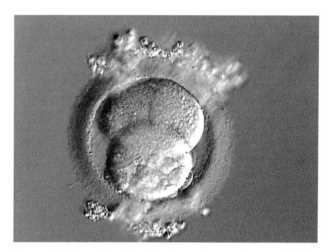

Figure 15 Two-cell embryo showing a cleavage furrow and a few fragments, grade 2

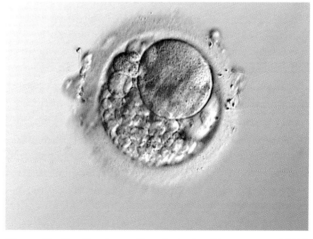

Figure 16 Day-2 embryo with a single clear blastomere and 50% fragmentation, grade 3

embryo as a means of determining the relationship between cell fragmentation and implantation potential, with the conclusion that not only the degree, but also the pattern of embryo fragmentation, determine its implantation potential.

Five distinct patterns of fragmentation which can be seen by day 3 were identified[52]:

(1) Less than 5% of the volume of the perivitelline space occupied by fragments;

(2) All or most fragments localized, concentrated in one area of the perivitelline space (PVS), with five or more normal cells visible;

(3) Fragments scattered throughout, and similar in size;

(4) Large fragments, indistinguishable from blastomeres, and scattered throughout the PVS; usually associated with very few cells;

(5) Fragments throughout the PVS, appearing degenerate such that cell boundaries are invisible, associated with contracted and granular cytoplasm.

Implantation potential was greatest in types (1) and (2), and diminished in types (3) and (4).

In 25 years of clinical embryology, there have been no definitive reports on the causes of blastomere fragmentation, although speculations include: high spermatozoal numbers and consequently high levels of free radicals, temperature or pH shock, and stimulation protocols. Observed through the scanning electron microscope, the surface of fragments is made up of irregularly shaped blebs and protrusions, very different to the regular surface of blastomeres, which is organized into short, regular microvilli. Interestingly, programmed cell death in somatic cells also starts with surface blebbing, and is caused, in part, by a calcium-induced disorganization of the cytoskeleton. We can speculate that similar mechanisms operate within human embryos, but we have so far no scientific evidence that this is the case. There appears to be an element of programming in this partial embryonic auto-destruction, since embryos from certain patients, irrespective of the types of procedure applied in successive IVF attempts, are always prone to fragmentation. Fragments may be removed during micromanipulation for assisted hatching, and there is growing evidence that fragment removal may improve implantation. Surprisingly, fragmented embryos, repaired or

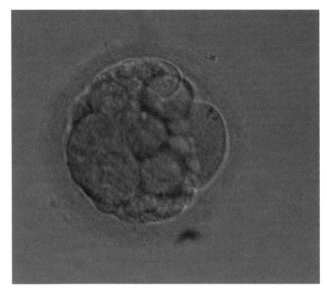

Figure 17 Grade 4 embryo, with > 50% fragmentation

not, do implant and often come to term. This demonstrates the highly regulative nature of the human embryo, as it can apparently lose over half of its cellular mass and still recover, and also confirms the general consensus that the mature oocyte contains much more material than it needs for development. The reasons why part, and only part, of an early embryo should become disorganized and degenerate are a mystery. Different degrees of fragmentation argue against the idea that the embryo is purposely casting off excess cytoplasm (somewhat analogous to the situation in annelids and marsupials that shed cytoplasmic lobes rich in yolk) and favors the idea of partial degeneration. Perhaps it involves cell polarization, where organelles gather to one side of the cell. It is certain that pH, calcium and transcellular currents trigger cell polarization, which may in certain cases lead to an abnormal polarization, and therefore to fragmentation. These areas are for the moment wide open to speculation, and continuing studies are in progress.

EMBRYO TRANSFER PROCEDURE

When selecting the 'best'-quality embryos for transfer, we must appreciate that the time during which this observation and judgment is made represents only a tiny instant of a rapidly evolving process of development. Embryos can be judged quite differently at two different periods in time, as may be seen if a comparison is made between assessments made in the morning, and later in the day immediately before transfer. Individual judgment should be exercised in determining which embryos are selected. In general, those embryos at later stages and of higher grades are preferred, but the choice is often not clear-cut. The grade 2 category covers a wide range of morphological states, but, provided the blastomeres are not grossly abnormal, a later-stage grade 2 embryo may be selected in preference to an earlier-stage grade 1 embryo. Attention should also be paid to the appearance of the zona pellucida and to the pattern of fragmentation. Embryos of grade 3 or 4 are transferred only where no better embryos are available. If only pronucleate embryos are available on day 2, they should be cultured further and transferred only if cleavage occurs. However, the application of preimplantation genetic diagnosis by FISH analysis of biopsied blastomeres has shown a surprising discrepancy between gross morphology and genetic normality of the embryos, in that even the most 'beautiful' embryos may have genetic abnormalities, whilst those with less esthetic qualities, including the presence of fragments, may in fact have normal implantation potential[75].

Remaining embryos

Embryos of grade 1 or 2 which remain after the embryo transfer procedure may be cryopreserved. Remaining cleaved embryos unsuitable for freezing can be kept in culture and scored daily until day 6. Those which develop to blastocyst stage on day 5 or 6 can also be cryopreserved (Figure 18).

Embryo transfer procedure (Figure 19)

Materials

(1) Pre-equilibrated, warmed culture medium;

(2) 1-ml disposable syringe;

(3) Embryo transfer catheter; Wallace

(4) Sterile disposable gloves (non-powdered);

(5) Clean Petri dish;

(6) Fire-polished Pasteur pipette and glass probe;

(7) Dissecting microscope with warm stage.

Although it may seem obvious that correct identification of patient and embryos is vital, errors in communication do happen and can lead to a disastrous mistake, especially should there be patients with similar names undergoing treatment at the same time. Therefore, a routine discipline of identification should be followed in order to avoid any possibility of mistake:

(1) Ensure that medical notes always accompany a patient who is being prepared for embryo transfer.

(2) The name and medical number on the medical notes and patient identity bracelet should be checked by two people, e.g. the clinician in charge of the procedure and the assisting nurse.

(3) The doctor should also check name and number verbally with the patient, and embryologist, nurse and the patient may sign an appropriate form confirming that the details are correct.

(4) The duty embryologist should check the same details with the embryology records, and also sign the same form in the presence of the doctor.

(5) The embryologist should check that the medical records and laboratory records correspond, and that the patient, doctor and nurse have all signed the identification form. The embryologist and a witness will also check that the identifying details on the culture dish correspond with the patient and the records.

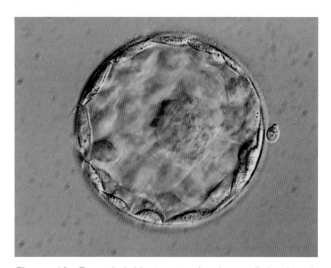

Figure 18 Expanded blastocyst, showing well-developed, centrally placed inner cell mass and single layer of trophectoderm cells

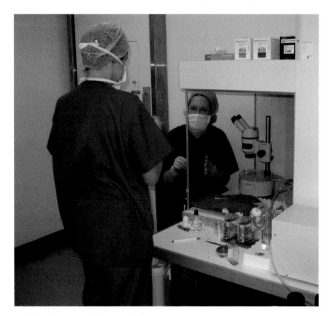

Figure 19 Embryo transfer procedure

Preparation of embryos for transfer

Legislation in the UK now states that no more than two embryos should be transferred in a single treatment cycle, although three may be transferred in selected patients over the age of 40, with documentation to justify the decision.

When the embryos for transfer have been identified and scored, and their details recorded, they are placed together in fresh medium in a single droplet under oil, or in a single well:

(1) After gently pushing the embryos together, leave them under low power on the heated stage of the microscope, in focus.

(2) Turn off the microscope light.

(3) Wash hands with a surgical scrub preparation, and don sterile gloves.

(4) Fill a 1-ml sterile syringe with warm medium, and eject any air bubbles.

(5) Check that the catheter to be used moves freely through its outer sheath, attach it to the syringe and eject the medium from the syringe through the catheter, discarding the medium.

(6) Draw up warm medium through the catheter into the syringe, and then push the piston down to the 10 μl mark, ejecting excess medium and again discarding it.

(7) Pour some clean warm medium into the warm Petri dish on the microscope stage (for rinsing the catheter tip).

(8) Place the end of the catheter carefully into the drop or well, away from the embryos, and inject a small amount of medium to break the boundary of surface tension that may appear at the end of the catheter. Aspirate the embryos into the catheter, so that the volume to be transferred is 15–20 μl.

(9) If the embryos have been loaded from a droplet under oil, rinse the tip of the catheter in the Petri dish containing clean warm medium.

Hand the catheter and syringe to the clinician for transfer to the patient. When the catheter is returned after the procedure, carefully inspect it, rotating under the microscope. It is especially important to ensure that no embryo is buried in any mucus present. The presence of mucus and/or blood on the catheter is noted. Loosen the Luer fitting, and allow the fluid in the catheter to drain into the clean Petri dish whilst continuing to observe through the microscope. Inform the doctor and patient as soon as you have confirmed that no embryos have been returned.

If any embryos have been returned, they should be re-loaded into a clean catheter, and the transfer procedure repeated. If difficulties arise during the transfer procedure causing delay, return the embryos to the culture drop in the interim, until the physician is confident that they can be safely transferred to the uterus of the patient.

Great strides have been made in terms of evaluating *in vitro* embryo competence over the past 25 years; many IVF units throughout Europe are now using careful embryo selection in order to employ single embryo transfer as a routine for the majority of patients[76–79]. Hopefully, further research over the next decade will lead us to the ultimate goal of assisted conception treatment: the delivery of a healthy baby as a result of each single embryo transferred.

REFERENCES

1. Quinn P, Warner GM, Klein JE, Kirby C. Culture factors affecting the success rate of in vitro fertilization and embryo transfer. Ann NY Acad Sci 1985; 412: 195

2. Purdy JM. Methods for fertilization and embryo culture in vitro. In Edwards RG, Purdy JM, eds. Human Conception In Vitro. London: Academic Press, 1982: 135

3. Elder KT, Baker DJ, Ribes JA. Infection and contamination control in the IVF laboratory. In Infections, Infertility and Assisted Reproduction. Cambridge: Cambridge University Press, 2004: Ch 13

4. Danforth RA, Piana SD, Smith M. High purity water: an important component for success in in vitro fertilization. Am Biotech Lab 1987; 5: 58

5. Rinehart JS, Bavister BD, Gerrity M. Quality control in the in vitro fertilization laboratory: comparison of bioassay systems for water quality. J In Vitro Fertil Embryo Transf 1988; 5: 335–42

6. Edwards RG, Brody SA. Human fertilization in the laboratory. In Principles and Practice of Assisted Human Reproduction. Philadelphia, PA: WB Saunders, 1995: 351–413

7. Critchlow JD. Quality control in an in-vitro fertilization laboratory: use of human sperm survival studies. Hum Reprod 1989; 4: 545–9

8. Wales RG. Effect of ions on the development of preimplantation mouse embryos in vitro. Aust J Biol Sci 1970; 23: 421–9

9. Biggers JD. Thought on embryo culture conditions. Reprod Biomed Online 2001; 4 (Suppl 1): 30–8

10. Bolton VN, Hawes SM, Taylor CT, Parsons JH. Development of spare human preimplantation embryos in vitro: an analysis of the correlations among gross morphology, cleavage rates, and development to the blastocyst. J In Vitro Fertil Embryo Transf 1989; 7: 186

11. Gardner DK, Lane M. Culture and selection of viable blastocysts: a feasible proposition for human IVF. Hum Reprod Update 1997; 3: 367–82

12. Ménézo Y, Veiga A, Benkhalifa M. Improved methods for blastocyst formation and culture. Hum Reprod 1998; 13 (Suppl) 4: 20

13. Ashwood-Smith MJ, Hollands P, Edwards RG. The use of Albuminar™ as a medium supplement in clinical IVF. Hum Reprod 1989; 4: 702–5

14. Staessen C, Van den Abeel E, Carle M, et al. Comparison between human serum and Albuminar-20™ supplement for in vitro fertilization. Hum Reprod 1990; 5: 336–41

15. Pickering SJ, Braude PR, Johnson MH, et al. Transient cooling to room temperature can cause irreversible disruption of the meiotic spindle in the human oocyte. Fertil Steril 1990; 54: 102–8

16. Almeida PA, Bolton VN. The effect of temperature fluctuations on the cytoskeletal organisation and chromosomal constitution of the human oocyte. Zygote 1996; 3: 357–65

17. Angell RR, Templeton AA, Aitken RJ. Chromosome studies in human in vitro fertilization. Hum Genet 1986; 72: 333

18. Plachot M, Veiga A, Montagut J, et al. Are clinical and biological IVF parameters correlated with chromosomal disorders in early life: a multicentric study. Hum Reprod 1988; 3: 627–35

19. Plachot M, de Grouchy J, Montagut J, et al. Multicentric study of chromosome analysis in human oocytes and embryos in an IVF programme. Hum Reprod 1987; 2: 29

20. Marquez C, Sandalinas M, Bahce M, et al. Chromosome abnormalities in 1255 cleavage-stage human embryos. Reprod Biomed Online 2001; 1: 17–26

21. Johnson C, Hofmann G, Scott R. The use of oil overlay for in vitro fertilization and culture. Assist Reprod Rev 1994; 4: 198–201

22. Veeck LL. Oocyte assessment and biological performance. Ann NY Acad Sci USA 1988; 541: 259–62

23. Plachot M, Mandelbaum J. Oocyte maturation, fertilization and embryonic growth in vitro. Br Med Bull 1990; 46: 675–94

24. Khan I, Staessen C, Van den Abeel E, et al. Time of insemination and its effect on in vitro fertilization, cleavage and pregnancy rates in GnRH agonist/HMG-stimulated cycles. Hum Reprod 1989; 4: 531–5

25. Alikani M, Palermo G, Adler A, et al. Intracytoplasmic sperm injection in dysmorphic human oocytes. Zygote 1995; 3: 283–8

26. Meriano JS, Alexis J, Visram-Zaver S, et al. Tracking of oocyte dysmorphisms for ICSI patients may prove relevant to the outcome in subsequent patient cycles. Hum Reprod 2001; 16: 2118–23

27. Homburg R, Shelef M. Factors affecting oocyte quality. In Grudzinskas JG, Yovich JL, eds. Gametes: the Oocyte. Cambridge: Cambridge University Press, 1995: 227–91

28. Regan L, Owen EJ, Jacobs H. Hypersecretion of luteinising hormone, infertility, and miscarriage. Lancet 1990; 336: 1141–4

29. Howles CM, Macnamee M, Edwards RG. Follicular development and early luteal function of conception and non-conceptual cycles after human in vitro fertilization. Hum Reprod 1987; 2: 17–21

30. Macnamee MC, Howles CM, Edwards RG, et al. Short term luteinising hormone agonist treatment, prospective trial of a novel ovarian stimulation regimen for in vitro fertilization. Fertil Steril 1989; 52: 264–9

31. Elder KT, Dale BD. In Vitro Fertilization. Cambridge: Cambridge University Press, 2001: Ch 12

32. Sultan KM, Munne S, Palermo GD, et al. Chromosomal status of uni-pronuclear human zygotes

following in-vitro fertilization and intracytoplasmic sperm injection. Hum Reprod 1995; 10: 132–6

33. Levron J, Munné S, Willadsen S, et al. Male and female genomes associated in a single pronucleus in human zygotes. J Assist Reprod Genet 1995; 12 (Suppl): 27s

34. Oehninger S, Acosta AA, Veek LL, et al. Delayed fertilization during in vitro fertilization and embryo transfer cycles: analysis of cause and impact of overall results. Fertil Steril 1989; 52: 991–7

35. Pampiglione JS, Mills C, Campbell S, et al. The clinical outcome of re-insemination of human oocytes fertilised in vitro. Fertil Steril 1990; 53: 306–10

36. Handyside AH, Kontogianni EH, Hardy K, Winston RML. Pregnancies from biopsied human preimplantation embryos sexed by Y-specific DNA amplification. Nature (London) 1990; 344: 768–70

37. Harper JC, Handyside AH. The current status of preimplantation diagnosis. Curr Obstet Gynaecol 1994; 4: 143–9

38. Harper JC, Coonan E, Ramaekers FCS. Identification of the sex of human preimplantation embryos in two hours using an improved spreading method and fluorescent in-situ hybridization (FISH) using directly labelled probes. Hum Reprod 1994; 9: 721–4

39. Gott AL, Hardy K, Winston RML, Leese HJ. Non-invasive measurement of pyruvate and glucose uptake and lactate production by single human preimplantation embryos. Hum Reprod 1990; 5: 104–10

40. Leese HJ. Analysis of embryos by non-invasive methods. Hum Reprod 1987; 2: 37–40

41. Cohen J, Inge KL, Suzman M, et al. Videocinematography of fresh and cryopreserved embryos: a retrospective analysis of embryonic morphology and implantation. Fertil Steril 1989; 51: 820

42. Bolton VN. Pregnancies after in vitro fertilization and transfer of human blastocysts. Fertil Steril 1991; 55: 830–2

43. Gregory L. Ovarian markers of implantation potential in assisted reproduction. Hum Reprod 1998; 13 (Suppl 4): 117–32

44. Gregory L, Leese HJ. Determinants of oocyte and pre-implantation embryo quality metabolic requirements and the potential role of cumulus cells. Hum Reprod 1996; 11 (Suppl): 96–102

45. Van Blerkom J. Can the developmental competence of early human embryos be predicted effectively in the clinical IVF laboratory? Hum Reprod 1997; 12: 1610–14

46. Van Blerkom J, Atczak M, Schrader R. The developmental potential of the human oocyte is related to the dissolved oxygen content of follicular fluid: association with vascular endothelial growth factor concentra-tions and perifollicular blood flow characteristics. Hum Reprod 1997; 12: 1047–55

47. Chui DKC, Pugh ND, Walker SM, et al. Follicular vascularity – the predictive value of transvaginal power Doppler ultrasonography in an in-vitro fertilization programme: a preliminary study. Hum Reprod 1997; 12: 191–6

48. Borini A, Maccolini A, Tallarini A, et al. Perifollicular vascularity and its relationship with oocytes maturity and IVF outcome. Ann NY Acad Sci 2001; 943: 64–7

49. Van Blerkom J, Davis P, Alexander S. Differential mitochondrial distribution in human pronuclear embryos leads to disproportionate inheritance between blastomeres: relationship to microtubular organization, ATP content and competence. Hum Reprod 2000; 15: 2621–33

50. Niemann H, Wrenzycki C. Alterations of expression of developmentally important genes in preimplantation bovine embryos by in vitro culture conditions: implications for subsequent development. Theriogenology 2000; 53: 21–34

51. Hardarson T, Lofman C, Coull G, et al. Internalization of cellular fragments in a human embryo: time-lapse recordings. Reprod Biomed Online 2002; 5: 36–8

52. Alikani M, Cohen J, Tomkin G, et al. Human embryo fragmentation in vitro and its implications for pregnancy and implantation. Fertil Steril 1999; 71: 836–42

53. Rosenbusch B, Schneider M, Glaser B, Brucker C. Cytogenetic analysis of giant oocytes and zygotes to assess their relevance for the development of digynic triploidy. Hum Reprod 2002; 17: 2388–93

54. Balakier H, Bouman D, Sojecki A, et al. Morphological and cytogenetic analysis of human giant oocytes and giant embryos. Hum Reprod 2002; 17: 2394–401

55. Ebner T, Yaman C, Moser M, et al. Prognostic value of first polar body morphology on fertilization rate and embryo quality in intracytoplasmic sperm injection. Hum Reprod 2000; 15: 427–30

56. Payne D, Flaherty SP, Barry MF, Matthews CD. Preliminary observations on polar body extrusion and pronuclear formation in human oocytes using time-lapse video cinematography. Hum Reprod 1997; 12: 532–41

57. Garello C, Baker H, Rai J, et al. Pronuclear orientation, polar body placement, and embryo quality after intracytoplasmic sperm injection and in vitro fertilization: further evidence of polarity in human oocytes? Hum Reprod 1999; 14: 2588–95

58. Triantafillous T. Polar body placement and pronuclear alignment as morphological criteria for the evaluation of 2PN zygotes: a computer based study. Thesis: MAS in Clinical Embryology, Krems, Austria, 2002

59. Clarke RN, Zaninovic N, Berrios R, Veek LL. The relationship between human prezygote morphology and subsequent preembryo development in culture. Fertil Steril 2001; 76: S101–2

60. Scott LA, Smith S. The successful use of pronuclear embryo transfers the day following oocyte retrieval. Hum Reprod 1998; 13: 1003–13

61. Sadowy S, Tomkin G, Munne S, et al. Impaired development of zygotes with uneven pronuclear size. Zygote 1998; 6: 137–41

62. Tesarik J, Greco E. The probability of abnormal preimplantation development can be predicted by a single static observation on pronuclear stage morphology. Hum Reprod 1999; 14: 1318–23

63. Tesarik J, Junca AM, Hazout A, et al. Embryos with high implantation potential after intracytoplasmic sperm injection can be recognized by a simple, noninvasive examination of pronuclear morphology. Hum Reprod 2000; 15: 1396–9

64. Lundqvist M, Johansson U, Lundkvist O, et al. Does pronuclear morphology and/or early cleavage rate predict embryo implantation potential? Reprod Biomed Online 2001; 2: 12–16

65. Lundin K, Bergh C, Hardarson T. Early embryo cleavage is strong indicator of embryo quality in human IVF. Hum Reprod 2001; 16: 2652–7

66. Sakkas D, Shoukir Y, Chardonnens PG, et al. Early cleavage of human embryos to the two-cell stage after ICSI as an indicator of embryo viability. Hum Reprod 1998; 13: 182–7

67. Sakkas D, Percival GB, D'Arcy Y, et al. Assessment of early cleaving in vitro fertilized human embryos to the 2-cell stage prior to transfer improves embryo selection. Fertil Steril 2001; 76: S89

68. Munne S, Weier HU, Grifo J, Cohen J. Chromosome mosaicism in human embryos. Biol Reprod 1994; 51: 373–9

69. Jackson KV, Ginsburg ES, Hornstein MD, et al. Multinucleation in normally fertilized embryos is associated with an accelerated ovulation induction response and lower implantation and pregnancy rates in in vitro fertilization embryo transfer cycles. Fertil Steril 1998; 70: 60–6

70. Kligman I, Benadiva C, Alikani M, Munné S. The presence of multinucleated blastomeres in human embryos is correlated with chromosomal abnormalities. Hum Reprod 1996; 11: 1492–8

71. Hardarson T, Hanson C, Sjögren A, Lundin K. Human embryos with unevenly sized blastomeres have lower pregnancy and implantation rates: indications for aneuploidy and multinucleation. Hum Reprod 2001; 16: 313–18

72. Giorgetti C, Terriou P, Auquier P, et al. Embryo score to predict implantation after in-vitro fertilization: based on 957 single embryo transfers. Hum Reprod 1995; 10: 2427–31

73. Van Royen E, Mangelschots K, De Neubourg D, et al. Characterization of a top quality embryo, a step towards single-embryo transfer. Hum Reprod 1999; 14: 2345–9

74. Alikani M, Calderon G, Tomkin G, et al. Cleavage anomalies in early human embryos and survival after prolonged culture in-vitro Hum Reprod 2000; 12: 2634–43

75. Delhanty JDA, Harper JC, Ao A, et al. Multicolour FISH detects frequent chromosomal mosaicism and chaotic division in normal preimplantation embryos from fertile patients. Hum Genet 1997; 99: 755–60

76. Gerris J, Van Royen E, De Neubourg D, et al. Impact of single embryo transfer on the overall and twin-pregnancy rates of an IVF/ICSI programme. Reprod Biomed Online 2001; 2: 172–7

77. Vilska S, Tiitinen A, Hyden-Granskog C, Hovatta O. Elective transfer of one embryo results in an acceptable pregnancy rate and eliminates the risk of multiple birth. Hum Reprod 1999; 14: 2392–5

78. Gerris J, De Neubourg D, Mangelschots K, et al. Prevention of twin pregnancy after in-vitro fertilization or intracytoplasmic sperm injection based on strict embryo criteria: a prospective randomized clinical trial. Hum Reprod 1999; 14: 2581–7

79. Gerris J, Van Royen E. Avoiding multiple pregnancies in ART. A plea for single embryo transfer. Hum Reprod 2000; 15: 1884–8

16

Laboratory techniques: sperm preparation for assisted conception

Leila M. Mitchell

INTRODUCTION

Prior to starting a treatment cycle, the semen sample will have been assessed and recommendations from the laboratory will have been taken into account. On the day of treatment the semen sample will be assessed and prepared accordingly. The choice of sperm preparation method will vary depending upon sperm density, motile count, percentage of immotile sperm, volume, presence of antisperm antibodies (ASABs), agglutination, white blood cells, viscosity and debris. All semen samples, even if normozoospermic, contain immotile (approximately 50%) and morphologically abnormal (approximately 70%) sperm that are unlikely to be involved in fertilization[1–4]. The purpose of preparing semen prior to insemination is to concentrate the motile, normal sperm and remove the seminal plasma. It has been shown that seminal plasma contains factors that inhibit capacitation and fertilization[5–8]. If capacitation is inhibited, then hyperactivation and the acrosome reaction will not occur, preventing zona binding and fertilization. Sperm used to be prepared by a simple wash and spin technique, but this concentrates immotile sperm as well as cells and debris in the insemination medium. The presence of large numbers of cells and debris has resulted in the reduction of fertilization[9]. It has been demonstrated that white blood cells and dead sperm in semen are a source of reactive oxygen species (ROS), which can initiate lipid peroxidation in the fatty acids present in the sperm membrane, and this can lead to inhibition of sperm fusion at fertilization[10]. However, for suboptimal samples to be prepared for intracytoplasmic sperm injection (ICSI), the high-speed centrifugation technique is still a valid preparation method, as sperm fusion events are bypassed and fertilization rates with ICSI are unaffected[11]. It has been shown that semen processed within 30 min after collection results in a higher pregnancy rate than that processed up to 60 min after collection[12].

COLLECTION OF SEMEN SAMPLES

The preparation of semen samples in the laboratory should be performed in a class II hood and with aseptic technique to reduce the risk of contamination during the culture of oocytes and embryos. At Bourn Hall, semen samples used to be collected as split ejaculates, as the majority of sperm are present in the first part of the ejaculate[13,14]. However, it was often found that the two pots contained similar sperm densities and motility, and therefore this collection technique was no longer deemed useful. Patients now produce into one pot, which makes it much easier for the patient, with less spillage reported.

Prior knowledge that a semen sample is positive for ASABs enables appropriate steps to be taken when the sample is produced and prepared, which may decrease the binding of antibody and therefore improve fertilization. If ASABs are detected at the assessment, then the semen sample is collected directly into 1 ml of 5% human serum albumin (HSA; Blood Products Laboratory, UK) and 1 ml of Universal *in vitro* fertilization (IVF) medium (Medicult, Denmark). The World Health Organization (WHO) quote levels of > 50% bound motile sperm as a significant result, but at Bourn Hall both medium and serum are added if any sperm binding is observed. The presence of albumin decreases the amount of sperm-associated antisperm antibody by binding to, and therefore decreasing, the amount of free antibody. It has been shown that the addition of serum to sample collection pots significantly improves fertilization rates, and is followed by a greater chance of conception for couples where the male partner has antisperm antibodies[8]. Agglutination occurs approximately 10–15 min after ejaculation, so the immediate processing of these samples on a density gradient helps to minimize antibody binding to sperm. If a sample is viscous at assessment, then collection of the sample into 2 ml of Universal IVF medium can help to reduce the viscosity.

With the recent introduction of witnessing in the United Kingdom by the Human Fertilisation and Embryology Authority (HFEA), a second embryologist or nurse (an independent witness) must observe any movement of gametes from one container to another, which means that during semen preparation a sample can be moved and witnessed up to four times. The Bourn Hall sperm preparation protocols can be found in full on the CD-ROM that accompanies this book.

MEDIUM FOR SPERM PREPARATION

At Bourn Hall, Universal IVF medium is used for sperm preparation, and this is also used at insemination. This medium is bicarbonate buffered, and must therefore be at the correct pH before it is used. The medium is gassed with 6% CO_2 before use, kept in sealed tubes and gassed between manipulations, when necessary.

SPERM PREPARATION METHODS

Direct swim-up

The direct swim-up technique is often used for normal samples. The neat semen sample is pipetted underneath fresh culture medium in a test-tube and allowed to stand at room temperature for an hour if the sample has good motility, and up to 4 h if the sample has poorer motility. Alternatively, 2 ml of medium can be layered over the semen sample in its pot, providing a larger surface area[15], which can also be achieved by using multiple tubes[16]. The motile sperm will swim into the clean medium, leaving the dead sperm and other cellular debris behind, resulting in a clean, motile sample. There will be an increase in the percentage of abnormal sperm the longer the sample is left to swim up. The top cloudy layer is carefully aspirated and placed into a clean test-tube, which can then be centrifuged at 200*g* for 5 min. The supernatant is removed and the pellet resuspended in fresh medium. The sample can then be assessed for count and motility. The swim-up technique is less successful for samples with low density, poor progression and increased viscosity and for those with significant levels of ASABs. Another variation of the swim-up technique involves centrifugation of the whole sample (for samples low in density and motility) in fresh culture medium with a layer of culture medium pipetted over the resulting pellet to allow the motile sperm to swim up. This technique has been recommended, as no extra chemicals are used, other than the culture medium, for the semen preparation[17].

Discontinuous buoyant density gradient

Density gradients are effective for most samples, but are particularly useful for viscous samples and samples positive for ASABs, and also help to remove debris and white blood cells. Percoll™ (Pharmacia, Belgium), a colloid of polyvinylpyrrolidone (PVP)-coated silica particles, was first used to prepare human sperm in 1984[18] in a continuous gradient at high-speed centrifugation. It was later found that using layers of different densities – known as a discontinuous buoyant density gradient – led to an increase in the number of functional sperm retrieved, and protected the sperm from the trauma of centrifugation[19]. Percoll was widely used in human semen preparation until its withdrawal for use in human IVF by the manufacturers in 1996. Many alternatives are now commercially available, which are based on silica particles or highly purified arabinogalactan. Reports have shown that there are no significant differences between the new kits and Percoll[20–22], although others report that using Percoll increases sperm concentrations, motility and morphology[23]. Sil-Select® (Fertipro, Belgium) is used at Bourn Hall, and has two gradients (40% and 80%) of silane-coated colloidal silica particles suspended in N-2-hydroxyethylpiperazine-N'-2-ethane-sulfonic acid (HEPES)-buffered Earle's balanced salt solution (EBSS). Sil-Select can be used for samples with greater than 2×10^6 motile sperm/ml, specimens with known ASABs and those with low progression. Care must be taken not to overload the sample on the density gradient as immotile sperm and debris can then pass through. A density gradient is performed for most normozoospermic samples at Bourn Hall Clinic (Figure 1). It has been shown that density gradients significantly decrease the percentage of abnormal sperm in the preparation compared with the ejaculate[24] and with swim-up preparations[25], although other results do not show this[17].

The lower layer (more dense gradient, often 80%) is placed into the bottom (1–2 ml) of a sterile conical tube with 1–2 ml of the upper layer (less dense gradient, often 40%) carefully layered over the top (Figure 1). The semen sample (1–2 ml) is layered over the density gradient and centrifuged according to the manufacturer's instructions (for Sil-Select, around 400g). The resulting pellet contains mostly motile sperm, as they are the densest particles, with the seminal plasma remaining at the top and the debris and immotile sperm stopped at the interface between the two gradients (Figure 1). Round cells and abnormal forms with amorphous heads and cytoplasmic droplets never reach the pellet because of their low density. The resulting pellet is carefully removed and resuspended in 1–2 ml of clean medium, then assessed using a Makler chamber. If the sample is clean and sufficiently motile (for an IVF sample > 80% motile), it is centrifuged for 5 min at 200g. The supernatant is removed and the pellet resuspended in fresh medium, and the final stock assessed. If there is a high percentage of immotile sperm present (< 80%), the sample should be centrifuged at 200g for 5 min as above, the supernatant removed, the pellet gently loosened and fresh medium layered over the pellet. This can be left for up to an

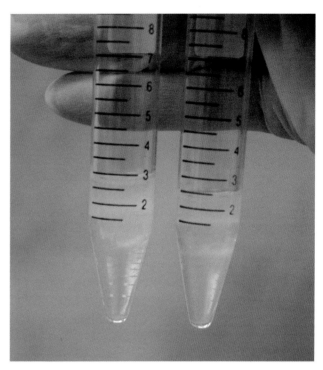

Figure 1 Discontinuous buoyant density gradients after semen samples have been centrifuged at 400g for 10 min

hour, after which the motile sperm can be taken off, care being taken not to dislodge the immotile sperm at the bottom of the tube.

Mini-density gradients have three layers (normally 0.3 ml of 50%, 70% and 95%), and are useful for oligozoospermic samples. They can improve filtration, because there is an increased loss of sperm the larger is the volume of the gradient. The procedure for the mini-gradient is exactly the same as for the two-step gradient above. It has been demonstrated that the mini-gradient recovers significantly more motile[26] and normal[27,28] sperm from the same semen sample, compared with the swim-up technique. It has also been demonstrated that fertilization[26] and pregnancy[27] rates were increased after sperm had been prepared using the mini-gradient, in comparison with swim-up prepared sperm. However, another group found the opposite, with gradients producing sperm with lower motility and normal forms, but the fertilization rates and embryo quality were similar[29].

It has been suggested that, in order to reduce semen-derived contamination in the culture system samples, they should be prepared by discontinuous buoyant density gradient. However, there are conflicting reports on this, with some clinics suggesting that gradients are not effective at separating out bacteria, and others finding that gradients prevent contamination of the final sperm stock[30–33].

High-speed centrifugation and washing

This method can be used for cryptozoospermic samples and those with very low density and motility counts, i.e. $< 0.1 \times 10^6$. The whole sample can be centrifuged or washed in fresh medium and then spun. The sample is centrifuged at $1800g$ for 5 min, the supernatant removed, the pellet washed with 1 ml of fresh medium and then spun at $200g$ for 5 min. The pellet should then be resuspended in a very small volume (50–200 µl). This technique is only ever used for ICSI samples at Bourn Hall, as these samples often have low counts that would be unsuccessful on a discontinuous buoyant density gradient. Obviously, any immotile and abnormal sperm as well as white blood cells and debris will also be concentrated, which can make ICSI more difficult.

Pellet and swim-up

This technique is similar to the high-speed centrifugation and wash technique and can be used when samples have been collected into medium and/or serum. It can also be used for viscous samples, but only after the viscosity has been decreased by pulling the sample through a needle and syringe twice. If the sample has not been collected into medium, then the sample should be mixed with an equal volume of fresh culture medium and centrifuged at $200g$. The supernatant is removed and 0.5–0.75 ml of fresh culture medium carefully layered over the pellet. This can be left at room temperature for the sperm to swim up into the clean medium for an hour or more. If the sample has lower motility, then leaning the tube on its side may improve the recovery of motile sperm by increasing the surface area of the pellet/medium interface. Once the fresh medium above the pellet has turned cloudy, indicating that the sperm have swum up, this layer can be carefully removed and placed into a clean centrifuge tube. The sample can be centrifuged again but this is often not necessary. This technique should probably be avoided for IVF cases as it is exposing motile sperm to peroxidative damage from concentrating dead sperm and white blood cells in the

pellet. It has also been shown that unselected sperm produce ROS in response to centrifugation[19,34,35]. It should not be used for samples with poor motility or with high amounts of debris or cellular contamination.

Layer under paraffin and sedimentation

This method can be useful for samples with low counts or poor motility and is quite effective at removing debris, but does require hours of preparation. This is similar to the high-speed centrifugation and wash technique (see above), with the pellet resuspended in a reduced volume of medium (approximately 200 µl). This final suspension is placed under mineral oil in a small culture dish and left in a desiccator (gassed with 6% CO_2) at room temperature for 3–24 h, but can be placed at 37°C if the sperm progression is poor. The upper part of the droplet, into which the motile sperm should have swum, is carefully removed using a sterile pipette, leaving behind the debris at the bottom of the drop. Aspiration is more accurate if a fine pipette is pulled and observed under a microscope to ensure as little debris as possible is also removed. The disadvantage of this technique is that it does not select for normal sperm, and it also concentrates the whole sample, including white blood cells and debris, therefore increasing the risk of ROS production and the possibility of lipid peroxidation. It is rarely necessary to perform this technique as it is possible to pick individual motile sperm during ICSI, even if there is a high amount of debris present.

Insemination concentration for standard IVF

Oocytes at Bourn Hall are routinely inseminated with a concentration of 100 000 normal motile sperm per ml. Approximately 200–250 µl of this dilution will be used to make a drop for each oocyte, giving a concentration of 20 000–25 000 motile sperm per oocyte. Other centers use from 20 000 to 500 000 sperm per oocyte for insemination[36,37]. Some suggest that increasing the insemination concentration can increase the fertilization rate[36]. Others have shown that varying the sperm concentration from 250 000 to 500 000 progressively motile sperm per oocyte made no significant difference to fertilization rates[38]. There is also the problem that increasing the sperm concentration may affect the incidence of polyspermy. Some researchers have shown that the incidence of polyspermia increases from 6% ($0.5–0.8\times10^6$ motile sperm per oocyte) to 20% (1.0×10^6 sperm per oocyte) and increases to 32% when using 1.5×10^6 sperm per oocyte[36]. Others have observed an increase in polyploidy when the sperm motility was greater than 70% and the percentage of normal morphology was more than 50%[39].

PESA/TESE samples

Percutaneous epididymal sperm aspiration (PESA) is performed at Bourn Hall for patients with irreversible obstructive azoospermia (i.e. multiple blockages, congenital bilateral absence of the vas deferens (CBAVD) or failed vasectomy reversal). A small drop of the retrieved fluid is examined on a slide under the microscope for the presence of motile/immotile sperm. Some PESAs are performed on the day of oocyte collection, known as 'hot' cases, and any excess sperm may be frozen for future use. The sample is washed then spun in fresh medium, and can be left at room temperature, if motile sperm are present. Some cases are 'cold', where the PESA is performed weeks before oocyte collection and all the sperm frozen for future use. A small amount of the frozen sample will be thawed in order to assess sperm survival following the freeze–thaw process. During treatment the thawed sample is analyzed on a microscope slide, washed in fresh medium and spun to remove the cryoprotectant and to concentrate the sperm. The pellet is resuspended in a small volume (approximately 0.2 ml). If the sperm are non-motile then the sample can be placed in the incubator at 37°C to encourage motility until ICSI is to be performed.

The primary consideration when processing epididymal sperm is to ensure that sperm loss is minimized at every preparation step so that repeat surgery is avoided. Epididymal sperm often contain high numbers of red blood cells. These can be reduced by thorough washing, as some blood cells will lyse when placed in fresh medium. Very occasionally, samples will have normal semen parameters of 20 million per ml and 50% motile, and can be placed on a density gradient, which removes the red blood cells.

Microsurgical epididymal sperm aspiration (MESA) is another procedure occasionally performed at Bourn Hall to obtain epididymal sperm. Sperm are removed from the epididymis by needle aspiration.

However, if no sperm are seen after MESA, then testicular sperm aspiration (TESA) or testicular sperm extraction (TESE) will be performed.

Testicular sperm extraction (TESE) and testicular sperm aspiration (TESA) can be performed if PESA has been unsuccessful, or was not appropriate, i.e. non-obstructive azoospermia. A needle is inserted and reinserted into the testicular parenchyma ten or more times before withdrawal. TESA is often unsuccessful as only very small amounts of testicular tissue are removed, and the focal areas where spermatogenesis occurs may not have been aspirated. If no sperm are found then TESE can be performed, where a larger testicular biopsy is taken through the scrotal skin. The testicular biopsy should be at least $5\,\text{mm}^3$ to facilitate sperm isolation, as spermatogenesis is located at foci within the testicle. The biopsy is placed into a sterile glass tissue homogenizer (also known as a macerator, Figure 2) with a small amount of culture medium (~0.3 ml), and thoroughly macerated to release the sperm. A drop of this tissue is placed onto a slide and viewed under the microscope for the presence of sperm. If only immotile sperm are present, the sample is placed in an incubator at 37°C and checked every hour to see if any sperm have become motile. Multiple biopsies from one or both testicles may be needed, and the search for sperm can take several hours. Any excess samples remaining after treatment can be frozen for future ICSI treatment.

Sperm retrieved from the testicles are immature, as epididymal maturation has not occurred. Therefore, they are unable to penetrate the oocyte, as the final maturation, fertilizing ability and motility are obtained in the duct system after release from the testes. It should be expected that sperm from testicular biopsies will have poor or no motility. If the post-thaw test of a testicular sample has taken several hours for motile sperm to be detected, this sample will require thawing the day before oocyte collection. This thawed sample is left in the incubator at 37°C overnight for sperm to become motile. If a sample has taken only an hour or two at 37°C for the sperm to become motile, then it will require thawing only on the day of oocyte retrieval. It has been suggested that incubation at 32°C rather than 37°C may also benefit TESA samples[40]. Testicular sperm samples are full of tissue and cellular debris, making the sperm difficult to retrieve. This often necessitates sperm harvesting using the ICSI equipment, where several motile sperm are transferred

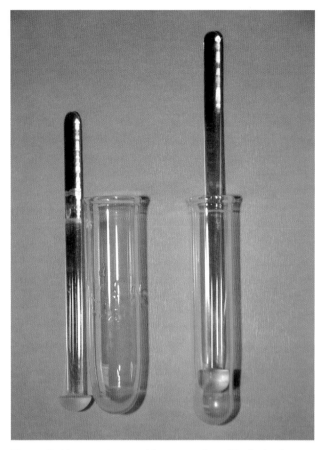

Figure 2 Homogenizer used for maceration of testicular tissue

into a drop before the oocytes are placed into the dish and ICSI performed.

Retrograde and electroejaculation

When the bladder neck fails to close during emission, ejaculation may occur in a retrograde manner and semen enters the bladder. Patients who experience retrograde ejaculation are given specific instructions on collection. On the morning of oocyte recovery, they are instructed to drink two teaspoons of bicarbonate of soda dissolved in 500 ml of water, 2–3 h before producing their samples, as this will increase the pH of the urine. Just before they produce, they are asked to urinate. For the sample collection they are given two containers (one semen pot and one 500-ml flask for urine) and told to ejaculate into the first pot and then to urinate into the flask immediately after ejaculation.

The urine sample must be processed straight away, as urine, even after administration of bicarbonate, may be acidic, and will kill sperm almost instantaneously.

Once the sample reaches the laboratory, the volume and pH of the urine should be measured and noted on the semen analysis sheet. The urine specimen must be mixed thoroughly, as any dead sperm present will sink to the bottom of the container. All the sperm present, even if immotile, need to be counted, so a drop of the urine sample should be viewed on a slide, and if enough sperm are present, a drop is analyzed on a Makler chamber. The urine sample should be centrifuged at 1500g for 10 min, with the pellets resuspended together in fresh culture medium. While the samples are being centrifuged, the antegrade sample (if there is one) should also be analyzed. The pellets obtained from the urine should be assessed on a slide or a Makler chamber, with the density, motility and morphology noted on the assessment sheet. Some retrograde samples analyzed at Bourn Hall are for diagnostic purposes, but if motile sperm are present the sample can be frozen for future treatment. Retrograde samples often contain a high percentage of immotile sperm, and therefore ICSI is often required.

Rectal electroejaculated samples, usually from spinal cord-injured men, will invariably contain a high percentage of immotile sperm cells and debris, due to the patient's inability to ejaculate regularly and, frequently, a very long period between ejaculations. These samples are usually just washed in fresh medium and spun. The pellet can be left to swim up if there are progressively motile sperm present. The majority of electroejaculation cases are performed before treatment and the samples frozen, which means that an even higher percentage of immotile sperm will be present, and therefore ICSI is usually performed using these samples. Because many of these patients have permanent catheters *in situ*, or perform regular self-catheterization, they are prone to urinary tract infections and the samples may therefore contain bacteria. It is useful for patients to produce a urine sample well before electroejaculation so as to determine whether infection is present, and, if so, prophylactic broad-spectrum antibiotics can be prescribed.

Use of chemicals to enhance sperm motility

Pentoxifylline (PTX) is a chemical that is known to increase spermatozoal intracellular levels of cyclic 3′5′-adenosine monophosphate (cAMP) *in vitro*, which plays a role in sperm motility[41]. It is thought that PTX enhances sperm motility in samples with poor progression by increasing intracellular adenosine triphosphate (ATP)[42]. Some clinics have found that PTX increases motility[43] and fertilization rate[44,45], whereas others have observed no differences in sperm parameters and fertilization rates after treatment with PTX and 2-deoxyadenosine[43,46–48]. The typical protocol for use of PTX involves a 30-min preincubation of prepared sperm with the stimulant (PTX at 1–5 mmol/l). The sperm is then washed to remove the stimulant and used immediately for insemination. It has been found that adding PTX and 2-deoxyadenosine to thawed testicular sperm increases the number of progressively motile sperm, when compared with culture *in vitro* alone, with normal babies being born as a result of treatment with stimulants[49,50].

Frozen sperm samples

Cryopreserved semen has been used successfully for intrauterine insemination (IUI) and IVF for many years. The cryoprotectant must be thoroughly removed from the semen sample before it is used. If the sample has more than 2 million motile sperm per ml, this can be performed by placing the sample on a discontinuous buoyant density gradient or by the wash and spin technique, with a swim-up if progressively motile sperm are present. ICSI should be performed if the sample has a low survival rate.

CONCLUSION

Individual laboratories should develop their own protocols in terms of how to process normozoopermic samples, as well as those with low density and/or motility, in order to obtain the most motile stocks with the best fertilizing ability. It is important to tailor the preparation method according to each sample produced on the day of treatment. A trial preparation can be performed prior to oocyte retrieval in order to ascertain how well a sample will perform. However, this can have limited use, as the sample produced on the day of treatment may vary greatly in quality from previous specimens. With the advent of ICSI, less rigorous techniques are required to obtain clean, motile sperm, as even samples with very low density and motility counts can produce good-quality embryos that can implant and result in the delivery of healthy babies.

REFERENCES

1. Fredricsson B, Bjork G. Morphology of postcoital spermatozoa in the cervical secretion and its clinical significance. Fertil Steril 1977; 28: 841–5
2. Mortimer D, Leslie EE, Kelly RW, et al. Morphological selection of human spermatozoa in vivo and in vitro. J Reprod Fertil 1982; 64: 391–9
3. Menkveld R, Stander FS, Kotze TJ, et al. The evaluation of morphological characteristics of human spermatozoa according to stricter criteria. Hum Reprod 1990; 5: 586–92
4. Liu DY, Baker HW. Morphology of spermatozoa bound to the zona pellucida of human oocytes that failed to fertilize in vitro. J Reprod Fertil 1992; 94: 71–84
5. Chang MC. A detrimental effect of seminal plasma in the fertilising capacity of sperm. Nature (London) 1957; 179: 258–9
6. Bedford JM, Chang MC. Removal of decapacitation factor from seminal plasma by high speed centrifugation. Am J Physiol 1962; 202: 179–81
7. Van der Ven H, Bhattacharya AK, Binor Z, et al. Inhibition of human sperm capacitation by a high molecular weight from human seminal plasma. Fertil Steril 1982; 38: 753–5
8. Elder KT, Wick KL, Edwards RG. Seminal plasma anti-sperm antibodies and IVF: the effect of semen sample collection into 50% serum. Hum Reprod 1990; 5: 179–84
9. Edwards RG, Fishel SG, Cohen J, et al. Factors influencing the success of in vitro fertilisation for alleviating human infertility. J In Vitro Fertil Embryo Transf 1984; 1: 3–23
10. Aitken RJ, Comhaire FH, Eliasson R, et al. WHO Manual for the Examination of Human Semen and Semen–Cervical Mucus Interaction, 2nd edn. Cambridge: Cambridge University Press, 1987
11. Elder K, Dale B, eds. Semen analysis and preparation for assisted reproductive techniques. In In Vitro Fertilisation, 2nd edn. Cambridge: Cambridge University Press, 2000: 130–51
12. Yavas Y, Selub MR. Intrauterine insemination (IUI) pregnancy outcome is enhanced by shorter intervals from semen collection to sperm wash, from sperm wash to IUI time, and from semen collection to IUI time. Fertil Steril 2004; 82: 1638–47
13. Cohen J, Fari A, Finegold WJ, et al. The split ejaculate. In Emperaire JC, Audebert A, Hafez ESE, eds. Clinics in Andrology, I. The Hague: Martinus Nijhoff Publishers, 1980: 112
14. Weeda AJ, Cohen J. Effects of purification or split ejaculation of semen and stimulation of spermatozoa

by caffeine on the motility and fertilizing ability with the use of zona-free hamster ova. Fertil Steril 1982; 37: 817–22

15. Cohen J, Edwards RG, Fehilly C, et al. In vitro fertilisation: a treatment for male infertility. Fertil Steril 1985; 43: 422–32

16. Mahadevan MM, Leeton JF, Tounson AO. Successful use of in vitro fertilisation for patients with persisting low quality semen. Ann NY Acad Sci 1985; 442: 293–300.

17. Soderland B, Lundin K. The use of silane-coated silica particles for density gradient centrifugation in in-vitro fertilisation. Hum Reprod 2000; 15: 857–60

18. Braude PR, Bolton VN. The preparation of spermatozoa for in vitro fertilisation by buoyant density centrifugation. In Feichtinger W, Kemeter P, eds. Recent Progress in Human In Vitro Fertilisation. Palermo Cofese: 1984; 125–34

19. Aitken RJ. Assessment of sperm function for IVF. Hum Reprod 1988; 3: 89–95

20. Centola GM, Herko R, Andolina E, et al. Comparison of sperm separation methods: effect on recovery, motility, motion parameters, and hyperactivation. Fertil Steril 1998; 70: 1173–5

21. Claassens OE, Menkveld R, Harrison KL. Evaluation of three substitutes for Percoll in sperm isolation by density gradient centrifugation. Hum Reprod 1998; 13: 3139–43

22. Mousset-Simeon N, Rives N, Masse L, et al. Comparison of six density gradient media for selection of cryopreserved donor spermatozoa. J Androl 2004; 25: 881–4

23. Chen MJ, Bongso A. Comparative evaluation of two density gradient preparations for sperm separation for medically assisted conception. Hum Reprod 1999; 14: 759–4

24. Tomlinson MJ, Moffatt O, Manicardi GC, et al. Interrelationships between seminal parameters and sperm nuclear DNA damage before and after density gradient centrifugation: implications for assisted conception. Hum Reprod 2001; 16: 2160–5

25. Hammadeh ME, Kuhnen A, Amer AS, et al. Comparison of sperm preparation methods: effect on chromatin and morphology recovery rates and their consequences on the clinical outcome after in vitro fertilisation embryo transfer. Int J Androl 2001; 24: 360–8

26. Sakkas D, Gianaroli L, Diotallevi L, et al. IVF treatment of moderate male factor infertility: a comparison of mini-percoll, partial zona dissection and sub-zonal sperm insertion techniques. Hum Reprod 1993; 8: 587–91

27. Van der Zwalmen P, Bertin-Segal G, Geerts L, et al. Sperm morphology and IVF pregnancy rate: comparison between Percoll gradient centrifugation and swim-up procedures. Hum Reprod 1991; 6: 581–8

28. Smith S, Hosid S, Scott L. Use of postpreparation sperm parameters to determine the method of choice for sperm preparation for assisted reproductive technology. Fertil Steril 1995; 63: 591–7

29. Englert Y, Van den Bergh M, Rodesch C, et al. Comparative auto-controlled study between swim-up and percoll preparation of fresh semen samples for in-vitro fertilisation. Hum Reprod 1992; 7: 399–402

30. Bolton VN, Warren RE, Braude PR. Removal of bacterial contaminants from semen for in vitro fertilization or artificial insemination by the use of buoyant density centrifugation. Fertil Steril 1986; 46: 1128–32

31. Sun LS, Gastaldi C, Peterson EM, et al. Comparisons of techniques for the selection of bacteria-free sperm preparations. Fertil Steril 1987; 48: 659–63

32. Elder K, Elliott T, eds. Problem Solving and Troubleshooting in IVF. Morley, Australia: Ladybrook Publishing, 1998

33. Nicholson CM, Abramsson L, Holm SE, et al. Bacterial contamination and sperm recovery after semen preparation by density gradient centrifugation using silane-coated silica particles at different g-forces. Hum Reprod 2000; 15: 662–6

34. Aitken RJ, Clarkson JS. Cellular basis of defective sperm function and its association with the genesis of reactive oxygen species by human spermatozoa. J Reprod Fertil 1987; 81: 459–69

35. Aitken RJ. Evaluation of human sperm function. Br Med Bull 1990; 46: 654–74

36. Van der Ven HH, Al-Hasani S, Diedrich K, et al. Polyspermy in in vitro fertilisation of human oocytes: frequency and possible causes. Ann NY Acad Sci 1985; 442: 88–95

37. Akerlof E, Fredricsson B, Gustafson O, et al. Sperm count and motility influence the results of human fertilisation in vitro. Int J Androl 1991; 14: 79–86

38. Diamond MP, Rogers BJ, Vaughn WK, et al. Effect of the number of inseminating sperm and the follicular stimulation protocol on in vitro fertilization of human oocytes in male factor and non-male factor couples. Fertil Steril 1985; 85: 499–503

39. Ho PC, Yeung WS, Chan YF, et al. Factors affecting the incidence of polyploidy in a human in vitro fertilisation program. Int J Fertil Menopausal Stud 1994; 39: 14–19.

40. Van den Berg M. In Elder K, Elliott T. eds. The Use of Epidemiological and Testicular Sperm in IVF. World Wide Conferences on Reproductive Biology. Morley, Australia: Ladybrook Publishing, 1998

41. Tash JS, Means AR. Cyclic adenosine 3′,5′ monophosphate, calcium and protein phosphorylation in flagellar motility. Biol Reprod 1983; 28: 75–104

42. Garbers DL, Lust WD, First NL, et al. Effect of phosphodiesterase inhibitors and cyclic nucleotides on sperm respiration and motility. Biochemistry 1971; 10: 1825–31

43. Dimitriadou F, Voutsina K, Rizos D, et al. The effect of pentoxifylline on sperm motility, oocyte fertilization, embryo quality, and pregnancy outcome in an in vitro fertilization program. Fertil Steril 1995; 63: 880–6

44. Yovich JM, Edirisinghe WR, Cummins JM, et al. Influence of pentoxifylline in severe male factor infertility. Fertil Steril 1990; 53: 715–22

45. Tarlatzis BC, Kolibianakis EM, Bontis J, et al. Effect of pentoxifylline on human sperm motility and fertilizing capacity. Arch Androl 1995; 34: 33–42

46. Tournaye H, Devroey P, Janssesns R, et al. In vitro fertilization in couples with previous fertilization failure using sperm incubated with pentoxifylline and 2-deoxyadenosine. Fertil Steril 1994; 62: 574–9

47. Tournaye H, Janssens R, Verheyen G, et al. An indiscriminate use of pentoxifylline does not improve invitro fertilization in poor fertilizers. Hum Reprod 1994; 9: 1289–92

48. Fountain S, Rizk B, Avery S, et al. An evaluation of the effect of pentoxifylline on sperm function and treatment outcome of male-factor infertility: a preliminary study. J Assist Reprod Genet 1995; 12: 704–9

49. Thomas TS, Howards SS, Bateman BG. Live births after ICSI with cryopreserved testicular sperm subjected to motility enhancement. Fertil Steril 2001; 96(Suppl 1): 59

50. Gonzalez-Utor A, Mendoza M, Casclaes O, et al. Pentoxifylline: an effective tool for ICSI with testicular sperm. Hum Reprod 2003; 18 (Suppl 1) 152–3 (abstr P–451)

17

Cryopreservation of embryos and spermatozoa

Martyn Blayney

EMBRYO CRYOPRESERVATION

Introduction

Since the first attempts to cryopreserve human embryos in the early 1980s[1-5], techniques have been modified, with a dramatic improvement in results. For example, using basically the same method as originally described by Lassalle and colleagues[4], post-thaw survival rates have risen from 19% of cleaved embryos to 87%[6], and more recently to as high as 92%[7] of zygotes, with corresponding pregnancy rates comparable to those using fresh *in vitro* fertilization (IVF).

This success has become well established. Embryo freezing now forms an integral part of routine IVF programs worldwide, with as many as 76% of IVF cycles yielding surplus embryos for cryopreservation (Bourn Hall data, 2003). This not only reduces wastage of valuable embryos, but also maximizes the number of conception attempts per stimulation cycle/oocyte collection[8], and significantly increases the cumulative pregnancy rate[9] and reduces the health risks, inconvenience and costs. The concept of freezing embryos can also be expanded and applied to the patient at risk of ovarian hyperstimulation syndrome (OHSS), as well as to the ovum recipient whose cycle is asynchronous with her donor, when all available embryos may be frozen. The 'freeze all' concept can be further used when embryos need to be quarantined to allow virology screening to take place before embryos are transferred – to a surrogate host, for example. Unexpected or emergency situations, such as failed embryo transfer, patient illness, endometrial unsuitability or any condition where implantation may be compromised, can also be rescued by freezing. In all of these cases cryopreservation not only avoids wastage of otherwise suitable embryos, but also allows time for further patient investigation and intervention, ensuring the embryos are only thawed and replaced when the uterine environment is at its most receptive.

Furthermore, this technology can be used to preserve the fertility of patients about to undergo sterilizing treatment for malignancy. However, this assumes that the patient has a partner, a non–estrogen sensitive tumor and sufficient time before treatment to allow an IVF cycle in which all embryos are frozen for later use when the patient is in remission.

Successful embryo cryopreservation programs have now been running for approaching 20 years, and in that time many couples have either completed their families or decided not to continue with treatment, whilst still having embryos in store. In such cases some couples have donated their embryos for use by those unable to produce normal or viable embryos themselves. Although the number of donated embryos each year is small, the success achieved from such a program makes it extremely worthwhile.

PRINCIPLES OF CRYOBIOLOGY

Cells are exposed to two major physicochemical stresses during freezing: those resulting directly from the reduced temperature, and the physical changes caused by ice formation. Damage to cell structure and function results from a sudden lowering of temperature; this so-called cold-shock injury is associated with membrane permeability and cytoskeletal structural changes. For a comprehensive guide to the factors that contribute to cellular injury and death in biological systems during cooling, see reference 10.

Physical changes associated with ice formation

During controlled slow freezing programs, such as those typically used for cryopreserving embryos, aqueous solutions have a tendency to cool well below their melting point before ice nucleation occurs spontaneously. After this, ice crystals form and the temperature increases to its melting point (the latent heat of fusion of ice) and plateaus, before dropping back rapidly to the ambient temperature. This phenomenon, known as under- or supercooling, is related to a number of factors, notably: temperature, rate of cooling, volume, purity of solution and particulate; therefore, embryo freezing systems have a strong tendency to supercool. This phenomenon makes it crucial that ice nucleation is initiated in a controlled manner, commonly referred to as 'seeding'. The temperature at which it is performed is important to achieve good rates of cryosurvival[11]. An experiment with mouse embryos published by Whittingham in 1977[12] showed similar survival rates when nucleation was performed between −4 and −6°C, after which survival rates fell to zero at −11°C. Optimum nucleation temperatures vary from system to system. Typically, for human embryos frozen with propanediol and sucrose as cryoprotectants, nucleation is performed at −7°C.

Ice formation effectively removes water from solution, forming a biphasic system where frozen and non-frozen fractions coexist. Removing water increases the concentration of any solutes in the liquid fraction; continued temperature reduction forms more ice and consequently raises the aqueous concentration still further. The net result of this effect causes a typical isotonic embryo culture medium to become lethally hypertonic. This consequence can be moderated by the addition of cryoprotective agents (CPAs), which reduce cellular damage simply by increasing the volume of the unfrozen fraction, thereby reducing the ionic concentration and osmotic stress on the cell.

Cryoprotectants

To reduce the damaging effects of cryopreservation on cells it is essential to equilibrate them in the presence of a suitable CPA. Such compounds need to be completely miscible, with water able to penetrate membranes rapidly and have a low toxicity. They are thought to protect cells by stabilizing intracellular proteins, reducing intracellular ice formation and moderating the impact of extracellular electrolytes[13].

CPAs can be divided into permeating and non-permeating groups, and as they are all hyperosmotic, it is accepted that CPAs themselves cause osmotic stress on the embryo. On initial exposure to 1.5 mol/l 1,2-propanediol (PROH), embryos shrink due to an efflux of water, then swell as the CPA enters, showing that embryos are more permeable to water than PROH. This shrink–swell effect is temperature dependent, and is less pronounced with PROH than with dimethyl sulfoxide (DMSO)[14,15]. These cell-volume excursions in response to CPA exposure can be reduced below ±30%, as recommended by Newton and colleagues[16], by adding PROH stepwise[15].

Effects of freezing on cells

Cells in suspension suffer no direct damage from ice crystal formation, but they do move into the hypertonic unfrozen fraction. Removing sufficient water from the cell is key to its cryosurvival. At slow cooling rates cells can remain in osmotic equilibrium with their surroundings. However, as the cooling rate is increased, there is less time for water to leave the cell, leading to supercooling and, ultimately, intracellular ice formation, which inevitably is lethal. The optimum cooling rate, which is cell-type-specific, derives from a balance of these two phenomena. A suboptimum cooling rate causes cell death by prolonged exposure to a hypertonic environment, whilst at a faster than optimum cooling rate, death is via intracellular ice formation.

The optimum cooling rate is determined by a number of biophysical factors[17]:

(1) Cell volume/surface area ratio;

(2) Permeability to water (Lp for human oocytes 0.44 μm/min/atm);

(3) Arrhenius activation energy (Ea 3.9 kcal/mol for human oocytes);

(4) Type and concentration of cryoprotective additives;

(5) Cooling rate.

Therefore, the optimum cooling rate leads to successful freezing–thawing by balancing the avoidance of intracellular ice formation against excessive exposure to a hypertonic post-ice-formation environment. When coupled with a suitable cryoprotectant this allows sufficient time for osmotic dehydration and a consequent altering of intracellular pH, while minimizing hypertonic exposure.

Cryopreservation techniques

In general terms, for successful cryopreservation, the larger is the cell the more slowly it must be cooled. The human oocyte is the largest cell in the body, with a volume of approximately $9 \times 10^5 \, \mu m^3$ and a surface area of $4.5 \times 10^4 \, \mu m^2$; this requires a lengthy equilibration period and hence an increased CPA exposure time. For this reason, many different cryopreservation techniques have been applied to the human embryo, including equilibrium and non-equilibrium protocols coupled with fast and slow cooling rates. Both penetrating cryoprotectants, such as glycerol, DMSO and PROH, and/or non-penetrating cryoprotectants, such as the sugars sucrose and raffinose, as well as amphipathic compounds, trehalose and praline, have been used. Over the years other cryo-additives have been tried in various combinations and concentrations and for various exposure times.

Non-equilibration freezing: vitrification

There are species of plants, insects and amphibians that survive in subzero environments through a natural form of vitrification. Arctic frogs have a special form of insulin which accelerates glycerol production as temperatures fall; this cryoprotectant enables them to survive with as much as 65% of their body water as ice. The arctic beetle *Peterostichus brevicornis* also utilizes sugars for their cryoprotective properties, enabling it to endure temperatures below −35°C. These beetles have been frozen to −87°C for 5 h before thawing, without any apparent ill-effects.

The attraction of vitrification lies in its simplicity; cells are placed in cryoprotectant and plunged into liquid nitrogen. The sample rapidly passes the glass transition point (−130°C for water), where the solution alters from liquid phase to an amorphous glassy solid or vitrified state. Clearly this process eliminates one of the major classes of cryoinjury, extracellular ice formation.

For successful vitrification it is necessary to balance a rapid cooling rate, typically > 2000°C/min, against the need for a small volume of highly concentrated cryoprotectant. The former may actually reduce damage of the zona pelluida compared with slow freezing methods, but the toxicity from highly concentrated cryoprotectants is the primary obstacle to vitrification. As well as using conventional straws[18,19], the necessity to reduce the volume of cryoprotectant to a minimum has led to some innovative cryostorage vessels: the open pulled straw[20], the cryoloop[21], the flexipet[22], the hemi-straw system[23] and electron microscope grids[24] have all been used successfully.

The long-term storage capabilities of such samples are as yet largely untested, and the glass-like state is not only fragile, but can break down over time, with the potential for cell damage. Of further concern are the safety issues resulting from the necessity for direct contact between samples and liquid nitrogen. A recent incident in a UK blood storage bank has highlighted that viable viral transmission between samples in a storage Dewar is indeed possible. Even if not contaminated with pathogens, liquid nitrogen is not supplied sterile, and therefore the potential for opportunistic infection of such samples must be considered. For a further discussion of these issues see the 'Safety of cryopreservation' section below.

Despite the differing post-thaw survival rates, successful pregnancies and deliveries after thawing of vitrified human embryos have been reported[25–28], and when considered with the convenience of the technique, further development and wider utilization of this method seems likely.

Equilibrium freezing: non-linear

A recent development in the field of cryopreservation comes with the development of a novel freezing machine, the Asymptote EF-100 (Asymptote, Cambridge, UK) (Figure 1). Previous attempts to improve cryosurvival of cells have focused mainly upon alterations to the methodologies and freezing solution composition, and trying to identify the optimal linear cooling rate. However, many of the physical changes that occur in an aqueous cryoprotectant post-ice formation are not linear in nature. Parameters such as pH, ice fraction, viscosity, ionic concentration and gas solubility all vary in a non-linear fashion with temperature[29,30], as do the biophysical characteristics of the cell which govern its response to cooling. Therefore, conventional freezing methods impose linear changes with time, while stresses experienced by the cell are all non-linear. Thus, it is appropriate to try specifically to manipulate the manner in which cells experience these changes, as a way of minimizing the stresses encountered during cryopreservation.

The unique Asymptote EF-100 (Figure 1) has specifically been designed with this in mind, as it is able to produce user-specific non-linear cooling rates and thereby control the physical gradients experienced by cells. Unlike conventional linear freezing machines, the sample holding plate is cooled by a reservoir of liquid nitrogen, and because the plate also houses individual heating elements, it is possible to balance the warming and cooling effects via a high-resolution thermometer, temperature controller and a computer to produce infinitely variable protocols. The cooling plate design also ensures intimate sample/plate contact, allowing excellent heat transfer to the samples, and thereby strict adherence to the programmed temperatures. The hypothesis was first tested by using this machine to cryopreserve human spermatozoa[31]. The conclusion was that cryosurvival rates could indeed be improved significantly by controlling the concentration gradients experienced by the spermatozoa during freezing.

The method giving the highest rates of survival (88% and 100%) was that which controlled the rate of change in extracellular concentration, such that the rate of change of concentration in the liquid phase decreased for more than 90% of the time taken to lower the temperature from −5°C to −45°C. This same approach was extended to denuded murine oocytes,

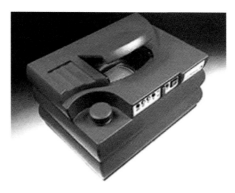

Figure 1 The Asymptote EF-100 freezing machine. Reproduced with permission of Asymptote

which were prepared in standard freezing solutions, loaded into straws and frozen by either linear or non-linear methods. As with spermatozoa, the non-linear group gave superior results to those of the linear group in all test parameters. Whilst this method should still be considered experimental, it shows that altering the fundamentals of how cells are frozen can be as effective in improving cryosurvival rates as adjusting the formulation of cryoprotective media.

Linear slow cooling

The first human pregnancy from a cryopreserved eight-cell embryo was reported in 1983 using dimethyl sulfoxide (DMSO) as a CPA[1], followed by the first birth from a frozen–thawed blastocyst 2 years later using glycerol[2]. Today, the most widespread method of freezing pronucleate and early cleavage stage embryos is a linear slow-cooling protocol in the presence of propanediol and sucrose, as described by Lassalle and colleagues in 1985[4]. Propanediol is a rapid-penetrating CPA, whilst sucrose ensures that water leaves the cell, thus reducing the potential for intracellular ice formation and minimizing the CPA exposure time needed for equilibration.

The first liquid nitrogen controlled-rate freezer (CRF) was produced in the UK by Planer plc in the early 1970s. It was developed following a request from Professor David Pegg, now of York University, UK, when it became apparent that rapid liquid nitrogen immersion methods gave poor results for delicate and valuable samples, such as human embryos. Stepwise cooling was required to allow embryo/cryoprotectant equilibration and user-definable programs which would enable researchers to identify the most effective cooling rates. The controlled-rate freezing process was a breakthrough in the preservation of biological samples, and Planer received the Queen's Award for Technology in 1984. The early freezer utilized the principle of a pulse-width modulated solenoid valve to admit liquid nitrogen into the freezing chamber, and this original Planer design forms the basis of most controlled-rate freezers used in the world today. The earliest freezers used a mechanical cam controller to achieve the freezing profiles, but in the late 1980s the company introduced its first fully digital controller, which has been continuously developed up to the present day. Building on 30 years' experience, the current MRV controller operates via a custom processor module dedicated solely to running the freezer, and is independent of all user-control and display interactions. The unit receives temperature data from high-resolution four-wire platinum resistance thermometer (PRT) sensors. An onboard computer is used solely to enhance the user interface and to archive run data and freezing programs; the system provides a printout of each run and also has a battery back-up in case of power failure (Figures 2 and 3).

Selecting embryos for freezing

At Bourn Hall, we currently freeze embryos at pronucleate, cleavage and blastocyst stages. Historically, our thawing and pregnancy rates from frozen pronucleate embryos have always been slightly better than from those frozen at the cleavage stage; therefore, we preferentially freeze zygotes. This includes patients who have all their embryos frozen. The thawing results from 1999 to 2002 show a 20.3% clinical pregnancy rate per transfer when pronucleate embryos were thawed, compared with 13.5% for cleavage stage embryos. It should be noted that we perform almost twice as many embryo transfers derived solely from thawed pronucleate than cleavage stage embryos.

Currently, four fertilized oocytes will be left to cleave to allow some embryo selection on day 2 at transfer. Any remaining zygotes showing two distinct clear pronuclei will be frozen. On day 2, after selecting

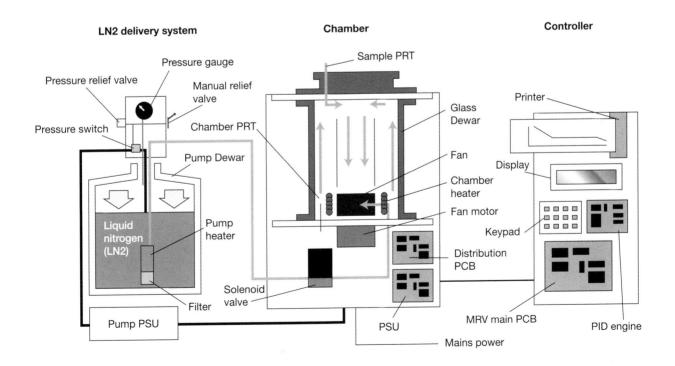

Figure 2 Schematic diagram of the Planer freezing system. PSU, power supply unit; PCB, printed circuit board; PID, proportional integral derivative. Reproduced with permission of Planer UK

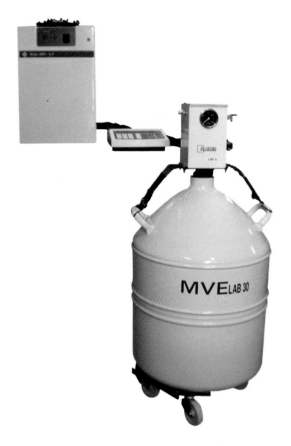

Figure 3 Planer freezing machine. Reproduced with permission of Planer UK

the two best-quality embryos for transfer, any surplus embryos of grade 2 or better (i.e. no more than 10% fragmentation with even, clear blastomeres) are also frozen. If, in the opinion of the embryologist, the zygotes or embryos do not appear to be freezable, they will all be left until embryo transfer to allow the maximum possible selection, and, if necessary, kept and frozen on day 3.

It is important to freeze only quiescent zygotes and embryos to avoid possible mitotic spindle damage and potential chromosomal chaos; for this reason, zygotes without distinct pronuclei and embryos which have divided asynchronously, or that appear to be in the process of cleaving, are not frozen. In the laboratory at Bourn Hall, freezing begins daily at 09.30, since timing may also play a part in embryo selection. We strive not only to have sufficient embryos available for transfer, but to have some frozen at both pronucleate and cleavage stages, thus allowing some flexibility when thawing.

Embryo freezing protocol

The freezing protocol used at Bourn Hall for pronucleate and cleavage embryos is based upon the three step propanediol/sucrose method described by Lassalle and colleagues[4]. The freezing solutions themselves are commercially produced and are available from several media manufacturers; the composition is as follows:

Solution A phosphate buffered saline (PBS) + 20% serum

Solution B PBS + 20% serum + 1.5 mol/l PROH

Solution C PBS + 20% serum + 1.5 mol/l PROH + 0.1 mol/l sucrose

As we believe that temperature control throughout the freezing process is important, the three freezing solutions are warmed to 37°C, then, in an attempt to achieve an equivalent cooling rate to room temperature, both solutions and embryos are removed from the incubator simultaneously.

The pre-selected embryos are next removed from their culture drops under oil and placed into well 1 of a Nunc four-well dish containing solution A. Both dishes are clearly labeled with patient identifiers and a second embryologist witnesses the transfer. If the embryos of several patients are being frozen, the embryos remain in solution A until all initial transfers have been made. The embryos are next transferred, in the same patient order that they were selected, into solution B and then solution C, spending 15 min in each. While the embryos are equilibrating in the freezing solutions, the paperwork will have been completed, storage location identified and the Planer MRV freezing machine prepared. The embryos are next loaded into the storage containers, be this in traditional plastic straws, CBS™ high-security straws or glass ampoules. At Bourn Hall we still favor the use of ampoules, as they are completely heat-sealable against potential contamination, and their large volume is an excellent buffer to temperature fluctuations, as shown in Figure 4.

Embryos are transferred from the Nunc dish into an ampoule containing 0.5 ml of solution C by means of a fine pulled Pasteur pipette and labeled with the patient's full name, number, embryo number and date. The whole procedure is witnessed and signed off by a second embryologist. The ampoules will contain

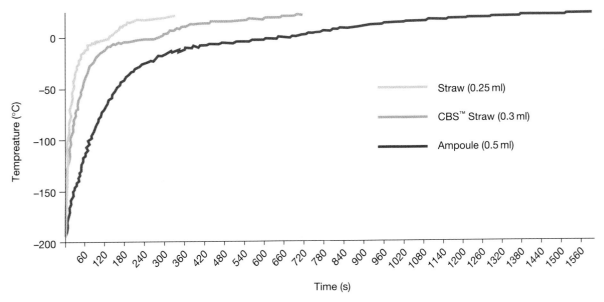

Figure 4 Graph showing warming rates from –196°C to 21°C for various cryovials

either one or two embryos, to allow choice when thawing, as we attempt only to thaw the number of embryos required for transfer. The ampoules are heat-sealed, and are loaded into the freezing machine when it has stabilized at room temperature, and the program started.

The details of the freezing program used at Bourn Hall are summarized in Table 1 and shown schematically in Figure 5.

When the freezing is complete, the ampoules are quickly transferred from the freezing machine into labeled visitubes, which are differently colored for each patient. These are then transferred to their allocated position in a storage Dewar and the dated printout of the run is archived for future reference.

Embryo thawing protocol

Pronucleate and cleavage stage embryos, having been identified for thawing by two embryologists, are removed from liquid nitrogen and rapidly thawed in a water bath at 37°C until the ice has just thawed. The embryos are aspirated into a labeled dish and spend 5 min in each of three dilution steps to remove the propanediol and sucrose, before being rinsed through several drops of culture medium under oil. The composition of the thawing media is as follows:

Table 1 Linear freezing program used in the Planer kryo-10

Cooling rate (°C/min)	To temperature (°C)	Hold period	Action
–1	21 (room temperature)	5 min	load
–2	–7	5 min	sample equilibration
0	–7	as required	seed
0	–7	5 min	sample equilibration
–0.3	–31	–	–
–50	–150	up to 1 h	remove samples to storage location

Solution D PBS + 20% serum + 1.0 mol/l PROH + 0.2 mol/l sucrose

Solution D/E PBS + 20% serum + 0.5 mol/l PROH + 0.2 mol/l sucrose

Solution E PBS + 20% serum + 0.2 mol/l sucrose

These steps are all witnessed. At this stage the embryos are scored for viability. The whole thawing process is performed at room temperature. Pronucleate embryos

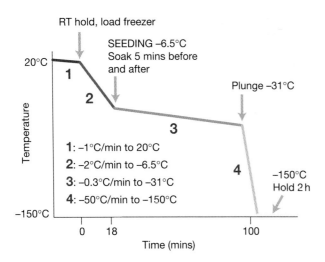

Figure 5 Schematic diagram of a typical freezing program. RT, room temperature

are thawed the day before embryo transfer. They are checked for cell lysis, intact zonae pellucidae and vitelline membranes, clear cytoplasm and the presence of two pronuclei. They are then transferred to an incubator at 37°C in an atmosphere of 6% CO_2. Embryo transfer is performed the following day if cleavage has occurred.

Cleavage stage embryos are thawed on the day of transfer and checked for intact zonae, clear cytoplasm and less than 50% cell lysis/damage. If thawed embryos have > 50% damaged blastomeres, more are thawed if available, otherwise they are cultured overnight and transferred only if further cleavage has occurred. Embryos with < 50% cell damage are cultured for a minimum of 1 h before being reassessed and transferred if they are still viable.

Excess good-quality blastocysts, as judged by the size of the blastocoel and the quality of the inner cell mass and trophectoderm, are also frozen, on either day 5 or day 6. Traditionally, glycerol has been the CPA of choice, but, as this penetrates the cell slowly, in order to speed the equilibration process, freezing is carried out at 37°C rather than at room temperature. The freezing protocol is based upon that described by Menezo and colleagues[32] and uses commercially prepared media. Blastocysts are transferred from culture into medium containing 5% glycerol for 10 min, followed by 10 min in 10% glycerol with 0.2 mol/l sucrose. All other aspects of the freezing process are the same as for zygote and cleavage stages. The procedure

is reversed to thaw blastocysts and is performed at room temperature on day 5. Blastocyst viability is difficult to assess, as they are often highly contracted upon thawing. Checks are made for gross cell lysis and the intactness of the zona pellucida, and are repeated after a minimum of 1 h in culture, at which point some re-expansion of the blastocoel should have occurred; if this is the case, transfer is performed. If no re-expansion has occurred, but the embryos still appear viable after 2 h in culture, embryo transfer will still be performed.

Embryo transfer cycles

To allow careful planning and management of frozen embryo transfers, patient cycles are controlled using pituitary down-regulation and hormone replacement therapy. A typical regimen would be:

(1) Down-regulate with luteinizing hormone-releasing hormone (LHRH) analogs for 14 days;

(2) Baseline ultrasound scan;

(3) If the endometrium is < 5 mm then:

(4) Start 2 mg estradiol valerate and analog for cycle days 1–5;

(5) 4 mg estradiol valerate and analog cycle days 6–9;

(6) 6 mg estradiol valerate and analog cycle days 10–15;

(7) Day-13 ultrasound scan;

(8) If endometrium is > 8 mm, arrange transfer;

(9) If endometrium is 6–8 mm, increase estradiol valerate + aspirin and repeat the scan in 2 days;

(10) Start Cyclogest® 400 mg b.d. 2 days before embryo transfer (ET);

(11) ET on days 15–21 (typically day 17).

Results

Tables 2 and 3 detail Bourn Hall frozen embryo transfer results from 2003. Early cleavage embryos made up 78% of transfers and were performed on day 2/3, and the remainder were blastocyst transfers on day 5/6, the average number of embryos replaced per patient was 1.77.

Table 2 Frozen embryo transfer results at Bourn Hall Clinic for 2003

Patients (*n*)	426
Transfers (*n* (%))	342 (80)
Clinical pregnancies per transfer (*n* (%))	70 (20.4)

Table 3 Frozen embryo transfer results at Bourn Hall Clinic for 2003 by patient age

Age (years)	Number of transfers	Clinical pregnancies per transfer (n (%))
<25	4	1 (25)
25–29	31	3 (9.7)
30–34	127	29 (22.8)
35–39	128	26 (20.3)
40+	52	11 (21.2)

Safety of embryo cryopreservation

It has been shown that embryos and spermatozoa do not deteriorate, even when stored for decades in liquid nitrogen[33,34]. It has been suggested that the only likely cause of damage to stored samples could come from the gradual build-up of background radiation. However, exposure to the equivalent of 2000 years of such radiation failed to induce any obvious mutation in mouse embryos[35].

The clear demonstration of the transmission of hepatitis B between bone marrow samples frozen in liquid nitrogen[36–38] has caused much concern in the field of IVF. Cross-contamination in an IVF storage facility could arise at various stages: in the freezing equipment, from other externally contaminated samples, in the same container and from the liquid nitrogen itself. Robust cryo-containers with liquid nitrogen-proof seals would ensure that any contamination was purely external, whereupon it could be removed; yet those that are damaged or which have poor or leaking seals could allow the ingress of contaminants.

At Bourn Hall, all patients are routinely screened for human immunodeficiency virus (HIV) and hepatitis B and C before treatment. Following the recommendations of a group convened by the Human Fertilisation and Embryology Authority (HFEA) to look into safe cryopreservation, such testing became mandatory on 31 December 2004 in the United Kingdom.

The level of microbial contamination in liquid nitrogen is generally low at the time of delivery; however, the precise levels vary widely with geographical region[38]. Furthermore, liquid nitrogen contamination in the Dewar could potentially increase every time the lid is removed, as the cloud of liquid nitrogen vapor released could potentially ensnare airborne microbes in ice crystals, only for them to fall into the open vessel. To counteract this effect, regular emptying and decontamination of Dewars would seem appropriate.

An infrequent, but unfortunately all too real, risk is the complete failure of a Dewar, resulting in total sample loss. Such failures generally occur without warning, and it is therefore important to take all reasonable precautions to minimize this risk.

At Bourn Hall the following steps are taken:

(1) As part of the laboratory quality control (QC) system Dewars are regularly checked and topped up. This procedure is signed off upon completion and a log maintained (the frequency of these checks is Dewar size-, capacity- and design-specific).

(2) Low nitrogen level alarms, with 24 h dial-out cover, are fitted to each vessel.

(3) Regular visual checks are made by security staff out of hours.

(4) An emergency back-up Dewar, capable of holding all samples from the largest Dewar, is kept full of liquid nitrogen.

(5) Dewars are replaced after 10 years of service.

The above system has recently been adopted by the HFEA, with all UK units being required to comply by June 2005. A further requirement is that samples from patients whose fertility may be impaired by medical treatment, such as those freezing semen prior to chemotherapy, are to be split between two separate Dewars. This action undoubtedly reduces the risk of total sample loss in the event of Dewar failure, but increases risks in other areas. Not only does it double the number of Dewars and consequently the amount of liquid nitrogen in the laboratory, but sample freezing, inventory and audit procedures are made all the more complicated as a result.

Safety of children born as a result of cryopreservation

The oldest children born from frozen embryos are now approaching their mid- to late teens, yet few reports following up these births have been published. There is currently no indication that babies born following the transfer of cryopreserved embryos show any increase in abnormalities[39–43], or that their well-being is anything other than satisfactory[44].

Work in one particular strain of mouse has shown an increase in developmental and learning difficulties from some offspring born from thawed embryos[45]. The authors concluded that cryopreservation is not severely detrimental, but indicated that it may not be absolutely free of long-term effects. This publication stimulated both criticism and debate[46], and the authors further stated that, of course, directly extrapolating from mice to humans was not appropriate[47].

Developmental problems, along with both minor and major congenital anomalies and malformations, were compared in a group of naturally conceived children and a group born from thawed embryos. The groups were matched for age, sex and social class. The results showed similar congenital anomaly and malformation rates and no developmental differences between the two groups[48].

Such conclusions are reassuring, but nevertheless, we should not be complacent about the outcomes, and it is important that continuing follow-up is performed on the children born as a result of these techniques.

Managing an embryo freezing program

The introduction and administration of a cryopreservation program is not without its difficulties, as it can raise both religious and ethical issues[49,50]. Legal issues also arise in countries such as Austria, Germany, Switzerland, Denmark, Italy and Sweden, where embryo cryopreservation is either banned or very strictly limited[51–53].

Clinics must ensure that patients are carefully counseled about the success rates and possible problems arising from the freezing of their embryos. Lengthy consent forms must be completed by both partners, indicating the number of years the embryos may be stored, and their wishes regarding the use or disposal of their embryos in the event of incapacity or death. Until a recent change in UK legislation it was

not possible for the genetic father to be registered on the birth certificate of any child born posthumously; this situation is now rectified, but requires signed consent from the male partner. Under the terms of the Human Fertilisation and Embryology Act (1990), embryos can be stored for up to 5 years in the first instance, and this can be extended to 10 years if, in the opinion of a medical expert, fertility is impaired. Rarely, where fertility is permanently impaired before the embryos can be used, as with oophorectomy for a malignancy, embryos may be stored until the female partner's 55th birthday.

Despite our best efforts to remain in contact with patients with embryos in our charge, and requests that they do likewise, contact is still frequently lost, and for this group the law dictates that their embryos must be discarded upon the expiry of their consented storage period. There is no doubt that, for some patients, the lack of communication is a deliberate act on their part knowing that it allows the UK law to make the difficult decision on disposal for them.

Our current procedure is to contact the 1000 or so patients who have embryos stored with us annually to ask them to reaffirm their wishes (the results from the 2003 mailing are summarized in Table 4). This not only serves as a reminder to the patients, but also satisfies the HFEA, who require clinics to hold up-to-date consents, and identifies changes of address. The form we send requires the signatures and agreement of both partners, as the withdrawal of consent by either must result in their embryos being removed from storage.

This schedule of the Human Fertilisation and Embryology Act has recently been challenged in the Appeal Court in the UK. A couple with stored embryos had separated and the male partner withdrew his consent for storage, whilst the female partner wanted to have the embryos implanted. The female party claimed that allowing the embryos to perish against her wishes was an infringement of her human rights. All three Court of Appeal Judges agreed that the 1990 Act represented a justified restriction on the human rights of the female, and dismissed the appeal.

Currently couples are given four choices each year:

(1) To continue storage for a further 12 months (for which a fee is raised);

(2) To donate the embryos to another infertile couple;

Table 4 Patient responses to 2003 questionnaire on their options for stored embryos

Option selected	Number of respondents	Respondents as a percentage
Continue storage	647	63
Donate to another couple	7	0.7
Donate to research	61	6
Dispose (before expiry)	120	11.3
Dispose (expired)	41	4
Letter returned	155	15

Table 5 Embryo donation program results 1995–2003 inclusive

Patients (n)	Cycles (n)	Clinical pregnancy rate (%)		Delivery rate (%)	
		Per cycle	Per patient	Per cycle	Per patient
5	119	33.6	53.3	30.2	48.0

(3) To donate the embryos for scientific research;

(4) To allow the embryos to perish.

The results from the 2003 consents are summarized in Table 4.

Of the 80 patients who were eligible to extend the storage of their embryos only 39 (49%) did. Unfortunately the number of patients donating their embryos for use by other couples was low, and showed a decrease of almost 50% from the 13 patients who donated in 2002. There are a number of factors that may deter couples from donating their embryos: the time-consuming screening and counseling process, the necessity to be registered with the HFEA or the imminent loss of anonymity of donors in the UK from 2005. Whether it is one single factor, or a combination, that affects their decision varies from couple to couple, but the number of potential embryo recipients in the past has outweighed the number of available donors. This situation is all the more frustrating when the results from our embryo donation program are studied (Table 5).

The success of this technique cannot be overstated, as almost half of the patients who received donated embryos achieved a live birth. Results such as these can only help to encourage more patients to donate their frozen embryos to such an effective and worthwhile program.

In addition to the annual patient contact, we are required by the Human Fertilisation Embryology Act to perform a yearly audit of all frozen embryos. At Bourn Hall, two embryologists check that the contents of the storage Dewars and each visitube with the names, dates and cycle numbers match the paper and computerized records. Each sheet is then signed and dated to provide an audit trail. With around 8000 embryos in storage, this is a major task, and, as such, is performed on a 'rolling' basis.

Conclusions

The efficacy and usefulness of embryo cryopreservation is now well accepted and established, yet the success rates vary widely. The goal of each laboratory offering this service is to achieve 100% post-thaw survival. There has been much research into the areas of cryoinjury, cryoprotectants and equipment used, combined with linear, non-linear slow and rapid freezing techniques. Nevertheless, aspirations of 100% cryosurvival may only be achieved when all the mechanisms for damage have been elucidated, and methods found to prevent them. Furthermore, it would seem probable that these multifactorial problems will require similarly complex solutions, and, were a universally successful freeze–thaw protocol possible, it might reasonably be expected to be a hybridization of the most effective parts of many methods.

Every laboratory has a duty of care to the patients for whom it stores embryos, and they should make all reasonable efforts to ensure the safety of the samples in their care. They should further ensure that the program is properly managed and that contact is maintained, to ensure an up-to-date record of the patients' wishes. When coupled with meticulous laboratory standards and careful embryo selection, such a program will give patients the best chance of achieving a pregnancy from any one oocyte recovery. To date, the limited published evidence suggests that, despite an increased incidence of preterm deliveries and multiple births, children born from frozen–thawed embryos are not adversely affected. However, follow-up studies must continue to be performed, coupled with the establishment of a multinational birth registry, to add weight to this conclusion[54].

SEMEN CRYOPRESERVATION

Introduction

Spallazani first proved the theory that sperm could be frozen in 1776, when he stored human, frog and stallion sperm on snow for 30 min before warming them, whereupon motility recovered. Nevertheless, it was not until 1953, when the first live births after insemination with cryopreserved human semen were reported, that the concept was proved[55].

Since those early successes, cryopreservation of sperm has become commonplace in IVF centers worldwide, although, unlike embryo freezing, methods and survival rates have not greatly improved.

Effects of cryopreservation

Human spermatozoa demonstrate unusual cryobiological behavior in that they appear indifferent to the rate at which they are cooled, and to which cryoprotectant is used; indeed it appears that seminal plasma itself has some cryoprotective properties. Typical post-thaw viability rates of spermatozoa average only 50% when using linear freezing protocols[56-58]. This is much lower than for many other mammalian cell types, and suggests that there are subpopulations that may differ in their freeze–thaw sensitivity. In support of this it has been shown that, unlike human erythrocytes that suffer a loss of viability with each repeated freeze–thaw cycle, human spermatozoa, under certain conditions, have a constant recovery rate, indicating a degree of freeze-tolerance[59].

By comparison with the amount of research into the effect of cooling rates upon human embryos, there are few such studies on spermatozoa, yet one publication suggests that cryosurvival can indeed be improved. Using an experimental non-linear freezing program, recovery rates of 88 and 100% have been reported[31].

A possible reason for the lack of progress with cryopreservation of spermatozoa is that, despite achieving suboptimal cryosurvival rates, overall fertilization and outcomes are not affected, regardless of whether ejaculated or surgically removed spermatozoa are used for standard IVF or intracytoplasmic sperm injection (ICSI)[60-62].

The atypical effects observed in frozen–thawed spermatozoa derive from the unique nature of the cell itself, as, unlike embryos, spermatozoa have several features that make them amenable to cryopreservation. They are relatively simple cells with a large surface area/volume ratio and high permeability to water, thus ensuring rapid osmotic equilibrium in the presence of cryoprotectants. They contain little cytoplasm, which has a low water, high protein content with few organelles that could be susceptible to cryoinjury, and, furthermore, the DNA is highly condensed, and hence in a protected state.

The lipid composition of sperm membranes is unusual compared with other mammalian membranes, not so much because of the types of lipids present (phospholipids, glycolipids and sterols), but more because of the relative ratios of these moieties. During cryopreservation, the lipid-rich sperm plasma membranes respond by undergoing reversible phase transitions from fluid to gel. However, such damage can be permanent, and has been associated with lower survival in post-thawed spermatozoa[63].

Cooling and rewarming sperm induces a capacitated-type behavior that may shorten their life span within the female tract, necessitating accurate timing of insemination[57]. Furthermore, there is a noticeable difference in cryosurvival rates between normal samples and those with abnormal parameters, such as count and percentage motility. Moreover, sperm DNA integrity from fertile men was unaffected by freeze–thawing, yet significant damage was sustained by sperm from infertile men. The same study showed that cryopreservation had a detrimental effect upon sperm morphology in both groups[64]. Despite these problems, many such spermatozoa are still capable of fertilizing an oocyte, and the technique has a number of useful applications for the assisted reproduction unit.

Freezing prior to cancer treatment

Recent improvements in the treatment of malignancies have led to greater long-term survival rates, which, in men with germ cell tumors, may reach 90%[65]. Iatrogenic oligozoospermia or azoospermia is a common side-effect of chemo- and radiotherapy, which not only affects the spermatogenic epithelium, but also can have mutagenic side-effects. Additionally, increased and persistent spermatozoal DNA damage was detected in a man after cytotoxic cancer treatment, although, thus far, no link between this observation and genetic disease in the children of these patients has been made[66]. Fertility preservation by banking sperm prior to treatment is now routine practice[67]. The service is well used and generally well tolerated by patients.

Samples from pre-chemotherapy patients are often poor and give a very low yield post-thaw. However, the advent of ICSI has meant that even severely olig-ozoospermic samples can now be stored and used successfully to achieve fertilization *in vitro*. The few studies reporting the number of patients returning to use their samples varies from 3.1%[67] to 8%[68] within 8 years of sample storage. However, a recent study is more encouraging, quoting a 27% return rate within 10 years[69]. The reasons for the low usage are unclear, although as many patients are reproductively young when they bank semen, it is likely that many will not have considered starting a family, even within the timescales quoted. When considered along with the legally permitted storage period for such samples (up to the patient's 55th birthday in the UK), it seems likely that extending the survey period would see more patients returning to use their samples.

Cryopreservation of surgically recovered sperm

Another group for whom cryopreservation has recently become significant are those men who require surgical sperm retrieval. Regardless of whether the sample is a testicular biopsy, or from percutaneous epididymal sperm aspiration (PESA), any sample left over after ICSI has been performed can be stored for future use, thus preventing the need for further invasive surgery. Similarly, if spermatozoa are found during an exploratory operation and the timing does not coincide with the partner's oocyte retrieval, cryopreservation at that point may prevent further surgery.

Other applications

Semen cryopreservation is also advantageous if the male partner has difficulty producing a semen sample. Having banked semen samples can reduce the

psychological pressure on the day of his partner's oocyte recovery and will often result in a fresh sample being provided, which is generally preferred by the embryologists.

Patients receiving anonymously donated oocytes often use frozen semen samples, as this not only reduces the risk of the couples meeting, but is also more convenient for the male partner, who does not need to attend the clinic at short notice. Similarly, patients who work away from home for extended periods may wish to freeze sperm for their wives to use in their absence.

In the case of sperm donors, cryopreservation allows samples to be quarantined for 6 months until negative virology screening tests are obtained and the samples can be released for use.

Methods of cryopreservation

Protocols for sperm cryopreservation differ widely in their detail from laboratory to laboratory, and are basic in comparison to the methods used for embryos; however, the fundamental methodology is the same.

Cryoprotectant media commonly used for sperm freezing are a tes and tris (TEST)-yolk buffer or human sperm preservation media (HSPM), both of which contain glycine and glucose with 10–15% glycerol as the cryoprotectant. Studies have shown TEST-yolk to give enhanced sperm survival[70] and improved acrosome protection[71] when compared with HSPM. However, as the egg-yolk component of TEST buffer is a possible source of contamination, safety concerns have been raised for samples frozen using this medium. There are now many commercially available sperm cryopreservation media, which are supplied sterile and ready for use.

At Bourn Hall, only samples from patients with up-to-date negative virology screening results for HIV, hepatitis B and hepatitis C are accepted for cryopreservation and valid Bourn Hall and HFEA consents to storage are a prerequisite. Under the terms of the Human Fertilisation and Embryology Act (1990), fertile men are permitted to store their samples for a maximum of 10 years. Only those whose infertility is permanently impaired, in the opinion of a medical practitioner, are allowed to keep their samples until their 55th birthday. Semen samples for freezing have a standard World Health Organization (WHO) assessment performed, and room temperature HSPM is then added in a drop-wise manner, with gentle agitation between each addition; a typical ratio of HSPM to semen is 1 : 1. Samples with a very high motile sperm count can be diluted 2 : 1 or even 3 : 1, and, conversely, samples with low numbers, especially if the ejaculate volume is high, can be centrifuged and the majority of the supernatant discarded to concentrate the sample. Following dilution, the sample is allowed a period of 10 min to equilibrate before being transferred to pre-labeled cryovials. The whole procedure is performed aseptically in a class II hood, and is witnessed by two embryologists. At Bourn Hall, semen is frozen in 1.8-ml Nunc ampoules, as there are fewer safety issues associated with them than with polyvinyl alcohol (PVA)-plugged straws, and they are more robust than heat-sealed straws. The ampoules are then cooled in vapor at approximately 10°C/min for 30 min by suspending them 18 cm above the level of liquid nitrogen in a wide-mouthed cryoflask with the lid on. Using a programmable freezer can enhance freeze–thaw survival rates[70], but as sufficient motile sperm are obtained from vapor-phase methods, machine freezing is generally unnecessary.

Surgically recovered sperm from PESA are frozen in the same manner as ejaculated samples, although post-thaw survival rates are usually very poor. Our experience has shown no difference in post-thaw survival rates from biopsies, whether disaggregated or not, prior to freezing; therefore, testicular biopsies are frozen whole in HSPM after rinsing free of blood. Due to the extreme variability in post-thaw survival rates achieved from surgically recovered samples, we consider it important to freeze a small aliquot for a post-thaw survival test. Biopsies will invariably need some incubation before motility is observed, and in some cases 24 h at 37°C is needed; this necessitates thawing the day before oocyte recovery. In cases of virtually zero survival post-thaw, having the results from a test sample allows time for the patient to consider what precautions to take if no viable sperm are located on the day of his partner's oocyte retrieval. The commonly considered options are: a repeat surgical sperm retrieval (SSR), using donor sperm or, as a last resort, oocyte freezing.

The safety issues regarding sperm storage are the same as for embryos; therefore, Dewars are subject to the same rigorous checking, filling and security procedures. At Bourn Hall the semen freezing program is managed in the same way as for embryos, in that Dewars are audited annually and patients asked if they wish to maintain their samples in storage (for which a charge is raised) or to have them discarded.

Conclusions

The advent of ICSI has enabled treatment using very low numbers of sperm, and, when used in conjunction with cryopreserved samples, the technique becomes all the more powerful. It has indeed proved farsighted that some 15 years ago we froze samples from pre-chemotherapy patients if they contained any sperm at all, as, unlike the time when they were first frozen, we are now able, to achieve fertilization, pregnancies and live births with ICSI. The reproductive potential of these patients has thus been preserved. Our ability to utilize such low numbers of sperm today should mean that we are no longer satisfied with mediocre cryosurvival rates, and further research into improving this situation should be urgently undertaken, perhaps with a view to helping the next 'ICSI generation'.

REFERENCES

1. Trounson A, Mohr L. Human pregnancy following cryopreservation, thawing and transfer of an eight-cell embryo. Nature (London) 1983; 305: 707–9
2. Cohen J, Simons RF, Edwards RG, et al. Pregnancies following the frozen storage of expanding human blastocysts. J In Vitro Fertil Embryo Transf 1985; 2: 59–64
3. Fehilly CB, Cohen J, Simons RF, et al. Cryopreservation of cleaving embryos and expanded blastocysts in the human: a comparative study. Fertil Steril 1985; 44: 638–44
4. Lassalle B, Testart J, Renard JP. Human embryo features that influence the success of cryopreservation with the use of 1,2 propanediol. Fertil Steril 1985; 44: 645–51
5. Cohen J, Simons RS, Fehilly CB, et al. Factors affecting the survival and implantation of cryopreserved human embryos. J In Vitro Fertil Embryo Transf 1986; 3: 46–52
6. Testart J, Lassalle B, Allart JB, et al. High pregnancy rate after early human embryo freezing. Fertil Steril 1986; 46: 268
7. Damario MA, Hammitt DG, Thornhill AR. Long-term results of an oocyte donation program which utilizes cryopreserved embryos exclusively. Fertil Steril 2001; 76: S84

8. Jones HW Jr, Jones D, Kolm P. Cryopreservation: a simplified method of evaluation. Hum Reprod 1997; 12: 548–53

9. Schroeder AK, Banz C, Katalinic A, et al. Counselling on cryopreservation of pronucleated oocytes. Reprod Biomed Online 2003; 6: 69–74

10. Shaw JM, Oranratnachai A, Trounson AO. Fundamental cryobiology of mammalian oocytes and ovarian tissue. Theriogenology 2000; 53: 59–72

11. Trad FS, Toner M, Biggers D. Effects of cryoprotectants and ice-seeding temperature on intracellular freezing and survival of human oocytes. Hum Reprod 1999; 14: 1569–77

12. Whittingham DG. Some factors affecting embryo storage in laboratory animals. The Freezing of Mamalian Embryos, Ciba Foundation Symposium. 1977; 52: 97–127

13. Mazur P, Kemp JA, Miller RH. Survival of fetal rat pancreases frozen to -78 and -196 degrees. Proc Natl Acad Sci 1976; 73: 4105–9

14. Paynter SJ, Cooper A, Gregory L, et al. Permeability characteristics of human oocytes in the presence of the cryoprotectant dimethylsulfoxide. Hum Reprod 1999; 14: 2338–42

15. Paynter SJ, O'Neil L, Fuller BJ, et al. Membrane permeability of human oocytes in the presence of the cryoprotectant propane-1,2-diol. Fertil Steril 2001; 75: 532–8

16. Newton H, Pegg DE, Barrass R, et al. Osmotically inactive volume, hydraulic conductivity, and permeability to dimethyl sulphoxide of human mature oocytes. Reprod Fertil 1999; 117: 27–33

17. Morris GJ. Physics of Freezing, Cool Guide to Cryopreservation. Cambridge, UK: Asymptote, 2000: 8–25

18. Rall WF, Fahy GM. Ice-free cryopreservation of mouse embryos at −196°C by vitrification. Nature (London) 1985; 313: 573–5

19. Rall WF. Factors affecting the survival of mouse embryos cryopreserved by vitrification. Cryobiology 1987; 24: 387–402

20. Vajta G, Holm P, Kuwayama M, et al. Open pulled straws (OPS) vitrification: a new way to reduce cryoinjuries of bovine ova and embryos. Mol Reprod Dev 1998; 51: 53–8

21. Lane M, Schoolcraft WB, Gardner DK. Vitrification of mouse and human blastocysts using a novel cryoloop container-less technique. Fertil Steril 1999; 72: 1073–8

22. Libermann J, Tucker MJ, Graham J, et al. Blastocyst development after vitrification of multipronucleate zygotes using the flexipet denuding pipette. Reprod Biomed Online 2002; 4: 146–50

23. Libermann J, Tucker MJ, Graham JR. The importance of cooling rate for successful vitrification of human oocytes: comparison of the cryoloop with the flexipet. Biol Reprod 2002; 66 (Suppl 1): 195 (abstr 240)

24. Kuwayama M, Kato O. Successful vitrification of human oocytes. Fertil Steril 2000; 74 (Suppl 3): S49 (abstr 0–127)

25. Hong SW, Chung HM, Lim JM, et al. Improved human oocyte development after vitrification: a comparison of thawing methods. Fertil Steril 1992; 72: 142–6

26. Yoon TK, Chung HM, Lim JM, et al. Pregnancy and delivery of healthy infants developed from vitrified oocytes in a stimulated in vitro fertilization-embryo transfer program. Fertil Steril 2000; 74: 180–1

27. Yokota Y, Yokota H, Yokota M, et al. Birth of healthy twins from in vitro development of human refrozen embryos. Fertil Steril 2001; 76: 1063–5

28. Son WY, Yoon SH, Yoon HJ, et al. Pregnancy outcome following transfer of human blastocysts vitrified on electron microscopy grids after induced collapse of the blastocoele. Hum Reprod 2003; 18: 137–9

29. Franks F. Biophysics and Biochemistry at Low Temperatures. Cambridge: Cambridge University Press, 1985: 657–67

30. Ashwood-Smith MJ, Morris GW, Fowler R, et al. Physical factors are involved in the destruction of embryos and oocytes during freezing and thawing procedures. Hum Reprod 1988; 3: 795–802

31. Morris GJ, Acton E, Avery S. A novel approach to sperm cryopreservation. Hum Reprod 1992; 14: 1013–21

32. Menezo Y, Nicollet B, Herbaut N, et al. Freezing cocultured human blastocysts. Fertil Steril 1999; 58: 977–80

33. Schuffner A, Stockler S, Costa S, et al. Long-term cryopreserved semen results in a live birth 12 years later. J Urol 2004; 171: 358

34. Fogarty NM, Maxwell WM, Eppleston J, et al. The viability of transferred sheep embryos after long-term cryopreservation. Reprod Fertil Dev 2000; 2: 31–7

35. Glenister PH, Whittingham DG, Lyon MF. Further studies on the effect of radiation during the storage of frozen 8-cell mouse embryos at −196 degrees C. J Reprod Fertil 1984; 70: 229–34

36. Tedder RS, Zuckerman AH, Goldstone AH. Hepatitis B transmission from contaminated cryopreservation tank. Lancet 1995; 346: 137–40

37. Fountain D, Ralston M, Higgins N, et al. Liquid nitrogen freezers: potential source of haematopoietic stem cell components. Transfusion 1997; 37: 585–91

38. Morris GJ. Cryopreservation and contamination. ART Sci 2002; 2: 1–3

39. Wada I, Matson P, Troup SA, et al. Outcome of treatment subsequent to the elective cryopreservation of all embryos from women at risk of the ovarian hyperstimulation syndrome. Hum Reprod 1992; 7: 962–6

40. Sutcliffe AG, D'Souza SW, Cadman J, et al. Outcome in children from cryopreserved embryos. Arch Dis Child 1995; 72: 290–3

41. Olivennes F, Schneider Z, Remy V, et al. Perinatal outcome and follow-up of 82 children aged 1–9 years conceived from cryopreserved embryos. Hum Reprod 1996; 11: 1565–8

42. Wennerholm UB, Hamberger L, Nilsson L, et al. Obstetric and perinatal outcome of children conceived from cryopreserved embryos. Hum Reprod 1997; 12: 1819–25

43. Wennerholm UB, Albertsson-Wikland K, Bergh C, et al. Post-natal growth and health in children born after cryopreservation as embryos. Lancet 1998; 351: 1085–90

44. Sutcliffe AG. Follow-up of children conceived from cryopreserved embryos. Mol Cell Endocrinol 2000; 27: 91–3

45. Dulioust E, Toyama K, Busnel MC, et al. Long term effects of embryo freezing in mice. Proc Natl Acad Sci USA 1995; 92: 589–93

46. Testart J. Safety of embryo cryopreservation: statistical facts and artifacts. Episcientific aspects of the epigenetic factors in artificial procreation. Hum Reprod 1998; 13: 783–8

47. Dulioust E, Busnel MC, Carlier M, et al. Embryo cryopreservation and development: facts, questions and responsibility. Hum Reprod 1999; 14: 1141–5

48. Sutcliffe AG, D'Souza SW, Cadman J, et al. Minor congenital abnormalities, major malformations and development in children conceived from cryopreserved embryos. Hum Reprod 1995; 10: 3332–7

49. Vidali A, Dani G, Antinori M, et al. Oocyte cryopreservation is a viable alternative option for patients who refuse embryo freezing. Fertil Steril 1988; 70 (Suppl 1): S138

50. Coticchio G, Garetti S, Bonu A, et al. Cryopreservation of human oocytes. Hum Fertil 2001; 4: 152–7

51. Wood C, Downing B, Trounson A, et al. Clinical implications of developments in in vitro fertilization. Br Med J 1984; 289: 978–80

52. Jones HW Jr. Cryopreservation and its problems. Fertil Steril 1990; 53: 780–4

53. Knoppers BM, Bris SL. Ethical and legal concerns: reproductive technologies 1990–1993. Curr Opin Obstet Gynaecol 1993; 5: 630–5

54. Sutcliffe AG. IVF Children: the First Generation. London: Parthenon Publishing, 2002: 39–59

55. Bunge RG, Sherman JK. Fertilizing capacity of frozen human spermatozoa. Nature (London) 1953; 172: 767–8

56. Esteves SC, Sharma RK, Thomas AJ, et al. Improvement in motion characteristics and acrosome status in cryopreserved human spermatozoa by swim-up processing before freezing. Hum Reprod 2000; 15: 2173–9

57. Holt WV. Basic aspects of sperm cryobiology: the importance of species and individual differences. Theriogenology 2000; 53: 47–58

58. Watson PF. The causes of reduced fertility with cryopreserved semen. Anim Reprod Sci 2000; 60: 481–92

59. Morris GJ. A new development in the cryopreservation of sperm. Hum Fertil 2002; 5: 23–9

60. Habermann H, Seo R, Cieslak J, et al. In vitro fertilization outcomes after intracytoplasmic sperm injection with fresh or frozen–thawed testicular spermatozoa. Fertil Steril 2000; 73: 955–60

61. Park YS, Lee SH, Song SJ, et al. Influence of motility on the outcome of in vitro fertilization/intracytoplasmic sperm injection with fresh vs. frozen testicular sperm from men with obstructive azoospermia. Fertil Steril 2003; 80: 526–30

62. Russell ST, Nehra A, Session DR, et al. 10 year experience of in vitro fertilization (IVF) outcomes using frozen semen at the mayo clinic. 2004; in press

63. Giraud MN, Motta C, Boucher D, et al. Membrane fluidity predicts the outcome of cryopreservation of human spermatozoa. Hum Reprod 2000; 15: 2160–4

64. Donnelly ET, Steele EK, McClure N, et al. Assessment of DNA integrity and morphology of ejaculated spermatozoa from fertile and infertile men before and after cryopreservation. Hum Reprod 2001; 6: 1191–9

65. Germa JR, Garcia Del Muro X, Maroto P, et al. Clinical pattern and therapeutic results obtained in germ cell testicular cancer in Spain based on a consecutive series of 1250 patients. Clin Med Barcelona 2001; 116: 481–6

66. Morris ID. Sperm damage and cancer treatment. J Androl 2002; 25: 255–61

67. Lass A, Akagbosu F, Abuhsheika N, et al. A programme of semen cryopreservation for patients with malignant disease in a tertiary infertility centre: lessons from 8 years' experience. Hum Reprod 1998; 13: 3256–61

68. Fossa SD, Aass N, Molne K. Is routine pre-treatment cryopreservation of semen worthwhile in the management of patients with testicular cancer? Br J Urol 1989; 64: 524–9

69. Blackhall FH, Atkinson AD, Maaya MB, et al. Semen cryopreservation, utilization and reproductive outcome in men treated for Hodgkin's disease. Br J Cancer 2002; 87: 381–4

70. Stanic P, Tandara M, Sonicki Z, et al. Comparison of protective media and freezing techniques for cryopreservation of human semen. Eur J Obstet Gynecol Reprod Biol 2000; 91: 65–70

71. Hammadeh ME, Georg T, Rosenbaum P, et al. Association between freezing agent and acrosome damage of human spermatozoa from subnormal and normal semen. Andrologia 2001; 33: 331–6

18

Assisted reproduction techniques for male-factor infertility: current status of intracytoplasmic sperm injection

Anick De Vos and André Van Steirteghem

INTRODUCTION

More than 20 years ago, a fruitful collaboration between Steptoe, a gynecologist, and Edwards, a physiologist, resulted in the birth of the first human baby after *in vitro* fertilization (IVF) and subsequent embryo transfer (ET)[1]. This report represented a major breakthrough in human infertility treatment, and, since then, IVF has become a well-established treatment procedure for certain types of infertility, including long-standing infertility due to tubal disease or endometriosis, unexplained infertility or infertility involving a male factor. It soon became obvious that certain couples with severe male-factor infertility could not be helped by conventional IVF. Extremely low sperm counts, impaired motility and/or poor morphology represent the main causes of failed fertilization in conventional IVF. In order to tackle this problem, several procedures of assisted fertilization based on micromanipulation of oocytes and spermatozoa have been established. The evolution of these techniques started with partial zona dissection (PZD)[2–5], followed by subzonal insemination (SUZI)[4,6–9], and finally led to the procedure of intracytoplasmic sperm injection (ICSI)[10]. The two former techniques were developed to circumvent the barrier to fertilization represented by the zona pellucida. PZD involves mechanical disruption of the zona pellucida so that inseminated sperm cells obtain direct access to the perivitelline space of the oocyte. In SUZI, several motile sperm cells (3–20) are immediately delivered into the perivitelline space by means of an injection pipette. ICSI is even more invasive, because a single spermatozoon is directly injected into the ooplasm, thereby crossing not only the zona pellucida but also the oolemma. ICSI had previously been used successfully to obtain live offspring in rabbits and cattle[11].

In 1992, our group reported the first human pregnancies and births after replacement of embryos generated by this novel procedure of assisted fertilization[12]. The use of PZD had become controversial and was subsequently abandoned by many workers. Fertilization rates after ICSI had been reported to be significantly better than after SUZI[13–16]. Moreover, ICSI resulted in the production of more embryos with higher implantation rates[13–16]. As a result, ICSI has been used worldwide and successfully to treat infertility due to impaired testicular function or obstruction of the excretory ducts resulting in severe oligo-, astheno- or teratozoospermia or even azoospermia in the ejaculate[13,15,17–20].

Since the first publications describing the ICSI procedure[9,12,13,15,16], minor modifications have contributed to reduced rates of oocyte degeneration, oocyte activation (one pronucleus or 1-PN) and abnormal fertilization (3-PN)[21]. Hyaluronidase may be responsible for oocyte activation. Therefore, the concentration used during oocyte denudation and the exposure time of oocytes to the enzyme have been reduced[22]. The moment of denudation relative to oocyte pick-up (immediately or 4 h later) does not influence the ICSI results[23]. The orientation of the polar body during injection has an influence on embryo quality[24]. Motile sperm cells are selected and immobilized prior to injection[25]. Cytoplasm aspiration to ensure oolemma rupture is critical for the ICSI procedure, and the method of rupture has been correlated with oocyte degeneration[24]. Furthermore, the morphology of the injected spermatozoon is related to the fertilization outcome of the procedure as well as to the pregnancy outcome[26].

This chapter surveys the current status of ICSI, emphasizing patient selection for ICSI, oocyte and sperm handling prior to microinjection, the procedure and outcome parameters of ICSI, its clinical application and overall results, including follow-up of the pregnancies and children.

PATIENT SELECTION: INDICATIONS FOR ICSI

Successful IVF depends on the presence in the ejaculate of a certain number of spermatozoa with good motility and morphology. Riedel and colleagues[27] reported minimal andrological requirements for conventional IVF: 5×10^6/ml total count, 30% progressive motility and 30% normal morphology. Men with sperm parameters below these values were considered to have a poor prognosis. Today, however, the most efficient procedure to treat this type of male infertility is ICSI: only one motile (live) spermatozoon is required per mature metaphase-II oocyte to be injected.

Before the era of ICSI, attempts were made to modify and refine conventional IVF in order to achieve increased rates of conception in cases of male infertility. The use of a high insemination concentration was shown to be beneficial for treating oligozoospermia and oligoasthenozoospermia[28–30]. However, sperm morphology has a major impact on the outcome of high insemination concentration in IVF. Oehninger and co-workers[31] reported improved

fertilization rates and pregnancy rates when using a high insemination concentration in cases with low numbers of morphologically normal spermatozoa. Nevertheless, significantly lower implantation and pregnancy rates were observed in patients with severe teratozoospermia[31]. Ombelet and colleagues[32] indicated that, whereas a 'normal' fertilization rate was restored in cases with moderate teratozoospermia using a high insemination concentration, the increased number of sperm cells added to the oocytes did not restore the fertilization rate if the sperm morphology was below 5% normal forms (scored according to strict Kruger criteria[33]). More recently, with the advent of ICSI, comparative studies between IVF with a high insemination concentration and ICSI in cases of severe teratozoospermia have been performed[34,35]. Higher fertilization rates[34] and significantly better embryo quality[34,35] were obtained by ICSI as compared with IVF with a high insemination concentration. A clear trend for better implantation and pregnancy rates was observed in the ICSI group[35]. Today, ICSI has clearly overshadowed the use of modified IVF procedures, including high insemination concentration, for the treatment of severe male-factor infertility. ICSI requires only one spermatozoon with a functional genome and centrosome for the fertilization of each oocyte.

Indications for ICSI are not restricted to impaired morphology of the spermatozoa but also include low sperm counts and/or impaired kinetic quality of the sperm cells. A summary of 4 years of ICSI practice indicated that similar results are achieved by ICSI with abnormal semen and by conventional IVF with normal semen parameters[36]. ICSI can also be used with spermatozoa from the epididymis or testis when there is an obstruction in the excretory ducts. Azoospermia caused by testicular failure can be treated by ICSI if enough spermatozoa can be retrieved in testicular tissue samples.

Table 1 gives an overview of the current indications for ICSI. ICSI with ejaculated spermatozoa can be used successfully in patients with fertilization failures after conventional IVF or other assisted fertilization procedures, and also for patients who cannot be accepted for these procedures because too few morphologically normal and progressively motile spermatozoa are present in the ejaculate (fewer than 500 000). High fertilization and pregnancy rates can be obtained when a motile spermatozoon is injected[16]. Injection

Table 1 Indications for intracytoplasmic sperm injection

Ejaculated sperm
Oligozoospermia ($< 20 \times 10^6$/ml)
Asthenozoospermia ($< 40\%$ progressive motility, of which at least 10% are of A type motility)
Teratozoospermia ($< 14\%$ normal forms according to strict Kruger cirteria[33])
Any combination of these three anomalies
Antisperm antibodies
Globozoospermia
Repeated fertilization failure after conventional IVF–ET
Ejaculatory disorders (electroejaculation, retrograde ejaculation)

Epididymal sperm
Young's syndrome
Congenital bilateral absence of the vas deferens
Failed vasoepididymostomy
Obstruction of both ejaculatory ducts

Testicular sperm
All indications for epididymal sperm
Failure of epididymal sperm recovery because of fibrosis
Azoospermia because of testicular failure (maturation arrest, germ-cell aplasia)
Necrozoospermia

IVF–ET, *in vitro* fertilization and embryo transfer

of only immotile or probably non-vital spermatozoa results in lower fertilization rates[37]. When only non-vital sperm cells are present in the ejaculate, the use of testicular sperm is indicated[38]. Other semen parameters, such as concentration, morphology (except for globozoospermia)[39] and high titers of antisperm antibodies[40], do not influence the success rates of ICSI[37]. Successful ICSI has also been described for patients with acrosomeless spermatozoa[41–43].

Any form of infertility due to obstruction of the excretory ducts can be treated by ICSI, with spermatozoa microsurgically recovered from either the epididymis[44–46] or the testis[47–49]. Obstructive azoospermia can result from congenital bilateral absence of the vas deferens (CBAVD), failed vasectomy reversal or vasoepididymostomy. Epididymal sperm is mainly obtained by microsurgical epididymal sperm aspiration (MESA) under general anesthesia. Less frequently used is percutaneous epididymal sperm aspiration (PESA) carried out under local anesthesia[50,51]. When no motile spermatozoa can be retrieved from the

epididymis, owing to epididymal fibrosis, testicular spermatozoa can be isolated from a testicular biopsy specimen[52]. Two approaches are used to obtain testicular tissue: an open excisional biopsy or fine-needle aspiration[53–55]. Testicular biopsy has also been useful in some cases of non-obstructive azoospermia[56–59]. In patients with severely impaired testicular function due to (incomplete) germ-cell aplasia (Sertoli-cell-only syndrome), hypospermatogenesis or incomplete maturation arrest, spermatozoa may be recovered, sometimes only after taking multiple biopsies. Testicular sperm recovery may not always be successful in all azoospermic patients[55]. Those factors correlated with a successful recovery procedure could allow objective counseling based on predictive factors. However, no strong predictors for successful testicular sperm recovery were determined except for testicular histopathology[60]. Optimal sperm recovery from a testicular biopsy can be obtained by finely mincing the tissue[61]. Very often, vital spermatozoa can be successfully recovered for ICSI only after processing the biopsy specimens with red blood cell lysis buffer[62] and/or an enzymatic collagen digestion medium[63,64]. Today, several reports show that lower fertilization and pregnancy results are obtained in cases of non-obstructive azoospermia, compared with obstructive cases[65–67].

Cryopreservation of supernumerary spermatozoa recovered from the epididymis[68–71] or the testis[72,73] is an important issue, because microinjection of frozen–thawed sperm cells can avoid repeated surgery in future ICSI cycles. Successful ICSI using frozen–thawed epididymal sperm has been described[68–71]. Although pregnancies resulting from ICSI with cryopreserved testicular sperm have been reported[73–75], cryopreservation of testicular sperm is more difficult, because only a very limited number of spermatozoa are present. Two groups described a method for cryopreserving limited numbers of single spermatozoa inside empty zonae pellucidae[76,77]; and the first births using this procedure were reported[78]. However, to adapt this method for testicular biopsies for non-obstructive cases would be cumbersome and extremely time-consuming.

It must be added that the ICSI procedure cannot be carried out in approximately 3% of scheduled cycles. Either no cumulus–oocyte complexes or metaphase-II oocytes are available, or no spermatozoa are found in testicular biopsies of patients with non-obstructive azoospermia.

OOCYTE HANDLING PRIOR TO MICROINJECTION

A successful ICSI program depends on ovarian stimulation, which is essentially similar to that for conventional IVF. Current ovarian stimulation regimens use a combination of gonadotropin releasing hormone (GnRH) agonists, human menopausal gonadotropin (hMG) or recombinant follicle stimulating hormone (r-hFSH) and human chorionic gonadotropin (hCG), which allows the retrieval of a high number of cumulus–oocyte complexes[79,80]. Administration of GnRH agonists allows for pituitary down-regulation to occur before the initiation of exogenous FSH. Gonadotropin preparations or r-hFSH are administered to stimulate multiple follicle development. Ovulation is induced by means of hCG (10 000 IU), which is administered when the serum estradiol level exceeds 1000 pg/ml and when at least three follicles of 18 mm or more in diameter are observed on ultrasound examination. The optimal time for ultrasound-guided transvaginal oocyte aspiration is 36 h after hCG administration[81]. On average, approximately 11 cumulus–oocyte complexes per cycle can be retrieved[82]. After cumulus and corona cell removal, this corresponds to approximately nine metaphase-II oocytes per cycle available for microinjection[82]. hCG may be used for luteal phase supplementation, although exogenous progesterone, administered intravaginally, is frequently applied in an attempt to avoid the risk of hCG stimulation of remaining growing follicles. More recently, the clinical introduction of GnRH antagonists[83,84] allows a powerful and immediate suppression of pituitary gonadotropin release and a rapid recovery of normal secretion of endogenous luteinizing hormone (LH) and FSH[85]. By making optimal use of endogenous FSH, the amount of exogenous FSH required for follicular growth could be substantially reduced. A rapid recovery of pituitary LH and FSH release after cessation of GnRH antagonist administration might permit the abandonment of additional luteal phase support.

In conventional IVF, oocytes are inseminated while they are lodged within the cumulus complexes. Prior to fertilization by means of micromanipulation, oocytes need to be denuded from the surrounding cumulus and corona cells, allowing not only precise injection of the oocytes, but also the assessment of their maturity, which is of critical importance for ICSI. Cumulus and corona cells are removed by a combination of enzymatic and mechanical procedures[22,86]. In a first step, oocytes are placed in a HEPES-buffered (4-(2-hydroxyethyl)-1-piperazineethanesulfonic acid) solution containing hylauronidase. The oocytes are repeatedly pipetted in and out of a Pasteur pipette. Both the enzyme concentration and the duration of exposure to the enzyme should be limited, because they can result in parthenogenetic activation of the oocytes[87]. Further mechanical denudation is carried out in the absence of the enzyme and by means of repeated aspiration into a finely pulled pipette.

Denuded oocytes can be observed under the inverted microscope (×200 magnification) in order to assess nuclear maturity. Observations include assessment of the zona pellucida and the oocyte, and the presence or absence of a germinal vesicle or a first polar body[86]. Ninety-five per cent of the retrieved cumulus–oocyte complexes contain an intact oocyte. The remaining 5% involve empty zonae, cracked zonae or morphologically abnormal oocytes. In Figure 1, three different stages of oocyte maturation are illustrated. On average, 3.7% of the retrieved oocytes are at the metaphase-I stage, having undergone breakdown of the germinal vesicle but not yet extrusion of the first polar body[82]. Approximately 9.8% of the oocytes are at the germinal vesicle (GV) stage, and about 81.5% of them are in the metaphase-II stage, showing the presence of the first polar body[82]. Because only metaphase-II oocytes have reached the haploid state and, thus, can be fertilized normally, ICSI is carried out only on such oocytes. Frequently, metaphase-I oocytes achieve meiosis after a few hours of *in vitro* culture and are available for ICSI on the day of oocyte retrieval. Despite somewhat lower fertilization rates (53% vs. 71%), injection of matured metaphase-I oocytes results in embryos of similar quality to that of metaphase-II oocytes at the moment of oocyte retrieval[88]. Germinal vesicle-stage oocytes require overnight culture in order to reach the metaphase-II stage. Only in rare cases, where too few, or no, metaphase-II oocytes are available or where the oocytes remained unfertilized after ICSI, *in vitro*-matured germinal vesical-stage oocytes are injected the day after oocyte pick-up. Only a few pregnancies[89,90] and deliveries[91,92] resulting from immature oocytes have been reported to date. Due to these poor results, the practice of injecting *in vitro* matured GV

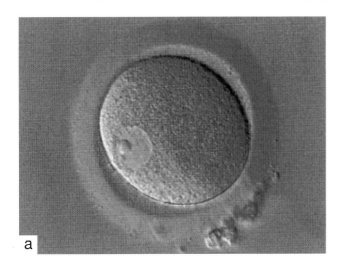

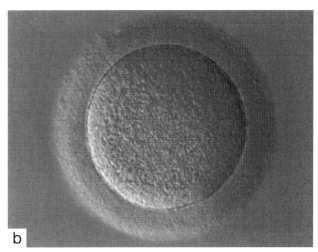

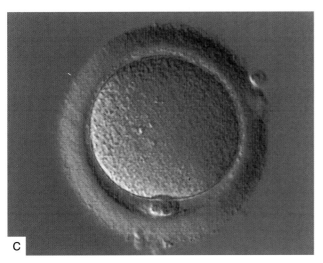

Figure 1 Oocyte maturity after cumulus and corona cell removal. Oocytes at the germinal vesicle stage are recognized by the presence of a typical germinal vesicle (a). Oocytes that have undergone germinal vesicle breakdown but have not yet extruded the first polar body are called metaphase-I oocytes (b). A typical metaphase-II oocyte displays the presence of a first polar body, which indicates that the oocyte is mature and has reached the haploid state (c). Only metaphase-II oocytes are submitted to intracytoplasmic sperm injection (ICSI)

oocytes may be abandoned in a routine ICSI program. Denuded and rinsed oocytes are incubated until the time of microinjection.

SPERM HANDLING PRIOR TO MICROINJECTION

For microinjection, spermatozoa from three different origins are processed: ejaculated sperm and surgically retrieved sperm from the epididymis or the testis. For all three catergories, ICSI in combination with sperm cryopreservation is currently used. Frozen ejaculated sperm has been useful for cured cancer patients, in cases of masturbation problems or for donor sperm. Injection of frozen–thawed epididymal sperm yields similar ICSI results to those with fresh epididymal sperm[68–71]. At present, the preclinical[72] and clinical[73–75] experience with frozen–thawed testicular sperm indicates satisfactory fertilization and pregnancy rates. Testicular sperm recovery after freezing may be improved by freezing testicular cell suspensions instead of whole biopsies[93].

All patients selected for ICSI with ejaculated semen undergo a preliminary semen assessment prior to the treatment cycle, in order to verify whether enough, preferably motile, spermatozoa are present to perform ICSI. Semen assessment is performed according to the recommendations of the World Health Organization (WHO)[94], except for sperm morphology, which is assessed by the strict criteria of Kruger and colleagues[33]. Semen values are considered normal if the volume of the ejaculate is at least 2 ml, sperm concentration is at least 20×10^6/ml, progressive motility is at least 40% and normal sperm morphology is at least 14%. In about 43% of ICSI patients with ejaculated sperm, all three semen parameters are abnormal. In one-third of patients, two semen parameters are impaired, and in one-fifth of them, one semen value is abnormal. The minority of patients with normal semen values (about 8%) involves those who had previously undergone conventional IVF treatments without success.

Routinely, sperm samples for ICSI are processed by density-gradient centrifugation (using silane-coated silica particle colloid solutions[95]), allowing an enrichment in the number of motile and morphologically normal sperm cells needed for assisted reproduction. Only in cases of extreme oligozoospermic samples, i.e. when gradient centrifugation results in an insufficient yield of sperm cells for ICSI, simple washing of the sperm sample is performed to reduce the loss of sperm cells for injection. Immediate injection of the oocytes is then indicated because sperm cells lose their initial motility and probably die when the sample is simply washed, which can be ascribed to the presence of reactive oxygen species and other damaging substances[96,97].

Epididymal sperm are usually recovered from the most proximal part of the caput of the epididymis in a microsurgical procedure[98,99]. During microsurgical epididymal sperm aspiration, several sperm fractions are collected into separate tubes. Sperm fractions with similar concentration and motility are pooled and then treated in the same way as extreme oligozoospermic ejaculated semen, i.e. a density-gradient centrifugation is performed. Because only a few spermatozoa are present, microdroplets of the resuspended pellet can be placed in separate medium droplets adjacent to the central polyvinylpyrrolidone (PVP) droplet in the injection dish. This facilitates the search for and the selection of single motile spermatozoa, which are then transferred to the PVP droplet and immobilized prior to injection. The presence of tissue debris and cells other than spermatozoa often blocks the injection pipette. In order to circumvent this problem, a pipette of larger diameter (testicular sperm extraction (TESE) pipette: outer diameter 8–10 µm instead of approximately 6–7 µm for an injection pipette) is used to collect the sperm cells. Whenever possible, some of the freshly recovered sperm should be frozen for later use in subsequent ICSI cycles, thereby avoiding repeated surgical procedures[98].

Testicular spermatozoa are isolated from a testicular biopsy specimen, which is usually obtained by means of surgical excisional biopsy performed under general anesthesia[48]. The testicular biopsy specimen is transferred to a Petri dish with HEPES-buffered Earle's medium, and shredded into small pieces with sterile microscope slides[61] on the heated stage of a stereomicroscope. The presence of spermatozoa is assessed on the inverted microscope, which determines whether the surgical procedure can be stopped or whether extra biopsy pieces need to be taken. The pieces of biopsy tissue are removed, and the medium is centrifuged at $300\,g$ for 5 min. The pellet is then resuspended for the ICSI procedure. The collection of single motile spermatozoa is similar to that for epididymal sperm, using separate medium droplets containing fractions of the testicular sperm suspension. If no sperm cells can be found, the tissue pieces can be treated with red blood cell lysis buffer[62] and/or an enzymatic collagen digestion medium[63]. Lysis of excess red blood cells may facilitate the search for sperm cells, and the use of enzymes may result in the recovery of sperm cells initially attached to the tissue and therefore inaccessible. It is well known that it is not always possible to retrieve testicular spermatozoa from biopsy specimens in patients with non-obstructive azoospermia due to germ-cell aplasia or maturation arrest[55,60]. In cases where testicular spermatozoa are retrieved under local anesthesia by means of the fine-needle aspiration approach, the aspirated fractions are immediately collected in the injection dish. No further sample processing, except collecting the single motile spermatozoa with a microneedle (TESE pipette), is needed prior to ICSI.

ICSI PROCEDURE

The equipment, requirements and skills in gamete handling and embryo culture *in vitro* in an established IVF laboratory are very similar, and thus very well applicable to an ICSI program. For the ICSI procedure itself, an inverted microscope equipped with micromanipulators and microinjectors should be available (Figure 2). Use of magnifications of ×200 and ×400 not only allows proper evaluation of oocyte fertilization (presence of pronuclei) and embryo quality, but is indeed a prerequisite for precise procedures such as ICSI. The inverted microscope can be modified in order to allow micromanipulation procedures. First of all, it is important that a heating stage is present, to allow the work to be carried out at 37°C. It has been shown that oocytes are sensitive to a decrease in temperature, which can cause irreversible damage to the meiotic spindle[100]. Therefore, the ambient temperature control is of vital importance for the survival of oocytes. Two identical sets of two manipulators are mounted on the microscope; this allows manipulation

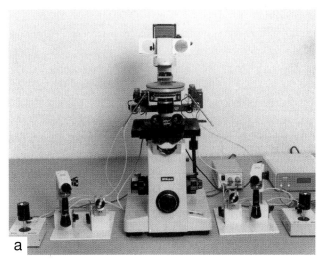
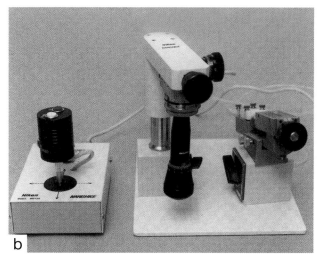

a

b

Figure 2 Equipment for intracytoplasmic sperm injection (ICSI). The equipment needed for microinjection involves an inverted microscope equipped with two identical sets of micromanipulators. Each set contains an electrically driven coarse positioning manipulator, a hydraulic remote control manipulator for fine movements and a micrometer-type injector allowing positive or negative pressure in the microtools. The inverted microscope is modified with a heating stage to allow manipulations at 37°C

of the holding and injection pipette on the left-hand and right-hand side, respectively. Both manipulators allow three-dimensional movements. An electrical manipulator allows coarse movements, whereas a hydraulic remote-control manipulator with a hanging joystick is used for fine movements. The microinjectors are used either to fix or to release the oocyte with the holding pipette or to aspirate and inject a spermatozoon with the injection pipette. The injectors consist of airtight glass syringes connected to the micropipette holders via flexible Teflon® tubing with airtight fitting. They are filled with mineral oil and the plunger is controlled by a micrometer. The whole set-up is placed on a vibration-proof table in order to avoid possible interfering vibration. Several companies supply microtools for holding and injection; however, some centers still prepare their own microtools, which demands much effort, time and extra equipment[21].

The ICSI procedure involves the injection of a single motile spermatozoon into the oocyte. The procedure is carried out in a plastic microinjection dish containing nine 10-μl droplets of HEPES-buffered medium covered with mineral oil (Figure 3). At the moment of injection, the central droplet is replaced by PVP and a fraction (approximately 1 μl) of the sperm suspension is added to the periphery of this droplet. The oocytes, denuded from their surrounding cumulus and corona cells, are then placed in the eight surrounding medium droplets. The viscous character

of the PVP solution slows down the motility of sperm cells, thereby facilitating the manipulation. It also allows better control of the fluid in the injection needle and it avoids sperm cells sticking to the pipette. Although microinjection without PVP is possible[101], and despite some concerns raised about the use of this potentially harmful agent[102], most centers continue to use PVP for microinjection.

During ICSI, special attention should be given to the following points:

(1) The selection and immobilization of a viable sperm cell;

(2) The correct positioning of the oocyte prior to injection;

(3) The rupture of the oolemma prior to the release of the sperm cell into the oocyte.

Figure 4 illustrates the whole injection procedure. In the injection pipette, which is filled with PVP, a single living morphologically normal-looking spermatozoon is aspirated. Viability is evidenced by the motility of the sperm cell, even if this is only a slight twitching of the tail. The sperm cell is then released in a perpendicular position to the injection pipette, which facilitates immobilization. Immobilization of a sperm cell involves rubbing the tail with the pipette against the bottom of the dish, which results in a breakage at one point, preferably below the midpiece. Immobilization

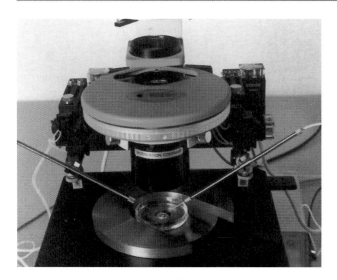

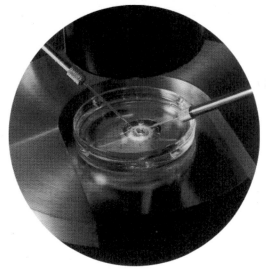

Figure 3 Microinjection dish. The intracytoplasmic sperm injection (ICSI) procedure is carried out on the heating stage of an inverted microscope at ×400 magnification. The holding and injection pipettes are fitted to a tool holder allowing three-dimensional movements and are connected to a micrometer-type microinjector. A typical injection dish contains a central droplet with polyvinylpyrrolidone to which a fraction of the sperm suspension is added. The eight surrounding droplets contain the oocytes

of spermatozoa has been proved to be important for oocyte activation, which is achieved by the release of sperm cytosolic factors via the ruptured membrane. Increased fertilization rates with ICSI have been reported following aggressive damage to the sperm tail plasma membrane[25,103].

After immobilization, the sperm cell is again aspirated, now tail-first, which will allow the injection of

a minimal volume of medium together with the sperm cell. The oocyte is held in position by means of minimal suction by the holding pipette. The polar body is located at the 6 o'clock position which avoids damage to the spindle[12,24]. Experiments in our laboratory using Hoechst colored oocytes for microinjection clearly showed no interference with the spindle if oocytes were injected with the polar body at the 6 o'clock position. If both the holding pipette and the oocyte are in perfect focus, the injection needle, containing the immobilized sperm cell near the tip, can be introduced in the equatorial plane of the oocyte at the 3 o'clock position. It is important to keep the tip of the injection pipette in permanent focus to ensure remaining in the equatorial plane of the oocyte. Passing through the zona pellucida is fairly easy and achieved by simply advancing the injection pipette. However, the oolemma is not always immediately pierced by simple injection of the needle, and often minimal suction needs to be applied. The ooplasm then enters into the injection pipette and sudden acceleration of the flow indicates membrane rupture. The aspiration is immediately stopped and the sperm cell is then slowly released into the oocyte with a minimal volume of medium, and the pipette can be withdrawn carefully.

Different patterns of oolemma breakage have been described depending on whether the ooplasm breaks during insertion of the pipette, whether slight or stronger aspiration of the ooplasm is needed or whether breakage of the oolemma in another place has to be attempted[24,104]. Immediate rupture of the oolemma without any aspiration has been associated with lower oocyte survival rates and a higher incidence of abnormal fertilization (≥ 3 pronuclei)[24,104]. Normal fertilization rates (two pronuclei) per number of intact oocytes after ICSI do not significantly differ for the different modes of oolemma rupture[24]. Developmental capacity, on the other hand, can be influenced by the type of oolemma breakage: the best embryos are more usually generated following breakage by only slight suction[24].

The moment of denudation relative to oocyte pick-up (immediately or 4 h later) does not influence the ICSI results[23]. However, the morphology of the injected spermatozoon is related to the fertilization outcome of the procedure as well as to the pregnancy outcome[26].

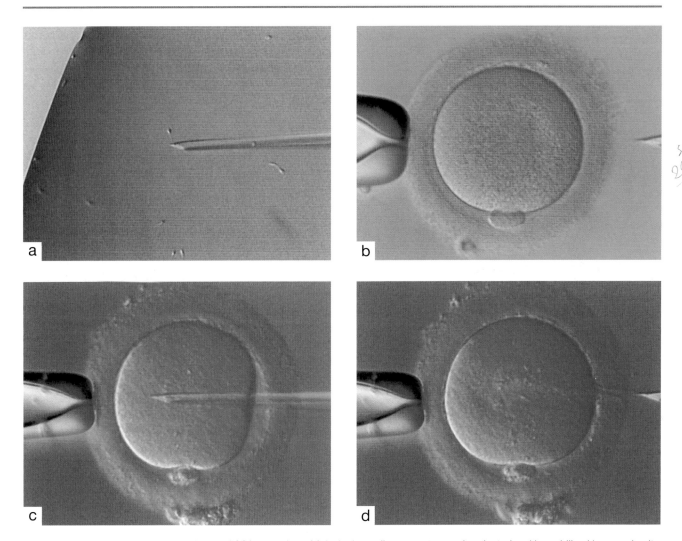

Figure 4 Intracytoplasmic sperm injection (ICSI) procedure. (a) A single motile spermatozoon is selected and immobilized by pressing its tail between the microneedle and the bottom of the dish. The sperm cell is then aspirated tail-first into the injection pipette. (b) A mature oocyte is fixed by the holding pipette with the polar body at the 6 o'clock position. The sperm cell is brought to the tip of the injection pipette. (c) The injection pipette is introduced at the 3 o'clock position and rupture of the oolemma is ascertained by slight suction. The sperm cell is delivered into the oocyte with a minimal volume of medium and the pipette can be withdrawn carefully. (d) A single sperm cell can be seen in the center of the ooplasm

OUTCOME PARAMETERS OF ICSI: FERTILIZATION AND EMBRYO CLEAVAGE

After the injection procedure, oocytes are rinsed and cultured in microdroplets covered with lightweight paraffin oil. The conditions are similar to those for IVF inseminated oocytes, i.e. they are kept at 37°C in an atmosphere of 5% O_2, 5% CO_2 and 90% N_2. The injected oocytes can be examined for intactness and fertilization at about 16–18 h after ICSI[105]. An average damage rate of approximately 10% of the injected oocytes can be expected, irrespective of the origin of the sperm used[68,82] (Figure 5). The number and aspect

of polar bodies and pronuclei are recorded (Figure 6). Oocytes are considered to be normally fertilized when two individualized or fragmented polar bodies are present together with two clearly visible pronuclei that contain nucleoli. The fertilization rate after ICSI using ejaculated spermatozoa can be expected to be 60–70% when expressed per number of injected oocytes[82]. The normal fertilization rate for ICSI using the three other types of sperm (fresh and frozen–thawed epididymal sperm and testicular sperm) is somewhat lower (55–60%) than with ejaculated sperm[82] (Figure 5). Abnormal fertilization may occur as one-pronuclear oocytes (approximately 3% of the injected oocytes)[82].

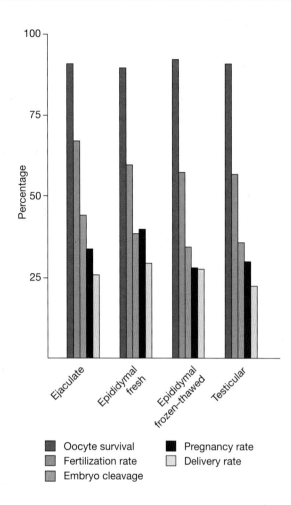

Figure 5 Sperm origin and outcome of intracytoplasmic sperm injection (ICSI). When sperm of different origins are used, similar results are obtained regarding oocyte intactness after ICSI, fertilization rates, embryo cleavage, pregnancy rates and delivery rates. The number of intact oocytes and the number of normally fertilized oocytes (two pronuclei) are expressed per number of oocytes injected. Embryo cleavage is expressed as the number of embryos that are transferred or frozen, as a percentage of the injected oocytes. Pregnancy rates are expressed per cycle with known human chorionic gonadotropin (hCG) outcome, and delivery rates are expressed per transfer with known pregnancy outcome. The data represent a summary of 7374 ICSI cycles performed between 1991 and 1997, except that the pregnancy rates were calculated for only the ICSI cycles performed between 1991 and 1996

If such abnormally fertilized one-pronuclear oocytes cleave, they are not transferred, because they are likely to be parthenogenetically activated as a result of mechanical or chemical factors[106,107]. The occasional finding of three-pronuclear oocytes (approximately 4%)[82] after injection of a single spermatozoon into the ooplasm is probably caused by non-extrusion of the

second polar body at the time of fertilization[107]. Embryos resulting from three-pronuclear oocytes are not transferred to patients. Abnormal fertilization occurs to a similar extent in the four different groups of spermatozoa[82]. Because one- and three-pronuclear oocytes may have similar potential to result in good-quality embryos as compared with two-pronuclear oocytes, it is of major importance to observe the presence of two pronuclei to ascertain normal fertilization. In order to meet this requirement, oocytes should be injected in the afternoon, followed by evaluation of fertilization in the early morning of the next day. However, within a busy ICSI program, including many difficult cases of extreme oligozoospermia and surgically retrieved spermatozoa, this tight schedule cannot always be respected.

Human embryos are selected for transfer using morphology at the cleaving and blastocyst stages. However, recently, additional zygote morphology has been related to implantation and pregnancy[108,109]. The zygotes are then scored according to the distribution, number and size of nucleoli within each nucleus (so-called zygote scoring or pronuclear scoring). Additionally, alignment and size of the pronuclei, as well as their location within the cytoplasm, seems to matter. Morphological analysis of both zygotes and embryos should of course be integrated with the *in vitro* growth rate in order to be highly predictable for IVF outcome[110]. Zygote scoring seems an efficient tool for embryo selection; however, different scoring systems have been published so far, and there is need for standardization[111].

The exceptional circumstances in which no injected oocytes fertilize normally are associated with only very few metaphase-II oocytes being available for ICSI, only totally immotile spermatozoa being available for the injection, gross abnormalities being present in the oocytes, round-headed spermatozoa being injected or all oocytes being damaged in the injection procedure. In these cases, most of the patients involved achieve fertilization in a subsequent cycle[112].

Post-fertilization, about 90% of 2-PN oocytes obtained by ICSI enter cleavage, resulting in multicellular embryos. Cleavage characteristics of the fertilized oocytes are evaluated daily. Normally developing, good-quality embryos reach the four- and eight-cell stage, respectively, on day 2 and in the morning of day 3 post-microinjection (Figure 7). Numbers and sizes of blastomeres and the presence of anucleate

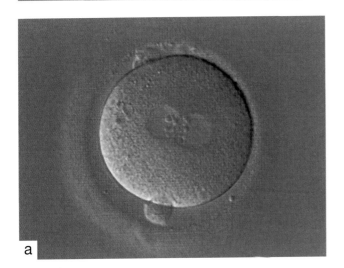

a

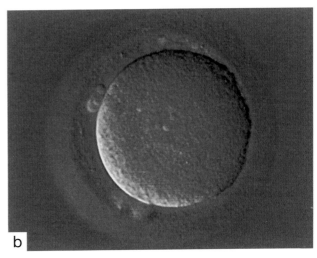

b

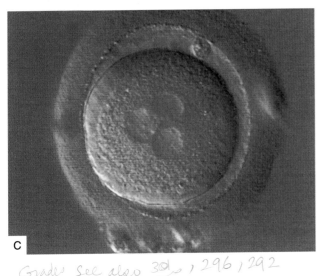

c

Gradu See also 301, 296, 292

Figure 6 Fertilization outcome after intracytoplasmic sperm injection (ICSI). Oocytes are considered to be normally fertilized when two individualized or fragmented polar bodies are present together with two clearly visible pronuclei that contain nucleoli (a). Abnormal fertilization may occur as one-pronuclear oocytes (b), probably owing to parthenogenetic activation. The occasional finding of three-pronuclear oocytes (c) after injection of a single spermatozoon into the ooplasmic is probably caused by non-extrusion of the second polar body at the time of fertilization

cytoplasmic fragments are recorded (Figure 8). Additional scoring criteria are the possible presence of vacuoles, cytoplasmic granulation and/or multinucleation. The cleaving embryos are scored according to equality of size of the blastomeres and proportion of anucleate fragments[113]. Four categories are distinguished within this scoring system. Type A or excellent-quality embryos are defined as embryos without anuclear fragments. This category includes embryos in which all blastomeres are of an equal size as well as embryos with non-equally sized blastomeres. Type B or good-quality embryos have blastomeres of non-equal size and a maximum of 20% of the volume of the embryo filled with anucleate fragments. In the third category, type C or fair-quality embryos, anucleate fragments represent 21–50% of the volume of the embryo. Type D or poor-quality embryos have anucleate fragments present in more than 50% of the

volume of the embryo. These embryos cannot be used for transfer to patients. Cleaved embryos with less than one-half of their volume filled with anucleate fragments (types A, B and C) are eligible for transfer. Supernumerary embryos with less than 20% of anucleate fragments (types A and B) can be cryopreserved on day 2 or day 3 after oocyte retrieval by means of a slow-freezing protocol with dimethylsulfoxide[114]. About two-thirds of the two-pronuclear oocytes after ICSI develop into cleaved embryos that are suitable for transfer or freezing[36,82]. Embryo replacement of at least one embryo is possible in approximately 90% of the treatment cycles and is not influenced by the source of spermatozoa used[36,82].

Nowadays, most centers perform embryo transfers on day 3 after oocyte retrieval. At that time, the embryos are expected to be at the eight-cell stage. As the embryonic genome is fully activated after the eight-cell stage[115], it may indeed be beneficial to evaluate embryos at least until after the transition from maternal to embryonic genome, making it possible to identify those embryos with a better developmental potential.

Today, a new generation of commercially available sequential culture media allows the culture of human

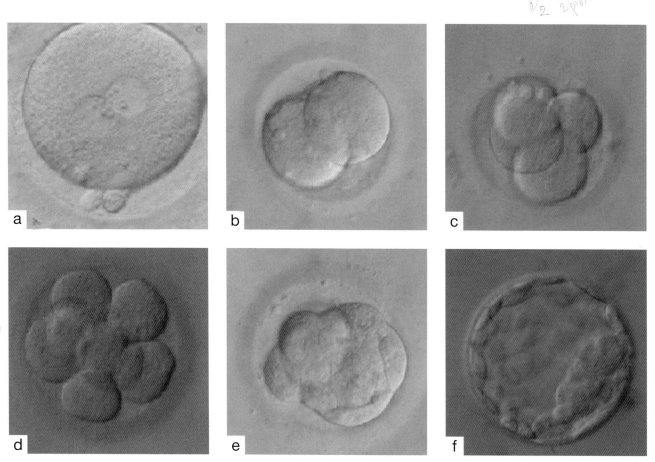

Figure 7 Embryo cleavage after intracytoplasmic sperm injection (ICSI). Only embryos resulting from normally fertilized oocytes (a) will be transferred to patients. Embryo cleavage is evaluated daily. Two-cell embryos (b), four-cell embryos (c) and eight-cell embryos (d) are usually obtained on day 1 (late afternoon), on day 2 and in the morning of day 3, respectively. The blastomere number is recorded and the embryos are scored according to equality of size of the blastomeres and the presence of anucleate cytoplasmic fragments[113]. On day 4 (sometimes already on day 3), a certain degree of compaction can be observed (e). For blastocyst (f) scoring, the classification system introduced by Gardner and Schoolcraft is used[122]. Embryo replacement can be done on day 3 (eight-cell stage) or on day 5 (blastocyst stage)

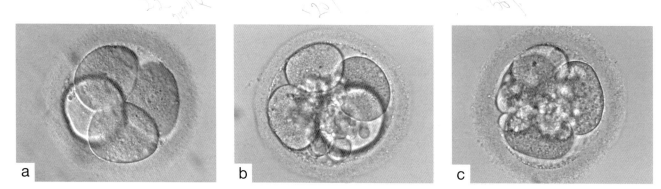

Figure 8 This figure illustrates a day-2 four-cell embryo. The embryos are scored according to equality of size of the blastomeres and proportion of anucleate cytoplasmic fragments[118]. (a) This represents a type A or excellent-quality embryo without anuclear fragments. Type B or good-quality embryos (b) have a maximum of 20% of the volume of the embryo filled with anucleate fragments. In type C or fair-quality embryos (c), anucleate fragments represent 21–50% of the volume of the embryo. Embryo replacement is usually carried out about 72 h after the microinjection procedure (day 3, eight-cell stage)

embryos up to the blastocyst stage (day 5 or 6)[116]. On day 4 (sometimes already on day 3), a certain degree of compaction can be observed. Compaction in the mammalian pre-embryo is a fundamental event that leads to the formation of the trophectoderm, the inner cell mass and the blastocoel. Full compaction (16- to 32-cell stage) is followed by immediate cavitation and blastocoel expansion[117]. For blastocyst scoring, the classification system introduced by Gardner and associates can be used[118]. A distinction between early and expanded blastocysts is made and the latter category is further scored according to the quality of the inner cell mass and the trophectoderm. The possibility of prolonged human embryo culture allows for day-5 or blastocyst transfers. Preferably, expanded blastocysts with a cohesive trophectoderm and a clear inner cell mass are transferred. Possible advantages of blastocyst transfer are a better embryo selection and a better synchronization between embryo and endometrium, which may result in higher implantation rates per blastocyst transferred[119,120]. This in turn would allow replacement of fewer embryos, thereby decreasing the number of multiple pregnancies[121]. Today, however, the superiority of blastocyst transfer as compared to early embryo transfer remains to be proven. Only a limited number of randomized controlled studies are available at present, some showing the benefit of blastocyst transfer, others showing no advantages of day 5 transfers over day-3 transfers[120–124].

As mentioned above, supernumerary embryos can be cryopreserved on day 2 or day 3 after oocyte retrieval[114]. Alternatively, embryos are frozen at the blastocyst stage on day 5 or day 6 using glycerol and sucrose as cryoprotectant agents[125].

Within an ICSI program, the embryo transfer policy is similar to that of conventional IVF. Most centers perform embryo transfers on day 3; however, day-5 or blastocyst transfers are well established as well, especially in combination with preimplantation genetic diagnosis (PGD)[126] or aneuploidy screening (PGD-AS)[127]. The number of embryos transferred depends on the age of the woman, on the rank of the trial and on the embryo quality. In women aged < 35 years having a first or second ICSI attempt, preference is given to transfer only one excellent or good-quality embryo. In other cases, two or more embryos may be replaced into the uterus. Higher pregnancy rates can be obtained when elective transfer of two or three embryos is possible[128]; however, it is important to limit

the number of embryos transferred to avoid multiple pregnancies. In both IVF and ICSI, the usual practice of transferring two or more embryos in order to achieve higher pregnancy rates results in a high incidence of multiple pregnancies and births. Of 2840 live-born ICSI children, 1499 children (52.8%) were from singleton pregnancies, 1228 (43.2%) were from twin pregnancies and 113 (4.0%) were from triplet pregnancies[129]. Multiple pregnancy carries additional risks for both mother and offspring and more elaborate monitoring of the pregnancy is required. Obstetric and neonatal complications associated with multiple pregnancy have been discussed by Hazekamp and colleagues[130]. Strategies for reducing the multiple pregnancies have been identified and debated[130–132]. Elective single embryo transfer for these patients with an increased risk of multiple birth would achieve the goal of a single healthy child as a result of IVF or ICSI treatment. Identification of high implantation embryos on the one hand and proper identification of patients at risk of a twin pregnancy after double embryo transfer on the other hand are equally important[131,132].

CLINICAL APPLICATION AND RESULTS

The number of ICSI cycles using ejaculated, epididymal and testicular sperm has increased significantly over the years since ICSI started to be used clinically. A world survey on overall ICSI results[133] illustrates the fast transition from an experimental procedure to a routinely applied clinical procedure. It indicates general acceptance and worldwide interest in the use of this procedure for the treatment of male-factor infertility.

Results of 7 years of ICSI practice (1991–97) have been reported before[82]. Here we present the results of 2000 and 2001, involving 2431 ICSI cycles in which 21 572 metaphase-II oocytes were injected. The ICSI procedure could not be carried out in 50 cycles (2.0%) because there were no cumulus–oocyte complexes or metaphase-II oocytes (22 cycles) or because no spermatozoa were available for the microinjection procedure (28 cycles, mainly testicular biopsy cases). The majority of cycles involved injection with ejaculated sperm (88.9%). Epididymal sperm was used in only 1.8% of the cycles, and in 9.4% of the cycles spermatozoa were retrieved from the testis. In total, 25 721 cumulus–oocyte complexes were retrieved, i.e. a mean of 10.6 per treatment cycle. Ninety-five per cent of the retrieved cumulus–oocyte complexes contained an intact oocyte. Of these, 8.7% were in the germinal-vesicle stage, 2.7% were in the metaphase-I stage and 88.6% represented mature metaphase-II oocytes. ICSI was performed on most of the mature oocytes (99.8%) and an oocyte survival rate of 92.6% was obtained. The oocyte survival rate was similar in the four categories of sperm cell origin (Table 2).

Normal fertilization (two pronuclei) was obtained in 80.1% of the intact oocytes or in 74.2% of the injected oocytes (Table 2). Normal fertilization rates with ejaculated sperm (75.7% per injected oocyte) were higher than with epididymal (72.1%) or testicular sperm (respectively 60.0% and 63.8% with fresh and frozen–thawed testicular sperm) (Table 2). Abnormal fertilization (one or ≥3 pronuclei) occurred, respectively, in 5.1% and 3.5% of the injected oocytes.

Embryo cleavage was evaluated on a daily basis. The percentages of 2-PN oocytes developing into excellent, good-quality and fair-quality embryos according to the different types of spermatozoa used for ICSI are summarized in Table 2. On day 2, 80.3% of the 2-PN oocytes resulted in excellent and good quality embryos. On day 3, this percentage was 72.9%. More excellent and good-quality embryos were obtained in the group using ejaculated spermatozoa than in the groups with epididymal and testicular sperm cells. The percentage of eight-cell embryos on day 3 (including >8-cell, compacting and compact embryos) varied between 34.8 and 47.5%. The total blastocyst formation rate per 2-PN oocytes was 44.7%; however, when including only good-quality blastocysts (i.e. expanded blastocysts with a cohesive trophectoderm and a clear inner cell mass), this formation rate was limited to 26.6%. More good-quality blastocysts were obtained when ejaculated (27.1%), epididymal (27.7%) and frozen testicular (26.2%) sperm cells were used for ICSI than when fresh testicular sperm cells were used for microinjection (14.1%). The percentages of embryos actually transferred were similar for the four types of spermatozoa and varied between 32.0 and 38.8%.

Cryopreservation of supernumerary embryos was postponed until day 5 and/or day 6, allowing a better selection of embryos actually frozen. More blastocysts were frozen when ejaculated (19.9%) or epididymal (19.0%) sperm cells were used for ICSI than when

testicular sperm cells were used (respectively, 11.2% and 11.9% with fresh and frozen–thawed testicular sperm). Overall, about half of the 2-PN oocytes (53.7%) resulted in embryos available for transfer or cryopreservation for the patients. This percentage did not differ between the different sperm categories (Table 2).

Replacement of at least one embryo was possible in 2293 of the 2431 ICSI treatment cycles (94.3%). As indicated in Table 3, the transfer rate was similar across the four sperm groups used for ICSI, varying from 92.5 to 95.3%. In 2000, mainly day-2 transfers were performed, whereas in 2001 we switched from day-2 to day-3 transfers. Of the 2293 embryo replacement cycles, 822 were on day 2, 1100 were on day 3 and 360 were on day 5. Only occasionally day-4 transfers (ten cycles) were performed, and one transfer involved a day-6 transfer. On average, 2.4 ± 0.8 embryos (range 1–8) were replaced per treatment cycle. Fourteen transfer cycles remained with an unknown serum hCG outcome, whereas for all other transfer cycles (*n* = 2279) the outcome was known. The overall pregnancy rates per transfer with known hCG outcome were similar for the four types of spermatozoa, varying from 32.4 to 35.7% per transfer (Table 3, see also Figure 5, ICSI cycles performed between 1991 and 1996). The overall pregnancy rate per treatment cycle was 32.8%. The implantation rate per embryo transferred was 15.1%, not different between the four sperm groups, except for the higher implantation rate obtained with embryos resulting from ICSI with epididymal sperm cells. All but 35 (27 in the ejaculated semen group, one in the epididymal spermatozoa group, four in the freshly collected testicular spermatozoa group and three in the frozen–thawed testicular spermatozoa group) embryo replacements with positive serum hCG resulted in a known outcome until delivery. Delivery rates per transfer varied from 23.4 to 28.2%.

FOLLOW-UP OF ICSI PREGNANCIES AND CHILDREN

The number of centers performing ICSI today and the number of ICSI cycles performed over the years indicates a general acceptance and worldwide interest in the use of this technique. However, the microinjection procedure remains invasive, and children are born

Table 2 Sperm origin, oocyte damage and pronuclear status and embryo development after intracytoplasmic sperm injection (ICSI) (results 2000–01)

| | Ejaculated semen | Epididymal semen | Testicular semen | | Total |
			Fresh	Frozen–thawed	
Number of cycles	2160	43	122	106	2431
Number of oocytes undergoing ICSI	19 027	373	1215	957	21 572
Intact oocytes (%)	92.5	93.8	92.1	94.1	92.6
Injected oocytes (%) with					
one pronucleus	4.8	9.1	8.3	5.9	5.1
two pronuclei	75.7	72.1	60.0	63.8	74.2
three or more pronuclei	3.5	2.1	3.3	3.9	3.5
Number of two-pronuclear oocytes	14 396	269	729	611	16 005
Embryonic development (day 2)					
excellent embryos (%)	18.8	10.0	14.5	14.2	18.3
good-quality embryos (%)	62.1	62.8	58.0	64.0	62.0
fair-quality embryos (%)	10.6	13.4	12.2	12.1	10.8
Embryonic development (day 3)					
excellent embryos (%)	15.0	5.3	11.5	9.9	14.5
good-quality embryos (%)	58.7	58.4	53.2	57.3	58.4
fair-quality embryos (%)	12.4	15.5	13.6	13.1	12.5
Embryonic development (day 5)					
blastocysts (%)	45.6	43.5	32.7	37.6	44.7
good-quality blastocysts (%)	27.1	27.7	14.1	26.2	26.6
Transfer and cryopreservation					
transferred embryos (%)	34.2	32.0	38.0	38.8	34.5
frozen embryos (%)	19.9	19.0	11.2	11.9	19.2

Table 3 Sperm origin and outcome of embryo transfers after intracytoplasmic sperm injection (ICSI) (results 2000–01)

| | Ejaculated semen | Epididymal semen | Testicular semen | | Total |
			Fresh	Frozen–thawed	
Number of cycles	2160	43	122	106	2431
Number of transfers	2040	41	114	98	2293
Transfer rate (%)	94.4	95.3	93.4	92.5	94.3
Number of embryos transferred					
mean ± SD	2.4 ± 0.9	2.1 ± 0.5	2.4 ± 0.8	2.4 ± 0.8	2.4 ± 0.8
range	(1–8)	(1–3)	(1–5)	(1–4)	(1–8)
Number of pregnancies	708	14	36	35	793
Number of transfers (known hCG outcome)	2030	40	111	98	2279
Pregnancy rate per transfer* (%)	34.9	35.0	32.4	35.7	34.8
Pregnancy rate per cycle* (%)	32.9	33.0	30.3	33.0	32.8
Implantation rate (%)[†]	15.0	21.4	14.0	15.1	15.1
Delivery rate per transfer[‡](%)	23.8	28.2	23.4	25.3	24.2

*With known human chorionic gonadotropin (hCG) outcome; [†]number of fetal heart beats (at 7 weeks) as a percentage of the number of embryos replaced; [‡]with known outcome until delivery after replacement of ICSI embryos using sperm (epididymal and testicular) which could never have been used successfully for spontaneous conception or any other form of assisted reproductive technologies (ART) treatment. The occasional use of immature sperm from the epididymis or testis may raise questions concerning genomic imprinting[134,135]. Another concern is the fertility status of the resulting offspring: if the spermatogenic defect is genetic in origin, there is a potential risk of transmitting this defect to future offspring[136]. To evaluate the safety of ICSI we compared neonatal outcome and the incidence of congenital malformations during pregnancy and at birth for 2955 IVF and 2840 ICSI children[129]. This follow-up study included genetic counseling and eventual prenatal karyotype analysis, followed by a physical examination of the children at 2 months, 1 year and 2 years. Prenatal testing was initially strongly recommended; nowadays, couples are informed about the risk factors and are free to choose prenatal testing or not. This comparison of IVF and ICSI children did not show any increased risk of major malformations and neonatal complications in the ICSI group. Major malformations (defined as those causing functional impairment or requiring surgical correction) occurred in 3.4% of the ICSI live-born children and in 3.8% of the IVF children (similar to that found in general population registries). The malformation rate in ICSI was not related to sperm origin or sperm quality. ICSI pregnancy complications such as increased risk for prematurity and low birth weight are related only to gestation multiplicity[137].

Abnormal fetal karyotypes were found in 47 cases out of 1586, i.e. 2.96%[138]. There were 25 (1.58%) *de novo* chromosomal aberrations: ten were sex-chromosomal aberrations (0.63%) and 15 were autosomal aberrations (0.95%), either numerical ($n = 8$) or structural ($n = 7$). In 17/22 inherited cases (21 balanced, one unbalanced), the chromosomal structural defect was inherited from the father. In comparison with a general neonatal population, these data indicate: first, a slight but significant increase in *de novo* sex chromosomal aneuploidy (0.6% instead of 0.2%) and structural autosomal abnormalities (0.4% instead of 0.07%), which was related to sperm concentration and motility; and second, an increased number of inherited (mostly from the infertile father) structural aberrations.

Initial reports of medical and developmental outcome of ICSI children at 1 and 2 years of age clearly indicate that ongoing developmental follow-up of children conceived by ICSI is needed[139–141].

While awaiting the results of other follow-up studies, patients should be informed – before starting treatment – of the existing data: the risk of transmitting chromosomal aberrations, the risk of *de novo* sex chromosomal and structural aberrations and the risk of transmitting fertility problems to the offspring. Patients should also be reassured that there seems to be no higher incidence of major congenital malformations in children born after ICSI.

As for conventional IVF, the major problem of ICSI outcome is the substantial number of multiple gestations and births. It is reasonable to assume that well over one million children have been born worldwide after IVF and ICSI. However, about half of these children are not from singleton pregnancies. Most multiple gestations are twin pregnancies, but triplet and higher-order gestations do occur. The most important challenge for all ART centers is a reduction in multiple pregnancies by limiting the number of transferred embryos to one or two. The magnitude of the problems generated by these multiple gestations is far superior in number compared with the occurrence of major malformations or chromosomal anomalies.

ACKNOWLEDGMENTS

The authors wish to acknowledge the assistance of the clinical, scientific, nursing and technical staff of the Centers for Reproductive Medicine and Genetics of the Medical Campus of the Dutch-speaking Brussels Free University. The work was supported by grants from the Fund for Scientific Research – Flanders.

REFERENCES

1. Steptoe PC, Edwards RG. Birth after the re-implantation of a human embryo. Lancet 1978; 2: 366
2. Cohen J, Malter H, Fehilly C, et al. Implantation of embryos after partial opening of oocyte zona pellucida to facilitate sperm penetration. Lancet 1988; 2: 162
3. Cohen J, Malter H, Wright G, et al. Partial zona dissection of human oocytes when failure of zona pellucida is anticipated. Hum Reprod 1989; 4: 435–42

4. Cohen J, Talansky BE, Malter HM, et al. Microsurgical fertilization and teratozoospermia. Hum Reprod 1991; 6: 118–23

5. Tucker MJ, Bishop FM, Cohen J, et al. Routine application of partial zona dissection for male factor infertility. Hum Reprod 1991; 6: 676–81

6. Laws-King A, Trounson A, Sathananthan H, et al. Fertilization of human oocytes by microinjection of a single spermatozoon under the zona pellucida. Fertil Steril 1987; 48: 637–42

7. Ng SC, Bongso A, Ratnam SS, et al. Pregnancy after transfer of sperm under zona. Lancet 1988; 2: 790

8. Bongso TA, Sathananthan AH, Wong C, et al. Human fertilization by microinjection of immotile spermatozoa. Hum Reprod 1989; 4: 175–9

9. Palermo G, Joris H, Devroey P, et al. Induction of acrosome reaction in human spermatozoa used for subzonal insemination. Hum Reprod 1992; 7: 248–54

10. Lanzendorf SE, Maloney MK, Veeck LL, et al. A preclinical evaluation of pronuclear formation by microinjection of human spermatozoa into human oocytes. Fertil Steril 1988; 49: 835–42

11. Iritani A. Micromanipulation of gametes for in vitro assisted fertilization. Mol Reprod Dev 1991; 28: 199–207

12. Palermo G, Joris H, Devroey P, et al. Pregnancies after intracytoplasmic injection of a single spermatozoon into an oocyte. Lancet 1992; 340: 17–18

13. Palermo G, Joris H, Devroey P, et al. Sperm characteristics and outcome of human assisted fertilization by subzonal insemination and intracytoplasmic sperm injection. Fertil Steril 1993; 59: 826–35

14. Van Steirteghem AC, Liu J, Nagy Z, et al. Use of assisted fertilization. Hum Reprod 1993; 8: 1784–5

15. Van Steirteghem AC, Liu J, Joris H, et al. Higher success rate by intracytoplasmic sperm injection than by subzonal insemination. Report of a second series of 300 consecutive treatment cycles. Hum Reprod 1993; 8: 1055–60

16. Van Steirteghem AC, Nagy Z, Joris H, et al. High fertilization and implantation rates after intracytoplasmic sperm injection. Hum Reprod 1993; 8: 1061–6

17. Payne D, Flaherty SP, Jefferey R, et al. Successful treatment of severe male factor infertility in 100 consecutive cycles using intracytoplasmic sperm injection. Hum Reprod 1994; 9: 2051–7

18. Redgment CJ, Yang D, Tsirigotis M, et al. Experience with assisted fertilization in severe male factor infertility and unexplained failed fertilization in vitro. Hum Reprod 1994; 9: 680–3

19. Mansour RT, Aboulghar MA, Serour GI, et al. The effect of sperm parameters on the outcome of intracytoplasmic sperm injection. Fertil Steril 1995; 64: 982–6

20. Van Steirteghem A, Verheyen G, Tournaye H, et al. Assisted reproductive technology by intracytoplasmic sperm injection in male-factor infertility. Curr Opin Urol 1996; 6: 333–9

21. Joris H, Nagy Z, Van de Velde H, et al. Intracytoplasmic sperm injection: laboratory set-up and injection procedure. Hum Reprod 1998; 13 (Suppl 1): 76–86

22. Van de Velde H, Nagy ZP, Joris H, et al. The effects of different hyaluronidase concentrations and mechanical procedures for cumulus–corona cell removal on the outcome of ICSI. Hum Reprod 1997; 12: 2246–50

23. Van de Velde H, De Vos A, Joris H, et al. Effect of timing of oocyte denudation and micro-injection on survival, fertilization and embryo quality after intracytoplasmic sperm injection. Hum Reprod 1998; 13: 3160–4

24. Nagy ZP, Liu J, Joris H, et al. The influence of the site of sperm deposition and mode of oolemma breakage at intracytoplasmic sperm injection on fertilization and embryo development rates. Hum Reprod 1995; 10: 3171–7

25. Palermo GD, Schlegle PN, Colombero LT, et al. Aggressive sperm immobilization prior to intracytoplasmic sperm injection with immature spermatozoa improves fertilization and pregnancy rates. Hum Reprod 1996; 11: 1023–9

26. De Vos A, Van de Velde H, Joris H, et al. Influence of individual sperm morphology on fertilization, embryo morphology and pregnancy outcome of intracytoplasmic sperm injection (ICSI). Fertil Steril 2003; 79: 42–8

27. Riedel HH, Hubner F, Ensslen SC, et al. Minimal andrological requirements for in vitro fertilization. Hum Reprod 1989; 4: 73–7

28. Fishel SB, Edwards RG. Essentials of fertilization. In Edwards RG, Purdy JM, eds. Human Conception In Vitro. London: Academic Press, 1982: 193–5

29. Edwards RG, Fishel SB, Cohen J, et al. Factors influencing the success of in vitro fertilization for alleviating human infertility. J In Vitro Fertil Embryo Transf 1984; 1: 3–23

30. Cohen J, Edwards RG, Fehilly C, et al. In vitro fertilization: a treatment for male infertility. Fertil Steril 1985; 43: 422–32

31. Oehninger S, Acosta AA, Morshedi M, et al. Corrective measures and pregnancy outcome in in vitro fertilization in patients with severe sperm morphology abnormalities. Fertil Steril 1988; 50: 283–7

32. Ombelet W, Fourie FL, Vandeput H, et al. Teratozoospermia and in vitro fertilization; a randomized prospective study. Hum Reprod 1994; 9: 1479–84

33. Kruger TF, Menkveld R, Stander FSH, et al. Sperm morphologic features as a prognostic factor in in vitro fertilization. Fertil Steril 1986; 46: 1118–23

34. Fishel S, Lisi F, Rinaldi L, et al. Intracytoplasmic sperm injection (ICSI) versus high insemination concentration (HIC) for human conception in vitro. Reprod Fertil Dev 1995; 7: 169–75

35. Oehninger S, Kruger TF, Simon T, et al. A comparative analysis of embryo implantation potential in patients with severe teratozoospermia undergoing in-vitro fertilization with high insemination concentration or intracytoplasmic sperm injection. Hum Reprod 1996; 11: 1086–9

36. Van Steirteghem A, Tournaye H, Van der Elst J, et al. Intracytoplasmic sperm injection three years after the birth of the first ICSI child. Hum Reprod 1995; 10: 2527–8

37. Nagy ZP, Liu J, Joris H, et al. The result of intracytoplasmic sperm injection is not related to any of the three basic sperm parameters. Hum Reprod 1995; 10: 1123–9

38. Tournaye H, Liu J, Nagy Z, et al. The use of testicular sperm for intracytoplasmic sperm injection in patients with necrospermia. Fertil Steril 1996; 66: 331–4

39. Liu J, Nagy Z, Joris H, et al. Successful fertilization and establishment of pregnancies after intracytoplasmic sperm injection in patients with globozoospermia. Hum Reprod 1995; 10: 626–9

40. Nagy ZP, Verheyen G, Liu J, et al. Results of 55 intracytoplasmic sperm injection cycles in the treatment of male-immunological infertility. Hum Reprod 1995; 10: 1775–80

41. Lanzendorf S, Maloney M, Ackerman S, et al. Fertilizing potential of acrosome defective sperm following microsurgical injection into eggs. Gamete Res 1988; 19: 329–37

42. Lundin K, Sjorgen A, Nilsson L, et al. Fertilization and pregnancy after intracytoplasmic microinjection of acrosomeless spermatozoa. Fertil Steril 1994; 62: 1266–7

43. Bourne H, Lui DY, Clarke GN, et al. Normal fertilization and embryo development by intracytoplasmic sperm injection of round headed acrosomeless sperm. Fertil Steril 1995; 65: 1329–32

44. Silber SJ, Nagy ZP, Liu J, et al. Conventional in-vitro fertilization versus intracytoplasmic sperm injection for patients requiring microsurgical sperm aspiration. Hum Reprod 1994; 9: 1705–9

45. Tournaye H, Devroey P, Liu J, et al. Microsurgical epididymal sperm aspiration and intracytoplasmic sperm injection: a new effective approach to infertility as a result of congenital bilateral absence of the vas deferens. Fertil Steril 1994; 61: 1045–51

46. Mansour RT, Aboulghar MA, Serour GI, et al. Intracytoplasmic sperm injection using microsurgically retrieved epididymal and testicular sperm. Fertil Steril 1996; 65: 566–72

47. Schoysman R, Vanderzwalmen P, Nijs M, et al. Successful fertilization by testicular spermatozoa in an invitro fertilization program. Hum Reprod 1993; 8: 1339–40

48. Silber SJ, Van Steirteghem AC, Liu J, et al. High fertilization and pregnancy rate after intracytoplasmic sperm injection with spermatozoa obtained from testicle biopsy. Hum Reprod 1995; 10: 148–52

49. Devroey P, Liu J, Nagy Z, et al. Normal fertilization of human oocytes after testicular sperm extraction and ICSI. Fertil Steril 1994; 62: 639–41

50. Shrivastav P, Nadkarni P, Wensvoort S, et al. Percutaneous epididymal sperm aspiration for obstructive azoospermia. Hum Reprod 1994; 9: 2058–61

51. Tsirigotis M, Pelekanos M, Beski S, et al. Cumulative experience of percutaneous epididymal sperm aspiration (PESA) with intracytoplasmic sperm injection. J Assist Reprod Genet 1996; 13: 315–19

52. Friedler S, Riedel A, Schachter M, et al. Outcome of first and repeated testicular sperm extraction and ICSI in patients with non-obstructive azoospermia. Hum Reprod 2002; 17: 2356–61

53. Bourne H, Watkins W, Speirs A, et al. Pregnancies after intracytoplasmic sperm injection of sperm collected by fine needle biopsy of the testis. Fertil Steril 1995; 64: 433–6

54. Tournaye H, Clasen K, Aytoz A, et al. Fine needle aspiration versus open biopsy for testicular sperm recovery: a controlled study in azoospermic patients with normal spermatogenesis. Hum Reprod 1998; 13: 901–4

55. Tournaye H. Surgical sperm recovery for intracytoplasmic sperm injection: which method is to be preferred? Hum Reprod 1999; 14 (Suppl 1): 71–81

56. Devroey P, Liu J, Nagy P, et al. Pregnancies after testicular extraction and intracytoplasmic sperm injection in non-obstructive azoospermia. Hum Reprod 1995; 10: 1457–60

57. Tournaye H, Camus M, Goossens A, et al. Recent concepts in the management of infertility because of non-obstructive azoospermia. Hum Reprod 1995; 10 (Suppl 1): 115–19

58. Kahraman S, Ozgur S, Alatas C, et al. Fertility with testicular sperm extraction and intracytoplasmic sperm injection in non-obstructive azoospermic men. Hum Reprod 1996; 11: 756–60

59. Silber S, Van Steirteghem AC, Nagy Z, et al. Normal pregnancies resulting from testicular sperm extraction and intracytoplasmic sperm injection for azoospermia due to maturation arrest. Fertil Steril 1996; 66: 110–17

60. Tournaye H, Verheyen G, Nagy P, et al. Are there any predictive factors for successful testicular sperm recovery in azoospermic patients? Hum Reprod 1997; 12: 80–6

61. Verheyen G, De Croo I, Tournaye H, et al. Comparison of four mechanical methods to retrieve spermatozoa from testicular tissue. Hum Reprod 1995; 10: 2956–9

62. Nagy P, Verheyen G, Tournaye H, et al. An improved treatment procedure for testicular biopsy specimens offers more efficient sperm recovery: case series. Fertil Steril 1997; 68: 376–9

63. Crabbé E, Verheyen G, Silber S, et al. Enzymatic digestion of testicular tissue may rescue the intracytoplasmic sperm injection cycle in some patients with non-obstructive azoospermia. Hum Reprod 1998; 13: 2791–6

64. Baukloh V. Retrospective multicentre study on mechanical and enzymatic preparation of fresh and cryopreserved testicular biopsies. Hum Reprod 2002; 17: 1788–94

65. Vernaeve V, Tournaye H, Osmanagaoglu K, et al. Intracytoplasmic sperm injection with testicular spermatozoa is less successful in men with nonobstructive azoospermia than in men with obstructive azoospermia. Fertil Steril 2003; 79: 529–33

66. Osmanagaoglu K, Vernaeve V, Kolibianakis E, et al. Cumulative delivery rates after ICSI treatment cycles with freshly retrieved testicular sperm: a 7-year follow-up study. Hum Reprod 2003; 18: 1836–40

67. Vernaeve V, Bonduelle M, Tournaye H, et al. Pregnancy outcome and neonatal data of children born after ICSI using testicular sperm in obstructive and non-obstructive azoospermia. Hum Reprod 2003; 18: 2093–7

68. Nagy P, Liu J, Janssenswillen C, et al. Using ejaculated, fresh and frozen–thawed epididymal and testicular spermatozoa gives rise to comparable results after intracytoplasmic sperm injection. Fertil Steril 1995; 63: 808–15

69. Friedel S, Raziel A, Soffer Y, et al. The outcome of intracytoplasmic injection of fresh and cryopreserved epididymal spermatozoa from patients with obstructive azoospermia – a comparative study. Hum Reprod 1998; 13: 1872–7

70. Tournaye H, Merdad T, Silber S, et al. No differences in outcome after intracytoplasmic sperm injection with fresh or with frozen–thawed epididymal spermatozoa. Hum Reprod 1999; 14: 90–5

71. Cayan S, Lee D, Conaghan J, et al. A comparison of ICSI outcomes with fresh and cryopreserved epididymal spermatozoa from the same couples. Hum Reprod 2001; 16: 495–9

72. Verheyen G, Nagy Z, Joris H, et al. Quality of frozen–thawed testicular sperm and its preclinical use for intracytoplasmic sperm injection into in vitro-matured germinal-vesicle stage oocytes. Fertil Steril 1997; 67: 74–80

73. Kupker W, Schlegel PN, Al-Hasani S, et al. Use of frozen–thawed testicular sperm for intracytoplasmic sperm injection. Fertil Steril 2000; 73: 453–8

74. Habermann H, Seo R, Cieslak J, et al. In vitro fertilization outcomes after intracytoplasmic sperm injection with fresh or frozen–thawed testicular spermatozoa. Fertil Steril 2000; 73: 955–60

75 Gil-Salom M, Romero J, Rubio C, et al. Intracytoplasmic sperm injection with cryopreserved testicular spermatozoa. Mol Cell Endocrinol 2000; 169: 15–19

76. Cohen J, Garrisi GJ, Congedo-Ferrara TA, et al. Cryopreservation of single human spermatozoa. Hum Reprod 1997; 12: 994–1001

77. Montag M, Rink K, Dieckmann U, et al. Laser-assisted cryopreservation of single human spermatozoa in cell-free zona pellucida. Andrologia 1999; 31: 49–53

78. Walmsley R, Cohen J, Ferrara-Congedo T, et al. The first births and ongoing pregnancies associated with sperm cryopreservation within evacuated egg zonae. Hum Reprod 1998; 13 (Suppl 4): 61–70

79. Diedrich K, Felberbaum R. New approaches to ovarian stimulation. Hum Reprod 1998; 13 (Suppl 3): 1–13

80. Macklon NS, Fauser BCJM. Regulation of follicle development and novel approaches to ovarian stimulation for IVF. Hum Reprod Update 2000; 6: 307–12

81. Mansour RT, Aboulghar MA, Serour GI, et al. Study of the optimum time for human chorionic gonadotropin–ovum pick-up interval in in vitro fertilization. J Assist Reprod Genet 1994; 11: 478–81

82. Bonduelle M, Camus M, De Vos A, et al. Seven years of intracytoplasmic sperm injection and follow-up of 1987 subsequent children. Hum Reprod 1999; 14 (Suppl 1): 243–64

83. Bouchard P, Fauser BCJM. Gonadotropin-releasing hormone antagonist: new tools vs. old habits. Fertil Steril 2000; 73: 18–20

84. Olivennes F, Cunha-Filho JS, Fanchin R, et al. The use of GnRH antagonists in ovarian stimulation. Hum Reprod Update 2002; 8: 279–90

85. Hall JE. Gonadotropin-releasing hormone antagonists: effects on the ovarian follicle and corpus luteum. Clin Obstet Gynecol 1993; 36: 744–52

86. Van Steirteghem AC, Joris H, Liu J, et al. Protocol for intracytoplasmic sperm injection. Hum Reprod Update 1995; 1 (3): CD-ROM

355

87. Pickering S, Johnson M, Braude P, et al. Cytoskeletal organization in fresh, aged and spontaneously activated human oocytes. Hum Reprod 1988; 3: 978–89

88. De Vos A, Van de Velde H, Joris H et al. In vitro-matured metaphase-I oocytes have a lower fertilization rate but similar embryo quality as mature metaphase-II oocytes after ICSI. Hum Reprod 1999; 14: 1859–63

89. Jaroudi KA, Hollanders JMG, Sieck UV, et al. Pregnancy after transfer of embryos which were generated from in-vitro matured oocytes. Hum Reprod 1997; 12: 857–9

90. Liu J, Katz E, Garcia JE, et al. Successful in vitro maturation of human oocytes not exposed to human chorionic gonadotropin during ovulation induction, resulting in pregnancy. Fertil Steril 1997; 67: 566–8

91. Nagy ZP, Janssenswillen C, Liu J, et al. Pregnancy and birth after intracytoplasmic sperm injection of in vitro matured germinal-vesicle stage oocytes: case report. Fertil Steril 1996; 65: 1047–50

92. Edirisinghe WR, Junk SM, Matson PL, et al. Birth from cryopreserved embryos following in-vitro maturation of oocytes and intracytoplasmic sperm injection. Hum Reprod 1997; 12: 1056–8

93. Crabbé E, Verheyen G, Tournaye H, et al. Freezing of testicular tissue as a minced suspension preserves sperm quality better than whole-biopsy freezing when glycerol is used as cryoprotectant. Int J Androl 1999; 22: 43–8

94. World Health Organization. WHO Laboratory Manual for the Examination of Human Semen and Sperm–Cervical Mucus Interaction, 4th edn. Cambridge: Cambridge University Press, 1999

95. Soderlund B, Lundin K. The use of silane-coated silica particles for density gradient centrifugation in in-vitro fertilization. Hum Reprod 2000; 15: 857–60

96. Griveau JF, Le Lannou D. Reactive oxygen species and human spermatozoa: physiology and pathology. Int J Androl 1997; 20: 61–9

97. Ford WC, Whittington K, Williams AC. Reactive oxygen species in human sperm suspensions: production by leukocytes and the generation of NADPH to protect sperm against their effects. Int J Androl 1997; 20 (Suppl 3): 44–9

98. Devroey P, Silber S, Nagy Z, et al. Ongoing pregnancies and birth after intracytoplasmic sperm injection with frozen–thawed epididymal spermatozoa. Hum Reprod 1995; 10: 903–6

99. Silber SJ, Nagy Z, Liu J, et al. The use of epididymal and testicular spermatozoa for intracytoplasmic sperm injection: the genetic implications for male infertility. Hum Reprod 1995; 10: 2031–43

100. Pickering S, Braude P, Johnson M, et al. Transient cooling to room temperature can cause irreversible disruption of the meiotic spindle in the human oocyte. Fertil Steril 1990; 54: 102–8

101. Harari O, Bourne H, McDonald M, et al. Intracytoplasmic sperm injection: a major advance in the management of severe male subfertility. Fertil Steril 1995; 64: 360–8

102. Jean M, Barriere P, Mirallie S. Intracytoplasmic sperm injection without polyvinylpyrrolidone: an essential precaution. Hum Reprod 1996; 11: 2332

103. Fishel S, Lisi F, Rimaldi L, et al. Systemic examination of immobilizing spermatozoa before intracytoplasmic sperm injection in the human. Hum Reprod 1995; 10: 497–500

104. Palermo GD, Alikani M, Bertoli M, et al. Oolemma characteristics in relation to survival and fertilization patterns of oocytes treated by intracytoplasmic sperm injection. Hum Reprod 1996; 11: 172–6

105. Nagy ZP, Liu J, Joris H, et al. Time-course of oocyte activation, pronucleus formation and cleavage in human oocytes fertilized by intracytoplasmic sperm injection. Hum Reprod 1994; 9: 1743–8

106. Sultan KM, Munné S, Palermo GD, et al. Chromosomal status of uni-pronuclear human zygotes following in-vitro fertilization and on intracytoplasmic sperm injection. Hum Reprod 1995; 10: 132–6

107. Staessen C, Van Steirteghem A. The chromosomal consitution of embryos developing from abnormally fertilized oocytes after an intracytoplasmic sperm injection and conventional in-vitro fertilization. Hum Reprod 1997; 12: 321–7

108. Scott L, Alvero R, Leondires M et al. The morphology of human pronuclear embryos is positively related to blastocyst development and implantation. Hum Reprod 2000; 15: 2394–403

109. Wittemer C, Bettahar-Leguble K, Ohl J, et al. Zygote evaluation: an efficient tool for embryos selection. Hum Reprod 2000; 15: 2591–7

110. DePlacido G, Wilding M, Strina I, et al. High outcome predictability after IVF using combined score for zygote and embryo morphology and growth rate. Hum Reprod 2002; 17: 2402–9

111. Zollner U, Zollner KP, Steck T, et al. Pronuclear scoring. Time for international standardization. J Reprod Med 2003; 48: 365–9

112. Liu J, Nagy Z, Joris H, et al. Analysis of 76 total fertilization failure cycles out of 2732 intracytoplasmic sperm injection cycles. Hum Reprod 1995; 10: 2630–6

113. Staessen C, Camus M, Khan I, et al. An 18-month survey of infertility treatment by in vitro fertilization, gamete and zygote intrafallopian transfer, and

replacement of frozen–thawed embryos. J In Vitro Fertil Embryo Transf 1989; 6: 22–9

114. Van Steirteghem AC, Van der Elst J, Van den Abbeel E, et al. Cryopreservation of supernumerary multicellular human embryos obtained after intracytoplasmic sperm injection. Fertil Steril 1994; 62: 775–80

115. Braude P, Bolton V, Moore S. Human gene expression first occurs between the four- and eight-cell stages of preimplantation development. Nature (London) 1988; 332: 459–61

116. Gardner DK, Lane M. Culture of viable human blastocysts in defined sequential serum-free media. Hum Reprod 1998; 13 (Suppl 3): 148–59

117. Hardy K, Warner A, Winston RM, et al. Expression of intracellular junctions during preimplantation development of the human embryo. Mol Hum Reprod 1996; 2: 621–32

118. Gardner DK, Lane M, Stevens J, et al. Blastocyst score affects implantation and pregnancy outcome: towards a single blastocyst transfer. Fertil Steril 2000; 73: 1155–8

119. Olivennes F, Hazout A, Lelaidier C, et al. Four indications for embryo transfer at the blastocyst stage. Hum Reprod 1994; 9: 2367–73

120. Scholtes MCW, Zeilmaker G. A prospective, randomized study of embryo transfer results after 3 or 5 days of embryo culture in in vitro fertilization. Fertil Steril 1996; 65: 1245–8

121. Karaki RZ, Samarraie SS, Younis NA, et al. Blastocyst culture and transfer: a step toward improved in vitro fertilization outcome. Fertil Steril 2002; 77: 114–18

122. Gardner DK, Schoolcraft WB, Wagley L, et al. A prospective randomized trial of blastocyst culture and transfer in in-vitro fertilization. Hum Reprod 1998; 13: 3434–40

123. Coskun S, Hollanders J, Al-Hassan S, et al. Day 5 versus day 3 embryo transfer: a controlled randomized trial. Hum Reprod 2000; 15: 1947–52

124. Rienzi L, Ubaldi F, Iacobelli M, et al. Day 3 embryo transfer with combined evaluation at the pronuclear and cleavage stages compares favourably with day 5 blastocyst transfer. Hum Reprod 2002; 17: 1852–5

125. Kaufman RA, Menezo Y, Hazout A, et al. Cocultured blastocyst cryopreservation: experience of more than 500 transfer cycles. Fertil Steril 1995; 64: 1125–9

126. Sermon K, Van Steirteghem A, Liebaers I. Preimplantation genetic diagnosis. Lancet 2004; 363: 1633–41

127. Wilton L. Preimplantation genetic diagnosis for aneuploidy screening in early human embryos: a review. Prenat Diagn 2002; 22: 512–18

128. Staessen C, Nagy ZP, Liu J, et al. One year's experience with elective transfer of two good quality embryos in the human in vitro fertilization and intracytoplasmic sperm injection programs. Hum Reprod 1995; 10: 3305–12

129. Bonduelle M, Liebaers I, Deketelaere V, et al. Neonatal data on a cohort of 2889 infants born after ICSI (1991–1999) and of 2995 infants born after IVF (1983–1999). Hum Reprod 2002; 17: 671–94

130. Hazekamp J, Bergh C, Wennerholm UB, et al. Avoiding multiple pregnancies in ART: evaluation and implementation of new strategies. Hum Reprod 2000; 15: 1217–19

131. Gerris J, Van Royen E. Avoiding multiple pregnancies in ART: a plea for single embryo transfer. Hum Reprod 2000; 15: 1884–8

132. Ozturk O, Bhattacharya S, Templeton A. Avoiding multiple pregnancies in ART: evaluation and implementation of new strategies. Hum Reprod 2001; 16: 1319–21

133. Tarlatzis BC, Bili H. Intracytoplasmic sperm injection. Survey of world results. Ann NY Acad Sci 2000; 900: 336–44

134. Manning M, Lissens W, Bonduelle M, et al. Study of DNA-methylation pattems at chromosome 15q11-q13 in children bom after ICSI reveals no imprinting defects. Mol Hum Reprod 2000; 6: 1049–53

135. Cox GF, Burger J, Lip V, et al. Intracytoplasmic sperm injection may increase the risk of imprinting defects. Am J Hum Genet 2002; 71: 162–4

136. Silber SJ, Repping S. Transmission of male infertility to future generations: lessons from the Y chromosome. Hum Reprod Update 2002; 8: 217–29

137. Tarlatzis BC, Grimbizis G. Pregnancy and child outcome after assisted reproduction techniques. Hum Reprod 1999; 14 (Suppl 1): 231–42

138. Bonduelle M, Van Assche E, Joris H, et al. Prenatal testing in ICSI pregnancies: incidence of chromosomal anomalies in 1586 karyotypes and relation to sperm parameters. Hum Reprod 2002; 17: 2600–14

139. Bowen JR, Gibson FL, Leslie GI, et al. Medical and developmental outcome at 1 year for children conceived by intracytoplasmic sperm injection. Lancet 1998; 351: 1529–34

140. Bonduelle M, Joris H, Hofmans K, et al. Mental development of 201 ICSI children at 2 years of age. Lancet 1998; 351: 1553

141. Sutcliffe AG, Taylor B, Saunders K, et al. Outcome in the second year of life after in-vitro fertilisation by intracytoplasmic sperm injection: a UK case–control study. Lancet 2001; 357: 2080–4

19

Alternative assisted conception techniques

William M. Buckett and Seang Lin Tan

INTRODUCTION

Assisted conception techniques have existed for several centuries. The first recorded successful birth of a child was following artificial insemination with husband's semen performed because of hypospadias, and was carried out by John Hunter in London in 1785. There were no further major developments in this field until 1954 when successful pregnancies were reported after insemination with frozen semen[1]. In the past three decades, since the birth of the first child conceived as a result of *in vitro* fertilization and embryo transfer (IVF–ET)[2], there has been an explosion of interest in methods of assisted reproduction, both within the medical profession and amongst the general public. The huge increase in the demand for assisted conception, particularly IVF, has led to a strain on both medical resources and also on the governmental or individual limited finances available for health-care.

As repeated IVF attempts may be necessary before achieving pregnancy[3] and live birth[4,5], a plethora of alternative techniques (all with their differing mnemonics) have emerged in an attempt to simplify treatment, improve the success rates or reduce some of the costs of treatment. Some of these alternative techniques are rarely used nowadays and others continue to stand the test of time.

Notwithstanding this, the principles underlying the management of most of these techniques are the same. In this chapter, we confine discussion to the following treatment methods:

(1) Direct intraperitoneal insemination (DIPI);

(2) Fallopian tube sperm perfusion (FSP) or intra-fallopian insemination (IFI);

(3) Peritoneal oocyte sperm transfer (POST) or follicle aspiration, sperm injection and assisted rupture (FASIAR);

(4) Zygote intrafallopian transfer (ZIFT), pronuclear stage tubal transfer (PROST), tubal embryo stage transfer (TEST), tubal embryo transfer (TET) or embryo intrafallopian transfer (EIFT);

(5) Transmyometrial embryo transfer (TM-ET) or surgical embryo transfer (SET);

(6) Direct oocyte transfer (DOT);

(7) Intravaginal culture (IVC).

Gamete intrafallopian transfer (GIFT), intracytoplasmic sperm injection (ICSI) and other micromanipulation techniques, surgical sperm retrieval such as microepididymal sperm aspiration (MESA), percutaneous sperm aspiration (PESA) and testicular sperm aspiration (TESA), gamete and embryo donation, surrogacy, preimplantation genetic diagnosis (PGD), aneuploidy screening, assisted hatching (AH), and immature and mature oocyte freezing and vitrification are discussed elsewhere.

DIRECT INTRAPERITONEAL INSEMINATION

Direct intraperitoneal insemination (DIPI) was first described by Manhes and Hermabessiere[6]. It involves ovarian stimulation, timed ovulation and the injection of a washed, capacitated sample of semen in the pouch of Douglas via the posterior vaginal fornix.

Indications for DIPI

DIPI has been used successfully for a number of indications, including unexplained infertility, cervical mucus hostility, minimal endometriosis, ovulatory disorders, mild male-factor infertility and failed donor insemination[6–9]. It has also been used in patients with patent Fallopian tubes undergoing *in vitro* fertilization who have ovulated prematurely[10].

Procedure

The steps involved in DIPI are:

(1) Ovarian stimulation;

(2) Monitoring follicular growth and timed human chorionic gonadotropin (hCG) administration;

(3) Preparation of semen sample;

(4) Intraperitoneal insemination with prepared sperm.

Ovarian stimulation

Although ovarian stimulation is not essential to the procedure, superovulation has been used in most of the studies reported. This increases the number of potential oocytes for fertilization. Various protocols, namely clomiphene citrate or tamoxifen alone or in combination with human menopausal gonadotropin (hMG) or urinary or recombinant follicle stimulating hormone (FSH), or hMG or FSH after pituitary desensitization with gonadotropin releasing hormone analogs (GnRH-a) have been used. In order to prevent an excessive number of follicles developing and the risk of high-order multiple pregnancy, it is essential

that controlled ovarian superovulation is monitored with serial ultrasound. Alternate-day hMG or FSH administration alone titrated against ovarian response or clomiphene citrate alone (provided that there is an adequate ovarian response of two or three mature follicles) gives the optimum pregnancy rates[9].

Monitoring of follicular growth and timing of hCG administration

Monitoring of follicular growth is achieved primarily by transvaginal ultrasound. Baseline ultrasound scans are performed ideally on day 2 of the menstrual cycle before ovarian stimulation is begun, to avoid ovarian stimulation in the presence of ovarian cysts. Monitoring ultrasound scans should then be performed from day 8 onwards, the frequency depending on the ovarian response. The sizes of the ovarian follicles should be measured in two planes, and the follicular growth serially recorded. Measurements of serum estradiol (E_2) and luteinizing hormone (LH) are no longer routinely necessary[11]. When the mean follicular diameter of the largest follicle reaches 18 mm, 5000 or 10 000 IU of hCG should be administered to preempt a spontaneous gonadotropin surge, and the DIPI planned 36 h later. If there are more than four follicles > 14 mm in size, there is a significant risk of high-order multiple pregnancy. In this case, as with other assisted conception techniques where oocytes and sperm fertilize *in vivo*, the cycle should either be abandoned with the couple avoiding intercourse or using contraception until the next menses, or be converted to an alternative procedure such as aspiration of the supernumery follicles[12], peritoneal oocyte sperm transfer (POST)[13], gamete intrafallopian transfer (GIFT)[14] or IVF[15].

Preparation of semen sample

A fresh sample of semen should be collected on the day of DIPI. The sperm are prepared by a standard 'swim-up' technique and diluted in Ham's F10 media with either 10%[9] or 20%[8] human serum albumin (although 10% wife's serum[16] has also been used). Initially, the sperm were suspended in a final volume of 2 ml[8], although more recent reports used 0.5 ml[16] for the DIPI.

Intraperitoneal insemination

The principle of DIPI is to place a sample of prepared semen in the pouch of Douglas at the time of ovulation (Figure 1). DIPI should be performed under ultrasound control with the patient in the 'sitting lithotomy position' to ensure that all the available peritoneal fluid gravitates to the pouch of Douglas. The vagina is cleansed with an antiseptic solution and transvaginal ultrasound scan performed to identify the fluid in the pouch of Douglas. There may be only a small amount of fluid in a narrow pool between the loops of bowel, so that identification of the optimal site into which to aim the needle may take a few minutes. A 19-gauge disposable needle is then passed through a needle guide attached to the vaginal probe, and the biopsy guide aligned to the peritoneal fluid. Having warned the patient that she will feel a sharp pain, the needle is passed with a single rapid movement into the pouch of Douglas. The needle tip should be easily identified within the fluid in the pouch of Douglas, and a small amount of peritoneal fluid aspirated to confirm that the needle is placed correctly. The syringe containing the prepared semen sample is then attached to the needle and the semen injected into the pouch of Douglas, which can be seen on the ultrasound screen. The procedure is quick and atraumatic. The patient requires no analgesia and is able to go home immediately.

Results

Since the original reports of DIPI, there have been many centers who have performed this procedure with pregnancy rates varying from 7%[8] per cycle to about 15%[9,16]. Both prospective and retrospective evidence[16,17] comparing DIPI versus intrauterine insemination (IUI) for unexplained infertility, cervical-factor infertility and minimal endometriosis conclude that the pregnancy rate is no better with DIPI. More recently, improved results using the GnRH-a long protocol for ovarian stimulation have been reported[18,19], although there have been no comparative studies.

Conclusions

Because the success rates for DIPI are no better than for superovulation and IUI[16], and because the procedure is more invasive, more expensive and less physiological, IUI should be used primarily.

There may be a very limited role for DIPI in cases of difficult IUI (for example, cervical stenosis) before

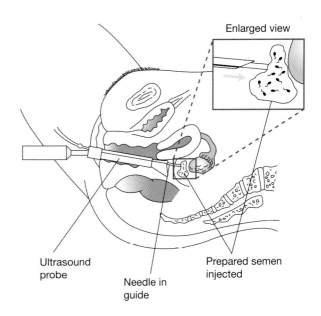

Figure 1 Direct intraperitoneal insemination. Prepared semen is injected into the pouch of Douglas via a needle mounted on the transvaginal ultrasound probe

resorting to more invasive treatments such as IVF–ET or GIFT, and some centers continue to offer this treatment.

FALLOPIAN TUBE PERFUSION/INTRATUBAL INSEMINATION

Direct Fallopian tube insemination was developed using the same rationale as for IUI, that is to increase the number of gametes at the site of fertilization. Following the first reports of transvaginal tubal catheterization[20], the first cases of intratubal insemination were reported[21]. Because of the difficulty and invasive nature of tubal catheterization, more recent techniques perfuse the tubes with larger volumes of sperm by preventing leakage through the cervix using a clamp[22] or a Foley catheter[23,24]. More recently, studies using the commercial device employed for hysterosalpingography (HSG) have also been reported[25].

The treatment involves ovarian stimulation, timed ovulation and the transvaginal and transcervical insemination of capacitated sperm into the Fallopian tube.

Indications for FSP

FSP (or IFI) has been successfully used as a treatment for non-tubal infertility including unexplained infertility, cervical mucus hostility, endometriosis, oligoasthenospermia and ovulatory disorders[21–23,26,27]. FSP has also been successfully used in patients with mild tubal disease[28], where the pressure of the injected sperm may open a partial tubal obstruction. Nevertheless, the highest pregnancy rates have been reported in couples with unexplained infertility[29].

Procedure

The steps involved in FSP or IFI are:

(1) Ovarian stimulation;

(2) Monitoring of follicular growth and timed hCG administration;

(3) Preparation of semen sample;

(4) Intrafallopian insemination.

The ovarian stimulation, monitoring of follicular growth, and timing and dose of hCG administartion are the same as used for DIPI.

Preparation of semen sample

Using a fresh sample of semen on the day of treatment, the preparation is similar to that used for DIPI. However, when intratubal catheterization is used, the sperm are resuspended in Ham's F10 medium to a volume of 0.3 ml[30], and when Fallopian tube sperm perfusion is done, the sperm are resuspended to a volume of 4.0 ml[27].

Intrafallopian insemination

Initial successes were performed using an ultrasound-guided coaxial catheter system[20,26,30] to enter the tube via a transvaginal, transcervical route where the inner catheter is loaded with the prepared sperm (Figure 2). A tactile technique for Fallopian tube catheterization has also been used with some success[21,30]. In both cases, the insemination is performed 2–4 cm distal to the tubal ostium on the side with the greater number of mature ovarian follicles.

The increased risk of complications related to tubal catheterization, namely tubal trauma, tubal infection and vasovagal sequelae, has led to the development of Fallopian tube sperm perfusion. Initial reports used

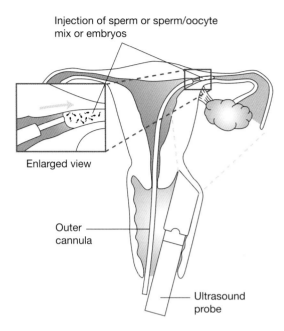

Figure 2 Intratubal insemination. The Fallopian tube is inseminated with prepared semen via transcervical catheterization of the tube, either with or without ultrasound guidance

large volumes of prepared semen and clamped the cervix to prevent leakage[22]. However, a simpler technique involves insertion of a pediatric Foley catheter into the uterine cavity to infuse a large volume (4 ml) of prepared semen to perfuse the Fallopian tubes, and the inflated balloon presses on the internal cervical os preventing reflux[23,24,27], or use of the device for infusion of radio-opaque dye at HSG[25]. Although mild discomfort is occasionally reported, the patient does not usually require analgesia and can go home after resting for about 10 min.

Results

Pregnancy rates of between 8 and 20% per cycle[20,25–27,29–32] are usually reported. Couples with unexplained infertility have the highest pregnancy rates. One study has reported pregnancy rates of 40% per cycle[28], although women in this study included 37% with 'partial tubal damage'. Although prospective, randomized studies have shown that FSP is well tolerated by patients, with the exception of two small studies[24,29], most report that there is no difference in results when FSP has been compared with IUI[23,25,31,32]. A recently presented Cochrane review[33] comparing FSP with IUI showed an odds ratio of 1.75 in favor of FSP, but the 95% confidence intervals were wide (0.83–3.67), suggesting that further prospective data are needed to determine whether indeed there is a benefit of FSP.

Conclusions

Because, at present, Fallopian tube insemination, whether by intrafallopian catheterization or by sperm perfusion, yields no better pregnancy rates than IUI, IUI should be used as the primary treatment where there is non-tubal pathology. The risks associated with intratubal catheterization preclude its use. There may be a possible role for Fallopian tube sperm perfusion in women with partial tubal disease prior to under-going IVF–ET where the large volume of inseminate may open a partial tubal obstruction, although only one center has reported high success with this. Evidence relating to perfusion pressures needed during transcervical tubal cannulation for proximal tubal disease[34] suggests that there may be such a role. Nevertheless, this indication requires further evaluation, and IVF–ET should be the treatment of choice.

PERITONEAL OOCYTE SPERM TRANSFER/FOLLICLE ASPIRATION, SPERM INJECTION AND ASSISTED RUPTURE

Peritoneal oocyte sperm transfer (POST) by the trans-abdominal route was originally described by workers in London[13,35], although this has since been super-seded by the transvaginal approach, which we pio-neered[36]. In this procedure a sample of prepared semen and up to four oocytes (retrieved from the ovary) are placed in the pouch of Douglas. POST avoids the lab-oratory costs of IVF–ET and the surgical costs and risks of GIFT. More recently, follicle aspiration, sperm injection and assisted rupture of the follicle (FASIAR) with only two or three follicles has been reported[37].

Indications for POST/FASIAR

The indications for POST have included cervical mucus hostility, antisperm antibodies, luteinized unruptured follicle (LUF) syndrome, oligoastheno-spermia, failed donor insemination and unexpl-ained infertility[13,35,36,38]. However, its most likely applications are in cases of demonstrable LUF syn-drome[37] or where more than four ovulatory follicles are generated in conjuction with IUI, thus rendering IUI inappropriate because of the risk of high-order multiple pregnancy[36].

Procedure

The steps involved in POST/FASIAR are:

(1) Ovarian stimulation;

(2) Monitoring of follicular growth and timed hCG administration;

(3) Oocyte retrieval;

(4) Preparation of sperm;

(5) Peritoneal transfer of prepared sperm and oocytes (through the ruptured follicle in the case of FASIAR).

Ovarian stimulation

The methods of ovarian stimulation used are similar to those described for DIPI. However, since POST/FASIAR involves aspiration of all the follicles and replacement of a maximum of four oocytes, larger doses of gonadotropins may be used either with or without prior pituitary desensitization with GnRH analogs[5].

Monitoring of follicular growth and timed hCG administration

Monitoring of follicular growth is similar to that used for DIPI. hCG is administered when there are more than three follicles with a mean diameter greater than 14 mm and the leading follicle is at least 17 mm diam-eter. If GnRH analogs with prior pituitary densensiti-zation or if GnRH antagonists are used, the timing of hCG can be delayed until three follicles have reached 18 mm diameter or more. The POST/FASIAR is scheduled 35–36 h after administration of hCG.

Oocyte retrieval

In the initial reports on the use of POST, oocytes were recovered by the transabdominal–transvesical route under ultrasound guidance[13,38]. However, nowadays most cases are performed transvaginally under ultrasound guidance[36]. Transvaginal oocyte recovery is performed in the same way as for conventional IVF–ET[39,40]. Because success is reduced when there is significant bleeding into the peritoneal cavity, a conscious effort should be made to keep trauma and therefore bleeding to a minimum. The collection needle should not be passed through the central hilum of the ovary where the main blood vessels are located. Once four oocytes have been aspirated, the remaining follicles should be emptied completely but not flushed, and small follicles < 12 mm should not be aspirated, to minimize spillage of blood into the pouch of Douglas.

Preparation of sperm

The semen sample is prepared in Earle's medium by a layering and swim-up technique to achieve a final concentration of 4×10^6/ml progressively motile sperm.

Peritoneal oocyte and sperm transfer

After oocyte recovery is complete, the pouch of Douglas should be completely aspirated and repeatedly rinsed with culture medium until the aspirate is clear. Occasionally, this may entail having to withdraw the needle from the vagina, localizing the fluid accurately and re-entering the pouch of Douglas in the most appropriate direction. When the aspirate is clear, the aspiration needle is left in position. Four million sperm in 1 ml Earle's medium together with a maximum of four oocytes are drawn into a long embryo transfer catheter. The catheter is passed through the aspiration needle and the oocyte–sperm mixture injected into the pouch of Douglas (Figure 3). The catheter and the needle are then withdrawn simultaneously. In FASIAR, the sperm and oocytes are injected through one of the follicles into the peritoneal cavity. The procedure lasts about 15 min and the patient is sent home after 1 h.

Results

Only four groups have reported successes with POST/FASIAR[36–38,41], and pregnancy rates per cycle from 3 to 20% have been reported. No comparative studies, either with IUI or with IVF–ET and GIFT, have been published.

Conclusions

The advantages of POST over IUI are that cycle cancelation in cases of ovarian overstimulation are

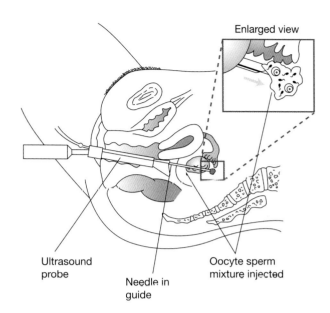

Figure 3 Peritoneal oocyte and sperm transfer. Oocytes with prepared sperm are injected into the pouch of Douglas via a needle mounted on the transvaginal ultrasound probe

avoided, and any spare embryos can be fertilized *in vitro* and cryopreserved for future use. The advantage over GIFT and IVF–ET is that the extra costs and intervention associated with these two procedures are avoided. Its major applications are for LUF syndrome or as a 'rescue' procedure where induction of ovulation results in too many follicles developing, thereby avoiding cycle cancelation. In both cases, IVF–ET should be the preferred option.

ZYGOTE INTRAFALLOPIAN TRANSFER

This procedure was initially described by Devroey and colleagues[42] in 1986, and it is essentially a modification of the GIFT procedure where fertilized embryos are transferred to the Fallopian tube, thereby reproducing a physiological step in *in vivo* fertilization, with the hope of possibly ameliorating the implantation rate. Currently, intratubal transfer of day-1 or day-2 embryos laparoscopically or transcervically is referred to as zygote intrafallopian transfer (ZIFT)[43]. This term has largely superseded pronuclear stage tubal transfer (PROST)[44], tubal embryo stage transfer (TEST)[45], tubal embryo transfer (TET)[46] or embryo intrafallopian transfer (EIFT)[47].

Indications for ZIFT

In the initial reports of ZIFT[42,44], the main indication was male-factor infertility where the Fallopian tubes were normal. This allowed an opportunity to select only the fertilized embryos for transfer. The absence of functioning Fallopian tubes was the only real contraindication, and ZIFT has been reported following ICSI[48] and also after assisted embryo hatching[49]. Other indications have included cervical stenosis and congenital cervical hypoplasia[50] and recurrent implantation failure[51]. ZIFT may also be beneficial when, in a given IVF–ET set-up, the *in vitro* culture systems are suboptimal for whatever reason[43].

Procedure

The steps involved in ZIFT are:

(1) Ovarian stimulation;

(2) Monitoring follicular growth and timed hCG administration;

(3) Oocyte retrieval;

(4) Sperm preparation and insemination;

(5) Intrafallopian transfer of embryos.

The techniques of ovarian stimulation, monitoring of follicular growth, hCG administration, oocyte retrieval, sperm preparation and oocyte insemination are all identical to those used for IVF–ET.

Intrafallopian transfer of embryos

Initially, intrafallopian transfer was performed laparoscopically[42,44] (Figure 4). However, following adaptation of the embryo catheter systems, transcervical intrafallopian transfer of embryos was made possible, initially by ultrasound guidance[52] and then by blind tactile tubal catheterization[53] (Figure 5). Although these techniques are less invasive and less expensive than laparoscopic ZIFT, there is a risk of damaging the endometrium and tubal mucosa, and case-controlled and prospective data demonstrate that transcervical ZIFT is inferior to laparoscopic ZIFT[54,55]. Hysteroscopic-guided transfer has been reported, but there is no evidence to sugggest that this technique is of any particular value[56]. Laparoscopic transfer is effected in a manner similar to the GIFT procedure, where the Fallopian tube is catheterized and up to three pronucleate, day-1 or day-2 embryos are loaded into the delivery catheter and injected into the Fallopian ampulla. The catheter is removed from the Fallopian tube and the procedure continued in exactly the same

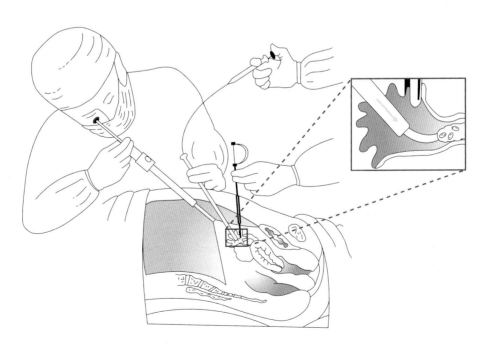

Figure 4 Laparoscopic zygote intrafallopian transfer. Day-1 or day-2 embryos are transferred to the ampullary portion of the Fallopian tube via laparoscopic catheterization of the tube under direct vision

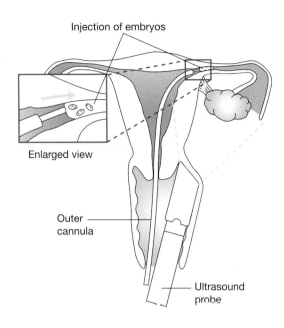

Figure 5 Transcervical zygote intrafallopian transfer. Day-1 or day-2 embryos are transferred to the ampullary portion of the Fallopian tube via transcervical catheterization of the tube, either with or without ultrasound guidance

manner as GIFT. The postoperative care and instructions are also the same.

Results

Pregnancy rates with ZIFT range from 25 to 55% per transfer and implantation rates from 13 to 20%[57]. Early retrospective studies comparing ZIFT with IVF reported higher pregnancy rates with ZIFT[44]. However, when the implantation rate was normal (i.e. > 10%) after day-2 uterine embryo transfer, no differences were noted[58]. Later, prospective studies[59–61] confirmed no advantage in pregnancy rate or implantation rate with ZIFT, and meta-analyses of all the studies so far also confirm this[62,63] and even show a trend toward ectopic pregnancy.

Conclusions

The need for general anesthesia and laparoscopy and their attendant risks are the major drawbacks to ZIFT. Since current evidence suggests no advantage over IVF, ZIFT cannot be recommended as a routine treatment. ZIFT may be useful if embryo culture systems are temporarily suboptimal in an IVF laboratory leading to low implantation rates. Whether there is any benefit in certain subgroups of patients (i.e. older women or those with recurrent implantation failure) remains to be proven, although no selection of the best embryos with true developmental potential can be expected from ZIFT.

TRANSMYOMETRIAL EMBRYO TRANSFER/SURGICAL EMBRYO TRANSFER

Whereas ovarian stimulation protocols, oocyte recovery techniques and embryological procedures have all undergone major changes since the advent of IVF–ET, the procedure for embryo transfer has remained essentially the same. The conventional technique consists of catheterization of the cervical canal with a special catheter, and injection of the embryos, with or without ultrasound guidance, into the uterine cavity. Occasionally, there may be some technical difficulty in inserting the catheter, especially in patients with cervical stenosis or cervical fibroids. Other disadvantages of the conventional approach to ET include a possible risk of infection, delayed expulsion of embryos from the uterine cavity and retention of embryos in the transfer catheter[64,65]. It is possible that some of the disadvantages associated with conventional transcervical ET may contribute to the relatively low pregnancy rate per ET. Surgical transmyometrial embryo transfer via the perurethral[66], transvaginal[66,67] and transabdominal[68] routes have been reported with some success.

Indications for transmyometrial embryo transfer

Although transmyometrial embryo transfer has proved to be superior to the transcervical technique in animal studies[69], the main indications in humans remain a history of previous difficult transcervical ET[67], known cervical stenosis[70], congenital atresia of the cervix[71] and difficult 'mock' transcervical ET immediately prior to the transfer itself[72].

Procedure

The steps involved in TM-ET are those of IVF prior to embryo transfer, and are discussed elsewhere.

Transmyometrial embryo transfer

Initial attempts at transmyometrial transfer at laparotomy or laparoscopy, which were not ultrasound-guided, failed to result in pregnancy[73,74]. Although subsequently, ultrasound-guided perurethral and transabdominal pregnancies have been reported[66,68], the transvaginal route is the approach of choice[67]. The patient is placed in the lithotomy position, the vagina cleansed and a transvaginal ultrasound probe, mounted with a biopsy guide, is inserted. The endometrial cavity is visualized and the biopsy guide aligned with a point 0.5 cm below the uterine fundus. The distance from the transducer head to the endometrial cavity is measured. A special needle with a stylet is inserted down the biopsy guide, and with a single movement, thrust precisely the distance measured into the myometrium and into the endometrium. The stylet is then removed, and a small amount of fluid injected via a long transfer catheter. A lack of resistance and the ultrasound identification of fluid appearing in the endometrial cavity confirms the position of the needle. Then the embryos are loaded in another catheter with a minimal amount of culture medium (about 20 µl). The catheter is passed through the needle and the embryos are transferred by gentle injection. Successful transfer is confirmed by echogenic brightness at the transfer site. The catheter is then withdrawn and checked for any returning embryos. The needle is then removed. Although this is an invasive procedure compared with transcervical ET, analgesia requirements are minimal, and the patient usually goes home after 20 min.

Results

Initial results were low following this technique[64], but success rates of around 30% per transfer have been reported[67,72]. However, these series are small and the only prospective study that has been done has shown no benefit of routine transmyometrial ET compared with transcervical ET in women who had a history of cervical stenosis or three previously failed transcervical transfers[70]. Transmyometrial embryo transfer has been shown to be associated with increased uterine contractility[75], which forms a theoretical objection to the procedure, although difficult transcervical embryo transfer is also associated with increased contractions.

Conclusions

Although TM-ET should not be routinely performed, even with a history of difficult insemination or cervical stenosis, in practice it may be the only possible route of transfer in a patient whose cervix does not allow conventional embryo transfer to be performed.

DIRECT OOCYTE TRANSFER

In an effort to reduce the need for prolonged oocyte and embryo culture, direct transfer of oocytes and sperm to the endometrial cavity was first described in 1982[76,77].

Indications for DOT

The technique can be used for all patients requiring IVF. Unfortunately, the limited success has prevented its widespread use.

Procedure

The steps involved in DOT are:

(1) Ovarian stimulation;

(2) Monitoring of follicular growth and timed hCG administration;

(3) Oocyte retrieval;

(4) Sperm preparation;

(5) Direct oocyte and sperm transfer.

The methods of ovarian stimulation, monitoring of follicular growth, hCG administration, oocyte transfer and sperm preparation are the same as those described for DIPI and POST.

Direct oocyte and sperm transfer

In the initial reports[76], the oocyte was incubated for 6 h in culture medium, prepared sperm were then added and the medium incubated for a further hour. The oocyte and about 20 000 sperm were then transferred into the uterine cavity in 20 µl culture medium with a normal embryo transfer catheter, 7 h after the oocyte retrieval. The modified technique involved mechanically stripping cumulus cells off all retrieved oocytes[77]. The oocytes were inseminated 3 h after retrieval. A maximum of four oocytes with tightly bound sperm were then transferred to the uterine cavity 5 h after oocyte retrieval.

Results

Pregnancy rates of 6.5% per cycle[76] were originally reported, although with the modification the results improved to 18.6% per cycle[77].

Conclusions

Although a simplification of the IVF procedure, the results of the original method do not warrant the extra intervention and cost. The modified procedure yields better results but requires more laboratory work and involves the transfer of four oocytes. There is little place for this technique today.

INTRAVAGINAL CULTURE

Intravaginal culture (IVC) of oocytes and sperm until embryo transfer using a cryotube was first described by Ranoux and colleagues[78]. The procedure is a simplification of IVF and reduces laboratory cost and time by avoiding direct manipulation of the gametes and the need for incubators.

Indications for IVC

The indications for IVC are essentially the same as those for IVF. Occasionally, a center performing GIFT without the ability to convert to IVF if necessary may use IVC to transport the gametes to a center where IVF–ET can be performed. A modification of IVC has allowed its use for the transport of oocytes and sperm to regional centers for ICSI or other micromanipulation techniques[79].

Procedure

The steps involved in IVC are:

(1) Ovarian stimulation;

(2) Monitoring of follicular growth and timed hCG administration;

(3) Oocyte retrieval;

(4) Sperm preparation;

(5) Mixing of gametes in the tube and insertion into the vagina;

(6) Removal, identification, grading and transfer or freezing of embryos.

The techniques of ovarian stimulation, monitoring of follicular growth, hCG administration, oocyte retrieval and sperm preparation are all identical to those described for IVF–ET. Occasionally the oocytes may be retrieved laparoscopically in a planned GIFT procedure.

Mixing of gametes

A small polypropylene tube is partly filled with IVF culture medium. It is maintained at 37°C and gassed with 5% CO_2 with air. Prepared sperm are added to the tube with up to four oocytes. If there are more oocytes, other tubes are prepared in the same way. The top of the tube is filled with medium and carefully screwed on, taking care that no air is trapped inside. The tube(s) are wrapped in clingfilm and placed inside the vagina (Figure 6). Usually a tampon or contraceptive diaphragm is used to keep the tubes in place.

Removal and transfer of embryos

After 48–50 h, the tube(s) are removed and transferred to the laboratory. The resultant embryos are then identified and the best-graded embryos transferred using standard ET techniques. Spare embryos may be cryopreserved.

Results

Initial results using IVC were comparable to those of IVF, with fertilization rates of 60% and pregnancy rates of 20%[78]. Pregnancy rates from 10 to 25% continue to be reported[80,81].

However, compared with conventional IVF, lower overall fertilization and pregnancy rates have been achieved. There have also been reported cases of lost tubes, as well as a case report of embryo yeast infection[82].

Conclusions

The main benefit of IVC is the lower cost to the patient by avoiding many of the laboratory costs, but this saving has to be weighed against a lower pregnancy rate. IVC is also a technique that is not readily

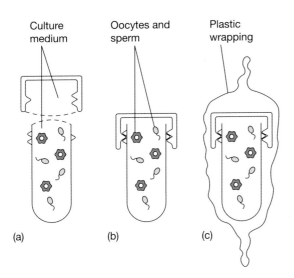

Figure 6 Intravaginal culture. (a) Oocytes and prepared sperm placed in a completely filled Nunc tube with the cap filled with medium; (b) cap screwed on with no air trapped; (c) tube wrapped in polythene or 'clingfilm' and placed in the vagina

acceptable to some women. Finally, the improvement in transport IVF programs and portable incubators[83] would facilitate transfer of gametes and/or embryos for ICSI or other micromanipulation techniques.

CONCLUSIONS

The increasing demand for assisted conception by patients has led to a veritable industry, and there remain a large number of different methods of assisted conception which have only marginal differences in success rates. Undoubtedly, new procedures and modifications will be introduced, and some will gain favor and be effective in the hands of their protagonists. While we must be receptive to any new developments, each technique must be carefully evaluated and compared with the existing and well-established reproductive technologies.

REFERENCES

1. Bunge RG, Sherman TK. Clinical use of frozen semen. Fertil Steril 1954; 5: 193–4

2. Steptoe PC, Edwards RG. Birth after reimplantation of a human embryo. Lancet 1978; 2: 366

3. Tan SL, Steer C, Royston P, et al. Conception rates and in vitro fertilisation. Lancet 1990; 2: 229

4. Tan SL, Royston P, Campbell S, et al. Cummulative conception and live birth rates after in vitro fertilisation. Lancet 1992; 1: 1390–4

5. Tan SL, Maconochie N, Doyle P, et al. Cumulative conception and live birth rates after in vitro fertilization with and without the use of long, short, and ultrashort regimens of the gonadotrophin-releasing hormone agonist buserelin. Am J Obstet Gynecol 1994; 171: 513–20

6. Manhes H, Hermabessiere J. Fecondation intra-peritoneal. Première grossese obtenu sur indication masculine. Presented at the 3rd International Forum on Andrology, Paris, France, 1985

7. Forrler A, Dellenbach P, Nisand I, et al. Direct intraperitoneal insemination in unexplained and cervical infertility. Lancet 1986; 1: 916

8. Curson R, Parsons J. Disappointing results with direct intraperitoneal insemination. Lancet 1987; 1: 112

9. Ben Rhouma K, Ben Miled E, Ben Marzouk A, et al. Direct intraperitoneal insemination and controlled ovarian hyperstimulation in subfertile couples. J Assist Reprod Genet 1994; 11: 189–92

10. Pampiglone J, Davies MC, Steer C, et al. Factors affecting direct intraperitoneal insemination. Lancet 1988; 2: 1336

11. Tan SL Simplifying in vitro fertilisation therapy. Curr Opin Obstet Gynecol 1994; 6: 111–14

12. DeGeyter C, DeGeyter M, Castro E, et al. Experience with transvaginal ultrasound-guided aspiration of supernumery follicles for the prevention of multiple pregnancies after ovulation induction and intra-uterine insemination. Fertil Steril 1996; 65: 1163–8

13. Sharma V, Mason BA, Pinker G, et al. Ultrasound guided peritoneal oocyte and sperm transfer. J In Vitro Fert Embryo Transf 1987; 4: 89–92

14. Buckett WM, Luckas MJM, Gazvani MR, et al. Conversion of intra-uterine insemination to gamete intra-fallopian transfer. J Gynecol Tech 1997; 3: 163–6

15. Nisker J, Tummon I, Daniel S, et al. Conversion of cycles involving ovarian hyperstimulation with intra-uterine insemination to in-vitro fertilization. Hum Reprod 1994; 9: 406–8

16. Hovatta O, Kurunmäki H, Tiitinen A, et al. Direct intraperitoneal or intrauterine insemination and superovulation in infertility treatment: a randomized study. Fertil Steril 1990; 54: 339–41

17. Gregoriou O, Papadias C, Konidaris S, et al. A randomized comparison of intrauterine and intraperitoneal insemination for the treatment of infertility. Int J Gynecol Obstet 1993; 42: 33–6

18. Misao R, Itoh M, Nakanishi Y, Tamaya T. Direct intraperitoneal insemination in ovarian hyperstimulation induced cycles induced with

gonadotrophin-releasing hormone agonist. Clin Exp Obstet Gynecol 1997; 24: 133–4

19. Minoura H, Tageuchi S, Shen X, et al. GnRH agonist: increasing the pregnancy rate after combined treatment with hMG/hCG and direct intraperitoneal insemination. J Reprod Med 1999; 44: 18–22

20. Jansen RBS, Anderson JC. Catheterization of the fallopian tubes from the vagina. Lancet 1987; 2: 309–10

21. Pratt DE, Bieber E, Barnes R, et al. Transvaginal intratubal insemination by tactile sensation: a preliminary report. Fertil Steril 1991; 56: 984–6

22. Kahn JA, von During V, Sunde A, Molne K. Fallopian tube sperm perfusion: first clinical experience. Hum Reprod 1992; 7: 19–24

23. Li TC. A simple, non-invasive method of Fallopian tube sperm perfusion. Hum Reprod 1993; 8: 1848–50

24. Maheshwari A, Jain K, Agarwal N. Fallopian sperm perfusion (FSP) using Foley's balloon system versus intrauterine insemination (IUI) in the treatment of infertility. Int J Gynaecol Obstet 1999; 65: 313–15

25. Ricci G, Nucera G, Pozzobon C, et al. A simple method for fallopian tube sperm perfusion using a blocking device in the treatment of unexplained infertility. Fertil Steril 2001; 76: 1242–8

26. Tzafettas J, Loufopoulos A, Stephanatos A, Mukherjee A. Tubal catheterization or intrafallopian insemination and transvaginal gamete (GIFT) or zygote intrafallopian transfer (ZIFT): our experience in a total of 1128 treatment cycles. J Assist Reprod Genet 1994; 11: 283–8

27. Nuojua-Huttunen S, Tuomivaara L, Juntunen K, et al. Comparison of fallopian tube sperm perfusion with intrauterine insemination in the treatment of infertility. Fertil Steril 1997; 67: 939–42

28. Fanchin R, Olivennes F, Righini C, et al. A new system for fallopian tube sperm perfusion leads to pregnancy rates twice as high as standard intrauterine insemination. Fertil Steril 1995; 64: 505–10

29. Trout SW, Kemmann E. Fallopian sperm perfusion versus intrauterine insemination: a randomized controlled trial and meta-analysis of the literature. Fertil Steril 1999; 71: 881–5

30. Oei ML, Surrey ES, McCaleb B, Kerin JF. A prospective, randomized study of pregnancy rates after transuterotubal and intrauterine insemination. Fertil Steril 1992; 58: 167–71

31. Ng EH, Makkar G, Yeung WS, Ho PC. A randomized comparison of three insemination methods in an artificial insemination program using husbands' semen. J Reprod Med 2003; 48: 542–6

32. Biacchiardi CP, Revelli A, Gennarelli G, et al. Fallopian tube sperm perfusion versus intrauterine insemination in unexplained infertility: a randomized,

prospective, cross-over trial. Fertil Steril 2004; 81: 448–51

33. Cantineau A, Heinemann MJ, Al Inany H, Cohlen B. Intra-uterine insemination versus fallopian sperm perfusion for non-tubal infertility: a Cochrane systematic review. Presented at the IFFS 18th World Congress on Fertility and Sterility, Montreal, Canada, 2004

34. Papaioannou S. A hypothesis for the pathogenesis and natural history of proximal tubal blockage. Hum Reprod 2004; 19: 481–5

35. Mason BA, Sharma V, Riddle A, Campbell S. Ultrasound guided peritoneal oocyte and sperm transfer. Lancet 1987; 1: 386

36. Tan SL, Pampiglione J, Steer C, et al. Transvaginal peritoneal oocyte and sperm transfer for the treatment of nontubal infertility. Fertil Steril 1992; 57: 850–3

37. Paulson RJ, Thornton MH. Follicle aspiration, sperm injection, and assisted rupture (FASIAR): a simple new assisted reproductive technique. Fertil Steril 1997; 68: 1148–51

38. Bongers MY, Bernadus RE, Schoemaker J, Vermeiden JW. Peritoneal oocyte sperm transfer: a prospective pilot study. Fertil Steril 1991; 56: 147–8

39. Tan SL, Waterstone J, Wren M, Parsons J. A prospective randomised trial comparing aspiration only with aspiration and flushing for transvaginal ultrasound directed oocyte recovery. Fertil Steril 1992; 58: 356–60

40. el Hussein E, Balen AH, Tan SL. A prospective study comparing the outcome of oocytes retrieved in the aspirate with those retrieved in the flush during transvaginal ultrasound directed oocyte recovery for in vitro fertilization. Br J Obstet Gynaecol 1992; 99: 841–4

41. Gentry W, Critser ES, Critser JK, Coulam CB. Pregnancy resulting from peritoneal ovum sperm transfer procedure. Fertil Steril 1989; 51: 179–81

42. Devroey P, Braekmans P, Smitz J, et al. Pregnancy after translaparoscopic zygote intrafallopian transfer in a patient with anti-sperm antibodies. Lancet 1986; 1: 1329

43. Tournaye H, Camus M, Ubaldi F, et al. Tubal transfer: a forgotten ART? Is there still an important role for tubal transfer procedures? Hum Reprod 1996; 11: 1815–22

44. Yovich JL, Yovich JM, Edrisinghe WR. The relative chance of pregnancy following tubal or uterine transfer procedures. Fertil Steril 1988; 49: 858–64

45. Yovich JL, Draper RR, Turner SR, Cummins JM. Transcervical tubal embryo transfer (TC-TEST). J In Vitro Fertil Embryo Transf 1990; 7: 137–40

46. Balmaceda JP, Gastaldi C, Remohi J, et al. Tubal embryo transfer as a treatment of infertility due to male factor. Fertil Steril 1988; 50: 476–9

47. Diedrich K, Bauer O. Indications and outcomes of assisted reproduction. Ballière's Clin Obstet Gynaecol 1992; 6: 373–88

48. Boldt J, Schnarr P, Ajame A, et al. Success rates following intracytoplasmic sperm injection are improved using ZIFT vs IVF for embryo transfer. J Assist Reprod Genet 1996; 13: 782–5

49. Castellotti DS, da Motta EL, Alegretti JR, et al. Successful birth after intrafallopian transfer of microhatched embryos. Fertil Steril 1997; 68: 267–369

50. Fluker MR, Bebbington MW, Munro MG. Successful pregnancy following zygote intrafallopian transfer for congenital cervical hypoplasia. Obstet Gynecol 1994; 84: 659–61

51. Levran D, Frahi J, Nahum H, et al. Prospective evaluation of blastocyst stage transfer versus zygote intrafallopian tube transfer in patients with repeated omplantation failure. Fertil Steril 2002; 77: 971–7

52. Jansen R, Anderson J, Sutherland P. Nonoperative embryo transfer to the fallopian tube. N Engl J Med 1988; 319: 288–91

53. Diedrich K, Bauer O, Werner A, et al. Transvaginal intratubal embryo transfer: a new treatment of male infertility. Hum Reprod 1991; 6: 672–5

54. Jansen R, Anderson J. Transvaginal versus laparoscopic gamete-intrafallopian transfer: case controlled retrospective comparison. Fertil Steril 1993; 59: 836–40

55. Scholtes M, Roozenburg B, Verhoeff A, Zeilmaker GH. A randomized study of transcervical intra-fallopian transfer of pronuclear embryos controlled by ultrasound versus intrauterine transfer of 4- to 8-cell embryos. Fertil Steril 1994; 61: 102–4

56. Seracchioli R, Possati G, Affara G, et al. Hysteroscopic gamete intrafallopian transfer: a good alternative to laparoscopic intrafallopian transfer. Hum Reprod 1991; 6: 1388–90

57. Ménézo YJR, Janny L. Is there a rationale for tubal transfer in human ART? Hum Reprod 1996; 11: 1818–20

58. Tournaye H, Camus M, Khan I, et al. In vitro fertilization, gamete or zygote intra-fallopian transfer for male infertility. Hum Reprod 1991; 6: 263–6

59. Tournaye H, Devroey P, Camus M, et al. Zygote intrafallopian transfer or in vitro fertilization and embryo transfer for the treatment of male factor infertility: a prospective randomised trial. Fertil Steril 1992; 58: 344–50

60. Fluker M, Zouves C, Bebbington M. A prospective randomised comparison of zygote intrafallopian transfer and in vitro fertilization–embryo transfer for non-tubal factor infertility. Fertil Steril 1993; 60: 515–19

61. Dale B, Fiorentino A, de Simone ML, et al. Zygote versus embryo transfer: a prospective randomized multicenter trial. J Assist Reprod Genet 2002; 19: 456–61

62. Tournaye H. Tubal embryo transfer [Letter]. Hum Reprod 1997; 12: 631–2

63. Habana AE, Palter SF. Is tubal embryo transfer of any value? A meta-analysis and comparison with the Society for Assisted Reproductive Technology database. Fertil Steril 2001; 76: 286–93

64. Tan SL, Bennett S, Parsons J. Surgical techniques of oocyte collection and embryo transfer. Br Med Bull 1990; 46: 628–42

65. Schulman JD. Delayed expulsion of transfer fluid after IVF–ET [Letter]. Lancet 1986; 1: 44

66. Parsons J, Bolton V, Wilson L, Campbell S. Pregnancies following in vitro fertilisation and ultrasound directed surgical embryo transfer by perurethral and transvaginal techniques. Fertil Steril 1987; 48: 691–3

67. Kato O, Takatsuka R, Asch RH. Transvaginal transmyometrial embryo transfer: the Towako method – experience of 104 cases. Fertil Steril 1993; 59: 51–3

68. Lenz S, Leeton J. Evaluating the possibility of uterine transfer by ultrasonically guided transabdominal puncture. J In Vitro Fertil Embryo Transf 1987; 4: 18–22

69. Iuliano MF, Squires EL, Cook VM. Effect of age of equine embryos and method of transfer on pregnancy rate. J Anim Sci 1985; 60: 258–62

70. Groutz A, Lessing JB, Wolf Y, et al. Comparison of transmyometrial and transcervical embryo transfer in patients with previously failed in vitro fertilization embryo transfer cycles and/or cervical stenosis. Fertil Steril 1997; 67: 1073–6

71. Anttila L, Penttila TA, Suikkari AM. Successful pregnancy after in-vitro fertilization and transmyometrial embryo transfer in a patient with congenital atresia of cervix: a case report. Hum Reprod 1999; 14: 1647–9

72. Sharif K, Afnan M, Lenton W, et al. Transmyometrial embryo transfer after difficult immediate mock transcervical transfer. Fertil Steril 1996; 65: 1071–4

73. Edwards RG, Steptoe PC, Purdy JM. Establishing full-term human pregnancies using cleaved embryos grown in vitro. Br J Obstet Gynaecol 1980; 87: 737–56

74. Leeton J, Kerin J. Embryo transfer. In Wood C, Trousson A, eds. Clinical IVF. New York, Springer-Verlag 1984: 117

75. Biervliet FP, Lesny P, Maguiness SD, et al. Transmyometrial embryo transfer and junctional zone contractions. Hum Reprod 2002; 17: 347–50

76. Craft I, Djahanbakhch O, McLeod F, et al. Human pregnancy following oocyte and sperm transfer to the uterus. Lancet 1982; 1: 1031–2

77. Tan SL, Brinsden PR. Alternative assisted conception techniques. In Brinsden PR, Rainsbury PA, eds. A Textbook of In Vitro Fertilization and Assisted Reproduction 1st edn. Carnforth, UK: Parthenon Publishing, 1991: 241–2

78. Ranoux C, Aubriot FX, Dubuisson JB. A new in vitro fertilization technique: intravaginal culture. Fertil Steril 1988; 49: 654–7

79. Sterzik K, Rosenbusch B, Noss U. First pregnancies after intravaginal transport and partial zona dissection of human oocytes. Fertil Steril 1993; 60: 582–4

80. Hewitt J. Intravaginal culture: present and potential uses. Br J Hosp Med 1990; 6: 182–8

81. Batres F, Mahadevan H, Morris M, et al. Stimulated cycle intravaginal culture fertilization in an office setting: a preliminary study. Fertil Steril 1997; 68 (ASRM Suppl): S168

82. Mahadevan H, Batres F, Miller MM, Moutis DM. Yeast infection of sperm, oocytes and embryos after intravaginal culture for embryo transfer. Fertil Steril 1996; 66: 481–3

83. Buckett WM, Fisch P, Dean NL, et al. In vitro fertilization and intracytoplasmic sperm injection pregnancies after successful transport of oocytes by airplane. Fertil Steril 1999; 71: 753–5

20.1

Oocyte donation

Neela Mukhopadhaya

Oocyte donation has brought new hope to many couples who otherwise would remain childless. Currently, there are about 67 clinics in the United Kingdom that have established oocyte donation programs. Thousands of women donate their oocytes each year, and of the 25 000 *in vitro* fertilization (IVF) cycles from 1 April 2000 to 31 March 2001, 1783 involved the use of donated oocytes (7–8%)[1].

HISTORY

Trounson and colleagues[2] from Australia first reported on oocyte donation in 1983, and in the following year the same group reported the achievement of a pregnancy in a patient with primary ovarian failure[3]. In 1987, Asch and colleagues[4] and Yovich and associates[5] reported the technique of tubal transfer of donated oocytes and donated zygotes.

Bourn Hall had its first oocyte donation success in 1985. In 1987, Serhal and Craft[6] reported successful pregnancies using a simplified hormone replacement protocol in recipients, and established the concept of a prolonged proliferative phase. In the same year, Van Steirteghem and colleagues[7] reported the first pregnancy from a frozen–thawed embryo transfer in a donated oocyte cycle.

In compliance with the Human Fertilisation and Embryology Authority (HFEA) regulations in the UK, all gamete donations must be altruistic, and by the 1990s, many clinics in the UK had established oocyte donation programs. In 1992, the UK regulatory body, the HFEA, issued directions 'permitting the provision of treatment services and sterilisation in exchange for Ovum Donation' (HFEA directions, 1992). Ahuja and co-workers[8] first reported 'egg-sharing' in 1996, following a pilot study, and in 1998, the HFEA announced that egg-sharing should be 'regulated, not banned'[9]. At its meeting in 1999, the Authority agreed that centers should be advised that 'allowing egg sharing to continue did not mean that the HFEA had given the practice its ethical approval'[10]. In the year 2000, however, guidance to centers was drawn up, and subsequently incorporated within the revised *Code of Practice* in 2001.

INDICATIONS FOR OOCYTE DONATION

During the late 1980s and early 1990s, most oocyte donation was carried out for premature ovarian failure. However, the high pregnancy and live birth rates achieved with oocyte donation led to its more widespread use in other groups of patients, primarily older patients and those with genetic diseases. Antinori[11],

Sauer[12] and Borini[13] and their groups showed that women in their 50s can establish successful pregnancies following egg donation, and that the uteri of menopausal women can respond adequately to steroid therapy, thus allowing implantation comparable in success to that in younger women. Oocyte donation is the most successful technique for achieving pregnancies in perimenopausal women[14]. While oocyte donation is becoming more accepted within the UK, its use remains controversial over the age of 45 years.

The main indications for oocyte donation are shown in Table 1.

Premature ovarian failure

In humans, the maximum number of primordial follicles is present at 20 weeks of intrauterine life[15], when it is approximately 6–7 million. Atretic processes within the ovary bring the total numbers of primordial follicles down to about 1–2 million at birth and 300 000 at puberty, at which time the hypothalamic–pituitary–ovarian axis is activated, and menstrual cycles start, with follicular growth and atresia each month. This process continues until the follicle pool is practically exhausted and menopause begins[16].

Almost 50% of oocyte recipients suffer from premature ovarian failure (POF). The most commonly accepted definition of POF is ovarian failure before the age of 40 years. Strictly, it is ovarian failure two standard deviations before the mean age of menopause of the study population. It is estimated that 1–3% of women experience premature menopause. This can present in 10–20% of women as primary amenorrhea and in up to 18% as secondary amenorrhea. The diagnosis of ovarian failure is based on the finding of raised follicle stimulating hormone (FSH) levels during the investigation of amenorrhea; a level of > 50 IU/l is generally accepted as the level of FSH for diagnosis of ovarian failure to be made. However, in terms of the realistic chances of achieving a pregnancy following IVF treatment, this level has a cut-off around 15 IU/l in most clinics. Pregnancy is very rare once the FSH levels exceed 20 IU/l.

The onset of autoimmune POF may occur in childhood, adolescence or adulthood, and, as a result, fertility may be compromised. Some 10–30% of women with POF have autoimmune disorders. Thus, a history of Addison's disease, hypothyroidism, diabetes and other less commonly associated conditions such as

Table 1 Main indications for oocyte donation

Premature ovarian failure
Idiopathic
Iatrogenic
　bilateral oophorectomy
　chemotherapy
　radiotherapy
Autoimmune
Raised FSH at initial presentation for ART
Poor ovarian response to gonadotropin therapy

Gonadal dysgenesis
Turner's syndrome
Small deletions of X-chromosome
Turner's variant
Turner's mosaic

Genetically transmissible diseases
Thalassemia, galactosemia

Repeated ART failure

ART, assisted reproductive technologies; FSH, follicle stimulating hormone

autoimmune thyroiditis and inflammatory bowel disease should be borne in mind when making the diagnosis. For example, APS II (autoimmune polyglandular syndrome) is characterized by autoimmunity against two or more endocrine organs. It is also important to elicit a family history of premature menopause; 13% of families with premature ovarian failure are at risk of transmitting fragile-X syndrome[17].

Rare inherited syndromes such as blepherophimosis and ptosis (BPES) and Perrault's syndrome (deafness and short stature) should be excluded by karyotyping when clinically indicated.

Resistant ovary syndrome

This syndrome is characterized by amenorrhea, normal secondary sexual characteristics and raised levels of FSH and lutenizing hormone (LH). It has been reasoned that a lack of sensitivity of the gonadotropin receptors, or a defect in the adenylate cyclase pathway, is the cause of this condition[18]. Pregnancies have been reported, suggesting the spontaneous reversal of receptor sensitivity[19]. Recent understanding of this condition suggests that it is an early phase of ovarian failure, rather than a separate entity.

Turner's syndrome

Turner's syndrome is characterized by an XO chromosome pattern, with an incidence of 1:3000 live births. Of these, 60% have a pure XO karyotype, 20% are mosaics (XO/XX) and the rest have deletions, rings or isochromosomes. Patients typically present with short stature, cubitus valgus, low intelligence quotient (IQ) and amenorrhea due to streak gonads. Congenital cardiac defects in the form of coarctation of the aorta, bicuspid aortic valve, ventricular septal defect and aortic root abnormalities are common. A small proportion of patients, particularly the mosaics and the variants, can be fertile, but premature ovarian failure is more common in this group. Nearly 40% of patients with primary amenorrhea are diagnosed with Turner's mosaic, Turner's variant or the presence of a Y chromosome.

Cytogenetic abnormalities are usually rare in women presenting with secondary amenorrhea; however, small deletions of the X chromosome have been found in women presenting with amenorrhea as late as 35 years of age.

Women with Turner's syndrome usually have a hypoplastic uterus with hypovascularization. Miscarriage rates can be as high as 40%[20]. Cardiovascular complications during pregnancy are potentially severe. There is a high risk of exacerbating pre-existing hypertension and dissection of aortic aneurysms. There is also a high incidence of birth by Cesarean section due to feto-pelvic disproportion, thereby leading to other maternal and neonatal complications. Elective single embryo transfer should be considered[20] in this group having oocyte donation. In an observational study, pregnancy rates in women with Turner's syndrome following oocyte donation were similar to those in women with other causes of primary ovarian failure[21].

Carriers of genetically transmissible diseases

Couples at risk of having children with fatal or severely disabling diseases may request oocyte donation. Although antenatal diagnosis is available for an increasing number of these conditions, for some couples termination of pregnancy is unacceptable. Recent advances in preimplantation genetic diagnosis have enabled couples to undergo IVF and transfer of normal embryos selected by embryo biopsy[22,23]. The high cost and complexity of the procedure puts it beyond the means of many.

X-linked diseases

Patients with X-linked diseases including hemophilia A and B, and some varieties of primary muscle-wasting diseases such as Becker's muscular dystrophy (X-linked recessive) and Duchenne's muscular dystrophy (X-linked recessive), should be offered genetic counseling. Oocyte donation may be an option for all such patients.

Galactosemia

This transferase deficiency is usually fatal by 4 weeks of life. A lactose-free diet is essential, and mild learning difficulties and infertility may be associated. Patients with galactosemia seeking fertility treatment may opt for donated oocytes to avoid transmission to the offspring.

Repeated IVF failure

Repeated IVF failure for the following reasons may indicate treatment with donor oocytes:

(1) Poor response to superovulation drugs;

(2) Repeated failure of oocyte recovery;

(3) Repeated failure of fertilization due to poor oocyte quality;

(4) Poor-quality embryos;

(5) Repeated implantation failure of apparently normal embryos.

SOURCE OF OOCYTE DONORS

The demand for donor oocytes far outstrips the supply of donors, who are generally recruited from two categories:

Known donors, where the donor donates specifically to a named recipient and is always altruistic;

Anonymous donors, where a donor donates her oocytes to a suitably matched recipient anonymously.

Anonymous donors can be unpaid, paid or egg-sharing donors.

Unpaid donors are those who donate directly to the waiting-list of oocyte recipients and are in the true sense altruistic.

Paid donors receive monetary benefits by donating their oocytes, which is allowed in the United States and some other countries. In the United Kingdom, the law states that 'no money or other benefit shall be given or received in respect of any supply of gametes or embryos unless authorised by directions'[24]. Any payment is therefore illegal.

In *egg sharing*, patients undergoing assisted reproductive technologies (ART) share half of their oocytes with an anonymous recipient. In lieu of this, they are offered treatment at a subsidized cost or no cost. This is the most widely practiced form of egg donation today in the UK.

ADVANTAGES OF THE SHARED-OOCYTE PROGRAM

(1) There is a reduced potential health hazard to non-patient donors;

(2) There is a shorter waiting time for recipients;

(3) Patients undergoing the shared-oocyte program are offered ART at a subsidized cost; this allows more women to receive treatment as, for many, the treatment becomes financially more viable;

(4) It can be utilized as a valuable research tool.

Sterilization patients

Some women undergoing tubal sterilization may, after suitable counseling, choose to have ovarian stimulation and oocyte retrieval at the time of sterilization, and to donate their oocytes to an anonymous recipient. This system has the advantage of using donors with proven fertility. This may be perceived to be against the altruistic principles of oocyte donation and is thus now rarely used in the UK.

RECRUITMENT AND SCREENING OF DONORS AND RECIPIENTS

Recruitment and screening of oocyte donors

(1) Donors should be between 19 and 35 years of age. There is a proven inverse relationship between age and birth rate[25]. Younger donors are known to achieve significantly higher pregnancy rates for recipients, suggesting that age should be a major factor in selecting prospective donors[26], and this also reduces the risk of aneuploidies in the off-spring[27,28].

(2) Previous known fertility has been shown to improve pregnancy success rates in recipients[29,30]; thus, prior gravidity is an important predictor of clinical pregnancy in donor oocyte cycles. In our own practice we try to recruit donors who already have children.

(3) Body mass index (BMI) should be < 30 kg/m² High BMI is detrimental to the outcome of IVF treatment[31].

(4) Ovarian reserve testing using early follicular phase FSH, LH and estradiol levels is carried out. The measurement of serum basal FSH and estradiol on day 2 or 3 of a menstrual cycle is often used to test for ovarian reserve. Common criteria for normal ovarian reserve are an early follicular phase FSH level of < 10 IU/l and an estradiol level of < 80 pg/ml. Elevated levels of FSH and estradiol are predictive of decreased ovarian response to stimulation with gonadotropins, requiring higher doses of gonadotropin and leading to higher IVF cancellation rates and lower pregnancy rates[32–35]. This is of particular relevance to egg-sharing patients.

(5) Full medical and family history is taken.

(6) Comprehensive general/physical and gynecological examination is conducted.

All patients are allowed a mandatory period of 1 month to make a considered decision before they visit the clinic for a review by the nurse co-ordinator. In-depth counseling by an independent counselor is considered to be essential. Consent forms are signed at this stage. Blood tests for screening are done. The 'cooling off' period allows couples to reconsider their decision before making the final commitment.

Recruitment of oocyte recipients

(1) There is as yet no upper age limit for oocyte recipients; however, at Bourn Hall, patients up to the age of 48–50 years are considered for treatment with donated oocytes.

(2) It is recommended that all recipients should be married or in a stable relationship.

(3) Detailed medical and family history is taken.

(4) General, physical and pelvic examinations are carried out. A pelvic ultrasound scan may be required to rule out pelvic pathologies such as ovarian cysts and fibroids. An assessment of endometrial thickness and quality is important in the late follicular or early luteal phase of the cycle. In the event of either a thin endometrium <6 mm or a thick irregular endometrium >14 mm an out-patient hysteroscopy should be considered. Hystero-contrast sonography using saline and galactose-based contrast medium has been used to assess endometrial cavity lesions, such as uterine polyps, submucous fibroids and congenital uterine anomalies. Doppler scans are used to assess uterine artery blood flow resistance, especially in women who have had previous pelvic radiation.

(5) Women with Turner's syndrome should have specialist cardiovascular and renal assessment.

(6) Women with hypertension, diabetes and heart disease should be managed appropriately.

(7) Amenorrheic oocyte recipients should be started on the standard cyclical combined hormone replacement therapy (HRT) preparation (see below).

Screening tests for oocyte donors

(1) Full blood count;

(2) Blood group and rhesus status;

(3) Tests for cystic fibrosis carrier status;

(4) Infection screen:

(a) Hepatitis B, hepatitis C, human immunodeficiency virus (HIV)-I and –II;

(b) Venereal Disease Research Laboratory/ *Treponema pallidum* hemagglutination assay (VDRL/ TPHA) for syphilis;

(c) Cytomegalovirus (CMV) antibody, immunoglobulins IgG and IgM;

(5) Cytogenetic analysis for karyotype;

(6) Enzymatic assay for Tay–Sachs disease carrier status (targeted screening, based on ethnic background)

(7) Sickle cell screen (targeted screening, based on ethnic background);

(8) Hemoglobin electrophoresis (targeted screening, based on ethnic background);

(9) Recent recipients of vaccinia vaccine and symptomatic contacts of smallpox vaccine recipients should defer treatment until their clinical status is clear. Although there is no definitive evidence linking vaccinia virus transmission through reproductive cells, good donor practice recommends deferring treatment for all such patients[36].

Rigorous screening strategies should be in place to avoid any genetic or infectious conditions being transmitted to the recipient or any offspring. Women testing positive to any of the screening tests are not eligible to act as donors. They should have the opportunity to discuss the results, and the implications on their own future medical and reproductive health, with the appropriate medical personnel.

If the prospective donor is found to be heterozygous for cystic fibrosis, the partner of the recipient should also be screened for cystic fibrosis. In this situation, the recipient has the option of rejecting the donor.

Written and verbal explanation should be provided at each step. Every clinic should aim to provide a dedicated team to guide these patients through their treatment. Women donating eggs are encouraged to keep their general practitioner involved.

Screening tests for oocyte recipients

(1) Blood group and rhesus status;

(2) Hemoglobin;

(3) Immunity to rubella;

(4) In-date cervical smear;

(5) Viral screening for HIV-I and -II, hepatitis B, hepatitis C and CMV antibodies.

The partner of the recipient should be negative for hepatitis B and C as well as HIV-I and -II antibodies, and also have a routine semen assessment. Advice on intracytoplasmic sperm injection (ICSI), if recommended, is provided at this stage.

COUNSELING OF DONORS AND RECIPIENTS

All prospective oocyte donors should be offered full counseling. Although the donor is not obliged to accept this, it is the duty of all involved in the program to ensure that the prospective donor is given enough information to make a fully informed decision. All patients and their partners will require a detailed explanation of the procedures involved and should have counseling on the moral, ethical and legal implications of oocyte donation. When dealing with oocyte recipients who have been exposed to chemotherapy in the past, their prognosis for long-term survival must be discussed before they consider treatment in order to become parents. Three distinct types of counseling should be made available:

(1) *Implications counseling*: this aims to help couples understand the implications or the effect of the proposed treatment on them, their family and any other children born as a result of the treatment.

(2) *Support counseling*: this aims to provide emotional support in times of stress during the treatment, e.g. an unsuccessful outcome.

(3) *Therapeutic counseling:* this aims to help couples understand and come to terms with the consequences of infertility and its treatment. It helps them to resolve any problems arising as result of treatment and to come to terms with the reality.

MATCHING PHYSICAL CHARACTERISTICS OF DONORS AND RECIPIENTS

The physical attributes compatible with the oocyte donor's phenotype are utilized in recruiting recipients. Blood group, rhesus status and CMV status are matched as closely as possible. Physical characteristics of the donor, such as skin color, eye color, height and weight are matched as closely as possible to the physical characteristics of the recipient couple. Ethnicity is an important aspect of matching, and most recipients prefer to have donors of their own ethnic origin. Some recipients, especially of certain religious faiths, may be specific in their choice of donors based on their religion. All clinics should endeavor to provide recipients with as close a match as possible and to comply with their specific requests. Once the recipient couple are satisfied with the match, they are obliged to sign an official acceptance form before the treatment can begin.

METHODS AND PROTOCOL FOR TREATMENT

Oocyte donors

Women undergoing treatment as oocyte donors are generally young, with regular cycles and without gynecological problems. The standard ovarian follicular stimulation protocol involves pituitary desensitization with a gonadotropin releasing hormone (GnRH) analog from the mid-luteal phase (day 21) in women with 28-day cycles and ovarian stimulation with gonadotropins, recombinant human FSH (r-hFSH) or human menopausal gonadotropin (hMG). The dose of gonadotropin will depend on the patient's age and ovarian reserve assessments. Long-acting GnRH analogs achieve the same results as those administered daily by nasal spray, but are more convenient for the patient[37]. GnRH antagonists can be used in cycling donors to reduce the total amount of gonadotropins and for shorter treatment times[38]. The first monitoring scan is performed on day 6 or 7 of stimulation and follicles > 12 mm in diameter are counted. Thereafter, scans are done at 1- or 2-day intervals, based on clinical observations. At each scan, estradiol levels are measured and interpreted in relation to follicular growth. When the leading follicle is between 16 and 18 mm in diameter, and usually on or about stimulation day 11–12, a surrogate LH surge is achieved with an injection of human chorionic gonadotropin (hCG). Oocyte retrieval is timed 36–40 h after hCG, under sedation or general anesthesia, as a day-case procedure. Under ultrasound guidance, transvaginal needle aspiration of all the follicles on both ovaries is performed (Chapter 20). The oocytes are then inseminated with a preparation of her partner's sperm.

Egg-sharing donors

With respect to the egg-sharing program, every clinic must have strict guidelines and protocols for recruitment of donors and treatment. In women donating in an egg-share arrangement, every clinic has a fixed number of oocytes that have to be collected in order for her to share with the recipient. Many studies have been done to identify a safe 'cut-off' number for both the donor and the recipient. It has been shown that decreasing the number of oocytes from a cut-off limit of 12 to eight, does not reduce the pregnancy rate in either the recipient or the donor, but reduces the cycle cancellation rate significantly[39]. Therefore, according to the standard protocol at Bourn Hall, if the donor has fewer than eight developing follicles on day 8 of stimulation, she is encouraged to have treatment for herself only. If on the day of oocyte retrieval seven or fewer oocytes are retrieved, then the donor retains all the oocytes and the recipient's cycle is canceled. When there are eight or more oocytes, they are divided equally between the donor and recipient and any odd number is allocated to the donor. Embryo transfer may be done on day 2 for the donor and day 3 for the recipient in an attempt to maintain anonymity. Although different centers vary in their protocol, the aim should be to achieve an adequate number of oocytes for both the donor and the recipient, with as few cycle cancellations as possible.

EMBRYO TRANSFER IN OOCYTE RECIPIENTS

Recipients without ovarian function (acyclic women)

Women without active ovaries are started on hormone replacement therapy (HRT) a few months prior to their planned treatment. They undergo careful assessment of the endometrium to rule out pathologies such as endometrial polyps, submucous fibroids impinging into the endometrial cavity, inadequate endometrial thickness or hyperplastic endometrium. An out-patient hysteroscopy may be indicated to confirm the diagnosis of the above (Chapter 6). The treatment is then synchronized with the donor's cycle. The follicular phase can be prolonged using HRT to achieve close synchrony[40]. The recipient's partner is required to produce a fresh semen sample on the day of donor's oocyte retrieval and embryo transfer is carried out 2 or 5 days later (Table 2).

Recipients with ovarian function (cyclic women)

Embryo transfer may be in a natural cycle or a hormone replacement cycle.

Embryo transfer in a natural cycle

Most recipients are older women and may have irregular cycles. Patients who have had recurrent failure of

previous IVF–embryo transfer (ET) treatment, or who have had poor responses to ovarian stimulation, will benefit from hormone replacement, rather than natural-cycle treatment. Natural cycles must be monitored closely by serial ultrasound scanning and estimations of plasma estradiol, progesterone and LH to determine the time of ovulation. Although in a natural cycle frozen ET is straightforward, fresh embryo transfer may be difficult due to the complexity of synchronizing donor and recipient cycles. ET is usually performed 3–4 days after the LH surge is detected. hCG may be administered to the donor within 24–48 h of the expected LH surge of the recipient.

Embryo transfer in a hormone replacement cycle

Women with regular menstrual cycles are 'down-regulated' with a GnRH analog, and receive estradiol valerate in incremental doses to achieve endometrial growth. Progesterone is added on the day of the donor's oocyte retrieval (Table 3). The present protocol at Bourn Hall is a modified form of the regimen used by Lutjen and colleagues in their original work[3]. The constant-dose protocol was introduced by Serhal and Craft[6]. They administered supraphysiological doses of estradiol valerate 6–8 mg orally daily for a variable length of time, and progesterone in the form of progesterone in oil 100 mg intramuscularly daily commencing on the day before the donor had her oocytes recovered. This protocol has the advantage of simplicity and of providing a larger window of time for transfer.

Synchronization of donor and recipient cycles is essential and can be achieved in various ways. The donor's menstrual period can be scheduled with pre-treatment with a combined oral contraceptive pill, or using norethisterone to postpone it. Alteration of the 'follicular phase' of estrogen replacement can help to synchronize the two cycles[40]. Administration of a GnRH analog to recipients with poor ovarian function can be used for synchronization. When pituitary down-regulation is achieved in both the donor and the recipient, the recipient starts her estrogen replacement, and the donor starts her ovarian stimulation regimen 5–6 days later. There is strong evidence that a temporal window of maximal endometrial receptivity exists[41]. Cryopreservation of the embryos and replacement at a later date may overcome any problem of dys-synchrony, but this may lead to a loss of embryos due to freezing and thawing.

Table 2 Embryo transfer protocol at Bourn Hall for acyclic women (with no ovarian function) receiving fresh embryos from donated oocytes

Day of week and date	Day of cycle	Tablets of estradiol valerate (Progynova®)	Luteal support with progesterone (Cyclogest®)
			IMPORTANT
Start of estradiol valerate	day 1	2 mg (1 tablet)	endometrial and Doppler scan is done on day 13
	day 2	2 mg (1 tablet)	in the event of inadequate endometrial thickness, i.e. <6 mm, increase Progynova to 8 mg daily and
	day 3	2 mg (1 tablet)	add aspirin 75 mg daily, rescan 2 days later
	day 4	2 mg (1 tablet)	the recipient's partner provides a fresh semen sample on the day of donor'
	day 5	2 mg (1 tablet)	oocyte retrieval
	day 6	4 mg (2 tablets)	the first pessary (Cyclogest 400 mg) will be used in the evening 2 days before the
	day 7	4 mg(2 tablets)	planned embryo transfer or evening of the donor's oocyte retrieval day and thereafter twice a day
	day 8	4 mg (2 tablets)	
	day 9	4 mg (2 tablets)	embryo transfer for day-2 or -3 cleaved embryos is done between days 15 and 21
	day 10	6 mg (3 tablets)	in the case of blastocyst transfer, the Cyclogest will be started 5–6 days prior to planned embryo transfer,
	day 11	6 mg (3 tablets)	i.e. transfer between days 19 and 23
	day 12	6 mg (3 tablets)	in the event of a pregnancy, Progynova is increased to 8 mg daily and progesterone is continued
Endometrial and Doppler scan	day 13	6 mg (3 tablets)	until day 77, after which the dose is tapered off over a week and then stopped
	day 14	6 mg (3 tablets)	
	day 15	6 mg (3 tablets)	
	transfer day	6 mg (3 tablets)	

RESULTS OF TREATMENT WITH DONATED OOCYTES

Excellent pregnancy and live birth rates have been achieved using oocyte donation. Table 4 summarizes the clinical pregnancy and live birth rates after oocyte donation. Paulson and co-workers reported an overall clinical pregnancy rate of 36.2%, with a cumulative pregnancy rate after four cycles of 87.9%. In addition, the overall delivery rate was 29.3% and the cumulative delivery rate was 86.1%. They showed that neither the recipient's age nor the diagnosis plays a substantial role in the success of oocyte donation[43]. Abdalla and colleagues reported that the decline in fecundity with age could not be explained by uterine factors alone[44]. In a separate study they concluded that oocyte donation should be considered as high risk, especially in those with ovarian failure, because of an increased incidence of small-for-gestational-age infants in these pregnancies. There is also a higher risk of pregnancy-induced hypertension and postpartum hemorrhage[45].

Edwards and colleagues[46] studied the comparative fertility of cyclic and acyclic women aged <50 years of age and found that, age for age, acyclic women were more fertile than those who received their own oocytes. Marcus and Edwards[47] reported high pregnancy rates in women who had amenorrhea for >4 months before their IVF treatment. They attributed

Table 3	Embryo transfer protocol for patients with regular cycles having embryo transfer as oocyte recipients			

Baseline scan	Day of HRT cycle	Start Synarel® or buserelin: luteal phase of previous cycle	Tablets of estradiol valerate (Progynova)	Luteal support with progesterone (Cyclogest)
	day 1	buserelin or Synarel	2 mg (1 tablet)	the first pessary (Cyclogest 400 mg) will be used on the evening 2 days before the planned embryo
	day 2	buserelin or Synarel	2 mg (1 tablet)	transfer, and thereafter twice a day
	day 3	buserelin or Synarel	2 mg (1 tablet)	in the case of blastocyst transfer, the Cyclogest will be started 5–6 days prior to planned
	day 4	buserelin or Synarel	2 mg (1 tablet)	embryo transfer
	day 5	buserelin or Synarel	2 mg (1 tablet)	the recipient's partner provides a fresh semen sample on the day of donor's oocyte retrieval
	day 6	buserelin or Synarel	4 mg (2 tablets)	
	day 7	buserelin or Synarel	4 mg (2 tablets)	the buserelin or Synarel continues until the day of donor's hCG
	day 8	buserelin or Synarel	4 mg (2 tablets)	if pregnancy test is positive, then Progynova and progesterone are continued until
	day 9	buserelin or Synarel	4 mg (2 tablets)	day 77 and then tapered off over a week
	day 10	buserelin or Synarel	6 mg (3 tablets)	
	day 11	buserelin or Synarel	6 mg (3 tablets)	
	day 12		6 mg (3 tablets)	
Endometrial and Doppler scan	day 13		6 mg (3 tablets)	
	day 14		6 mg (3 tablets)	
	day 15		6 mg (3 tablets)	
	transfer day		6 mg (3 tablets	

HRT, hormone replacement therapy; hCG, human chorionic gonadotropin

Table 4	Clinical pregnancy rate (CPR) and live births (LB) after oocyte donation				

Source	Status of embryos	Patients (n)	ET cycles (n)	CPR/ET	LB/ET
HFEA	fresh	826	916	226 (24.7%)	180 (19.7%)
HFEA	frozen	298	331	64 (19.3%)	48 (14.5%)
Bourn Hall*	frozen	104	107	37 (34.6%)	29 (27.1%)
Bourn Hall†	fresh	82	97	30 (30.9%)	29 (29.8%)
	frozen	82	98	27 (27.5%)	21 (21.4%)

HFEA, Human Fertilisation and Embryology Authority. Sixth Annual Report for the year 1995[42]; *Bourn Hall Clinic data during the period 1985–95; †Bourn Hall Clinic data during the period 1996–2003; ET, embryo transfer the higher pregnancy rates in agonadal women to the possible effect of uterine rest, which may restore the function of steroid-sensitive structures, such as the pinopodes[48,49], after a long period of constant menstrual cycling[50,51].

There are no reports of increased fetal abnormalities following oocyte donations, although data are scanty. Agonadal women can breast-feed their babies, and suckling is sufficient to maintain the milk supply.

LEGAL, MORAL AND ETHICAL ISSUES

It is important that both oocyte recipients and their donors have appropriate counseling and a clear understanding of the legal, moral and ethical issues related to oocyte donation.

Legal

In the UK, donors are not paid, thus, 'gametes cannot be sold'. However, reasonable expenses can be paid to a maximum of £15, plus other costs incurred from loss of work or travel during the treatment. This is in contrast to the USA, where payment of gamete donors is allowed.

Although the legal status of oocyte donation is clear in most countries, conflicting opinions about the rights and interests of oocyte donors still persist in some countries. Oocyte donation is not allowed in Austria, Bangladesh, Egypt, El-Salvador, Germany, Japan, Jordan, Morocco, Norway, Portugal, Saudi Arabia, Switzerland, Tunisia and Turkey. In Denmark, egg-sharing is the only form of oocyte donation allowed.

Until recently, all gamete donations (except known donation) in the UK were on an anonymous basis. Concerns were, however, expressed by experts about the rights of children born from gamete donation to find out more about their genetic parents. Golombok and colleagues raised some pertinent issues in 1996[52], and highlighted the views and concerns relating to disclosure and secrecy in couples who conceived using donated gametes. A study by Söderström-Antilla in 1995, from Finland, reported that almost 42% of oocyte donors preferred not to receive any information concerning either the child or the recipient couple[53]. The Department of Health in the UK aims to abolish anonymity from sperm, egg and embryo donors from April 2005. Children born from donor gametes produced after this date, on attaining the age of 18 years, will have access to information identifying their genetic parents.

Moral

The vulnerability of oocyte recipients is an important issue. Gentle but professional implications counseling is mandatory. This should address anonymity issues and the forthcoming change in the law. Women awaiting their turn on the waiting list to receive donated oocytes are often willing to accept anything on offer. They should thus be given all information relevant to their treatment and any other information on legal issues that may affect them. The recipient couple should be aware that they would become the legal parents of any resulting children. They will thus be responsible for all costs relating to rearing the child, including those which may arise in the event of any disability that the child may have. Clear explanations should be given about the likelihood of a successful pregnancy, risks of multiple pregnancy, ectopic pregnancy, miscarriage and welfare of the child issues. In accordance with the Human Fertilisation and Embryology Act (1990), the clinic has a statutory obligation to take account of the welfare of the child, and of any other children that may be affected by treatment.

Egg-share donors are usually better informed than altruistic donors, as many have undergone treatment before and have suffered the agony of being infertile. However, donor counseling should include the change in the law of anonymity and the frustration in the event of several failed attempts at treatment. The potential risks to altruistic donors, such as ovarian hyperstimulation and infection, should be explained. All altruistic donors should use adequate contraception during the treatment.

Ethical

To some couples, donated oocytes are unacceptable, and this may be due to their religious beliefs. Ethical dilemmas are always being raised in relation to gamete donation and the debate will continue. The ethical argument about egg-sharing, which, in effect, defies the law in the UK that 'no money or other benefit in kind shall be given or received in respect of any supply of gametes or embryos', continues. The possible feelings of 'coercion', especially with sister-to-sister donation and the family stresses in known donations, remain. Arguably, as the demand for oocytes far outweighs the supply, a compromise between the ethical concerns and beliefs and the practical issues has to be found.

CONCLUSION

Oocyte donation remains one of the ways of bringing the joy of parenthood to many couples who cannot conceive naturally. The ethical, moral, legal and medical issues have been addressed time and time again, yet the debate goes on. Strict guidelines and protocols are necessary. Within the complexity of these issues, continued efforts have to be made to improve the outcome of oocyte donation programs for both the recipients and the oocyte donors.

REFERENCES

1. Human Fertilisation and Embryology Authority. Annual Report (1 April 2000–31 March 2001). London: HFEA, 2001

2. Trounson A, Leeton J, Besanko M, Wood C. Pregnancy established in an infertile recipient after transfer of a donated embryo fertilised in vitro. Br Med J 1983; 286: 835–8

3. Lutjen P, Trounson A, Leeton J, et al. The establishment and maintenance of pregnancy using in vitro fertilization and embryo transfer in a patient with primary ovarian failure. Nature (London) 1984; 307: 174–5

4. Asch R, Balmaceda J, Ord T, et al. Oocyte donation and gamete intrafallopian transfer as treatment for premature ovarian failure. Lancet 1987; 1: 687

5. Yovich JL, Blackledge DG, Richardson PA, et al. PROST for ovum donation. Lancet 1987; 1: 1209–10

6. Serhal PF, Craft IL. Ovum donation – a simplified approach. Fertil Steril 1987; 48: 265–9

7. Van Steirteghem AC, Van den Abeel E, Braeckmans P, et al. Pregnancy with a frozen–thawed embryo in a woman with primary ovarian failure. N Engl J Med 1987; 317: 113

8. Ahuja KK, Simons EG, Fiamanya W, et al. Egg sharing in assisted conception: ethical and practical considerations Hum Reprod 1996; 11: 1126–31

9. Human Fertilisation and Embryology Authority. Paid egg sharing to be regulated, not banned. [Press release]. London: HFEA, 10 December 1998

10. Human Fertilisation and Embryology Authority. Notes of meeting July 1999. http://www.hfea.gov.uk/frame .htm

11. Antinori S, Versaci C, Gholami GH, et al. Oocyte donation in menopausal women. Hum Reprod 1993; 8: 1487–90

12. Sauer MV, Paulson RJ, Lobo RA. Pregnancy after age 50: application of oocyte donation to women after natural menopause. Lancet 1993; 341: 321–3

13. Borini A, Bafaro G, Violini F, et al. Pregnancies in postmenopausal women over 50 years old in an oocyte donation program. Fertil Steril 1994; 63: 258–61

14. Weiss G. Fertility in the older woman. Clin Consult Obstet Gynaecol 1996; 8: 56–9

15. Baker TG. A quantitative and cytological study of germ cells in the human ovary. Proc R Soc (London) 1963; 158: 417–33

16. Faddy MJ, Gosden RG. A model conforming the decline in follicle numbers to the age of menopause in women. Hum Reprod 1996; 11: 1484–6

17. Conway GS, Payne NN, Webb J, et al. Fragile X premutation screening in women with premature ovarian failure. Hum Reprod 1998; 13: 1184–7

18. Jones JS, DeMoraes-Rheusen M. A new syndrome of amenorrhoea with hypergonadotropism and apparently normal follicular apparatus. Am J Obstet Gynecol 1969; 104: 597–600

19. Jewelewicz R, Schwartz M. Premature ovarian failure. Bull NY Acad Med 1986; 62: 219–36

20. Foudilla T, Söderström-Antilla V, Hovatta O. Turner's syndrome and pregnancies after oocyte donation. Hum Reprod 1999; 14: 532–5

21. Press F, Shapiro FM, Cowell CA, Oliver GD. Outcome of ovum donation in Turner's syndrome patients. Fertil Steril 1995; 64: 99

22. Liu J, Lissens W, Silber SJ, et al. Birth after preimplantation diagnosis of cystic fibrosis delta F508 mutation by polymerase chain reaction in human embryos resulting from intracytoplasmic sperm injection with epipidymal sperm. J Am Med Assoc 1994; 23: 1858–60

23. Sermon K, Van Steirteghem A, Liebaers I. Preimplantation genetic diagnosis Lancet 2004; 363: 1633–41

24. Human Fertilisation and Embryology Act (1990) Section 12. London: HMSO, 1990

25. Harris SE, Faddy M, Levett S, et al. Analysis of donor heterogeneity as a factor affecting the clinical outcome of oocyte donation. Hum Fertil (Camb) 2002; 5: 193–8

26. Cohen MA, Lindheim SR, Sauer MV. Donor age is paramount to success in oocyte donation. Hum Reprod 1999; 14: 2755–8

27. American College of Obstetricians and Gynaecologists. Genetic screening of gamete donors. ACOG

Committee Opinion Number 192, October 1997. Committee on genetics. Int J Gynaecol Obstet 1998; 60: 190–2

28. Aird I, Barratt C, Murdoch A, et al. BFS recommendation for good practice on screening of egg and embryo donors. Hum Fertil (Camb) 2003; 3: 162–5

29. Darder MC, Epstein YM, Treiser SL, et al. The effects of prior gravidity on the outcomes of ovum donor and own oocyte cycles. Fertil Steril 1996; 65: 578–82

30. Abdalla HI, Barber R, Kirkland A, et al. A report on 100 cycles of oocyte donation; factors affecting the outcome. Hum Reprod 1990; 5: 1018–22

31. Salha O, Dada T, Sharma V. Influence of body mass index and self administration of hCG in the outcome of IVF cycles: a prospective cohort study. Hum Fertil (Camb) 2001; 4: 37–42

32. Smotrich DB, Widra EA, Gindoff PR, et al. Prognostic value of day 3 estradiol on in vitro fertilization outcome. Fertil Steril 1995; 64: 1136–40

33. Frattarelli JL, Bergh PA, Drews MR, et al. Evaluation of basal estradiol levels in assisted reproductive technology cycles. Fertil Steril 2000; 74: 518–24

34. Licciardi FL, Liu HC, Rosenwaks Z. Day 3 estradiol serum concentrations as prognosticators of ovarian stimulation response and pregnancy outcome in patients undergoing in vitro fertilization. Fertil Steril 1995; 64: 991–4

35. Toner JP, Philput CB, Jones GS, Muasher SJ. Basal follicle–stimulating hormone level is a better predictor of in vitro fertilization performance than age. Fertil Steril 1991; 55: 784–91

36. The Practice Committeee of American Society for Reproductive Medicine and the Society for Assisted Reproductive Technology. Society for Assisted Reproductive Technology position statement on donor suitability of recipients of smallpox vaccine (vaccinia virus). Fertil Steril 2004; 81: 1172–3

37. Neuspiller F, Levy M, Remohi J, et al. The use of long- and short-acting forms of gonadotropin-releasing hormone analogues in women undergoing oocyte donations. Hum Reprod 1998; 13: 1148–51

38. Sauer MV, Paulson RJ, Lobo RA. Comparing the clinical utility of GnRH antagonist to GnRH agonist in an oocyte donation program. Gynaecol Obstet Invest 1997; 43: 215–18

39. Kolibianakis EM, Tournaye H, Osmanagaoglu K, et al. Outcome of donors and recipients in two egg-sharing policies. Fertil Steril 2003; 79: 69–73

40. Remohi J, Gutierrez A, Cano K, et al. Long oesrogen replacement in an oocyte donation programme. Hum Reprod 1995: 10: 1387–91

41. Devroey P, Pados G. Preparation of endometrium for egg donation. Hum Reprod Update 1998; 4: 856–61

42. Human Fertilisation and Embryology Authority. Sixth Annual Report for the Year 1995. London: HFEA, 1997

43. Paulson RJ, Hatch IL, Lobo RA, Sauer MV. Cumulative conception and live birth rates after oocyte donation: implications regarding endometrial receptivity. Hum Reprod 1997; 12: 835–9

44. Abdalla HI, Wren ME, Thomas A, Korea L. Age of the uterus does not affect pregnancy or implantation rates; a study of egg donation in women of different ages sharing oocytes from the same donor. Hum Reprod 1997; 12: 827–9

45. Abdalla HI, Billett A, Kan AK, et al. Obstetric outcome in 232 ovum donation pregnancies. Br J Obstet Gynaecol 1998; 105: 332–7

46. Edwards RG, Marcus S, MacNamee M, et al. High fecundity of amenorrhoeic women in embryo transfer programmes. Lancet 1991; 238: 292–4

47. Marcus S, Edwards RG. High rates of pregnancy after long-term down-regulation of women with severe endometriosis. Am J Obstet Gynecol 1994; 171: 812–17

48. Psychoyos A. The high fertility of agonadal and amenorrhoeic women after oocyte donation [Letter]. Hum Reprod 1993; 8: 498–9

49. Nikas G, Drakakis P, Loutradis D, et al. Uterine pinopodes as a marker of the nidation window in cyclic women receiving exogenous estradiol and progesterone. Hum Reprod 1995; 10: 1208–13

50. Edwards RG. Why are agonadal and post-menopausal women so fertile after oocyte donation [Editorial]. Hum Reprod 1992; 7: 733–4

51. Edwards RG, Marcus SF. Does a period of amenorrhoea raise subsequent chances of implantation in women? Curr Sci 1995; 68: 386–91

52. Golombok S, Brewaeys A, Cook R, et al. The European study of assisted reproduction families: family functioning and child development. Hum Reprod 1996; 11: 2324–31

53. Söderström-Antilla V. Follow-up study of Finnish volunteer oocyte donors concerning their attitudes to oocyte donation. Hum Reprod 1995; 10: 3073–6

20.2

Embryo donation

Thomas Matthews

Ever since controlled ovarian hyperstimulation was first used in *in vitro* fertilization (IVF) practice for producing multiple follicular development, couples have had 'spare' embryos, after selection of those to be transferred. In the early days of IVF, there was anxiety amongst clinicians, scientists and patients about the safety of freezing these spare embryos, and many of them were allowed to perish. The first successful pregnancy from a frozen–thawed embryo was reported in Melbourne in 1983[1]. Since then, others, including Wada and colleagues[2] from Bourn Hall, have shown that there is no increase in fetal abnormalities in babies born from frozen–thawed embryos, when compared with babies born from fresh embryos.

The donation of their 'spare' embryos by a couple, for the use of another infertile couple, has always been a rather emotive topic, and there are a number of specific issues to be considered in such a situation. Treatment with donated embryos has, however, become a very real, and sometimes the only, viable option for some infertile couples. This treatment option was first carried out successfully in Australia, and reported by Trounson[3] and Leeton[4] and co-workers in 1983. The procedure is now legal and widely practiced in the United Kingdom, and has been offered at Bourn Hall Clinic for more than two decades.

As embryo freezing and thawing became more successful and more widespread, couples increasingly requested that their spare embryos be cryopreserved. The obvious reason for freezing spare embryos was that, if the initial treatment was not successful, the couple could return a few months later to have frozen–thawed embryos transferred, without going through the whole process of ovarian stimulation and oocyte collection again. Better still, if the couple were successful at their first attempt in achieving a pregnancy and live birth, they could return a year or more later to try for another baby from the same batch of embryos. By this time, the forerunners of the Human Fertilisation and Embryology Authority (HFEA), and later the HFEA, had ruled that embryos could be kept cryopreserved for 5 years initially, and that this storage period could be extended by another 5 years to a maximum of 10 years. The safety of long-term storage of embryos was demonstrated by Avery and colleagues[5].

For couples who then decided to limit their family size after the first one or two live births following IVF, the question of what was to be done with their cryopreserved 'spare' embryos became a serious ethical and moral issue. The alternative to having more treatment, and possibly more babies, was to authorize the destruction of their embryos, or to allow scientific research with their embryos. The first option was unacceptable to many infertile couples after they had been to such lengths to achieve these embryos. The second option of donating supernumerary embryos for research has always been available to patients, but the acceptability of this varies around the world. In the USA, according to Hoffman and associates[6], there were about 400 000 embryos stored nationwide, based on statistics from the Society for Assisted Reproductive Technology (SART), but only 2.8% of these were available for research. In contrast to this, reports from other countries have varied, from 30% in Australia[7], 54% in the United Kingdom[8], 60% in Denmark[9] and 92% in Sweden[10].

There was then a third option – that of donating these embryos for the treatment of another infertile couple. This option is, however, only acceptable to a small percentage of couples with frozen/stored supernumerary embryos. Van Voorhis and colleagues[11] from the United States reported that at the University of Iowa Hospitals and Clinics, only 11% of couples elected to donate their embryos to other infertile couples, while Kovacs and co-workers[12] from Monash University IVF clinic in Melbourne, Australia, reported that 89.5% of couples opted to discard rather than donate their embryos.

Donors of embryos

Donors are healthy young couples who have had IVF or intracytoplasmic sperm injection (ICSI) therapy, and who have supernumerary embryos in storage. Most of these couples have had their own gametes used in their treatment, but occasionally the embryos may have been created from donated sperm or from donated eggs. In the United Kingdom, the female partner who produced the eggs used in the creation of these embryos would have been under 36 years of age at the time of their creation. Before the IVF procedure that resulted in the creation of these embryos, both genetic parents would have been screened for human immunodeficiency virus (HIV) antibodies, hepatitis B surface antigen and hepatitis C antibodies. Before assigning these embryos to another couple, and at least 6 months from the date of the original tests, the HIV test is repeated for both partners. They are, in addition, screened for syphilis by Venereal Disease Laboratories (VDRL) test and/or *Treponema pallidum* hemagglutination assay (TPHA). They are also screened for cytomegalovirus (CMV, immunoglobulins IgG and IgM antibodies) and for cystic fibrosis carrier status, and their blood group and karyotype are confirmed.

Other screening tests, e.g. for sickle cell disease, thalassemia, Tay–Sachs disease, etc. are done in specific ethnic groups.

Both partners are given a detailed questionnaire (Appendix A) asking for details of their ethnic background, physical characteristics, occupation, religion, personal and family history, and in particular the medical details of any children that they have. They are also invited to write details of their hobbies and interests, their strengths and weaknesses, and a description of their own personalities. They are strongly urged to have free and independent counseling from one of the clinic counselors, although they have the right to decline this. Their original consent to the duration of embryo storage is checked, and, if necessary, they are requested to consent to extension of that storage for the maximum permitted period of 10 years.

Recipients of donated embryos

For these couples, receiving donated embryos is often far easier to accept psychologically than receiving donated gametes (sperm or oocytes). Although the resulting child will not be genetically related to either parent, both partners accept an equal responsibility for their infertility, and the element of 'blame' of one partner by the other is eliminated. Receiving donated embryos is, in a way, the earliest form of 'adoption', without having to go through all the legal difficulties that the normal adoption process entails. Furthermore, by going through a pregnancy and delivery, the recipient couple have the opportunity to 'bond' with their baby from a very early stage.

Receiving donated embryos is far safer than IVF for the female partner, as it eliminates the risk of ovarian hyperstimulation syndrome (OHSS) and the surgical and anesthetic risks (albeit small) associated with oocyte retrieval. Finally, the cost of treatment with donated embryos is less than the cost of IVF, inclusive of the cost of the drugs needed for ovarian stimulation.

For a couple to be accepted on the waiting-list for donated embryos, both partners must have a significant degree of impairment of gametogenesis. In the female partner, this is usually menopause, or incipient menopause, whether natural or premature. Premature menopause may be idiopathic, or may be part of the sequelae of pelvic surgery, radiotherapy or chemotherapy. In the male partner, there is either total azoospermia, or grossly deficient sperm parameters, where even intracytoplasmic sperm injection (ICSI) would be considered unlikely to succeed. In rare situations, embryo donation is indicated where gametogenesis is normal, but where one (or both) partner has a genetic condition that would make it highly likely that any fetus resulting from their own gametes would be seriously affected.

Both partners in the recipient couple undergo detailed medical screening, including physical examination, blood tests for HIV antibodies, hepatitis B surface antigens and hepatitis C antibodies. The blood group of each partner is checked, and the female partner is screened for CMV IgM and IgG antibodies. If the woman has a raised IgM antibody titer, suggesting current or recent infection, the test is repeated 6 months later, and treatment is deferred until she has converted to being positive for IgG antibodies, and negative for IgM antibodies.

They are then required to complete a form (Appendix B) detailing their ethnic origin, occupation, religion or belief system (if any), physical characteristics, blood groups and the female partner's CMV status.

Counseling

Both partners are required to see an independent counselor (usually together, but could be separately) for in-depth counseling before embarking on this major decision to accept donated embryos. Counseling is an important and integral part of all assisted conception therapy, but is of even greater relevance when donated gametes or donated embryos are being used. Counseling can never be mandatory, but when the importance of counseling is carefully explained to couples, very few refuse outright. Counseling should be offered free of cost, and ideally the counselor should be an independent practitioner, with no direct financial or other connection to the clinic where the treatment is being carried out. The couples should have access to the counselor before, during and at any time after treatment.

The treatment cycle

Once all these preparations have been completed, and the appropriate consent forms signed, arrangements are made to match the prospective recipient couple with donor couples whose embryos are in storage. Care is taken to match the ethnic groups, physical characteristics and blood groups as closely as possible. A CMV-negative recipient woman is matched only to a CMV-negative donor couple, whilst a CMV-positive recipient woman may be matched to a CMV-positive or -negative donor couple.

The endometrium of the recipient woman has to be carefully prepared before donated embryos are placed within it. If the woman has regular menstrual cycles, it is advisable to down-regulate her pituitary with a standard preparation of gonadotropin releasing hormone (GnRH) agonist, and to then build up her endometrium with estradiol valerate tablets, starting with 2 mg daily, increasing gradually to a maximum of 6 mg daily (see Table 3 in Chapter 20.1). Within 2 weeks of starting this regimen, the endometrium should be 8 mm or more in thickness when measured by ultrasound scan, which should be favorable for implantation of embryos. In a menopausal woman, or one with irregular infrequent menstruation, one should prescribe three cycles of a suitable combined preparation of estradiol valerate and a progestogen to induce regular endometrial build-up and shedding, followed by estradiol valerate tablets alone as for the woman with regular menstrual cycles.

When the endometrium is considered to be sufficiently thick for embryo transfer, the GnRH agonist is stopped, and the patient begun on a course of a suitable progesterone preparation, usually as a vaginal pessary. The progesterone pessaries and the estrogen tablets are continued until a pregnancy test 2 weeks after embryo transfer. If the test is negative, both medications are discontinued, but if it is positive, these are both continued through the first trimester of pregnancy, and gradually tapered down in dosage during the last (13th) week of their use.

Results

Embryo donation is still a very uncommon treatment option in many countries, and in many clinics within the United Kingdom. Statistics regarding success rates are scarce, because the numbers of patients are usually very low. In 1992 Asch[13] reported a success rate of 77% (13/17) for patients receiving donated embryos. In 2001 Söderström-Anttila and colleagues[14] from Finland reported a clinical pregnancy rate of 27.8% (15/54) per embryo transfer, and in 2003 Kovacs and co-workers[12] from Australia reported a pregnancy rate of 17.4% (16/92) per embryo transfer and 32% (16/50) per patient.

At Bourn Hall Clinic, for the years 1995 to 2003, a total of 75 patients had 119 cycles of treatment with donated embryos. There were 40 clinical pregnancies (i.e. a fetal heartbeat seen on ultrasound scan on day 35 after embryo transfer) and 36 live births in this group, giving a clinical pregnancy rate of 33.6% per embryo transfer, and 53.3% per patient. The live birth rate was 30.2% per embryo transfer and 48.0% per patient.

CONCLUSION

Treatment with donated embryos is a valid and viable treatment option, with a high success rate, for carefully selected couples where gametogenesis is severely compromised in both partners. The program must be carefully organized and monitored, and more young couples who have had successful treatment by IVF and who have completed their own families should be encouraged to donate their embryos to other patients, rather than allowing them to perish.

The importance of counseling patients who donate embryos, and those who receive donated embryos, cannot be overemphasized. They must be made fully aware of the recent change in legislation in the United Kingdom, by which children born from donated gametes or embryos have the right, on attaining the age of 18, to identify their genetic parents.

REFERENCES

1. Trounson A, Mohr L. Human pregnancy following cryopreservation, thawing and transfer of an eight-cell embryo. Nature (London) 1983; 305: 707–9

2. Wada I, Macnamee M, Wick K, et al. Birth characteristics and perinatal outcome of babies conceived from cryopreserved embryos. Hum Reprod 1994; 9: 543–6

3. Trounson A, Leeton J, Besanko M. Pregnancy established in an infertile patient after transfer of a donated embryo fertilised in vitro. Br Med J 1983; 286: 835–8

4. Leeton J, Trounson A, Conti A, et al. Pregnancy established in an infertile recipient after transfer of a donated embryo fertilised in vitro. Fertil Steril 1983; 39: 414–15

5. Avery S, Marcus S, Spillane S, et al. Does the length of storage time affect outcome of frozen embryo replacements? J Assist Reprod Genet 1995; 12 (Suppl): 675

6. Hoffman D, Zellman G, Fair C, et al. Cryopreserved embryos in the United States and their availability for research. Fertil Steril 2003; 79: 1063–9

7. Burton P, Sanders K. Patient attitudes to donation of embryos for research. Med J Aust 2004; 180: 559–61

8. Choudhary M, Haimes E, Herbert M, et al. Demographic, medical and treatment characteristics associated with couples' decisions to donate fresh spare embryos for research. Hum Reprod 2004; 19: 2091–6

9. Bangsbøll S, Pinborg A, Andersen C, Andersen A. Patients' attitudes towards donation of surplus cryopreserved embryos for treatment or research. Hum Reprod 2004; 19: 2415–19

10. Bjuresten K, Hovatta O. Donation of embryos for stem cell research – how many couples consent? Hum Reprod 2003; 18: 1353–5

11. Van Voorhis B, Grinstead D, Sparks A, et al. Establishment of a successful donor embryo program: medical, ethical and policy issues. Fertil Steril 1999; 71: 604–8

12. Kovacs G, Breheny S, Dear M. Embryo donation at an Australian university in-vitro fertilisation clinic: issues and outcomes. Med J Aust 2003; 178: 127–9

13. Asch R. High pregnancy rates after oocyte and embryo donation. Hum Reprod 1992; 6: 733–4

14. Söderström-Anttila V, Foudila T, Ripatti U-R, Siegberg R. Embryo donation: outcome and attitudes among embryo donors and recipients. Hum Reprod 2001; 16: 1120–8

APPENDIX A

MEDICAL NUMBER ....

BOURN HALL
CLINIC

CHARACTERISTICS FORM FOR DONORS

Please can you complete this summary sheet, in addition to some or all of the enclosed HFEA Donor Information Form. Guidelines for completion of that form are herewith, and you will be able to talk to a member of staff about the form at the Clinic. However, there are some sections (25, 26 and 27) which may require some preparation before completion. A form has to be completed by each donor.

SURNAME _____

Forename _____

Date of birth _____

The items below are also on the enclosed green form, but for ease of use in the Clinic, please can you complete them on this form and on the green form.

ETHNICITY: Please refer to this list and then complete the box below regarding ethnicity.

National descriptions and ethnic codes					
A	White British	D	White & Black Caribbean	M	Black Caribbean
B	White Irish	E	White & Black African	N	Black African
C	Any other White background	F	White & Asian	P	Other Black b/ground
CF	Greek	G	Any other mixed background	PA	Somali
CG	Greek Cypriot	H	Indian	PE	Black British
CH	Turkish	J	Pakistani	R	Chinese
CJ	Turkish Cypriot	K	Bangladeshi	S	Another other ethnicity
CY	Other White European	L	Any other Asian background	Z	Not stated

What is your ethnic group? _____

What is your current height? _____ What is your current weight? _____

What is your eye colour?   Blue ☐   Brown ☐   Green ☐   Grey ☐   Hazel ☐

Other: _____

What is your natural hair colour: Black ☐   Brown, dark ☐   Brown, light ☐
Blonde, light ☐   Blonde, dark ☐   Red ☐

What is your skin colour?   Light/fair ☐   Medium ☐   Dark ☐   Freckles ☐   Olive ☐

To be completed by Clinic staff:

Blood / rhesus group _____   CMV status _____

Signature _____

Date _____

Form No: D.1.8   Version No: 7.0.   08.09.04

APPENDIX B

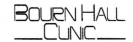

MEDICAL NUMBER ....

CHARACTERISTICS REQUEST FORM FOR RECIPIENTS

Please circle: **donor semen**   **donor oocytes**   **donated embryos**

	FEMALE	MALE
SURNAME		
Forenames		
Date of birth		
Height		
Weight		
Occupation		
Do you have children of your own?	YES / NO	YES / NO
What is your religion / belief system?		
Ethnic group – please refer to key overleaf		

In the 'female' and 'male' columns, please complete your own characteristics. In the 'alternative acceptable characteristics' column, please enter any different characteristics that a donor may have that you both agree are acceptable to you.

	FEMALE (please complete)		MALE (please complete)	Alternative acceptable characteristics
Skin colour *please tick*		Light/fair		
		Medium		
		Dark		
		Freckles		
		Olive		
Natural hair colour *please tick and be specific*		Black		
		Brown, dark or light		
		Blonde, dark or light		
		Red		
Eye Colour *please tick*		Blue		
		Brown		
		Green		
		Grey		
		Hazel		
		Other		
Blood / rhesus group		Blood test or copy report required		
Cytomegalovirus		Blood test at Bourn Hall if necessary	NOT REQUIRED FOR MALE	NOT RELEVANT

Female Partner's Signature ....   Date ....

Male Partner's Signature ....   Date ....

For Clinic use only

IS THIS FOR SIBLING USE? Yes / No IF SO, GIVE APPROPRIATE DONOR NUMBER						
DONOR ASSIGNED						
USE BY DATE						
DATE ASSIGNED						
SIGNATURE						

Form No: D.1.7   Version No: 10.0   Date: 22.09.04   **Continued...**

APPENDIX B2 continued

PLEASE USE THIS KEY TO DESCRIBE YOUR ETHNIC BACKGROUNDS:
(The options below are taken from the current HFEA donor registration form).

ETHNICITY: Please enter the appropriate code overleaf.

National descriptions and ethnic codes					
A	White British	D	White & Black Caribbean	M	Black Caribbean
B	White Irish	E	White & Black African	N	Black African
C	Any other White background	F	White & Asian	P	Other Black b/ground
CF	Greek	G	Any other mixed background	PA	Somali
CG	Greek Cypriot	H	Indian	PE	Black British
CH	Turkish	J	Pakistani	R	Chinese
CJ	Turkish Cypriot	K	Bangladeshi	S	Another other ethnicity
CY	Other White European	L	Any other Asian background	Z	Not stated

21

Surrogacy

Peter R. Brinsden

INTRODUCTION

Surrogacy has been accepted as an answer to certain forms of childlessness for centuries. The earliest mention is in the Old Testament of the Bible[1]. The story goes that Sarai, at the age of 80, was unhappy that she had been unable to bear Abram a child, and she suggested to Abram that he 'go in unto my maid (Hager); it may be that I may obtain children by her'. He did as he was bid, at the age of 90, and Ishmael was born as a result. It was even more extraordinary that later, when Sarai was herself 90, the Lord God allowed her to have her own child by Abram, who by then was 100 years old. Isaac was later born to Sarai – an exceptionally 'elderly primigravida'!

Before the advent of modern assisted conception techniques, 'natural surrogacy' was the only means of helping certain barren women to have children. Before artificial insemination, babies were conceived the 'natural way', as practiced by Abram. Later, as artificial insemination (AI) was accepted, this became the usual means of achieving pregnancy, being more socially acceptable than the 'natural way'. When assisted conception methods such as *in vitro* fertilization (IVF) became available, it was a natural step to use the eggs of the woman wanting the baby and, with the sperm of her husband, to create their own unique embryos *in vitro* and transfer these to a suitable host, thus enabling them to have their own genetic children.

IVF surrogacy is now accepted in the United Kingdom, and a limited number of other countries, as a treatment option for infertile women with certain clearly defined medical problems. A report, commissioned by the British Medical Association (BMA)[2], was published in 1990, the first time that surrogacy was formally accepted by the medical establishment as legitimate treatment. Previously, in 1984, the 'Warnock report'[3] had recommended that surrogacy should not be allowed. Opinions started to change in 1985, when the annual representative meeting of the BMA passed a resolution that 'this meeting agrees with the principle of surrogate births in selected cases with careful controls'[4]. However, the BMA published another report in 1987[5], stating that surrogacy should not be accepted. Later that year, at the annual general meeting, the concept of surrogacy was again rejected, in spite of the 1985 resolution. This report made it clear that doctors 'should not participate in any surrogacy arrangements'. The BMA then established a working party that produced the 1990 report[2], and they concluded that: 'It would not be possible or desirable to seek to prevent all involvement of doctors in surrogacy arrangements, especially as the Government does not intend to make the practice illegal'. This report proposed guidelines for doctors which make it clear that only after intensive investigation and counseling, and very much as a last resort, should this particular form of treatment be used to overcome a couple's infertility problems. In the same year, the Human Fertilisation and Embryology Act (1990)[6] was passed by the UK Parliament; this did not ban surrogacy.

The most recent report from the BMA[7] states that 'Surrogacy is an acceptable option of last resort in cases where it is impossible or highly undesirable for medical reasons for the intended mother to carry a child herself'. In most other European countries, surrogacy is still prohibited[8]. The first baby to be born by an IVF surrogacy arrangement was in the United States[9], from where the largest series on both natural and IVF surrogacy have been reported[10,11].

At Bourn Hall in 1985, despite opposition from the BMA, Mr Patrick Steptoe and Professor Robert Edwards, the pioneers of IVF, first proposed treating a patient by IVF surrogacy. After extensive discussions with the independent Ethics Committee, they undertook treatment of the first couple in the UK. Following an IVF treatment cycle, embryos from the 'genetic couple' were transferred to the sister of the woman and a child was born to them in 1989. In the same year, the Ethics Committee to Bourn Hall drew up guidelines for the treatment of women by IVF surrogacy, and the full program was formalized in 1990. The first 10 years of our experience was reported in 2000[12]. This chapter describes the experience of this clinic and others in the management of this special group of women whose only chance of having a child was treatment by IVF surrogacy.

DEFINITION OF TERMS

In this chapter, the couple who provide both sets of gametes are known as 'the genetic couple'; they have also been known as 'the commissioning couple' or 'intended parents'[7]. The woman receiving the embryos created from the gametes of the genetic couple is known as the 'surrogate host' or 'host'. All of the couples in our series, except two, have been treated by 'IVF surrogacy' (otherwise known as 'gestational surrogacy' or 'full surrogacy'), in which both sets of gametes have come from the genetic couple. In two couples, 'natural surrogacy' (otherwise known as 'straight surrogacy' or partial surrogacy'') was carried

out under medical supervision. This involved insemination of the host (in both cases sisters of the wives) with the sperm of the husband of the genetic couple.

INDICATIONS FOR TREATMENT

The principal indications for treatment by IVF surrogacy are clear-cut, but there are a few indications that are less obvious and are therefore more contentious:

(1) Patients without a uterus, but with one or both ovaries functioning, are the most obvious group that may be suitable for surrogacy. These include:
   (a) Women with congenital absence of the uterus;
   (b) Women who have had a hysterectomy for carcinoma;
   (c) Women who have had a hysterectomy for severe hemorrhage or ruptured uterus.

(2) Women who suffer repeated miscarriage, and for whom the prospect of carrying a baby to term is deemed to be very remote, are considered. In this group, those who have repeatedly failed to achieve a pregnancy following IVF treatment may also be considered.

(3) Women with certain medical conditions, which may make pregnancy life-threatening, but for whom the long-term prospects for health are good, are also considered for treatment.

(4) Requests for career or social reasons are not considered as reasonable indications.

The large majority of women who have requested help by surrogacy have had clear-cut and valid reasons (Table 1). The Ethics Committee to Bourn Hall considers each request after a full report has been presented to them by a clinician and the counselor to the Clinic. Guidelines, which are regularly reviewed, have been issued by the Ethics Committee to assist patients, doctors and counselors (see Appendix).

PATIENT SELECTION

In our practice, all genetic couples are referred by their local consultant gynecologist or general practitioner, and are therefore already preselected as probably suitable for this treatment. The genetic couple are usually

Table 1 Indications for the treatment of 37 couples requiring treatment by *in vitro* fertilization (IVF)-surrogacy at Bourn Hall Clinic. From reference 13, with kind permission of Oxford University Press

Indications	Number of cases	%
Following cancer surgery	10	27
Congenital absence of the uterus	6	16
Postpartum hysterectomy	6	16
Repeated failure of IVF	6	16
Recurrent abortion	5	13
Hysterectomy for menorrhagia	2	5
Severe medical conditions	2	5

Table 2 Relationship of the 'genetic mother' to the 'surrogate host'. From reference 13, with kind permission of Oxford University Press

Relationship	Number	%
Related	15	36.6
Sister	9	22
Sister-in-law	5	12
Stepmother	1	2.5
Non-related	26	63.4
Friend	4	10
Agency introduction	6	14.5
Found through own initiative	16	39

seen alone in the first instance, and an in-depth consultation and counseling of all the medical aspects of the treatment takes place. If the couple are considered to be medically suitable for treatment and fall within the guidelines laid down by the Ethics Committee, and of the *Code of Practice* of the Human Fertilisation and Embryology Authority[14]. Particular attention is paid to the clause about the welfare of any child born as a result of treatment. The couple are informed that they are required (by UK law) to find their own host. They are given some guidance on finding a host for themselves, being told that the host could be a member of the family or a close friend; alternatively, they may be able to find a suitable host through one of the major patient infertility support groups or through specific surrogacy support groups in the UK, such as COTS (Childlessness Overcome Through Surrogacy) and SurrogacyUK. The relationships between the genetic couples and their selected hosts who have been treated at Bourn Hall are shown in Table 2.

When the genetic couple have found someone they believe will be a suitable host, she and her partner are interviewed at length and a full explanation of the implications of acting as a surrogate host is given to them. If the host is thought to be suitable, both couples are counseled in depth, usually in the home of the genetic couple, by an independent counselor to this Clinic. If the counseling process is satisfactory and if there are no apparent reasons that the arrangement should not proceed, a combined medical and counseling report is prepared and the case discussed anonymously at the next meeting of the independent Ethics Committee. At this meeting the surrogacy arrangements are approved or held over pending further information and discussion, or a recommendation may be made that the arrangement should not proceed.

COUNSELING

The role of counseling in surrogacy is to help to prepare all parties contemplating this last-resort treatment and to consider all the factors that will have an influence on the future lives of each of them. Counseling also ensures that all parties to the arrangement are confident and comfortable with their decisions, and have trust in each other, so that no one party is felt to be taking advantage of the other, or to be exploiting the regulations that Parliament laid down in 1990[6]. The BMA in its 1990 report[2] produced a very useful statement: 'The aggregate of foreseeable hazards should not be so great as to place unacceptable burdens on any of the parties – including the future child'. Couples will often have other hazards in their lives which can potentiate the pressures that surrogacy can impose.

There are very many issues that must be discussed with both the genetic couple and the proposed host surrogate. These have been abstracted from the recommendations of the BMA (1996)[7] and include the following.

For the genetic couple:

(1) A review of all alternative treatment options;

(2) The need for in-depth counseling;

(3)   The need to find their own host (UK);

(4)   The practical difficulty and cost of treatment by gestational surrogacy;

(5)   The medical and psychological risks of surrogacy;

(6)   The potential psychological risk to the child;

(7)   The chances of having a multiple pregnancy;

(8)   The degree of control that the host should have over the child of the genetic couple both during the pregnancy and after;

(9)   The possibility that a child may be born with a handicap;

(10) The risks to the baby of the host smoking and drinking during a pregnancy;

(11) The possibility that the host may wish to retain the child after birth and the fact that surrogacy contracts in the UK are not enforceable;

(12) The importance of obtaining legal advice;

(13) The genetic couple are advised to take out insurance cover for the surrogate host;

For the host:

(1)   The full implications of undergoing treatment by IVF surrogacy;

(2)   The possibility of multiple pregnancy;

(3)   The possibility of family and friends being against such treatment;

(4)   The need to abstain from unprotected sexual intercourse during and just before the treatment;

(5)   The normal medical risks associated with pregnancy and the possibility of Cesarian section;

(6)   The implications and feelings of guilt on both sides if the host should spontaneously abort a pregnancy;

(7)   The possibility that the host will feel a sense of bereavement when she gives the baby to the genetic couple;

(8)   The possibility that the child may be born with a handicap;

(9)   The fact that hosts in the United Kingdom are expected to only claim 'reasonable expenses'

– commonly ranging between £7000 and £10 000 ($10 000–$15 000).

Other issues that must be discussed in depth with both parties to a surrogacy arrangement include whether and what both parties will tell the children born as a result of treatment in the future about their origins, and also what the host mother will tell any children she has. There is an increasing willingness of all couples involved with treatment by assisted reproductive technologies (ART) to be more open about their treatment, whether this be by IVF, the use of donor gametes or surrogacy. It is felt by most workers in the area that it is better for couples to be open with their children about their origins rather than to try and cover it up.

Another issue that is often raised in counseling is whether the genetic mother may be able to breast-feed her baby when it is given to her by the host surrogate. There is a belief that the genetic mother may be able to provide some breast-milk, which will almost certainly require bottle supplementation, if she puts the child to the breast regularly. It has been proposed that the genetic mother who receives the baby should prepare for the possibility of breast-feeding by stimulating secretion of milk manually, or with a breast-pump, in the few weeks leading up to the delivery of her child. If there is an enthusiasm to breast feed then it is worth an attempt, but there is a strong possibility of disappointment.

Counseling of couples in our own practice invariably has taken place in the homes of the genetic couples by an independent fertility counselor to the Clinic; it often takes several hours and frequently several visits. With the consent of all involved, the counsellor then seeks permission to share that confidence anonymously with the independent Ethics Committee who advise the Clinic. Although there is no requirement under the Human Fertilisation and Embryology Act 1990 to refer such cases to an ethics committee, the views and support of a wider group of people drawn from many disciplines, and with a lay majority, has been very valuable to the clinic staff, and is appreciated by the patients themselves. Counseling is made available for as long as required by any of the parties – including any existing or future children.

If treatment fails, it may have a profound effect on the commissioning couple and their families, as well as the host, her husband or partner and their children.

Many of those who have not succeeded in surrogacy have nevertheless been grateful that they have at least tried. They have been better able to adjust to their situation, knowing that they have explored all the possibilities and have made every possible effort.

PATIENT MANAGEMENT

Treatment of the genetic mother

Most of the work-up of a woman referred for IVF surrogacy will normally have been carried out by the referring consultant. This should include laparoscopy if there are congenital anomalies; however, if the uterus has been removed for carcinoma or hemorrhage, then laparoscopy may not be necessary. The serum follicle stimulating hormone (FSH), luteinizing hormone (LH) and prolactin levels should be assayed in most cases, as some women suffer premature ovarian failure after hysterectomy. There are occasional indications to confirm ovarian activity by serial ultrasound scanning. These tests are considered to be the minimum required before proceeding with treatment; there may be others that are indicated on an individual basis. The blood groups of the genetic parents are requested if the group of the host is found to be rhesus negative. Finally, both genetic parents have their hepatitis B (HBV), hepatitis C (HCV) and human immunodeficiency virus (HIV) status checked. Regulations in the UK require that the sperm of the commissioning or genetic husband/partner must be 'quarantined' for 6 months before being used, or the embryos created with his sperm must be frozen and quarantined for 6 months[12]. The genetic husband/partner then has a further test of his HIV status and the embryos may be transferred or the sperm thawed and used to create 'fresh' embryos for transfer to the surrogate host. This policy is governed by the rule which states that sperm used in surrogacy arrangements must be treated in the same way as donor sperm, which, by law in the UK, must be frozen and quarantined for 6 months before it can be used.

In view of the fact that most women requesting surrogacy are normal, apart from not having a uterus, the management of their treatment cycles is usually straightforward. Even though the majority will not be experiencing menstruation, many women without a uterus, but with normally functioning ovaries, will experience some cyclical symptoms – often at the time of ovulation or in the equivalent 'premenstrual' phase. These patients will usually be treated with a period of long down-regulation[15] with the gonadotropin releasing hormone analog naferelin (Synarel®; Searle, High Wycombe, UK) or buserelin (Suprecur®; Shire Pharmaceuticals, Andover, UK), for up to 2 weeks, after which the serum levels of LH, progesterone and estrogen are measured. If they have achieved baseline levels, then follicular stimulation with gonadotropins can begin as described in Chapter 6. Vaginal ultrasound oocyte recovery, as described in Chapter 11, is the preferred method, as it is less stressful and does not require general anesthesia. The genetic father is asked to produce a specimen of sperm before his wife proceeds to the operating room. This is prepared in the normal manner as for IVF (see Chapter 13). As many oocytes as possible are recovered and are inseminated after about 4 h, depending upon their maturity (see Chapter 12) The next day, any normal-appearing zygotes with two pronuclei are frozen. The embryos are kept frozen for a minimum period of 6 months, to comply with the UK regulations as described above, or the alternative is to freeze the sperm of the male partner of the genetic couple for 6 months before starting treatment, recheck his HIV status and inseminate the freshly collected oocytes of his wife/partner.

Treatment of the host mother

The major part of the investigation of the host mother is her medical and psychological assessment, as well as by means of the counseling process. Host mothers will always be normal, fit women, usually less than 38 years of age and who have had at least one child. We prefer that they should be in a stable marriage or relationship, and the husband or partner should be fully aware of the implications for both his partner and himself of what acting as a host mother involves. It is desirable to keep invasive testing to a minimum; preliminary laparoscopy is certainly not considered to be necessary. Testing of the blood group and HBV, HCV and HIV status of both the husband and the wife are the minimum requirements. If the host mother is on the oral contraceptive pill, then it is recommended that this be discontinued one or two cycles before the treatment cycle and barrier methods of contraception used.

The host may be treated in one of the two following ways.

Embryo replacement in a natural cycle

This method is considered most suitable for women who have been sterilized, or whose husbands have had a vasectomy and who have been confirmed azoospermic. Initially, replacement in a natural cycle was not considered suitable for women practicing barrier contraception because of the risk to themselves of conceiving in the replacement cycle and the awful consequences of either giving their own child away, in the belief that it was from the transferred embryo, or there being a twin mixed conception. More recently, however, we believe the risks of this happening, with proper contraceptive advice, are very small indeed, and some well-motivated hosts have been treated in natural cycles.

Embryo replacement in a hormone-controlled cycle

Control of the host's replacement cycle by down-regulation with a gonadotropin releasing hormone analog and replacement estrogen therapy, as described in Chapter 25, may be recommended for two main reasons:

(1) If the menstrual cycles of the host are irregular, if they are found not to be ovulating regularly or if luteal phase insufficiency is suspected;

(2) If the host is fertile and has to rely on barrier contraception (but see above).

The preparation and treatment of couples for treatment by IVF surrogacy at Bourn Hall, as described above, is very similar to that practiced by other centers[11,16–18]. All the procedures are as for normal IVF cycles, but with transfer of the embryos to another woman, who has been suitably prepared.

RESULTS OF TREATMENT

Through treatment by IVF surrogacy, satisfactory 'delivered baby rates' can be achieved, both per genetic couple and per surrogate host. In our own published series, a live birth rate of 37% per genetic couple and 34% per surrogate host was achieved, in a mean of 1.6 cycles with two embryos transferred[12]. In another UK series, studying only women who had had a

hysterectomy, a pregnancy rate of 37.5% per surrogate host and 27.3% (6/22) per cycle of treatment begun was achieved[16]. The same group reported a series of six women, all with the Rokitansky– Kuster–Hauser syndrome; three had babies through their hosts[19].

In the 1989 series of Utian and colleagues[10] a clinical pregnancy rate of 18% (7/39) per cycle initiated and a 23% clinical pregnancy rate per embryo transfer were reported. Other series from the United States reported ongoing or delivered pregnancy rates of 36% (172 of 484 surrogate hosts)[20] with a mean of 5 ± 1.3 embryos transferred, and Corson and colleagues reported a clinical pregnancy rate of 58% per commissioning couple and 33.2% per embryo transfer in women where the genetic women were less than 40 years of age[17].

It was remarked as far back as 1986 by the Ethics Committee of the American Fertility Society[21] that very little investigation of the immediate and long-term outcome of the babies born as a result of gestational surrogacy has been carried out. It is only recently that studies have been published looking at the outcome of the babies and of couples entering into surrogacy arrangements. Parkinson and colleagues[22] reviewed the perinatal outcome of pregnancies from IVF surrogacy and compared it with the outcome of pregnancies resulting from standard IVF. As would be expected, the surrogate hosts who carried twin and triplet gestations delivered substantially earlier than those who gestated singleton pregnancies, and the twin newborns were significantly lighter than singleton infants born through IVF surrogacy. Interestingly, the occurrence of pregnancy-induced hypertension and bleeding in the third trimester of pregnancy was up to five times lower in the surrogate hosts than in the standard IVF patient controls. Apart from birth weights and prematurity, little other information is given about the outcome of the babies. The few long-term follow-up studies of women who have acted as surrogate hosts indicate that there is little to suggest any long-term harm or regret among them[23–26].

COMPLICATIONS ASSOCIATED WITH IVF SURROGACY

Most of the major problems that are related to surrogacy have been in natural surrogacy arrangements and are mostly legal issues. These problems have largely arisen because these arrangements are unsupervised by clinicians, counselors and often lawyers, whereas all IVF surrogacy arrangements require the active participation of these professionals. In our own experience of 15 years, no serious clinical, ethical or legal problems have arisen. The few other large published series have reported no major complications. The following are the major problems that could arise during treatment, and which are invariably discussed with couples as part of the counseling process before treatment:

(1) The issue which causes most concern to commissioning couples is that the host may wish to retain custody of the child. This has occurred, but is very rare, particularly in gestational surrogacy arrangements where there is no genetic link to the surrogate mother.

(2) The prospective parents often express concerns about what would happen if the child were born abnormal. To our knowledge, this has not yet occurred, but it is an issue that must be discussed openly with both parties to a surrogacy arrangement. The fear is that both couples might reject any grossly abnormal child.

(3) In spite of the reassuring studies that have been carried out on the effects of surrogacy on the host and on the commissioning couples, further large follow-up studies are required, especially regarding the long-term effects on the children born as a result of surrogacy arrangements.

Issues that were highlighted in our own previously reported series[12] include:

(1) A few of the commissioning women responded poorly to follicular stimulation and achieved relatively small numbers of oocytes following a standard stimulation regimen. The mean number of oocytes recovered in our series was ten, but the range has been between two and 24. Similarly, Meniru and Craft[16] reported that three of their 11 patients who had previously had a hysterectomy failed to respond to stimulation at all, and two other patients produced very few oocytes, which failed to fertilize. The reduced response to stimulation has been attributed to disruption of the vascular supply to the ovaries following surgery[16]. Ovarian function after hysterectomy may be compromised in up to 50% of women[27], but the responses can be variable[19].

(2) Unlike post-hysterectomy patients, young women with Rokitansky–Kuster–Hauser (RKH) syndrome usually respond to ovarian follicular stimulation remarkably well[18]. Ben-Rafael and coworkers[28] reported four patients who undertook ten stimulation cycles in their program with standard doses of human menopausal gonadotropin (hMG) and achieved a mean of 14.6 oocytes (range 8–24), with a fertilization rate of 71%. Wood and colleagues[29] retrieved a mean of 8.7 oocytes with a 53% fertilization rate. Also reassuring to young women with RKH syndrome are the findings of Petrozza and associates[30] that congenital absence of the uterus and vagina was not transmitted as a dominant genetic trait.

A survey carried out on behalf of the British Fertility Society (BFS)[31] of all licensed clinics performing surrogacy in the UK showed that 29 of the 113 licensed clinics in the UK had carried out surrogacy treatments. The most significant of the problems reported were:

(1) There was one report of a host who failed to surrender the baby immediately after birth, but did so subsequently, without legal intervention.

(2) One commissioning couple separated just before treatment started.

(3) There was unwelcome newspaper publicity in one case.

(4) A number of couples withdrew from treatment following initial counseling. (We believe that this is not a negative outcome of counseling, rather a positive one, in that they had been made fully aware of the full implications of the treatment.)

(5) Poor responses to follicular stimulation were noted, particularly after a Wertheim's hysterectomy.

(6) Most clinics stated that there should be greater control of surrogacy, particularly of natural surrogacy, and that, if it was to be performed only within licensed clinics, the appropriate health screening and counseling could be provided and fewer complications would occur.

THE LEGAL STATUS OF SURROGACY

In the UK, the Surrogacy Arrangements Act 1985, which was hastily drafted following concerns raised by the 'baby Cotton case'[32], prohibits commercial (but not voluntary) surrogacy agencies and outlaws advertising for or about surrogacy. Only the commissioning parents and the host surrogate may initiate, negotiate or compile information to make a surrogacy arrangement. Non-commercial voluntary agencies are permitted, and remain unmonitored and unregulated. The Act does not prohibit payments to surrogate mothers. The Surrogacy Arrangements Act 1985 was supplemented by clauses relating specifically to surrogacy in the Human Fertilisation and Embryology Act 1990. These restrict 'licensable activity' to premises licensed by the Authority (HFEA). These activities include the creation or use of an embryo outside the body and the use of donated eggs, sperm or embryos.

The Human Fertilisation and Embryology Act 1990 also clarified uncertainties about the legal status of surrogacy contracts by unambiguously declaring them unenforceable in law (section 36). It also clarified the issue of legal parentage by defining the child's legal mother as the woman carrying it, regardless of whether mother and child are genetically related (section 27). These two sections of the Act ensure that, if the surrogate host changes her mind and decides to keep the child, she is legally entitled to do so. If the commissioning couple decide to reject the child, it remains the legal responsibility of the host. The Act also defines the legal paternity of the child.

Until the Human Fertilisation and Embryology Act 1990, commissioning couples had to adopt their own child and all the provisions of the Adoption Acts (1976, 1985) applied. Section 30 of the 1990 Act, however, allows for the parentage to be changed by the issue of 'parental orders', with the following conditions:

(1) The applicants (the genetic or commissioning couple) must be married;

(2) They must be over age 18;

(3) One or both must be genetically related to the child;

(4) One or both must be domiciled in the UK, Channel Islands or Isle of Man;

(5) The child must already be in their care;

(6) The birth mother and birth father (if applicable) must have given their consent;

(7) No money (other than expenses approved by the courts) must have been paid;

(8) Application is made within 6 months of the birth of the child.

In the United States, different legislation has been enacted in different states. Generally, the courts have placed increasing importance on the genetic relationship of the child over that of the birth mother, but many states still consider the birth mother to be the legal mother of the child – as in the UK. Some states allow the payment of hosts (e.g. Nevada, Virginia) while others do not (e.g. New York, Nebraska, Utah). Shuster has reviewed the complex differences between states very clearly[33,34]. By the year 2000, twenty-three US states had laws on the practice of surrogacy, but they still differ widely[35].

Like the United States, Australia has different regulations in different states. In New South Wales, Western Australia and the Australia Capital Territory surrogacy is freely available. In Victoria, South Australia and Tasmania, it is not illegal, but the very strict controls on payment and the lack of any binding legal arrangements make surrogacy almost impossible to carry out there[36]; couples requiring surrogacy therefore tend to move from state to state.

The only countries in Europe which allow surrogacy are the United Kingdom, Belgium, Holland and Finland[37].

ETHICAL CONSIDERATIONS

It is a requirement of the United Kingdom's Human Fertilisation and Embryology Act 1990 that the welfare of any child born as a result of treatment and the welfare of any existing children must at all times be taken into account when considering licensed treatment. This tenet guides the management of all couples undertaking treatment by surrogacy in the UK. In our own practice, the advice of the independent Ethics Committee to Bourn Hall Clinic is sought on every surrogacy arrangement. The Bourn Hall Ethics Committee guidelines for surrogacy are given in the Appendix. The Ethics Committee discuss each arrangement on its merits and believes that the guidelines should be there for the guidance of the Committee, but that they should be reasonably flexible.

RELIGIOUS CONSIDERATIONS

The Catholic Church is strongly against all forms of assisted conception, particularly those associated with gamete donation and surrogacy[38]. The Anglican Church is less rigid in its views and has not condemned the practice of surrogacy.

Surrogacy is not forbidden in the Jewish religion, which is very much family-oriented and which puts a duty to have children onto Jews[39]. Any child born as a result of surrogacy will belong to the father who gave the sperm and to the woman who gave birth[40,41].

The Islamic view appears to be absolute in that, in the same way as the use of donor sperm is strictly forbidden in all schools of Islamic law, so egg donation and surrogacy would not be allowed, except, perhaps, that it might be permissible between wives with the same husband, but debate continues and there are differences in the degree to which some Muslims will adhere to the faith[42].

CONCLUSIONS

IVF surrogacy is now an accepted form of medical treatment in the UK for a small group of infertile women with unique causes of their infertility, although it remains controversial and is not practiced in most other European countries. The indications for treatment are limited to a small group of women who have no uterus, suffer recurrent abortions or suffer from certain medical conditions which would threaten the life of a woman were she to become pregnant.

The treatment process is in itself straightforward. In a normal stimulated IVF cycle, any embryos are frozen and later transferred to a selected surrogate host, or fresh embryos are transferred that have been created from freshly collected oocytes fertilized with sperm that have been quarantined (in the UK) for the statutory 6 months. The difficult aspect of the treatment is the extreme care with which the surrogate hosts must be selected by the genetic couple to ensure complete compatibility, and also the in-depth counseling that is

required, in both the short and the long term, on all aspects of the treatment.

In the UK, the Surrogacy Arrangements Act 1985 does not make it illegal for a host to receive payment for her services, but section 30 of the Human Fertilisation and Embryology Act 1990 does, other than for reasonable expenses. It is therefore all the more impressive that women will carry another woman's child for mainly altruistic reasons. The system is simpler in the USA, where in some states it is legal to pay a woman to carry a child, and there is therefore a greater availability of hosts. Our experience over the past 15 years, however, shows that an 'altruistic system' can work and work well. The only substantial disadvantage is that some women are unable to find hosts at all, and are therefore denied the opportunity of even attempting treatment.

We believe that the support and advice of an independent ethics committee is invaluable, indeed essential, in assessing the suitability of individual cases. As clinicians, counselors and scientists, we are inclined to become so involved in the problems of individual couples that some of the more obvious pitfalls in the social, religious or ethical aspects of treating a particular couple are easily overlooked.

There are a number of instances where problems have been reported in surrogacy cases; although, when related to the number of surrogacy arrangements that have taken place, with more than 250 births known to have occurred with natural and IVF surrogacy arrangements in the UK, these are relatively few. The majority of the problems that have occurred are related to natural surrogacy. Only one case of IVF surrogacy in the UK has ended in court because of a 'tug-of-love' dispute between the genetic and host mothers.

During the past 15 years of our series, no serious clinical, ethical or legal problems have been encountered. In one sister-to-sister arrangement, failure of the treatment caused disagreement and unhappiness between the sisters, and support counseling was required for more than 3 years. A more minor problem encountered has been that both parties to the arrangement frequently have had unreasonably high expectations of success, in spite of very frank information and counseling being provided to them. Because the host is fit, young and known to be fertile, she and the genetic parents expect success and feel badly let down if this is not achieved. Another problem that has arisen is a host achieving a pregnancy and then miscarrying. This has been more common than expected (33% of the pregnancies in our series aborted spontaneously)[18], and causes severe stress to both parties. The host has felt guilt that she lost the genetic couple's hard-won pregnancy, and the genetic couple has felt guilt that the host has been through the stress of a miscarriage and possible curettage. Full support counseling for both couples is essential.

We have shown that treatment by IVF surrogacy of young women without a uterus, or for other clear indications, is successful and relatively free of the complications associated with natural surrogacy. We believe that, if couples requesting treatment are carefully selected clinically, counseled in depth and provided with support throughout treatment, the incidence of complications will be minimal. Surrogacy arrangements should not be undertaken lightly, or without the full support of an experienced fertility team, an experienced counselor and recourse to advice and support from an independent ethics committee.

At Bourn Hall we believe that a limited IVF surrogacy service should be part of the comprehensive infertility treatment program that most larger centers should offer, now that it is an ethically accepted form of treatment. At present IVF surrogacy only accounts for about 1% of all assisted conception cycles that are carried out at Bourn Hall. We will continue to have a policy of very careful selection and screening of both genetic and host couples, with intensive independent counseling playing an essential part in the process. It is to be hoped that the high success rates of treatment that have been achieved initially will continue. Indeed, this is likely, since in effect neither party is truly infertile; the genetic mother invariably has perfectly normal ovaries and the host is fertile.

APPENDIX: BOURN HALL ETHICS COMMITTEE GUIDELINES FOR SURROGACY

Introduction

Bourn Hall Ethics Committee is prepared to consider IVF surrogacy in cases where an embryo or embryos from the commissioning couple are transferred to the uterus of the host. The use of donor eggs or donor sperm and natural surrogacy may be considered in exceptional circumstances. It considers that surrogacy should only be undertaken as a last resort. The need to safeguard the welfare of any children born as a result of a surrogacy arrangement and the welfare of any existing children of the commissioning couple and host will be the paramount principle.

The Committee considers that every case must be looked at by the Ethics Committee on its own merit, based on information provided by the Clinic. Following discussion the Committee may recommend approval or rejection of a request for treatment. Alternatively the Committee may request further information and the opportunity for reconsideration at a later date.

Procedures

Following examination by a clinician, the prospective genetic parents and host and partner must be counseled by a professional counselor. If the clinician and counselor, who must not be members of the Ethics Committee, are satisfied they will prepare a report, a copy of which must be submitted to each member of the Ethics Committee. The case will then be considered by the Ethics Committee, who will make their recommendations to the Clinic. The genetic parents and host and her partner are recommended to take independent legal advice and encouraged to take out insurance.

Cases will not be considered if the genetic couple does not comply with the requirements for a parental order under section 30 of the Human Fertilisation and Embryology Act 1990 or subsequent legislation.

Categories acceptable for treatment

(1) Total or partial absence of the uterus either of congenital origin or after surgery;

(2) Repeated miscarriage;

(3) Multiple failure of infertility treatment; the clinicians must be satisfied that there is no reasonable prospect of success in the future.

Motives considered unacceptable

(1) Social reasons;

(2) Prospective genetic parents with severe health problems; clinicians and the Committee will need

to be satisfied that the strain of bringing up a child is unlikely to damage the mother's health so seriously as to jeopardize the welfare of that child.

Considerations which apply to all cases

(1) The Clinic must not be involved in initiating or making arrangements between genetic and host couples.

(2) The relationship between the genetic couple and the host must be carefully considered to avoid creating conflicting family relationships.

(3) Counseling must be available to both genetic and host couples.

(4) The age of the genetic mother and of the host is important. In view of the HFEA Code of Practice, the Committee considers that 35 should be the maximum age of the genetic mother unless there are exceptional circumstances. The host should generally be below 40.

(5) The principal motive of a prospective host should always be to help an infertile couple.

(6) A prospective host should have had at least one child before becoming a surrogate.

(7) The commissioning couple in a surrogacy arrangement should be married. The Committee prefers that the host is in a stable relationship; if the host is single then she should be adequately supported.

REFERENCES

1. Genesis. 16: 1–15; 17: 15–19; 21: 1–4
2. British Medical Association. Surrogacy: Ethical Considerations. Report of the Working Party on Human Infertility Services. London: BMA Publications, 1990
3. Report of the Committee of Inquiry into Human Fertilisation and Embryology. London: Her Majesty's Stationery Office, 1984
4. British Medical Association. Annual Representative Meeting Report. London: British Medical Association, 1985
5. British Medical Association. Surrogate Motherhood. Report of the Board of Science and Education. London: British Medical Association Publications, 1987
6. Human Fertilisation and Embryology Act 1990. London: Her Majesty's Stationery Office, 1990
7. British Medical Association. Changing Conceptions of Motherhood. The Practice of Surrogacy in Britain. London: British Medical Association Publications, 1996
8. Cohen J, Jones H. Assisted reproduction. Rules and laws. International comparisons. Contracept Fertil Sex 1999; 27: I–VII
9. Utian WH, Sheehan L, Goldfarb JM, et al. Successful pregnancy after in vitro fertilization and embryo transfer from an infertile woman to a surrogate. N Engl J Med 1985; 313: 1351–2
10. Utian WF, Goldfarb JM, Kiwi R, et al. Preliminary experience with in vitro fertilization – surrogate gestational pregnancy. Fertil Steril 1989; 52: 633–8
11. Marrs RP, Ringler GE, Stein AL, et al. The use of surrogate gestational carriers for assisted reproductive technologies. Am J Obstet Gynecol 1993; 168: 1858–63
12. Brinsden PR, Appleton TC, Murray E, et al. Treatment by in vitro fertilisation with surrogacy: experience of one British centre. Br Med J 2000; 320: 924–8
13. Brinsden PR. Gestational surrogacy. Hum Reprod Update 2003; 9: 483–91
14. Human Fertilisation and Embryology Authority. Code of Practice, 6th edn. London: HFEA, 2003
15. Marcus SF, Brinsden PR, Macnamee MC, et al. Comparative trial between an ultra-short and long protocol of luteinising hormone-releasing hormone agonist for ovarian stimulation in in-vitro fertilization. Hum Reprod 1993; 8: 238–43
16. Meniru GI, Craft IL. Experience with gestational surrogacy as a treatment for sterility resulting from hysterectomy. Hum Reprod 1997; 12: 51–4
17. Corson SL, Kelly M, Braverman A, et al. Gestational carrier pregnancy. Fertil Steril 1998; 69: 670–4
18. Beski S, Gorgy A, Venkat G, et al. Gestational surrogacy: a feasible option for patients with Rokitansky syndrome. Hum Reprod 2000; 15: 2326–8
19. Metcalf MG, Braiden V, Livesey JH. Retention of normal ovarian function after hysterectomy. J Endocrinol 1992; 135: 597–602
20. Batzofin J, Nelson J, Wilcox J, et al. Gestational surrogacy: is it time to include it as part of ART? Fertil Steril 1999; (ASRM Annual Meeting Program Suppl): Abstr P-017
21. Report of the Ethics Committee of the American Fertility Society. Fertil Steril 1986; 3 (Suppl): 62–8
22. Parkinson J, Tran C, Tan T, et al. Perinatal outcome after in-vitro fertilization-surrogacy. Hum Reprod 1999; 14: 671–6
23. Fischer S, Gillman I. Surrogate motherhood: attachment, attitudes and social support. Psychiatry 1991; 54: 13–20

24. Blyth E. Interviews with surrogate mothers in Britain. J Reprod Infert Psychol 1994; 12: 189–98

25. MacCallum F, Lycett E, Murray C, et al. Surrogacy: the experience of commissioning couples. Hum Reprod 2003; 18: 1334–42

26. Jadva V, Murray C, Lycett E, et al. Surrogacy: the experience of surrogate mothers. Hum Reprod 2003; 18: 2196–204

27. Siddle N, Sarrel P, Whitehead M. The effect of hysterectomy on the age at ovarian failure: identification of a subgroup of women with premature loss of ovarian function and literature review. Fertil Steril 1987; 47: 94–100

28. Ben-Rafael Z, Bar-Hava I, Levy T, et al. Simplifying ovulation induction for surrogacy in women with Mayer–Rokitansky–Kuster–Hauser syndrome. Hum Reprod 1998; 13: 1470–1

29. Wood E, Batzen F, Corson S. Ovarian response to gonadotrophins, optimal method for oocyte retrieval and pregnancy outcome in patients with vaginal agenesis. Hum Reprod 1999; 14: 1178–81

30. Petrozza JC, Gray MR, Davis AJ, et al. Congenital absence of the uterus and vagina is not commonly transmitted as a dominant genetic trait: outcomes of surrogate pregnancies. Fertil Steril 1997; 67: 387–9

31. Balen AH, Hayden CA. British Fertility Society survey of all licensed clinics that perform surrogacy in the UK. Hum Fertil (Camb) 1998; 1: 6–9

32. Cotton K. Surrogacy should pay. Br Med J 2000; 320: 928–9

33. Shuster E. Non-genetic surrogacy: no cure but problems for infertility? Hum Reprod 1991; 6: 1176–80

34. Shuster E. When genes determine motherhood: problems in gestational surrogacy. Hum Reprod 1992; 7: 1029–33

35. Andrews LB, Elster N. Regulating reproductive technologies. J Legal Med 2000; 21: 35–65

36. Leeton J. The current status of IVF surrogacy in Australia. Aust NZ J Obstet Gynaecol 1991; 31: 260–2

37. Soderstrom-Anttila V, Blomqvist T, Foudila T, et al. Experience of in virto fertilization surrogacy in Finland. Acta Obstet Gynecol Scand 2002; 81: 747–52

38. McCormick RA. Surrogacy: a Catholic perspective. Creighton Law Rev 1992; 25: 1617–25

39. Hirsh AV. Infertility in Jewish couples, biblical and rabbinic law. Hum Fertil (Camb) 1998; 1: 14–19

40. Benshushan A, Schenker JG. Legitimizing surrogacy in Israel. Hum Reprod 1997; 12: 1832–4

41. Schenker JG. Infertility evaluation and treatment according to Jewish law. Eur J Obstet Gynecol Reprod Biol 1997; 71: 113–21

42. Hussain FA. Reproductive issues from the Islamic perspective. Hum Fertil 2000; 3: 124–8

22

Regulation of embryo–endometrial interactions at implantation

J. Robert A. Sherwin and Andrew M. Sharkey

INTRODUCTION

Successful implantation requires the production of a hatched blastocyst capable of implanting, and the simultaneous development of an endometrium that is receptive to the embryo. Following fertilization, the zygote passes down the Fallopian tube where it is exposed to soluble factors in secretions from the oviduct and the uterus, which can influence its development. The embryo in turn produces growth factors that act in an autocrine fashion or on the endometrium. At the same time under the influence of ovarian steroids, the endometrium undergoes cyclical changes, resulting in a tissue receptive to embryo implantation. These changes involve complex interactions between stromal cells, the overlying epithelium and the embryo itself. Our understanding of the molecular dialog that occurs during embryo–endometrial interactions comes mainly from studies of murine implantation.

THE RECEPTIVE ENDOMETRIUM

Classical embryo transfer studies in rodents have shown that the endometrium becomes receptive to implantation only for a very limited period of time. In rats and mice this receptive phase occurs between days 3 and 5 after mating, after which the endometrium becomes refractory to implantation[1]. Embryos transferred to the endometrium outside this time fail to implant. In humans and primates, embryo transfer experiments have confirmed the existence of a receptive phase that extends from day 5 to day 10 after the luteinizing hormone (LH) surge, although the exact duration of this receptive period is less well defined than in rodents[2].

The initial step in implantation is hatching of the blastocyst, followed by attachment to a receptive uterine epithelium. This apposition triggers local stromal edema, followed by the process of decidualization, in which stromal cells undergo transformation to large glycogen-rich decidual cells. Electron microscopy shows dramatic changes in membrane morphology that occur in the luminal epithelium during the period of uterine receptivity[3]. In particular, pinopodes, which are large cytoplasmic projections from the uterine epithelium, are expressed during the period of endometrial receptivity, and their expression persists for 24–48 h between days 19 and 21 of the menstrual cycle[4]. In rodents the appearance of pinopodes is regulated by progesterone, and, although their function is unknown, they coincide with the receptive state. *In vitro* studies of implantation show that blastocysts in culture adhere to pinopode-rich areas of endometrial strips, further emphasizing the potential importance of pinopode expression[5] (Figure 1).

Analogy has been drawn between the initial attachment of the embryo to the apical surface of the uterine luminal epithelium and the attachment of leukocytes to the endothelial lining of blood vessels at the site of tissue injury. The multistep process of leukocyte rolling and margination is mediated in a sequential manner by chemokines and adhesion molecules of the selectin, integrin and immunoglobulin supergene families[6]. It is likely that a similar multistep process involving many different adhesion and signaling molecules is involved in embryo attachment.

The carbohydrate chains of glycoproteins expressed on the apical surface of the uterine luminal epithelium extend beyond membrane-bound protein or lipid cores, and are therefore probably the first structures encountered by the apposing blastocyst[7]. In preparation for implantation, luminal epithelium undergoes a change in the expression of a number of surface glycoproteins. The unmasking, modification or relocation of adhesion factors on the apical uterine luminal epithelial surface is believed to result in a sticky surface that fixes the slowly moving blastocyst, prior to a more permanent attachment and invasion. The role of carbohydrates has been studied in mice, which lack specific carbohydrate species. All of these knock-out mice have been fertile[8]. Many carbohydrate moieties exist, and so functional redundancy is to be expected. The mucin MUC-1 is a large glycoprotein, expressed by human luminal epithelium, which carries charged carbohydrate residues such as Sialyl Le^x and Sialyl Le^y, which are able to bind selectins. Implantation-competent human embryos express L-selectin[9], and so it has been hypothesized that the initial attachment of the embryo to the luminal epithelium is mediated by L-selectin binding to ligand receptors expressed on the luminal epithelium (Figure 2).

Further data implying a role for MUC-1 in implantation come from studies of the MUC-1 gene in a cohort of infertile women. These women were found to have a reduced variable number of tandem repeats (VNTR) in the MUC-1 gene, which is associated with a reduction of glycosylation sites in the MUC-1 protein[10]. It is suggested that the loss of these glycosylation sites reduces the ability of the MUC-1 protein to bind selectins, and hence may reduce the likelihood of embryo attachment. Other groups have

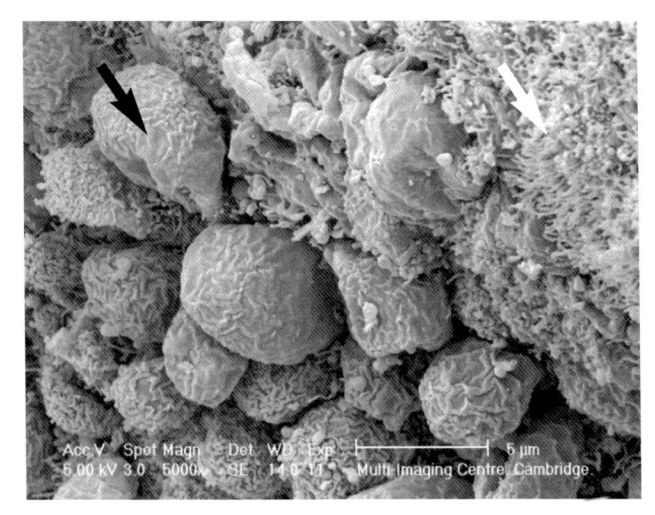

Figure 1 Pinopode expression by secretory phase endometrium. Scanning electron micrograph of the apical surface of uterine luminal epithelium 8 days after the luteinizing hormone surge (LH + 8) in a normal cycle. Fully developed pinopodes (black arrow) cover the surface, which also has microvilli (white arrow) present (× 4278)

been unable to confirm an association between infertility and polymorphism of the MUC-1 gene[11]. Interestingly, Muc-1 is down-regulated in murine luminal epithelium during the implantation window[12], and transgenic mice carrying a null mutation for Muc-1 are fertile[13]. In rodents, however, there may be redundancy, as Muc-4, another large glycoprotein, is progesterone-regulated in rat luminal epithelium[14].

ROLE OF STEROID HORMONES IN THE REGULATION OF EMBRYO–ENDOMETRIAL INTERACTIONS

The development of uterine receptivity depends upon the sequential exposure of endometrium to estrogen and progesterone. Estrogenic and progestogenic actions on target cells are mediated by steroid hormones binding, respectively, to specific, high-affinity estrogen (ER-α, ER-β) and progesterone receptors (PRA, PRB)[15]. These receptors act as ligand-modulated transcription factors, and transactivate genes via estrogen and progesterone response elements[16]. Mice carrying null mutations for the PRB gene (PRBKO) are fertile, although PRB is required for normal mammary ductal morphogenesis[17]. Therefore, in mice carrying null mutations for both PRA

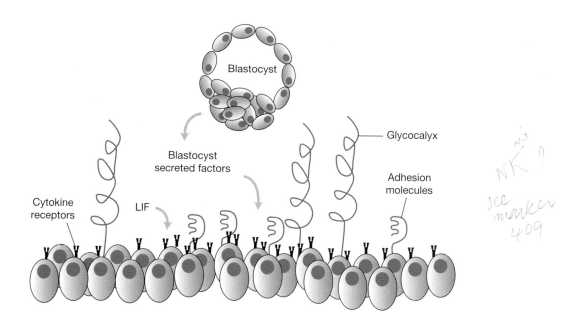

Figure 2 A schematic representation of blastocyst attachment. Carbohydrate moieties of glycoproteins, expressed on endometrial luminal epithelium, form an initial interaction with the blastocyst, which is later reinforced by adhesion molecules. The paracrine actions of cytokines, such as leukemia inhibitory factor (LIF), prepare steroidally primed endometrium to receive blastocyst-derived factors, which initiate localized endometrial receptivity

and PRB (PRKO), the reproductive phenotype of ovulatory failure and hyperplastic uteri, which fail to decidualize[18], is due to the absence of PRA[19]. Injection of neutralizing antibodies to progesterone or antiprogestins shows that implantation requires progesterone action on days 3 and 4 of implantation[20]. Immunohistochemical analysis of PR expression in the mouse uterus shows low expression in the luminal epithelium and stroma on day 2 of pregnancy[21]. There is a marked increase in PR expression in luminal epithelium on day 3, which subsequently reduces on day 4, and this is accompanied by a rise in stromal PR expression. PR is known to be estrogen-regulated in many cell types, via estrogen response elements in the PR gene promoter[22]. However, elegant tissue recombination experiments show that in mouse uterine luminal epithelium, the action of estrogen on stromal cells induces paracrine gene regulation in the overlying luminal epithelium[23]. Thus, estrogen-induced down-regulation of PR expression, in luminal epithelium derived from ER-α null mutants, occurs only if the luminal epithelium is in contact with stromal cells that express functional ER-α. Estrogen-induced uterine epithelial cell proliferation and secretory protein synthesis is mediated via ER-α[24,25]. ER-α is expressed in epithelial and stromal cell compartments of the uterus throughout early pregnancy[23].

In human endometrium the action of PR is also essential for normal implantation. Immunohistochemistry of LH + 3 (pre-receptive) endometrium has shown the expression of estrogen receptors in epithelial and stromal cells[26,27]. The expression levels of both receptors reduces at the opening of the implantation window under the influence of progesterone. Although endometrium is brought to a receptive state by estrogen and progesterone, in mice, implantation is initiated by a short burst of estrogen on day 4 of pregnancy. This nidatory estrogen may induce endometrial receptivity by triggering the expression of a set of 'receptivity' genes, in a progesterone-primed endometrium, which permit embryo attachment. There is no evidence for the requirement of a nidatory estrogen surge in humans. The possible mediators of sex hormone action are discussed below.

IMPLANTATION IN THE MOUSE

It is now clear that many of the actions of steroids in regulating endometrial function and preparation for implantation are mediated by locally acting growth factors and cytokines. These are secreted proteins that control cell function such as proliferation, differentiation and secretion in a paracrine or autocrine manner. Although the expression patterns of many growth factors and their receptors have been described in endometrium of several species, for most, their function is unclear. Recently, gene targeting studies that produce mice lacking in a specific growth factor or receptor have been used to identify genes that are important in implantation. At present this technique is restricted to mice (Table 1). A surprising finding is that for many factors which affect embryo development or endometrial function *in vitro*, no deleterious effect is seen in animals totally lacking these genes. Alternatively, injection of antibodies or antisense oligonucleotides into the uterus to reduce the expression of target genes in luminal epithelium has successfully identified genes that play a central role in implantation.

LEUKEMIA INHIBITORY FACTOR

Leukemia inhibitory factor (LIF) belongs to a group of related cytokines, which includes interleukin-6 (IL-6), interleukin-11 (IL-11), cardiotropin (CT-1), oncostatin-M (OSM), ciliary neurotrophic factor (CNTF), cardiotropin-like cytokine (CLC) and neuropoietin (NP)[43]. These molecules all share the gp130 protein as part of the signal transduction complex, which may account for the functional redundancy of some of their effects. The first evidence that LIF plays an important role in implantation came when LIF mRNA was shown to be transiently expressed at high levels in the mouse uterine epithelium on day 4 of pregnancy, just prior to blastocyst attachment. Female mice lacking LIF (LIF–/–) produce normal embryos, but these fail to implant[28]. Implantation is restored in LIF–/– mice by an intraperitoneal infusion or intrauterine injection of LIF protein[28]. The site of action of LIF has been defined by localization of the LIF receptor (LIFR)/gp130 complex in the mouse uterus. LIFR has been localized both by *in situ* hybridization and immunohistochemistry to the luminal epithelium on day 4 of pregnancy[44,45]. LIF is not required to act directly on the embryo, since embryos lacking LIFR or gp130 do implant, although later embryo development is affected[46,47]. Recently,

the generation of mice with a mutation in gp130 that abolishes signal transducer and activator of transcription (STAT) but not mitogen-activated protein kinase (MAPK) signaling has shown that embryo attachment depends on the activation by LIF of the Janus kinase (JAK)/STAT signaling pathway in luminal epithelium. Taken together, these data suggest that maternal expression of LIF on day 4 of pregnancy is necessary to sensitize the endometrium to recognize or respond to the implanting embryo. Although the mechanism by which LIF brings the luminal epithelium to a receptive state remains elusive, several molecules which are up-regulated by LIF have been identified. These include cochlin, immune response gene 1 (IRG1), insulin-like growth factor binding protein 3 (IGFBP3) and amphiregulin[48,49]. However, of these molecules, only IRG1 has been shown to be essential for implantation[42,50]. The function of IRG1 is unknown.

In human endometrium, LIF mRNA levels are low in the proliferative phase, but rise dramatically in the mid- to late-luteal phase[51–53]. LIF immunoreactivity is detectable primarily in the glandular epithelium at this time, and epithelial cells secrete much more LIF than stromal cells *in vitro*, confirming that they are the major site of LIF secretion. The components of the LIF receptor complex (LIFR) and gp130 are expressed mainly on the luminal epithelium[52], throughout the menstrual cycle, indicating that, as in the mouse, this is the primary site of LIF's actions in human endometrium.

Evidence for a role for LIF in human implantation comes from a number of sources. Delage and colleagues showed that LIF secretion by endometrial explants, cultured for 5 days, was reduced in patients with unexplained infertility[54]. Laird and associates showed that concentrations of LIF in endometrial flushings were also reduced in patients with unexplained infertility[55]. However, these studies measured the secretion of LIF in isolation from its naturally occurring agonist sLIFR and antagonist sgp130. The possibility that the naturally occurring agonists could interfere with the enzyme-linked immunosorbent assays (ELISAs) used for LIF, or could affect the bioactivity of LIF, was not addressed. Cullinan and colleagues identified two infertile patients, out of their study group of 49, who showed no endometrial LIF immunostaining in secretory phase biopsies[52]. Treatment of women with RU486, which is known to

Table 1   Molecules of known importance in rodent implantation

Gene	Phenotype	Reference
LIF	LIF–/– mice, normal embryo development but embryo attachment fails	28
gp130	mice with gp130 lacking STAT binding site show same phenotype as LIF–/– mice	29
Hmx3	Hmx3–/– mice, embryo development normal, LIF not up-regulated and attachment fails	30
IL-1	intraperitoneal injection of an inhibitor to IL-1 inhibits implantation, but IL-1R knock-out mice are fertile	31,32
IL-11R	IL-11R–/– decidualization gradually fails	33
Hoxa10, Hoxa11	mice lacking Hoxa10 or Hoxa11 show reduced attachment and decidualization	34,35
Cox-2	Cox-2–/– show impaired ovulation and fertilization failure with delayed implantation	36
Lox 12/15	competitive inhibition of Lox 12/15 expression causes an 80% reduction in implantation sites	37
HB-EGF	induced in LE prior to implantation; beads soaked in HB-EGF induce decidualization	38
Integrin $\alpha_v\beta_3$	expressed in LE and blastocyst, disruption of $\alpha_v\beta_3$ function reduces implantation	39
Calcitonin	reduced calcitonin expression by antisense oligonucleotides inhibits implantation by 50%	40
Calbindin D_{9k}	inhibition of Calbindin D_{9k} and D_{28k} expression obliterates implantation	41
IRG1	intrauterine transfection with IRG1 antisense oligonucleotide reduces implantation by up to 90%	42

LIF, leukemia inhibitory factor; STAT, signal transducer and activator of transcription; Hmx3, homeobox 3; IL-1, interleukin-1; IL-11R, interleukin-11 receptor; Hoxa10 and 11, homeobox a 10 and 11; Cox-2, cyclo-oxygenase 2; Lox 12/15, leukocyte 12/15 lipoxygenase; HB-EGF, heparin binding-epidermal growth factor; IRG1, immune response gene 1; LE, luminal epithelium

prevent implantation, has been shown to reduce LIF immunoreactivity in endometrial glands in both women and primates. The best evidence for the role of LIF in primate implantation comes from experiments in which anti-LIF antibodies were injected into the uteri of rhesus monkeys on day 8 of pregnancy (post-coital day 8)[56]. The pregnancy rate was significantly reduced from 12/18 animals (66.7%) to 4/18 animals (22.2%).

In summary, there is some evidence for reduced secretion of LIF in women with unexplained infertility and of altered LIF secretion in response to RU486. However, in women, a critical role for LIF in implantation is not proven.

Interleukin-11

Interleukin-11 is a member of the IL-6 family of cytokines. It has well-characterized actions on hemopoietic cells, on the gastrointestinal tract and on the nervous system[57]. Until recently, no role in implantation was suspected. However, mice lacking the IL-11 receptor (IL-11R) are infertile[33]. RNAse protection assays showed that IL-11R mRNA was maximal in the uterus on days 5–8 of pregnancy, which is immediately after implantation. *In situ* hybridization studies in normal animals showed that IL-11 expression was induced after implantation in the primary decidual zone, immediately adjacent to the implanting blastocyst, with the IL-11R expression in the surrounding secondary decidual zone. Examination of the IL-11R–/– females revealed normal numbers of blastocysts and implantation sites, but that by day 5.5 the decidual response was reduced and by day 10.5 all embryos were resorbed. These defects were not due to problems in embryo development. The IL-11R–/– embryos were found to develop normally to term upon transfer to the uterus of normal mice, demonstrating that the deficiency was in the maternal IL-11R–/– uterine environment. Artificial decidualization induced by oil injection into the uterine lumen was also impaired. The failure to produce live young in the IL-11R–/– animals was therefore due to fetal resorption because of abnormal decidualization.

Epidermal growth factor family

Recent studies have suggested that the epidermal growth factor family, which includes epidermal growth factor (EGF), transforming growth factor

(TGFα), heparin binding-EGF (HB-EGF), amphiregulin (AR), betacellulin, epiregulin and the heregulins/neu-differentiation factors, might mediate in embryo/endometrial signaling[58,59]. All of these cytokines are proteolytically cleaved from integral membrane protein precursors. They interact with members of the ErbB tyrosine kinase receptor family, namely ErbB1 (EGF-R), ErbB2, ErbB3 and ErbB4. EGF and TGFα are expressed in the luminal epithelium of the preimplantation uterus, following the nidatory burst of estrogen, on day 4 of pregnancy. HB-EGF appears to be induced in the luminal epithelium at the site of blastocyst apposition at approximately 1600 h on postcoital day 4 (84 h), some 6–7 h prior to the estimated time of increased vascular permeability and trophectoderm/luminal epithelium interaction[60]. HB-EGF expression is not seen in the luminal epithelium surrounding dormant blastocysts, but is induced following estrogen treatment. This implies that estrogen primes the endometrium to be receptive to blastocyst-derived factors that are necessary for attachment and subsequent invasion. In contrast, AR is expressed throughout the luminal epithelium on day 4 of pregnancy under the control of maternal progesterone. After attachment, AR expression is further up-regulated in the luminal epithelium surrounding the apposing blastocyst and down-regulated between the implantation sites[58].

Epiregulin and betacellulin gene expression is up-regulated in both luminal epithelium and stromal cells underlying the attaching blastocyst[61], and also EGF-R is expressed on the blastocyst[62]. Therefore these ligands have the potential to signal to the attaching embryo. However, mice deficient in AR, EGF or TGFα, or double knock-outs for EGF and TGFα, are fertile[63]. The phenotype of EGF-R-deficient mice depends upon genetic background[64]. These mice have multiple abnormalities and varying implantation rates, as compared with heterozygote and wild-type littermates[65]. The precise function of HB-EGF is unknown; however, beads soaked in HB-EGF and placed into the uterus on day 4 induce localized vascular permeability, decidualization and the expression of bone morphometric protein (BMP-2)[38]. The expression of BMP-2 is normally up-regulated in the stroma, at the site of blastocyst attachment[38]. Therefore, the up-regulation of HB-EGF by the activated blastocyst may induce the expression of genes such as BMP-2 whose function in implantation may be to initiate decidualization.

Hoxa10 and Hoxa11

Hox (homeobox) genes are highly conserved in evolutionary development, and act as regulators of embryonic differentiation (see reference 66 for review). The differential expression of Hoxa9, Hoxa10, Hoxa11 and Hoxa13 genes along the undifferentiated paramesonephric duct in the mouse is essential for the appropriate formation of the tubes, uterus, cervix and upper vagina[67]. These transcription factors are also expressed in the mature murine reproductive tract[34,68]. A shift from luminal and glandular expression of Hoxa10 on postcoital days 0.5 and 1.5 to stromal expression from postcoital day 3.5 occurs. Females deficient in Hoxa10 or Hoxa11 show reduced fertility, which may result from altered uterine patterning during development. Recently, a role for Hoxa10 in implantation itself has been demonstrated. Uterine gene transfection with antisense oligonucleotides to reduce Hoxa10 or Hoxa11 was shown to reduce implantation rates[66,69]. Fecundity in these gene-deleted animals is reduced but not obliterated, which suggests that there is some redundancy in terms of gene regulation by these transcription factors.

Calcitonin

Calcitonin is a peptide hormone, secreted by the C cells of the mammalian thyroid, which lowers blood calcium by inhibiting bone mineral resorption and increasing urinary excretion of calcium and phosphate. Secretion from the thyroid is regulated by the levels of ionized calcium in the blood[70]. The binding of calcitonin to a G protein-coupled receptor (CR-1) activates adenylate cyclase and elevates cytosolic Ca^{2+} levels. Recently, calcitonin has been shown to be expressed in the glands of the rat uterus, from postcoital day 2 to day 6, in a progesterone-induced manner[71]. Intrauterine injection of calcitonin antisense oligodeoxynucleotides results in a reduction in implantation rates[40]. The uterine site of the calcitonin receptor expression is unknown. The effects of calcitonin antisense treatment on the embryo have not been addressed. However, blastocysts treated with calcitonin differentiate *in vitro* at an accelerated rate[72]. Calcitonin is expressed in human and baboon endometrium during the implantation window and shows progesterone regulation[73,74]. There have been no studies testing the functional importance of calcitonin in primate implantation.

Interleukin-1

IL-1 exists in two distinct molecular forms (IL-1α and IL-1β), which, in the mouse, share only 23% amino acid homology[75]. Despite this, they bind to the same receptors, IL-1R (types I and II), and exhibit very similar biological actions. IL-1α is mostly intracellular and IL-1β is cleaved from the cell surface by IL-1 converting enzyme (ICE). A naturally occurring antagonist to IL-1β (IL-1Ra) is also secreted by many IL-1 producing cells. IL-1R type I is located in mouse endometrial luminal epithelium, with increased intensity in the peri-implantation period[31]. Intraperitoneal injection with recombinant human (r-h) IL-1Ra has been shown to reduce implantation. This effect was not due to any toxic effect of the r-hIL-1Ra on the embryo. However, mice deficient in IL-1R type I or double knock-outs of both IL-1α and IL-1β are fertile; therefore, the mechanism of the effect on implantation is unclear[32,76].

Cyclo-oxygenase

Cyclo-oxygenase (COX) is the rate-limiting enzyme that mediates the conversion of arachadonic acid to prostaglandins[77]. COX exists as two isoforms that are encoded by specific genes[78,79]. COX-1 is localized to the endoplasmic reticulum and is constitutively expressed. COX-2 is inducible during inflammation and is localized to the nuclear envelope, suggesting a role in gene regulation. Cox-1 is expressed in the uterine luminal epithelium on the morning of postcoital day 4, but is undetectable at the time of blastocyst attachment[80]. Cox-2 is expressed in uterine luminal epithelium and underlying stromal cells at the site of blastocyst attachment. COX-1-deficient mice are fertile[36]. Cox-2-deficient mice appear to show reduced implantation rates when wild-type blastocysts are transferred into pseudopregnant Cox-2−/− mice. However, a more detailed analysis shows a delay in the timing of implantation of some 24 h in Cox-2−/− mice rather than a failure of implantation[81].

Calbindin-D$_{9k}$

Three genes, calbindin-D$_{9k}$, mouse monoclonal non-specific suppressor factor beta (MNSFβ) and SC35, have been recently cloned in experiments designed to identify genes whose expression differs between implantation sites and the interimplantation zone. Calbindin-D$_{9k}$ is a calcium binding protein, and its expression has been shown to be progesterone-regulated and localized to the uterine luminal epithelium[82]. Calbindin-D$_{9k}$ expression at implantation sites increases during early pregnancy, and then is significantly reduced on days 4.5 and 5.5. In mice that are deficient for calbindin-D$_{28k}$, inhibition of calbindin-D$_{9k}$ expression on day 4 of pregnancy results in a dramatic reduction in the number of implantation sites[41]. Clearly this illustrates the issue of redundancy in which one gene can compensate for the absence of another. Reduction of calbindin-D$_{9k}$ in normal mice where calbindin-D$_{28k}$ is still present has no effect.

Leukocyte 12/15 lipoxygenase

Leukocyte 12/15 lipoxygenase (Alox15) is a lipid-metabolizing enzyme that generates hydroxyeicosatetraenoic acids, which are known to act as cell differentiation signals. The two known isoforms of this enzyme are expressed in luminal epithelium only on the day of implantation, and this is accompanied by a marked increase in their metabolites, such as 12-HETE. Blockade of uterine Alox15 activity by the specific inhibitor AA-861 reduces implantation by more than 80%[37]. Since metabolites such as 12-HETE can function as activating ligands of the peroxisome proliferation-activated receptor gamma (PPARγ), it has been hypothesized that PPARγ could be a downstream target. Administration of rosaglitazone, a potent PPARγ agonist, restored implantation in animals treated with the Alox15 inhibitor[37]. Therefore, pathways that converge or regulate directly lipid metabolism in the luminal epithelium may play a crucial role in implantation.

Immune response gene 1

IRG1 is highly conserved in vertebrates, and strongly resembles the bacterial enzyme methylcitrate dehydratase. IRG1 is expressed in luminal epithelium with peak expression coinciding with implantation on day 4 of pregnancy[83]. This expression is primarily regulated by P4, since IRG1 expression in the mouse uterus on day 4 is reduced eight-fold by prior treatment with the antiprogestin RU486, and mice deficient for PR fail to express IRG1. Treatment with antisense oligodeoxynucleotides to IRG1 on day 3 of pregnancy decreases its expression on day 4, and reduces implantation by up to 90%[42,50]. Chen and colleagues propose that IRG1 may play a role in odd-chain lipid metabolism[50]. This may explain the effect of IRG1 on implantation, since several other enzymes that affect fatty acid metabolism are also known to be important in implantation. More recently, we have shown that the full physiological expression of IRG1 on day 4 requires the combined action of PR and LIF[49]. This illustrates how several signal transduction pathways are integrated to regulate specific genes.

CONCLUSIONS

Data from rodent models show that, although many genes are regulated by steroid hormones and are located in the luminal epithelium or around the blastocyst, most of them do not appear to be essential for implantation. This may be due to redundancy, as illustrated by the calbindins. Alternatively, where several signal transduction pathways converge to regulate a gene, removal of one of these may not have a significant impact. In humans, no genes other than PR have been proved to be essential in implantation. Based on the results above, a scheme can be proposed for murine implantation, which incorporates the best-documented steps in the implantation process. This can serve as a template for the investigation of implantation in humans (Figure 3).

PREIMPLANTATION EMBRYO DEVELOPMENT

Preimplantation embryo development requires activation of the embryonic genome. This occurs at the two-cell stage in mice and the four-cell stage in human embryos[84]. Activation of the embryonic genome results in secretion of paracrine factors, which are able to signal to the endometrium and also influence the maternal endocrine system, as well as the expression of growth factor and cytokine receptors on the trophectoderm. As the embryo does not respond directly to sex hormones, peptides and growth factors present in endometrial secretions, which are regulated by estrogen and progesterone, can only affect embryo function if the appropriate receptor is expressed on the trophectoderm.

Many assisted reproduction techniques require a period of embryo culture *in vitro*; there is evidence that even short periods of culture may result in developmental delay and reduced implantation rates[85]. Embryos cultured together in the same drop, or in conditioned medium from feeder cell layers, exhibit improved growth and reduced delay. The best results have been obtained following embryo culture with epithelial cell lines, supporting the hypothesis that soluble factors secreted by reproductive tract epithelium can enhance embryo development. A drawback with the use of feeder cell layers of primary cells or even cell lines is that these methods are cumbersome to apply in clinical practice. The availability of highly purified recombinant growth factors and other proteins has stimulated efforts to identify individual proteins in the conditioned media, which might have beneficial effects on embryos *in vitro*. In order for a growth factor to act on a preimplantation embryo, the corresponding receptor must be expressed. However, demonstrating receptor expression on single embryos is technically demanding. Recently, the technique of reverse transcriptase polymerase chain reaction (RT-PCR) has provided a highly sensitive method to screen for growth factor and receptor mRNAs in single embryos. cDNA from a single embryo can be used to examine the expression of mRNA encoding many different genes. We have previously used this method to examine the expression of interleukin-6 (IL-6) and the IL-6 receptor (IL-6R) in human preimplantation embryos[86]. mRNA for both ligand and receptor were detected only at the blastocyst stage. Therefore, prior to this, the embryo cannot make or respond to IL-6. This experiment shows that co-culture of human embryos prior to the blastocyst stage with IL-6 would be fruitless. This type of analysis has allowed a phenotypic expression map to be developed for human embryos[87].

These results are important because they indicate which cytokines cannot act on embryos directly, as the receptor is never expressed. They also identify which stages can respond to particular cytokines because the receptor is present. The ultimate aim of such an analysis is to identify growth factors whose receptors are expressed on embryos and which enhance embryo development when added to *in vitro* culture medium.

It is difficult to assess the relative contributions that blastocyst and endometrium make to successful implantation, or indeed to implantation failure. Data

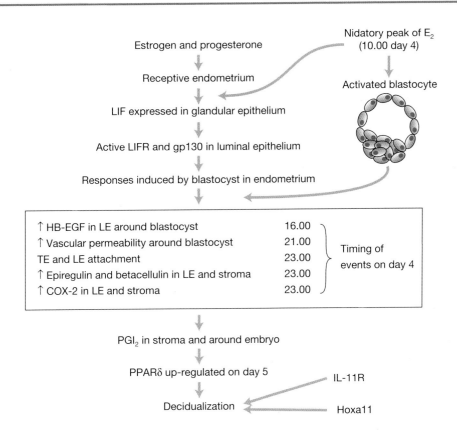

Figure 3 Summary of peri-implantation changes in the mouse uterus. Scheme outlining the morphological and molecular changes in early mouse implantation. Timings are approximate and are taken from the day of plug detection (day 1). LIF, leukemia inhibitory factor; HB-EGF, heparin binding-epidermal growth factor; E_2 estrogen; TE, trophectoderm; LE, uterine luminal epithelium, COX-2, cyclo-oxygenase 2; IL-11R, interleukin-11 receptor; Hoxa11, homeobox a 11; PPARδ, peroxisome proliferator-activated receptor delta; PGI$_2$, prostaglandin I$_2$

from oocyte or embryo donation programs suggest that implantation rates in older recipient mothers can be up to 45%[88]. This suggests that the fall in fecundity that occurs with age may be mainly due to embryo and not endometrial quality. Furthermore, the importance of the embryo can be seen, as embryos selected after blastomere aneuploidy studies or embryos cultured in sequential media have a high probability of implanting. This implies that embryo quality is a very important factor in implantation success. However, it is clear that endometrial quality also contributes to implantation success. Pregnancy rates in women undergoing multiple IVF cycles are relatively constant for up to three cycles of embryo replacement. After three cycles, the likelihood of pregnancy starts to decline, implying that in these women, as embryo quality is constant, a significant endometrial factor is present. The murine implantation studies clearly show that a fertile endometrial phenotype requires the synchronized expression of specific endometrial genes.

The key question is, to what extent does failure to develop a receptive endometrium contribute to low implantation rates in women?

EMBRYO-INDUCED RECEPTIVITY

Evidence that the development of functional receptivity by the endometrium depends in part upon signals from the embryo comes from experiments in rodents and primates. We know that preimplantation embryos secrete many soluble factors that may act on the endometrium. Chorionic gonadotropin, which is known to exhibit a luteotrophic effect on the ovary, also acts on both luminal and stromal cells of the endometrium. Intrauterine infusion of chorionic gonadotropin in baboons causes increased secretion of PP14 (glycodelin) and α smooth muscle actin, and also induces in the luminal epithelium the appearance of endometrial plaques, which are an early maternal response to pregnancy[89]. In humans, infusion of chorionic gonadotropin (hCG) via a microdialysis catheter inserted into the uterus results in an increased secretion of matrix metalloproteinase 9 (MMP9), a tissue remodeling peptide, as well as the secretion of IGFBP1, a marker of decidualization. IL-1 secretion by the blastocyst into culture medium induces the expression of integrin β_3 on the epithelial surface of co-cultured endometrium[90]. This integrin has been shown to be expressed in glandular epithelium during the period of the implantation window, and also to be dysregulated in some cases of infertility[91,92]. In experimental animals the ability of the embryo to modulate receptivity has been clearly demonstrated[93,94]. The most convincing data come from *in situ* hybridization experiments in mice, where HB-EGF mRNA expression is up-regulated at the site of blastocyst attachment some 6 h before physical contact between the trophectoderm and the uterine epithelium is made[60]. Therefore, a state of functional receptivity may only be fully established when the primed endometrium receives a signal from the attachment-competent blastocyst, which triggers the attachment process. It is worth noting that for obvious ethical reasons, almost all the studies on endometrial receptivity in humans have been conducted on non-pregnant endometrium.

MARKERS OF HUMAN ENDOMETRIAL RECEPTIVITY

The search for endometrial markers of receptivity has proved elusive for various reasons. There are great variations in both the site and the level of expression of individual genes in the endometrium, even in a cohort of carefully monitored normally cycling women[95]. Also, the endometrium shows a remarkable degree of plasticity in its differentiation. Endometrial morphology and gene expression can be shown to have 'caught up', as an initially aberrant gene expression and tissue architecture in an early secretory phase biopsy can become normalized in a subsequent biopsy from the same patient in the same menstrual cycle[96]. Finally, inadvertent endometrial biopsy during a conception cycle has demonstrated that endometrium displaying abnormal architecture is able to support implantation successfully[97].

Attempts to define markers of a receptive endometrium have focused mainly on the expression of integrins. Lessey and colleagues showed that the co-expression of two integrin complexes ($\alpha_4\beta_1$) and ($\alpha_v\beta_3$), in glandular epithelium, frames the implantation window[98], and that this expression is altered in women with unexplained infertility[92]. It is probable that the lack of co-expression of these integrins reflects a dysfunctional endometrial response to progesterone, and is not the cause *per se* of an individual's infertility. The expression of other proteins including progesterone receptor[99,100] and placental protein 14 (PP14)[101] have been suggested as potential markers of uterine receptivity. PP14 can be assayed in serum, but serum levels have a low positive-predictive value for subsequent pregnancy. All of these markers require endometrial biopsies, which precludes their use in actual implantation cycles, and there is a substantial overlap in expression levels between subfertile patient groups and normal controls. Unfortunately, non-invasive assays of endometrial receptivity such as the assessment of endometrial thickness or endometrial volume by ultrasound are not useful in predicting fertility[102]. There are significant patient-to-patient variations in the levels of proteins secreted from the endometrium, such as IL-18[103] and sgp130[95]. This means that although a statistical difference in protein secretion between fertile and infertile patient groups is demonstrable, assays of these markers are not useful clinically.

Identification of markers of human receptivity

An alternative approach has been to seek a combination of markers, which could reliably differentiate receptive and non-receptive endometrium. Microarrays allow the measurement of expression levels of thousands of RNA species simultaneously. Several recent studies have sought to define a gene expression profile that distinguishes the receptive and non-receptive states. Using advanced bioinformatics techniques, this has shown that endometrium from different patient groups can be clearly distinguished[104] (Figure 4).

Similarly, it has been shown that microarray data can be used to date endometrial biopsies or monitor changes in the endometrium throughout the menstrual cycle[105]. These methods hold great promise, and it is likely that high-throughput techniques such as microarrays will become routine diagnostic tools for

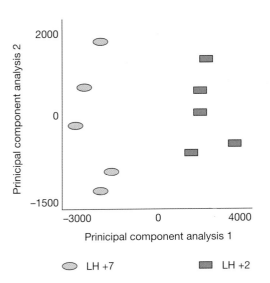

Figure 4 Principal component analysis (PCA) of ten endometrial biopsies taken at 2 and 7 days after the luteinizing hormone surge (LH + 2 and LH + 7), using 2000 randomly chosen genes. The PCA successfully clustered the samples into distinct groups. After reference 104

physicians treating endometrial dysfunction. These approaches have been shown to work in principle; what is now required are the appropriate clinical studies to provide an evidence base for their use.

SUMMARY

(1) Genes have been identified in mice that are essential for endometrial receptivity.

(2) The presence of a functional progesterone receptor is known to be essential for implantation in humans.

(3) The embryo may locally induce receptivity in appropriately primed endometrium.

(4) Microarray analysis of endometrial gene expression may allow classification of endometrium into receptive and non-receptive phenotypes.

REFERENCES

1. Psychoyos A. Hormonal control of ovoimplantation. Vitam Horm 1973; 31: 201–56

2. Bergh PA, Navot D. The impact of embryonic development and endometrial maturity on the timing of implantation. Fertil Steril 1992; 58: 537–42

3. Murphy CR, Rogers PAW, Hosie MJ, et al. Tight junctions of human uterine epithelial cells change during the menstrual cycle: a morphometric study. Acta Anat 1992; 144: 36–8

4. Psychoyos A, Nikas G. Uterine pinopodes as markers of uterine receptivity. Assist Reprod Rev 1994; 4: 26–32

5. Bentin-Ley U, Lopata A. In vitro models of human blastocyst implantation. Baillière's Best Pract Res Clin Obstet Gynaecol 2000; 14: 765–74

6. Ebnet K, Vestweber D. Molecular mechanisms that control leukocyte extravasation: the selectins and the chemokines. Histochem Cell Biol 1999; 112: 1–23

7. Kimber SJ, Stones RE, Sidhu SS. Glycosylation changes during differentiation of the murine uterine epithelium. Biochem Soc Trans 2001; 29: 156–62

8. Kimber SJ, Spanswick C. Blastocyst implantation: the adhesion cascade. Semin Cell Dev Biol 2000; 11: 73–86

9. Genbacev OD, Prakobphol A, Foulk RA, et al. Trophoblast L-selectin-mediated adhesion at the maternal–fetal interface. Science 2003; 299: 405–8

10. Hardy K, Spanos S, Becker D, et al. From cell death to embryo arrest: mathematical models of human preimplantation embryo development. Proc Natl Acad Sci USA 2001; 98: 1655–60

11. Goulart LR, Vieira GS, Martelli L, et al. Is MUC1 polymorphism associated with female infertility? Reprod Biomed Online 2004; 8: 477–82

12. Braga VM, Gendler SJ. Modulation of Muc-1 mucin expression in the mouse uterus during the estrus cycle, early pregnancy and placentation. J Cell Sci 1993; 105: 397–405

13. DeSouza MM, Surveyor GA, Price RE, et al. MUC1/episialin: a critical barrier in the female reproductive tract. J Reprod Immunol 1999; 45: 127–58

14. Idris N, Carraway KL. Sialomicin complex (Muc4) expression in the rat female reproductive tract. Biol Reprod 1999; 61: 1431–8

15. Evans RM. The steroid and thyroid hormone receptor superfamily. Science 1988; 240: 889–95

16. O'Malley BW, Tsai MJ. Molecular pathways of steroid receptor action. Biol Reprod 1992; 46: 163–7

17. Mulac-Jericevic B, Mullinax RA, DeMayo FJ, et al. Subgroup of reproductive functions of progesterone mediated by progesterone receptor-B isoform. Science 2000; 289: 1751–4

18. Lydon JP, DeMayo FJ, Funk CR, et al. Mice lacking progesterone receptor exhibit pleiotropic reproductive abnormalities. Genes Dev 1995; 9: 2266–78

19. Conneely OM, Mulac-Jericevic B, DeMayo F, et al. Reproductive functions of progesterone receptors. Recent Prog Horm Res 2002; 57: 339–55

20. Whyte A, Wang MW, King IS, et al. Biotinylated anti-progesterone monoclonal antibodies specifically target the uterine epithelium and block implantation in the mouse. J Reprod Immunol 1992; 21: 127–38

21. Cheon YP, Li Q, Xu X, et al. A genomic approach to identify novel progesterone receptor regulated pathways in the uterus during implantation. Mol Endocrinol 2002; 16: 2853–71

22. Kraus WL, Montano MM, Katzenellenbogen BS. Identification of multiple, widely spaced estrogen-responsive regions in the rat progesterone receptor gene. Mol Endocrinol 1994; 8: 952–69

23. Kurita T, Lee KJ, Cooke PS, et al. Paracrine regulation of epithelial progesterone receptor by estradiol in the mouse female reproductive tract. Biol Reprod 2000; 62: 821–30

24. Couse JF, Curtis SW, Washburn TF, et al. Disruption of the mouse oestrogen receptor gene: resulting phenotypes and experimental findings. Biochem Soc Trans 1995; 23: 929–35

25. Couse JF, Curtis SW, Washburn TF, et al. Analysis of transcription and estrogen insensitivity in the female mouse after targeted disruption of the estrogen receptor gene. Mol Endocrinol 1995; 9: 1441–54

26. Moutsatsou P, Sekeris CE. Estrogen and progesterone receptors in the endometrium. Ann NY Acad Sci 1997; 816: 99–115

27. Matsuzaki S, Fukaya T, Suzuki T, et al. Oestrogen receptor alpha and beta mRNA expression in human endometrium throughout the menstrual cycle. Mol Hum Reprod 1999; 5: 559–64

28. Stewart CL, Kaspar P, Brunet LJ, et al. Blastocyst implantation depends on maternal expression of leukaemia inhibitory factor. Nature (London) 1992; 359: 76–9

29. Ernst M, Inglese M, Waring P, et al. Defective gp130-mediated signal transducer and activator of transcription (STAT) signaling results in degenerative joint disease, gastrointestinal ulceration, and failure of uterine implantation. J Exp Med 2001; 194: 189–203

30. Wang W, Van De Water T, Lufkin T. Inner ear and maternal reproductive defects in mice lacking the Hmx3 homeobox gene. Development 1998; 125: 621–34

31. Simon C, Frances A, Piquette GN, et al. Embryonic implantation in mice is blocked by interleukin-1 receptor antagonist. Endocrinology 1994; 134: 521–8

32. Glaccum MB, Stocking KL, Charrier K, et al. Phenotypic and functional characterization of mice that lack the type I receptor for IL-1. J Immunol 1997; 159: 3364–71

33. Robb L, Li R, Hartley L, et al. Infertility in female mice lacking the receptor for interleukin 11 is due to a defective uterine response to implantation. Nat Med 1998; 4: 303–8

34. Benson GV, Lim H, Paria BC, et al. Mechanisms of the reduced fertility in the Hoxa-10 mutant mice: uterine homeosis and loss of maternal Hoxa-10 expression. Development 1996; 122: 2687–96.

35. Gendron RL, Paradis H, Hsieh-Li HM, et al. Abnormal uterine stromal and glandular function associated with maternal reproductive defects in Hoxa-11 null mice. Biol Reprod 1997; 56: 1097–105

36. Lim H, Paria BC, Das SK, et al. Multiple female reproductive failures in cyclooxygenase 2-deficient mice. Cell 1997; 91: 197–208

37. Li Q, Cheon YP, Kannan A, et al. A novel pathway involving progesterone receptor, 12/15-lipoxygenase-derived eicosanoids, and peroxisome proliferator-activated receptor gamma regulates implantation in mice. J Biol Chem 2004; 279: 11570–81

38. Paria BC, Ma W, Tan J, et al. Cellular and molecular responses of the uterus to embryo implantation can be elicited by locally applied growth factors. Proc Natl Acad Sci USA 2001; 98: 1047–52

39. Illera MJ, Cullinan E, Gui Y, et al. Blockade of the alpha(v)beta(3) integrin adversely affects implantation in the mouse. Biol Reprod 2000; 62: 1285–90

40. Zhu LJ, Bagchi MK, Bagchi IC. Attenuation of calcitonin gene expression in pregnant rat uterus leads to a block in embryonic implantation. Endocrinology 1998; 139: 330–9

41. Luu KC, Nie GY, Salamonsen LA. Endometrial calbindins are critical for embryo implantation: evidence from in vivo use of morpholino antisense oligonucleotides. Proc Natl Acad Sci USA 2004; 101: 8028–33

42. Cheon YP, Xu X, Bagchi MK, et al. Immune-responsive gene 1 (Irg1) is a novel target of progesterone receptor and plays a critical role during implantation in the mouse. Endocrinology 2003; 144: 5623–30

43. Derouet D, Rousseau F, Alfonsi F, et al. Neuropoietin, a new IL-6-related cytokine signaling through the ciliary neurotrophic factor receptor. Proc Natl Acad Sci USA 2004; 101: 4827–32

44. Nichols J, Davidson D, Taga T, et al. Complementary tissue-specific expression of LIF and LIF-receptor mRNAs in early mouse embryogenesis. Mech Dev 1996; 57: 123–31

45. Yang ZM, Le SP, Chen DB, et al. Leukaemia inhibitory factor (LIF), LIF receptor and gp130 in the

416

mouse uterus during early pregnancy. Mol Reprod Dev 1995; 42: 407–14

46. Ware CB, Horowitz MC, Renshaw BR, et al. Targeted disruption of the low-affinity leukemia inhibitory factor receptor gene causes placental, skeletal, neural and metabolic defects and results in perinatal death. Development 1995; 121: 1283–99

47. Yoshida K, Taga T, Saito M, et al. Targeted disruption of gp130, a common signal transducer for the interleukin 6 family of cytokines, leads to myocardial and hematological disorders. Proc Natl Acad Sci USA 1996; 93: 407–11

48. Rodriguez CI, Cheng JG, Liu L, et al. Cochlin, a secreted VWA domain containing factor, is regulated by LIF in the uterus at the time of embryo implantation. Endocrinology 2003; 145: 1410–18

49. Sherwin JR, Freeman TC, Stephens RJ, et al. Identification of genes regulated by leukemia-inhibitory factor in the mouse uterus at the time of implantation. Mol Endocrinol 2004; 18: 2185–95

50. Chen B, Zhang D, Pollard JW. Progesterone regulation of the mammalian ortholog of methylcitrate dehydratase (immune response gene 1) in the uterine epithelium during implantation through the protein kinase C pathway. Mol Endocrinol 2003; 17: 2340–54

51. Charnock-Jones DS, Sharkey AM, Fenwick P, et al. Leukaemia inhibitory factor mRNA concentration peaks in human endometrium at the time of implantation and the blastocyst contains mRNA for the receptor at this time. J Reprod Fertil 1994; 101: 421–6

52. Cullinan EB, Abbondanzo SJ, Anderson PS, et al. Leukemia inhibitory factor (LIF) and LIF receptor expression in human endometrium suggests a potential autocrine/paracrine function in regulating embryo implantation. Proc Natl Acad Sci USA 1996; 93: 3115–20

53. Vogiagis D, Marsh MM, Fry RC, et al. Leukaemia inhibitory factor in human endometrium throughout the menstrual cycle. J Endocrinol 1996; 148: 95–102

54. Delage G, Moreau JF, Taupin JL, et al. In-vitro endometrial secretion of human interleukin for DA cells/leukaemia inhibitory factor by explant cultures from fertile and infertile women. Hum Reprod 1995; 10: 2483–8

55. Laird SM, Tuckerman EM, Dalton CF, et al. The production of leukaemia inhibitory factor by human endometrium: presence in uterine flushings and production by cells in culture. Hum Reprod 1997; 12: 569–74

56. Yue ZP, Yang ZM, Wei P, et al. Leukemia inhibitory factor, leukemia inhibitory factor receptor, and glycoprotein 130 in rhesus monkey uterus during menstrual cycle and early pregnancy. Biol Reprod 2000; 63: 508–12

57. Nandurkar HH, Robb L, Begley CG. The role of IL-11 in hematopoiesis as revealed by a targeted mutation of its receptor. Stem Cells 1998; 16 (Suppl 2): 53–65

58. Das SK, Chakraborty I, Paria BC, et al. Amphiregulin is an implantation-specific and progesterone-regulated gene in the mouse uterus. Mol Endocrinol 1995; 9: 691–705

59. Paria BC, Reese J, Das SK, et al. Deciphering the cross-talk of implantation: advances and challenges. Science 2002; 296: 2185–8

60. Das SK, Wang XN, Paria BC, et al. Heparin-binding EGF-like growth factor gene is induced in the mouse uterus temporally by the blastocyst solely at the site of its apposition: a possible ligand for interaction with blastocyst EGF-receptor in implantation. Development 1994; 120: 1071–83

61. Das SK, Das N, Wang J, et al. Expression of betacellulin and epiregulin genes in the mouse uterus temporally by the blastocyst, solely at the site of its apposition is coincident with the 'Window' of implantation. Dev Biol 1997; 190: 178–90

62. Wiley L, Jie-Xin W, Harari I, et al. Epidermal growth factor receptor mRNA and protein increase after the four cell preimplantation stage of murine development. Dev Biol 1992; 149: 247–60

63. Stewart CL, Cullinan EB. Preimplantation development of the mammalian embryo and its regulation by growth factors. Dev Genet 1997; 21: 91–101

64. Threadgill DW, Dlugosz AA, Hansen LA, et al. Targeted disruption of mouse EGF receptor: effect of genetic background on mutant phenotype. Science 1995; 269: 230–4

65. Iwamoto R, Yamazaki S, Asakura M, et al. Heparin-binding EGF-like growth factor and ErbB signaling is essential for heart function. Proc Natl Acad Sci USA 2003; 100: 3221–6

66. Taylor HS. The role of HOX genes in human implantation. Hum Reprod Update 2000; 6: 75–9

67. Taylor HS, Vanden Heuvel G, Igarashi P. A conserved Hox axis in the mouse and human reproductive system: late establishment and persistent expression of the Hoxa cluster genes. Biol Reprod 1997; 57: 1338–45

68. Satokata I, Benson GV, Maas RL. Sexually dimorphic sterility phenotypes in Hoxa10-deficient mice. Nature (London) 1995; 374: 460–3

69. Bagot CN, Troy PJ, Taylor HS. Alteration of maternal Hoxa10 expression by in vivo gene transfection affects implantation. Gene Ther 2000; 7: 1378–84

70. Hardy RN, Hobsley M, Saunders KB. Endocrine Physiology. London: Edward Arnold, 1981

71. Ding Y-Q, Zhu L-J, Bagchi MK, et al. Progesterone timulates calcitonin gene expression in the uterus during implantation. Endocrinology 1994; 135: 2265–74

72. Wang J, Rout UK, Bagchi IC, et al. Expression of calcitonin receptors in mouse preimplantation embryos and their function in the regulation of blastocyst differentiation by calcitonin. Development 1998; 125: 4293–302

73. Kumar S, Zhu LJ, Polihronis M, et al. Progesterone induces calcitonin gene expression in human endometrium within the putative window of implantation. J Clin Endocrinol Metab 1998; 83: 4443–50

74. Kumar S, Brudney A, Cheon YP, et al. Progesterone induces calcitonin expression in the baboon endometrium within the window of uterine receptivity. Biol Reprod 2003; 68: 1318–23

75. Callard R, Gearing A. The Cytokine Facts Book. London: Academic Press, 1994

76. Mizushima H, Zhou CJ, Dohi K, et al. Reduced postischemic apoptosis in the hippocampus of mice deficient in interleukin-1. J Comp Neurol 2002; 448: 203–16

77. Smith WL, Marnett LJ, DeWitt DL. Prostaglandin and thromboxane biosynthesis. Pharmacol Ther 1991; 49: 153–79

78. Funk CD, Funk LB, Kennedy ME, et al. Human platelet/erythroleukemia cell prostaglandin G/H synthase: cDNA cloning, expression, and gene chromosomal assignment. FASEB J 1991; 5: 2304–12

79. Jones DA, Carlton DP, McIntyre TM, et al. Molecular cloning of human prostaglandin endoperoxide synthase type II and demonstration of expression in response to cytokines. J Biol Chem 1993; 268: 9049–54

80. Chakraborty I, Das SK, Wang J, et al. Developmental expression of the cyclo-oxygenase-1 and cyclo-oxygenase-2 genes in the peri-implantation mouse uterus and their differential regulation by the blastocyst and ovarian steroids. J Mol Endocrinol 1996; 16: 107–22

81. Cheng JG, Stewart CL. Loss of cyclooxygenase-2 retards decidual growth but does not inhibit embryo implantation or development to term. Biol Reprod 2003; 68: 401–4

82. Nie GY, Li Y, Wang J, et al. Complex regulation of calcium-binding protein D9k (calbindin-D(9k)) in the mouse uterus during early pregnancy and at the site of embryo implantation. Biol Reprod 2000; 62: 27–36

83. Li Q, Zhang M, Kumar S, et al. Identification and implantation stage-specific expression of an interferon-alpha-regulated gene in human and rat endometrium. Endocrinology 2001; 142: 2390–400

84. Artley JK, Braude PR, Johnson MH. Gene activity and cleavage arrest in human pre-embryos. Hum Reprod 1992; 7: 1014–21

85. Sellens MH, Sherman MI. Effects of culture conditions on the developmental programme of mouse blastocysts. J Embryol Exp Morphol 1980; 56: 1–22

86. Sharkey AM, Dellow K, Blayney M, et al. Stage-specific expression of cytokine and receptor messenger ribonucleic acids in human preimplantation embryos. Biol Reprod 1995; 53: 974–81

87. Hardy K, Spanos S. Growth factor expression and function in the human and mouse preimplantation embryo. J Endocrinol 2002; 172: 221–36

88. Paulson RJ, Boostanfar R, Saadat P, et al. Pregnancy in the sixth decade of life: obstetric outcomes in women of advanced reproductive age. J Am Med Assoc 2002; 288: 2320–3

89. Cameo P, Srisuparp S, Strakova Z, et al. Chorionic gonadotropin and uterine dialogue in the primate. Reprod Biol Endocrinol 2004; 2: 50

90. Simon C, Gimeno MJ, Mercader A, et al. Embryonic regulation of integrins beta 3, alpha 4, and alpha 1 in human endometrial epithelial cells in vitro. J Clin Endocrinol Metab 1997; 82: 2607–16

91. Lessey BA, Castelbaum AJ, Sawin SW, et al. Aberrant integrin expression in the endometrium of women with endometriosis. J Clin Endocrinol Metab 1994; 79: 643–9

92. Lessey BA, Castelbaum AJ, Sawin SW, et al. Integrins as markers of uterine receptivity in women with primary unexplained infertility. Fertil Steril 1995; 63: 535–42

93. Godkin JD, Bazer FW, Thatcher WW, et al. Proteins released by cultured day 15–16 conceptuses prolong luteal maintenance when introduced into the uterine lumen of cyclic ewes. J Reprod Fertil 1984; 71: 57–64

94. Shiotani M, Noda Y, Mori T. Embryo-dependent induction of uterine receptivity assessed by an in vitro model of implantation in mice. Biol Reprod 1993; 49: 794–801

95. Sherwin JR, Smith SK, Wilson A, et al. Soluble gp130 is up-regulated in the implantation window and shows altered secretion in patients with primary unexplained infertility. J Clin Endocrinol Metab 2002; 87: 3953–60

96. Damario MA, Lesnick TG, Lessey BA, et al. Endometrial markers of uterine receptivity utilizing the donor oocyte model. Hum Reprod 2001; 16: 1893–9

97. Rogers PA, Murphy CR, Leeton J, et al. Ultrastructural study of human uterine epithelium from a patient with a confirmed pregnancy. Acta Anat (Basel) 1989; 135: 176–9

98. Lessey BA, Ilesanmi AO, Lessey MA, et al. Luminal and glandular endometrial epithelium express integrins differentially throughout the menstrual cycle: implications for implantation, contraception, and infertility. Am J Reprod Immunol 1996; 35: 195–204

99. Lessey BA, Yeh I, Castelbaum AJ, et al. Endometrial progesterone receptors and markers of uterine receptivity in the window of implantation. Fertil Steril 1996; 65: 477–83

100. Ilesanmi AO, Hawkins DA, Lessey BA. Immunohistochemical markers of uterine receptivity in the human endometrium. Microsc Res Tech 1993; 25: 208–22

101. Klentzeris LD, Bulmer JN, Seppala M, et al. Placental protein 14 in cycles with normal and retarded endometrial differentiation. Hum Reprod 1994; 9: 394–8

102. Sterzik K, Grab D, Rosenbusch B, et al. Receptivity of the endometrium: comparison of ultrasound and histologic findings after hormonal stimulation. Geburtsh Frauenheilkd 1991; 51: 554–8

103. Ledee-Bataille N, Olivennes F, Kadoch J, et al. Detectable levels of interleukin-18 in uterine luminal secretions at oocyte retrieval predict failure of the embryo transfer. Hum Reprod 2004; 19: 1968–73

104. Riesewijk A, Martin J, van Os R, et al. Gene expression profiling of human endometrial receptivity on days LH+2 versus LH+7 by microarray technology. Mol Hum Reprod 2003; 9: 253–64

105. Ponnampalam AP, Weston GC, Trajstman AC, et al. Molecular classification of human endometrial cycle stages by transcriptional profiling. Mol Hum Reprod 2004; 10: 879–93

23

Cryopreservation of human oocytes and ovarian tissue

Roger G. Gosden and Lucinda L. Veeck Gosden

INTRODUCTION

Low-temperature preservation of cells occupies a key role among modern reproductive technologies. Some cell types are more robust during freezing and thawing than others. Spermatozoa are relatively tolerant and were the first mammalian cells to be successfully cryopreserved for reproductive purposes; subsequently, embryo cryopreservation was introduced to augment pregnancy rates when IVF became established as a routine clinical procedure. However, mammalian cells are not well adapted to the stresses of freezing and thawing, and some cell types are sensitive even to the effects of chilling to a few degrees below physiological temperatures. There are ectothermic organisms, however, that have evolved to withstand freezing temperatures, and some will even tolerate freeze-drying as part of their life cycle. Cryobiologists may yet learn much from the survival strategies of invertebrates and amphibians which provide natural examples of cryoprotective agents (CPAs). The rate of cooling is generally more important than the degree to which temperatures are lowered, and is at least as important as the choice of CPA. The lower the storage temperature the better, and cells remain genetically stable long-term in liquid nitrogen. The delayed arrival of oocyte cryopreservation as a routine reproductive technology indicates the greater technical problems encountered with these cells. They are highly sensitive to cooling, and can also be injured by exposure to CPAs, although their vulnerability varies with the stage of oogenesis and between species. Whilst progress towards routine banking of mature or immature oocytes has been slow, it has been accelerating recently as a result of technological innovations.

Oocytes: a limited resource

The female gamete is probably the rarest cell in the body. Normally, only one oocyte is ovulated per menstrual cycle, and there are no more than 450 cycles in an average reproductive life-span of 35 years. More oocytes can be ovulated per cycle after hyperstimulation with gonadotropins, but repeated treatment is limited by cost, patient acceptability, safety and age. Moreover, the effects of aging on gamete quality are more striking in females than in males, and oocytes have a remarkably high rate of aneuploidy[1]. Natural fertility populations and sperm donation programs have revealed that the time taken to conception (as a relative measure of fertility) doubles approximately every 5 years after 30 years of age. Hence, reproductive medicine units are usually reluctant to provide IVF services to patients beyond their mid-40s because the prospects of a successful pregnancy are very slim. Since oocyte quality and number are diminished in reproductive-aged women, cryopreservation of oocytes is not a realistic proposition because the procedures further compromise the chances of reproductive success.

Oocytes can be recovered from unstimulated cycles at the germinal vesicle (GV) stage, but the harvest is usually smaller than after controlled ovarian stimulation, except in the case of polycystic ovaries when a large yield of variable quality can be obtained. There are some theoretical advantages with GV oocytes, as noted later, but the outcome of cryopreservation is, in practice, even less satisfactory than with the metaphase II stage.

There are some notable advantages of obtaining oocytes from even earlier stages, namely, the preantral and primordial follicle stages. For one thing, they are far more abundant than fully-grown oocytes. An ovarian biopsy measuring only 2 mm in diameter from a woman in her early 30s contains a variable number of up to about 300 follicles, mainly at the primordial stage[2]. One day, oocytes from these stages may become preferred for oocyte banking, at least for some groups of patients, but at present the technology is limited by our ability competently to culture oocytes to maturity *in vitro*[3].

The case for preserving oocytes

Technologies that are now taken for granted and considered to be necessities of life, such as refrigerators and computers, were once regarded as luxuries for the few or served as curious gizmos. At first, they often encountered resistance to commercial introduction for philosophical reasons or because they crossed time-honored traditions. However, history records that successful technologies eventually overcome social and/or financial thresholds to become generally desirable, and later become virtually mandatory services and applications. Some novelties (witness the Segway human transporter) do not live up to commercial expectations, but that is sometimes because they were invented before a suitable 'niche' has fully evolved. Such examples have parallels in the history of reproductive cryobiology.

Embryo cryopreservation is a technology that has reached a mature stage of development[4]. It is well established in many centers, highly reliable and considered by most authorities to be safe. Apart from a minority of people who have fundamental ethical objections to *in vitro* fertilization (IVF) technologies, embryo banking is regarded as a responsible way to safeguard precious cells and augment pregnancy rates in the best interests of patients. Oocyte cryopreservation has not yet reached the same stage, although it may cross the threshold from experimental to routine service in a few years. Some practitioners of ART argue that the crossing has already been made, at least for mature oocytes, and a few welcome the imminent arrival of commercial egg banks. Frozen storage of ovarian tissue preceded oocyte banking by several decades, but, like the Segway, has not found a large application yet.

The controversy about egg banking is changing, although there are cases which provoke little debate. For instance, cryopreservation of oocytes when a man is unexpectedly unable to produce sperm on the day that oocytes are collected from his partner is justified if the alternative is to waste the female gametes. Furthermore, in countries where only a limited number of oocytes can be inseminated legally (because all embryos must be freshly transferred to the patient), it is desirable to cryopreserve the spare ones for future fertilization attempts. What is more, egg banking could play an important role in the future of oocyte donation programs by optimizing the distribution of cells and overcoming the problems associated with transportation and quarantine.

More controversially, when the technology allows, eggs banks will undoubtedly be used by young women seeking greater assurance of late fertility should they need to postpone child-bearing for professional or social reasons. There are also an increasing number of young women and children who need fertility preservation for medical reasons. With the dramatic increase in survival rates after cancer, greater emphasis is now being placed on quality-of-life issues, including fertility. It has been estimated that by the end of this decade as many as one in 250 people will be a survivor of childhood cancers, and, in addition, there are about 50 000 women in the USA annually who are under 40 years of age at diagnosis with invasive cancer[5]. A significant number of these are now sterilized or have ovaries compromised by the effects of chemotherapy, radiotherapy or surgery[6]. Oocyte and ovarian tissue banking may ultimately help such individuals to realize their genetic potential for reproduction. This would be a welcome development, because there are few options for preserving fertility in females, and embryo banking only meets the needs of those who already have a male partner.

History of cryopreservation

Attempts to cryopreserve mammalian cells during the early part of the 20th century were unsuccessful because the nature of freezing damage was not understood and CPAs had not yet been identified. A breakthrough was made in 1949 by a chance discovery in a laboratory in London, England. Researchers discovered that glycerol was able to preserve the spermatozoa of cockerels and bulls after cooling to $-79°C$ and re-warming[7]. Like other CPAs, glycerol is a low-molecular-weight compound which is highly soluble in water and permeable to cell membranes, and has relatively low toxicity at high concentrations. This discovery led to sperm banking for the dairy-cow industry and soon spread worldwide. A few years later, the first tentative attempts were made to store human spermatozoa at liquid nitrogen temperatures[8]. The same laboratory, headed by Sir Alan Parkes, subsequently extended the successful protocols to other cell types, as well as to tissues and organs. They were first to demonstrate that fragments of rat ovaries can produce estrogens after transplantation to ovariectomized host animals, and, in 1960, reported the first successful pregnancy in mice after cryopreserving ovarian tissue[9]. It has taken over 40 years to reach the stage at which similar success has been obtained with human ovarian tissue.

During the intervening decades up to 1980, little attention was given to the cryopreservation of the female gamete. IVF did not become established as a routine clinical procedure until the early 1980s, and controlled-rate freezers were not widely available at first. However, an important paper published by Whittingham in 1977[10] demonstrated that the mature mouse oocyte could be successfully cryopreserved. His work formed the basis of protocols for other species. However, ovarian tissue banking attracted little interest until the 1990s, since there appeared to be no application for the technology. This was in spite of the fact that striking progress was being made in the treatment of common malignant diseases in young patients. For example, the 5-year survival rate for acute lymphoblastic leukemia rose 2–3-fold between 1960 and 1990. While this success was a cause for rejoicing, the drugs and radiation treatment that were responsible for

long-term remission or cure from potentially fatal diseases were often gonadotoxic and in many cases triggered ovarian failure. The dose of ionizing radiation that destroys 50% of human ovarian oocytes (LD-50) has been estimated to be as low as $2\,Gy$[11], and these cells are also highly vulnerable to alkylating agents such as busulfan and cyclophosphamide[12]. The probability of irreversible ovarian failure after total body irradiation for bone transplant approaches 100%, although it is somewhat lower in very young women[6]. Moreover, patients whose menstrual cycles recover spontaneously have a high risk of an early menopause and truncated reproductive life-span. For these reasons, ovarian tissue banking has emerged as a promising procedure for preserving fertility in patients with cancer or other diseases requiring high-dose cytotoxic treatment. The recent history of cryopreservation therefore confirms the old saying that necessity is the mother of invention.

Principles of cryoprotection

When cells are cooled to the temperature of liquid nitrogen they are stable. Successful insemination has been possible from human sperm specimens stored for at least 21 years, and there was no evidence of increased mutation rates in mouse embryos stored for even longer. It is likely that female germ cells will also prove to be stable, but the challenge is to freeze them without damage, and then reverse the process safely.

The main danger to cells cooled to sub-zero temperatures is intracellular ice formation, which is usually lethal. Successful cryopreservation protocols avoid, or at least minimize, ice crystal growth. This can theoretically be achieved by very high rates of cooling, although conventional slow-cooling methods, often called 'equilibrium cooling' and developed in the Parkes laboratory, have proved to be versatile for different cell types and are well controlled.

When a cell is cooled slowly, ice crystals are first formed extracellularly. Since the water is preferentially removed from solution, the ionic strength of the solution increases and, hence, there is net water movement down its chemical gradient from inside the cell and across the plasma membrane[13]. This process continues until little water remains within the cell, and the viscosity rises to a level at which the intracellular substance can vitrify (i.e. form a glass-like solid). Accompanying this change is an increase in the intracellular salt concentration, which can harm cells by modifying protein structure and function. Choline has been used to replace sodium ions to minimize this risk, and this strategy has recently been tested with some favorable results in animal and human oocytes[14,15].

There is, however, no single protocol that is ideal for all cell types. The rate of cell cooling must be tailored to the hydraulic permeability of the cell membrane, which differs between cells[16]. Too fast a rate of cooling puts the cell in jeopardy of intracellular crystallization, whereas too slow risks damaging the cell during prolonged exposure to CPAs at relatively high temperatures. During the cooling process, the liquid phase tends to supercool, which is an unstable state that can exist to below −40°C before crystals start to appear. For this reason, controlled ice nucleation ('seeding') is usually carried out by grasping the straw or cryovials with forceps after dipping them into liquid nitrogen. Early studies with mouse embryos revealed that nucleation is optimal between −5 and −7°C, a finding that has been applied to many other species and cell types[17]. While glycerol was the first effective CPA and is a natural substance, it is no longer the only one available, nor is it always the best. Some cells, including oocytes, have membranes that are relatively impermeable to glycerol, and better results have been obtained using dimethyl sulfoxide (DMSO), 1,2-propanediol (PROH) and ethylene glycol (EG), all of which equilibrate more rapidly[18–20]. Some cell types, such as sperm or mouse embryo stem cells, are relatively tolerant, and finely controlled freezing rates are not necessary to obtain satisfactory outcomes. These cells are either abundant (sperm) or can replace damaged cells rapidly (stem cells), while oocytes are rare and precious. Consequently, it is vital to optimize cryopreservation protocols for oocytes that are frozen for clinical use.

Although volume changes accompany cooling as a result of osmotic movement of water, this is not the first volume excursion that cells undergo. When immersed in high concentrations of CPAs (which is normally done at 0–4°C to reduce toxicity), cells are subjected to osmotic stress[21] because their membranes are more permeable to water than to solute. Water is withdrawn and the cells shrink (Figure 1). Subsequently, cell volume returns to near normal values as the CPA diffuses into the cell and replaces the lost water. Knowledge of membrane permeability to water and to the CPA, as well as the activation energy, can serve as a basis for predicting volume changes over

time using the Kedem–Katchalsky model[22,23]. Such mathematical models can help to refine cryopreservation protocols to minimize volume changes, although the character of cryoinjury is far more complex than existing models, and empirical studies are necessary to define optimal conditions for cryopreservation.

CPAs lower the freezing point of the medium and replace cell water and, when a critical viscosity is reached, they promote intracellular vitrification[24]. A mixture of CPAs is sometimes used so that the concentration and toxicity of each compound can be reduced. This precaution may be more important with the vitrification technique, which employs CPAs at approximately three-fold higher molar concentration (5–6 mol/l), than with equilibrium cooling methods (see below). The CPAs must be washed out rapidly after thawing to avoid exposing the cells at high temperatures. This is normally carried out step-wise to reduce volume changes, and protocols can be refined using the aforementioned mathematical models. Osmotic buffers are also used to minimize volume excursions. These buffers are normally mono- or disaccharides, which are impermeable to cell membranes and serve as secondary CPAs[25]. The CPAs are dissolved in a buffered salt solution containing albumin or serum. Antioxidant compounds are often omitted because some CPAs and other constituents in the medium have the same property, but they can be helpful during the transportation of tissue[26].

Cooling and re-warming curves of cryopreservation protocols are not symmetrical. If re-warming is carried out at too slow a rate, there is a further risk that intracellular ice crystals form as the temperature ascends. Hence, most cells are warmed as quickly as possible (> 100°C per minute). Rates of cooling and re-warming are also affected by the type of vessel. Thin-walled straws allow rapid heat transfer, but the temperature of medium within plastic cryovials lags significantly behind the cooling chamber because of greater thermal insulation.

The seminal article reporting successful cryopreservation by slow cooling of fowl spermatozoa[7] used the expression 'vitrification'. This may strike modern readers as inappropriate because we now apply this word to a method of rapid freezing which contrasts with standard, slow cooling methods[27]. The authors were, however, correct because successful cryopreservation involves intracellular vitrification, as indicated above. We now generally use the word 'vitrification'

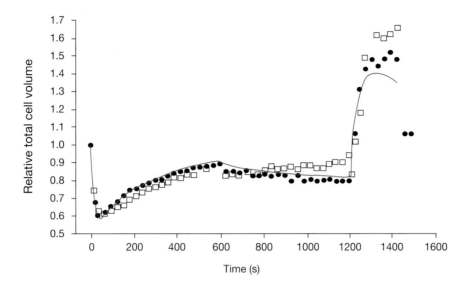

Figure 1 Volume changes estimated by curve fitting for fresh (solid circles) and failed-to-fertilize (open boxes) human oocytes during immersion in 1.5 mol/l dimethyl sulfoxide (DMSO). Reprinted from reference 22. Calculating from the Kedem–Katchalsky model, the hydraulic conductivity was 1.3×0^{-6} cm atm^{-1} s^{-1} and the solute permeability was 3.15×10^5 cm s^{-1} for these cells

for methods in which the entire medium is vitrified. When a medium of sufficiently high CPA concentration is cooled very rapidly, the medium forms a vitreous-like solid rather than forming ice. This strategy is promising for a range of cell types, including oocytes and embryos.

All technologies are interim and current methods will, eventually, be succeeded by better ones. Over 40 years ago, Parkes speculated about freeze-drying as an alternative for preserving cells. In recent years, mouse spermatozoa have been successfully preserved in this manner, as demonstrated by the production of viable pups after inseminating oocytes using the intracytoplasmic sperm injection (ICSI) technique[28]. Whether freeze-drying can be applied to other cell types is more doubtful, especially for oocytes and other cells with abundant cytoplasm. The condensed nuclei of sperm are peculiarly adapted to this extreme form of preservation, although some organisms regularly withstand this treatment and still manage to avoid lethal chromosomal damage.

CRYOPRESERVATION OF FULLY GROWN OOCYTES

It is probably, and unfortunately, true that oocytes are among the most difficult cell types to freeze and thaw successfully. Their large size, complex cytoplasm, specialized membrane and transitory status present problems for developing effective protocols. The first successful pregnancies were reported in the mid-1980s, a couple of years after the breakthrough with embryo cryopreservation[29–31]. However, the success rates were low and concerns over disruption or damage to cellular components that emerged toward the end of the decade halted further attempts. The problems of oocyte cryopreservation are compounded by the limited numbers that are available and the variable quality. There may even be significant variations between patients in the ability of their oocytes to withstand the multiple stresses imposed on them during cryopreservation, as is the case with spermatozoa[8]. If true, it implies that no single protocol will be optimal for cryopreserving oocytes in all patients. Most experience has been based on mature oocytes.

Metaphase II-stage oocytes

Equilibrium cooling

The first protocols used for cryopreserving oocytes were based on slow freezing/rapid re-warming using DMSO as the CPA, and then fertilizing the eggs using standard IVF techniques[29–31]. When it became apparent that zona hardening occurs after cooling (probably because of exocytosis of cortical granules), conventional IVF was abandoned until ICSI bypassed the problem. At the same time, alternative CPAs were being tested, and PROH, which had become standard for banking embryos, began to replace DMSO, which was considered to be more toxic and likely to affect the cytoskeleton[32]. Thus, the almost simultaneous introduction of ICSI and PROH (some authorities advocate EG) was welcomed as a new dawn for oocyte cryopreservation. However, randomized controlled trials have not been performed to compare CPAs in large-scale studies. Every compound used at the high concentrations required by a CPA is likely to have some adverse effects, and PROH raises intracellular calcium and may induce parthenogenetic development in oocytes[33]. Nevertheless, the aforementioned developments laid the basis for current methods, such as that summarized in Protocol 1 in the Appendix[34]. Recently, it was reported that higher survival rates can be obtained by increasing the concentration of the secondary CPA to 0.3 or even 0.5 mol/l[35]. Sucrose is frequently used, although equimolar concentrations of a monosaccharide, such as fructose, should provide the same osmotic buffering with less viscosity. Live births have also been reported after the partial substitution of sodium by choline prior to oocyte cooling[15], and intracellular injection of trehalose is another novel strategy that has been claimed to improve oocyte freezing tolerance[36]. Trehalose is a disaccharide with interesting properties: it has a high glass transition temperature and stabilizes proteins during freezing and desiccation.

Vitrification

A number of theoretical and practical considerations have encouraged a wave of interest in vitrification, and have encouraged speculation about whether this technique will replace equilibrium cooling[27]. The chief advantages of vitrification lie in its speed and simplicity and the avoidance of intracellular ice crystal formation. This method does not require an expensive freezer, although automated vitrification is now becoming available to produce greater control and higher rates of cooling. However, the apparent simplicity of vitrification is perhaps deceptive because the margins of error are narrower and there can be large variations in success between operators. Indeed, there are other drawbacks with vitrification. It requires direct immersion of the cells in liquid nitrogen, which

is not normally supplied sterile, and the concentrations of CPAs are very high. The latter problem is more acute with tissues than single cells, because outer parts are exposed to the vitrifying medium for longer than the inner ones. Nevertheless, encouraging results have been obtained, even with vitrification of mouse ovaries and ovarian biopsies from larger species[37].

A number of modified protocols for vitrification have emerged recently, and studies are now needed to compare their merits. In each case, the goal is to lower the temperature as rapidly as possible by direct immersion in liquid nitrogen. Three basic methods have been introduced, and others are under development (Figure 2):

(1) After equilibration for a few minutes in the vitrifying medium, the cells are placed on electron microscope copper grids for immersion[38].

(2) A plastic straw is drawn out narrow for taking up the cells. This is then immersed directly in liquid nitrogen and transferred to a storage tube. This 'open pulled straw' method also facilitates rapid thawing and is becoming widely used for farm-animal embryos[39].

(3) The CryoLoop™ (Hampton Research, Aliso Viejo, CA) is a simple device, which after dipping into medium creates a film into which the cells can be placed. The thin, nylon loop is directly immersed into liquid nitrogen[40].

Germinal vesicle-stage oocytes

When viewed under the PolScope™ (SpindleView™, Cambridge Research & Instrumentation, Woburn, MA), the spindle apparatus of oocytes disappears during cooling as a result of microtubule depolymerization. Surprisingly, the chromosomes do not disperse throughout the cytoplasm and the spindle can reform after the temperature is restored. But there is a risk of infidelity of chromosome segregation at anaphase and, hence, of aneuploidy[41–43] (Figure 3). Can this problem be avoided by cryopreserving cells at the germinal vesicle stage? Initial optimism was misplaced because it has turned out to be more difficult to preserve cells at this stage even if spindles are not always compromised by the treatment[44,45], because they have to achieve effective cytoplasmic maturation in culture once the cells are thawed. Cryopreservation not only affects the

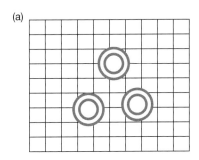 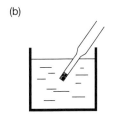 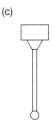

Figure 2 Three common methods for vitrifying oocytes and embryos: (a) open pulled straw, (b) electron microscope grid, (c) cryoloop

spindle and zona pellucida, but undoubtedly has other deleterious effects, such as membrane lipid phase changes[46]. Since oocytes of humans and some animals (e.g. cows) are highly sensitive to chilling by even a few degrees below normal, vitrification has raised hopes of greater success[47]. To date, the germinal vesicle stage has received less attention with this particular methodology, and, generally, the standard protocols used for mature oocytes have been applied to these cells. A main limitation is the need to preserve physiological interactions between the oocyte and the surrounding cumulus granulosa cells, which extend transzonal projections through the zona to contact the oocyte. It would be surprising if both cell types have the same optimal rates of cooling. Besides, osmotic stress may break the cell–cell junction associations and impair nuclear maturation and/or cytoplasmic maturation. Hence, cryopreservation compounds the relatively low pregnancy success rates obtained after *in vitro* maturation of immature oocytes, although these will surely improve[48,49]. The germinal vesicle stage is very attractive for oocyte banking for a patient's own use or for egg donation and it is hoped that the obstacles to success will be overcome.

Efficiency

The efficiency of oocyte cryopreservation is still difficult to quantify, with few notable exceptions such as the groups in Bologna which have extensive clinical experience[34,50]. In most other centers, few treatment cycles have been performed and it is often unclear how the subjects were selected and what were the rates of cycle cancellation and miscarriage. Frequently, the data have only been published as brief reports without full details[18,51–55].

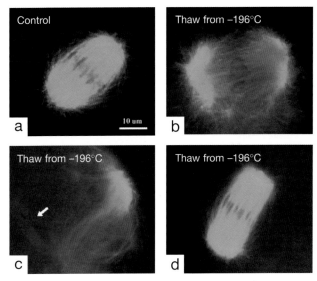

Figure 3 Spindle formation and chromosome behavior in freshly isolated (a) or slowly frozen–rapidly thawed (b, c and d) metaphase II mouse oocytes. Oocytes (a) and (d) possessed a normal barrel-shaped bipolar spindle with chromosomes well aligned at the equatorial plate. On the other hand, oocytes (b) and (c) had damaged spindles and displaced chromosomes (arrow in c) after cryopreservation to liquid nitrogen temperatures. 4′,6-Diamidino-2-phenylindole (DAPI) was used to stain chromosomes (blue) and fluorescein isothiocyanate (FITC) to label tubulin (green). Bar = 10 μm. (Photographs courtesy of Hang Yin, PhD)

A chief limitation in the early studies was a low survival rate, which was often in the region of 30% or even lower. Improved protocols have raised survival rates to 60%, and some centers now report in the region of 80% oocyte survival[35]. Yet survival is not the only arbiter of normality, and the quality of embryos, rates of biochemical and continuing pregnancies should be published. Without these data, it is difficult to evaluate claims that pregnancy rates after thaw are comparable to those obtained with fresh oocytes.

Table 1 Summary of clinical outcome of cryopreserving human oocytes by equilibrium cooling

Reference	Fertilized by	Number of oocytes	Pregnancies (n)	Number of live babies
Chen (1986)[29]	IVF	40	—	1
van Uem (1987)[30]	IVF	28	—	1
Al-Hasani (1987)[31]	IVF	182	—	2
Siebzehnrübl (1986)[56]	IVF	38	—	1
Tucker (1996)[18]	ICSI	81	3	0
Porcu (1997)[19]	ICSI	12	1	1
Tucker (1998)[48]	ICSI	13	1	1
Borini (1998)[57]	ICSI	129	3	—
Porcu (1998)[58]	ICSI	709	9	6
Young (1998)[52]	ICSI	9	1	(3)
Polak de Fried (1998)[51]	ICSI	10	1	1
Donaldson (2000)[59]	ICSI	18	2	—
Porcu (2000)[50]	ICSI	1840	19	12
Winslow (2001)[20]	ICSI	324	—	16
Chen (2002)[53]	ICSI	8	1	—
Porcu (2002)[60]	ICSI	124	—	3
Yang (2002)[54]	ICSI	158	11	14
Quintans (2002)[15]	ICSI	109	5	2
Fosas (2003)[61]	ICSI	88	—	5
Boldt (2003)[62]	ICSI	90	—	5
Porcu (2004)[34]	ICSI	?	60	33

IVF, *in vitro* fertilization; ICSI, intracytoplasmic sperm injection

Table 1 summarizes most of the available published data based on equilibrium cooling methods for oocytes. Evidently, there is considerable variation between centers as well as in the numbers of observations (some are very low). Undoubtedly, there are many cases that have gone unrecorded in the literature, and a worldwide database is a desirable objective, although we are aware of fewer than 100 reported live births so far. There is a reassuring lack of reports of excess congenital abnormalities. Regrettably, one of the important denominators of success that is often omitted from reports is the total number of oocytes. If we consider, for example, a young woman who wishes to store oocytes from a single controlled ovarian stimulation cycle, she will want to know her chances of success with the 10–15 oocytes normally available. Unfortunately, we cannot yet provide her with clear advice, except about the disadvantages of delaying the procedure until an advanced reproductive age. If we consider the data published in Table 1, it appears that for every 100 oocytes that have been cryopreserved for assisted reproduction there are only one or two babies born. This estimate of efficiency may be too pessimistic because of variations between centers and recent improvements in technology, but it is a clear warning against undue optimism.

Fewer data are available for vitrification, and the relative merits of this strategy will become clearer in the next few years as more studies are published (Table 2). The results to date are encouraging[63,66,68], but it is premature to draw any firm conclusions about the efficiency compared with other methods or reproductive safety or the best method of vitrification.

CRYOPRESERVATION OF PRIMORDIAL FOLLICLES

These stages are advantageous for germ cell banking for several reasons. As a consequence of their smaller size, they have a larger surface area to volume ratio than that of mature eggs, and this facilitates equilibration of water and solutes across the membranes. What is more, they are relatively undifferentiated and their

Table 2 Summary of clinical outcome of cryopreserving human oocytes by vitrification

Reference	Fertilized by	Number of oocytes	Pregnancies (n)	Number of live babies
Kuleshova (1999)[63]	ICSI	17	1	1
Yoon (2000)[64]	ICSI	90	3	2
Kuwayama (2000)[65]	ICSI	?	1	1
Wu (2001)[66]	IVF	—	1	—
Katayama (2003)[67]	ICSI	46	2	—
Yoon (2003)[68]	ICSI	474	—	7

ICSI, intracytoplasmic sperm injection; IVF, *in vitro* fertilization

cytoplasm contains fewer organelles. Because the cells are in prophase I there is no spindle apparatus that can be affected by cooling, and primordial follicles do not possess oocytes with zonae pellucidae. The main disadvantage is that they require a period of prolonged growth to become competent for maturation, and they have to be grown with granulosa cells within a follicular structure. Small follicles may be stored in two ways. First, they may be harvested as individual units after being isolated from surrounding stromal tissue[69]. Thus, they present a minimal mass for chemical and thermal equilibration, as well as the possibility for monitoring the number of units and even their quality. Second, the follicles can be stored *in situ*, without removing them from the stroma[70,71]. The attraction of this strategy lies in its simplicity and because intact structural relationships between cell types are preserved. On the other hand, the numbers of follicular units within intact living tissue cannot be determined, and the lack of a blood supply encourages the accumulation of toxic products of metabolism.

Isolated follicles

Isolation techniques

Small follicles can be rapidly obtained, and in large numbers, from rodent ovaries by enzymatic digestion. Immature ovaries are bisected whereas adult organs must be chopped into small pieces no larger than about 1 mm³. These pieces are then incubated in medium containing collagenase. To prevent the cells from sticking to one another or to the vessel, DNase I is added to the medium[69]. Pipetting speeds up the process of isolation. Follicles should be removed to enzyme-free medium as quickly as possible after they

are isolated to prevent further damage. Even so, damage is often extensive: the basement membrane is eroded, the granulosa layer is often disrupted, and some oocytes may be completely denuded. Primordial follicles are most severely affected, although this may not be apparent immediately. Since the pregranulosa cells are loosely attached to the oocyte, they tend to round up and fall away from the oocyte after the basement membrane is lost. Naked oocytes can be successfully cryopreserved, but the 'Humpty-Dumpty' feat of putting the cells back together again *in vitro* has not yet been achieved. It is possible, however, to recombine the cells for grafting.

Follicle isolation from the fibrous ovaries of humans and farm animals is not very successful except by the laborious and slow yielding method of manual dissection[70]. The time taken to disaggregate the organ using enzymes is extensive and few follicles survive, although partial digestion is helpful. If a thin cortical strip of tissue is prepared, it is possible to adjust the submicroscopic illumination to visualize the follicles. Dissection is carried out using fine needles (25–28 gauge according to the size of the follicles and the type of stroma). Growing follicles usually contain some adherent stroma-theca, but this may be beneficial to the culture process. Human primordial follicles can be visualized as tiny, pearl-like structures attached to collagen fibers. They are 50–100-fold more abundant than growing follicles, but the efficiency of recovery is low.

Follicle culture

There are a number of options for culturing isolated follicles from rodent ovaries. In each case, the objective is to enable small, undifferentiated oocytes to grow to full size and become competent to undergo meiosis.

The length of culture depends on the starting stage, and is 16–20 days for primordial follicles from mouse ovaries. The basic requirement is to maintain the structural and physiological integrity of the unit. Damaged follicles tend to adhere to the plastic Petri dish, causing the granulosa cells to migrate away and expose the oocyte. However, intact follicles can be cultured successfully and produce pseudo-antral follicles which spread on the plastic substratum[71]. More spherical structures can be produced if the follicles are suspended in collagen gel or transferred daily between microdroplets of medium[72]. A high proportion of these follicles (>75%) can be ovulable under these conditions, and even produce viable oocytes. While culture methods for growing follicles have been established in many laboratories, the Eppig group has produced fertile oocytes from primordial follicles of mouse ovaries, but this requires a multi-step process and stage-specific media[73]. First, the follicles are allowed to initiate their growth in ovarian tissue explants. When they have generated two layers of granulosa cells, they are disseggregated from the tissue and transferred to collagen membranes for culturing for a further 7–10 days. Finally, having reached full size, the oocytes are removed from the granulosa cells to undergo maturation *in vitro*, a process that requires 12–16 h in this species.

Despite the exciting progress being made with these models, it has turned out to be extremely difficult to adapt these methods to follicles from primate and farm-animal ovaries. For one thing, we have already noted that the follicles are more difficult to harvest in good condition and number. For another, the corresponding culture period is much longer (many weeks or even months), and suitable conditions have not yet been defined. There appears to be little prospect of an early breakthrough for growing oocytes *in vitro* for clinical purposes, although small follicles are readily cryopreserved.

Ovarian tissue

Source and preparation of tissue

Since the initial breakthrough with cryopreservation of ovarian tissue during the 1950s, the emergence of automated freezers and alternative CPAs have fostered progress. Surprisingly good results have been obtained when the technologies have been applied to organs of larger species, including humans. The goal has been to optimize the survival of follicles and maximize the number of gametes that can be generated after transplantation or in culture. The plasticity and tissue architecture of the ovary are favorable because primordial follicles are close to the ovarian surface, facilitating rapid thermal and chemical equilibration. Small ovaries of laboratory animals can be cryopreserved intact or after bisection, if they are no more than 2–3 mm in the longest dimension. For larger ovaries, the cortical 'skin' can be prepared by dissection within 30 min using a scalpel and forceps. The product should be no thicker than 1–2 mm and must be kept moist with culture medium at all times (e.g. Leibovitz-L15). It can then be cut into pieces of suitable size for accommodating in cryovials or bags after equilibration with the freezing mixture. Equilibration can be carried out in 20-ml roller tubes (approximately 2 Hz) at 0–4°C.

If a whole ovary is not available, biopsies measuring 3–4 mm may be used. Unfortunately, there are no reliable external markers to predict which cortical regions are dense with small follicles, although the hilus, large follicles and former corpora lutea should be avoided, and specimens are collected during the follicular phase of the ovarian cycle.

Progress has also been made with the cryopreservation of intact ovaries from rats and sheep[74,75]. In theory, whole-ovary cryopreservation and transplantation using vascular surgery should restore natural fertility for a normal span of reproductive life, although this goal has yet to be attained in any species. In the rat model, the animals are first heparinized and then the ovarian vessels are dissected back to the aorta and vena cava to produce short cuffs (the donor animal must be sacrificed). Because the calibers of vessels are minute, it is necessary to dissect the ovary together with its Fallopian tube and the upper third of the uterine horn. The organs may then be removed *en bloc* for perfusion with a cryoprotective medium by slow infusion to minimize stressing the vasculature. The organs can then be transferred to medium in a cryo-bag and loaded into an automated freezer for slow cooling. After thawing, the process is reversed, taking care not to damage the delicate vessels and to remove the CPA slowly. The organs are transplanted to ovariectomized host animals, by end-to-side anastomosis of vessels and uterouterine anastomosis. After removal of the clamps the flow of blood into the organ can be observed. This procedure has resulted in the restoration of ovarian cyclicity and even fertility. The surgery tends to be more straightforward with larger animals, but the cryopreservation of bulky organs is likely to be more problematic. If progress with farm-animal models continues, the possible application of whole-ovary transplantation in humans as an alternative to tissue slices will have to be considered.

Cryopreservation protocols

There are several protocols that are currently used for human tissue, and they are derived from methods developed for mouse oocytes. Protocol 2 (see the Appendix) illustrates a method which is currently in use at Cornell University[76] and has proved to be successful for cryopreserving tissue of large animals, including sheep[77].

A growing number of centers have begun to bank ovarian tissue for patients, but few have any clinical or experimental experience of its post-thaw application. At present, it is not feasible to culture follicular oocytes to maturity for reproductive purposes, except in small animal models. Consequently, the only option is auto-transplantation, for which there is a long history of animal research[78]. Only the salient points are mentioned here.

Ten years ago, we showed that cryopreserved tissue slices from sheep ovaries could restore estrous cycles and fertility after orthotopic transplantation[77]. It was surprising that a dense tissue could tolerate a series of physical and metabolic stresses during these procedures, but the results augured well for human applications[72]. The first attempts to transplant thawed human ovarian tissue were modestly successful in demonstrating follicular survival, if not long-term restoration of spontaneous menstrual cycles[79,80]. Better outcomes might have been obtained if the patients had been younger and/or had not received chemotherapy previously. To minimize surgery, Oktay and subsequently others transplanted fresh and cryopreserved tissue to heterotopic sites, including forearm, belly and breast tissue[81]. Based on studies of sheep and other species, it was already known that apparently normal follicular growth with steroidogenesis can occur heterotopically, with oocyte recovery for IVF[82]. Whilst the harvest of oocytes was small, and some of them required in vitro maturation even after gonadotropin stimulation, they may fertilize and cleave. Oktay and colleagues recovered 20 oocytes from eight

percutaneous harvests, and one of eight oocytes suitable for ICSI reached the four-cell stage, but it did not produce a pregnancy after transfer[83]. It is likely that this procedure will eventually succeed in establishing a viable pregnancy. Recently, two viable pregnancies have been reported after orthotopic ovarian transplantation of frozen and fresh ovarian grafts, respectively. A former Hodgkin's disease patient required IVF to establish pregnancy[84], whereas a graft between the two healthy monozygotic twins enable natural conception[85]. All these results should be encouraging for the hundreds of patients worldwide who, during the past decade, have stored ovarian tissue before iatrogenic sterilization.

SAFETY CONSIDERATIONS

There are safety measures that apply to the child-to-be as well as to the mother. Indeed, it was concerns about the cytogenetic effects of CPAs and/or cooling on oocytes that led to a voluntary suspension of the technology during the late 1980s and early 1990s. While fresh human oocytes are prone to aneuploidy, cryopreservation may increase the risk. According to some studies of mouse oocytes, there is also an increase in polypoidy[86], and an unconfirmed report suggests that the frequency of sister chromatid exchange is raised, implying that cryopreservation can cause DNA damage[86]. Accordingly, some authorities have recommended that preimplantation genetic diagnosis (PGD) should be required for screening chromosomes by fluorescent in situ hybridization (FISH) when applying this technology. However, FISH cannot reveal the full karyotype, and fortunately the reproductive system appears to be 'forgiving', because the uterine environment is highly efficient at eliminating conceptuses with abnormal karyotypes. With the introduction of improved protocols and more encouraging data these concerns have diminished, although continuing vigilance is still needed. Storage of immature oocytes at either germinal vesicle or earlier stages may generate other problems, although most animal studies have been reassuring. The larger concern is not the cryopreservation per se but rather the culture technologies to grow the oocytes to maturity. The stress of culture alters housekeeping gene expression and perhaps affects the function of imprinted genes, with possible consequences for embryo viability and child health.

But, since the technology of *in vitro* growth of oocytes is still in its infancy, safety issues are not yet pressing concerns for clinical practice.

Ovarian autotransplantation is currently the only available strategy for realizing the fertile potential of stored ovarian tissue. This carries risks of surgery when recovering and grafting the tissue. Whilst these risks are well known, there are other risks, specific to former cancer patients who have their ovarian tissue re-implanted. If any malignant stem cells were resident in the ovarian tissue when it was cryopreserved, they may rekindle disease after transplantation to the patient[87]. Transplantation, therefore, requires the utmost prudence and the involvement of a clinical team, including oncologists, gynecologists, laboratory personnel and patient counselors, when treatment strategies are decided. The risks of harboring cancer cells in ovarian tissue vary between diseases. For example, they are high with a peripheral disease such as acute leukemia, and low with Hodgkin's disease[88]. Breast cancer carries an intermediate, but significant, risk of ovarian metastases[89]. Further research is needed to define these risks more precisely using histopathology, xenograft models and, where appropriate, molecular markers. The possibility of purging ovarian tissue of malignant cells prior to transplantation is also under consideration[90].

Finally, there are safety issues that are common to all reproductive cells and tissues that are stored at low temperatures. Occasional reports have emerged from bone marrow transplant centers of cross-infection by viruses between specimens stored in the same liquid nitrogen Dewar[91]. Screening of patients and quarantining of specimens are important safeguards, but various devices and double-bagging have also been introduced to avoid leakage from frozen straws and cryovials. Contamination can also be avoided by storage in the vapor phase of a Dewar, although the specimens are at greater risk of temperature fluctuations.

ETHICAL AND LEGAL ISSUES

Preservation of fertility by long-term storage of gametes and germ cells raises ethical and legal issues which have been discussed in detail elsewhere[92]. While many of them are similar to those encountered with sperm and embryo cryopreservation, long-term fertility preservation for young women and children raises some new issues. One of the main ones arises from the storage of ovarian tissue for children[93]. There are well-established procedures for obtaining surrogate consent from parents or guardians of children undergoing surgery or medical treatment, and the principle of Gillick competence is established in the United Kingdom (where adolescents of sufficient understanding and intelligence can make a medical decision independent of parental consent). Nevertheless, this is a thorny issue and compounded by the experimental nature of the technologies and the likelihood of storing for many years. There is also the sensitive question of obtaining consent for the disposal of tissues that are not required for fertility treatment. In case the patient dies or no longer requires the tissue for other reasons, full consideration must be given in advance to its ultimate fate: destruction or donation to research or (for mature oocytes) donation to other patients. It is also worth bearing in mind that experience with semen cryopreservation has shown that only a minority of patients ever elect to use their banked specimens. If this turns out to be true for egg banking, the decision to undergo the procedures should be even more circumspect because they are invasive and more costly.

Controversy is likely to continue to surround these technologies for some years, until they become accepted into routine clinical practice. For the present, we believe that cryopreservation of oocytes, and especially ovarian tissue, should be considered as experimental procedures, and are not ripe for commercialization. The borderline between experimental and conventional medical practices is not easily defined and professional opinions vary. Since fewer than 100 babies have been reported after oocyte cryopreservation and only one after ovarian tissue cryopreservation, it is too early to be declarative about the clinical efficiency or reproductive safety of either procedure. There are many factors that need to be taken into account when considering which patients should be offered these procedures: age, male partner, survival prospects, chances of premature ovarian failure, risk of disease recurrence, risk of metastases to the gonads, costs of the medical procedures and of long-term banking, uterine competence and time available for a fertility-sparing preserving procedure. Each patient presents a unique set of circumstances, and decisions are reached after weighing the risks and benefits[94]. It is worth noting that attempts have been made in related fields to develop objective and quantifiable criteria for medical decision-making. Thornton and colleagues[95] created a 'decision-tree' for patients with cervical cancer based on the primary question of whether they should have a radical hysterectomy (first branch of the tree). A corresponding decision-tree can be devised for patients considering their options for preserving fertility[96] (Figure 4). In the future, data may become available to make this device serviceable. Nevertheless, there are so many uncertainties surrounding the banking of germ cells and gametes that decision-making will continue to be difficult for these vulnerable patients. Litigation is likely to shape practices in some countries.

Sönmezer and Oktay[94] propose a comprehensive approach to counseling patients, and advocate that procedures that are not routinely carried out should be referred to specialized centers that have gained the most experience. That is wise advice for uncommon procedures, such as ovarian tissue banking. It is likely, however, that oocyte cryopreservation will become widely applied in both small and large assisted reproduction centers, just as embryo banking is today. Scientific progress towards identifying the most effective

and safe procedures will require cooperation between centers to gather sufficient numbers of cases and expertise for clinical trials to determine which procedures are most effective and who can benefit.

CONCLUSIONS

The rising number of research reports about low-temperature preservation of female germ cells, including mature oocytes, reveals growing optimism in this option for fertility preservation. There has been much debate about the greater technical hurdles for cryopreserving oocytes rather than embryos, and concerns about low efficiency and cytogenetic risks. Egg banking is obviously an attractive alternative to embryo banking and provides an opportunity for single women to preserve their genetic potential for reproduction. Moreover, banking of immature germ cells provides a prospect for prepubertal girls to preserve their fertility if it is jeopardized by sterilizing treatment. These techniques will remain experimental until more data are available and consistent success rates can be obtained. Concerns about the safety of these techniques may have been overestimated and,

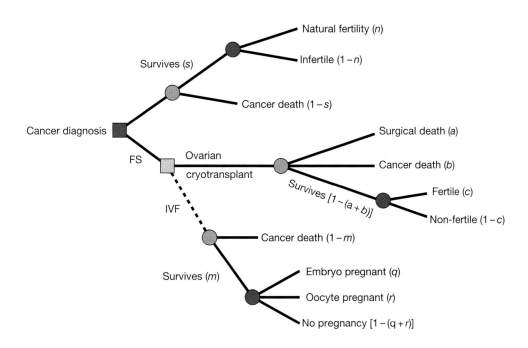

Figure 4 A decision analysis tree for cancer patients undergoing potentially sterilizing treatment and needing fertility sparing procedures (FS). IVF, *in vitro* fertilization

hopefully, new protocols and targeting selected groups of patients will enable continuing improvements. Most reports to date have been based upon standard methods of slow cooling and rapid thawing of oocytes or ovarian tissue, although there are increasing reports of the use of vitrification. Vitrification has a number of practical advantages as well as disadvantages, but we expect this procedure will gain more attention, at least for mature oocytes, and possibly even for ovarian tissue banking. It is highly unlikely, however, that a single cryopreservation protocol will be optimal for every stage of oocyte development, and a compromise will probably have to be struck for cryopreserving germ cells versus their granulosa cells in ovarian tissue and intact follicles. Small oocytes, and particularly primordial follicles, appear to be robust, but small follicle banking is limited by the challenge of maturing the oocytes to the metaphase II stage and the viability of embryos. The problems of growing small follicles to maturity in culture are still overwhelming for patient care, and progress is likely to come slowly and for germinal vesicle stages first. At present, ovarian transplantation provides the only realistic option for realizing the fertile potential of frozen–thawed ovarian tissue. This procedure, while having potential for restoring natural fertility, carries greater uncertainties than with mature oocytes. But it must be borne in mind that none of the protocols currently in use have been fully optimized, and most are based upon methods that were originally obtained from mouse oocytes, which may not be the best model. Oocytes from different species vary in size, sensitivity to chilling, robustness of the meiotic spindle and their lipid content. The limited numbers of good-quality oocytes from patients for research, or indeed from subhuman primate models, is a major impediment to progress toward defining optimal conditions. Major progress awaits coordinated, multicenter, clinical trials in which common protocols, expertise and cases can be pooled in an effort to define the best methods and realistic success rates.

ACKNOWLEDGMENTS

We would like to thank our many colleagues and collaborators who have shared with our endeavors to develop cryopreservation technologies for the female germ cell. Among the many people with whom we have worked on these projects we would particularly like to acknowledge the following: David Baird, Kutluk Oktay, Dror Meirow, Samuel Kim, Hang Yin, Jacob Mayer, Nikica Zaninovic, Richard Bodine and Zev Rosenwaks. It is a pleasure to record the financial support provided in the early stages of our research in the United Kingdom by the Leukemia Research Fund. We would also like to take this opportunity of thanking Nancy Garcia for help with this manuscript and her cheerful support and cooperation for us both over the years.

APPENDIX

Protocol 1

This protocol is modified from Porcu et al.[34] for cryopreserving human oocytes by slow cooling and rapid re-warming using 1,2-propanediol as the CPA.

Freezing protocol

Two to three hours after collection, the cumulus–corona complex of each oocyte is removed by exposure for 30–40 s to a HEPES-buffered (4-(2-hydroxyethyl)-1-piperazineethane sulfonic acid) culture medium (made on-site) containing 40 IU/ml hyaluronidase (SynVitro® Hyadase, MediCult, Denmark). Cumulus– corona cells are completely removed by aspiration and expulsion through a hand-drawn glass pipette. Mature oocytes are cryopreserved using a slow freeze–rapid thaw protocol as follows:

(1) Oocytes are equilibrated for 10 min in a HEPES-buffered version of phase I sequential medium supplemented with 1.5 mol/l 1,2-propanediol (PROH; Sigma-Aldrich, St Louis, MO) and 30% Plasmanate® (Bayer Corporation, Elkhart, IN).

(2) After equilibration, oocytes are transferred briefly into HEPES-buffered phase I sequential medium supplemented with 1.5 mol/l PROH/30% Plasmanate/0.2 mol/l sucrose.

(3) Oocytes are then loaded into sterile cryovials (Nunc™; Nalge Nunc International, Rochester, NY) containing 0.3 ml of the same solution and placed into an automated Planer Series III biological freezer (TS Scientific, Perkasie, PA) with a starting chamber temperature of 22.0°C.

(4) The temperature within the freezer is slowly reduced from 22.0 to −7.0°C at a rate of −2.0°C/min. The freezer is held at −7.0°C for 5 min (soak time).

(5) Manual seeding is performed at −7.0°C by grasping and holding the cryovial at the level of the medium meniscus using forceps that have been dipped into liquid nitrogen. Once seeding is accomplished and verified by formation of an ice crystal, the cryovial is gently lowered back into the freezing unit.

(6) The temperature is held at the same value for 10 min before being allowed to drop further.

(7) After 10 min, the temperature within the freezing chamber is gradually reduced to −30.0°C at a rate of −0.3°C/min, and then rapidly lowered to −150.0°C at a rate of −50.0°C/min.

(8) After 10 min of temperature equilibration at −150.0°C, the cryovial is plunged into liquid nitrogen and subsequently stored in a liquid nitrogen-filled Dewar until thawing.

Thawing protocol

(1) Cryovials are removed from liquid nitrogen storage, air-warmed for 30 s, and then placed into a 30°C water bath until all ice has dispersed. Cryoprotectant is removed in a stepwise manner as follows.

(2) Oocytes are transferred into HEPES-buffered sequential phase I medium with 1.0 mol/l PROH/0.3 mol/l sucrose/30% Plasmanate.

(3) After 5 min, oocytes are transferred to medium with 0.5 mol/l PROH/0.3 mol/l sucrose/30% Plasmanate.

(4) After another 5 min, oocytes are transferred to medium with only 0.3 mol/l sucrose/30% Plasmanate.

(5) After 10 min, oocytes are transferred to medium with 30% Plasmanate (no sucrose) for 10 min at room temperature, and then for an equal period at 37.5°C.

Oocytes are cultured within fresh culture medium in a routine manner at 37.5°C under 5.5% CO_2 for 3–4 h before ICSI is performed.

Protocol 2

This is a protocol for cryopreserving ovarian tissue (modified from Oktay)[76].

Thin ovarian cortical biopsies are obtained in the operating room and placed into normal saline for transport to the laboratory; alternatively, whole ovaries may be transported and processed within the laboratory. At room temperature, tissue is diced with a scalpel into pieces less than 0.4 mm^2 and up to five pieces are placed into Nunc cryovials (Nalge-Nunc International, Rochester, NY) containing 0.5 ml of HEPES-buffered sequential phase I medium (made on-site) with 20% Plasmanate (Bayer Corporation, Elkhart, IN), 1.5 mol/l DMSO (Sigma-Aldrich, St Louis, MO) and 0.1 mol/l sucrose. Cryovials are equilibrated for 30 min on ice.

After equilibration, tissues are frozen as follows:

(1) Using a Planer Series III biological freezer (TS Scientific, Perkasie, PA) and a start temperature of 0°C, begin cooling at a rate of −2.0°C/min until reaching −7.0°C.

(2) Soak for 10 min before performing manual seeding.

(3) Perform manual seeding and hold at −7.0°C for an additional 5 min.

(4) Continue cooling at a rate of −0.3°C/min to −40.0°C.

(5) Cool rapidly at a rate of −10.0°C/min from −40.0 to −140.0°C.

(6) Plunge into liquid nitrogen and transfer cryovials to liquid nitrogen storage.

Thawing protocol

(1) Thaw rapidly in a 30.0°C waterbath until all ice is dispersed.

(2) Wash tissue in progressively lower concentrations of cryoprotective medium:

(3) 1.0 mol/l DMSO/0.1 mol/l sucrose for 5 min.

(4) 0.5M DMSO/0.1 mol/l sucrose for 5 min.

(5) Medium with 0.1 mol/l sucrose only for 5 min.

(6) Transfer to fresh sequential phase I culture medium (no HEPES buffers) and incubate at 37.5°C under 5.5% CO_2 until tissue transplantation.

REFERENCES

1. Pellestor F, Andreo B, Arnal F, et al. Maternal ageing and chromosomal abnormalities: new data drawn from in vitro unfertilized human oocytes. Hum Genet 2003; 112: 195–203

2. Lambalk CB, de Koning CH, Flett A, et al. Assessment of ovarian reserve. Ovarian biopsy is not a valid method for the prediction of ovarian reserve. Hum Reprod 2004; 19: 1055–9

3. Gosden RG, Mullan J, Picton HM, et al. Current perspective on primordial follicle cryopreservation and culture for reproductive medicine. Hum Reprod Update 2002; 8: 105–10

4. Avery S. Embryo cryopreservation. In Brinsden PR, ed. Textbook of In Vitro Fertilization and Assisted Reproduction, 2nd edn. Carnforth:, UK: Parthenon Publishing, 1999: 211–17

5. American Cancer Society. Cancer Facts and Figures 2001, Atlanta, GA: American Cancer Society, 2001

6. Sanders JE, Buckner CD, Amos D, et al. Ovarian function following marrow transplantation for aplastic anemia or leukemia. J Clin Oncol 1988; 6: 813–18

7. Polge C, Smith AU, Parkes AS. Revival of spermatozoa after vitrification and dehydration at low temperatures. Nature (London) 1949; 169: 626–7

8. Leibo SP, Picton HM, Gosden RG. Cryopreservation of human spermatozoa. In Current Practices and Controversies in Assisted Reproduction, Report of a World Health Organization meeting. Geneva: WHO,

9. Parrott DVM. The fertility of mice with orthotopic ovarian derived from frozen tissue. J Reprod Fertil 1960; 1: 230–41

10. Whittingham DG. Fertilization in vitro and development to term of unfertilized mouse oocytes previously stored at −196 degrees C. J Reprod Fertil 1977; 49: 89–94

11. Wallace WH, Thomson AB, Kelsey TW. The radiosensitivity of the human oocyte. Hum Reprod 2003; 18: 117–21

12. Meirow D, Nugent D. The effects of radiotherapy and chemotherapy on female reproduction. Hum Reprod Update 2001; 7: 535–43

13. Mazur P. Kinetics of water loss from cells at subzero temperatures and the likelihood of intracellular freezing. J Gen Physiol 1963; 47: 347–69

14. Stachecki JJ, Willadsen SM. Cryopreservation of mouse oocytes using a medium with low sodium content: effect of plunge temperature. Cryobiology 2000; 40: 4–12

15. Quintans CJ, Donaldson MJ, Bertolino MV, et al. Birth of two babies using oocytes that were cryopreserved in a choline-based freezing medium. Hum Reprod 2002; 17: 3149

16. Leibo SP. Cryobiology: preservation of mammalian embryos. In Evans JW, Hollaender A, eds. Genetic Engineering of Animals. New York: Plenum Publishing Corp, 1986: 251–72

17. Trad FS, Toner M, Biggers JD. Effects of cryoprotectants and ice-seeding temperature on intracellular freezing and survival of human oocytes. Hum Reprod 1999; 14: 1569–77

18. Tucker M, Wright G, Morton P, et al. Preliminary experience with human oocyte cryopreservation using 1,2-propanediol and sucrose. Hum Reprod 1996; 11: 1513–15

19. Porcu E, Fabbri R, Seracchioli R, et al. Birth of a healthy female after intracytoplasmic sperm injection of cryopreserved human oocytes. Fertil Steril 1997; 68: 724–6

20. Winslow KL, Yang D, Blohm PL, et al. Oocyte cryopreservation: a three year follow up of sixteen births. Fertil Steril 2001; 76: P28

21. Mullen SF, Agca Y, Broermann DC, et al. The effect of osmotic stress on the metaphase II spindle of human oocytes, and the relevance to cryopreservation. Hum Reprod 2004; 19: 1148–54

22. Newton H, Pegg DE, Barrass R, et al. Osmotically inactive volume, hydraulic conductivity, and permeability to dimethyl sulphoxide of human mature oocytes. J Reprod Fertil 1999; 117: 27–33

23. Paynter SJ, Cooper A, Gregory L, et al. Permeability characteristics of human oocytes in the presence of the cryoprotectant dimethylsulphoxide. Hum Reprod 1999; 14: 2338–42

24. Meryman HT. Cryoprotective agents. Cryobiology 1971; 8: 173–83

25. Leibo SP, Mazur P. Methods for the preservation of mammalian embryos by freezing. In Daniel JC Jr, ed. Methods in Mammalian Reproduction. New York: Academic Press, 1978: 179–201

26. Kim SS, Yang HW, Kang HK, et al. Quantitative assessment of ischemic tissue damage in ovarian cortical tissue with or without antioxidant (ascorbic acid) treatment. Fertil Steril 2004; 82: 679–85

27. Fahy GM, MacFarlane DR, Angell C, et al. Vitrification as an approach to cryopreservation. Cryobiology 1984; 21: 407–26

28. Wakayama T, Yanagimachi R. Development of normal mice from oocytes injected with freeze-dried spermatozoa. Nat Biotech 1998; 16: 639–41

29. Chen C. Pregnancy after human oocyte cryopreservation. Lancet 1986; 2: 884–6

30. Van Uem JFHM, Siebzehnrübl ER, Schuh B, et al. Birth after cryopreservation of unfertilized oocytes. Lancet 1987; 1: 752–3

31. Al-Hasani S, Diedrich K, van der Ven H, et al. Cryopreservation of human oocytes. Hum Reprod 1987; 2: 695–700

32. Pickering SJ, Braude PR, Johnson MH. Cryoprotection of human oocytes: inappropriate exposure to DMSO reduces fertilization rates. Hum Reprod 1991; 6: 142–3

33. Litkouhi B, Winlow W, Gosden RG. Impact of cryoprotective agent exposure on intracellular calcium in mouse oocytes at metaphase II. Cryo-Letters 1999; 20: 353–62

34. Porcu E, Fabbri R, Damiano G, et al. Oocyte cryopreservation in oncological patients. Eur J Obstet Gynecol Reprod Biol 2004; 113 (Suppl 1): S14–16

35. Fabbri R, Porcu E, Marsella T, et al. Human oocyte cryopreservation: new perspectives regarding oocyte survival. Hum Reprod 2001; 16: 411–16

36. Eroglu A, Russo MJ, Bieganski R, et al. Intracellular trehalose improves the survival of cryopreserved mammalian cells. Nature Biotech 2000; 18: 163–7

37. Hasegawa A, Hamada Y, Mehandjiev T, et al. In vitro growth and maturation as well as fertilization of mouse preantral oocytes from vitrified ovaries. Fertil Steril 2004; 81 (Suppl): 824–30

38. Park S-K, Kim EY, Kim DI, et al. Simple, efficient and successful vitrification of bovine blastocysts using electron microscope grids. Hum Reprod 1999; 14: 2828–43

39. Vajta G, Holm P, Kuwayama M, et al. Open pulled straw (OPS) vitrification: a new way to reduce cryoinjuries of bovine ova and embryos. Mol Reprod Dev 1998; 51: 53–8

40. Mauatides A, Morrou D. Cryopreservation of bovine oocytes: is cryoloop vitrification the future to preserving the female gamete? Reprod Nutr Dev 2002; 42: 73–80

41. Pickering SJ, Braude PR, Johnson MH, et al. Transient cooling to room temperature can cause irreversible disruption of the meiotic spindle in the human oocyte. Fertil Steril 1990; 54: 102–8

42. Songsasen N, Yu IJ, Ratterree MS, et al. Effect of chilling on the organization of tubulin and chromosomes in rhesus monkey oocytes. Fertil Steril 2002; 77: 818–25

43. Eichenlaub-Ritter U, Vogt E, Yin H, Gosden R. Spindles, mitochondria and redox potential in ageing oocytes. Reprod BioMed Online 2003; 8: 45–58

44. Baka SG, Toth TL, Veeck LL, et al. Evaluation of the spindle apparatus of in-vitro matured oocytes following cryopreservation. Hum Reprod 1995; 10: 1816–20

45. Zenzes MT, Bielecki R, Casper RF, et al. Effects of chilling to 0 degrees C on the morphology of meiotic spindles in human metaphase II oocytes. Fertil Steril 2001; 75: 769–77

46. Arav A, Pearl M, Zeron Y. Does lipid profile explain chilling sensitivity and membrane lipid phase transition of spermatozoa and oocytes. Cryo-Letters 2000; 21: 179–86

47. Vajta G. Vitrification of the oocytes and embryos of domestic animals. Anim Reprod Sci 2000; 60–61: 357–64

48. Tucker MJ, Wright G, Morton PC, et al. Birth after cryopreservation of immature oocytes with subsequent in vitro fertilization. Fertil Steril 1998; 70: 578–9

49. Saunders KM, Parks JE. Effects of cryopreservation procedures on the cytology and fertilization rate of in vitro-matured bovine oocytes. Biol Reprod 1999; 61: 178–87

50. Porcu E, Fabbri R, Damiano G, et al. Clinical experience and applications of oocyte cryopreservation. Mol Cell Endocrinol 2000; 169: 33–7

51. Polak de Fried E, Notrica J, Rubinstein M, et al. Pregnancy after human donor oocyte cryopreservation and thawing in association with intracytoplasmic sperm injection in a patient with ovarian failure. Fertil Steril 1998; 69: 555–7

52. Young E, Kenny A, Puigdomenech E, et al. Triplet pregnancy after intracytoplasmic sperm injection of cryopreserved oocytes: case report. Fertil Steril 1998; 70: 360–1

53. Chen SU, Lien YR, Tsai YY, et al. Successful pregnancy occurred from slowly freezing human oocytes using the regime of 1.5 mol/l 1,2-propanediol with 0.3 mol/l sucrose. Hum Reprod 2002; 17: 1412

54. Yang D, Winslow KL, Blohm PL, et al. Oocyte donation using cryopreserved donor oocytes. Fertil Steril 2002; 78: S14–S15

55. Gook DA, Osborn SDM, Bourne H, et al. Fertilization of human oocytes following cryopreservation; normal karyotypes and absence of stray chromosomes. Hum Reprod 1994; 9: 684–91

56. Siebzehnruble E, Trotnow S, Weigel M, et al. Pregnancies after in vitro fertilsation, cryopreservation and embryo transfer. J Vitro Fert Embryo Transf 1986; 3: 261–3

57. Borini A, Bafaro MG, Bonu MA, et al. Pregnancies after oocyte freezing and thawing. Hum Reprod 1998; 13: 124–5 (Abstract book)

58. Porcu E, Fabbri R, Seracchioli R, et al. Birth of six healthy children intracytoplasmic sperm injection of crypreserved human oocytes. Hum Reprod 1998; 13: 124 (Abstract book)

59. Donaldson Pregnancies achieved after the transfer of embryos obtained by IVF of humans oocytes cryopreserved in low sodium

60. Porcu E, Fabbri R, Ciotti Pm, et al. Oocytes of embryo storage? Fertil Steril 2002; 78: S15

61. Fosas N, Marina F, Torres PJ, et al. The borths of five Spanish babies from cryopreserved donated oocytes. Hum Reprod 2003; 18: 1417–21

62. Boldt J, Cline D, McLaughlin D. Human oocyte cryopreservation as an adjunct to IVF–embryo transfer cycles. Hum Reprod 2003; 18: 1250–5

63. Kuleshova L, Gianaroli L, Magli C, et al. Birth following vitrification of a small number of human oocytes. Hum Reprod 1999; 14: 3077–9

64. Yoon TK, Chung HM, LIm JM, et al. Pregnancy and the delivery of hea;thy infants developed from vitrified oocytes in a stimulated in vitro ferlization–embryo transfer program. Fertil Steril 2000; 74: 180–1

65. Kuwayama M, Kato O. Successful vitrification of human oocytes. Fertil Steril 2000; 74: 549

66. Wu J, Zhang L, Wang X. In vitro maturation, fertilization and embryo development after ultrarapid freezing of immature human oocytes. Reproduction 2001; 121: 389–93

67. Katayama KP, Stehlik J, Kuwayama M, et al. High survival rate of vitrified human oocytes results in clinical pregnancy. Fertil Steril 2003; 80: 223–4

68. Yoon TK, Kim TJ, Park SE, et al. Live births after vitrification of oocytes in a stimulated in vitro fertilization–embryo transfer program. Fertil Steril 2003; 79: 1323–6

69. Oktay K, Nugent D, Newton H, et al. Isolation and characterization of primordial follicles from fresh and cryopreserved human ovarian tissue. Fertil Steril 1997; 67: 481–6

70. Telfer EE. The development of methods for isolation and culture of preantral follicles from bovine and porcine ovaries. Theriogenology 1996; 45: 101–10

71. Smitz T, Corturindt R. Follicle culture after ovarian cryostorage. Maturitas 1998; 30: 171–9

72. Spears N, Boland NI, Murray AA, et al. Mouse oocytes derived from in vitro grown primary ovarian follicles are fertile. Hum Reprod 1994; 9: 527–32

73. O'Brien MJ, Pendola, J. Eppig JJ. A revised protocol for in vitro development of mouse oocytes from primordial follicles dramatically improves their developmental competence. Biol Reprod 2003; 68: 1682–6

74. Yin H, Wang X, Kim SS, et al. Transplantation of intact rat gonads using vascular anastomosis: effects of cryopreservation, ischaemia and genotype. Hum Reprod 2003; 18: 1165–72

75. Bedaiwy MA, Jeremias E, Gurunluoglu R, et al. Restoration of ovarian function after autotransplantation of intact frozen-thawed sheep ovaries with microvascular anastomosis. Fertil Steril 2003; 79: 594–602

76. Oktay K. New horizons in assisted reproductive technologies. Assist Reprod Rev 1998; 8: 51

77. Gosden RG, Baird DT, Wade JC, Webb R. Restoration of fertility to oophorectomized sheep by ovarian autographs stored at −196 degrees C. Hum Reprod 1994; 9: 597–603

78. Nugent D, Meirow D, Brook PF, et al. Transplantation in reproductive medicine: previous experience, presented knowledge and future prospects. Hum Reprod Update 1997; 3: 267–80

79. Oktay K, Karlikaya G. Ovarian function after transplantation of frozen, banked autologous ovarian tissue. N Engl J Med 2000; 42: 1919

80. Radford JA, Lieberman BA, Brison DR, et al. Orthotopic reimplantation of cryopreserved ovarian cortical strips after high-dose chemotherapy for Hodgkin's lymphoma. Lancet 2001; 357: 1172–5

81. Oktay K, Economos K, Kan M, et al. Endocrine function and oocyte retrieval after autologous transplantation of ovarian cortical strips to the forearm. J Am Med Assoc 2001; 286: 1490–3

82. Aubard Y, Piver P, Cogni Y, et al. Orthotopic and heterotopic autografts of frozen-thawed ovarian cortex in sheep. Hum Reprod 1999; 14: 2149–54

83. Oktay K, Buyuk E, Veeck L, et al. Embryo development after heterotopic transplantation of cryopreserved ovarian tissue. Lancet 2004; 363: 832–3

84. Donnez J, Dolmans MM, Demylle D, et al. Livebirth after orthotopic transplantation of cryopreserved ovarian tissue. Lancet 2004; 364: 1405–10

85. Silber S, Lenahan KM, Levine D, et al. Ovarian transplantation between monozygotic twins discordant for premature ovarian failure. N Engl J Med 2005; in press

86. Bouquet M, Selva J, Auroux M. Cryopreservation of mouse oocytes: mutagenic effects in the embryo? Biol Reprod 1993; 49: 764–9

87. Shaw JM, Bowles J, Koopman P, et al. Fresh and cryopreserved ovarian tissue samples from donors with lymphoma transmit the cancer to graft recipients. Hum Reprod 1996; 11: 1668–73

88. Kim SS, Radford J, Harris M, et al. Ovarian tissue harvested from lymphoma patients to preserve fertility may be safe for autotransplantation. Hum Reprod 2001; 16: 2056–60

89. Gagnon SS, Tetu B. Ovarian metastases of breast carcinoma. Cancer 1989; 64: 892–8

90. Schroder CP, Timmer-Bosscha H, Wijchman TG, et al. An in vitro model for purging of tumour cells from ovarian tissue. Hum Reprod 2004; 19: 1069–75

91. Tedder RS, Zuckerman MA, Goldstone AH, et al. Hepatitis B transmission from contaminated cryopreservation tank. Lancet 1995; 346: 137–40

92. Bahadur G. Ethical issues of fertility preservation. In Tulandi T, Gosden RG, eds. Preservation of Fertility. London: Taylor & Francis Medical, 2004: 257–69

93. Grundy R, Larcher V, Gosden RG, et al. Fertility preservation for children treated for cancer (2): ethics of consent for gamete storage and experimentation. Arch Dis Child 2001; 84: 360–2

94. Sönmezer M, Oktay K. Fertility preservation in female cancer patients: a comprehensive approach. In Tulandi T, Gosden RG eds. Preservation of Fertility. London: Taylor & Francis Medical, 2004: 177–90

95. Thornton JG, Lilford RJ, Johnson N. Decision analysis in medicine. Br Med J 1992; 304: 1099–103

24

In vitro maturation of oocytes

William M. Buckett and Seang Lin Tan

See 2070

INTRODUCTION

In the past three decades, since the birth of the first child conceived as a result of *in vitro* fertilization (IVF) and embryo transfer[1], there has been an explosion of interest in assisted conception and in the practice of IVF particularly. IVF is now performed in nearly every country of the world, and hundreds of thousands of babies have been born worldwide.

Most IVF protocols use ovarian stimulation to achieve multiple follicular development because this enables a larger number of oocytes to be retrieved and more embryos to be generated and transferred, thereby resulting in higher pregnancy rates[2].

The generation of greater numbers of embryos also allows selection of embryos for cryopreservation[3]. This provides the opportunity for repeated attempts at embryo transfer and pregnancy without the costs and risks of repeated cycles of hormone stimulation and oocyte retrieval. Similarly, the generation of greater numbers of embryos also may allow continued embryo culture and blastocyst development, leading to the selection of embryos with better reproductive potential, and therefore improve overall pregnancy rates[4]. Finally, the generation of greater numbers of embryos also enables embryo biopsy and preimplantation embryo testing for genetic disease and aneuploidy, and therefore selection of non-affected embryos for transfer[5].

However, there are several potential problems with ovarian stimulation. The drugs are often costly and there is an increased need for biochemical and ultrasound monitoring. As well as the direct costs of treatment and medication, the increased time off work and additional hospital/clinic visits increase the indirect cost of treatment.

Side-effects of ovarian stimulation include pain and irritation at the site of injection; although this has been ameliorated by the subcutaneous use of more highly purified or recombinant preparations, the risk of allergic response still remains[6]. Other commonly reported side-effects include hot flushes, tiredness, breast or nipple tenderness, pelvic discomfort or pain, and emotional lability. Ovarian cyst formation is also well recognized[7]. This can further increase the time of treatment and necessary monitoring.

Ovarian hyperstimulation syndrome (OHSS) is the most serious complication of ovarian stimulation[8] and is discussed elsewhere. Prevention of severe OHSS remains the primary aspect of management in patients at risk of developing OHSS.

Following reports of ovarian cancers in women who have undergone ovarian stimulation or ovulation induction[9,10], continued concern remains. However, the available data from epidemiological studies and case reports do not support a direct causal relationship[11,12]. Nevertheless, because any possible long-term

441

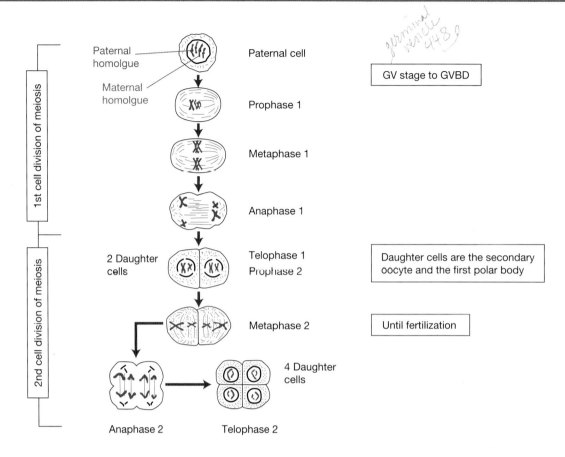

Figure 1   Schematic representation of meiosis and the relevant changes pertaining to oocyte maturation. GV, germinal vesicle; GVBD, germinal vesicle breakdown

consequences are not absolutely known, many women would prefer not to have hormonal stimulation of the ovaries, if this could be avoided.

Natural-cycle IVF has been used, with varying degrees of success, for women who for various reasons seek to avoid the risks of ovarian stimulation[13,14], although the success rates per cycle are low. Problems associated with natural-cycle IVF include an increased risk of cycle cancellation due to a premature luteinizing hormone (LH) surge[15], poor follicle development[16] and no oocyte at collection or embryo for transfer[17]. Furthermore, women with anovulatory infertility will not develop a dominant follicle and subsequent LH surge; therefore, for these women the retrieval of mature oocytes in the context of natural-cycle IVF will not be possible.

During the follicular phase of the menstrual cycle, within the cohort of antral follicles from which a single dominant follicle develops, there are also many immature oocytes[18]. The ability to collect these immature oocytes and effect their maturation *in vitro* allows the generation of multiple embryos[19–21], which therefore provides similar benefits to those with conventional IVF, while avoiding the problems associated with ovarian stimulation.

CONTROL AND INITIATION OF OOCYTE MATURATION *IN VIVO*

Human oocytes are arrested in prophase I of meiosis during fetal life. These immature oocytes can be found in the non-growing follicles. As each cohort is recruited and follicular dominance is established, the oocyte acquires the ability to reinitiate meiosis[22] (Figure 1).

Following resumption of meiosis, the nuclear membrane dissolves and the chromosomes progress from metaphase I to telophase I. The dissolution of the nuclear membrane is known as germinal vesicle breakdown (GVBD). Following completion of the first meiotic division and extrusion of the first polar body, the second meiotic division starts and is arrested at metaphase II (MII) until ovulation and fertilization. Immature oocytes (i.e. those which have not reached MII) are unable to undergo fertilization and subsequent embryo cleavage. Oocyte maturation, therefore, can be defined as the reinitiation and completion of the first meiotic division from the germinal vesicle (GV) stage to the MII stage, with the accompanying cytoplasmic maturation.

Nuclear maturation begins with GVBD. This is initiated *in vivo* either by the atretic degeneration of the follicle or by the preovulatory gonadotropin surge (follicle stimulating hormone (FSH) and primarily LH). The LH surge provides the classic hormonal endocrine trigger for ovulation and luteinization of the follicle, as well as leading to the resumption of oocyte meiosis[23,24]. The establishment of pregnancies following *in vitro* fertilization (IVF) of oocytes aspirated from the ovary required identification of the LH surge prior to collection before yielding mature oocytes capable of fertilization[25], and the use of human chorionic gonadotropin (hCG) has subsequently been used pharmacologically as a homolog for the LH surge to produce mature oocytes for many forms of assisted reproduction treatment[26]. However, there are no LH receptors on the oocyte[27]; therefore, nuclear maturation must be mediated either through the granulosa cells and follicular fluid, or via the cumulus cells which are intimately connected with the oocyte through numerous gap junctions.

Many factors and regulatory molecules have been shown either to inhibit or to promote nuclear and cytoplasmic oocyte maturation[28], either directly or via the cumulus cells (Figure 2).

MATURATION OF OOCYTES *IN VITRO*

Oocytes from stimulated ovaries

Isolation and maturation of human oocytes *in vitro* was first reported as long ago as the 1960s[29,30], and this was followed by the first reports of fertilization *in vitro*[31] and the first successful pregnancy and live birth[1]. Although these oocytes were derived from natural ovulatory cycles, as a result of better oocyte retrieval rates and pregnancy rates with multiple follicular

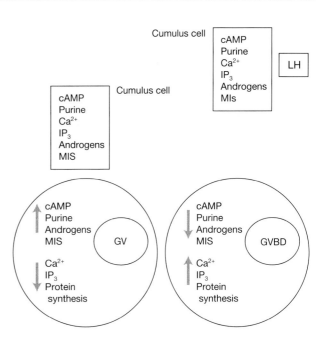

Figure 2 Schematic representation of hypothetical model for the participation of various factors involved in the initiation of germinal vesicle breakdown (GVBD). Luteinizing hormone (LH) binding to the cumulus cells leads to a loss of cumulus–oocyte communication and a change in cytoplasmic oocyte factors. MIS, Mullerian inhibiting substance; IP$_3$, inositol 1,4,5-triphosphate; cAMP, cyclic adenosine monophosphate

development it quickly became standard practice to stimulate ovaries with various hormone protocols. This superovulation led to follicular asynchrony[32], where most oocytes were MI or MII at oocyte retrieval but some remained GV-stage oocytes.

These GV oocytes retrieved from stimulated ovaries are capable of undergoing spontaneous nuclear maturation and subsequent fertilization *in vitro*, although the rates of maturation and fertilization are low (35% and 12%, respectively). This is improved (to 65% and 45%, respectively) with the addition of human menopausal gonadotropin (1 : 1 FSH : LH) to the usual Ham's F-10 media[33].

When immature oocytes from stimulated and unstimulated ovaries are compared in culture, the time from GV stage through GVBD to MII is accelerated in immature oocytes derived from stimulated ovaries[34]. This would imply that the *in vivo* ovarian stimulation and subsequent gonadotropin surge has an effect on oocyte maturation before the oocytes are retrieved and studied. It is well recognized that different ovulation induction protocols have led to variations in mature oocyte quality as well as fertilization and embryo cleavage rates[35].

Because the vast majority of oocytes (> 90%) retrieved from stimulated cycles in women undergoing IVF are MI or MII, the differences in immature oocyte quality and subsequent *in vitro* maturation have little impact on overall fertilization and pregnancy rates.

Oocytes from unstimulated ovaries

Oocytes from unstimulated ovaries have been obtained from women undergoing tubal surgery, cesarean section and oophorectomy as part of an organized oocyte donation program[36] or as an adjunct to natural-cycle IVF (i.e. with unstimulated or minimally stimulated ovaries)[37]. However, maturation rates, fertilization rates (even with intracytoplasmic sperm injection) and ultimately pregnancy rates initially were disappointingly low[34], although improvements in retrieval technique and maturation culture have led to significantly improved clinical pregnancy rates[38].

Factors which have been reported to affect the maturational competence of aspirated immature oocytes include the timing of retrieval and the size of the ovarian follicles. Early evidence suggested that immature oocytes collected in the luteal phase had significantly higher maturation rates[39]. However, it has been found that there is a decreased maturation rate in oocytes from small follicles (3–4 mm) when compared with those from larger follicles (9–15 mm)[40], and similarly there is a decreased chance of obtaining oocytes as the follicle becomes mature/dominant in the absence of a spontaneous gonadotropin surge or administered hCG[41]. More recent evidence suggests that aspiration in the mid-follicular phase in women with regular menstrual cycles of the antral follicles (8–10 mm) prior to the emergence of the dominant follicle offers the best oocytes for maturation and ultimately pregnancy[42].

Initial *in vitro* culture of immature human oocytes was with standard TCM-199 or Ham's F-10 media supplemented with 10% fetal calf serum, and this resulted in maturation rates (to MII) of around 30%[43]. Maturation rates improved to around 60% when this was substituted with human follicular fluid or peritoneal fluid[36], and currently maturation rates of around 80% are achieved with *in vitro* maturation (IVM) oocyte medium with human serum albumin

(HSA) or IVM oocyte medium without HAS, which needs a supplemented protein source (usually inactivated maternal serum) as well as FSH and LH (either urinary or recombinant preparations)[34,42,44]. Some authors also routinely use antibiotic supplements in the culture media.

Oocytes from women with polycystic ovaries or polycystic ovarian syndrome

Polycystic ovarian syndrome (PCOS) is characterized by chronic anovulation and mild hyperandrogenemia, and the typical surgical, histological and ultrasound findings are of an increased number of peripheral medium-sized ovarian follicles (2–10 mm). Immature oocytes from these follicles retain their maturational and developmental competence[45], and pregnancies have been reported[19,45,46]. Although early studies suggested that the developmental capacity of immature oocytes seemed higher in regularly cycling women compared with women with irregular and anovulatory cycles[34,47], later studies showed comparable maturation and fertilization rates[48,49], and the success of many IVM programs in treating women with polycystic ovaries and PCOS demonstrates that indeed the reverse may be true[38].

CLINICAL APPLICATION OF *IN VITRO* MATURATION

Development of IVM as a clinical treatment for infertility

The first successful IVM birth was in Korea. In this case, immature oocytes were collected at cesarean section for oocyte donation[36]. Following this, the first pregnancy in a woman with anovulatory infertility using her own immature oocytes was reported in Australia[45], and a further pregnancy in a woman with PCOS was reported by the same group, using IVM combined with intracytoplasmic sperm injection, assisted hatching and blastocyst culture[46]. In addition, immature oocytes have also been retrieved from ovaries during either follicular or luteal phases of ovulatory cycles[39].

As women with polycystic ovaries or PCOS undergoing IVF have an increased risk of OHSS from gonadotropins, compared with women with normal ovaries[50], these women are an obvious group who may benefit from IVM and thereby avoid ovarian stimulation. Initial studies indicated that, although immature oocytes recovered from unstimulated patients with polycystic ovaries or PCOS could be matured, fertilized and developed *in vitro*, the implantation rate of these cleaved embryos was disappointingly low[47,51,52]. However, recent data indicate that IVM using FSH or hCG priming before immature oocyte retrieval leads to clinical pregnancy and implantation rates of 30–35% and 10–15%, respectively[28]. Further studies and current data show that pregnancy rates of 30–40% are achieved in women with the higher numbers of antral follicles associated with polycystic ovaries or PCOS[20].

Pre-retrieval priming with human chorionic goandotropin

Although germinal vesicle-stage oocytes have been retrieved from the standard stimulated cycles 36 h after hCG administration, and successful pregnancies have been established using such *in vitro* matured oocytes[53–56], the pregnancy rates are low.

However, in women undergoing IVM without ovarian stimulation, it has been demonstrated that the time course of oocyte maturation *in vitro* is hastened and the rate of oocyte maturation is increased by priming with 10 000 IU hCG 36 h before retrieval of immature oocytes from women with polycystic ovaries or PCOS[57,58].

Initial reports also suggested that pregnancy rates may be improved by priming with hCG prior to immature oocyte retrieval[19], and this has been confirmed by subsequent reports[59–62].

Based on more than 1000 IVM cycles in a multicenter study with hCG priming before immature oocyte retrieval from women with polycystic ovaries or PCOS, the pregnancy and implantation rates reached 30–35% and 10–15%, respectively[38]. Interestingly, recent findings show that in women with polycystic ovaries or PCOS, the time course and maturation rates are different when germinal vesicle-stage oocytes are divided into different groups based on the morphology of cumulus cells after hCG priming[63]. Therefore, it seems that hCG priming both promotes some oocytes to undergo maturation to the metaphase-I stage, when derived from the relatively larger follicles (> 10 mm in diameter), and also

enhances some germinal vesicle-stage oocytes from small follicles to acquire maturational and developmental competence *in vivo*.

Priming with follicle stimulating hormone

As an alternative approach, a truncated course of ovarian stimulation with FSH before immature oocyte retrieval has been applied, suggesting that FSH pretreatment promotes efficient recovery of immature oocytes and maturation *in vitro*[64]. It has been reported that the immature oocytes from stimulated cycles from normal-cycling women without hCG can be matured and fertilized *in vitro*, and pregnancies and live births have been reported[65].

Some data[42] showed that low-dose FSH priming with a fixed dose (150 IU/day) for 3 days from day 3 of the menstrual cycle does not increase the number of oocytes obtained per aspiration, and does not improve oocyte maturation, cleavage rates or embryo development when women with normal cycling ovaries are treated. On the other hand, other data[48] showed that low-dose FSH priming started from the previous luteal phase improves the efficiency of immature oocyte recovery, *in vitro* maturation and fertilization.

Nevertheless, it has been reported that priming with recombinant FSH during the follicular phase before harvesting of immature oocytes from patients with PCOS improves the maturational potential of the oocytes, leading to increased implantation and pregnancy rates (21% and 29%, respectively)[66].

Indications for IVM

As detailed above, both IVM protocols currently used report the highest pregnancy rates in women with polycystic ovaries or PCOS. Therefore, women with PCOS, ultrasound-only polycystic ovaries or a combined antral follicle count of greater than 20, who need IVF, are the best candidates for IVM. The antral follicle count is the best clinical predictor of the number of immature oocytes that may be retrieved and the best predictor of clinical pregnancy[20] (Figure 3). These women are also at increased risk of OHSS, and therefore would benefit most from avoiding ovarian stimulation, as well as having the highest success rates with IVM.

Another indication for IVM is a patient who repeatedly produces a majority of poor-quality

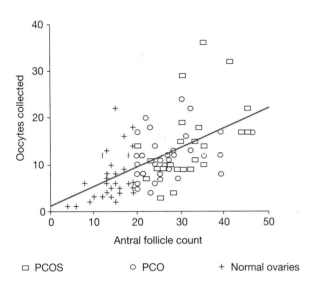

□ PCOS   ○ PCO   + Normal ovaries

Figure 3 Number of immature oocytes collected and early follicular phase antral follicle count. Data from reference 20. PCOs, polycystic ovarian syndrome; PCO, polycystic ovaries

embryos through conventional IVF. Indeed, one of our first IVM pregnancies was in a young woman who produced mostly poor-quality embryos in three different IVF cycles with different protocols and gonadotropins. When she underwent IVM, the majority of embryos were of good quality, and she had a live birth following her first IVM attempt. Following her departure from Montreal, she underwent a further two conventional IVF cycles elsewhere, and again produced embryos of poor quality. She therefore returned to our center for IVM and had a second pregnancy and live birth. In our experience there is a small group of women who repeatedly produce mostly poor-quality embryos for no apparent reason. When IVM is performed for these women, their embryos are of good quality and they are able to achieve successful pregnancies. It would appear that gonadotropin stimulation for multiple follicular development may have an adverse effect on the embryos in these women.

Other indications for IVM include women undergoing ovarian stimulation for conventional IVF, who develop an over-response and would otherwise be canceled because of the risk of developing OHSS. Initially, one live birth was reported from immature oocytes that were collected from a patient at risk of developing OHSS[67]. More recently, eight clinical pregnancies (out of 17 cycles) were achieved from

patients with potential risk of developing OHSS followed by immature oocyte retrieval and IVM[68].

Similarly, women with poor ovarian response to ovarian stimulation may benefit from IVM. Two pregnancies were reported following IVM when GV- or MI-stage oocytes were retrieved after hCG administration from poor responders. More recently, three pregnancies (out of eight cycles) were obtained following immature oocyte retrieval and IVM without hCG administration before oocyte collection[69], suggesting that IVM may be a viable alternative to cancellation in poor responders undergoing conventional IVF.

Avoiding the cost, increased monitoring and time associated with ovarian stimulation in conventional IVF is appealing to many women. However, the scarcity of altruistic oocyte donors makes IVM an attractive option for these women, and pregnancies have been reported following IVM for oocyte donation[70,71].

Finally, the increasing survival rates following cancer treatment have led to attempts through cryopreservation to try to preserve fertility in young women who need potentially sterilizing chemo- or radiotherapy. Ovarian tissue cryopreservation[72] is associated with increased anesthetic and surgical morbidity, unless laparotomy is indicated, and conventional IVF with ovarian stimulation followed by oocyte or embryo cryopreservation is a prolonged treatment, and not indicated in hormone-dependent cancers[73]. IVM is less invasive than ovarian biopsy or resection, and avoids the time and risks associated with ovarian stimulation. IVM and oocyte vitrification to preserve fertility in a woman with breast cancer have been reported[74].

PROCEDURE OF *IN VITRO* MATURATION

The steps involved in clinical IVM cycles are:

(1) Cycle initiation;

(2) Immature oocyte retrieval;

(3) *In vitro* oocyte maturation;

(4) Fertilization;

(5) Embryo transfer;

(6) Endometrial preparation and luteal support.

Cycle initiation

In women with oligo- or amenorrhea, the treatment cycle is initiated by the administration of oral, intravaginal or intramuscular progesterone, and the timing of the start of treatment can be planned. Withdrawal bleeding usually occurs within 3 days after the last dose. On day 2–4 following the onset of menstrual bleeding, the women undergo a baseline ultrasound scan to ensure that there are no ovarian cysts. Women with spontaneous or regular menstruation should have the baseline ultrasound scan in the early follicular phase as detailed above.

Transvaginal ultrasound scans should be repeated on day 7–9 to plan the immature oocyte retrieval. In women with ovulatory cycles this should be performed before day 9–11 of the cycle, and in women with anovulatory cycles the retrieval can be performed on day 10–14 of the cycle. Prior to immature oocyte retrieval, women are primed with 10 000 IU hCG subcutaneously 36 h before oocyte retrieval.

Immature oocyte retrieval

Transvaginal ultrasound-guided oocyte collection is performed using a specially designed 17-gauge single-lumen aspiration needle (K-OPS-1235-Wood; Cook, Australia) with an aspiration pressure of 7.5 kPa. Aspiration of all small follicles is performed under intravenous sedation with paracervical block, or under spinal anesthesia. A multiple puncture technique is used. Oocytes are collected in 10-ml culture tubes containing 2 ml warm 0.9% saline with 2 IU/ml heparin. The collection needle should be flushed regularly to prevent blockage with debris or blood clot. All aspirates are examined under the microscope for cumulus–oocyte complexes (COCs). Prior to discarding the fluid, it should be poured through a filter (Cell Strainer 352350; Falcon, USA) then rinsed with IVM washing medium and re-examined under the microscope for further COCs.

In vitro oocyte maturation

Following oocyte collection, the oocytes are evaluated for the presence or absence of a germinal vesicle (GV) in the cytoplasm of the oocyte (Figure 4), and the immature oocytes are then transferred into the maturation medium for culture. If no GV is seen in an immature oocyte, the oocyte is defined as germinal vesicle breakdown (GVBD) (Figure 5). The mature (MII) oocytes are determined by the presence of a first polar body (Figure 6). All oocyte handling procedures are conducted on warm stages and plates at 37°C. Cumulus–oocyte complexes are rinsed in IVM washing medium. Immature oocytes are then incubated in an organ tissue culture dish (60×15 mm; Falcon) containing 1 ml of IVM oocyte medium supplemented with 75 mIU/ml FSH and 75 mIU/ml LH at 37°C in an atmosphere of 5% CO_2 and 95% air with high humidity. Following culture, the maturity of the oocytes is determined under the microscope at 12-h intervals for up to 48 h following the retrieval.

Fertilization

Oocytes which are mature at the time of checking are then denuded of cumulus cells using finely drawn glass pipettes, following 1 min of exposure to 0.1% hyaluronidase solution, ready for intracytoplasmic sperm injection (ICSI). Spermatozoa for ICSI are prepared by mini-Percoll separation (45% and 90% gradients) at 560g for 20 min. Following Percoll separation, the sperm pellet is washed twice (200g) with 2 ml of Medi-Cult IVF medium. A single spermatozoon is then injected into each metaphase II oocyte. Following ICSI, each oocyte is transferred into a 20 μl droplet of Medi-Cult IVF medium in a tissue culture dish (35×10 mm; Falcon) under mineral oil. Fertilization is assessed 18 h after ICSI for the appearance of two distinct pronuclei and two polar bodies.

Embryo transfer

Following fertilization, embryos with two pronuclei are transferred into 1.0 ml of Medi-Cult IVF medium in the organ tissue culture dish (60×15 mm; Falcon) for further culture. Because implantation rates are lower with IVM, compared with ovarian stimulation and conventional IVF, we recommend transferring 1–2 more embryos at IVM than would be transferred for conventional IVF in the same age group. Since oocytes are not necessarily mature and inseminated at the same time following maturation in culture, the developmental stages of embryos may be variable both within and between patients. Before transfer, all embryos for each patient are pooled and selected for

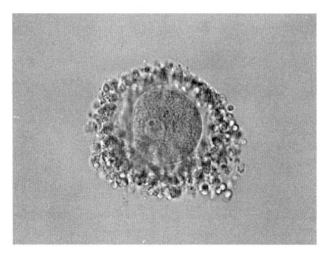

Figure 4 A germinal vesicle (GV)-stage immature oocyte

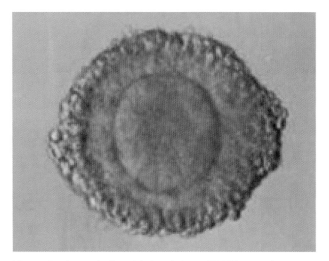

Figure 5 A germinal vesicle breakdown (GVBD)-stage immature oocyte

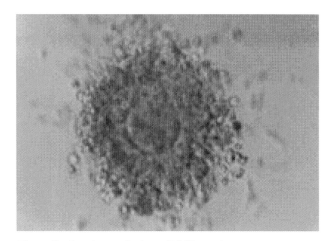

Figure 6 A mature metaphase-II (MII) oocyte

transfer. The embryo transfer technique is the same as that employed for conventional IVF.

Endometrial preparation and luteal support

For preparation of the endometrium, women are given estradiol valerate of a dosage depending on endometrial thickness on the day of oocyte retrieval in divided doses, starting on the day of oocyte retrieval. If endometrial thickness on the day of oocyte retrieval is < 4 mm, a 10–12-mg dose is administered daily; if it is between 4 and 6 mm, a dose of 8 mg is given, and if it is > 6 mm, a 6-mg dose is given.

Luteal support is started on the day that MII maturation is achieved and ICSI is performed. Previously this was provided by 400 mg intravaginal progesterone twice daily for 16 days, although 50 mg intramuscular progesterone is currently given.

On the day of embryo transfer, the endometrial thickness is measured again by transvaginal ultrasound scan. If the endometrial thickness is < 8 mm, the couple are offered embryo cryopreservation and transfer in a subsequent cycle.

DISADVANTAGES OF *IN VITRO* MATURATION

Although the clinical application of IVM is an exciting development in the field of assisted reproductive technologies, there have been several concerns regarding potential disadvantages associated with IVM. Although the clinical use of IVM is practiced in many European, Asian and North American countries, at present the Human Fertilisation and Embryology Authority (HFEA) have not licensed IVM for clinical use in the United Kingdom.

Increased cost

IVM represents a significant reduction in the cost of IVF to the couple seeking treatment by virtue of avoiding the costs of ovarian stimulation. These can be significant, particularly when gonadotropin releasing hormone analog long protocols are used either with or without recombinant gonadotropins, typically ranging from $2000 to $2500 per cycle started[75].

However, there are increased laboratory costs. These include the direct and indirect costs of oocyte maturation, ICSI and often assisted hatching. As the immature oocytes need to be checked every 12 h, this also increases laboratory costs.

Finally, there is a need for training, both for clinicians to learn the immature oocyte retrieval, which may be technically more demanding than conventional IVF because the follicles are smaller and the ovaries are often more mobile, and for embryologists to learn the maturation techniques.

Lower success rates

At present, many centers report clinical pregnancy rates with conventional IVF in excess of 40% per oocyte retrieval[76], and HFEA data[77] show live birth rates per cycle started in excess of 20%. Although some IVM programs report success rates approaching this[38], many do not. The only study to have tried to compare IVM with conventional IVF was a case-matched controlled study of women with polycystic ovaries or PCOS. This showed clinical pregnancy rates of 38% with conventional IVF and 26% with IVM[78], although obviously there were no cases of OHSS in the IVM group.

All centers which perform conventional IVF as well as IVM report higher clinical pregnancy and implantation rates with conventional IVF, although IVM has a much higher clinical pregnancy rate per cycle compared with natural cycle IVF[14]. The reduced costs, monitoring and risks associated with IVM still make this treatment an attractive alternative to conventional IVF with ovarian stimulation.

Chromosomal abnormalities

Some authors have concern regarding the risk of karyotypic abnormalities in *in vitro* matured oocytes, particularly as there may be higher rates of karyotypic abnormalities amongst immature oocytes[79]. More recent evidence, however, suggests that there is no increase in the karyotypic abnormality rates in successfully matured oocytes, although these data are still preliminary[80].

Lack of outcome data

The successful establishment of effective IVM programs for the treatment of infertility is still relatively new. Therefore, the number of babies born worldwide is still relatively small. The two studies so far have shown no increase in adverse obstetric, perinatal and neonatal outcomes in women who conceived following IVM[81,82].

Nevertheless, caution and appropriate counseling are needed regarding the unknown long-term effects of IVM on any children conceived as a result of treatment, and continued follow-up is advised.

CONCLUSIONS

In vitro maturation has been shown to be an effective treatment for infertility in women with polycystic ovaries or PCOS who have not conceived following ovulation induction or who need IVF for other indications. IVM has also proved effective in women with regular cycles, either with FSH priming or when combined with natural-cycle IVF.

IVM avoids the costs, monitoring and risks associated with ovarian stimulation. This makes it an attractive treatment option not only for many women undergoing treatment themselves, but also for women wishing to donate oocytes.

IVM followed by oocyte or embryo cryopreservation is also an appropriate treatment option for women wishing to preserve their fertility, prior to potentially sterilizing chemotherapy or radiotherapy. It may even open the door to young women who wish to defer child-bearing to a later age, to preserve their fertility by undergoing IVM with vitrification of the oocytes retrieved.

Although IVM is a relatively new treatment, early evidence from *in vitro* studies and from pregnancy-outcome studies suggests that there is unlikely to be significant risk associated with this treatment.

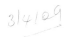

REFERENCES

1. Steptoe PC, Edwards RG. Birth after reimplantation of a human embryo. Lancet 1978; 2: 366
2. Tan SL, Maconochie N, Doyle P, et al. Cumulative conception and live-birth rates after in vitro fertilization with and without the use of long, short, and ultrashort regimens of the gonadotropin-releasing hormone agonist buserelin. Am J Obstet Gynecol 1994; 171: 513–20
3. Trounson A, Dawson K. Storage and disposal of embryos and gametes. Br Med J 1996; 313: 1–2

4. Gardner DK, Schoolcraft WB, Wagley L, et al. A prospective randomized trial of blastocyst culture and transfer in in vitro fertilization. Hum Reprod 1998; 13: 3434–40

5. Dean NL, Tan SL, Ao A. The development of pre-implantation genetic diagnosis for myotonic dystrophy using multiplex fluorescent polymerase chain reaction and its clinical application. Mol Hum Reprod 2001; 7: 895–901

6. Engmann L, Shaker A, White E, et al. A prospective randomized study to assess the clinical efficacy of gonadotrophins administered subcutaneously and intramuscularly. Hum Reprod 1998; 14: 167–71

7. Biljan MM, Mahutte NG, Dean N, et al. Pretreatment with an oral contraceptive is effective in reducing the incidence of functional ovarian cyst formation during pituitary suppression by gonadotropin-releasing hormone analogues. J Assist Reprod Genet 1998; 15: 599–604

8. Rizk B, Smitz J. Ovarian hyperstimulation syndrome after superovulation using GnRH antagonists for IVF and related procedures. Hum Reprod 1992; 7: 320–7

9. Shushan A, Paltiel O, Iscovich J, et al. Human menopausal gonadotropin and the risk of epithelial ovarian cancer. Fertil Steril 1996; 65: 13–18

10. Salle B, de Saint Hilaire P, Devouassoux M, et al. Another two cases of ovarian tumours in women who had undergone multiple ovulation induction cycles. Hum Reprod 1997; 12: 1732–5

11. Tarlatzis BC, Grimbizis G, Bontis J, Matalenakis S. Ovarian stimulation and ovarian tumours: a critical reappraisal. Hum Reprod Update 1995; 1: 284–301

12. Potashnik G, Lerner-Geva L, Genkin L, et al. Fertility drugs and the risk of breast and ovarian cancers: results of a long-term follow-up study. Fertil Steril 1999; 71: 853–9

13. Lenton EA, Cooke ID, Hooper M, et al. In vitro fertilization in the natural cycle. Ballière's Clin Obstet Gynaecol 1992; 6: 229–45

14. Nargund G, Waterstone J, Bland J, et al. Cumulative conception and live birth rates in natural (unstimulated) IVF cycles. Hum Reprod 2001; 16: 259–62

15. Claman P, Domingo M, Garner P, et al. Natural cycle in vitro fertilization – embryo transfer at the University of Ottawa: an inefficient therapy for tubal infertility. Fertil Steril 1993; 60: 298–302

16. Svalander P, Green K, Haglund B. Natural versus stimulated cycles in IVF–ET treatment for tubal infertility. Hum Reprod 1991; 9 (Suppl 4): 101

17. Lenton EA, Woodward B. Natural cycle versus stimulated cycle IVF: is there a role for IVF in the natural cycle? J Assist Reprod Genet 1993; 10: 406–8

18. Chian RC, Buckett WM, Abdul Jalil AK, et al. Natural-cycle in vitro fertilization combined with in vitro maturation of immature oocytes is a potential approach in fertility treatment. Fertil Steril 2004; 82: 1675–8

19. Chian RC, Gulekli B, Buckett WM, Tan SL. Priming with human chorionic gonadotrophin before retrieval of immature oocytes in women with infertility due to polycystic ovary syndrome. N Engl J Med 1999; 341: 1624–6

20. Tan SL, Child TJ, Gulekli B. In vitro maturation and fertilization of oocytes from unstimulated ovaries: predicting the number of immature oocytes retrieved by early follicular phase ultrasonography. Am J Obstet Gynecol 2002; 186: 684–9

21. Buckett WM, Chian RC, Tanl SL. Human chorionic gonadotrophin for in vitro oocyte maturation: does it improve the endometrium or implantation? J Reprod Med 2004; 49: 93–8

22. Pincus G, Enzmann EV. The comparative behaviour of mammalian eggs in vivo and in vitro I: The activation of ovarian eggs. J Exp Med 1935; 62: 655–75

23. Channing CP, Hillensjo T, Schaerf FW. Hormone control of oocyte meiosis, ovulation and luteinization in mammals. Clin Endocrinol Metab 1978; 7: 601–24

24. Seibel MM, Smith DM, Levesque L, et al. The temporal relationship between the luteinizing hormone surge and human oocyte maturation. Am J Obstet Gynecol 1982; 142: 568–72

25. Edwards RG, Steptoe PC, Purdy JM. Establishing full term human pregnancies using cleaved embryos grown in vitro. Br J Obstet Gynaecol 1980; 87: 737–46

26. Steptoe PC, Edwards RG. Laparoscopic recovery of pre-ovulatory human oocytes after priming the ovaries with gonadotrophins. Lancet 1970; 2: 880–2

27. Dekel N. Spatial relationship of follicular cells in control of meiosis. In Haseltine FP, First HL, eds. Meiotic Inhibition and Molecular Control of Meiosis. New York: Alan Liss, 1990: 87–101

28. Chian RC, Buckett WM, Tan SL. In vitro maturation of human oocytes. Reprod Biomed Online 2004; 8: 148–66

29. Edwards RG. Maturation of in vitro mouse, sheep, cow, pig, rhesus monkey, and human ovarian oocytes. Nature (London) 1965; 208: 349–51

30. Edwards RG. Mammalian in vitro maturation of human ovarian oocytes. Lancet 1965; 2: 926–9

31. Edwards RG, Bavister BD, Steptoe PC. Early stages of fertilization in vitro of human oocytes matured in vitro. Nature (London) 1969; 221: 632–5

32. Laufer N, Tarlatzis BC, DeCherny AH, et al. Asynchrony between human cumulus–corona cell

complex and oocyte maturation after human menopausal gonadotropin treatment for in vitro fertilization. Fertil Steril 1984; 42: 366–72

33. Prins GS, Wagner C, Weidel L, et al. Gonadotropins augment maturation and fertilization of human immature oocytes cultured in vitro. Fertil Steril 1987; 47: 1035–7

34. Cha KY, Chian RC. Maturation in vitro of immature human oocytes for clinical use. Hum Reprod Update 1999; 4: 103–20

35. De Sutter P, Dhont M, vanLuchene E, Vandekerckhove D. Correlations between follicular fluid steroid analysis, maturity, and cytogenic analysis of human oocytes which remained unfertilized after in vitro fertilization. Fertil Steril 1991; 55: 958–63

36. Cha KY, Koo JJ, Ko JJ, et al. Pregnancy after in vitro fertilization of human follicular oocytes collected from nonstimulated cycles, their culture in vitro and their transfer in an oocyte donation program. Fertil Steril 1991; 55: 109–13

37. Paulson RJ, Sauer MV, Francis MM, et al. Factors affecting pregnancy success of human in vitro fertilization in unstimulated cycles. Hum Reprod 1994; 9: 1571–5

38. Chian RC, Lim JH, Tan SL. State of the art in in vitro oocyte maturation. Curr Opin Obstet Gynecol 2004; 16: 211–19

39. Cha KY, Do BR, Chi HJ. Viability of human follicular oocytes collected from unstimulated ovaries and matured and fertilized in vitro. Reprod Fertil Dev 1992; 4: 695–701

40. Tsuji K, Sowa M, Nakano R. Relationship between human oocyte maturation and different follicular sizes. Biol Reprod 1985; 32: 413–17

41. Templeton AA, Van Look P, Angell RE, et al. Oocyte recovery and fertilization rates in women at various times after the administration of hCG. J Reprod Fertil 1986; 76: 771–8

42. Mikklesen AL, Smith SD, Lindenberg S. In vitro maturation of human oocytes from regular menstruating women may be successful without FSH priming. Hum Reprod 1999; 14: 1847–51

43. Shea BF, Baker RD, Latour JP. Human follicular ocytes and their maturation in vitro. Fertil Steril 1975; 26: 1075–82

44. Smith SD, Mikklesen A, Lindenberg S. Development of human oocytes matured in vitro for 28 or 36 hours. Fertil Steril 2000; 73: 541–4

45. Trouson A, Wood C, Kausche A. In vitro maturation and fertilization and developmental competence of oocytes recovered from untreated polycystic ovarian patients. Fertil Steril 1994; 62: 353–62

46. Barnes FL, Crombie A, Gardener DK, et al. Blastocyst development and birth after in vitro maturation of human primary oocytes, intracytoplasmic sperm injection, and assisted hatching. Hum Reprod 1995; 10: 3243–7

47. Barnes FL, Kausche A, Tiglias J, et al. Production of embryos from in vitro matured primary human oocytes. Fertil Steril 1996; 65: 1151–6

48. Suikkari AM, Tulppala M, Tuuri T, et al. Luteal phase start of low-dose FSH of follicles results in an efficient recovery, maturation and fertilization of immature human oocytes. Hum Reprod 2000; 15: 747–51

49. Cavilla JL, Kennedy CR, Baltsen M, et al. The effects of meiosis activating sterol on in vitro maturation and fertilization of human oocytes from stimulated and unstimulated ovaries. Hum Reprod 2001; 16: 547–55

50. MacDougall MJ, Tan SL, Jacobs HS. In vitro fertilization and ovarian hyperstimulation syndrome. Hum Reprod 1992; 7: 597–600

51. Trounson A, Anderiesz C, Jones GM, et al. Oocyte maturation. Hum Reprod 1998; 13 (Suppl 3): 52–62

52. Cha KY, Han SY, Chung HM, et al. Pregnancies and deliveries after in vitro maturation culture followed by in vitro fertilization and embryo transfer without stimulation in women with polycystic ovary syndrome. Fertil Steril 2000; 73: 978–83

53. Veeck LL, Wortham JW Jr, Witmyer J, et al. Maturation and fertilization of morphologically immature human oocytes in a program of in vitro fertilization. Fertil Steril 1983; 39: 594–602

54. Nagy ZP, Cecile J, Liu J, et al. Pregnancy and birth after intracytoplasmic sperm injection of in vitro matured germinal-vesicle stage oocytes: case report. Fertil Steril 1996; 65: 1047–50

55. Edirisinghe WR, Junk SM, Matson PL, Yovich JL. Birth from cryopreserved embryos following in-vitro maturation of oocytes and intracytoplasmic sperm injection. Hum Reprod 1997; 12: 1056–8

56. Check ML, Brittingham D, Check JH, Choe JK. Pregnancy following transfer of cryopreserved–thawed embryos that had been a result of fertilization of all in vitro matured metaphase or germinal stage oocytes. Case report. Clin Exp Obstet Gynecol 2001; 28: 69–70

57. Chian RC, Buckett WM, Too LL, Tan SL. Pregnancies resulting from in vitro matured oocytes retrieved from patients with polycystic ovary syndrome after priming with human chorionic gonadotropin. Fertil Steril 1999; 72: 639–42

58. Chian RC, Buckett WM, Tulandi T, Tan SL. Prospective randomized study of human chorionic gonadotrophin priming before immature oocyte

retrieval from unstimulated women with polycystic ovarian syndrome. Hum Reprod 2000; 15: 165–70

59. Lin YH, Hwang JH, Huang LW, et al. Combination of FSH priming and hCG priming for in-vitro maturation of human oocytes. Hum Reprod 2003; 18: 1632–6

60. Hwang JL, Lin YH, Tsai YL, et al. Oocyte donation using immature oocytes from a normal ovulatory woman. Acta Obstet Gynecol Scand 2002; 81: 274–5

61. Nagele F, Sator MO, Juza J, Huber JC. Successful pregnancy resulting from in-vitro matured oocytes retrieved at laparoscopic surgery in a patient with polycystic ovary syndrome. Hum Reprod 2002; 17: 373–4

62. Son WY, Yoon SH, Lee SW, et al. Blastocyst development and pregnancies after IVF of mature oocytes retrieved from unstimulated patients with PCOS after in-vivo HCG priming. Hum Reprod 2002; 17: 134–6

63. Yang S, Son W, Lee S, et al. Expression of luteinizing hormone receptor (LH-R), follicle stimulating hormone receptor (FSH-R) and epidermal growth factor receptor (EGF-R) in cumulus cells of the oocytes collected from PCOS patients in hCG-priming IVM/F–ET program. Fertil Steril 2001; 76 (Suppl 3S): S38–S100

64. Wynn P, Picton HM, Krapez J, et al. Pretreatment with follicle stimulating hormone promotes the number of human oocytes reaching metaphase II by in vitro maturation. Hum Reprod 1998; 13: 3132–8

65. Liu J, Katz E, Garcia JE, et al. Successful in vitro maturation of human oocytes not exposed to human chorionic gonadotropin during ovulation induction, resulting in pregnancy. Fertil Steril 1997; 67: 566–8

66. Mikkelsen AL, Lindenberg S. Benefit of FSH priming of women with PCOS to the in vitro maturation procedure and the outcome: a randomized prospective study. Reproduction 2001; 122: 587–92

67. Jaroudi KA, Hollanders JMG, Elnour AM et al. Pregnancy after transfer of embryos which were generated from in-vitro matured oocytes. Hum Reprod 1997; 12: 857–9

68. Lim KS, Son WY, Yoon SH, et al. IVM/F–ET in stimulated cycles for the prevention of OHSS. Fertil Steril 2002; 76 (Suppl 3S): S11–S25

69. Liu J, Lu G, Qian Y, et al. Pregnancies and births achieved from in vitro matured oocytes retrieved from poor responders undergoing stimulation in in vitro fertilization cycles. Fertil Steril 2003; 80: 447–9

70. Gulekli B, Child TJ, Chian RC, Tan SL. Immature oocytes from unstimulated polycystic ovaries: a new source of oocytes for donation. Reprod Technol 2001; 10: 295–7

71. Scharf E, Chian RC, Abdul-Jalil K, et al. In vitro maturation of oocytes: a new option for donor oocyte treatment. Fertil Steril 2004; 82 (Suppl 2): 514

72. Oktay K, Buyuk E, Veeck L, et al. Embryo development after heterotopic transplantation of cryopreserved ovarian tissue. Lancet 2004; 363: 837–40

73. Prest SJ, May FE, Westley BR. The estrogen-regulated protein, TFF1, stimulates migration of human breast cancer cells. FASEB J 2002; 16: 592–4

74. Rao GD, Chian RC, Son WS, et al. Fertility preservation in women undergoing cancer treatment. Lancet 2004; 363: 1829–30

75. Silverberg K, Daya S, Auray JP, et al. Analysis of the cost effectiveness of recombinant versus urinary follicle-stimulating hormone in in vitro fertilization/intracytoplasmic sperm injection programs in the United States. Fertil Steril 2002; 77: 107–13

76. Society for Assisted Reproductive Technology/American Society for Reproductive Medicine. Assisted reproductive technology in the United States: 2000 results generated from the American Society for Reproductive Medicine/Society for Assisted Reproductive Technology Registry. Fertil Steril 2004; 81: 1207–20

77. Human Fertilisation and Embryology Authority. The Patient's Guide to IVF Clinics. London: HFEA, 1999

78. Child TJ, Phillips SJ, Abdul-Jalil AK, et al. A comparison of in vitro maturation and in vitro fertilization in women with polycystic ovaries. Obstet Gynecol 2002; 100: 665–70

79. Hardy K, Wright CS, Franks S, Winston RM. In vitro maturation of oocytes. Br Med Bull 2000; 56: 588–602

80. Picton H, Platteau P, Grondhal C. The impact of different culture environments on the in vitro maturation potential and genetics of human oocytes. Presented at the 11th World Congress on Human Reproduction, Montreal, Canada 2002: 20

81. Mikkelsen AL, Ravn SH, Lindenberg S. Evaluation of newborns delivered after in vitro maturation. Hum Reprod 2003; 18 (Suppl 1): O–018

82. Buckett WM, Chian RC, Barrington K, et al. Obstetric, neonatal and infant outcome in babies conceived by in vitro maturation (IVM): initial five year results 1998–2003. Fertil Steril 2004; 82 (Suppl 2): 5133

25

Preimplantation genetic diagnosis and its role in assisted reproduction technology

Yury Verlinsky and Anver Kuliev

INTRODUCTION

Preimplantation genetic diagnosis (PGD) is becoming an established approach to detect and avoid transferring embryos with genetic abnormalities as an alternative to the transfer of embryos based on morphological criteria, which is currently practiced in *in vitro* fertilization (IVF)[1–4]. PGD was first performed for X-linked disorders using blastomere biopsy and gender determination[5], and for autosomal recessive conditions using polar body (PB) removal and specific genetic diagnosis[6]. At present, PGD may be performed by

three major approaches, including first and second PB (PB1 and PB2) removal following maturation and fertilization of oocytes (Figure 1), blastomere biopsy at the cleavage stage (Figure 2) and blastocyst biopsy. The biopsied material is tested for single gene disorders using polymerase chain reaction (PCR) analysis, or for chromosomal abnormalities using fluorescence *in situ* hybridization (FISH) analysis[7,8].

Each of these PGD methods has advantages and disadvantages, and their choice depends on circumstances; however, in some cases the combination of two or three methods may be required. Despite a

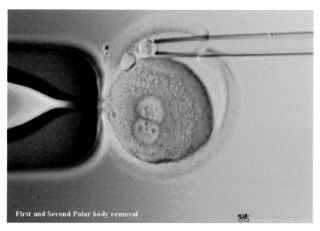

Figure 1 Procedure of simultaneous first and second polar body sampling

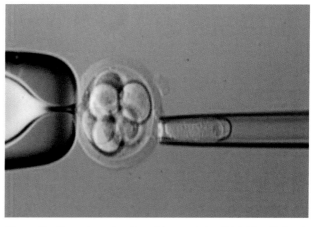

Figure 2 Procedure of embryo biopsy at day 3 (eight-cell stage)

possible embryo cell number reduction, which might have a potential influence on embryo viability, blastomere biopsy allows the detection of paternally derived abnormalities. Removal of PB1 and PB2, on the other hand, should not have any effect on embryo viability, as they are naturally extruded from oocytes as a result of maturation and fertilization; however, they provide no information on paternally derived anomalies, even if this constitutes less than 10% of chromosomal errors in preimplantation embryos.

To perform PGD for chromosomal aneuploidies, both PB1 and PB2 are removed simultaneously the next day after insemination of the matured oocytes or intracytoplasmic sperm injection (ICSI) (Figure 1), and analyzed by FISH, as described elsewhere[7,8]. PB1 is the by-product of the first meiotic division and normally contains a double signal for each chromosome, each representing a single chromatid (Figure 3). Accordingly, in case of meiosis I error, instead of a double signal, four different patterns might be observed, ranging from no or one signal to three or four signals, suggesting either chromosomal non-disjunction, evidenced by no or four signals, or chromatid mis-segregation, represented by one or three signals. The genotype of the oocytes will, accordingly, be opposite to the PB1 genotype, i.e. missing signals will suggest extra chromosome material in the corresponding oocyte, while an extra signal (or signals) will indicate monosomy or nullisomy status of the tested chromosome. In contrast to PB1, the normal FISH pattern of PB2 is represented by one signal for each chromosome (chromatid), so any deviation from this, such as no or two signals instead of one, will suggest a meiosis II error.

The method of blastomere biopsy (Figure 2) has been extensively used, despite its limitation due to a high mosaicism rate in cleaving embryos[9-13]. The FISH pattern of blastomeres is represented by two signals for each chromosome tested (Figure 3), so any deviation from this pattern suggests the chromosomal abnormality. The same pattern applies to blastocyst analysis, which has the advantage of analyzing not one but a group of cells, obviating the problem of mosaicism, at least to some extent.

Although more data have to be collected to exclude short-term and/or long-term side-effects completely, the data currently available show no evidence of any detrimental effect of PB, blastomere or blastocyst biopsy[4,14,15]. Overall, PGD for aneuploidy has been applied in more than 5000 clinical cycles, and

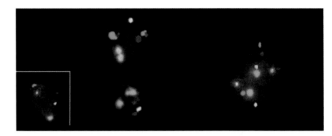

Figure 3 Normal pattern of fluorescence *in situ* hybridization (FISH) signals for chromosomes 13, 16, 18, 21 and 22 in the first (middle) and second (left) polar bodies and blastomeres (right). Left panel shows double signals for each chromosome in the first polar body (middle panel), and single signals for each chromosome in the second polar body (left panel)

resulted in the birth of at least 1000 unaffected children, showing a comparable prevalence of congenital abnormalities to that in the general population[14], which suggests that there is no detrimental effect of any of the biopsy procedures mentioned above.

CHROMOSOMAL ANEUPLOIDIES IN PREIMPLANTATION DEVELOPMENT

The majority of chromosomal abnormalities originate from female meiosis, which, according to DNA polymorphism studies, derive mainly from meiosis I[16-19]. Common trisomies were shown to increase with maternal age, which may be due to the age-related reduction of meiotic recombination[17-19]. However, these data are inferred from the study of aneuploidies compatible with birth or recognized pregnancies, while only limited data are available on direct testing of the outcome of the first and second meiotic divisions[20].

The usefulness of PGD in assisted reproduction is obvious from data on the prevalence of chromosomal abnormalities in oocytes obtained from women of 35 years and older (average age 38.5 years)[20]. In a large series of 6733 oocytes obtained from 1297 PGD cycles, 3509 (52%) were aneuploid, based on FISH analysis using specific probes for chromosomes 13, 16, 18, 21 and 22. Overall, 41.8% oocytes were demonstrated to be with meiosis I errors, and 37.3% with meiosis II errors (Figure 4). So in contrast to the expected predominance of chromosomal abnormalities of female meiosis I origin, the above results suggest that chromosomal errors originate comparably in meiosis I and meiosis II (Figure 4). These results are of

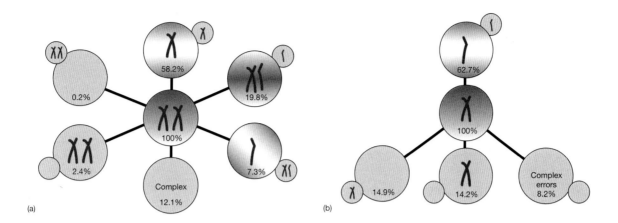

Figure 4 Meiosis I and meiosis II errors. (a) Meiosis I errors observed in fluorescence *in situ* hybridization (FISH) analysis of oocytes in women of advanced reproductive age. Upper center: normal segregation of homologs in the first meiotic division, resulting in extrusion of the first polar body (PB1) (smaller circle) containing one of the homologs (58.2%). Accordingly, the resulting secondary (metaphase II) oocyte contains the remaining homolog with two chromatids (bigger circle). Upper left: chromosomal non-disjunction in meiosis I resulting in nullisomy in metaphase II (MII) oocyte. Lower left: chromosomal non-disjunction in meiosis I resulting in disomy in MII oocyte. Upper right: chromatid malsegregation in meiosis I resulting in extrusion of only one chromatid instead of two, which leads to formation of MII oocyte with extra chromatid. Lower right: chromatid malsegregation in meiosis I resulting in extrusion of three instead of two chromatids, which leads to formation of MII oocyte with missing chromatid. Lower center: complex errors, resulting from different types of errors involving different chromosomes. (b) Meiosis II errors in FISH analysis of oocytes from women of advanced reproductive age. Upper center: overall proportion of oocytes with normal (62.7%) patterns following meiosis II. Normal segregation of chromatids, resulting in extrusion of the second polar body (PB2) (smaller circle) containing one of the chromatids (62.7%). Accordingly, the resulting oocyte contains the remaining single chromatid (bigger circle). Lower part of figure: abnormal segregation in meiosis II detected through PB2 testing (37.3%), including extrusion of both chromatids with PB2, resulting in nullisomy in oocyte (lower left); chromatid mis-segregation leading to extrusion of PB2 containing no chromosome material, with both chromatids remaining in oocyte, resulting in disomic oocyte (34.6%) (lower middle); and different types of errors of different chromosomes (lower right)

clinical significance, as the genotype of the resulting zygotes cannot be predicted without testing of the outcome of both meiotic divisions. For example, testing of meiosis I errors alone should reduce the aneuploidy rate in embryos by at least two-thirds[20]. Despite the fact that approximately one-third of these oocytes will be aneuploid following the second meiotic division, PB1 testing could still improve implantation and pregnancy rates sufficiently in poor-prognosis IVF or ICSI patients, by applying ICSI selectively to oocytes with aneuploidy-free PB1[21]. On the other hand, only half of the abnormalities deriving from second meiotic division may be detected by PB1 analysis, so to avoid transfer of all embryos resulting from aneuploid oocytes, testing of both PB1 and PB2 will still be required. As PB1 and PB2 have no biological significance in pre- and postimplantation development, their removal and testing may become a useful tool in assisted reproduction practices to identify the aneuploidy-free oocytes, which should help in preselecting oocytes with the highest potential for

establishing viable pregnancies and thus improving IVF efficiency.

The above aneuploidy rate in oocytes is comparable to that in preimplantation embryos, which was shown to be approximately 60%[13,22–24]. Types of chromosomal abnormalities, however, are different, mainly attributable to a high frequency of mosaicism in embryos, constituting up to half of chromosomal abnormalities at the cleavage stage. A significant proportion of mosaic embryos may originate from aneuploid zygotes, through mitotic non-disjunction in the first cleavage divisions. A possible higher rate of mitotic errors in cleaving embryos, deriving from oocytes with complex errors, may also explain a phenomenon of chaotic embryos, which make up almost half of the embryos with mosaicism.

More than 40% of abnormal oocytes from women of advanced reproductive age were found to have complex errors, including an error of the same chromosome in both meiotic divisions (21.5%), or an error of different chromosomes (78.5%)[20]. In addition to the age-related alterations in recombination rates, this may also be due to spindle formation errors, which were reported to increase with age[25,26]. Because more than one-third of aneuploidies in oocytes and preimplantation embryos are of a complex nature, testing for only five chromosomes could probably contribute to detecting the majority of aneuploid oocytes and embryos.

However, there is still need for the development of methods for full karyotyping of oocytes and embryos, which currently include the use of nuclear transfer techniques for PB or blastomere nuclear conversion[27–29] combined with FISH analysis or spectral karyotyping[30], and the application of comparative genome hybridization (CGH)[31–34]. These methods may enable the detection and exclusion from transfer of aneuploid embryos, of which a certain proportion could have been misdiagnosed as normal by the commercially available FISH probes, although there are still important limitations to these highly labor-intensive procedures.

Even with possible progress in full karyotyping, the accuracy of PGD for aneuploidies will depend on avoiding misdiagnosis due to mosaicism at the cleavage stage. Assuming that every second embryo may be mosaic at the cleavage or blastocyst stage, it will be of importance to obtain the meiosis information for each embryo, so that false-negative diagnosis may be avoided. A few misdiagnoses observed in PGD for aneuploidy performed at the cleavage stage may be explained by false-negative diagnosis determined by mosaicism[35].

To investigate whether day-3 blastomere analysis accurately represents the numerical status of embryos, a few follow-up studies have recently been performed by reanalysis of the embryos on day 5[36,37]. In one of these studies 660 embryos from 94 PGD cycles were biopsied, removing a single blastomere, which was tested using FISH probes specific for chromosomes 13, 18, 21, X and Y. Of 367 embryos free from aneuploidy, 213 were transferred, while 86 of them, as well as 281 aneuploid embryos, were further cultured to day 6. Those reaching the blastocyst stage, including 54 (62.8%) with predicted normal and 74 (26.3%) with aneuploidies, were reanalyzed, demonstrating concordance in only 60.7% of embryos, with the remaining being misdiagnosed[36]. In the other study, a two-blastomere biopsy from 17 day 3-embryos was performed and tested using FISH probes specific for

chromosomes 1, 7, 13, 15, 16, 18, 21, 22, X and Y, and the embryos were then followed up on day 5. The initial diagnosis was confirmed in only ten of 17 embryos, while the remaining had a false positive (six embryos) or a false-negative (one embryo) diagnosis[37].

Thus, testing of one and even two blastomeres at the cleavage stage might not represent the actual chromosome number in the embryo, with the possibility of misdiagnosis due to mosaicism. For example, a normal karyotype of an embryo deriving from an oocyte with missing or extra chromosome material will mean that the embryo is mosaic for this particular chromosome, so the transfer of this embryo may result in spontaneous abortion or birth of a chromosomally abnormal baby. In contrast, missing or extra chromosomes in an embryo originating from a chromosomally normal oocyte will suggest either a paternally derived abnormality, or aneuploidy deriving primarily from mitotic errors. Therefore, the diagnostic accuracy may be improved by a combination of PB and blastomere testing.

CHROMOSOMAL TRANSLOCATIONS

Because carriers of translocations have an extremely poor pregnancy outcome, translocations have been one of the most important indications for PGD, which was first performed by PB1 analysis using whole painting probes in a combination of centromeric and/or subtelomeric probes[38,39]. However, because without PB2 the meiotic outcome of translocations cannot be accurately established, especially in cases of chromatid exchange[40], interphase blastomere analysis was used in most cases, despite a limited availability of probes and an inability to distinguish normal from balanced translocation embryos[13,41,42].

In our experience of 162 PGD cycles for translocations, the majority were performed utilizing the nuclear conversion method, involving fusion of single blastomeres with enucleated or intact mouse zygotes, followed by fixing the resulting heterokaryons at the metaphase of the first cleavage division, or treating them with okadaic acid to induce premature chromosome condensation. Overall, the technique was applied to 437 blastomeres, which included 333 for reciprocal and 104 for Robertsonian translocations, resulting in successful nuclear metaphase conversion in as many as 383 (88%) blastomeres. This made possible the preselection of normal embryos or those with a balanced chromosomal complement for transfer in 73% of the cycles, yielding a 29% pregnancy rate.

In 38 PGD cycles from couples with maternally derived translocations, testing was performed using PB1 and PB2 FISH analysis. Of 446 oocytes from these cycles tested, FISH results were available in 351 (79%), allowing preselection of normal or balanced embryos for transfer in 71.4% of the cycles, resulting in a 36% clinical pregnancy rate and births of healthy children. The confirmatory testing was possible in two of three spontaneously aborted embryos, showing the presence of *de novo* translocations different from the expected meiotic outcomes.

The proportion of abnormal oocytes and embryos detected varied, depending on the type of translocations and their origin. The results of testing for maternally or paternally derived reciprocal or Robertsonian translocations showed that testing of 382 embryos from 44 PGD cycles for maternally derived reciprocal translocations resulted in the prediction of 76.4% unbalanced embryos, leaving only 23.6% suitable for transfer, among which 11.3% were determined to be balanced and 12.3% normal. On the other hand, the testing of 214 embryos from 32 PGD cycles for paternally derived reciprocal translocations resulted in the prediction of 68.2% unbalanced embryos, leaving 31.8% embryos suitable for transfer, among which 13.1% were determined to be balanced and 18.7% normal.

Testing of 101 embryos obtained from 12 PGD cycles for maternally derived Robertsonian translocations resulted in the prediction of 71.3% unbalanced embryos, with the remaining 28.7% embryos suitable for transfer, which included 15.8% balanced and 12.9% normal embryos. Similarly, the testing of 50 embryos obtained from six PGD cycles for paternally derived Robertsonian translocations allowed identification of 56% unbalanced embryos, with the remaining 44% suitable for transfer, including 22% balanced and 22% normal ones.

The overall results for the total of 162 PGD cycles for translocation show that normal/balanced embryos were available for transfer in 112 (69%) of the clinical cycles. Thirty-nine (35%) clinical pregnancies resulted from 112 transfer cycles in which the mean number of embryos transferred was 1.7, of which 27 resulted in the delivery of 30 healthy children. Data on pregnancy

outcomes prior to undertaking PGD were available in more than 100 couples with translocations, suggesting a tremendous positive impact of PGD on the clinical outcome of pregnancies in couples carrying both reciprocal and Robertsonian translocations (see below).

The detection rate of embryos suitable for transfer clearly depends on the type of translocation tested. For example, the clinical outcome is poorer in reciprocal than in Robertsonian translocations, with pregnancy rates of 23% and 33%, respectively, based on the analysis of data from PGD cycles for maternally derived translocations. As may be predicted, there is also a correspondence between poorer clinical outcome and the proportion of unbalanced embryos in these PGD cycles.

Although application of the conversion technique to visualize chromosomes in single blastomeres improves the accuracy of diagnosis by analysis of metaphase chromosomes using a combination of commercially available probes, a high frequency of mosaicism in cleavage stage embryos, arising from anaphase lag or nuclear fragmentation, still presents problems for diagnosis. Follow-up analysis of 78 unbalanced embryos, including those in which chromatid malsegregation or recombination was identified by the analysis of PB1, and subsequent testing of PB2 implied a balanced or normal embryo, revealed a mosaicism rate of 41%. Different cell lines were present, including normal or balanced, which, if investigated only by embryo biopsy, may have led to misdiagnosis. Therefore, for maternally derived translocations the PGD strategy may still be based on PB1 and PB2 testing, applying the blastomere nucleus conversion technique only if further testing is required.

We have also observed that embryos with unbalanced chromosome complements have the potential to reach the blastocyst stage of embryo development in extended culture. Of 538 (76%) unbalanced embryos identified from 707 embryos with FISH results, 250 were cultured for a further period, of which many (78; 3%) reached the blastocyst stage, confirming our previous results, that some of the detected chromosomal rearrangements may not be lethal in preimplantation development, but are eliminated, during either implantation or postimplantation development[43], explaining an extremely high spontaneous abortion rate in couples carrying translocations.

Because PGD is practically the only hope for couples with translocations to have an unaffected child without fear of repeated spontaneous abortions, increasing numbers of PGD cycles for this indication have been performed. Approximately 500 clinical cycles have been undertaken to date, resulting in more than 100 clinical pregnancies and births of unaffected children[44].

The presented data suggest that PGD is of special relevance for poor-prognosis IVF patients carrying translocations, as these patients are at an extremely high risk for implantation failure or spontaneous abortion, if they become pregnant. Awareness of the availability of PGD will permit these couples to establish pregnancies which are unaffected from the onset, and offer them the opportunity to have children of their own, instead of multiple unsuccessful attempts of prenatal diagnosis and subsequent termination of pregnancy.

THE IMPACT OF PGD ON IVF OUTCOME

As shown above, more than half of embryos obtained from poor-prognosis IVF patients are chromosomally abnormal from the outset, so PGD for chromosomal aneuploidy should allow avoidance of these embryos for transfer, and contribute to an improvement of the pregnancy outcome of IVF patients of advanced reproductive age. The majority of these chromosomally abnormal embryos seem to be eliminated before implantation, as only one in ten of recognized pregnancies are chromosomally abnormal. Incidental transfer of these embryos in the absence of chromosomal testing could lead to implantation and pregnancy failures in IVF patients of advanced reproductive age, or may compromise the pregnancy outcome by leading to spontaneous abortions. To 2004, PGD for chromosomal disorders had been applied in approximately 5000 IVF cycles[44], resulting in improved implantation and pregnancy rates in patients of advanced reproductive age and those with translocations.

The clinical impact of aneuploidy testing, in terms of improved outcome of pregnancies through the reduction of spontaneous abortions, has been observed not only for IVF patients with advanced reproductive age, but also for other poor-prognosis patients, including those with repeated IVF failures and repeated spontaneous abortions[22,23,35,45–49]. Although

randomized controlled studies will still be required to quantify further the clinical impact of preselection of aneuploidy-free zygotes for embryo transfer, the available results suggest the clinical relevance of the preselection of aneuploidy-free oocytes and embryos. It is obvious, however, that an improvement of the outcome of PGD may be expected only when the number of embryos biopsied is equal to or higher than the number of embryos expected to be replaced without PGD[13,49].

The positive impact of PGD is particularly obvious from comparison of reproductive outcomes in the same patients with and without PGD, as previous reproductive experience of the patients is the best control for PGD impact. In one such series, in which the outcome of transfer of 318 FISH-normal embryos was analyzed, an implantation rate of 65.1% in pregnant patients was observed, with a total of 161 clinical pregnancies generated. These resulted in the birth of 153 children from 125 couples, and 26 spontaneous abortions, giving a take-home-baby rate of 82.3%[50]. Of 161 couples involved in the study, 41 were in their first cycle; 14 had experienced 31 spontaneous pregnancies, with 29 abortions and two deliveries; and there was only one birth in the remaining 27 couples. A total of 367 cycles were completed by 120 of these couples before undertaking PGD, with 30 pregnancies; five went to term and 25 aborted. These couples had also experienced 50 spontaneous pregnancies; three carried to term and 47 aborted. The overall implantation rate derived from their previous reproductive experience was 13.0% and the take-home-baby rate 6.8%. These data make obvious the clinical usefulness of PGD for IVF patients with poor reproductive performance.

In a similar study, we analyzed 431 outcomes of pregnancies obtained from PGD cycles performed in 432 patients (mean patient age 37 years), involving a combined PB1, PB2 and blastomere FISH analysis for 5–9 chromosomes (chromosomes 13, 15, 16, 17, 18, 21, 22, X and Y), resulting in the transfer of 1462 aneuploidy-free embryos. The data were compared with the outcome of all previous pregnancies of the same patients, whether achieved following IVF (239 pregnancies) or spontaneous (529 pregnancies). Implantation, spontaneous abortions and take-home-baby rates were analyzed before and after PGD; rates appeared to be significantly improved after PGD. For example, the implantation rate prior to PGD was only

7.2%, in contrast to 34.8% after PGD, an almost five-fold improvement. As expected, there was also a significant reduction in the spontaneous abortion rate, which was 80% before and 26.9% after PGD. Accordingly, this contributed to a more than two-fold increase in the take-home-baby rate after PGD, which was as high as 65.7% in PGD cycles compared with 27.9% without PGD (Figure 5; Verlinsky *et al.*, unpublished data).

The impact was even higher in translocation patients, with an implantation rate after PGD as high as 61.6%. A comparison of spontaneous abortion rates before and after PGD revealed an almost six-fold reduction: 87.8% before and 15.6% after PGD. The take-home-baby rate in these patients was only 11.5% before PGD and was 79.4% after PGD application (Verlinsky *et al.*, unpublished data).

In the light of these data, the current IVF practice of selection of embryos for transfer based on morphological criteria may hardly be an acceptable procedure for IVF patients of advanced reproductive age in the future. In addition to an extremely high risk of establishing an affected pregnancy from the outset, this will significantly compromise the very poor chances of these patients becoming pregnant, especially with the current tendency of limiting the number of transferred embryos to only two, thus leaving only a single embryo on average with a potential chance of reaching a term pregnancy. Although culturing embryos to day 5 (blastocyst) before transfer may allow, to some extent, preselection of developmentally more competent embryos, compared with day 3, at least some aneuploid embryos will still be capable of developing to the blastocyst stage[51–53]. Thus, these abnormal embryos will not be eliminated in the current trend of blastocyst transfer, and may implant and lead to spontaneous abortions, compromising the outcome of pregnancies resulting from normal implanted embryos in multiple gestations. In fact, multiple pregnancies represent a severe complication of IVF, which may in future be avoided by the preselection and transfer of a single blastocyst with the greatest developmental potential to result in a healthy pregnancy. Such testing is currently possible for nuclear abnormalities, and may soon become realistic for cytoplasmic disorders as well.

Avoiding multiple pregnancies through the use of PGD may contribute to avoiding low-birth-weight babies and congenital malformations, reported

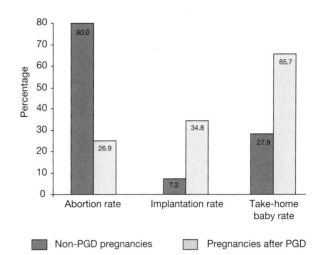

Figure 5 Outcome of 432 pregnancies before and after preimplantation genetic diagnosis (PGD) (see explanation in text): mean age 37 ± 3.3 years

recently in association with IVF[54,55]. It could also be expected that PGD may allow the prevention of at least some imprinting disorders, which have also recently been reported to be associated with assisted reproductive technologies (ART)[56–61]. Although the causative relationship between imprinting disorders and ART is still not understood, avoiding the transfer of embryos originating from meiotic errors may also reduce the chances of transferring embryos with uniparental disomies, one of the possible contributors to imprinting disorders.

While it may be predicted that PGD will soon become standard practice for IVF patients of advanced reproductive age, it cannot be excluded that preselection of aneuploidy-free embryos may appear of even higher value for younger IVF patients, because of the higher number of oocytes available for testing. This may contribute to improving overall standards of assisted reproduction practice, by substituting the present practice of selection of embryos for transfer using morphological parameters with the preselection of chromosomally normal embryos with a higher potential of resulting in a normal pregnancy.

CONCLUSION

There is clear evidence of the clinical usefulness of PGD for assisted reproduction, as more than half of preimplantation embryos are chromosomally abnormal from the outset, and should be avoided for transfer to IVF patients of advanced reproductive age. Therefore, further improvement of IVF efficiency seems to be unrealistic without application of the preselection of aneuploidy-free oocytes and embryos. With the current tendency towards blastocyst transfer and limiting the number of transferred embryos to only two or one, preselection of aneuploidy-free embryos may soon become standard IVF practice, since there is no sense in deliberately transferring aneuploid embryos, thus compromising the IVF outcome in the traditional setting. Information on the availability of PGD should therefore be provided to at least women of advanced reproductive age or poor-prognosis IVF patients, so that they may have the opportunity of improving their chances of becoming pregnant and avoiding the establishment of a pregnancy destined to be lost due to aneuploidy. The clinical outcomes currently available for hundreds of pregnancies resulting from PGD of aneuploidies demonstrate its positive impact on implantation and pregnancy rates, as well as on the improvement of pregnancy outcomes.

REFERENCES

1. Verlinsky Y, Kuliev A. Preimplantation Diagnosis of Genetic Diseases: a New Technique in Assisted Reproduction. New York: Wiley-Liss, 1993
2. International Working Group on Preimplantation Genetics. Preimplantation genetic diagnosis – experience of three thousand clinical cycles. Report of the 11th Annual Meeting International Working Group on Preimplantation Genetics, in conjunction with 10th International Congress of Human Genetics, Vienna, May 15, 2001. Reprod Biomed Online 2001; 3: 49–53
3. Munné S, Cohen J, Sable D. Preimplantation genetic diagnosis for advance maternal age and other indications. Fertil Steril 2002; 78: 234–36
4. Verlinsky Y, Cohen J, Munné S, et al. Over a decade of preimplantation genetic diagnosis experience – a multicenter report. Fertil Steril 2004; 82: 292–4
5. Handyside AH, Kontogiani EH, Hardy K, Winston RML. Pregnancies from biopsied human preimplantation embryos sexed by Y-specific DNA amplification. Nature (London) 1990; 344: 768
6. Verlinsky Y, Ginsberg N, Lifchez A, et al. Analysis of the first polar body: preconception genetic diagnosis, Hum Reprod 1990; 5: 826–9
7. Verlinsky Y, Cieslak J, Kuliev A. Preimplantation FISH diagnosis of aneuploidies. In Fan Y, ed. Molecular Cytogenetics: Protocols and Applications. Totowa, NJ: Humana Press, 2002: 259–73
8. Verlinsky Y, Kuliev A. Atlas of Preimplantation Genetic Diagnosis. Carnforth, UK: Parthenon Publishing, 2004
9. Munné S, Weier HUG, Grifo J, Cohen J. Chromosome mosaicism in human embryos. Biol Reprod 1994; 51: 373–9
10. Delhanty JDA, Griffin DK, Handyside AH. Detection of aneuploidy and chromosomal mosaicism in human embryos during preimplantation sex determination by fluorescent in situ hybridisation (FISH). Hum Mol Genet 1993; 2: 1183–5
11. Harper JC, Coonen E, Handyside AH, et al. Mosaicism of autosomes and sex chromosomes in morphologically normal monospermic preimplantation human embryos. Prenat Diagn 1994; 15: 41–9
12. International Working Group on Preimplantation Genetics. Current status of preimplantation diagnosis. J Assist Reprod Genet 1997; 14: 72–5
13. Munné S. Preimplantation genetic diagnosis of numerical and structural chromosome abnormalities. Reprod Biomed Online 2002; 4: 183–96
14. Kuliev A, Verlinsky Y. Current feature of preimplantation genetic diagnosis. Reprod Biomed Online 2002; 5: 296–301
15. ESHRE Preimplantation Genetic Diagnosis Consortium. Data Collection III, May 2002. Hum Reprod 2002; 17: 233–46
16. Peterson MB, Mikkelsen M. Nondisjunction in trisomy 21: origin and mechanisms. Cytogenet Cell Genet 2000; 91: 199–203
17. Sherman SL, Peterson MB, Freeman SB, et al. Nondisjunction of chromosome 21 in maternal meiosis I: evidence for a maternal age-dependent mechanism involving reduced recombination. Hum Mol Genet 1994; 3: 1529–35
18. Hassold T, Merril M, Adkins K, et al. Recombination and maternal age-dependent nondisjunction: molecular studies of trisomy 16. Am J Hum Genet 1995; 57: 867–74
19. Lamb NE, Freeman S, Savage-Austin A, et al. Susceptible chiasmate configurations of chromosome 21 predispose to nondisjunction in both maternal meiosis I, and meiosis II. Nat Genet 1996; 14: 400–5
20. Kuliev A, Cieslak J, Illkewitch Y, Verlinsky Y. Chromosomal abnormalities in a series of 6733 human oocytes in preimplantation diagnosis of age-related aneuploidies. Reprod Biomed Online 2003; 6: 54–9
21. Munné S, Sepulveda S, Bolmaceda J, et al. Selection of the most common chromosome abnormalities in

oocytes prior to ICSI. Prenat Diagn 2000; 7: 582–6

22. Gianaroli L, Magli MC, Ferraretti AP, et al. Preimplantation genetic analysis increases the implantation rate in human in vitro fertilization with poor prognosis by avoiding the transfer of chromosomally abnormal embryos. Fertil Steril 1997; 68: 1128–91

23. Gianaroli L, Magli MC, Ferraretti AP, Munné S. Preimplantation diagnosis for aneuploidies in patients undergoing in vitro fertilization with poor prognosis: identification of the categories for which it should be proposed. Fertil Steril 1999; 72: 837–44

24. Kahraman S, Benkalifa M, Donmez E, et al. Overall results of aneuploidy screening in 276 couples undergoing assisted reproductive techniques. Prenat Diagn 2004; 24: 307–11

25. Eichenlaub-Ritter U, Shen Y, Tinneberg U. Manipulation of the oocytes: possible damage to the spindle apparatus. Reprod Biomed Online 2002; 5: 117–24

26. Battaglia DE, Goodwin P, Klein NA, Soules MR. Influence of maternal age on meiotic spindle assembly in oocytes from naturally cycling women. Hum Reprod 1996; 11: 2217–22

27. Verlinsky Y, Evsikov S. Karyotyping of human oocytes by chromosomal analysis of the second polar body. Mol Hum Reprod 1999; 5: 89–95

28. Verlinsky Y, Evsikov S. A simplified and efficient method for obtaining metaphase chromosomes from individual human blastomeres. Fertil Steril 1999; 72: 1–6

29. Willadsen S, Levron J, Munné S, et al. Rapid visualization of metaphase chromosomes in single human blastomeres after fusion with in-vitro matured bovine eggs. Hum Reprod 1999; 14: 470–5

30. Marquez C, Sandalinas M, Bahce M, et al. Chromosomal abnormalities in 1255 cleavage-stage human embryos. Reprod Biomed Online 2000; 1: 17–27

31. Voullaire L, Slater H, Williamson R, Wilton L. Chromosome analysis of identified blastomeres from human embryos by using comparative genomic hybridization. Hum Genet 2000; 106: 210–17

32. Wells D, Delhanty DA. Comprehensive chromosomal analysis of human preimplantation embryos using whole genome amplification and single cell comparative genomic hybridization. Mol Hum Reprod 2000; 6: 1055–62

33. Wilton L, Williamson R, McBain J, et al. Birth of healthy infant after preimplantation confirmation of euploidy by comparative genomic hybridization. N Engl J Med 2001; 345: 1537–41

34. Voullaire L, Wilton L, McBain J, et al. Chromosome abnormalities identified by comparative genomic hybridization in embryos from women with repeated

implantation failure. Mol Hum Reprod 2002; 11: 1035–41

35. Gianaroli L, Magli MC, Ferraretti AP. The in vivo and in vitro efficiency and efficacy of PGD for aneuploidy. Mol Cell Endocrinol 2001; 183: S13–18

36. Li M, Hill D, Danzer H, Surrey M. FISH reanalysis on day 6 blastocysts diagnosed as aneuploidy on day 3: does day 3 single cell analysis accurately represent the numerical chromosomeal status of the embryo? Fertil Steril 2004; 81(Suppl): S11

37. Baart EB, Van Opstal D, Los FL, et al. Fluorescent in situ hybridization analysis of two blastomeres from day 3 frozen-thawed embryos followed by analysis of the remaining embryo on day 5. Hum Reprod 2004; 19: 685–93

38. Munné S, Scott R, Sable D, Cohen J. First pregnancies after preconception diagnosis of translocations of maternal origin. Fertil Steril 1998; 69: 675–81

39. Munné S, Morrison L, Fung J, et al, Spontaneous abortions are significantly reduced after preconception genetic diagnosis of translocations. J Assist Reprod Genet 1998; 15: 290–6

40. Munné S, Bahce M, Schimmel T, et al. Case report: chromatid exchange and predivision of chromatids as other sources of abnormal oocytes detected by preimplantation genetic diagnosis of translocations. Prenat Diagn 1998; 18: 1450–8

41. Munné S, Sandalinas M, Escudero T, et al. Outcome of premplantation genetic diagnosis of translocations. Fertil Steril 2000; 73: 1209–18

42. Verlinsky Y, Cieslak J, Evsikov S, et al. Nuclear transfer for full karyotyping and preimplantation diagnosis for translocations. Reprod Biomed Online 2002; 4: 300–5

43. Evsikov S, Cieslak J, Verlinsky Y. Survival of unbalanced translocations to blastocyst stage. Fertil Steril 2000; 74: 672–6

44. Kuliev A, Verlinsky Y. Thirteen years' experience of preimplantation diagnosis: report of the Fifth International Symposium on Preimplantation Genetics. Reprod Biomed Online 2004; 8: 229–35

45. Munné S, Magli C, Cohen J, et al. Positive outcome after preimplantation diagnosis of aneuploidy in human embryos. Hum Reprod 1999; 14: 2191–9

46. Kahraman S, Bahce M, Samli H, et al. Healthy births and ongoing pregnancies obtained by preimplantation genetic diagnosis in patients with advanced maternal age and recurrent implantation failures. Hum Reprod 2000; 15: 2003–7

47. International Working Group on Preimplantation Genetics. Tenth Anniversary of Preimplantation Genetic Diagnosis: Report of the 10th Annual Meeting International Working Group on Preimlantation Genetics, in association with 3rd International

Symposium on Preimplantation Genetics, Bologna, Italy, June 23, 2000. J Assist Reprod Genet 2001; 18: 66–72

48. Verlinsky Y, Cieslak J, Ivakhnenko V, et al. Chromosomal abnormalities in the first and second polar body. Mol Cell Endocrinol 2001; 183: S47–9

49. Munné S, Sandalinas M, Escudero T, et al. Improved implantation after preimplantation genetic diagnosis of aneuploidy. Reprod Biomed Online 2003; 7: 91–7

50. Ginaroli L, Magli MC, Ferraretti A. Preimplantation genetic diagnosis for aneuploidies: clinical outcome. Presented at the Fifth International Symposium on Preimplantation Genetics, Antalya, Turkey, 5–7 June 2003: 25

51. Magli MC, Jones GM, Gras L, et al. Chromosome mosaicism in day 3 aneuploid embryos that develop to morphologically normal blastocysts in vitro. Hum Reprod 2000; 15: 1781–6

52. Sandalinas M, Sadowy S, Alikani M, et al. Developmental ability of chromosomally abnormal human embryos to develop to the blastocyst stage. Hum Reprod 2001; 16: 1954–8

53. Munné S, Bahce M, Sandalinas M et al. Differences in chromosome susceptibility to aneuploidy and survival to first trimester. Reprod Biomed Online 2004; 8: 81–90

54. Hansen M, Kurinczuk JJ, Bower C, Webb S. The risk of major birth defects after intracytoplasmic sperm

injection and in vitro fertilization. N Engl J Med 2002; 346: 725–30

55. Anthony S, Buitendijk SE, Dorrepaal CA, et al. Congenital malformations in 4224 children conceived after IVF. Hum Reprod 2002; 17: 2089–95

56. Cox GF, Burger J, Lip V, et al. Intracytoplasmic sperm injection may increase the risk of imprinting defects. Am J Hum Genet 2002; 71: 162–4

57. DeBaun MR, Niemitz EL, Feinberg AP. Association of in vitro fertilization with Beckwith–Wiedemann syndrome and epigenetic alterations of LIT1 and H19. Am J Hum Genet 2003; 72: 156–60

58. Ostavic KH, Eiklid K, van der Hagen CB, et al. Another case of imprinting defect in a girl with Angelman syndrome who was conceived by intracytoplasmic spem injection. Am J Hum Genet 2003; 72: 218–19

59. Gickel C, Gaston V, Mandelbaum J, et al. In vitro fertilization may increase the risk of Beckwith–Wiedemann syndrome related to the abnormal imprinting of the KCN1OT gene. Am J Hum Genet 2003; 72: 1338–41

60. Maher ER, Brueton LA, Bowdin SC, et al. Beckwith–Wiedemann syndrome and assisted reproduction technology (ART). J Med Genet 2003; 40: 62–4

61. Niemitz L, Feinberg AP. Epigenetics and assisted reproductive technology: a call for investigation. Am J Hum Genet 2004; 74: 599–609

26

The role of sex selection techniques in an assisted reproductive technologies program

Zaid Kilani, Mohammed Shaban and Lamia Haj Hassan

INTRODUCTION

In 1902, John Beard of the University of Jena declared that: 'Any interference with or alteration of the determination of sex is absolutely beyond human power'. However, today, due to the progress of technology and the need of mankind, this has proved not to be true, as scientific methods have developed to determine the gender of progeny.

Sex selection is a term currently used when a couple try to determine the sex of their offspring. The motive for gender selection is geared by medical and non-medical issues including cultural, religious, psychological and economic factors, and by attempts not to undermine the importance of inheritance, which in many cultures is to the advantage of the male. In ancient mythology, several methods were practiced for that purpose. The ancient Greeks believed that male-determining sperm came from the right testicle; a man could produce a son while lying on his right side. In the 18th century in France, it was recommended that men who wished to have a son should tie off their left testicle during intercourse. The old advice to wear boots to bed was recommended to husbands keen to have a boy, or that women who desired to have a daughter should eat sweets (sour food for a son)[1]. In medieval times the suggested formula became even more bizarre: to have a son alchemists recommended

drinking the blood of a lion and then having intercourse under a full moon[2]. The Chinese calendar method that relates the age of the wife with the month of conception has been adopted by many. In the Jewish tradition, on the other hand, gender selection is believed to be influenced by the sequence of orgasm: 'A male child is likely to be conceived if the woman emits her semen first, whereas if the man emits his semen first it is more likely that the child will be a female'[3]. Ancient Egyptians believed that women of dark complexion were destined to have boys[4].

The above-mentioned examples show how desperate mankind was, willing to tolerate unpleasant procedures, and to commit unusual and senseless practices in the hope of conceiving a male. However, man was even more aggressive in using criminal acts to get rid of females, challenging the psychological and ethical implications, and ignoring rules and laws.

Infanticide has been practiced by the Chinese, Indians[5,6] and ancient Arabs, and this was later condemned by Islam[7]. Sex-selective abortion has been made possible through the introduction of prenatal diagnostic techniques, in particular ultrasonography, which ironically was introduced in part to save babies and to assure their well-being. Instead, it was used to diagnose the gender of the fetus and subsequently to terminate a pregnancy of unwanted gender, which is usually female. It is estimated that in Asia, several million female fetuses were aborted in the last two decades of the 20th century[8,9].

In this chapter the methods currently available for sex selection are discussed, whether used for medical or non-medical indications, based on scientific grounds. Their strengths and effectiveness, in addition to their risks and limitations, are also addressed. Furthermore, we touch on the ethical and religious aspects, but concentrate mainly on 'the role of sex selection in an assisted reproductive technologies program'.

SEX-SELECTION METHODS

Sex selection in an assisted reproduction program can be done at two levels:

(1) Preconception (prefertilization): sperm sorting techniques;

(2) Preimplantation: preimplantation genetic diagnosis (PGD).

Preconceptional sperm separation techniques

In assisted reproduction, sperm separation must fulfill three criteria:

(1) Viability: sperm obtained must be viable;

(2) Number: sufficient sperm of each type must be obtained;

(3) Accuracy: sperm separation must be complete.

A reliable and accurate method for sex selection in humans at the preconceptional level has been sought by researchers for many years. Scientists have attempted to separate X- from Y-bearing sperm using different methods based on physical, biochemical or immunological differences. An efficient and reliable method for the separation of X- and Y-bearing sperm should rely on an identifiable distinction between these two living cells. Currently, the difference in total DNA content between living X- and Y-bearing sperm is the only recognizable distinction due to the larger size of the X chromosome[10]. Sperm separation methods can be divided into two main techniques:

(1) Gradient methods;

(2) Flow cytometry.

Gradient methods

Early attempts to separate X- from Y-bearing sperm focused on the use of gradient methods. In 1973, Ericsson and colleagues were the first to report that, when sperm were layered in columns of liquid albumin of different concentrations, approximately 85% of the sperm in the lowermost portions of the columns were Y-bearing[11]. Later, other gradient methods for X- and Y-sperm separation, in addition to albumin gradients[11–13], were developed, such as Sephadex™ columns[12,14,15], discontinuous Percoll™[16] and swim-up[17,18] procedures. All these methods involve processing the sperm through different concentrations of the material used, although the exact mechanism(s) underlying these methods are not well defined. Different physical features of X- and Y-bearing sperm have been suggested to account for the separation qualities, e.g. the high negative charge on the X-bearing sperm might explain the enrichment with 80% Percoll[19]. On the other hand, Beernink and colleagues[13] and Sumner and Robinson[20] suggested that the faster swimming ability and the smaller head of the Y-bearing sperm might be responsible for their separation using other gradient methods.

A description of the human albumin gradient follows, focusing on the human serum albumin method[13].

Human albumin gradient method for sperm separation

One volume of semen is diluted with an equal volume of Tyrode's salt solution. The sample, is centrifuged at $300g$ for 10 min. The pellet is re-suspended in Tyrode's solution at a concentration of 30×10^6 sperm/ml. Human serum albumin (HSA) is diluted with Tyrode's solution to the appropriate concentration for the individual column. The albumin columns are prepared by layering different HSA concentrations, with the highest concentration being at the bottom of the column. The prepared semen sample is then layered over the albumin gradient column.

Three protocols are described below.

Protocol A

(1) The albumin column gradient is prepared with 0.5 ml of 17.5% HSA at the bottom and 1.0 ml of 7.5% HSA at the top.

(2) The washed sperm sample (0.5 ml) is then layered at the top of the albumin gradient column.

(3) This is followed by incubation for 1.5 h at room temperature.

The sorted sperm are used for female sex selection in conjunction with clomiphene citrate treatment for the woman[13].

Protocol B
(1) 0.5 ml of the washed semen sample is layered at the top of 1.0 ml of 7.5% HSA for 1 h at room temperature.

(2) The lower HSA layer is aspirated after the incubation period, and centrifuged at $300g$ for 10 min.

(3) The pellet is re-suspended in a 1:1 ratio in Tyrode's solution, and then 0.5 ml of the re-suspension is layered on top of a column of 0.5 ml of 20% HSA at the bottom and 1.0 ml of 12.5% HSA at the top for 1.5 h at room temperature.

Modified protocol B
(1) The washed semen sample (0.5 ml) is layered at the top of 1.0 ml of 10% HSA for 45 min at room temperature.

(2) The lower HSA layer is aspirated after the incubation period, and centrifuged at $300g$ for 10 min.

(3) The pellet is re-suspended in a 1:1 ratio in Tyrode's solution, and then 0.5 ml of the re-suspension is layered on top of a column of 0.5 ml of 20% HSA at the bottom and 1.0 ml of 12.5% HSA at the top for 1 h at room temperature.

The sorted sample from protocol B and modified protocol B can be used for male sex selection[13]. However, modified protocol B works best when the total semen count is 150×10^6.

A sample of the pellet can be evaluated to confirm the sorting efficiency of the above technique using either fluorochrome quinacrine or fluorescent *in situ* hybridization (FISH); however, this would render the evaluated sample unfit for clinical use.

Sperm obtained by albumin gradient methods can be used for intrauterine insemination (IUI) at the time of ovulation, or even in assisted reproduction to obtain embryos of the desired gender, either to prevent X-linked diseases or for non-medical reasons. The use of albumin gradients was reported to enrich the sorted sample with 85% of Y-bearing sperm[11]. Other studies have supported Ericsson's data [12,21–23], while yet others have reported failure of this technique in sperm

separation[14,15,24]. The use of FISH on the sorted sperm fraction obtained after use of the albumin gradient method showed a slight increase in the percentage of Y-bearing chromosomes[22], while Vidal and colleagues[14] reported failure of this technique to separate Y-rich sperm.

Using albumin gradient sperm separation, Beernink and colleagues reported 85% enrichment of the Y-bearing chromosomes. However, only 76% of the children born after sperm separation using the albumin gradient method followed by IUI were males[13].

Other gradient methods such as Sephadex and Percoll have been reported to show inconsistent results. For Sephadex, some authors have reported a sorting efficiency reaching up to 75% for X-bearing sperm[12,14,15,24,25], while others have reported the failure of Sephadex to increase the X-bearing sperm fraction[14,18,26–28]. In addition, the use of different preparations of discontinuous Percoll showed an increase in X-bearing sorted sperm in some studies[19], while others were unable to show a significant difference in the sorted sperm samples[17,29,30]. Furthermore, although many studies found the swim-up technique to be inefficient in Y-bearing sperm separation[29,30], Check and Katsoff [17] claimed an 88.5% male delivery rate using the modified swim-up technique, compared with a 50% male delivery rate with a Percoll preparation or in a control group.

Because the outcome of these methods is variable and inconsistent, and the sorting efficiency is not 100% reliable either for X- or for Y-bearing sperm in the treated sample, the application of such techniques for the purpose of preconceptional sex selection, whether for prevention of X-linked diseases or for non-medical reasons, is not justified.

Flow cytometry

This technique was introduced in animals in the late 1980s[31] by Johnson and colleagues for the separation of viable X- and Y-bearing sperm[32]. Development of the method for human use was first reported by Johnson's group in 1993[33]. It is a complex, time- and cost-consuming procedure. The technique depends on the fact that the Y-bearing sperm contain 2.8% less DNA, compared with the X chromosome[20]. The sorted sperm can be used in IUI or *in vitro* fertilization/intracytoplasmic sperm injection (IVF/ICSI) programs; nevertheless, so far the accuracy is not absolute.

The technique is described below.

Intact sperm preparation Sperm are suspended at a concentration of 10×10^6/ml in modified Tyrode's medium (117.5 mmol/l NaCl, 0.3 mmol/l NaH$_2$PO$_4$, 8.6 mmol/l KCl, 2.5 mmol/l CaCl$_2$, 0.4 mmol/l MgCl$_2$.6H$_2$O, 2.0 mmol/l glucose, 25 mmol/l HEPES (4-(2-hydroxyethyl)-1-piperazineethanesulfonic acid), 19 mmol/l sodium lactate, 0.25 mmol/l sodium pyruvate, 100 IU/ml penicillin).

(1) The sperm are stained by adding a vital fluorochrome, bisbenzimide (Hoechst 33342), to a concentration of 9 μmol/l.

(2) Samples are incubated at 35°C for 1 h.

(3) Sperm are then sorted using a flow/cell sorter modified especially.

(4) The sperm are excited with ultraviolet (351–364 nm) lines of a 5-W 90-5 Innova argon-ion laser operating at 175 mW, and fluorescence detected through 418-nm long-pass filters.

(5) Sperm are sorted directly onto a standard coded microscope slide to be evaluated.

(6) The spermatozoa are probed for X or Y chromosomes.

(7) The resultant sorted sperm are then treated with a special liquid and centrifuged as required.

The sorted sperm can be used for IUI or IVF/ICSI to attain embryos of the required gender.

Flow cytometry for sperm separation: safety, accuracy and limitations There have been concerns regarding the safety of sorting sperm by flow cytometry for clinical use, because the technique employs two mutagenic substances: near ultraviolet light and a DNA-binding agent, Hoechst 33342. Ultraviolet light has been reported to produce an increase in chromosome structural abnormalities in mouse sperm[34], whereas at concentrations about ten times less than those necessary for cytometry separation, Hoechst 33342 was shown to cause inhibition of DNA synthesis in V79 cells[35]. Furthermore, exposure to Hoechst 33342 was reported to result in decreased cell survival[35]. The first human clinical pregnancy resulting from X-enriched sorted sperm for the prevention of X-linked hydrocephalus was reported by Levinson and colleagues in 1995[36].

Sorting by flow cytometry results in a lower number of sperm available for assisted reproduction. It yields 20–40 sperm from each 1000[36]. The method cannot produce enough sperm for artificial insemination purposes in oligospermic patients. Therefore, to obtain reasonable pregnancy rates it has to be used in conjunction with IVF or ICSI. Sorting efficiency for X-bearing sperm can reach up to 90% at 6 million sperm sorting per hour, and around 75–80% if 20 million sperm are sorted per hour[36,37]. In addition, Vidal and colleagues[14] showed by using the FISH technique that the efficiency of sorting was 80–90% for X-bearing sperm and 60–70% for Y-bearing sperm. Using MicroSort® XSORT® for flow cytometry, Fugger and associates[38] reported 208 IUI cycles in which 22 clinical pregnancies (10.6%) were achieved. In that study, a total of 29 clinical pregnancies were achieved using MicroSort XSORT for IUI, IVF or ICSI. Of the 14 pregnancies with known fetal or birth gender, 13 were female conceptions (92.9%).

Preimplantation genetic diagnosis

Preimplantation genetic diagnosis (PGD) is a technique that was introduced originally and mainly as an alternative to prenatal testing in order to avoid pregnancy termination for couples who are at risk of transmitting certain genetic diseases. Since Handyside and colleagues reported the first pregnancy using PGD in 1990[39], more than 4000 PGD cycles have been performed, suggesting that PGD is no longer a research tool. It offers a relatively accurate and reliable way to identify more than 100 different genetic diseases in human embryos obtained through *in vitro* fertilization (IVF), before transferring them to the uterus. PGD is of particular help for: carriers of balanced translocations[40]; aneuploidy screening (PGD-AS); couples with poor prognosis in assisted reproductive technologies (ART) treatment such as those with advanced maternal age; repeated implantation failure; and repeated pregnancy loss[41–43]. A novel feature of PGD is its application for conditions which previously were never considered indications for prenatal testing, such as late-onset disorders with genetic predisposition[44,45] and PGD for human leukocyte antigen (HLA) matching, not only for the purpose of having an unaffected child, but also for future stem-cell transplantation from a potential donor sibling[46].

The availability of PGD as the most reliable method for X- and Y-chromosome identification, to avoid X-linked diseases[39,47–49], made it an attractive option for couples seeking gender selection, either as a byproduct of testing for genetic disorders or aneuploidy screening, or when it is done purely for the purpose of social gender selection[50–53].

Steps of PGD for sex selection

(1) Superovulation;

(2) Oocyte collection;

(3) IVF or ICSI;

(4) Cleavage-stage embryo biopsy;

(5) Genetic analysis of the biopsied blastomeres;

(6) Selective embryo(s) transfer of the desired gender.

There are two techniques that can be used for gender preimplantation diagnosis:

(1) Polymerase chain reaction (PCR);

(2) Fluorescent *in situ* hybridization (FISH).

Currently, FISH is used for sex selection and analysis of structural and numerical chromosomal abnormalities, while the PCR technique is applied for the diagnosis of monogenic disorders.

Cleavage-stage embryo biopsy

Cleavage-stage embryo biopsy is usually performed on day 3 of normally developing embryos (Figure 1). A hole of 15–20 μm is made in the zona pellucida (ZP) using a laser, acid Tyrode's or mechanical drilling. One or two blastomeres are removed with a glass polished needle introduced in the perivitelline space through the breach in the ZP. The biopsied blastomere(s) are then subjected to either FISH or PCR.

The PCR technique   This is used to amplify sufficient DNA from the blastomeres, usually to diagnose monogenic disorders. The biopsied blastomere(s) are placed in a solution that lyses the cell and releases the DNA, then a PCR reaction mix is added and PCR begins.

In 1990, Handyside and co-workers[39,54] were the first to report use of the PCR technique to determine the sex of an embryo. X-linked recessive disorders, such as Duchenne's muscular dystrophy and hypoxanthine–guanine phosphoribosyl-transferase (HPRT) deficiency, were among the first disorders for which PGD was applied, in order to avoid affected offspring (Table 1).

The PCR testing in the above report was based on amplification of a specific sequence derived from the Y chromosome. A misdiagnosis occurred due to amplification failure of the Y-specific sequence[54]. To minimize incorrect assignment of gender, other PCR techniques were developed. Kontogiani and colleagues reported on the application of simultaneous amplification of X- and Y-specific sequences[55]. Nakahori's group used coamplification of related homologous X- and Y-linked genes or pseudogenes with the same primers, yielding final X- and Y-specific products that differered in length[56,57].

However, the PCR technique has the following drawbacks and limitations: occasional failure of

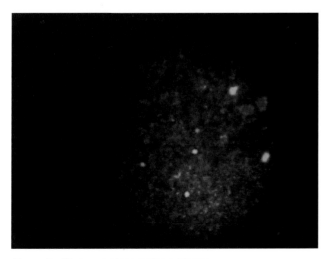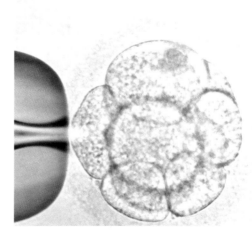

Figure 1   Cleavage-stage embryo biopsy

Table 1   X-linked diseases diagnosed by preimplantation genetic diagnosis (PGD)

Duchenne's and Becker's muscular dystrophy
Hemophilia
Fragile-X syndrome
Mental retardation
Wiskott-Aldrich syndrome
Charcot–Marie–Tooth
Coffin–Lowry syndrome
Granulomatous disease
Hydrocephalus
FG syndrome
Agammaglobulinemia
Anderson–Fabry disease
Ataxia
Autism
Barth's syndrome
Goltz's syndrome
Hunter's syndrome
Hypohydrotic ectodermal dysplasia
Incontinentia pigmenti
Kennedy's disease
Lowe's syndrome
Pelizaeus–Merzbaher syndrome
Proliferative disease
Retinitis pigmentosa
Retinoschisis

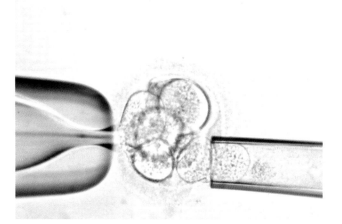

Figure 2 Fluorescent *in situ* hybridization (FISH) for X, Y chromosomes

amplification of the target nucleotide sequence; risk of contamination by sperm or foreign DNA; and it cannot detect an abnormal number of sex chromosomes, e.g. 45,X and 46,XX may yield indistinguishable results.

The FISH technique   The biopsied blastomeres are transferred to a hypotonic solution and the nucleus is fixed on a glass slide using Carnoy's fixative (3 : 1 methanol : acetic acid). After dehydration in ethanol for 2 min each at concentrations of 70%, 85% and 100%, consecutively, the fixed blastomeres are analyzed using FISH probes for chromosomes X and Y, labeled with orange and green spectra respectively (Vysis Inc., Downers Grove, IL)(Figure 2).

FISH probes for chromosomes 13, 18, 21, X and Y are labeled with red, aqua, green, blue and yellow spectra respectively (Vysis Inc., Downers Grove, IL) (Figure 3).

The fixed blastomeres and the probes on the slides are co-denatured in HYBrite (Vysis Inc., Downers

Grove, IL) at 73°C for 5 min, then hybridized consecutively at 42°C for 30 min and 37°C for 90 min. The excess probe is washed off with 0.7% standard saline citrate (SSC)/0.3% NP40 and the slides are observed under a fluorescent microscope.

The FISH technique is viewed as the method of choice for preimplantation gender determination of human embryos for many reasons: it is relatively accurate and reliable; simultaneous identification of the X and Y chromosomes can be done in two different colors (Figure 2[58]; and ploidy status (Figure 3) and mosaicism of the sex and other tested chromosomes can be detected[59]. Accurate sex determination can be available within a few hours[60]. Furthermore, the risk of contamination is negligible.

PGD: safety and accuracy

The technique of PGD is now well established, and has shown a high degree of safety and accuracy[61]. Reports of misdiagnoses are anecdotal. The European Society of Human Reproduction and Embryology (ESHRE) PGD consortium reported on the occurrence of eight misdiagnoses in 450 (2%) pregnancies using FISH or PCR. Using PCR, misdiagnosis was reported in five cases out of 145 (3%) pregnancies, two for sexing for X-linked diseases (one retinitis pigmentosa, and the other Duchenne's muscular dystrophy), and one each for cystic fibrosis, β-thalassemia and myotonic dystrophy. On the other hand, applying the FISH technique, misdiagnosis was reported in three out of 305 (1%) pregnancies, one for trisomy 21, one

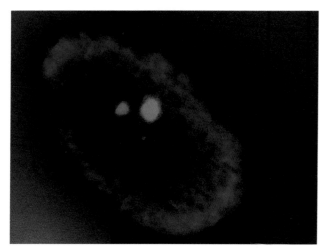

Figure 3 Fluorescent *in situ* hybridization (FISH) for 13, 18, 21, X, Y chromosomes

Table 2 Pregnancy outcome* by embryo transfer cycles

Transferred cycles (*n*)	354 (278 patients)
Age (years) (mean ± SD)	34.7 ± 4.8
Embryos transferred (mean ± SD)	1.7 ± 0.8
Pregnancies (*n*)	92 (26%)
miscarriages (*n*)	33
ectopics (*n*)	2
delivered (*n*)	53
lost contact (*n*)	4

*A total of 68 babies were born: 39 singleton, 13 twins and one triplet were of the wanted gender. One male had Beckwith–Wiedemann syndrome. In four cases follow-up was not possible after confirmation of pregnancy

for translocation and one for sexing for social reasons[62]. The biopsy procedure does not seem to have an adverse effect on further embryo development[63]. Data on the clinical outcome of PGD indicate that around 3000 PGD transfer cycles have been performed, with more than 600 unaffected children born, suggesting the accuracy, reliability and safety of the technique[64]. Verlinsky and Kuliev and their group at the Chicago center[65,66] have reported the largest single series, where 1416 PGD embryo transfer cycles resulted in 338 (23.9%) clinical pregnancies, and the birth of 260 unaffected children. In addition, data collected from 25 different centers[62] showed that out of 1670 PGD transfer cycles, 309 (18.5%) clinical pregnancies were achieved, and a total of 269 unaffected children born. The overall congenital malformation rate was not different from the population prevalence, at 5.4% for the Chicago center, and 6.6% for the ESHRE group. Major malformations accounted for 2.25% and 3.9%, respectively.

The application of PGD using the FISH technique for gender determination for non-medical reasons has been reported by Malpani[51], where 42 PGD cycles initiated resulted in 14/39 (35.8%) clinical pregnancies and nine live births, all of which were the desired gender. In our series[53] 354 PGD transfer cycles using the FISH technique resulted in 92 (26%) clinical pregnancies, and the birth of 68 children. All were of the desired gender, normal and healthy, except for one male baby affected by Beckwith–Wiedemann syndrome (Table 2). Beckwith–Wiedemann syndrome is

an imprinting disorder resulting from mutations or epimutations affecting imprinted genes in chromosome 11p15.5. Classical clinical features are macroglossia, pre- and postnatal overgrowth and anterior abdominal wall defects. A total of six cases have been reported following ICSI/IVF procedures[67]; nevertheless, this is the only case reported following PGD for gender selection[53].

PGD for sex selection: risks and limitations

The PGD program for sex selection is a complex, stressful and costly one. It might be associated with potential problems and disappointments at each and every step, such as: ovarian hyperstimulation syndrome (OHSS), a well-known, potentially life-threatening iatrogenic complication of superovulation; poor follicular response; fertilization failure; embryo development arrest; and damage to the embryo(s) during the biopsy procedure. Obviously it is impossible to guarantee that the desired-gender embryo(s) will be obtained, or even be available for transfer. In our series, embryos of both genders were diagnosed in 349 (74.5%) cycles, while in 56 (12%) cycles only male embryos were diagnosed, and in 63 (13.5%) cycles only female embryos were diagnosed (Table 3).

Out of 495 initiated cycles, embryo transfer was canceled in 141 (30.7%) cycles: in 89 (63.1%) cycles the desired gender was not available, and in 52 (36.9%) cycles the cancellation was due to the presence of aneuploid embryos only. Furthermore, the overall aneuploidy rate using FISH for either X or Y

Table 3 Distribution of XX and YY embryos in preimplantation genetic diagnosis cycles for gender selection

	XY only	XX only	XX and XY
Cycles (n = 468)	56 (12%)	63 (13.5%)	349 (74.57%)
100% abnormal Y cycles	13 (23%)	—	68 (19.5%)

Table 4 Aneuploidy rate using fluorescent *in situ* hybridization in diagnosed embryos[53]

Embryos analyzed (n)	2216
Normal using X and Y probes only (n)	1575 (71%)
Abnormality using X and Y probes (n)	484 (21.8%)
Normal using X, Y and other probes (n)	1325 (59.8%)
Abnormality using X, Y and other probes (n)	734 (33.1%)
No diagnosis (n)	157 (7.1%)

chromosomes, or when combined with FISH for other chromosomes (13, 16, 18, 21, 22), was 21.8% or 33.1%, respectively (Table 4).

In view of the complexity, limitations, risks and the high expectations related to the issue of sex selection through PGD, thorough counseling should be carried out before starting the IVF cycle for sex selection. In addition, a consent form should be signed.

The ethics committee at our institute adopted the following guidelines in considering a PGD service for non-medical reasons: the presence of three children or more of the same gender *and* the desire to have the opposite sex; the presence of a mentally or physically handicapped child of a certain gender with the desire to have a healthy child of the same gender; the loss of a child of certain gender and the desire to have another child of the same gender; maternal age > 35 years, with one or more children of the same gender, and the desire to have a child of the opposite sex; or late marriage with a special need to have a certain gender[50].

GENDER SELECTION: RELIGIOUS ASPECTS

In several countries, practices of assisted reproduction, including PGD for sex selection, are strongly influenced by the attitude of religious doctrine. A frequently asked question by couples seeking preconceptional or preimplantation gender selection is whether such techniques are permissible from a religious point of view. Herewith, we mention the views of three religions from that aspect: Judaism, Christianity and Islam.

In *Judaism*, the presence of at least one son is an essential prerequisite to fulfill the criteria of procreation; accordingly, the use of either preconceptional or preimplantation methods can be justified and may be of certain practical importance. For Christianity on

the other hand, and as viewed by the *Catholic Church*, the concept of sex selection is totally forbidden, even for medical purposes. However, in the *Islamic* religion, although the attitude toward sex selection is guarded, its practice is not banned. The decision to allow sex selection whether using preconceptional or preimplantation methods should be individualized and based on the premise that there is no harm to the community[68].

GENDER SELECTION: ETHICAL CONSIDERATIONS AND THE VIEW OF INTERNATIONAL ORGANIZATIONS

In 1997, the International Federation of Gynecology and Obstetrics (FIGO) offered a somewhat lenient conclusion. It rejected sex-selection abortion on the grounds that 'no fetus should be sacrificed because of its sex alone'. However, it reached the conclusion that 'pre-conceptional sex selection can be justified on social grounds in certain cases for the objective of *allowing children of the two sexes to enjoy the love and the care of parents*' (authors' italics)[69].

The Ethics Committee of the American Society for Reproductive Medicine (ASRM) explored the issue of sex selection for non-medical reasons in its 1999 and 2001 reports. In 1999, the ASRM criticized the use of PGD exclusively for the purpose of sex control, and claimed that it is '*morally inappropriate*'[70]. The Ethics Committee of the ASRM concluded that '*PGD* for sex selection for *non-medical* reasons should be discouraged because it poses a risk of unwarranted gender bias, social harm, and results in diversion of medical resources from genuine medical needs.' *Significantly*, the report noted that the ethical objection would apply *equally* to other sperm-sorting techniques. Although the Committee acknowledges that individuals have the right to enjoy procreative liberty and that serious reasons must be provided if a limitation on reproductive freedom is to be justified, it claims that the social risks of sex selection for non-medical reasons outweigh the social benefits. The Committee did not favor its legal prohibition. In 2001, the ASRM reviewed the concept of *preconception* gender selection for non-medical reasons, and further explored the issues that arise from preconception (prefertilization) methods of gender selection. The ASRM concluded that it is permissible to use the technology of sperm sorting for sex control but not yet the technology of PGD for the same purpose, and raised concerns about both gender bias and the *moral status* of the embryo. The Committee concluded that 'the use of preconception methods of gender selection for creating gender variety in a family would *not* necessarily be *unethical* when certain other conditions are met, including establishment of safety and efficacy of the preconception methods that at present are still experimental'[71]. However, the issue is still controversial and it is currently under revision again by the ASRM Ethics Committee.

The ESHRE Task Force on Ethics and Law, in 2001, expressed certain concerns related to the technique of PGD: 'We are aware of the *risks of abuse* for non-medical reasons. Information and consent of the couple, public transparency and the respect of professional guidelines will limit abuse'[72]. Furthermore, the Task Force, in its statement in 2003, has *not* been able to reach a *unanimous* decision regarding the application of PGD for gender selection for non-medical reasons. Two positions can be distinguished: those opposed to every application of sexing for non-medical reasons, and those who accept sex selection for family balancing[73].

The Human Fertilisation and Embryology Authority (HFEA) in the UK in 2003 stated, regarding the issue of sex selection, 'We found this a difficult issue. It has taken us over a year to reach conclusions because of their far-reaching nature. But it is clear that most people are against sex selection for social reasons. The HFEA has to balance the potential benefit of any technique against the potential harm. We are not persuaded that the likely benefits of permitting sex selection for social reasons are strong enough to outweigh the possible harm that might be done.' Furthermore, the HFEA added that, 'The HFEA cannot stop people from going abroad for sex selection.'

CONCLUSION

This chapter summarizes the different scientific techniques currently available for the purpose of sex selection, including sperm-sorting methods and PGD, in ART programs. Nowadays, choosing the gender of offspring for either medical or non-medical reasons is no longer a fantasy. However, the availability of relatively reliable, and accurate, methods for gender selection such as PGD has raised not only hopes and expectations, but also serious moral, legal, ethical, social and religious concerns. The issue of using new medical technologies for non-medical purposes, such as gender selection for social reasons, is an intricate one that involves tackling issues such as gender *stereotyping*, *procreative liberty* and, for some, the *misallocation* of medical resources, in addition to issues related to *respect* for the earliest stages of human life.

Although a growing number of clinics offer PGD for social sex selection in different parts of the world, there is a paucity of published data, presumably because, in the view of many, this is a guarded practice and is still a controversial issue. Gender selection for non-medical indications could lead to dire consequences if it is left without tight medical regulations and guidelines. With the rapid progress in technology and the eagerness of mankind, a simple, convenient, accurate and cheap method will soon be available. The medical profession then will be confronted with the implications of such a practice if it is left unregulated. Therefore, gender selection services should be limited to specialized, licensed, highly qualified centers, subject to *strict* monitoring by health authorities. This will assure high scientific standards and high-quality professional care, and will enable detailed research. A proper follow-up of the outcomes of such ART procedures, and their immediate and long-term impact on the different aspects, including the distribution of sex ratio, can be evaluated.

ACKNOWLEDGMENTS

The authors thank Sanad Kilani, a medical student at The Royal College of Surgeons in Dublin, for his comments, input and critical reading, and Miss Rene Juha for her patience in preparing the manuscript.

REFERENCES

1. The President's Council on Bioethics, Human Cloning and Human Dignity: An Ethical Inquiry. Washington, DC: Government Printing Office, 2003
2. Kaplan L, Tong R. Controlling Our Reproductive Destiny: A Technological and Philosophical Perspective. Cambridge, MA: MIT Press, 1994
3. Stolkowski J, Choukroun J. Preconception selection of sex in man. Isr J Med Sci 1981; 17: 1061–7
4. Serour GI. Transcultural issues in gender selection. International Congress Series. Adv Fertil Reprod Med 2004; 1266: 21–31
5. Chan CL, Yip PS, Ng EH, et al. Gender selection in China, its meanings and implications. J Assist Reprod Genet 2002; 19: 426–30
6. Bhargava PM. Ethical issues in modern biological technologies. Reprod BioMed Online 2003; 7: 276–85
7. Holy Qur'an, Sura Al-Takweer, 8–9
8. Miller BD, Female selective abortion in Asia: patterns, policies, and debates. Am Anthropol 2001;103: 1083–95
9. Allahbadia GN. The 50 million missing women J Assist Reprod Genet 2002; 19: 411–16
10. Pinkel D, Lake S, Gledhill BL, et al. High resolution DNA content measurements of mammalian sperm. Cytometry 1982; 3: 1–9
11. Ericsson RJ, Langevin CN, Nishino M. Isolation of fractions rich in human Y sperm. Nature (London) 1973; 246: 421–24
12. Quinlivan WL, Preciado K, Long TL, et al. Separation of human X and Y spermatozoa by albumin gradients and Sephadex chromatography. Fertil Steril 1982; 37: 104–7
13. Beernink FJ, Dmowski WP, Ericsson RJ. Sex preselection through albumin separation of sperms. Fertil Steril 1993; 59: 382–6
14. Vidal F, Moragas M, Catala V, et al. Sephadex filtration and human serum albumin gradients do not select spermatozoa by sex chromosome: a fluorescent in-situ hybridization study. Hum Reprod 1993; 8: 1740–3
15. Steeno O, Adimoelja A, Steeno J. Separation of X and Y bearing human spermatozoa with the Sephadex gel-filtration method. Andrologia 1975; 7: 95–7
16. Kaneko S, Yamaguchi J, Kobayashi T, et al. Separation of human X and Y bearing sperm using Percoll density gradient centrifugation. Fertil Steril 1983; 40: 661–5
17. Check JH, Katsoff D. A prospective study to evaluate the efficacy of modified swim-up preparation for male sex selection. Hum Reprod 1993; 8: 211–14
18. Han TL, Flaherty SP, Ford JH, et al. Detection of X- and Y-bearing human spermatozoa after motile sperm isolation by swim-up. Fertil Steril 1993; 60: 1046–51
19. Wang HX, Flaherty SP, Swann NJ, et al. Discontinuous Percoll gradients enrich X-bearing human spermatozoa: a study using double-label fluorescent in-situ hybridization. Hum Reprod 1994; 9: 1265–70
20. Sumner AT, Robinson JA. A difference in dry mass between the heads of X- and Y-bearing human spermatozoa. J Reprod Fertil 1976; 48: 9–15
21. Corson SL, Batzer FR, Alexander NJ, et al. Sex selection by sperm separation and insemination. Fertil Steril 1984; 42: 756–60
22. Claassens OE, Oosthuizen CJ, Brusnicky J, et al. Fluorescent in situ hybridization evaluation of human Y-bearing spermatozoa separated by albumin density gradients. Fertil Steril 1995; 63: 417–18
23. Dmowski WP, Gaynor L, Rao R, et al. Use of albumin gradients for X and Y sperm separation and clinical experience with male sex preselection. Fertil Steril 1979; 31: 52–7
24. Adimoelja A, Hariadi R, Amitaba IG, et al. The separation of X- and Y- spermatozoa with regard to the possible clinical application by means of artificial insemination. Andrologia 1977; 9: 289–92
25. Porstmann T, Schmechta H. Separation of human X- and Y-chromosome-bearing spermatozoa by column chromatography. Dermatol Monatsschr 1979; 165: 28–35
26. Schilling E, Lafrenz R, Klobasa F. Failure to separate human X- and Y-chromosome bearing spermatozoa by Sephadex gel-filtration. Andrologia 1978; 10: 215–17
27. Gawecka-Szczygiel M, Kurpisz M. X- and Y-chromosome-bearing sperm selection and detection methods. A review. Folia Histochem Cytobiol 1995; 33: 219–27
28. Lin SP, Lee RK, Tsai YJ, et al. Separating X-bearing human spermatozoa through a discontinuous Percoll density gradient proved to be inefficient by double-label fluorescent in situ hybridization. J Assist Reprod Genet 1998; 15: 565–9
29. Samura O, Miharu N, He H, et al. Assessment of sex chromosome ratio and aneuploidy rate in motile spermatozoa selected by three different methods. Hum Reprod 1997; 12: 2437–42
30. Check JH, Kwirenk D, Katsoff D, et al. Male : female sex ratio in births resulting from IVF according to swim-up versus Percoll preparation of inseminated sperm. Arch Androl 1994; 33: 63–5

31. Johnson LA, Flook JP, Hawk HW. Sex preselection in rabbits. Live births from X and Y sperm separated by DNA and cell sorting. Biol Reprod 1989; 41: 199–203

32. Johnson LA, Pinkle D. Modification of a laser-based flow cytometer for high resolution DNA analysis of mammalian spermatozoa. Cytometry 1986; 7: 268–73

33. Johnson LA, Welch GR, Keyvanfa K, et al. Gender preselection in humans? Flow cytometric separation of X and Y spermatozoa for the prevention of X-linked diseases. Hum Reprod 1993: 8: 1733–9

34. Matsuda Y, Tobari I. Chromosomal analysis in mouse eggs fertilized in vitro with sperm exposed to ultraviolet light (UV) and methyl and ethyl methanesulfonate (MMS and EMS). Mutat Res 1988; 198: 131–41

35. Durand RE, Olive PL. Cytotoxicity, mutagenicity and DNA damage by Hoechst 33342. J Histochem Cytochem 1982; 30: 111–16

36. Levinson G, Keyvanfar K, Wu JC. DNA based X-enriched sperm separation as an adjunct to preimplantation genetic testing for the prevention of X-linked disease. Hum Reprod 1995; 10: 979–82

37. Johnson LA, Welch GR. Sex selection: high-speed flow cytometric sorting of X and Y sperms for maximum efficiency. Theriogenology 1999; 52: 1323–41

38. Fugger EF, Black SH, Keyvanfarl K, et al. Births of normal daughters after MicroSort sperm separation and intrauterine insemination, in-vitro fertilization, or intracytoplasmic sperm injection. Hum Reprod 1998; 13: 2367–70

39. Handyside AH, Kontogianni EH, Hardy K, et al. Pregnancies from biopsied human preimplantation embryos sexed by Y-specific DNA amplification. Nature (London) 1990; 244: 768–70

40. Munne S, Sandalinas M, Escudero T. Outcome of preimplantation genetic diagnosis of translocations. Fertil Steril 2000; 73: 1209–18

41. Gianaroli L, Magli MC, Ferrareti AP. Preimplantation genetic diagnosis increases the implantation rate in human in vitro fertilization by avoiding the transfer of chromosomally abnormal embryos. Fertil Steril 1997; 68: 1128–31

42. Gianaroli L, Magli C, Ferraretti AP, et al. Preimplantation diagnosis for aneuploidies in patients undergoing in vitro fertilization with poor prognosis: identification of the categories for which it should be proposed. Fertil Steril 1999; 72: 837–44

43. Munne S, Sandalinas M, Escudero T, et al. Improved implantation after preimplantation genetic diagnosis of aneuploidy. Reprod BioMed Online 2003; 7: 91–7

44. Verlinsky Y, Rechitsky S, Verlinsky O, et al. Preimplantation diagnosis for p53 tumor suppressor gene mutations. Reprod BioMed Online 2001; 2: 102–5

45. Rechitsky S, Verlinsky O, Chistokhina A, et al. Preimplantation genetic diagnosis for cancer predisposition. Reprod BioMed Online 2002; 5: 148–55

46. Verlinsky Y, Rechitsky S, Schoolcraft W, et al. Preimplantation diagnosis for Fanconi anemia combined with HLA matching. J Am Med Assoc 2001; 285: 3130–33

47. Griffin DK, Handyside AH, Harper JC et al. Clinical experience with preimplantation diagnosis of sex by dual fluorescent in situ hybridization. J Assist Reprod Genet 1994; 11: 132–43

48. Munne S, Tang YX, Grifo J, et al. Sex determination of human embryos using the polymerase chain reaction and confirmation by fluorescence in situ hybridization. Fertil Steril 1994; 61: 111–17

49. Staessen C, Van Assche E, Joris H. Clinical experience of sex determination by fluorescent in situ hybridization for preimplantation genetic diagnosis. Mol Hum Reprod 1999; 5: 382–9

50. Kilani Z, Haj Hassan L. Sex selection and preimplantation genetic diagnosis at The Farah Hospital. Reprod BioMed Online 2001; 4: 68–70

51. Malpani A. The use of preimplantation genetic diagnosis in sex selection for family balancing in India. Reprod BioMed Online 2002; 4: 16–20

52. Malpani A, Malpani A. Preimplantation genetic diagnosis for gender selection for family balancing: a view from India. Reprod Bio Med Online 2002; 4: 7–9

53. Kilani Z. Controversies in gender selection. In Fertility and Reproductive Medicine Proceedings of the 18th World Congress on Ferility and Sterility, 2004; 4: 245–8

54. Handyside AH, Delhanty JDA. Cleavage stage biopsy of human embryos and diagnosis of X-linked recessive disease. In Edwards RG, ed. Preimplantation Diagnosis of Human Genetic Disease. Cambridge: Cambridge University Press, 1993: 239–70

55. Kontogiani EH, Hardy K, Handyside AH. Co-amplification of X- and Y-specific sequences for sexing preimplantation human embryos. In Verlinsky Y, Storm C, eds. Preimplantation Genetics. New York: Plenum Press, 1991: 139–45

56. Nakahori Y, Hamanoa K, Iwaya M, Nakagome Y. Sex identification by polymerase chain reaction using X–Y homologous primers. Am J Med Genet 1991; 39: 472–3

57. Nakahori Y, Takenaka O, Nakagome Y. A human X–Y homologous region encodes 'amelogenin'. Genomics 1991; 9: 264–9

58. Griffin DK, Wilton LJ, Handyside AH, et al. Dual fluorescent in situ hybridization for simultaneous detection of X and Y chromosome-specific probes for the sexing of the human preimplantation embryonic nuclei. Hum Genet 1992; 89: 18–22

59. Delhanty JDA, Griffin DK, Handyside AH, et al. Detection of aneuploidy and chromosomal mosaicism in human embryos during preimplantation sex determination by fluorescent in situ hybridization (FISH). Hum Mol Genet 1993; 2: 1183–5

60. Harper JC, Coonen E, Ramaekers CS, et al. Identification of the sex of human preimplantation embryos in two hours using an improved spreading method and fluorescent in situ hybridization (FISH) using directly labeled probes. Hum Reprod 1994; 9: 721–4

61. ESHRE Preimplantation Genetic Diagnosis Consortium. Data collection II. Hum Reprod 2000; 15: 2673–83

62. ESHRE Preimplantation Genetic Diagnosis Consortium. Data Collection III. Hum Reprod 2002; 17: 233–46

63. Hardy K, Martin KL, Leese HJ, et al. Human preimplantation development in vitro is not adversely affected by biopsy at the 8-cell stage. Hum Reprod 1990; 5: 708–14

64. International Working Group on Preimplantation Genetic Diagnosis. Experience of 3000 clinical cycles. Report of the 11th Annual Meeting of International Working Group on Preimplantation Genetics in association with the 10th International Congress of Human Genetics, Vienna, May 15. Reprod BioMed Online 2001; 3: 49–53

65. Verlinsky Y, Cieslak J, Evsikov S. Nuclear transfer for full karyotyping and preimplantation diagnosis for translocations. Reprod BioMed Online 2002; 5: 300–5

66. Kuliev A, Cieslak J, Ilkevitch Y, Verlinsky Y. Chromosomal abnormalities in a series of 6733 human oocytes in preimplantation diagnosis for age-related aneuploidies. Reprod BioMed Online 2003; 6: 54–9

67. Maher ER, Brueton LA, Bowdin SC, et al. Beckwith–Wiedemann syndrome and assisted reproduction technology (ART). J Med Genet 2003; 40: 62–4

68. Schenker JG. Gender selection: cultural and religious perspective. J Assist Reprod Genet 2002; 19: 400–19

69. FIGO. Recommendations on the Ethical Issues in Obstetrics and Gynecology by the FIGO committee for the study of Ethical Aspects of Human Reproduction and Women's Health. 2003 www.figo.org

70. Ethics Committee of the ASRM. Sex selection and preimplantation genetic diagnosis. Fertil Steril 1999; 72: 595–8

71. Ethics Committee of the ASRM. Preconception gender selection for nonmedical reasons. Fertil Steril 2001; 75: 861–4

72. ESHRE Task Force on Ethics and Law. The moral status of the pre-implantation embryo. Hum Reprod 2001; 16: 1046–8

73. ESHRE Ethics Task Force. Taskforce 5: preimplantation genetic diagnosis. Hum Reprod 2003; 18: 649–51

27

Recent scientific developments in assisted reproduction

Jacques Cohen, James Stachecki, Henry Malter and Dagan Wells

INTRODUCTION

With the birth of the second millionth baby born from assisted reproduction approaching, researchers are more often than not barred from the normal process of funding and review along the lines of traditional medical investigation. In part, this is the result of the inability of funding agencies and governments to accept the notion that the processes in early human reproduction are species-specific and animal models are only rarely attainable. During the development of assisted reproductive technologies (ART), reproductive scientists in most countries have been outspoken about their quest for answers to clinical problems, yet they have been denied access to public funding time and again. This state of affairs has been severely complicated by the position of some of the larger organized religions who consider the embryo morally equivalent to human life. This flawed perception has often led to conditions prohibiting certain reproductive technologies, and in some countries all forms of ART have been outlawed or criminalized. If there was any doubt about the link between church and state even in the most liberal of nations, then certainly the attitude towards reproductive medicine testifies to the contrary. Good examples of these are the laws now in place in Italy and Germany. Research into the mechanism underlying erroneous embryo development has

been embargoed because of these pressures, even in countries where laws are absent or moderate. Clinically, assisted reproduction has developed in this largely unsupported environment in spite of the opposition. Imagine what advances would have been made if support had been the norm rather than the exception! In this chapter we review aspects of embryological research that have been emphasized in recent years, in both clinical experimentation and molecular biology.

First, there has been a revival of cryopreservation technology, with particular emphasis on freezing unfertilized oocytes and blastocysts. This development is fascinating, since the technology often follows paths taken decades earlier, yet with some relatively simple new tools, and the field is now also being supported by biotechnology corporations, and it is likely therefore that this new position will revolutionize the way we freeze. This may initially result in technologies with minimal effects, if any, on cryopreserved cells. Second, micromanipulation procedures have improved the treatment of male factor associated infertility through intracytoplasmic sperm injection (ICSI), while biopsy allows geneticists to look into aspects of genetic disease or chromosomal disorders prior to embryo transfer. Such processes are discussed elsewhere in this volume. Some new micromanipulation technologies may still be relevant for the treatment of certain conditions or for the diagnosis of others, yet it is likely that there are limits to some applications such as nuclear transplantation. Here we discuss some of the potential uses associated with nuclear and cytoplasmic transplantation for treatment of infertility, as well as for treating other disorders. Third, the largest new contribution still to come may be from molecular biology. Tools will be developed that will permit transfer of single embryos after assessment of gene expression or gene product analyses, and from findings related to the understanding of molecular processes in the developing embryo. Progress in these fields is still hampered by prohibitive legislation and lack of funding, but is nevertheless advancing.

CRYOPRESERVATION OF OOCYTES AND EMBRYOS

Cryopreservation of gametes and embryos is an attractive option for the future prevention of infertility and the postponement of pregnancy. Much more commonly it has been applied as an extender of treatment during assisted reproduction, since it allows the ability ethically to remove embryos from the transfer process, thereby diminishing the chance of high-order multiple pregnancy. In this respect, embryo freezing has revolutionized *in vitro* fertilization, even though it is associated with some embryo loss. It is interesting to observe that current cryopreservation technology is still based on the notion that biological activity ceases at subzero temperature. Indeed, one wonders why there are no other modes of arresting cellular processes without affecting future viability. As it is, there simply seems to be no way around the basic biophysical balancing of processes such as hydration, dehydration, osmotic pressure, pH and ionic stress management. With every so-called development of new cryopreservation technology, the same basic principles are still being reshuffled. It is imperative to understand the physics of the technology, particularly if human oocytes are going to be frozen on a massive scale as a preventive measure to delay reproduction deliberately. In the USA, there are now several organizations aiming to promote exactly that. This may cause the preservation of perhaps millions of oocytes from very young women in ways that may prove to be suboptimal decades later. This is very different to using cryopreservation technology when there is no other

solution, such as during conventional assisted reproduction, when preventing the risk of multiple pregnancy is not an optional process. Embryos are usually removed from storage because of failed implantation of fresh embryos, or when patients return to opt for more siblings. Length of storage rarely exceeds 5 years (Cohen, unpublished data).

There has been renewed interest in oocyte cryopreservation because of the prohibitive nature of some legislation, such as the recent law change in Italy which prohibits embryo freezing, but also because some studies suggest that the procedure can be more successful than initially thought[1]. Clinical oocyte freezing was probably seriously hindered by reports more than 15 years ago that the spindle of mouse eggs could disassemble at low temperature[2–4]. The notion that egg freezing could cause chromosomal anomalies became a 'fact of the trade', and was shown to be only moderately accurate years later[5]. Another interesting turn-around, simple in retrospect, was that fertilization could be more precise using ICSI[6]. Until then, polyspermy was common after egg freezing. Several laboratories started carefully reintroducing egg freezing, and by 2000 an estimated 20 children had been born from the procedure[7]. This number is now likely to exceed 300 babies, indicating that the first hurdles hindering wide application of this technology have been removed.

Some cryopreservation protocols use the conventional slow-cooling approach, which, with the addition of high sucrose, may be quite promising[1]. Others use rapid freezing and vitrification. A third experimental approach involves technology developed in our laboratory[8]. This involves new media from which sodium chloride has been removed. A fourth proposal is based on studies of organisms that survive extreme conditions of cold. Several species have demonstrated the ability to accumulate intracellular sugars to survive in extreme conditions. The catch to this is that the sugars may not permeate mammalian cells rapidly enough. So researchers have suggested circumventing the problem by microinjection[9]. There have been no clinical reports yet of this technology. A fifth system looks at the cell cycle and proposes to freeze interphase nuclei. One of the alternatives involves freezing immature germinal vesicle eggs, which is complicated because it also involves egg maturation[10]. An alternative to this would be to freeze activated oocytes and cryopreserve female pronuclei separately from male karyoplasts[11]. Thawing of both pronuclei could then reconstitute the zygote. Although elegant, the approach is cumbersome. However, mice have been born from this procedure.

Even with modification of freezing protocols and an improvement in survival rates, it still appears complicated to obtain a high percentage of fertilized and normally dividing embryos after oocyte cryopreservation. Initial survival rates for frozen–thawed human oocytes are around 50–70%, but that number can be significantly reduced after pronuclear formation (fertilization), and cleavage beyond the two-cell stage. As a notable exception, Marina and Marina reported similar pregnancy rates for oocytes and embryos after cryopreservation, but this work requires further confirmation[12].

Chromosomal condition of oocytes

The reason why oocytes are more sensitive to cryopreservation than embryos is uncertain; hence investigators have been trying to determine the differences between the two cell types. The most obvious is the difference in cell cycle, as the DNA of mature, unfertilized oocytes is compacted into chromosomes that are aligned on a metaphase plate, while the majority of DNA in embryos exists as decondensed chromatin at interphase. It was therefore assumed early on that the physical state of the DNA could be altered by cryopreservation, and investigators analyzed the chromatin and spindle structure and cryoprotectant exposure before and after cooling. They found that the spindle became disorganized and the genetic integrity of the resulting embryos suspect[13].

Physical conditions, including temperature and cryoprotectants, can affect microtubule polymerization[14]. Specific alterations, including the depolymerization of microtubules during the cryopreservation of metaphase II oocytes, pose a potential problem for normal spindle function after storage. Some reports suggest that the spindle apparatus of cryopreserved metaphase II oocytes depolymerizes and can only rarely reform properly. Other studies suggest the contrary, arguing that the spindle does repolymerize correctly[15–18]. In general, the differences between these reports lie in the details of cryopreservation. There appears to be agreement about the depolymerization of microtubules of mammalian oocytes during cryopreservation.

Besides the microtubules that make up the spindle apparatus, other cytoskeletal elements, particularly those associated with cell membrane, have been shown to play a role in oocyte survival following cryopreservation. Compounds including the cytochalasins, ethylene glycol tetraacetic acid (EGTA) and taxol which affect the cytoskeleton have been used as stabilizers prior to or during cryopreservation, and have had, in some cases, beneficial effects. However, these and similar compounds have not made their way into clinical protocols.

Many papers analyzing the effect of cryopreservation on spindle reformation report relatively low oocyte survival rates of 50–70% (mouse and human). It is reasonable to assume that spindle reformation and functionality would benefit from a protocol where oocytes survived at a high frequency[19]. Unpublished data from our laboratory on mouse, bovine and human oocytes also show that, if the oocytes are frozen and thawed properly, the spindle can and will reform[20]. It is important to remember that in fresh, non-cryopreserved oocytes the percentage of normal spindles is only around 90%. Functionality after spindle reformation must be considered as well. Of the births resulting from frozen–thawed oocytes, no abnormalities have yet been reported, despite the concerns raised above[12,21].

Some other studies on zona hardening, digyny, cooling sensitivity and osmotic tolerance have simply raised more questions rather than provided answers[22–24]. Since 1970, only minor modifications to clinical cryopreservation practice have occurred, with no significant breakthroughs, except for vitrification. It has therefore become obvious that oocytes need a different approach to cryopreservation than embryos, although the ground rules of cryopreservation are fundamentally similar.

Optimizing cryopreservation

The observation that oocytes and embryos can survive freezing to subzero temperatures, storage for extended periods of time and rewarming to physiological temperatures, is remarkable. The difficulties in learning about the process are vastly increased by the fact that, during cooling and storage, the cells are inside containers under extreme conditions that do not allow for any type of analysis. This means that for the most part we make visual observations of gross morphology only prior to and after the entire cryopreservation process. In order to improve survival rates and development to healthy offspring significantly we have to understand the entire process, including understanding the stresses which cells can tolerate when subjecting them to cryopreservation. Oocytes and embryos are incredibly complicated, highly organized living structures that respond only to a limited extent to environmental changes. Each step in the cryopreservation process is critically important when trying to obtain a high survival and birth rate. For a new approach to cryopreservation of oocytes, we must keep an open mind and take nothing for granted, unless specifically tested with appropriate controls.

MICROMANIPULATION OF CELLULAR PROCESSES PRIOR TO IMPLANTATION

Advanced assisted reproductive techniques are being proposed for new applications involving the creation of embryos with selected genomes for use in medical scenarios that fall outside standard infertility treatment. These techniques are often misguidedly lumped together under the umbrella of 'cloning', but the physical manipulation of cellular and nuclear components in the oocyte or early embryo can be used for a large variety of reasons, ranging from therapeutic nuclear transplantation for human leukocyte antigen (HLA) matching of embryonic stem cells, to cytoplasmic transplantation in zygotes for avoiding transmission of mitochondrial disease. Such manipulation and any other manipulation of cellular processes during the critical early stages of development is a complicated matter, with potentially negative consequences for subsequent development. The limited basic and applied scientific knowledge available suggests that application in the human of nuclear transplantation may be at least problematic, and possibly have effects on offspring. Furthermore, such manipulation is seen by many as inherently unethical and taboo.

There currently exists a wide range of opinion and action within the pursuit and application of such techniques. Some human ART workers suggest that even the most extreme scenarios involving human nuclear transfer are well within the grasp of current or near-future technology[25,26]. Others conclude that any manipulative intervention for the establishment of pregnancy will forever be out of the question because

of safety issues, while the use of such techniques for so-called 'therapeutic' intervention (stem cell development) should be pursued. Interestingly, this position regarding one revered experimental concept seems to be held by the majority of the basic science community. Constructive analysis must be maintained here, since the possibility of adverse imprinting shown after reproductive cloning probably applies to other forms of nuclear transplantation as well. Some suggest a complete restriction on all interventional strategies, including most treatments for human infertility. This is obviously a complex matter, one that is intricately connected to morality as enforced by organized religion, a prime example being the recent Italian law, called Legge 40[27]. The attitude towards manipulation of germ cells and embryos is a defining issue for the future of reproductive medicine and ART. A critical and honest understanding of these techniques and their potential problems and benefits is therefore vital. The technologies under consideration fall into three main types: diagnostic, ART-related and stem cell-related.

Diagnostic techniques

Diagnostic scenarios have already successfully used nuclear transfer-based techniques for facilitating the genetic assessment of gametes and embryos. An example of this involves obtaining condensed chromosomes from germ-cell or embryonic nuclei[28–30]. These techniques involve the combination (by injection or electrofusion) of the cell to be analyzed with the oocytes or early embryos of experimental animals, directing the injected nucleus to undergo cell-cycle changes subject to the controlling cytoplasm. In this scenario, introduced nuclei may be redirected by the cell cycle, leading to the production of condensed chromosomes, which are usually only seen at metaphase. Such techniques, using readily available bovine or mouse material, allow for a complete chromosomal analysis as necessary in the case of certain complex translocations. These techniques have been applied both in the assessment of human spermatozoa and in the assessment of individual blastomeres from human embryos during ART. Recently, a similar technique, termed 'gamete duplication', has been suggested by Willadsen (unpublished data) for creating two haploid chromosome complements from one spermatozoon. This would theoretically allow one set of genetic material to be used for analysis while the other could be used in a nuclear transfer-based clinical scenario (Willadsen, unpublished data). The metaphase diagnostic techniques perhaps fall outside what is currently considered invasive clinical nuclear manipulation, since, apart from a standard biopsy procedure, the actual clinical embryos are not disturbed. However, these are still experimental protocols involving nuclear manipulation of human material, and could be extended in the future to become part of more invasive interventional strategies. The current trend among many lawmakers is to generalize any technology involving nuclei. This attitude has outlawed perfectly acceptable diagnostic approaches in many countries. Fortunately, there are exceptions to this devastating anti-scientific trend, such as the UK and Belgium, where reproductive technology is debated in an open-minded and intelligent manner.

Clinical ART-related techniques

Interventional ART techniques could potentially address a variety of clinically relevant deficits in the gametes or preimplantation embryos of infertile patients or of those with heritable genetic lesions. Conceptually, these techniques range from mildly invasive strategies for 'improving' oocytes to full-fledged somatic cell nuclear transfer for the creation of gametes or embryos. In addressing cases of poor development and implantation failure associated with dysfunctional or genetically abnormal oocytes, such compromised oocytes can simply be replaced by donor substitutes, but at the price of losing the patient's genetic contribution. A variety of potentially controversial strategies, initially proposed by Willadsen, have been examined to get around this problem, including oocyte to donor ooplast nuclear transfer and the creation of functional 'oocytes' from the patient's somatic cells[31–33]. Another concept involves attempts to 'improve' the patient's own eggs by infusion of theoretically healthy ooplasm or ooplasmic components from a donor egg[34,35].

Known anomalies in the oocyte fall into two main categories, those directly related to oocyte aneuploidy and those related to oocyte dysfunction. The incidence of chromosomal abnormalities such as aneuploidy is one of the biggest challenges facing the treatment of infertility in patients of advanced age[36]. Cytoplasmic deficits related to poor oxidative conditions or the lack

of critical meiotic components have been proposed as causative factors in the generation of such meiotic abnormalities[37–39]. Theoretically, a correction of these cytoplasmic deficits could result in promoting correct spindle behavior and chromosome segregation. Since the majority of aneuploidy in the human apparently arises in the meiotic divisions involved in the generation of the mature metaphase II oocyte, manipulative intervention would need to occur prior to the completion of meiosis[40]. The main manipulative strategy that has been proposed is the transfer of the oocyte nucleus at the germinal vesicle (GV) stage from a theoretically compromised patient egg to an enucleated donor oocyte[41]. In this way, the entire cytoplasmic component is exchanged between the patient and the donor. Experimental protocols in the mouse and human have demonstrated that such GV stage nuclear transfer can be performed, and that reconstituted oocytes can exhibit successful maturation and subsequent fertilization by ICSI. However, to date, the extent of such studies is still very limited, and a complete and satisfactory evaluation of even the physical aspects of these methods in the human is lacking. Furthermore, the overall concept that such cytoplasmic exchange can correct spindle function and lead to a reduced rate of meiosis-associated aneuploidy remains to be established.

The second area in which manipulative techniques could be used is for ooplasmic deficits. Ooplasmic-mediated activities are critical in setting up much of the subsequent developmental program, with stable and heritable downstream effects[42,43]. There can be little question that dysfunction in ooplasmic components is a causative factor in human infertility. Preliminary work in the mouse demonstrated the lack of a detrimental effect for cytoplasmic transfer and suggested the presence of a positive effect under some scenarios[44]. A variety of other animal research also supports such a positive effect[45–47]. Based on these experiments and others, the direct transfer of synchronous cytoplasm from donor to patient eggs was attempted in patients with recurring developmental deficits and implantation failure[34,48]. This technique is based on the concept that healthy donor cytoplasm contains components that are lacking or compromised in patient oocytes, and that an infusion of such components will have a positive effect on development. The initial results from applying this experimental technique in a defined group of patients seemed to be moderately positive. Implantation was improved, with a 43% clinical pregnancy rate (and several births) in 27 couples with a consistent combined history of almost 100 failed assisted reproduction cycles[49]. To date, several variations on the oocyte infusion concept have been reported, including the use of cryopreserved oocytes or polyspermic zygotes for donor cytoplasm and the injection of purified mitochondria from the patient's own cumulus cells[35,50,51]. This approach has led to the birth of a number of babies in Taiwan, yet issues such as accumulation of mutations in somatic mitochondria and the fact that mitochondrial DNA replication is passive in oocytes, but not in the injected mitochondria, requires further basic studies. Following its initial clinical trial, the United States Food and Drug Administration (FDA) issued an order stating that ooplasmic transfer and similar protocols are subject to approval under an Investigational New Drug application. This intervention was based solely on the issue of genomic transfer, since mitochondrial genomes were shown to be transferred from the donor to the patient oocyte during the procedure. This matter is currently under analysis and review, and will no doubt have an impact on the future applications of similar manipulative human clinical protocols. Recently, cytoplasmic 'correction' has been attempted, involving the transfer of pronuclei between patient zygotes and donor zygote-stage cytoplasts[52]. This procedure was used in a patient exhibiting consistent developmental failure during ART, and led to the establishment of a complicated triplet pregnancy which failed prior to 30 weeks' gestation. The fetuses derived from this procedure were shown to carry the patient's genome, overtly normal karyotypes and mitochondrial genotype derived solely from the donor zygote cytoplasts.

The most invasive manipulative techniques proposed for ART-related treatment concern the use of genomic manipulation to create gametes or embryos for individuals who lack functional germ cells. A variety of strategies might be possible based on nuclear transfer scenarios using premature or non-functional germ cells or somatic cells as the genome source. One strategy would involve the creation of patient-derived haploid cells that could be combined with an ooplast to create a functional 'oocyte'. A possibility is to use stem cell-derived gamete development[53]. A second strategy would be simply to create an embryo through nuclear transfer from a patient-derived somatic cell.

This would constitute true somatic cell nuclear transfer (SCNT) 'cloning', and the resulting offspring would harbor the identical genome of their parent. Such proposals are highly controversial from both scientific and ethical standpoints even though for some individuals this may be the only reproductive option available.

Creating artificial gametes from the diploid germline or somatic cells via nuclear transfer would require the additional step of haploidizing the source genome to allow for compatible combination with a germ cell genome or second haploidized genome. Experiments in the mouse and human have demonstrated limited development following protocols with diploid somatic cells[54,55]. An issue that must be addressed is the incomplete or absent crossing-over phenomenon that naturally shuffles genes during the early stage in meiosis. In the human, somatic cells injected into enucleated oocytes apparently underwent haploidization by the emission of a polar body, yet it is not known whether crossing-over gene reorganization happened. It is also not known whether the processes of erasure and acquisition of imprint took place. The resulting artificial 'oocytes' could be fertilized, and fluorescent *in situ* hybridization analysis of the second polar body indicated a haploid complement. Haploid pronuclei have also been observed following diploid cell injection into enucleated human oocytes[56]. Theoretically, a variety of techniques are possible based on the premise of allowing diploid chromosomes to segregate in an oocyte. The resulting pronuclei or polar bodies can theoretically be retransferred to a second enucleated oocyte or to a zygote from which the appropriate pronucleus has been removed. To date, experimental protocols inducing haploidization have been very limited, and a definitive demonstration that only chromosome reduction is sufficient for normal development is lacking.

A secondary application for some of the cellular transplantation techniques would be to circumvent inheritance of deleterious mitochondrial genotypes associated with several rare but serious human diseases. Individuals harboring such genotypes transmit them to their offspring through the ooplasm. Theoretically, by manipulation or exchanging compromised ooplasm with healthy donor ooplasm, such inheritance could be prevented. This might be possible either via ooplasmic injection or through nuclear transfer. In this regard, it is interesting to note that donor mitochondrial genomes could be detected in a limited subset of offspring produced from ooplasmic transfer[57]. Conversely, the patient's mitochondrial genome could not be detected in pronuclear transfer-derived fetuses which harbored at least a majority donor mitochondrial genotype[52]. Mitochondrial inheritance is still not fully understood, and further work will be needed to establish the basis for such interventional strategies.

Therapeutic 'cloning' techniques

A final category for invasive manipulation involves the use of nuclear transfer for the creation of embryonic stem cell lines. This has been phrased 'therapeutic cloning', vernacular that is inflammatory from a public relations point of view.

'Therapeutic cloning' would be technically similar to the previously discussed techniques for use in germinal vesicle (GV) or somatic cell nuclear transfer. However, in this case such nuclear transplantation methods would be applied in achieving the creation of patient-specific embryonic stem cell lines for use in HLA-compatible cellular-replacement therapies[58,59]. Blastocysts created by patient SCNT to an enucleated donated oocyte would be used as the source for the derivation of such cell lines[60]. In this way, the stem cells or derived tissues, such as neurons, muscle or blood cells, would be immunologically identical with the patient and would not be subject to rejection[61–63]. Recently, the first successful demonstration of the derivation of human embryonic stem cells from cloned embryos has been reported[64].

Safety and clinical application of cell cycle-related micromanipulation

Nuclear transfer and related techniques have been applied in mammalian embryology for over 20 years. Although much has been learned, the process and developmental consequences of nuclear transfer are still poorly understood. One clear aspect that has emerged from this work is that critical genomic 'remodeling' and processing occurs during early development, and this process can be perturbed by manipulative intervention. For the most part, development following nuclear transfer experiments of somatic nuclei has been compromised. Problems with the efficiency of nuclear transfer cloning technology

have been associated with aberrant epigenetic processing and altered genomic imprinting[65–67]. However, this connection is complicated by the fact that simple *in vitro* culture is known to result in certain epigenetic effects in animal models as well[68–70]. The connection between altered imprinting, gene expression and developmental consequences is far from defined, although developmental abnormalities, pathological conditions and other phenotypic consequences of imprinting defects are clearly present in mammals, including the human[71,72]. However, it is also recognized that differences in epigenetic processing exist between model species and the human[73]. These differences suggest that epigenetically derived abnormalities observed following *in vitro* manipulation in experimental animals may not be fully relevant to the human. In primates, a secondary issue may arise from depletion of critical maternal ooplasmic proteins during enucleation[74]. This phenomenon has been suggested to underlie a failure to obtain experimental primate offspring from SCNT. However, the recent success of SCNT in producing apparently normal human blastocysts and embryonic stem cells (which used a unique enucleation technique) indicates that this problem may be avoidable and is possibly of a technical nature[64].

The identified and potential developmental problems that could arise from inadequate genetic programming, imprinting deficits and other developmental perturbations make the immediate clinical application of invasive manipulative techniques questionable. However, as stated before, there are clear differences in genetic, developmental and physical aspects between the experimental animal systems in which techniques such as SCNT have been developed and the human. Obviously, much basic research remains to be done in the human. For instance, the simple expression analysis of imprinted genes in experimental nuclear transfer human embryos (as has already been accomplished in normal oocytes and embryos) would be a critical step in assessing potential aberrant epigenetic aspects[75]. There is reason to hope that the problematic aspects of nuclear transfer can be successfully addressed in the human. A consistent lesson from the past 15 years of human oocyte micromanipulation, including the development of enucleation techniques and ICSI, is that human oocytes and early embryos exhibit much greater tolerance of physical manipulation compared with rodent and possibly even non-human primate material. Furthermore, other critical differences may exist that will facilitate nuclear transfer in the human. This has recently been supported by the identification of clear differences in the imprinting process between human and rodent/large animal species, and in the successful production of blastocysts and stem cells following human SCNT[64,73].

It is at the very least premature to suggest that success with these or related techniques in clinical applications will be impossible. As in any medical practice issue, examining this should involve an honest recognition of potential benefits and risks. The potential of such invasive manipulative techniques needs to be recognized, while accepting that safety and efficacy remain to be determined. Individuals, organizations and governments are currently involved in considerable debate as to the proper course to take in regulating human research and medical practice in this area. It is clear that considerable further research, including human experiments and clinical trials, will be necessary to begin to answer many questions, answers to which will help to define this assessment. Hopefully, the coming years will see an increase in support for such basic research, while the ethical debate continues.

GENE EXPRESSION ANALYSIS IN HUMAN OOCYTES AND EMBRYOS

Gene activity is responsible for the co-ordination of cellular processes throughout life, regulating features such as cell division and differentiation as well as having an important function in the control of homeostatic and metabolic mechanisms. Precise control of gene activity is of particular significance during preimplantation development, a phase at which the first cellular differentiation begins and the embryo switches from a dependence on maternal RNA, derived from the oocyte, to expression of its own genome. Given the importance of gene activity, it is perhaps surprising that few data concerning gene expression in human preimplantation embryos currently exist.

The characterization of gene activity at given phases of development provides an indication of the biochemical and cellular pathways active or repressed at specific stages. This information is of great scientific interest, revealing the mechanisms underlying key developmental events. Additionally, it is becoming increasingly clear that the analysis of gene expression also has the potential to become a powerful clinical tool, assisting in the optimization of assisted reproductive technologies, yielding information concerning embryo viability and providing clues to optimizing environmental conditions.

Recent data from our laboratory have shown that human preimplantation embryos exhibit patterns of gene expression that are highly characteristic of their developmental stage. Each new phase of preimplantation development is accompanied by predictable fluctuations in gene expression. Our study concentrated on nine genes that function in a range of important cellular processes, including cell cycle regulation, DNA repair, apoptosis, maintenance of accurate chromosome segregation and construction of the cytoskeleton. The activity of nine genes was quantified in each of over 50 embryos at various stages of pre-implantation development, using real-time reverse transcriptase-polymerase chain reaction (RT-PCR)[76,77].

The detailed analysis of preimplantation gene expression revealed that mRNA levels in oocytes are generally high, but fall dramatically after fertilization, an observation that has been previously reported[78–80]. For most genes a small recovery in expression was seen in embryos composed of 4–8 cells, although some genes, such as *BRCA1*, sometimes displayed massive expression at this stage. In most cases (although not all), expression continued to increase at the morula stage, with the greatest expression levels usually observed in blastocysts[76].

The stage-specific activation or repression of genes that function in specific metabolic pathways can be taken as an indicator of a change in nutritional requirements. Additionally, the activation of genes expressed in response to a variety of stresses, including nutrient deprivation and other suboptimal culture conditions, may reveal deficiencies of *in vitro* methods. For these reasons, data on gene expression can provide clues that assist in the optimization of media formulations and embryo culture protocols.

Although our research indicates that embryos at specific stages of preimplantation development have characteristic profiles of gene expression, a few embryos with atypical patterns of gene activity were observed. Interestingly, embryos with unusual gene expression profiles were frequently morphologically abnormal. A careful analysis of morphological notes and gene expression data revealed that up-regulation or repression of certain genes was correlated with specific abnormalities, many of which are negatively correlated with embryo implantation[77].

One morphological abnormality that was found to be associated with altered expression of several genes was cellular fragmentation. The proportion of the embryo volume composed of fragments and the temporal and spatial patterns of fragment distribution have been shown to influence embryo implantation rate[81–83]. For this reason, fragmentation is routinely evaluated at infertility clinics, and serves as a useful indicator of developmental competence.

Our analyses suggest that the number of transcripts from the *BRCA1* gene tended to be lower than average in fragmented embryos, while the *ATM*, β-*actin* and *TP53* genes were frequently overexpressed relative to morphologically normal embryos[77]. Up-regulation of *TP53* was the change most strongly associated with fragmentation. The protein product of *TP53* (p53) is a transcription factor, activated in response to a variety of cellular stresses, including DNA damage, mitotic spindle aberrations, hypoxia, nitric oxide and ribonucleotide depletion. Not only does this finding hint at possible causes of fragmentation, which currently remain elusive, but also suggests that it may be possible to devise embryo viability assays based on genes such as *TP53*.

Currently, assessments of embryo viability are based, for the most part, on morphological observation, a useful but far from perfect approach, as individual parameters are rarely predictive in an absolute sense. In some cases, viability screening has been improved by the supplementation of morphological examination with information on chromosomal status determined using preimplantation genetic diagnosis (PGD)[84,85]. We think it likely that the pattern of genes expressed by an embryo also reveals important information concerning its viability. It is reasonable to expect that characteristic patterns of expression will be observed in embryos suffering from problems such as thermal shock or abnormal chromosome numbers, or in embryos initiating pathways leading to developmental arrest or apoptosis. The early stages of such processes are likely to be invisible to morphological examination, but may be revealed by gene expression analysis.

We suggest that an embryo displaying an expression profile that is appropriate for its developmental stage and is not associated with abnormal morphology is much more likely to be viable than an embryo showing atypical expression and/or activation of stress-related genes. If such patterns could be assessed prior to embryo transfer they could assist embryologists and clinicians in deciding which embryos to transfer to the uterus. However, the question of how gene expression can be assessed without destruction of the embryo still remains. Also, it is likely that early clinical work will involve biopsy procedures that can provide an accurate analysis of cellular dysfunction, yet may not be predictive of accompanying domains.

Previous studies have indicated that meaningful expression data can be obtained by the biopsy and analysis of single blastomeres[86,87]. However, it is likely that some genes display significant variation in transcript number between different blastomeres of the same embryo[88]. Consequently, any tests based on embryo biopsy can only be applied to genes that have relatively homogeneous expression throughout preimplantation embryos. Additionally, the precise stage at which analysis is attempted will be critical, as the gene in question must be expressed to detectable levels and not obscured by oocyte-derived maternal mRNA transcripts[89]. Ultimately, it may prove more feasible to assess prognostically relevant genes (or other elements/products of the pathways they influence) via methods that do not depend on blastomere biopsy.

In the future, it may be possible to design a new generation of PGD tests, combining analysis of genes or their products that serve as indicators of embryo viability with an assessment of mRNA from genes responsible for single gene disorders, thus permitting simultaneous PGD and embryo evaluation. An approach to PGD based on single blastomere biopsy and mRNA analysis has been suggested previously[86]. Theoretically, such tests should be resistant to allele drop-out (ADO), a phenomenon unique to single-cell PCR, whereby only one of the two alleles in a heterozygous cell successfully amplifies[90,91]. ADO has caused several PGD misdiagnoses, but only occurs if the copy number of the target DNA sequence is very low (e.g. only one copy of each allele is present per cell). Expressed genes often produce thousands of mRNA copies per cell, and consequently amplification of the resultant cDNA should not be affected by ADO.

In recent years there have been growing concerns over the safety of certain assisted reproductive techniques, such as ICSI. While it is important to note that the vast majority of children born following ICSI are as healthy as their naturally conceived counterparts, there is evidence to suggest an elevated risk of certain disorders caused by the aberrant expression of specific genes, such as Angelman's syndrome[92,93]. The genes involved are known as 'imprinted genes', and are unusual in that only one of the two copies in each somatic cell is active. The active copy of the gene is determined by the parent from whom it was derived. Some imprinted genes are only expressed from the maternally inherited copy, the paternally inherited copy remaining silent, while for other imprinted genes the reverse is true. It seems that the 'imprint', a chemical modification of the DNA that distinguishes genes of maternal and paternal origin, may be lost as the result of certain *in vitro* techniques, thus leading to aberrant expression.

By analyzing the expression of imprinted genes in ART-derived embryos, the frequency of problems induced by assisted reproductive methods can be determined. Furthermore, if techniques used for the analysis of gene expression and methods used for preimplantation genetic diagnosis are combined, it should be possible to screen for abnormal expression of imprinted genes prior to embryo transfer. This seems particularly interesting, as the maternal imprint has been implicated in most cases in children born from ART.

One of the most recent developments in the field of gene expression analysis has been the application of microarray technology, methods that permit the simultaneous analysis of many thousands of genes in a single experiment. We have recently succeeded in adapting microarray protocols to the analysis of single oocytes and embryos, a step which should greatly accelerate the rate at which genes relevant to embryo viability are identified[94]. Microarray technology is a relatively new technique that provides the investigator with the ability to monitor and quantify the expression of thousands of genes simultaneously. This technological breakthrough has the potential to provide detailed insight into cellular processes involved in the regulation of gene expression. Bermudez and colleagues used microarray methods to examine the expression of linearly amplified RNA from individual and pooled ($n = 5$) human oocytes[94]. The amplification

strategy consistently produced a complex representative cDNA population. A catalogue of 1361 transcripts expressed in human oocytes was identified, of which 406 have been independently confirmed.

REFERENCES

1. Fabbri R, Porcu E, Marsella T. Human oocyte cryopreservation: new perspectives regarding oocyte survival. Hum Reprod 2001; 16: 411–16
2. Pickering SJ, Braude PR, Johnson MH. Transient cooling to room temperature can cause irreversible disruption of the meiotic spindle in the human oocyte. Fertil Steril 1990; 54: 102–8
3. Pickering SJ, Johnson MH. The influence of cooling on the organization of the meiotic spindle of the mouse oocyte. Hum Reprod 1987; 2: 207–16
4. Sathananthan AH, Ng SC, Trounson AO. The effects of ultrarapid freezing on meiotic and mitotic spindles of mouse oocytes and embryos. Gamete Res 1988; 21: 385–401
5. Gook DA, Osborn SM, Bourne H. Fertilization of human oocytes following cryopreservation; normal karyotypes and absence of stray chromosomes. Hum Reprod 1994; 9: 684–91
6. Tucker MJ, Morton PC, Wright G, et al. Clinical application of human egg cryopreservation. Hum Reprod 1998; 13: 3156–9
7. Stachecki JJ, Cohen J. An overview of oocyte cryopreservation. Reprod Biomed Online 2004; 9: 152–63
8. Stachecki JJ, Cohen J, Willadsen SM. Cryopreservation of unfertilized mouse oocytes: the effect of replacing sodium with choline in the freezing medium. Cryobiology 1998; 37: 346–54
9. Wright DL, Eroglu A, Toner M, Toth TL. Use of sugars in cryopreserving human oocytes. Reprod Biomed Online 2004; 9: 179–86
10. Zhang J, Wang CW, Krey L, et al. In vitro maturation of human preovulatory oocytes reconstructed by germinal vesicle transfer. Fertil Steril 1999; 71: 726–31
11. Levron J, Willadsen SM, Shimmel T, Cohen J. Cryopreservation of activated mouse oocytes and zygote reconstitution after thaw. Hum Reprod 1998; 13 (Suppl 4): 109–16
12. Marina F, Marina S. Comments on oocyte cryopreservation. Reprod Biomed Online 2003; 6: 401–2
13. Kola I, Kirby C, Shaw J, et al. Vitrification of mouse oocytes results in aneuploid zygotes and malformed fetuses. Teratology 1988; 38: 467–74
14. Vincent C, Johnson MH. Cooling, cryoprotectants, and the cytoskeleton of the mammalian oocyte. Oxf Rev Reprod Biol 1992; 14: 73–100

15. Zenzes MT, Bielecki R, Casper RF. Effects of chilling to 0 degrees C on the morphology of meiotic spindles in human metaphase II oocytes. Fertil Steril 2001; 75: 769–77

16. Boiso I, Marti M, Santalo J. A confocal microscopy analysis of the spindle and chromosome configurations of human oocytes cryopreserved at the germinal vesicle and metaphase II stage. Hum Reprod 2002; 17: 1885–91

17. Saunders KM, Parks JE. Effects of cryopreservation procedures on the cytology and fertilization rate of in vitro-matured bovine oocytes. Biol Reprod 1999; 61: 178–87

18. Wu B, Tong J, Leibo SP. Effects of cooling germinal vesicle-stage bovine oocytes on meiotic spindle formation following in vitro maturation. Mol Reprod Dev 1999; 54: 388–95

19. Gook DA, Osborn SM, Bourne H. Fertilization of human oocytes following cryopreservation; normal karyotypes and absence of stray chromosomes. Hum Reprod 1994; 9: 684–91

20. Stachecki JJ, Willadsen SM. 2004; in press

21. Fosas N, Marina F, Torres PJ. The births of five Spanish babies from cryopreserved donated oocytes. Comments on oocyte cryopreservation. Hum Reprod 2003; 18: 1417–21

22. Carroll J, Wood MJ, Whittingham DG. Normal fertilization and development of frozen-thawed mouse oocytes: protective action of certain macromolecules. Biol Reprod 1993; 48: 606–12

23. George MA, Johnson MH. Use of fetal bovine serum substitutes for the protection of the mouse zona pellucida against hardening during cryoprotectant addition. Hum Reprod 1993; 8: 1898–900

24. Pickering SJ, Johnson MH. The influence of cooling on the organization of the meiotic spindle of the mouse oocyte. Hum Reprod 1987; 2: 207–16

25. Zavos PM. Human reproductive cloning: the time is near. Reprod Biomed Online 2003; 6: 397–8

26. Zhan J, Zhuang G, Zeng Y, et al. Pregnancy derived from human nuclear transfer. Fertil Steril 2003; 80: S56

27. Benagiano G, Gianaroli L. The new Italian IVF legislation. Reprod Biomed Online 2004; 9: 117–25

28. Lee JD, Kamiguchi Y, Yanagimachi R. Analysis of chromosome constitution of human spermatozoa with normal and aberrant head morphologies after injection into mouse oocytes. Hum Reprod 1996; 11: 1942–6

29. Verlinsky Y, Evsikov S. A simplified and efficient method for obtaining metaphase chromosomes from individual human blastomeres. Fertil Steril 1999; 72: 1127–33

30. Willadsen SM, Levron J, Munné S, et al. Rapid visualization of metaphase chromosomes in single human blastomeres after fusion with in-vitro matured bovine eggs. Hum Reprod 1999; 14: 470–5

31. Willadsen SM. Observations on the behavior of foreign nuclei introduced into in-vitro matured oocytes. Presented at a Symposium on 'cloning mammals by nuclear transfer', International Embryo Transfer Society, Colorado, USA, 1992

32. Takeuchi T, Gong J, Veek LL, et al. Preliminary findings in germinal vesicle transplantation of immature human oocytes. Hum Reprod 2001; 16: 730–6

33. Nagy PZ, Bourg de Mello MR, Tesarik J, et al. Fertilizable bovine oocytes reconstructed using somatic cell nuclei and metaphase-II oocytes. Hum Reprod 2001; 16 (Suppl 1): abstr O–009

34. Cohen J, Scott R, Schimmel T, et al. Birth of an infant after transfer of anucleate donor cytoplasm into recipient eggs. Lancet 1997; 350: 186–7

35. Tzeng C, Hsieh S, Chang N. Pregnancy derived from mitochondrial transfer (MIT) into oocyte from patient's own cumulus cells (cGCs). Fertil Steril 2001; 76 (Suppl 3S): abstr O–180

36. Munné S, Alikani M, Tomkin G. Embryo morphology, developmental rates, and maternal age are correlated with chromosome abnormalities. Fertil Steril 1995; 64: 382–91

37. Gaulden ME. Maternal age effect: the enigma of Down syndrome and other trisomic conditions. Mutat Res 1992; 296: 69–88

38. Tarin JJ. Aetiology of age-associated aneuploidy: a mechanism based on the 'free radical theory of ageing'. Hum Reprod 1995; 10: 1563–5

39. Van Blerkom J, Antczak M, Schrader R. The developmental potential of the human oocyte is related to the dissolved oxygen content of the follicular fluid: association with vascular endothelial growth factor levels and peri-follicular blood flow characteristics. Hum Reprod 1997; 12: 1047–55

40. Hassold T, Chiu D. Maternal age-specific rates of numerical chromosome abnormalities with specific reference to trisomy. Hum Genet 1985; 70: 11–17

41. Zhang J, Wang CW, Krey LC. In vitro maturation of human pre-ovulatory oocytes reconstructed by germinal vesicle transfer. Fertil Steril 1999; 71: 726–31

42. Kono T, Obata Y, Yoshimzu T. Epigenetic modifications during oocyte growth correlates with extended parthenogenetic development in the mouse. Nat Genet 1996; 13: 91–4

43. Roemer I, Reik W, Dean W, Kloase J. Epigenetic inheritance in the mouse. Curr Biol 1997; 7: 277–80

44. Levron J, Willadsen S, Bertoli M, Cohen J. The development of mouse zygotes after fusion with

synchronous and asynchronous cytoplasm. Hum Reprod 1996; 11: 1287–92

45. Muggleton-Harris A, Whittingham D, Wilson L. Cytoplasmic control of preimplantation development in vitro in the mouse. Nature (London) 1982; 299: 460–2

46. Pratt H, Muggleton-Harris A. Cycling cytoplasmic factors that promote mitosis in the cultured 2-cell mouse embryo. Development 1988; 104: 115–20

47. Flood JT, Chillik C, van Uem JFHM. Ooplasmic transfusion: prophase germinal vesicle oocytes made developmentally competent by microinjection of metaphase II egg cytoplasm. Fertil Steril 1990; 53: 1049–54

48. Cohen J, Scott R, Alikani A. Ooplasmic transfer in mature human oocytes. Mol Hum Reprod 1998; 4: 269–80

49. Barritt JA, Tomkin G, Sable DB, Cohen J. Effects of cytoplasmic transfer on embryo quality are post-genomic. Fertil Steril 2001; 76 (Suppl 3S): abstr O–14

50. Huang C, Cheng T, Chang H. Birth after the injection of sperm and the cytoplasm of tripronucleate zygotes into metaphase II oocytes in patients with repeated implantation failure after assisted fertilization procedures. Fertil Steril 1999; 72: 702–6

51. Lanzendorf SE, Mayer JF, Toner J. Pregnancy following transfer of ooplasm from cryopreserved–thawed donor oocytes into recipient oocytes. Fertil Steril 1999; 71: 575–7

52. Zhang J, Zhuang G, Zeng Y, et al. Pregnancy derived from human nuclear transfer. Fertil Steril 2003; 80: S56

53. Hubner K, Fuhrmann G, Christenson LK, et al. Derivation of oocytes from mouse embryonic stem cells. Science 2003; 300: 1251–6

54. Lacham-Kaplan O, Daniels R, Trounson A. Fertilization of mouse oocytes using somatic cells as male germ cells. Reprod Biomed Online 2001; 3: 205–11

55. Tesarik J, Nagy ZP, Sousa M. Fertilizable oocytes reconstructed from patient's somatic cell nuclei and donor ooplasts. Reprod Biomed Online 2001; 2: 160–4

56. Takeuchi T, Kaneko M, Veek LL. Creation of viable human oocytes using diploid somatic nuclei. Are we there yet? Hum Reprod 2001; 16: 5 (abstr O–011)

57. Barritt J, Brenner C, Malter, H, Cohen J. Mitochondria in human offspring derived from ooplasmic transplantation. Hum Reprod 2001; 16: 513–16

58. Thomson JA, Itskovitch-Eldor J, Shapiro SS, et al. Embryonic stem cell lines derived from human blastocysts. Science 1998; 282: 1145–7

59. Lanza RP, Cibelli JB, West MD. Prospects for the use of nuclear transfer in human transplantation. Nat Biotechnol 1999; 17: 1171–4

60. Keller G, Snodgrass HR. Human embryonic stem cells: the future is now. Nat Med 1999; 5: 151–2

61. Solter D, Gearhart J. Putting stem cells to work. Science 1999; 283: 1468–70

62. Cibelli JB, Kiessling AA, Cuniff K, et al. Somatic cell nuclear transfer in humans: pronuclear and early embryonic development. J Regen Med 2002; 2: 25–31

63. Lanza RP, Cibelli JB, West MD. Human therapeutic cloning. Nat Med 1999; 5: 975–7

64. Hwang WS, Ryu YJ, Park ES, et al. Evidence of a pluripotent human embryonic stem cell line derived from a cloned blastocyst. Science 2004; 303: 1669–74

65. Young LE, Sinclair KD, Wilmut I. Large offspring syndrome in cattle and sheep. Rev Reprod 1998; 3: 155–63

66. Ogonuki N, Inoue K, Yamamoto Y, et al. Early death of mice cloned from somatic cells. Nat Genet 2002; 30: 253–4

67. Rideout W, Eggan K, Jaenisch R. Nuclear cloning and epigenetic reprogramming of the genome. Science 2001; 293: 1093–8

68. Dean W, Bowden L, Aitchison A. Altered imprinted gene methylation and expression in completely ES cell-derived mouse fetuses: association with aberrant phenotypes. Development 1998; 125: 2273–82

69. Stojanov T, O'Neill C. In vitro fertilization causes epigenetic modifications to the onset of gene expression from the zygotic genome in mice. Biol Reprod 2001; 64: 696–705

70. Young LE, Fernandes K, McEvoy TG. Epigenetic change in IGF2R is associated with fetal overgrowth after sheep embryo culture. Nat Genet 2001; 27: 153–4

71. Reik W, Walter J. Genomic imprinting: parental influence on the genome. Nat Rev Genet 2001; 2: 21–32

72. Reik W, Walter J. Evolution of imprinting mechanisms: the battle of the sexes begins in the zygote. Nat Genet 2001; 27: 255–6

73. Killian J, Nolan C, Wylie AA, et al. Divergent evolution in M6P/IGF2R imprinting from the Jurassic to the Quaternary. Hum Mol Genet 2001; 10: 1721–8

74. Simmerly C, Dominko T, Navara C, et al. Molecular correlates of primate nuclear transfer failures. Science 2003; 300: 297

75. Salpekar A, Huntriss J, Bolton V, Monk M. The use of amplified cDNA to investigate the expression of seven imprinted genes in human oocytes and preimplantation embryos. Mol Hum Reprod 2001; 7: 839–44

76. Wells D, Bermudez MG, Steuerwald N, et al. Expression of genes regulating chromosome segregation, the cell cycle and apoptosis during human preimplantation development. Hum Reprod 2005; in press

77. Wells D, Bermudez MG, Steuerwald N, et al. Association of abnormal morphology and altered gene expression in human preimplantation embryos. Hum Reprod 2004; in press

78. Telford NA, Watson AJ, Schultz GA. Transition from maternal to embryonic control in early mammalian development: a comparison of several species. Mol Reprod Dev 1990; 26: 90–100

79. Bachvarova R, De Leon V. Polyadenylated RNA of mouse ova and loss of maternal RNA in early development. Dev Biol 1980; 74: 1–8

80. Clegg KB, Piko L. PolyA length, cytoplasmic adenylation and synthesis of poly(A)+ RNA in early mouse embryos. Dev Biol 1983; 95: 331–41

81. Ziebe S, Petersen K, Lindenberg S, et al. Embryo morphology or cleavage stage: how to select the best embryos for transfer after in-vitro fertilization. Hum Reprod 1997; 12: 1545–9

82. Alikani M, Cohen J, Tomkin G, et al. Human embryo fragmentation in vitro and its implications for pregnancy and implantation. Fertil Steril 1999; 71: 836–42

83. Ebner T, Yaman C, Moser M, et al. Embryo fragmentation in vitro and its impact on treatment and pregnancy outcome. Fertil Steril 2001; 76: 281–5

84. Munné S, Sandalinas M, Escudero T, et al. Improved implantation after preimplantation genetic diagnosis of aneuploidy. Reprod Biomed Online 2003; 7: 91–7

85. Munné S, Magli C, Cohen J, et al. Positive outcome after preimplantation diagnosis of aneuploidy in human embryos. Hum Reprod 1999; 14: 2191–9

86. Eldadah ZA, Grifo JA, Dietz HC. Marfan syndrome as a paradigm for transcript-targeted preimplantation diagnosis of heterozygous mutations. Nat Med 1995; 1: 798–803

87. Hansis C, Tang YX, Grifo JA, Krey LC. Analysis of Oct-4 expression and ploidy in individual human blastomeres. Mol Hum Reprod 2001; 7: 155–61

88. Krussel JS, Huang HY, Simon C, et al. Single blastomeres within human preimplantation embryos express different amounts of messenger ribonucleic acid for beta-actin and interleukin-1 receptor type I. J Clin Endocrinol Metab 1998; 83: 953–9

89. Taylor DM, Handyside AH, Ray PF, et al. Quantitative measurement of transcript levels throughout human preimplantation development: analysis of hypoxanthine phosphoribosyl transferase. Mol Hum Reprod 2001; 7: 147–54

90. Findlay I, Ray P, Quirke P, et al. Allelic drop-out and preferential amplification in single cells and human blastomeres: implications for preimplantation diagnosis of sex and cystic fibrosis. Hum Reprod 1995; 10: 1609–18

91. Piyamongkol W, Bermudez MG, Harper JC, Wells D. Detailed investigation of factors influencing amplification efficiency and allele drop-out in single cell PCR: implications for preimplantation genetic diagnosis. Mol Hum Reprod 2003; 9: 411–20

92. Cox GF, Burger J, Lip V, et al. Intracytoplasmic sperm injection may increase the risk of imprinting defects. Am J Hum Genet 2003; 71: 162–4

93. Orstavik KH, Eiklid K, van der Hagen CB, et al. Another case of imprinting defect in a girl with Angelman syndrome who was conceived by intracytoplasmic semen injection. Am J Hum Genet 2003; 72: 218–19

94. Bermudez MG, Wells D, Malter H, et al. Expression profiles of individual human oocytes using microarray technology. Reprod Biomed Online 2004; 8: 325–37

28

Complications in assisted reproductive technology treatment

Michael Ludwig

INTRODUCTION

Assisted reproductive technologies (ART) have become a very successful treatment over the past 25 years. Patients, however, have to be counseled not only about their chances of success, but also about the possibility of complications arising, which depend on: individual factors of the medical history, and the chosen treatment.

This chapter does not address the issue of ovarian hyperstimulation syndrome, since this is discussed elsewhere (Chapter 12). The main focus is on:

(1) Complications during oocyte pick-up;

(2) The risk of spontaneous abortion;

(3) The risk of extrauterine and heterotopic pregnancies;

(4) The risk of pregnancy complications, such as pregnancy-induced hypertension (PIH), pre-eclampsia, placental insufficiency, etc.;

(5) The risks for the newborn child, with special emphasis on intrauterine growth restriction (IUGR) and premature birth;

(6) The risk of major malformation.

The postpartum development of children is the topic of another chapter in this book. Since there are only scanty data on pregnancy and birth outcomes following intrauterine insemination (Chapter 31), this chapter focuses mainly on pregnancies established after *in vitro* fertilization (IVF) and intracytoplasmic sperm injection (ICSI).

THE RISK OF COMPLICATIONS DURING AND AFTER OOCYTE PICK-UP

Oocyte pick-up nowadays is almost always carried out using a transvaginal ultrasound-guided approach. This can be done even without anesthesia; it is still, however, a surgical procedure. Possible complications include:

(1) The risk of bleeding from the ovaries;

(2) The risk of infection and abscesses;

(3) The risk of damage to organs (bladder, bowel, blood vessels, etc).

Besides some anecdotal reports on complications after oocyte pick-up, only a limited number of series have been published[1,2]. Bleeding from a vaginal source occurs quite frequently, but mostly can be managed just by compression or, rarely, by suture.

Tubo-ovarian abscesses are an especially severe complication, but are described only rarely[2-12]. In two larger series the incidence was suggested to be as frequent as 0.24–0.30% of all cycles[1,2].

Bennett and colleagues[1] did not provide prophylactic administration of antibiotics. The vagina was prepared by chlorhexidine and cetrimide. Abscess formation was the most frequent complication after bleeding. Others have suggested that antibiotics should be given before oocyte pick-up[2]. Since, however, the same number of abscesses has been observed following administration of prophylactic antibiotics as without, this approach is questionable. Prospective, randomized studies regarding this topic have not yet been performed.

One must be aware that the diagnosis of abscesses was made with a latency of 4–56 days in one[1] and 7–43 days in the second above series[2]. This is consistent with other case reports. The latency is caused by various accompanying factors, related to ovarian stimulation and the IVF procedure itself. Enlarged ovaries and abdominal pain are frequently observed situations after oocyte pick-up, and therefore do not lead to immediate intervention in daily clinical practice.

Patients who undergo only frozen embryo transfer or oocyte donation cycles are also at risk of developing inflammatory complications[3,8]. The treating physician must keep this in mind when patients present with symptoms which otherwise cannot be explained.

THE RISK OF EXTRAUTERINE AND HETEROTOPIC PREGNANCIES

The chance of having an ongoing pregnancy is different after ART compared with spontaneously conceived pregnancies. There is a higher rate of extrauterine pregnancies, especially after IVF, and a higher incidence of heterotopic pregnancies, both due to the high prevalence of tubal factor infertility[13]. Extrauterine pregnancies may occur in 4–5% of patients after IVF[14]. Worldwide, the incidence is estimated to be in the range of 1 : 250 to 1 : 87 per live-born child[15]. Heterotopic pregnancies – the occurrence of at least two different implantation sites at two different locations (e.g. uterus–tube, left tube–right tube, cervix–uterus, etc.) – occur in natural conceptions in 1 : 30 000 pregnancies, and are increased up to 300-fold after IVF and multiple embryo transfer[16].

Patients, therefore, must be monitored closely up to the time when an intrauterine gestational sac with a viable embryo is seen. After that, even in patients with an intrauterine viable singleton pregnancy, the possibility of heterotopic pregnancy must be kept in mind in patients who present wth unexplainable symptoms.

SPONTANEOUS ABORTION AFTER ART

The risk of spontaneous abortion following IVF is increased[13,17,18]. Data for the counseling of patients who achieve pregnancy after IVF are shown in Figure 1. This increased risk, however, seems not to be a result of the technique, but a result of infertility itself. This can be shown from two studies in which patients on a waiting list for infertility treatment who achieved a pregnancy after either spontaneous conception or infertility treatment of any kind showed no difference in clinical abortion rates (Table 1)[17]. This finding has been confirmed by another recent analysis, which clearly shows the major impact of the risk factors in infertility patients, as compared with patients without fertility problems[18]. Infertile patients are not comparable – for various reasons – to women without fertility problems! In this study, three prospectively collected data cohorts were compared with each other. One cohort included 1945 pregnancies following ART, another included 549 and a third 4265 pregnancies following spontaneous conception (historical control cohorts). In fact, there was a slight increase in spontaneous abortions in ART pregnancies compared with one of the control cohorts, even after adjustment for risk factors; the difference, however, was only small (Table 2).

In conclusion, patients should be counseled of a possible slight increased risk of spontaneous abortions after ART, which primarily seems to be related to their own risk factors.

PREGNANCY COURSE AFTER ART

Ongoing pregnancies are, of course, endangered by the high rate of multiples following ART. This very special situation is not analyzed specifically in this chapter, since the risks are outlined elsewhere in obstetric textbooks. Recent studies have also shown that the risk of neurologic disorders in children born after IVF is mainly due to the problem of multiples and not to the IVF procedure itself[19].

In singleton pregnancies also, however, the risk of premature birth, intrauterine growth restriction,

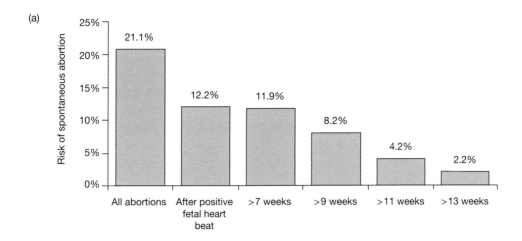

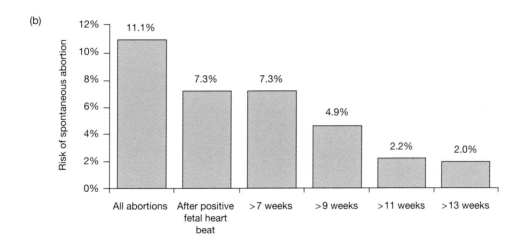

Figure 1 The risk of spontaneous abortion following *in vitro* fertilization (IVF) in singletons (a) and twins (b). Data are from a prospective study including 1200 singleton pregnancies and 397 twin pregnancies, according to reference 20

Table 1 The risk of spontaneous abortion (*n*(%)) in a cohort of patients in an infertility program. The patients became pregnant either with infertility treatment or spontaneously (waiting-list). There was no significant difference between abortion rates depending on the method of conception. Data according to reference 17

Age (years)	Ovulation induction	Method of conception		
		IVF	Other treatments	Spontaneous
< 35	36 (18.8%)	13 (18.8%)	12 (27.3%)	15 (19.5%)
35–39	11 (26.8%)	3 (15.8%)	3 (30.0%)	8 (44.4%)
≥ 40	4 (50.0%)	3 (37.5%)	3 (100.0%)	5 (41.7%)
Total	51 (21.3%)	19 (19.8%)	18 (31.6%)	28 (26.2%)

IVF, *in vitro* fertilization

Table 2 The risk of spontaneous abortion (n(%)) in two prospectively collected data cohorts after either assisted reproductive technologies (ART) or spontaneous conception. Data according to reference 18

| | Age (years) | | | | |
Cohort	<25	25–29	30–34	35–39	≥40
ART cohort	59 (19%)	492 (17%)	899 (18%)	433 (24%)	62 (40%)
Control cohort	68 (23%)	265 (12%)	191 (15%)	57 (25%)	8 (50%)
Relative risk (95% CI)	0.83 (0.42–1.67)	1.51 (1.01–2.28)	1.23 (0.85–1.78)	0.95 (0.60–1.52)	0.81 (0.34–1.90)

CI, confidence interval

Table 3 Risks for pregnancy complications after intracytoplasmic sperm injection (ICSI). Results of a prospective, controlled study[22]

| | ICSI cohort (n = 2055) | | Control cohort (n = 7861) | | | |
Pregnancy complication	n	%	n	%	RR	95% CI
Placenta previa	47	2.3	28	0.4	6.42	4.03–10.22
Placental insufficiency	79	3.8	82	1.0	3.69	2.72–5.00
Abruptio placentae	42	2.0	89	1.1	1.81	1.26–2.60
PIH or pre-eclampsia	193	9.4	569	7.2	1.30	1.11–1.52
Premature birth	248	12.1	524	6.7	1.80	1.56–2.08

PIH, pregnancy-induced hypertension; RR, relative risk; CI, confidence interval

small-for-gestational-age birth and pre-eclampsia seems to be increased[13,21–23] (Table 3). These risks could not be correlated with the kind of ART (IVF or ICSI)[22]. Even if some, in a retrospective study, have suggested that the risk of pre-eclampsia may be related to surgical retrieval of sperm as compared with the use of ejaculated sperm[21], others have not confirmed this in a prospective study of a larger cohort of patients[24] (Table 4).

To conclude on this issue, the risk of a more complicated pregnancy is increased after IVF and ICSI. No results concerning pregnancies after hormonal treatment or intrauterine insemination are yet available; however, at the moment, these patients should be counseled in the same way.

OBSTETRIC OUTCOME AFTER IVF AND ICSI

As already mentioned, children born after IVF and ICSI more often will be premature, with a lower birth weight as compared with those conceived in a natural way. Several recent studies have confirmed this[14].

Schieve and colleagues[25], in a registry-based analysis, showed that the risk for low and very low birth weight was independent of the presence of a male factor (Table 5). Bonduelle and colleagues[26] and Katalinic and co-workers[23] confirmed this for ICSI with data from prospectively controlled trials (Table 6). Katalinic and Ludwig could not demonstrate an influence of the severity of male factor in an ICSI program on obstetric outcome parameters[24]. However, others, in a small number of patients in a prospective ongoing study comparing non-obstructive (n = 70) and obstructive azoospermia (n = 204), demonstrated a slightly increased risk of prematurity and low gestational age in the group treated for non-obstructive azoospermia[27]. Further studies must be done in the future, with more patients, to prove this assumption.

However, there is an increased incidence of prematurity in children born after ART. This prematurity, even in singletons, explains the higher incidence of

Table 4 The risk of pre-eclampsia associated with the origin of sperms, according to a retrospective analysis of Wang and colleagues[21] (a). In that study the odds ratio (OR) and 95% confidence interval (CI) were adjusted for age and body mass index. Also results of a prospective controlled study in pregnancies achieved after either intracytoplasmic sperm injection (ICSI) or spontaneous conception are shown[24] (b)

(a)

| | Ejaculation | | Surgery | |
	IVF	ICSI	ICSI	p Value
Pregnancies (n)	1075	464	82	
PIH (n)	123	54	18	0.02
(%)	11	12	22	
OR (95% CI)	1	1.03 (0.75–1.40)	2.10 (1.30–3.62)	
Pre-eclampsia (n)	40	18	9	0.01
(%)	4	4	11	
OR (95% CI)	1	1.02 (0.62–1.81)	3.10 (1.59–6.73)	

(b)

	Ejaculate	TESE	MESA
Pregancies (n)	2339	187	19
Children (n)	2944	229	26
PIH or pre-eclampsia (n)	113	9	1
% (95% CI)	4.8 (4.1–5.6)	4.8 (2.5–8.2)	5.3 (0.3–22.6)
RR (95% CI)	1	1.00 (0.53–1.89)	1.09 (0.16–7.34)

PIH, pregnancy-induced hypertension; RR, relative risk; IVF, *in vitro* fertilization; TESE, testicular sperm extraction; MESA, microsurgical epididymal sperm aspiration

Table 5 The risk of low and very low birth weight in pregnancies achieved after *in vitro* fertilization (IVF) or intracytoplasmic sperm injection (ICSI). There was no increased risk of low or very low birth weight after surrogate motherhood[24]

	Total number	Standardized risk ratio	(95% Confidence interval)
Low birth weight			
Pregnancies with one fetal heart	16 730	1.8	1.7–1.8
Use of donor oocytes, no male factor	1397	1.6	1.4–1.8
Male-factor infertility	2759	1.7	1.5–1.8
Pregnancies in surrogate motherhood	180	1.2	0.6–1.8
Very low birth weight			
Pregnancies with one fetal heart	16 730	1.7	1.5–1.9
Use of donor oocytes, no male factor	1397	2.1	1.5–2.7
Male-factor infertility	2759	2.0	1.6–2.5
Pregnancies in surrogate motherhood	180	—*	

*No cases observed but 2.6 cases expected

neurological sequelae[19]. There is also a higher risk for delivery by cesarean section in ART, compared with spontaneous pregnancies[13,22]. One possible explanation for this phenomenon may be that the obstetrician, as well as the parents, are more concerned about the risks and problems for the unborn child. On the other hand, the higher rate of cesarean section might reflect the *per se* higher rate of placental insufficiency, premature birth, pre-eclampsia, etc. and may be more a multicausal result than a simple epiphenomenon.

THE RISK OF MAJOR MALFORMATION

Studies in the 1980s and 1990s found that the risk of major malformation after ART was not increased above the normal risk. The studies to evaluate this risk, however, were not of good quality. They were, mostly, not prospective, not properly controlled or too small to estimate accurately the relative risk of major malformations. Even today, there are problems which cannot be overcome by even the most complicated study design. These problems are in the recruitment of a proper control cohort, the blinding of the examiner and, especially in long-term follow-up studies, the problem of high drop-out rates.

In the past 5 years, studies have been conducted with the focus on the major malformation risk in children born after ICSI, as well as after IVF. Bonduelle and colleagues[26] have published an increasing amount of prospective data from an ongoing study comparing the risks of children born after IVF and ICSI, who were evaluated using the same protocol. There was a non-significantly different risk of major malformation in children born after IVF of 4.7% (135/2895), as compared with 4.2% after ICSI (122/2889).

A group from Australia published data collected from registries including children with major malformations; the study design was retrospective. A significantly increased risk of major malformation at the age of 1 year for children born after IVF (relative risk (RR) 2.0, 95% confidence interval (CI) 1.5–2.9) as well as ICSI (RR 2.0, 95% CI 1.3–3.2) was described[28]. This risk was confirmed after logistic regression analysis including maternal age, parity and gender of the child. In total, 301 children born after ICSI, 837 born after IVF and 4000 children born following spontaneous conception were included.

A third prospective, controlled study confirmed an increased risk of malformation for pregnancies established after ICSI (8.7%, 295/3372) as compared with those after spontaneous conception (6.1%, 488/8016) (RR 1.44, 95% CI 1.25–1.65)[23]. This study included all pregnancies from the 16th week of gestation onwards, including spontaneous abortions, induced abortions, stillbirths and live-births. The risk remained significantly increased after adjustment for maternal

Table 6 Obstetric outcome after intracytoplasmic sperm injection (ICSI). Results of a prospective controlled study[22]

Children/fetuses	ICSI (n = 2055)	Controls (n = 7861)	p Value
Gestational age (weeks)	38.4 ± 3.4	39.2 ± 2.3	< 0.01
Birth weight (g)	3214 ± 714	3368 ± 580	< 0.01
Birth weight < 2500 g (%)	10.9	5.3	< 0.01
Birth weight < 1500 g (%)	3.2	1.1	< 0.01
Mode of delivery (%)			< 0.01
cesarean section	33.5	13.9	
forceps/vacuum	7.5	8.7	
spontaneous	58.6	74.7	
others/unknown	0.4	2.7	

age, malformations in the parents and previous pregnancies with a stillborn or malformed child[25,29,30]. This increased risk was not related to the rate of multiple pregnancies, the indication for ICSI, the sperm count or the origin of sperm used for the ICSI treatment[23,24,30]. There is therefore no special subgroup of couples undergoing ICSI who can be counseled about an increase (or not) of malformation.

Other studies have confirmed a higher risk for major malformations overall, or for individual entities, in pregnancies established after ICSI, as compared with those after IVF or spontaneous conception[31,32].

To date, the increased risk cannot be sufficiently explained. The confirmed similarity between malformation rates in pregnancies after IVF and ICSI indicates that a major influence of the ICSI technique is unlikely[33]. On the other hand, a minimal influence of the techniques themselves cannot be excluded[22].

In the past few years, reports have been published of a higher risk of errors in genomic imprinting in children born after IVF and ICSI. Those errors may lead to diseases such as Beckwith–Wiedemann syndrome or Angelman's syndrome[34]. Changes in the *in vitro* culture conditions of animals may explain changes in gene expression[35]. Some have suggested a relation of imprinting errors to the severity of the male factor[36]. However, it is not yet clear whether there is really an increased risk for those diseases or not, since their incidence is very rare, in the range of 1 : 15000 to 1 : 30000[33,34]. Since these diseases are important in the counseling of couples asking for infertility treatment, more data are needed to clarify this question.

Besides the influence of *in vitro* culture or the fertilization techniques used, it may also be that infertility or subfertility *per se* has an impact on the incidence of major malformations or imprinting errors. A similiar or the same cause might, on the one hand, lead to a problem becoming pregnant, and on the other hand, result in a higher risk of major malformations. This theory is supported by data regarding pregnancy course and obstetric outcome.

INFERTILITY AS A RISK FACTOR

All the described risks have been shown for conventional IVF, as well as ICSI. The ICSI technique itself seems not to be one of the major risk factors. On the other hand, it cannot be concluded that it has no impact overall, since, of course, it means an additional factor in manipulation of the oocyte.

Furthermore, some have argued that *in vitro* culture must have a major impact on this risk. On the other hand, there are no adequate data on the less invasive techniques, such as hormonal treatment or intrauterine insemination, regarding pregnancy course and obstetric outcome. Good-quality data from larger cohorts on intrauterine insemination cycles would help to elucidate the question whether *in vitro* treatment of sperm might contribute to the risks, or whether even less severe forms of infertility may have an impact. Even more important would be data on pregnancy course and obstetric outcome after hormonal treatment only, since in these cases no handling of gametes *in vitro* could influence the outcome.

Since all these data do not yet exist, the answer cannot be given to whether the *in vitro* conditions are actually responsible for the outcome, whether the severeness of infertility factors might have an impact or whether infertility *per se* is a factor in high-risk pregnancy. There is some evidence from the literature that the last should be considered in these circumstances.

Another issue is the risk of spontaneous abortion. This risk is increased in infertile patients, independently, whether they become pregnant spontaneously (after a long time to pregnancy) or following any kind of infertility treatment (Tables 1 and 2)[17]. Yet another issue is the risk of pregnancy complications. Pandian and colleagues[37] have studied 877 couples suffering from idiopathic infertility, defined as more than 12

months' infertility of unknown cause. Of these couples, 498 became pregnant. The study cohort consisted of 372 singleton pregnancies established either naturally or following infertility treatment. Over the same time period, i.e. 10 years, 32 969 singleton pregnancies were delivered in the institution of the authors; this cohort was included in the study as a control group. In the study group, independent of the method of conception, the risks of abruptio placentae (RR 3.05, 95% CI 1.4–6.2), pre-eclampsia (RR 5.61, 95% CI 3.3–9.3), cesarean section (RR 1.46, 95% CI 1.1–1.8) and induction of labor (RR 1.24, 95% CI 1.0–1.5) were significantly increased[37].

Even more important are data from Scandinavian countries. Data from the Danish National Birth Cohort demonstrated a significantly increased risk for pre-eclampsia which depended only on the time to pregnancy in spontaneously conceived pregnancies (Figure 2)[38]. Similarly, for two other population-based studies, there was a significantly increased risk for premature birth in singleton pregnancies without infertility treatment, but with more than 12 months' time to pregnancy[39]. The risk was increased by 1.6-fold (95% CI 1.0–2.7) and 1.8-fold (95% CI 1.2–2.2), respectively, in the two different studies included in this publication[39].

Finally, the data of Schieve and colleagues showed an increased risk for low- and very-low-birth-weight babies for all patients treated by IVF or ICSI, but not for those with a surrogate mother (Table 5)[25]. This also confirms that it is not the *in vitro* culture but the presence of infertility which seems to contribute to the risk of pregnancy complications, since *in vitro* culture is also applied in surrogate motherhood.

Why should infertility *per se* be a risk factor for pregnancy and obstetric outcome? Mainly genetic problems could be responsible for this phenomenon. Male-factor infertility, for example, is well known to be associated with genetic risks such as chromosome abnormalities[40–42], mutations in the cystic fibrosis transmembrane conductance regulator (CFTR) gene[43] or microdeletions of the Y chromosome[44]. Other genetic factors might also be present which have not yet been identified. Furthermore, the risk that sperm might be aneuploid is higher with the more severe forms of oligozoospermia[45].

It should also be kept in mind that infertility is always a problem of a couple – a problem of two individuals coming together. A subfertile male with a

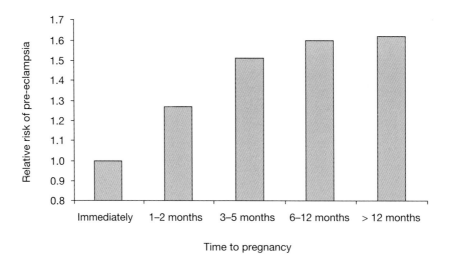

Figure 2 Risk of pre-eclampsia depending on the time to pregnancy without infertility treatment. Shown are data for singletons only in primiparas. In women with more than 12 months' time to pregnancy the risk was increased significantly (relative risk 1.62, 95% confidence interval 1.14–2.30). The risk showed no major changes after adjustment for the presence of irregular cycles, age, body mass index and smoking[38]

'superfertile' female might induce a pregnancy, and vice versa, but the same male with a different female partner may require infertility treatment. Recently, it has been shown that the prevalence of subfertility in males with or without a pregnancy in a previous partnership does not vary[46]. There are also reports that have shown a higher prevalence of chromosomal abnormalities in female partners when ICSI treatment is planned[47–49]. One possible explanation for this phenomenon may be that these abnormalities might slightly reduce the fertility of these females, but not be clinically detectable, and therefore lead to the need for ICSI treatment.

In animal models, other examples have been published that can be translated to infertility. The retinoblastoma-knockout mouse is an animal which dies *in utero*[50]. It shows abnormalities of the placenta, with a severe reduction in vascularization. The chimera with a retinoblastoma-intact genome in the trophoblast, but retinoblastoma-knockout genome in the embryoblast, can survive, which underlines a problem restricted to placentation[50]. Others have shown abnormalities in the placentas of mice with paternal uniparental disomy 12, a genetic model for imprinting on chromosome 12[51]. In this model, again, problems in placentation were the most apparent failure of development. These changes add support to the discussion on genomic imprinting problems in

children born following ART procedures, as described above[35].

All these issues are, of course, assumptions; some might be theoretical, others have to be proved with more supporting data in the future. However, from all the data available to date, a theoretical model can be suggested which might explain, on the one hand, the problem of infertility, but also, on the other hand, observed problems in pregnancy and children's health.

Principally, it may be possible that infertile patients have a predisposition to imprinting problems. This predisposition might also lead to implantation failure or implantation problems. It is also possible that other genetic causes exist in parallel. Taking together all the facts discussed in this chapter, one might consider Figure 3, which shows a logic sequence in the development of the various abnormalities observed in pregnancies following ART. One of the first signs may be the higher risk of clinical abortions; a second sign might be the abnormal hormone synthesis, which is well known from pregnancies after IVF and ICSI cycles[52–59]. Further details are given in Figure 3.

CONCLUDING REMARKS

Patients undergoing infertility treatment, and especially ART, must be counseled about the risks of

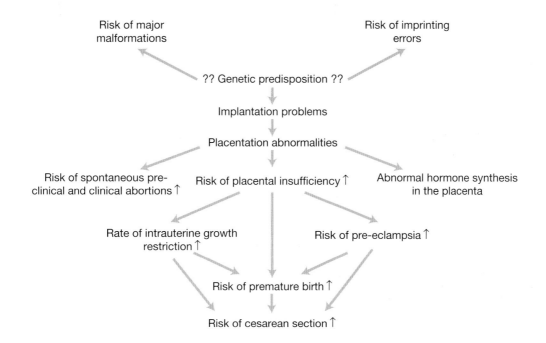

Figure 3 The figure shows the consequences of implantation problems which might be responsible for at least some cases of infertility. These implantation problems might delay the possibility of pregnancy and lead to many of these couples attending for infertility treatment. Others may become pregnant spontaneously, but the consequences of implantation problems remain. A direct consequence might be abnormal placentation, which leads to the increased risk of pre-eclampsia, intrauterine growth restriction and premature birth. It also might explain the higher frequency of cesarean section due to signs of fetal hypoxia during delivery. There is, to date, no evidence for a genetic predisposition of infertile couples to develop implantation problems. This predisposition, however, might be related to genomic imprinting or single gene disorders, which are also responsible for a slightly increased risk of major malformations

treatment (e.g. the risks involved in oocyte pick-up) as well as risks in pregnancies established after ART. Similiar risks to those described for infertile patients are prevalent for couples with a longer time to pregnancy (> 12 months). The risks seem to be lower when fertile women undergo infertility treatment, as, for example, in the case of surrogate mothers. This confirms that the risks for the course of pregnancy and obstetric outcome are associated with being infertile.

Whether the same factors, which may explain these risks, are also responsible for the slightly increased risk of major malformations cannot yet be answered. Future studies should also concentrate on data from pregnancies following intrauterine insemination, since the embryos resulting from these treatment cycles will never have been exposed to *in vitro* culture.

Future, prospective, perhaps multinational and multicentric studies should also concentrate on the issue of imprinting errors. The question of whether these

special abnormalities are also found with an increased frequency has yet to be answered.

REFERENCES

1. Bennett SJ, Waterstone JJ, Cheng WC, Parsons J. Complications of transvaginal ultrasound-directed follicle aspiration: a review of 2670 consecutive procedures. J Assist Reprod Genet 1993; 10: 72–7
2. Dicker D, Ashkenazi J, Feldberg D, et al. Severe abdominal complications after transvaginal ultrasonographically guided retrieval of oocytes for in vitro fertilization and embryo transfer [see Comments]. Fertil Steril 1993; 59: 1313–15
3. Dicker D, Dekel A, Orvieto R, et al. Ovarian abscess after ovum retrieval for in-vitro fertilization. Hum Reprod 1998; 13: 1813–14
4. Friedler S, Ben-Shachar I, Abramov Y, et al. Ruptured tubo-ovarian abscess complicating transcervical cryopreserved embryo transfer. Fertil Steril 1996; 65: 1065–6

5. Ludwig M, Felberbaum RE, Bauer O, Diedrich K. Ovarian abscess and heterotopic triplet pregnancy: two complications after IVF in one patient. Arch Gynecol Obstet 1999; 263: 25–8

6. Marlowe SD, Lupetin AR. Tuboovarian abscess following transvaginal oocyte retrieval for in vitro fertilization: imaging appearance. Clin Imaging 1995; 19: 180–1

7. Padilla SL. Ovarian abscess following puncture of an endometrioma during ultrasound-guided oocyte retrieval. Hum Reprod 1993; 8: 1282–3

8. Sauer MV, Paulson RJ. Pelvic abscess complicating transcervical embryo transfer. Am J Obstet Gynecol 1992; 166: 148–9

9. Shulman A, Fejgin M, Ben-Nun I. Transvaginal ultrasound-guided drainage of an ovarian abscess following in vitro fertilization [Letter]. Int J Gynaecol Obstet 1995; 49: 69–70

10. Wei CF, Chen SC. Pelvic abscess after ultrasound-guided aspiration of endometrioma: a case report. Chung Hua I Hsueh Tsa Chih (Taipei) 1998; 61: 603–7

11. Younis JS, Ezra Y, Laufer N, Ohel G. Late manifestation of pelvic abscess following oocyte retrieval, for in vitro fertilization, in patients with severe endometriosis and ovarian endometriomata. J Assist Reprod Genet 1997; 14: 343–6

12. Zweemer RP, Scheele F, Verheijen RH, et al. Ovarian abscess during pregnancy mimicking a leiomyoma of the uterus: a complication of transvaginal ultrasound-guided oocyte aspiration. J Assist Reprod Genet 1996; 13: 81–5

13. Ludwig M. Pregnancy and Birth after Assisted Reproductive Technologies, 1st edn. Berlin, Heidelberg, New York: Springer-Verlag, 2002

14. Diedrich K, Weiss J, Felberbaum R. In-vitro fertilisation. In Diedrich K, ed. Weibliche Sterilität. Berlin, Heidelberg, New York: Springer-Verlag, 1998: 380–407

15. Schneider J, Berger CJ, Cattell C. Maternal mortality due to ectopic pregnancy. A review of 102 deaths. Obstet Gynecol 1977; 49: 557–61

16. Ludwig M, Kaisi M, Bauer O, Diedrich K. The forgotten child – a case of heterotopic, intra-abdominal and intrauterine pregnancy carried to term. Hum Reprod 1999; 14: 1372–4

17. Pezeshki K, Feldman J, Stein DE, et al. Bleeding and spontaneous abortion after therapy for infertility. Fertil Steril 2000; 74: 504–8

18. Wang JX, Norman RJ, Wilcox AJ. Incidence of spontaneous abortion among pregnancies produced by assisted reproductive technology. Hum Reprod 2004; 19: 272–7

19. Strömberg B, Dahlquist G, Ericson A, et al. Neurological sequelae in children born after in-vitro fertilisation: a population based study. Lancet 2002; 359: 461–5

20. Tummers P, De Sutter P, Dhont M. Risk of spontaneous abortion in singleton and twin pregnancies after IVF/ICSI. Hum Reprod 2003; 18: 1720–3

21. Wang JX, Knottnerus A-M, Schuit G, et al. Surgically obtained sperm, and risk of gestational hypertension and pre-eclampsia. Lancet 2002; 359: 673–4

22. Helmerhorst FM, Perquin DA, Donker D, Keirse MJ. Perinatal outcome of singletons and twins after assisted conception: a systematic review of controlled studies. Br Med J 2004; 328: 261

23. Katalinic A, Rösch C, Ludwig M. Pregnancy course and outcome after intracytoplasmic sperm injection (ICSI) – a controlled, prospective cohort study. Fertil Steril 2004; 81: 1604–16

24. Ludwig M, Katalinic A. Pregnancy course and health of children born after ICSI depending on parameters of male factor infertility. Hum Reprod 2003; 18: 351–7

25. Schieve LA, Meikle SF, Ferre C, et al. Low and very low birth weight in infants conceived with use of assisted reproductive technology. N Engl J Med 2002; 346: 731–7

26. Bonduelle M, Liebaers I, Deketelaere V, et al. Neonatal data on a cohort of 2889 infants born after ICSI (1991–1999) and of 2995 infants born after IVF (1983–1999). Hum Reprod 2002; 17: 671–94

27. Vernaeve V, Bonduelle M, Tournaye H, et al. Pregnancy outcome and neonatal data of children born after ICSI using testicular sperm in obstructive and non-obstructive azoospermia. Hum Reprod 2003; 18: 2093–7

28. Hansen M, Kurinczuk JJ, Bower C, Webb S. The risk of major birth defects after intracytoplasmic sperm injection and in vitro fertilization. N Engl J Med 2002; 346: 725–30

29. Ludwig M, Diedrich K. Follow up of children born after assisted reproductive technologies. Reprod Biomed Online 2002; 5: 317–22

30. Ludwig M, Katalinic A. Malformation rate in fetuses and children conceived after intracytoplasmic sperm injection (ICSI): results of a prospective cohort study. Reprod Biomed Online 2002; 5: 171–8

31. Ericson A, Kallen B. Congenital malformations in infants born after IVF: a population-based study. Hum Reprod 2001; 16: 504–9

32. Wennerholm UB, Bergh C, Hamberger L, et al. Incidence of congenital malformations in children born after ICSI. Hum Reprod 2000; 15: 944–8

33. Edwards RG, Ludwig M. Are major defects in children conceived in vitro due to innate problems in

patients or to induced genetic damage? Reprod Biomed Online 2003; 7: 131–8

34. Gosden R, Trasler J, Lucifero D, Faddy M. Rare congenital disorders, imprinted genes, and assisted reproductive technology. Lancet 2003; 361: 1975–7

35. Sollars V, Lu X, Xiao L, et al. Evidence for an epigenetic mechanism by which Hsp90 acts as a capacitor for morphological evolution. Nat Genet 2003; 33: 70–4

36. Marques CJ, Carvalho F, Sousa M, Barros A. Genomic imprinting in disruptive spermatogenesis. Lancet 2004; 363: 1700–2

37. Pandian Z, Bhattacharya S, Templeton A. Review of unexplained infertility and obstetric outcome: a 10 year review. Hum Reprod 2001; 16: 2593–7

38. Basso O, Weinberg CR, Baird DD, et al. Subfecundity as a correlate of preeclampsia: a study within the Danish National Birth Cohort. Am J Epidemiol 2003; 157: 195–202

39. Henriksen TB, Baird DD, Olsen J, et al. Time to pregnancy and preterm delivery. Obstet Gynecol 1997; 89: 594–9

40. De Braekeleer M, Dao T-N. Cytogenetic studies in male infertility: a review. Hum Reprod 1991; 6: 245–50

41. Pauer H-U, Engel W. Die Bedeutung chromosomaler Anomalien bei der männlichen Infertilität. Gynäkologe 2000; 33: 88–93

42. Van Assche E, Bonduelle M, Tournaye H, et al. Cytogenetics in infertile men. Hum Reprod 1996;11 (Suppl 4):1–24

43. Stuhrmann M, Dork T. CFTR gene mutations and male infertility. Andrologia 2000; 32: 71–83

44. Foresta C, Moro E, Ferlin A. Y chromosome microdeletions and alterations of spermatogenesis. Endocr Rev 2001; 22: 226–39

45. Egozcue J, Blanco J, Vidal F. Chromosome studies in human sperm nuclei using fluorescence in-situ hybridization (FISH). Hum Reprod Update 1997; 3: 441–52

46. Lucidi PS, Kavoussi S, Witz CA. Prior fertility in the male partner: a predictor of normal semen analysis? Fertil Steril 2003; 80 (Suppl 3): S234–S235

47. Meschede D, Lemcke B, Exeler JR, et al. Chromosome abnormalities in 447 couples undergoing intracytoplasmic sperm injection - prevalence, types, sex distribution and reproductive relevance. Hum Reprod 1998; 13: 576–82

48. Peschka B, Leygraaf J, van der, Montag V, et al. Type and frequency of chromosome aberrations in 781 couples undergoing intracytoplasmic sperm injection. Hum Reprod 1999; 14: 2257–63

49. Scholtes MC, Behrend C, Dietzel-Dahmen J, et al. Chromosomal aberrations in couples undergoing intracytoplasmic sperm injection: influence on implantation and ongoing pregnancy rates. Fertil Steril 1998; 70: 933–7

50. Wu L, de Bruin A, Saavedra HI, et al. Extra-embryonic function of Rb is essential for embryonic development and viability. Nature (London) 2003; 421: 942–7

51. Georgiades P, Watkins M, Surani MA, Ferguson-Smith AC. Parental origin-specific developmental defects in mice with uniparental disomy for chromosome 12. Development 2000; 127: 4719–28

52. Ghisoni L, Ferrazzi E, Castagna C, et al. Prenatal diagnosis after ART success: the role of early combined screening tests in counseling pregnant patients. Placenta 2003; 24 (Suppl B): S99–103

53. Hui PW, Lam YH, Tang MH, et al. Amniotic fluid human chorionic gonadotrophin and alpha-fetoprotein levels in pregnancies conceived after assisted reproduction. Prenat Diagn 2003; 23: 484–7

54. Liao AW, Heath V, Kametas N, et al. First-trimester screening for trisomy 21 in singleton pregnancies achieved by assisted reproduction. Hum Reprod 2001; 16: 1501–4

55. Maymon R, Shulman A. Serial first- and second-trimester Down's syndrome screening tests among IVF- versus naturally-conceived singletons. Hum Reprod 2002; 17: 1081–5

56. Muller F, Dreux S, Lemeur A, et al. Medically assisted reproduction and second-trimester maternal serum marker screening for Down syndrome. Prenat Diagn 2003; 23: 1073–6

57. Ribbert LS, Kornman LH, de Wolf BT, et al. Maternal serum screening for fetal Down syndrome in IVF pregnancies. Prenat Diagn 1996; 16: 35–8

58. Wald NJ, White N, Morris JK, et al. Serum markers for Down's syndrome in women who have had in vitro fertilisation: implications for antenatal screening. Br J Obstet Gynaecol 1999; 106: 1304–6

59. Wojdemann KR, Larsen SO, Shalmi A, et al. First trimester screening for Down syndrome and assisted reproduction: no basis for concern. Prenat Diagn 2001; 21: 563–5

29

Quality management in reproductive medicine

Christoph Keck, Robert Fischer, Vera Baukloh, P. Sass and Michael Alper

INTRODUCTION

Reproductive medicine is a field in which the scientific achievements over the past 10–15 years have led to major changes in diagnostic and therapeutic procedures. Whereas until 15 years ago intrauterine insemination (IUI) and *in vitro* fertilization (IVF) were the major treatment options in assisted reproductive technologies (ART), today complex techniques such as intracytoplasmic sperm injection (ICSI) or testicular sperm extraction/microepididymal sperm aspiration (TESE/MESA) have become routine procedures for almost all centers offering ART.

The awareness of potential problems and risks associated with these treatments has led to the need to develop techniques to control treatment quality. This is most notable in countries (such as Germany) where laws have been established that require quality management systems for medical institutions[1–3]. Even though the primary concern of any health-care system is, and will continue to be, medical performance[4], health-care systems need to be seen as 'service corporations' dealing with patients, referring doctors and employees. This means that other qualities – in addition to medical performance – must be taken into consideration.

Quality management (QM) systems offer the possibility for a medical organization to document the quality of its services to its customers and cost-bearers. In addition, applying QM instruments helps to provide services in a cost-effective, high-quality manner[5–7].

QUALITY MANAGEMENT SYSTEMS

There are several different QM systems, which are discussed in this chapter. The quality to be managed in a medical organization refers mainly to the diagnostic and therapeutic processes performed. In addition, all administrative and paramedical processes must be included. The sum of all these elements and how they relate to each other is called the quality management system[8–10].

A major concern for people starting to establish a QM system is that they have the feeling that they are 'reinventing the wheel'; this is certainly not the case, as a QM system can and should be based on rules, guidelines and strategies that already exist within the center. Commonly, most IVF centers already work according to a number of guidelines, so the primary step in establishing a QM system is to find out which guidelines already exist. When an IVF center contemplates a QM system, it is important to develop a baseline of existing elements of the QM system. This is important to establish the scope of the project.

Examples of quality standards used in ART laboratories around the world are:

(1) 'Guidelines for human embryology and andrology laboratories', the American Fertility Society[11];

(2) 'Guidelines for good practice in IVF laboratories', the European Society of Human Reproduction and Embryology (ESHRE), 2000, http://www.eshre.com;

(3) 'Reproductive Laboratory Accreditation Standards', the College of American Pathology, 2002, http://www.cap.org/lap/rlap.html;

(4) 'Accreditation standards and guidelines for IVF laboratories', the Association of Clinical Embryologists, 2000, http://www.ivf.net/ace/.

The above-mentioned guidelines and standards describe the specific requirements for reproductive laboratories, and include various aspects of the implementation of a quality management system. These well-defined standards describe the minimum conditions that should be met. However, a proper QM system covering the whole clinic is far more powerful than that defined in laboratory standards and guidelines[12–14]. Furthermore, most guidelines are not applicable to many areas of the IVF center such as clinical, administrative and other areas[15].

ISO STANDARDS

Although several QM systems have come into existence for various industries all over the world[16,17], those following the manuals of the International Standards Organization (ISO 9000 series) have become the most popular (ISO 9001:2000; ISO/Draft International Standard (DIS) 15189:2002; ISO/International Electrotechnical Comission (IEC) 17025:1999; ISO/IEC Guide 25:1990). The ISO standard defines the basic elements of a QM system in a relatively abstract and non-specific manner. This means that the standard can be used for any type of company, including health-care organizations. However, the ISO standard needs to be adapted to the specific requirements of the respective organization. This process is usually assisted by employing an ISO consultant who

is experienced in adapting the standard to a widely diverse number of companies.

CERTIFICATION/ACCREDITATION

Once a QM system has been developed and implemented in a hospital or medical practice, an independent certification body must approve whether or not the QM system is functioning properly and meets the criteria defined in the ISO standard. This approval is called 'certification', and can be performed on the basis of the German (DIN) European Standard (EN) ISO 9001 or DIN EN ISO 9004[18,19].

The ISO standard 9001:2000 is process- and outcome-oriented. In simple terms, ISO requires that you 'say what you do' and that you 'do what you say'. A certification body must confirm that the organization is complying with its own directives. Certification according to ISO 9001:2000 can be performed for an IVF organization as a whole (including the laboratory)[20,21].

The laboratory is certainly a key element in every IVF center. Applying ISO 9001:2000 ensures that all procedures are standardized in the laboratory. However, this does not necessarily mean that the latest and most successful laboratory technology is used. This is the reason why laboratories may also want to consider additional standards governing qualification and competence. The current ISO standard relevant for ART laboratories is ISO/IEC 17025:1999. This standard is entitled 'General requirement for the competence of testing and calibration laboratories', and replaces both the ISO/IEC Guide 25 and the European standard EN 45001. The establishment of a standard directed to the specific requirements of medical laboratories is currently in process (DIN EN ISO 15189:2003).

Compliance with the ISO 9001:2000 standard can lead to certification, as already mentioned above. In contrast to this, compliance with the ISO 17025 standard can lead to accreditation (accreditation is defined as 'a procedure by which an authoritative body gives formal recognition that a body or person is competent to carry out specific tasks'), which exceeds certification (defined as 'a procedure by which a third party gives written assurance that a product, process or service conforms to specific requirements'). ART laboratories may want to consider ISO 17025 accreditation to supplement ISO 9001:2000 certification[8,22].

HOW TO PROCEED

One of the questions most frequently asked is: 'What is the first step in implementing a QM system at our center?' Of course this question cannot be answered uniformly, as the situation is different at any given IVF center. However, to implement fully the ISO 9001:2000 system in a medical institution, 20 elements must be considered. These are listed in Table 1. Thus, which element to start with must be agreed, and the way in which these elements are implemented must be clearly documented in QM manuals, handbooks, instructions and standard operating procedures.

For many centers the decision is to start with the quality policy[23], which is defined as a group of principles according to which the medical institution works. This quality policy of any medical organization should be developed as a consensus between management and employees and should be reviewed periodically to make sure that the principles are still valid and that both management and employees still agree with them. The policy should be simple and concise. The quality policy at Boston IVF can be taken as an example. The Boston IVF team decided that the quality policy is 'CARE', which is an acronym for 'compassionate, advanced, responsive, experienced'.

The ISO standard requires that management responsibility is clearly defined. Despite that the responsibility of management (or the governing structure) can be defined differently in various medical organizations, according to ISO standards, certain generally valid aspects can be defined[24]:

(1) The hierarchy of the institution has to be defined and outlined clearly.

(2) Descriptions of authority must be available for all positions within the organization.

(3) The more complex are the hierarchical structures within a medical institution, the more precisely these structures have to be defined for the system to work effectively and robustly at all times and under all (extraordinary) conditions.

(4) The 'decision' of the head of the organization must be available at any time, even if he or she is absent. Therefore, it must be absolutely clear to everyone within the organization which person has the competency and authority to make decisions.

Table 1 Elements/criteria of the DIN EN ISO 9001:2000 standard
(1) Responsibility
(2) Quality management system
(3) Contract control
(4) Design management
(5) Document and data management
(6) Measures
(7) Management of products provided by customers
(8) Designating and retrospective observation
(9) Process management
(10) Revision
(11) Control of revision resources
(12) Evidence of revisions
(13) Defective product management
(14) Corrections and preventive measures
(15) Handling, storage, packaging, conservation, distribution
(16) Quality report management
(17) Internal quality audits
(18) Training
(19) Maintenance
(20) Statistical methods

There are different methods of making these structures as transparent as possible. One easy way is the development of an organizational chart.

As already stated above, the ISO 9001:2000 standard is very much a process-oriented undertaking. This means that the management of processes is a key element. Therefore, early in the process of implementing a QM system, it is necessary to define and describe precisely all relevant processes, and to structure them according to QM guidelines[15,25]. For medical facilities, the most important 'processes' are those of diagnostic and therapeutic procedures. Certainly for IVF centers, one of the most important processes is the IVF procedure itself, so we can take this as an example of how individual processes can be structured (Figure 1).

In addition to purely medical aspects, many other administrative and organizational processes are involved in the care of patients. Sometimes these 'secondary' processes affect the patient's (= customer's) perspective much more than do the pure medical processes. It is difficult for the patient to judge the quality of medical care, but the patient clearly knows

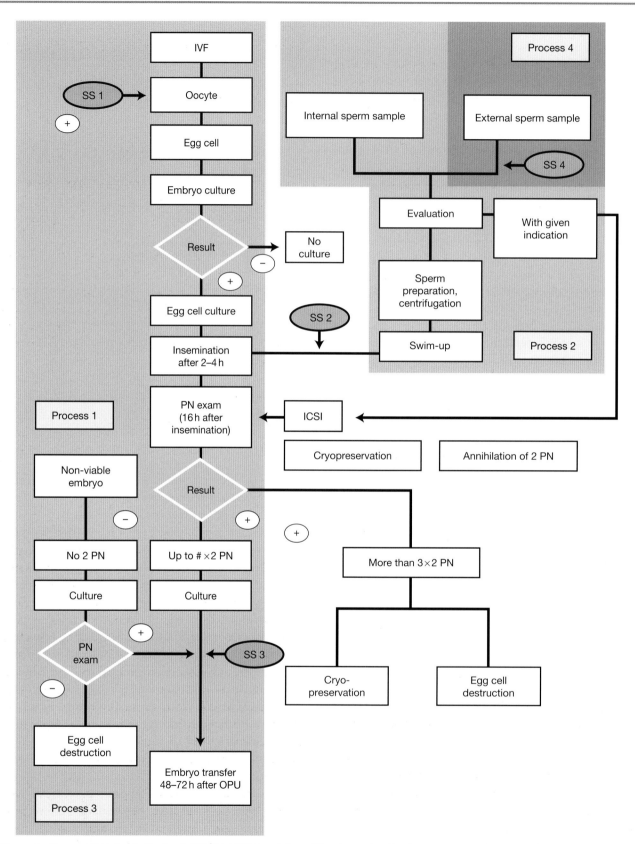

Figure 1 Process flow for an *in vitro* fertilization (IVF) procedure. SS, process interfaces; PN, pronucleate; OPU, oocyte pick-up; ICSI, intracytoplasmic sperm injection (From reference 23)

whether the treatment service is inadequate. People have to be aware that sometimes poor communication processes can ruin a patient's experience, despite the best medical care within the IVF center. In fact, it is more likely that a patient will leave a medical facility because of an organizational problem, such as substandard secretarial or administrative abilities, than because of a medical deficiency[26].

The inter-relationship of different processes can be defined by 'interfaces' or 'boundaries'. We can differentiate between internal and external interfaces[1]. Two processes that are performed within the medical institution are connected by 'internal interfaces'[2]. 'External interfaces' connect the institution to referring doctors, external institutions, suppliers (inputs) and patients (outputs). Communication is critical for the optimization of both internal and external interfaces.

DOCUMENTATION IN A QM SYSTEM

As with all QM systems, the ISO standard clearly defines the type of documentation that is required. Expressed in a simple way, you must 'say what you do' for every process within the organization. It has to be decided in what detail documentation should be conducted. Basically, the owners of processes (those people who perform the respective procedures) must decide in how much detail the process should be documented in the system. Nevertheless, detailed descriptions are essential for all key processes.

For the ISO standard, different levels of documentation are necessary:

(1) Quality manual;

(2) Handbooks;

(3) Standard operating procedures (SOPs).

The quality manual is the 'bible' of the QM system. It contains the quality policy of the institution as well as a brief description of the manner in which the work processes are governed. Furthermore, it also describes the most important staff members and their positions. Whereas the quality manual contains more general information, the individual processes and procedures are described in a more detailed way in handbooks/ job instructions or SOPs. These SOPs go through the processes step by step and describe the materials/

methods used and the way each process is performed. Standard operating procedure manuals should be available to all personnel. In these manuals, every single procedure must be fully documented with signature and date, and reviewed regularly.

APPLYING ISO STANDARDS TO THE ART LABORATORY

For ART centers, certainly the laboratory is the most critical part in terms of quality control and quality assurance[27]. The main goal of the quality assurance system in an ART laboratory is to guarantee a constant level of success for every step of every procedure by every staff member involved[28–30]. This requires the implementation of methods for system checks and detailed training plans for new team members, as well as a plan for regular and relevant evaluation of the performance of staff members[31,32].

Quality assurance within the ART laboratory comprises two main elements:

(1) Control of relevant equipment;

(2) Recruitment, training, development and control of staff involved.

Control of relevant equipment

In the control of relevant equipment one has to differentiate between routine checks and 'extreme conditions'. For routine work, daily control and documentation of working conditions should be performed. In addition, the performance of equipment under extreme conditions – for example, electrical failure, frequent opening of incubators, low and high loading of analyzers with samples, etc. – should be tested[33]. If, for example, the temperature and gas concentration of an incubator decrease very slowly and steadily after interruption of the electrical supply, it may be advisable to leave samples inside the incubator rather than try to evacuate them to another incubator, if correction of the problem is to be expected within 1–2 h (Figure 2).

In principle, all relevant equipment in the IVF laboratory, such as incubators, pH meters, osmometers, microscopes, etc., should undergo similar testing. It has to be decided who is responsible for making sure that appropriate methods for system checks are applied and

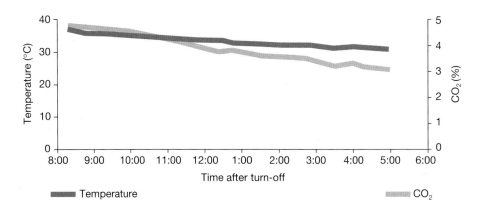

Figure 2 Control of temperature and CO_2 content of a standard incubator after turn-off

that the results of these checks are documented and followed[30,34]. In most IVF centers this responsibility lies with the laboratory director.

Staff development in the ART center

Results in an ART center cannot be achieved by a single person, such as a medical doctor just 'doing it all himself'. ART involves teamwork. Therefore, all the positive attributes – efficiency, effectiveness, productivity, creativity and, ultimately, good results – are best achieved by everyone working effectively both as a team and as individuals[5,7,35]. Thus, everyone needs to be good at his or her own job. This requires proper training and staff development. Other issues such as motivation go hand-in-hand with staff development. However, development has a particular and significant role to play[36]. This sounds logical and simple, but does not happen easily. There are too many potential difficulties:

(1) Lack of time;

(2) Inadequate resources;

(3) Under-funded training budgets;

(4) Conflicting priorities;

(5) Lack of clarity about what should be done;

(6) Failure to identify or accept the need;

(7) Shortfall in training skill or experience.

ART centers frequently do not properly fund the training of staff activities. However, one should keep the following in mind: 'If you think training is expensive, try ignorance...'

If one accepts that proper staff development makes a difference, then the job of doing it and making it work must be tackled. It is a striking phenomenon, which can be observed in ART centers, that doctors think staff development is not their responsibility but that of the laboratory manager or administration department. However, it should be very clear that the responsibility for staff development lies with the person responsible for the ART center. That need not mean he must personally provide all the development that takes place, but it is likely to mean he initiates most of it[37,38].

The following focuses on key elements of staff development in the ART center and gives examples of how instruments of quality management can be used to plan, perform and monitor development activities.

Staff requirements

ART centers offer highly specific treatments. The therapeutic procedures offered are typically complex and sophisticated. There is a lot of pressure on IVF team members to perform this treatment as efficiently and as successfully as possible. This can only be done by highly qualified people. Therefore, it is one of the most important tasks of management to recruit the right people to do the job, to train these people properly, to motivate them adequately and to monitor their performance precisely.

The first question you have to ask yourself is: 'What is the appropriate number of qualified people to do the job?' This question cannot be answered uniformly.

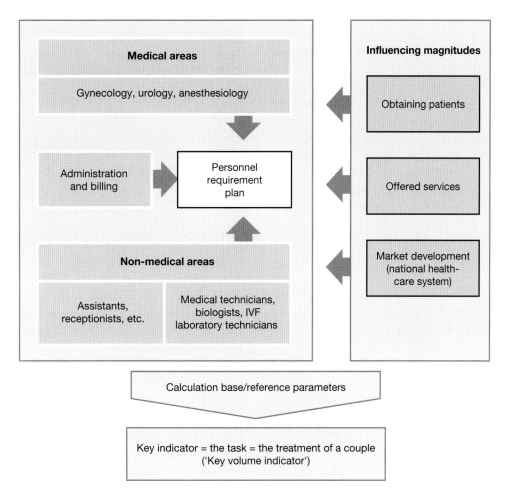

Figure 3 Staff requirement plan. IVF, *in vitro* fertilization. (From reference 23)

However, the way to deal with this question is to set up a staff requirement plan[23].

In most medical institutions it is recommended that one must define the levels for which the number of staff should be planned. Thus, the top level (management) and other levels (which can be further divided according to qualification) are defined. The number of employees should be determined for particular fields according to their tasks and range of techniques offered. This is why regulation for the equalization of staff must be created. This system makes planning easier and emphasizes the qualifications needed and, for instance, the rule of substitution.

The development of job descriptions is crucial for this system. Descriptions must be created for particular positions and must state, among other things, what a job-holder's qualifications are and what experience is required. In addition to this formal information, the work description should also contain information about the employee's personal attributes. For various positions a combination of abilities are important:

(1) Social competence;

(2) Organizational abilities;

(3) Communication skills, etc.

The staff requirement plan must be set up in a way that makes it possible to react adequately to unexpected situations. Furthermore, absence from work for holidays, illness and educational conferences needs to be considered. The minimum number of employees who must be present at any time should be determined for certain departments, which does not depend on the actual workload (Figure 3).

For the development of a staff requirement plan in an ART center, the medical as well as the non-medical areas have to be defined and considered. The question of how many people are needed to do the job properly can be answered on the basis of calculating the 'influence magnitudes'. The type of services offered strongly influences the number of people required. Thus, the staff requirements are different in a center in which predominantly conservative treatments and intrauterine inseminations are performed, compared with a center in which predominantly IVF/ICSI and cryopreservation cycles are performed. For an IVF center with a 'typical' distribution of procedures, estimates for staff requirement are given in Table 2.

Staff recruitment

If the management realizes that the work volume demands an increase in the number of staff, this cannot be solved just by hiring the first person who comes along. Recruitment and selection processes must be conducted carefully and demand a systematic approach[39]. Many people think that the processes involved in recruitment are wasted time, including the seemingly endless interviews. Worse may be that they assume that they are able to assess people 'as they walk through the door'. Most doctors have not been trained in these matters. However, good recruitment is an essential prerequisite to ensuring that a team keeps on functioning well. Getting it wrong has direct consequences: certainly the time and cost of getting rid of a candidate who should never have been appointed in the first place, and also the dilution of effectiveness (at worst, damage) they may cause while in office. It is worth the time and trouble necessary to make the best appointments possible.

Several issues should be defined before you start screening people for a new job.

A job definition

This is a clear statement of what the job entails, spelling out the objectives, responsibilities and the tasks to be undertaken. Without thinking this through carefully, sensible recruitment is impossible.

A candidate profile

A matching of, and clear statement about, the kind of person required to do the job (experience, knowledge, qualifications, background capabilities, etc.) completes this picture.

Table 2 Number of positions for different functions in the *in vitro* fertilization (IVF) center per number of treatment cycles performed per year (positions in the laboratory include laboratory director)

Cycles per year	Laboratory	Medical professional	Nursing
<250	1.5	2	3
250 to <500	2.5	—	4
500 to <750	3.0	2.5	4.5
750 to <1000	4.0	3	5
1000 to <1500	5.0	—	5.5
1500 to <2000	6.0	3.5	6
2000 to <2500	7.0	—	6.5
2500 to <3000	8.0	4	7

If the above two aspects are taken into account this may be sufficient to aid the recruitment and selection process, helping to produce any necessary job advertisements, focus interviews and guide the final selection. However, other issues may also be necessary. For instance, a job description which goes beyond the job definition is critical. The job description may be regarded as having two distinct roles: a formal one (linked to personnel systems, appraisal, etc.) and an informal one providing a working reference, and a document that acts day-to-day to help ensure that the correct focus is maintained, both in the job and around an organization or department.

SYSTEMATIC TRAINING OF EMPLOYEES
General remarks

In principle, the staff of an ART team can be subdivided into the following specialties:

(1) Nurses and/or physician assistants (care during and after medical procedures, operating theater);

(2) Laboratory team members (hormone, andrology and ART laboratories);

(3) Administration employees (billing, financial affairs, staff administration, information technology).

These special areas of work have to be taken into account when training plans specific to a center are being established.

It is important to define the needs of the center, and to check these against the skills that the employees have already mastered. Immediate action has to be taken only if there is a striking discrepancy between the two. Usually, this is true for beginners in their respective fields, and for these beginners a detailed training plan must be established, which is followed and supervised by a senior member of the specific team. It is advisable to set out some kind of follow-up of the learning curves of the trainees to evaluate and judge their progress in the methods that they are taught.

In the interest of continuous improvements, the performance of the more experienced team members should be followed to identify weak points in the course of work flow or in the abilities of individuals. Therefore, characteristic and measurable performance figures for the specific duties of a department must be identified and used to estimate objectively the abilities of persons and the efficiencies of processes. These data have to be analyzed and the results used to initiate appropriate improvements by specific training actions or remodeling of processes. Then the efficiency of these measures has to be evaluated, based upon the same parameters, in order to check the success of the improvement process.

It is of vital importance that every team member knows exactly his or her competences, responsibilities and authorities within the system, and that this assessment is also known to all other members of the team. Regular and structured communication between the top management and the employees is a must for an organization to function smoothly. For staff development, this implies obtaining knowledge about underutilized abilities of an individual that may be developed to the benefit of both the center and the employee.

In order to characterize the specific abilities of staff members working in a department, the assignment of individuals to the following levels may be helpful:

(1) Introduction to the basics;

(2) Practicing under supervision/training stage;

(3) Working independently;

(4) Instructing beginners.

These levels should be shown in an overview for every department in the center, stating also the name of the person responsible for the department and the stand-in regulations. An example of such a scheme is shown in Figure 4.

Nurses and/or physician assistants

The paramedical personnel are the part of the team who, in addition to the treating gynecologist, have the most intimate contact with patients. Therefore, their spectrum of abilities has to cover not only their professional skills, but also their social competence. The receptionist is the first person that a patient will meet on entering an ART center. The impression they get from that person will influence their opinion of the whole center. Later, many personal problems which may emerge during a treatment cycle are typically discussed while, for example, blood is being drawn by the nurse for hormone determination. During the time of oocyte retrieval and embryo transfer, careful attention towards the patient's needs and concerns helps them through the most demanding of the treatment phases.

This type of competence is very often a personal talent, and is very difficult to teach or to evaluate. However, team members may benefit from communication skills training in order to prepare them for dealing with the emotional needs of patients.

Developing a training plan for beginners

Nurses or physician assistants starting work in an IVF center need to be familiarized with their duties by an experienced team member. A detailed plan helps them to become oriented and to check their improvement for themselves. In order to characterize their progress within the center, a report should be written by the supervisor and be discussed with the trainee at reasonable intervals.

The training plan should be structured according to the following:

Patient communication and care

(1) Organization of appointments;

(2) Information about therapy details and treatment costs, in person or on the phone;

(3) Blood drawing;

(4) Injections.

Department:

In charge:				Quality assurance:	
Stand in:					

Staff members

	x...	y...	z...

Processess and test procedures

	Introduced to basics	Training stage	Working independently	May instruct beginners	Introduced to basics	Training stage	Working independently	May instruct beginners	Introduced to basics	Training stage	Working independently	May instruct beginners
1	✓	✓	✓	✓	✓	✓	✓	✓	✓	✓	✓	—
2	✓	✓	✓	✓	✓	✓	✓	✓	✓	✓	✓	—
3	✓	✓	✓	✓	✓	✓	✓	—	✓	✓	—	—
4	✓	✓	✓	✓	✓	✓	✓	✓	✓	✓	—	—
5	✓	✓	✓	✓	✓	✓	✓	✓	✓	✓	—	—
6	✓	✓	✓	✓	✓	✓	✓	✓	✓	✓	—	—
7	✓	✓	✓	✓	✓	—	—	—	✓	✓	—	—

Figure 4 Example of departmental overview of levels of achievement of procedures. 1–7, different team members

Organizational duties

(1) Preparation of consultation units;

(2) Cleaning and sterilization of instruments;

(3) Hygiene standards;

(4) Maintenance and control of equipment;

(5) Ordering and storage of material;

(6) Preparation and actualization of patient files in written and/or electronic form.

Assistance in the operation theater

(1) Assistance during oocyte retrievals;

(2) Assistance during embryo transfers;

(3) Care and supervision of patients after oocyte retrieval/embryo transfer.

Monitoring the performance of team members

The professional performance of nurses and/or physician assistants' duties can be monitored by several approaches, which of course have to be adjusted to the specific needs of individual ART centers (Table 3).

From key figures relating to all experienced team members, a mean value of performance can be established and the standard deviation calculated. The range obtained by mean plus/minus two standard deviations (mean $\pm 2\,SD$) will represent the performance of 95.5% of the respective staff. Individuals falling below this range should be considered for specific training in the field identified by these means. Special care should be taken to communicate to the team that this approach is not perceived as a control and punishment policy, but an improvement option for individuals and the whole process they are involved in.

Table 3 Monitoring of nurses' and/or physician assistants' performance of routine duties

Activity	Measurement of performance	Key figure
Correct adherence to hygiene regulations	swab tests	proportion of positive tests
Cleaning and sterilization of instruments	sterilization protocols	incidence of incorrect handling
Preparation of patient files	test every 10th file, error list	proportion of incorrect files
Record-keeping and documentation	number of mistakes, error list	proportion of mistakes per file
Incidence of hematoma or complaints by patients after blood drawing/injections	list of complaints	proportion of complaints per number of patients treated
Preparation of instruments for oocyte retrieval or embryo transfer	personal check by gynecologist	incidence of corrections
Assistance during procedures	personal check by gynecologist	incidence of corrections

Measuring training effects

Short-term assessments

During the training phase, learning progress has to be carefully followed by the supervisor performing the training. Once it is begun, a short period of time (i.e. a month or as appropriate) of close follow-up should be conducted to make sure the training was effective.

Long-term assessments

The further progress of trained persons can be monitored during the routine follow-up of staff performance. The data collected have to be edited in a way to give quick and reasonable comparison of all team members' outcomes.

Laboratory staff

The importance of a well-organized and effective laboratory team needs no further elucidation. This part of the ART center is an important partner with the medical staff, and the achievements of which are an important contribution to achieving high pregnancy rates. Quality assurance measures within the laboratory should be in the hands of an experienced and motivated team member, educated in the basics of quality management procedures.

Every assisted reproduction technique offered by the center has to be covered by at least two members of the laboratory team to assure availability at any given time. The performance of every team member must be at the same high quality level to ensure the same efficiency of techniques for every patient treated. To guarantee this, a detailed quality assurance system needs to be established and maintained for all decisive procedures in the laboratory. The performance figures applied have to be adjusted to the exclusive activities of the laboratory, independent of intervention by the medical side (i.e. provider differences in pregnancy rates).

A good electronic database system should be in place for fast and regular evaluation of results, as well as for the long-term retrospective follow-up of individual performances of laboratory techniques. For this purpose, every data set for each specific procedure must include identification of the person completing the step.

Developing a training plan for beginners in the laboratory

It is advisable to have a standardized training plan ready for everybody starting as a new team member in an ART laboratory, irrespective of any previous experience. The sequence of techniques to be learned may be fixed, or can be adjusted to the needs of the laboratory. The number of cases that a person must be trained on before being allowed to work independently should be defined for every procedure. A tutor should be nominated who is responsible for the practical and theoretical training and monitoring of the success of a new employee, and who is also authorized to judge the level of performance reached, i.e.:

Table 4 Training plan for new staff members in the *in vitro* fertilization (IVF) laboratory

Procedure	Observation of an experienced staff member	Practice under supervision, at least		Allowance to work independently, after	May instruct beginners, after
Preparation of culture material	5 cases	5 cases		20 cases correctly prepared	60 cases
Oocyte retrieval	5 cases	30 cases		50 cases	400 cases
Culture and scoring fertilization	5 cases	10 cases or 70 oocytes		50 cases, <10% loss of oocytes	500 cases
embryo development	5 cases	30 cases		30 cases with correct scoring	500 cases
Embryo transfer	5 cases	20 cases		50 cases with <5% losses	300 cases
Cryopreservation and thawing	sperm: 3 cases	5 cases		10 cases, survival rate ≥30%	20 cases
	PN stages: 5 cases	10 cases		20 cases, survival rate ≥55%	50 cases
Assisted hatching	5 cases	5 unfertilized oocytes	10 actual cases	no degeneration in 10 cases	50 cases
ICSI	5 cases	20 unfertilized oocytes	50 oocytes of actual cases	fertilization rate ≥50%, degeneration rate <15%	100 cases
Andrology	ejaculates: 5 cases	25 cases		50 cases, ≥10% recovery, ≥20% increase in motility	150 cases
	TESE specimen: 3 cases	5 cases		10 cases	30 cases

ICSI, intracytoplasmic sperm injection; PN, pronucleate; TESE, testicular sperm extraction

(1) Introduced to the basics;

(2) Practice under supervision/training stage;

(3) May work independently;

(4) May instruct beginners.

The following schedule outlines the approach applied in our own laboratory, which may serve as an example since it has proved to be of value in our hands for several years. Every procedure is explained to the trainee in detail and the specific manual chapter read for theoretical and practical background before the start of training. The values given define the minimum number of cases that must be accomplished before the next level can be reached. These numbers may of course need modification for individual differences in learning abilities (Table 4).

The performance on specific techniques should be monitored and discussed to give the beginner a chance to adjust the technique where possible. An example of training success in the ICSI procedure for three new

team members as observed in our center is illustrated for the period July 2001 to December 2002 in Figure 5. Individuals '4' and '5' showed similar learning curves, with high degeneration rates and low fertilization rates during the first periods, which normalized gradually to levels similar to those of the experienced staff. In individual '6' a common phenomenon for beginners was observed for the first quarter: that person was very anxious about damaging oocytes and therefore the degeneration rate was low, but so was the fertilization success. After being told to be a bit more aggressive, that trainee also performed like the other two.

Monitoring the performance of team members

The performance of experienced team members should be followed regularly according to a fixed schedule of assurance procedures. The key figures to be evaluated must be specific for the laboratory procedures exclusively. Such parameters could be:

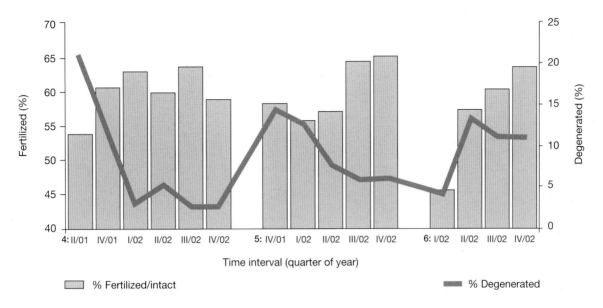

Figure 5 Intracytoplasmic sperm injection (ICSI) results for new team members in training phase

Short-term scheme (at least two team members in comparison, at least weekly):

(1) Evaluation of a semen specimen for concentration, motility and morphology;

(2) Evaluation of oocyte quality, fertilization rates, embryo scores.

Long-term scheme (individual evaluations for all team members, monthly to quarterly):

(1) Recovery rates and final motility in sperm samples after preparation;

(2) Degeneration and fertilization rates after ICSI;

(3) Survival rates after cryopreservation.

The results obtained may be summarized in graphical form to allow quick estimation of trends or deviations. For long-term follow-ups, calculation of mean values and standard deviations or standard errors of the means of results are helpful for clearly identifying team members with superior or inferior performance.

Some examples of test series for laboratory personnel obtained in our own laboratory are given below.

Short-term scheme The mean deviation between two individuals determining sperm motility (Figure 6) was around 5% for both the original sample and the

fraction prepared after density gradient centrifugation; only exceptional deviations larger than 10% were observed.

The greatest difficulties in judging embryo quality obviously occurred with day-4 embryos (Figure 7), when cell numbers cannot be determined exactly and the rate of fragmentation is hard to estimate without knowing the embryo's morphology on the preceding days.

Long-term scheme Long-term evaluation of performance may show important trends. The results shown in Figure 8 caused an important team discussion, since it became evident that individuals '1' and '5' obviously had put less effort into obtaining a sufficient concentration of spermatozoa in the final prepared volume, compared with the other three, especially in very severely impaired specimens. Interestingly, these two colleagues worked exclusively in the andrology laboratory, while individuals '2', '3' and '4' also had to do ICSIs with the prepared spermatozoa. These three team members made the other two watch the procedure and explained to them the difficulties associated with very low sperm numbers for ICSI. After receiving this information, the preparation efficiency of all five team members became comparable (Figure 9).

These results are a good example of the need to analyze the obtained data carefully for confounding factors. If only fertilization rates are considered,

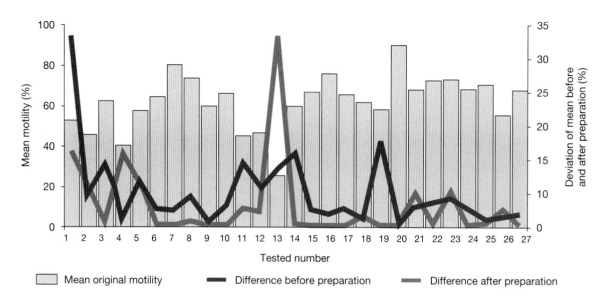

Figure 6 Comparison of motility determination in semen samples (2003). $n = 27$ tests, before preparation: 5.96 ± 1.28 (SE), after preparation: 3.59 ± 1.35 %(SE) deviation

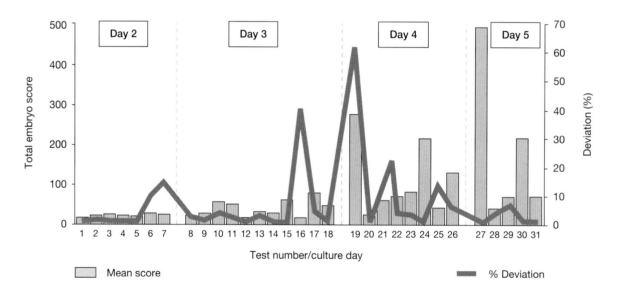

Figure 7 Comparison of total embryo scores (sum of cell stages×fragmentation ranking; 2003, two team members). Total mean deviation: $n = 31$ tests, 6.5 ± 2.38% (SE) (day 2: 3.7%, day 3: 5.00%, day 4: 13.9%, day 5: 2.2%)

individuals '1', '2' and '3' clearly seem to have performed worse than the others. These people, however, were the most experienced in our laboratory. Because of their experience they had to deal with the problem cases. Technician '2', for example, took over the cases with low numbers of mature oocytes, and '1' and '3' handled the majority of cases requiring testicular sperm

extraction, which were therefore also associated with a slight increase in the degeneration rates (Figure 10).

The evaluation of these data made clear that the impact of the person doing the cryopreservation procedure and that of the one responsible for the thawing process are both important for the cryo-survival of pronuclear stage embryos.

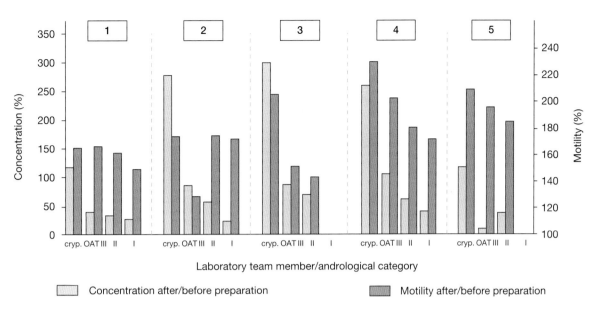

Figure 8 Efficiency of preparation in the andrology laboratory (2002). Andrological categories: cryp., cryptozoospermia < 1, oligoasthenoteratozoospermia (OAT) III < 5, OAT II < 10, OAT I < 20 million spermatozoa per ml

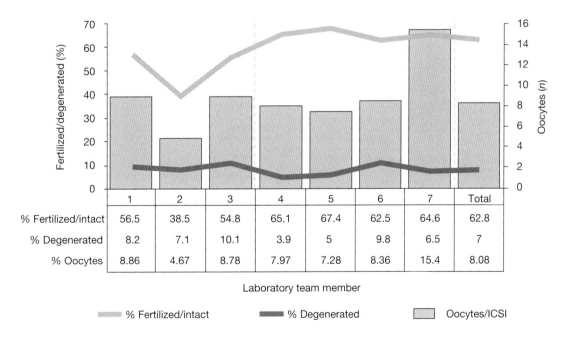

	1	2	3	4	5	6	7	Total
% Fertilized/intact	56.5	38.5	54.8	65.1	67.4	62.5	64.6	62.8
% Degenerated	8.2	7.1	10.1	3.9	5	9.8	6.5	7
% Oocytes	8.86	4.67	8.78	7.97	7.28	8.36	15.4	8.08

Laboratory team member

Figure 9 Intracytoplasmic sperm injection (ICSI) results according to team member (2003). $n = 7$ individuals, % fertilized: 58.5 ± 3.76, % degenerated: 7.2 ± 0.88 (mean ± SE)

Identifying training needs

The results of the tests described need to be discussed with the team members on a regular basis to ensure benefit for everybody participating. Emphasis should be put on the results of the top performers in the group. By declaring their level, the goal for every team member will be realized. Charts such as those shown allow quick orientation in cases when results for an individual differ greatly from those of others. The

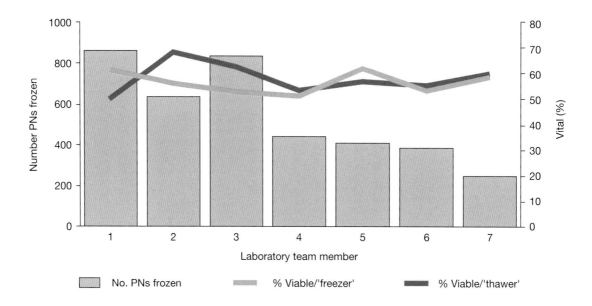

Figure 10 Survival rates according to team member performing cryopreservation or thawing of pronuclear stages (2000–03). $n = 7$ individuals, $56.6 \pm 1.57\%$ (SE) (freezing) and $57.8 \pm 2.35\%$ (SE) (thawing) survival rate. PN, pronucleate

normal level of successful performance may be defined as the range characterized by the mean value obtained by all people involved with a specific method plus/minus two standard deviations, which will cover 95.5% of all values, as mentioned above. Anybody reaching test levels below this margin more than once should be trained specifically by one of the top performers or a senior team member. Nevertheless, the work of that person should be investigated thoroughly for confounding factors before initiation of further steps, since quite often the difficult cases (i.e. low oocyte numbers in ICSI cycles, poor zygote morphology for cryopreservation) are handled by specific members.

Another method of tracking performance, which is used in industry, is 'P-charts'. These charts are used to measure 'out of control' occurrences. An example of this is illustrated in Figure 11 which shows the pregnancy rate per doctor performing an embryo transfer.

Measuring training effects

After specific training periods, the key figures identified for the process in question have to be monitored at short-term intervals for the trained person until the desired level is attained. The evaluation of training effects should be done by the supervisor or the person responsible for quality assurance in the laboratory.

Special arrangements must be made for team members to attend external courses or conferences. The knowledge gained by these activities should be communicated to all colleagues in a structured way, and the scientific value of that training should also be judged by the person attending it.

In order to estimate the overall abilities of an ART laboratory, it is an advisable policy to participate in comparisons between similar laboratories. This can be done by exchanging documented material (photos, videos, etc.) and scoring it according to defined criteria, or by undergoing audits, exchanging the specialists between laboratories.

Administration employees

The following fields can be allocated to the department of administration and financial management:

(1) Accounting;

(2) General administration;

(3) Human resources management;

(4) Purchasing department;

(5) Business management/controlling;

(6) Organization/information technology

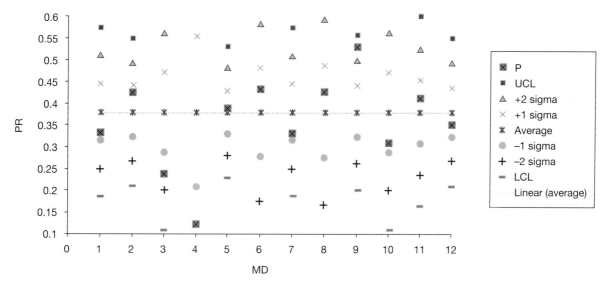

'P-charts: out of control'
(1) 1 point above 3 sigma line (UCL) or 1 point below –3 sigma line (LCL)
(2) 2 of 3 consecutive points above 2 sigma line or 2 of 3 consecutive points below –2 sigma line
(3) 4 of 5 consecutive points above 1 sigma line or 4 of 5 consecutive points below –1 sigma line
(4) 8 consecutive points above or below center line (average)
(5) 6 consecutive increasing or decreasing points

Figure 11 Pregnancy rate (PR) per doctor (MD) per embryo transfer

Increasingly intense competition between units makes the roles of administration and information technology (IT) vitally important to the success of a clinic. This is a consequence of the fact that, within an ART center, a manpower-intensive service is offered (with a corresponding significance of the human/human resource factor), and increases in efficiency are only obtained through an intelligent IT-assisted organization. Last, but not least, an informative controlling system is needed to master the economic necessities efficiently and to be goal-oriented. Furthermore, it has to be decided to what extent these functions may be covered by in-house facilities, or may be purchased. It could, for example, be advantageous to delegate 'salary accounting' to an external party, in view of the multi-faceted legal regulations and the modifications caused by them. The same may be true for specific projects in the IT sector.

Developing a training plan for beginners in administration

In order to train new team members a standardized training plan is executed. This is composed of the following two main areas.

ART treatment   First of all the basic medical interrelations are explained, followed by the specific treatment methods. As a completion of this block, control questions may be answered in order to acquire some feed back about the learning achievement. In a second step an overview has to be gained about the collaboration of the specific departments of the ART center. This implies the definition of their duties, responsibilities and interfaces. Again, the answering of control questions will reflect the progress in understanding of the trainee.

Specific assignments   Once the basics are achieved, training for the specific area of working is started, i.e. financial accounting or staff administration. For this, specialized knowledge has to be imparted such as the organization of the accounts structure within the accounting department, or the allocation directives.

Monitoring the performance of team members   As a prerequisite for this, the availability of meaningful criteria for measuring the efficiency must be provided and performance standards be agreed upon. The following measurement categories are mentioned as examples.

Enumerable performances:

(1) Number of account positions per time unit;

(2) Number of bookings per time unit;

(3) Obtained abatements of prices in comparison with previous year;

(4) Regarding projects: adherence to appointed time/milestones.

Non-enumerable performance:

(1) Customer satisfaction.

Identifying training needs and measuring training effects If efficiency criteria have been defined and measurements and adjustments against predefined performance standards have been obtained, then negative deviations will indicate any needs for further training. After accomplishment of the respective action and the subsequent measurement of procedures, the result of this training can be controlled.

The best instrument for this is the so-called 'score card', which can be adjusted individually for their particular requirements.

Calculating a budget for training activities

The following information has to be made available in order to calculate an adequate budget:

(1) The number of persons in whom deviations between the evaluated personal capacity and the specification have been identified: these discrepancies will determine the training requirements for particular persons.

(2) After identifying the persons in need of training, and the individual discrepancy between personal efficiency and demand, a profile is produced with individual training needs.

(3) After this, quotations on costs are solicited. Where applicable, the time expenditure and the resulting internal expense ratio are calculated when the training is by internal specialists.

(4) After collating all the information, a training plan is produced containing the names of participants, the individual training measures and the prospective costs. The date of the respective measure should also be determined within the training plan.

CONCLUSIONS

No internationally accepted standards exist for quality mangement in ART laboratories and ART centers. In order to ensure high quality and continuous improvement, it is recommended that all ART centers striving for excellence should develop a QM system. In some countries, such as Germany, there is now already a legal requirement to implement a QM system in medical institutions.

A functioning QM system allows the organization to gain control of its procedures and their documents, and to monitor and document the clinical and non-clinical outcomes[40]. Furthermore, the issues of staff recruitment and staff development can be addressed systematically and thereby, again, the overall outcome will be improved. The ISO standard offers the medical facility access to an internationally endorsed and proven QM system. ART practitioners in particular have a unique opportunity to set the standard in medicine for quality management principles.

REFERENCES

1. Eckert H, Bohmer K. Reform of the Law DIN EN ISO 9001:2000. Commentary on the new requirements on quality management systems. Z Ärztl Fortbild Qualitätssich 2000; 94: 669–75

2. Birkner B. Certification of an ambulatory gastroenterologic service fulfilling ISO Law 9001 – criteria and national guidelines of the Gastroenterologic Association. Z Ärztl Fortbild Qualitätssich 2000; 94: 639–43

3. Beholz S, Koch C, Konertz W. Certification and quality management of a complex university cardiac center according to law EN ISO 9001:2000. Z Ärztl Fortbild Qualitätssich 2003; 97: 141–4

4. Field MJ, Lohr KN. Guidelines for Clinical Practice. From Development to Use. Washington: National Academy Press, 1992

5. Collings J. An international survey of the health economics of IVF and ICSI. Hum Reprod Update 2002; 8: 265–77

6. Garceau L, Henderson J, Davis LJ, et al. Economic implications of assisted reproductive techniques: a systematic review. Hum Reprod 2002; 17: 3090–109

7. Alper MM, Brinsden PR, Fischer R, Wikland M. Is your IVF programme good? Hum Reprod 2002; 17: 8–10

8. Duvauferrier R, Rolland Y, Philippe C, et al. Comparison of accreditation procedures, ISO 9000 certification procedures and total quality management. Personal experiences and application of quality assurance in a department of radiology and medical imaging. J Radiol 1999; 80: 363–7

9. Fritze B, Amon U. The 'Hersbruck Model'. Application and integration of the DIN EN ISO 9001 quality norms with criteria of the European Foundation for Quality Management in a clinic. Z Ärztl Fortbild Qualitätssich 1999; 93: 701–7

10. Edelstein ME. ISO 9001:2000 – setting the standard for quality management. J Am Health Int Manage Assoc 2001; 72: 34–9

11. American Fertility Society. Guidelines for human embryology and andrology laboratories. Fertil Steril 1992; 58 (Suppl 1): S1–10

12. Yasin MM, Meacham KA, Alavi J. The status of TQM in healthcare. Health Mark Q 1998; 15: 61–84

13. Bloor G. Organisational culture, organisational learning and total quality management: a literature review and synthesis. Aust Health Rev 1999; 22: 162–79

14. Geraedts HP, Montenarie R, Van Rijk PP. The benefits of total quality management. Comput Med Imaging Graph 2001; 25: 217–20

15. Weiler T, Hoffmann R, Strehlau-Schwoll H. Quality management and certification. Optimizing hospital procedures. Unfallchirurg 2003; 106: 692–7

16. Shaw CD. External quality mechanisms for health care: summary of the ExPeRT project on visitatie, accreditations, EFQM and ISO assessment in European Union countries. External Peer Review Techniques. European Foundation for Quality Management. International Organization for Standardization. Int J Qual Health Care 2000; 12: 169–75

17. Guillain H. Four models for external quality assessment in the health sector. Rev Med Suisse Romande 2001; 121: 791–3

18. Ollenschlager G. Thoughts on certification on ambulatory care – exemplified by DIN EN ISO certification. Z Ärztl Fortbild Qualitätssich 2000; 94: 645–9

19. Staines A. Benefits of an ISO 9001 certification – the case of a Swiss regional hospital. Int J Health Care Qual Assur Inc Leadersh Health Serv 2000; 13: 27–33

20. Setti Bassanini MC. Accreditation and certification. Int J Artif Organs 1998; 21: 730–5

21. Plebani M. Role of inspectors in external review mechanisms: criteria for selection, training and appraisal. Clin Chim Acta 2001; 309: 147–54

22. Honsa JD, McIntyre DA. ISO 17025: practical benefits of implementing a quality system. J Assoc Offic Anal Chem Int 2003; 86: 1038–44

23. Keck C. Quality Management in Assisted Reproduction. Prague: KAP Ltd, 2003; 23–4

24. Bron MS, Salmon JW. Infertility services and managed care. Am J Manag Care 1998; 4: 715–20

25. Moore LM. High standards: ISO 9000 comes to health care. Trustee 1999; 52: 10–14

26. Gondringer NS. Benchmarking: friend or foe. Am Assoc Nurs Anesth J 1997; 65: 335–6

27. De Jonge C. Commentary: forging a partnership between total quality management and the andrology laboratory. J Androl 2000; 21: 203–5

28. Brown RW. Errors in medicine. J Qual Clin Pract 1997; 17: 21–5

29. Colton D. The design of evaluations for continuous quality improvement. Eval Health Prof 1997; 20: 265–85

30. Matson PL. Internal quality control and external quality assurance in the IVF laboratory. Hum Reprod 1998; 13 (Suppl): 156–65

31. Lehmann HP. Certification standards transfer: from committee to laboratory. Clin Chim Acta 1998; 278: 121–44

32. Libeer JC. Effect of accreditation schemes on the setting of quality specifications by laboratories. Scand J Clin Lab Invest 1999; 59: 575–8

33. Padden H. Instrument calibration. Occup Health Saf 2002; 71: 66–70

34. Gianaroli L, Plachot M, Van Kooij R, et al., and committee of the Special Interest Group on Embryology. ESHRE guidelines for good practice in IVF laboratories. Hum Reprod 2000; 15: 2241–6

35. Squires A. New graduate orientation in the rural community hospital. J Contin Educ Nurs (United States) 2002; 33: 203–9

36. Sigrudsson HO. Career development programs at Landspitali University Hospital. Nurs Leadersh Forum (United States) 2003; 8: 40–4

37. Kissel C, Keck C. Introduction of a structured training course for medical doctors in training in the field of reproductive medicine. Geburtsh Frauenheilk 2004; 64: 160–3

38. Rose JL. Developing new and current employees. Mich Health Hosp (United States) 2003; 39/3: 22–3

39. O'Brodovich H, Pleinys R, Laxer R, et al. Evaluation of a peer-reviewed career development and compensation program for physicians at an academic health science center. Pediatrics (United States) 2003; 111: 26–31

40. Metz-Schimmerl S, Schima W, Herold CJ. Certification according to ISO 9001 – waste of time or necessity? Radiologe 2002; 42: 380–6

FURTHER READING

ISO/DIS 15189:2: 2002. Medical Laboratories – Particular requirements for quality and competence.
ISO/IEC 17025:1999. General requirements for the competence of testing and calibration laboratories.
ISO/IEC Guide 25:1990. General requirements for the competence of testing and calibration laboratories.
ISO 9001:2000. Quality management systems – Requirements.

Internet addresses related to the subject of quality management

http://www.asrm.com/
http://www.ferti.net/
http://www.iso.ch/
http://www.isoeasy.org/
http://www.guideline.gov/
http://www.praxion.com

30

Quality control in the *in vitro* fertilization laboratory

Adam Burnley

INTRODUCTION

The *in vitro* fertilization (IVF) laboratory plays a fundamental role in the delivery of treatment to infertile couples. IVF centers must ensure that they provide a consistently high-quality service. The quality of service is of the utmost importance to companies who want to be successful in what is recognized as a competitive marketplace. But what exactly is quality? Currently, many national registries focus on pregnancy rate or live birth rate as their sole outcome measure. However, these can be misleading, as higher pregnancy rates may be associated with the exclusion of patients less likely to become pregnant, excessive numbers of cases of hyperstimulation and multiple pregnancies; IVF treatment may even be recommended to those who might conceive using simpler approaches. 'The use of pregnancy rates as the sole or most important criteria for the measure of quality in an IVF center is misguided'[1].

In the United Kingdom, there are few standards, other than the Human Fertilization and Embryology Authority (HFEA) league tables, that enable patients to compare IVF programs. In light of this, when deciding which center to choose for their IVF treatment, the consumer is not able to base their decision on quality of treatment provided. The consumer's choice must therefore be based on the existing published information that comprises nationally reported clinic-specific pregnancy rates. Whilst a low pregnancy rate might indicate a laboratory that is performing poorly, it might also be due to other factors, such as a high proportion of patients who have a poor prognosis. In such cases the laboratory may be performing to an excellent standard, but without any acknowledgment of this in the information that is available to patients.

International Standards for laboratory accreditation (ISO 17025 and ISO 15189) have been developed recently. Adherence to these Standards may be suitable for those laboratories acting as the supplier of test results. However, participation has financial implications and is not compulsory; therefore, participation throughout the UK is variable. Most people working in an IVF laboratory acknowledge the need for an adequate quality control (QC) system to help ensure optimal quality of treatment.

It is the clinical embryologist who bears the responsibility for the standard of treatment provided by his or her own laboratory. Much effort has been dedicated to promoting knowledge of techniques, procedures and strategies in order to ensure use of the highest-quality practices in reproductive medicine. Therefore, it is not unreasonable to suggest that every IVF laboratory should implement a quality management system to establish and maintain strict QC[2].

The main aim of a QC system is to ensure the consistency and reproducibility of all procedures conducted in the laboratory by evaluating the effectiveness of policies and procedures, detecting and correcting problems and monitoring the performance and competency of equipment and staff. By using a structured and comprehensive QC system it should be possible to ensure that a laboratory will be successful and guarantee optimum standards of treatment and care for its patients.

All aspects of work in laboratories involved in the diagnosis and treatment of human infertility can benefit from internal QC and external quality assurance (QA), moving the work from being a subjective art form to an objective science[3]. Due to the lack of a recognized accreditation scheme, such programs have tended to rely on the motivation of the individual laboratory.

WHAT IS A QUALITY SYSTEM?

Many books and articles have been published that describe quality systems. These systems usually comprise the same principles and techniques, but can be known by different names, such as total quality management (TQM) and total quality improvement (TQI).

Quality systems are frequently divided into three distinct levels: total quality management, quality assurance and quality control. There are fundamental differences between the three levels that are often confused[4].

Total quality management

The British Quality Association describes TQM as:

> ...a business management philosophy which recognises that customer needs and business goals are inseparable...it ensures maximum effectiveness and efficiency...by putting in place processes and systems which will promote excellence, prevent errors and ensure that every aspect of the business is aligned to customer needs and advancement of business goals. ...It involves every department, function and process in a business and the active involvement of all employees.

TQM can be applied to any type of organization and represents a philosophy of continuously striving to improve every aspect of a service. This is achieved through comprehensive monitoring in order to detect any problems, ongoing refinements in response to continuous customer feedback and constant exploration of ways to increase the effectiveness of the service. TQM activity is, as stated, not restricted to the IVF laboratory but includes every function within the assisted conception unit (ACU). TQM encompasses quality assurance and quality control.

Quality assurance

Quality assurance has been described as the sum of all activities required in order to establish confidence that the product or service meets the determined quality requirements[2]. QA involves monitoring and evaluating a whole process to ensure the highest standard of treatment. Elements of a QA program are a written procedure manual and all quality control activities.

Quality control

QC is any activity designed to ensure that a specific element within the laboratory is functioning correctly[4]. For individual elements of the laboratory, e.g. personnel, equipment and supplies, measurements are taken which can be compared with previously established thresholds and acceptable limits. In this way it is possible to maintain the optimal standard of results.

The relationship between the three levels of a quality system is illustrated in Figure 1.

Whilst it has been recognized that TQM activity is not restricted to the IVF laboratory, this chapter concentrates solely on the laboratory aspects of such a program.

IMPLEMENTING A QUALITY SYSTEM

Staff

An IVF laboratory is only as good as the personnel it employs. Laboratory management should ensure that there are appropriate numbers of staff, with the required education and training to meet the demands of the service and appropriate national legislation and regulations[5].

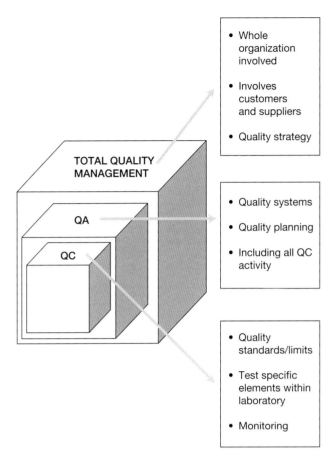

- Whole organization involved
- Involves customers and suppliers
- Quality strategy

- Quality systems
- Quality planning
- Including all QC activity

- Quality standards/limits
- Test specific elements within laboratory
- Monitoring

Figure 1 Diagram to illustrate the three levels of a quality system. QA, quality assurance; QC, quality control (adapted from Aston University MBA Resource Pack 2001)

Table 1 Survey of staffing levels of *in vitro* fertilization (IVF) clinics in the United Kingdom related to total number of cycles (IVF + intracytoplasmic sperm injection) performed. The Association of Clinical Embryologists (ACE) conducted the survey during 2002[6]

Total number of cycles	Full-time staff (average)	Full-time staff (range)
1–200	1.5	1–2
201–400	2.7	1–4.5
401–600	3.8	2.5–5
601–800	5.1	4.5–5.5
801–1000	5.5	4–6.5
>1000	7.25	6–8.5

cases and 200–400 cases per embryologist were quoted[7].

In order to assure medical colleagues and patients that every embryologist within an IVF laboratory is performing laboratory procedures to a high and similar standard, and to ensure consistency of results, it is important that staff members undergo personal audits of their performance. This is covered in greater detail later in this chapter.

The staffing requirements must include a comprehensive orientation and induction program, a job description that specifies duties and responsibilities, and the opportunity to increase their knowledge and competence through continuing educational programs.

What is the appropriate staffing level for an IVF laboratory? This is dependent upon the numbers of IVF, intracytoplasmic sperm injection (ICSI) and frozen-embryo cycles conducted, as well as any additional work such as research projects, external activities and administrative duties. The Association of Clinical Embryologists (ACE) of the United Kingdom conducted a survey of UK IVF centers during 2002 to establish existing staffing levels[6] (Table 1).

A significant difference in staffing levels between IVF centers was highlighted during a recent worldwide conference on IVF, when ratios of between 110

Procedures

An essential element of a quality program is the establishment and documentation of standard operating procedures (SOPs). There should be a detailed written procedure that describes each laboratory process and which includes the relevant equipment, materials and standard required for each process. A file containing all SOPs should be located in a prominent place in the laboratory and be available for all laboratory personnel. All laboratory staff should sign that they have read and understood the procedures[8]. SOPs should be reviewed annually and, if necessary, be amended to take into account any legal requirements and changes in practice. Mechanisms need to be in place for recording the creation of, and updates to, existing SOPs, incorporating the date and signature of the relevant manager. Outdated procedures should be stored in a separate archive section of the procedures file with a date indicating when it was taken out of service.

Table 2 Selected quality control activities within the *in vitro* fertilization (IVF) laboratory			
Parameter	Frequency	Pass level	Action required on failure
Incubator temperature (°C) (digital display)	daily (tick-sheet)	36.5–37.5°C	test using independent thermocouple, recalibrate if necessary
Incubator CO_2 (%) (digital display)	daily (tick-sheet)	5.5–6.5% CO_2	test using independent CO_2 monitor, recalibrate if necessary
Fridge temperature (°C)	daily (tick-sheet)	4.0–8.0°C	test using independent thermocouple, contact engineer
Sterilizing oven temperature (°C)	×2 per month	≥180°C for 1 h	recalibrate and retest
Microscope heated stages and tube heater (°C)	monthly	maintain Petri dish at 37°C ± 1°C for 1 h	recalibrate and retest
Incubator temperature (°C)	×2 per month	maintain Petri dish at 37°C ± 0.5°C for 1 h	recalibrate and retest
Incubator CO_2 concentration (°C)	×2 per month	5.5–6.5%	recalibrate and retest
LN_2 Dewar alarms	×2 per month	—	contact engineer

LN_2, liquid nitrogen

Laboratory equipment

A fundamental element of the laboratory QA program is regular QC for every piece of equipment involved in the IVF process, including those devices that are used for the purpose of calibrating other instruments. The objective of the QC program is to ensure that the equipment being used is of suitably high quality, is frequently quality controlled and is maintained at regular intervals. In this way it should be possible to ensure reproducibility of results from each item.

The program may be organized using a document that lists each item to be tested together with a schedule detailing the frequency of testing and a range of acceptable limits for each piece of equipment (Table 2). This document needs to incorporate the procedure to be followed if an item of equipment fails to fall within the acceptable range and needs recalibrating.

Equipment for which QC procedures and protocols are required include:

(1) Incubators;

(2) Microscopes and heated stages;

(3) Flow hoods;

(4) Fridges;

(5) Sterilizing oven;

(6) Liquid nitrogen Dewars;

(7) Calibration equipment;

(8) Tissue culture/plastic ware/culture media.

Incubators

The incubator is arguably the most important item of equipment used in any IVF laboratory. Good embryo culture conditions and subsequent embryonic development are dependent upon a correctly maintained incubator temperature and pH.

Temperature and CO_2 readings should be recorded on a daily basis. Use of a tick-sheet located on the front door of each incubator may be helpful. The use of tick-sheets allows the early identification of any change in the reported values and therefore early management of any problems that occur. It is, however, insufficient to rely solely on the digital display of the incubator. The readout should be verified as being correct, at regular intervals, through the use of an independent thermocouple and CO_2 monitor as seen in Figure 2.

Any deviations from the acceptable ranges should be recorded and the instrument recalibrated.

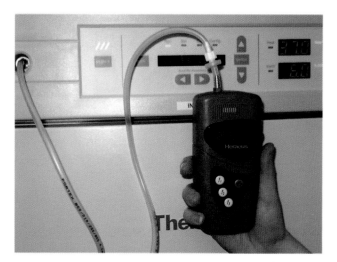

Figure 2 Verification of incubator CO_2 concentration using an independent CO_2 monitor

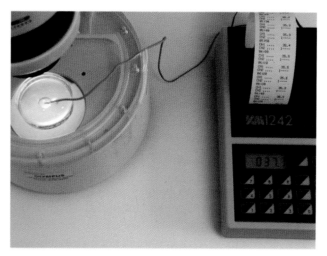

Figure 3 Verification of heated stage temperature using an independent thermocouple

It is often assumed that if the concentration of CO_2 measured in an incubator falls within the acceptable range that the pH of the culture drops inside that incubator is also at the optimal level. This is not necessarily the case. Therefore, the pH of the culture medium within an incubator should be tested independently and regularly using a microprobe attached to a pH meter.

Microscopes and heated stages

The microscope is a fundamental tool for the identification and scoring of gametes and embryos. These must be regularly maintained and serviced to ensure ease of use and accuracy. Embryology procedures inevitably involve the removal of Petri dishes, containing patient oocytes and embryos, from the optimal culture conditions of the incubator for microscopic examination. It is almost impossible, even when culturing under mineral oil, to avoid small changes in temperature of the contents of the dishes. It has been shown that fluctuations in temperature have a negative effect upon the developmental potential of embryos, and the exposure of human oocytes, even to room temperature, can cause irreversible damage to the meiotic spindle[9]. It is therefore imperative that, once the Petri dish is in place, the integrated heated stage maintains the temperature of the dish as close to 37°C as possible throughout the duration of any microscopic procedure.

This can be evaluated by placing the probe of an independent thermocouple into a Petri dish on a heated stage (Figure 3). The temperature should be maintained at 37°C ($\pm\,0.5$°C) for a fixed time period, e.g. 1 h.

Flow hoods

These need to be regularly serviced and maintained by an independent contractor to ensure that they are performing effectively and offering protection to both the sample being examined and the operator performing the task.

Refrigerators

Most culture media used in an IVF laboratory will be stored in a refrigerator. This maintains the stability of components and prevents the growth of contaminants. A simple thermometer can be placed within the refrigerator to establish the inner temperature. Tick-sheets recording acceptable limits may be attached to the door of each refrigerator in order to monitor fluctuations of temperature. Records should be archived for the appropriate length of time.

Sterilizing oven

In order to guarantee the sterility of reusable glass or metal products, a laboratory needs to be sure that the sterilizing oven being used is heating the instruments to the correct temperature for a measured length of time. In the author's laboratory the level has been set at ≥ 180°C for a minimum of 1 h.

Again, it is not sufficient to rely on the integral display of the oven, but to verify the readout, on a regular basis, with the use of a calibrated, independent thermocouple.

Liquid nitrogen Dewars

The provision for safe storage of patient gametes and embryos is critical for any IVF center offering a cryo-preservation service. The consequences of liquid nitrogen (LN_2) falling below the acceptable level within a Dewar would be catastrophic for patients and possibly therefore for the future of the unit.

Storage Dewars must be filled with LN_2 according to a schedule which should be located in a highly visible position. Low-level alarms must be in place for the early detection of changes to the level of nitrogen (Figure 4).

The alarms used should have a visual display of current status as well as an inbuilt dial-out facility that attempts to contact the nominated telephone(s) until the call is acknowledged and the Dewar has been checked. Frequent testing of the alarm system is necessary to ensure that each alarm unit is functioning correctly. In the event that a Dewar malfunctions and the amount of nitrogen drops to a level that activates the Dewar alarm, there should be provision for the transfer of all stored material to a separate storage container, i.e. an 'emergency Dewar', which also requires filling according to the Dewar filling schedule.

Calibration equipment

The equipment used for calibrating any instruments used in the laboratory, e.g. incubators and microscope heated stages, cannot be relied upon to give an accurate reading without sufficient maintenance and recalibration, preferably by an independent contractor.

Tissue culture/plastic ware/culture media

Many of the products used in the preparation and culture of human gametes and embryos are disposable and for single use only. Recording batch numbers and the start-of-use dates for new batches of disposable products enables a laboratory to trace a particular batch should the need arise. This approach can also be adopted for batches of media used during the culture and cryopreservation of gametes and embryos, such as IVF culture media, mineral oil, hyaluronidase, and freezing and thawing solutions. Although some products may have been embryo tested by the supplier, a standard 48-h sperm survival test can be performed

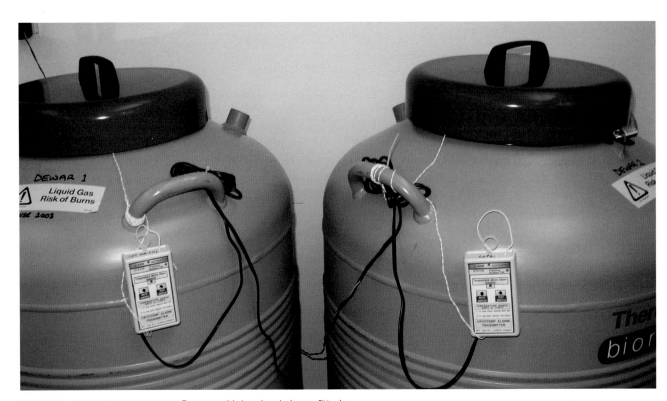

Figure 4 Liquid nitrogen storage Dewars with low-level alarms fitted

upon new products or new batches of existing products to confirm their suitability for use in the laboratory.

Audit

An ongoing audit of laboratory results will provide evidence of the effectiveness of the quality control program. A logbook or computerized records are useful for recording patient details and outcomes. A range of performance measures can then be examined at frequent intervals and compared with the expected range of results or confidence limits. Measures frequently include:

(1) Oocyte maturity (ICSI cases);

(2) Fertilization rate;

(3) ICSI damage rate;

(4) Embryo cleavage rate;

(5) Pregnancy rate.

Using the information gathered during an audit, downward trends in performance can be identified quickly and investigated. Detection of a decline in performance will occur retrospectively, as results of just a few days' laboratory work will not be sufficient to provide any statistical differences. More often, differences will only be noticed after the analysis of results based on several weeks' work in the laboratory. Outcomes can be influenced by unknown factors. This emphasizes the need to work to strict procedures and undertake quality control activities on a regular basis. It should then be possible to eliminate all the variables that are tested as being those responsible for any changes in results.

Personal performance audits are an important element of any QA program within the IVF laboratory. These may include the audit of the number of oocytes collected per embryologist, the survival and fertilization rate of ICSI oocytes, pregnancy rates per embryologist and any procedure that is performed by a single operator. These audits provide the following benefits:

(1) Highlight differences between operators;

(2) Enable identification of specific areas where retraining is required;

(3) Act as an early indicator of changes in overall laboratory performance;

(4) The laboratory can ensure that the required standard of work is attained by all members of the team.

For centers treating only a small number of patients, a difference in performance between embryologists is unlikely to be properly identified until after a period of a few weeks, or even months. Insufficient numbers will not provide statistically significant data, but may still provide an early indication of future performance.

Figure 5 shows the average number of oocytes collected per embryologist over the course of 2003 at Bourn Hall. During this period 760 oocyte collections were performed. The average number of oocytes collected per patient was 10.6. For every variable analyzed an acceptable range can be calculated. For this particular variable the range was set at plus or minus ten per cent of the average, i.e. 9.5–11.2. If an embryologist's performance fell below the accepted range the reasons for this would need to be investigated, and, if necessary, further training provided.

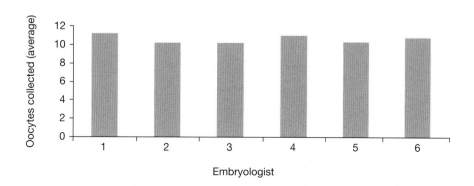

Figure 5 Graph showing the average number of oocytes collected per embryologist at Bourn Hall Clinic during 2003

Due to the relatively high number of oocyte collections performed by all operators, the fact that embryologists are randomly assigned to conduct oocyte collections and the long time period covered by the graph, no significant differences can be observed between embryologists. However, audits should be performed on a more frequent basis, enabling any change in performance to be identified early and extra training provided as soon as possible. In this instance there were no deviations from this range and therefore no remedial action was necessary.

CONCLUSIONS

The quality of service provided by the IVF laboratory has a profound effect upon the success of IVF treatment. Therefore the IVF laboratory must ensure that it consistently provides a high-quality service. The existing recognized standard of quality continues to be pregnancy rates, usually in the form of league tables. Whilst the information contained within these tables provides an indication of the overall quality of a service, it can be misleading. There are other factors associated with higher pregnancy rates in addition to the work performed in the IVF laboratory. Therefore, patients cannot base their choice of treatment provider on the quality of treatment provided by the IVF laboratory alone.

Due to the lack of a recognized standard system of accreditation, the manager of each individual laboratory determines the extent of participation in quality control activities. The importance of the implementation of a quality control program in the laboratory cannot be over stressed. Reproducibility of results, evaluation of the effectiveness of policies and procedures, the detection and correction of problems, and the monitoring of the performance and competency of equipment and staff benefits both patients and the IVF center itself.

A comprehensive schedule of quality control testing should enable the IVF laboratory to perform to a consistently high standard, providing that the recorded quality measurements consistently fall within the approved control range.

Development of a quality program is time-consuming and requires commitment and organization from every member of the laboratory for it to succeed. By using a structured and comprehensive quality system it is possible to ensure that a laboratory is successful and guarantees an optimal standard of treatment and care for its patients.

(Note: the detailed procedures and protocols used by the laboratory at Bourn Hall are shown in the CD-ROM that accompanies this book.)

REFERENCES

1. Alper MM, Brinsden P, Fischer R, et al. Is your IVF program good? Hum Reprod 2002; 17: 8–10
2. Kastrop P. Quality management in the ART laboratory. Reprod Biomed Online 2003; 7: 691–4
3. Matson PL. Internal quality control and external quality assurance in the IVF laboratory. Hum Reprod 1998; 13 (Suppl 4): 156–65
4. Mayer J. Total quality improvement in the IVF laboratory: choosing indicators of quality. Reprod Biomed Online 2003; 6: 695–9
5. Professional Bodies Joint Consultation. Quality Assurance and Accreditation of Assisted Conception Units. London, 2000
6. Workforce Planning Questionnaire 2002. Embryologist 2002; 32: 6–8
7. Elder K, Elliott T, eds. World Wide Conferences on Reproductive Biology. West Leederville, Australia: Ladybrook Publishing, 1998: 33–5
8. Association of Clinical Embryologists. Accreditation standards and guidelines for IVF laboratories. London: ACE, March 1999
9. Pickering S, Braude P, Johnson M, et al. Transient cooling to room temperature can cause irreversible disruption of the meiotic spindle in the human oocyte. Fertil Steril 1990; 54: 102–8

31

The health of children born after assisted reproductive technologies

Alastair G. Sutcliffe

This chapter provides a synopsis of the known literature concerning what is surely the most important outcome of assisted reproductive technologies (ART), the well-being of children thus conceived. Omitted from this chapter is an overview of studies of the psychological development of ART-conceived children, as these are the subject of a separate chapter by Professor Golombok (Chapter 32).

The first generation of ART-conceived children are now growing up, and ART practice has changed much during this period. The initial method of *in vitro* fertilization (IVF) has been supplemented by embryo cryopreservation and more recently intracytoplasmic sperm injection (ICSI), and following on from these procedures such as testicular sperm aspiration (TESA) and testicular biopsy, which have resulted in a less and less naturally selective form of reproduction. These developments and also such methods as extended culture, blastocyst transfers, etc. are often introduced without explicit consideration of the risks for the child. However, many positive practice developments are appearing now, including a genuine effort (underpinned by legislation) to reduce the risk of higher-order births (still the main risk to children born after ART), and to consider the well-being of the child more formally from the start of new therapies. For example, I have recently been involved as an adviser to a trial which investigates the efficacy of a treatment to enhance embryo implantation. The study designers, from the outset, sought advice on how to assess the health of any children born after successful pregnancies, both at birth and at 1 year with possibly longer-term plans.

Studies can reasonably be divided up into categories based on whether they investigate perinatal health, toddlers or older children, and also by other considerations, such as the nature of the ART procedure and whether the study looked at singleton births or twin births.

Typically, studies of perinatal health have investigated congenital anomalies. It should be said at this stage that the perfect study has yet to be done in this important area of outcome. Issues surrounding study designs include the quality of the ascertainment of anomalies in birth registries, and possible confounders such as ascertainment bias due to the examining clinician's awareness that the baby in question has been conceived by ART.

An anecdote from my own clinical institution illustrates this well. A single woman was expecting a baby conceived with donor sperm and with the use of ICSI. The obstetrician had read somewhere vaguely that there was a higher risk of sex chromosomal aneuploidy after ICSI, and suggested that an amniocentesis for fetal karyotyping was performed. The literature underpinning this advice is weak, and far from sufficient to justify giving this advice to a pregnant woman. She refused the amniocentesis but then became concerned. After the birth she requested a karyotype on her child, and this was done. The karyoptype was XYY. Subsequently, this nice little boy (who is now 7 years) is living with this 'label', with the largest literature on this topic suggesting that most children with this 'variant' are normal and indeed grow up to be healthy adults. It could be argued that this bad advice and indeed the subsequent testing contravened the well-established guidelines concerning the clinical testing of children for genetic conditions. These should be rigidly applied and clearly state that, where a condition has no health implications during childhood or an intervention cannot ameliorate the condition, there is no ethically justifiable reason for the child to be tested. Indeed, this child may well have refused such a test when grown up. I am sure that the reader does not need to be convinced that the whole scenario would not have arisen if the child was not ART-conceived, and if Dr Bonduelle's work on the subject of aneuploidy after ICSI had been carefully checked beforehand.

PERINATAL AND CONGENITAL ANOMALY STUDIES OF CHILDREN CONCEIVED AFTER ART

Herein lies the greatest short-term risk for children born after ART, largely but not entirely due to the risk of higher-order births, well described after all types of ART. In developed nations the rate of twinning has doubled in the past 25 years. This is thought to be 90% attributable to ART and 10% to rising maternal age at first pregnancy. Some 50% of twins are born at less than 2500 g and 50% are born at less than 38 weeks' gestation[1]. Yet the risk of higher-order births (multiple pregnancies) after ART is 20–30%. Allegedly, there is one clinic in the USA where the service is 'no pregnancy, no fee', but that fee is alleged to be $20 000. The clinic replaces large numbers of embryos, despite the evidence that, above two embryos, the only risk of three embryo replacement is a triplet birth, not an higher overall pregnancy rate. To a pediatrician this is irresponsible. However, recently published guidelines in the United States, which are consistent with those in other countries, may well impact on such practice[2].

What is the overall message from the literature concerning the risk of congenital anomalies and ART? While one major study suggested a higher risk (a doubling[3]) of anomalies after ICSI generally, other large studies suggest that, while there is a broadly increased risk of anomalies post-ART, that risk is modest. A large prospective study is needed, and such a study has not been performed. Such studies are very expensive, and all studies to date can be criticized due to the inescapable fact that there may be ascertainment bias.

It is unsurprising that such a small increased risk of anomalies exists in view of the nature of the ART couple. Genetic factors come to bear on all types of infertility; furthermore, since the advent of ICSI, couples in whom there is predominantly male-factor subfertility are now able to reproduce, some of whom clearly have known genetic defects, resulting in the non-obstructive oligozoospermia underpinning the need for ICSI. Then there are other possible factors which may increase the risks from ART, such as culture media, which may be relevant, especially to the recently described increased risk of genomically imprintable disorders after ART such as Beckwith–Wiedemann syndrome.

A summary of the three major studies of congenital anomalies after different types of ART is provided in Table 1. Also, further commentary allows consideration of studies in different categories.

Evaluation of the major published studies

IVF compared with the general population

Different studies based on registry data have yielded contradictory results. After allowance of confounders, the difference in the studies, by Westergaard and colleagues[7], Ericson and Kallen[8] and Anthony and colleagues[9], disappeared. However, the study by Hansen and associates, even after adjusting for confounders such as maternal age, parity and sex, still showed an increased risk with an odds ratio of 2[3]. However, Hansen's study did not control for a number of variables, which could have been different in the two populations and could have led to different results.

ICSI compared with the general population

Retrospective studies   In the Australian study of Hansen and colleagues[3] concerning congenital malformations at the age of a year, the odds ratio remained 2, after

Table 1 Three major studies of congenital anomalies after different forms of assisted reproductive technologies (ART)

Authors	Study group	Study type	Outcome	Comments
Bonduelle et al.[4]	the follow-up study included agreement to genetic counseling and eventual prenatal diagnosis, followed by a physical examination of the children after 2 months, after 1 year and after 2 years; 2840 ICSI children (1991–99) and 2955 IVF children (1983–99) were live-born after replacement of fresh embryos; ICSI was carried out using ejaculated, epididymal or testicular sperm	ongoing retrospective cohort study	major malformations (defined as those causing functional impairment or requiring surgical correction) were observed at birth in 3.4% of the ICSI live-born children and in 3.8% of the IVF children ($p = 0.538$); malformation rate in ICSI was not related to sperm origin or sperm quality; the number of stillbirths (born ≥ 20 weeks of pregnancy) was 1.69% in the ICSI group and 1.31% in the IVF group; total malformation rate taking into account major malformations in stillborns, in terminations and in live-borns was 4.2% in ICSI and 4.6% in IVF ($p = 0.482$)	a superb series of papers on this cohort, hindered only by the comparison group being IVF and not natural conception
Katalinic et al.[5]	3372 children and fetuses and 8016 children and fetuses after the 16th week of gestation in pregnancies after ICSI and natural conception, respectively	prospective controlled study	the major malformation rate was 8.7% (295/3372) for the ICSI cohort and 6.1% (488/8016) for the population-based control cohort (relative risk 1.44 (1.25–1.65)); after adjustment for risk factors, the risk declined (adjusted odds ratio 1.24 (95% CI 1.02–1.50)); regarding singletons, there was a significant difference for birth weight and gestational age, with a higher number of preterm and low-birth weight children in pregnancies achieved after ICSI	in my view the best study so far due to its prospective nature
Bergh et al.[6]	the medical records were retrieved for 1139 infants, 736 singletons, 200 sets of twins and one set of triplets. The total number of infants with an identified anomaly was 87 (7.6%), 40 of which were minor; the incidence of malformations in children born after ICSI was also compared with all births in Sweden using data from the Swedish Medical Birth Registry and the Registry of Congenital Malformations	retrospective case–control study in which a smaller number of infants was compared with the Swedish Medical Birth Registry	for ICSI children, the odds ratio (OR) for having any major or minor malformation was 1.75 (95% confidence interval (CI) 1.19–2.58) after stratification for delivery hospital, year of birth and maternal age; if stratification for singletons/twins was also done, the OR was reduced to 1.19 (95% CI 0.79–1.81); the increased rate of congenital malformations is thus mainly a result of a high rate of multiple births; the only specific malformation which was found to occur in excess in children born after ICSI was hypospadias (relative risk 3.0, exact 95% CI 1.09–6.50) which may be related to paternal subfertility	good-quality retrospective data compared with an acknowledged high-quality national registry; disadvantage could be ascertainment bias in the index cases

ICSI, intracytoplasmic sperm injection; IVF, in *vitro* fertilization adjustments. However, there was no allowance for years of infertility or sociodemographic factors, such as ethnic background, which may have been different in the two populations. Two Swedish analyses[10,11] showed an increase in congenital malformations in ICSI and IVF; however, the adjustments for maternal age and other adjustments resulted in the differences disappearing.

Prospective studies There is only one prospective study, which was an excellent one, by a German group[5]. ICSI children ($n = 3372$) were compared with a select control group ($n = 8016$). This prospective study compared major malformations in ICSI and a naturally conceived population base. Here the risk, as stated in Table 1, was slightly above that of the natural population, at 1.24.

ICSI compared with IVF

Bonduelle's excellent series of papers[4,12–15] give valid comments on this topic, and no difference in malformation rates has been found between ICSI and IVF children, the largest cohort being 2995 IVF versus 2899 ICSI.

Malformations in different organ systems

None of the published studies are sufficiently substantive to comment on this; however, there is emerging evidence from Bonduelle's work, and that of others, to suggest that urogenital malformations in ICSI are more common. This is surely unsurprising, in view of the parental genetic background and the increased risk of male subfertility when there are genitourinary defects in the father. Various subanalyses have been performed to look at whether sperm quality and sperm source are relevant, but no clear message is available for this because of the limited number of children in the subgroups.

DEVELOPMENTAL OUTCOME STUDIES OF IVF AND ICSI CHILDREN

(See Table 2 for an overview of some earlier IVF studies.)

ICSI-CFO, an international collaborative study of intracytoplasmic sperm injection–child and family outcomes, is by far the largest (and most recent) study

on IVF/ICSI children[22]. It was performed in five European countries. Approximately 500 singleton ICSI, 500 IVF and 500 naturally conceived (NC) children aged 5 years were each assessed, with observer blinding to conception status. Confounders were avoided by ensuring that all children were born at > 32 weeks' gestation, singletons, matched for sex and social class and Caucasian. These children were comprehensively assessed. This study showed no effect whatsoever of conception status on neurodevelopment, and, although there was greater use of health-service resources by ICSI and IVF children in relation to NC children, when examined in a comprehensive manner 'top to toe', these children were not found to be physically different from NC children, with the exception of congenital anomalies.

Developmental differences in an ICSI-conceived group of children, when compared with conventional IVF and naturally conceived controls, were reported by Bowen and colleagues in 1998[23]. They found an increase in mild developmental delay using the Bayley scales of infant development to derive a mental development index. However, the study used comparison groups of IVF- and naturally conceived children who were already enrolled in a separate study and had differing demographics to the ICSI group. There was also no blinding of the assessors, and the number of participants in the study was small with 89 ICSI, conceived children.

Bonduelle and colleagues have published several papers investigating congenital malformation rates and physical development of ICSI children[4,12–15]. Several of these papers allude to the fact that developmental milestones were assessed, but formal assessments of these children, undertaken between 1995 and 1998, were published in a research letter to the *Lancet* in 1998[14]. This article reported 201 ICSI children and 131 IVF children who were assessed using Bayley, and the results were compared with those for a subset of children representing the Dutch population. The age of the children was not corrected for gestational age, but the ICSI and IVF children were found to have similar scores to the general population. The twins scored slightly lower than the singletons.

Sutcliffe and co-workers studied 208 singleton ICSI, conceived children at around 18 months and compared them with a matched naturally conceived control group[24,25]. The children were assessed by a single observer using the Griffiths scales of mental

Table 2 Developmental outcome studies for conventional *in vitro* fertilization (IVF) children (modified from unpublished thesis of C. Peters with kind permission)

Authors	Study group	Study type	Outcome	Key results	Comments
D'Souza et al.[16]	278 IVF and 278 naturally conceived UK children. IVF singletons mean 25.5 months (SD 7.9). IVF multiple births mean 24.8 months (SD 5.1)	prospective case–control study; matched for sex and social class	results of Griffiths scales of development	mean developmental quotient (DQ): IVF singletons 116.9 (SD 12.6), IVF multiple births 106.9 (SD 10.9), not stated for controls*; developmental delay (DQ <70) noted in two multiple birth IVF children only	46% IVF children from multiple births; all controls were singletons; no matching for prematurity, birth weight or gestation
Cederblad et al.[17]	99 Swedish IVF children (age 33–85 months)	single cohort compared with Swedish and American norms	results of Griffiths scales of development	developmental quotient (DQ) above Swedish norm	no matched control group; high numbers of multiple births and prematurity
Brandes et al.[18]	116 Israeli (Hebrew-speaking) IVF children and 116 matched non-IVF children (age 12–45 months)	case–control study; matched for birth weight, gestational age, birth order, order in multiple births, mode of delivery, sex, age, maternal age and education	Bayley scales for infants up to 30 months; Stanford–Binet scales for children >30 months; scales mean 100 ± 16	MDI Bayley scores: IVF 106 ± 19.6, non-IVF 110.6 ± 19.3; composite index for Stanford–Binet: IVF 106.2 ± 8, non-IVF 104.4 ± 10.2	no correction for prematurity because children all >12 months
Morin et al.[19]	83 IVF children from Norfolk, USA and 93 matched non-IVF children (age 12–30 months)	case–control study; matched for age, sex, race, multiple births and maternal age	results of Bayley scales: mean develop mental index (MDI) and physical developmental index (PDI); mean score 100	MDI scores: IVF 115 ± 13, non-IVF 111 ± 13 ; PDI scores: IVF 114 ± 14, non-IVF 108 ± 15	study had power of 99% to detect difference; strongly suggests no difference; however, scores corrected for prematurity
Mushin et al.[20]	33 Australian children (age 12–37 months)	single cohort from first 52 infants conceived at Monash IVF center; no matched controls	results of Bayley scales; one child (37 months) assessed using McCarthy scales	overall MDI of 111 (SD = 15) and PDI of 105 (SD = 23); 4 children with physical and developmental problems had lower scores	high numbers of multiple births and prematurity; of 4 children with poor scores; 2 were VLBW, 1 severe CHD
Yovich et al.[21]	20 Australian children (age 12–13 months)	single cohort of first 20 infants conceived after IVF in Western Australia	results of Griffiths scales of development	general developmental quotient (GQ) was greater than mean of 100 in 19/20 children after correction for gestational age	no matched control group; increased rate of multiple births, IUGR, prematurity and cesarean section

SD, standard deviation; VLBW, very low birth weight; CHD, congenital heart disease; IUGR, intrauterine growth restriction development. No differences in developmental outcome were found between the two groups.

Table 3 summarizes developmental studies for ICSI children.

PHYSICAL ASSESSMENTS OTHER THAN FOR CONGENITAL ANOMALIES

Use of medical services

IVF children are more likely to need neonatal care, primarily because of the prematurity related to multiple pregnancies.

Initial reports suggested that IVF children did not require extra medical attention after the neonatal period[25,26]. Leslie and colleagues[27] studied 95 IVF children and compared them with 79 naturally conceived children matched for maternal age and parity. IVF children were also less likely to be breast-fed by the time of discharge. However, ICSI–CFO has disagreed with these findings and has clearly shown higher use of medical resources amongst IVF/ICSI children, including surgery.

The point to emphasize here is that the ICSI–CFO study was performed with older children and was ten times as large as any of these early studies, and thus far more likely to detect a difference.

Growth

Saunders and colleagues published a case-matched control study of children conceived after assisted reproduction, and found that the physical outcomes: weight, head circumference and malformation rates, were no different between groups[28]. The IVF group had a greater mean length centile and the twins in each group had poorer physical outcomes with an increase in prematurity and lower birth weights, and reduced height and weight, at age 2, when compared with singletons in each group. Here the ICSI–CFO study[22] concurs, in showing that the growth standard deviation scores (SDS) for both IVF and ICSI are higher than for NC children. This latter finding needs verification, but is somewhat alarming as, so far, nobody has accurately charted growth of ART children, and larger children have been 'buried' in the effects of prematurity and higher-order births.

Retinopathy of prematurity

The increase in multiple births and premature births related to assisted conception has led to an increase in conditions such as retinopathy that are directly related to early births and low birth weights[29,30].

Anteby and colleagues[31] reported the ocular manifestations in children born after IVF and referred for ophthalmological assessment. Major ocular malformations were found in 12 (26%) of the small cohort of 47 children studied. Seven major malformations were listed, including congenital cataract, optic atrophy and retinoblastoma. The study was limited in power due to the small numbers of children involved, and, because the study was conducted in a tertiary hospital, it is possible that the numbers were skewed owing to the type of patients referred.

Childhood cancer

There have been case reports of children conceived after assisted conception developing neuroectodermal tumors[32,33], but no large study has confirmed this finding. Bruinsma and associated used a record-linkage cohort design to link assisted reproduction births to a population-based cancer registry in Australia[34]. This study included 5249 births, and found no increase in the incidence of cancers in the assisted reproduction groups. However, these groups were relatively small and underpowered for the outcomes measured. The mean length of follow-up was only 3 years 9 months, although neuroblastomas tend to occur within the first year of life. These findings were supported by a smaller, similar Israeli study[35].

More recently, Klip and associates[36] examined a large population-based historical cohort, established to investigate gynecological disorders in women undergoing IVF. This cohort included 9484 children whose mothers had been given IVF or related fertility treatments and 7532 children whose mothers were subfertile, but had conceived naturally. The mothers were mailed questionnaires enquiring about cancer in their children. There was a 67% response rate and no difference between the groups was noted, implying that IVF and related treatments do not increase the cancer risk to the child.

The cancer incidence in IVF children studied for the UK Medical Research Council (MRC) working party[35] and a Swedish national cohort study of IVF

Table 3 Developmental outcome studies for intracytoplasmic sperm injection (ICSI) children (modified from unpublished thesis of C. Peters with kind permission)

Authors	Study group	Study type	Outcome	Key results	Comments
Ponjaert-Kfristofferson et al.[37]	1515 children, 538 naturally conceived (NC), 437 IVF, 540 ICSI; aged 5 years	population control study; singletons, > 32 weeks, Caucasian	results of WPPSI, McCarthy motor scales; laterality, full physical check, growth, audiometry, ophthalmic checks	normal IQ, normal laterality, normal motor skills (in press); taller than NC peers, higher anomalies; ability at age 5 is predictive of ability in adult life	the most important study in the medical literature
Sutcliffe et al.[26]	208 UK children conceived after ICSI compared with 221 naturally conceived controls; age 12–24 months	case–control study; matched for social class, maternal educational level, region, sex and race	results of Griffiths scales of infant development	griffiths quotients: ICSI 98.08 (S10.93), controls 98.69 (SD 9.99)	no correction for gestational age in Griffiths scales; single observer; 90% follow-up
Bowen et al.[23]	89 Australian ICSI children compared with 84 conventional IVF children and 80 naturally conceived; assessed at birth and at corrected age of 12 months	prospective case–control study; matched for parental age, parity and multiplicity of the pregnancy; conventional and IVF children were recruited through separate study	results of Bayley scales of infant development	98% follow-up at 1 year; MDI Bayley scores: ICSI 95.9 (SD 10.7), IVF 101.8 (SD 8.5), non-IVF 102.5 (SD 7.6)	included frozen embryos (39% ICSI, 31% IVF); lack of blinding and differences in sociodemographic factors, particularly between parents of the ICSI group and other groups
Bonduelle et al.[214]	201 Belgian (Dutch-speaking) ICSI children compared with 131 conventional IVF children; assessment age 22–26 months	blinded prospective case–control trial	results of Bayley scales; test results scored by subtracting chronological age from test age; test age calculated from subset of 1283 Dutch children aged 2–30 months	scored mean age differences: ICSI singleton +2.11 (SD 3.12), IVF singleton +2.30 (SD 2.63), ICSI twin +1.67 (SD 3.06), IVF twin +0.31 (SD 3.75); lower scores for triplets with males scoring lower than females	no correction for gestational age; higher scores for singletons; matching not discussed in this letter; single observer; 60% follow-up

IVF, in vitro fertilization; WPPSI, Weshler primary and preschool score of intelligence; IQ, intelligence quotient; SD, standard deviation; MDI, mean developmental index

children[6] also found no increase in cancer rates, but the power of these studies was limited by too small a number of children studied. Doyle and colleagues[38] estimated that 20 000 children would be required to observe a doubling or halving of the risk of childhood cancer in children conceived after assisted reproduction, compared with the general population. This would provide 95% significance and 90% power if children were followed up for 5 years.

Neurological outcomes

There has been some suggestion from a Swedish study that children born after IVF have an increased risk of developing neurological problems, particularly cerebral palsy[39]. The authors found a four-fold increase in the risk of cerebral palsy in children born after IVF compared with matched controls, odds ratio (OR) 3.7 (95% confidence interval (CI) 2.0–6.6). The risk in singletons was nearly three times, OR 2.8 (95% CI 1.3–5.8). After adjusting for birth weight and a gestation of > 37 weeks, the risk remained with an OR of 2.5 (95% CI 1.1–5.2). The authors admitted that the frequency of cerebral palsy in controls was lower than the Swedish norm. Calculations using their data indicate a prevalence of cerebral palsy in the control group as 1.5/1000 compared with an accepted prevalence rate of 2.0–2.5/1000[40]. The increased risk was shown to be mainly with multiple births, and was associated with low birth weight and low gestational age. Leviton and colleagues[41] noted that there is some overaggregation of the data, with children less than 30 weeks' gestation grouped together. This does not allow for the effect of decreasing risk of cerebral palsy with increasing gestation, particularly in those infants born after 30 weeks. Also, in a commentary by Sutcliffe[42], it was noted that the study used proxy measures for disability, and it was unexplained why the rate of problems seemed higher in the singleton group than in the IVF group, in contradiction to the entire twin literature!

GENOMIC IMPRINTING

Genomic imprinting is the mechanism that determines the expression or repression of genes from maternal or paternal chromosomes. This modification of genetic material is epigenetic, i.e. reversible between generations, and is not a mutation. Maternal and paternal germ-lines confer an imprint or sex-specific mark on certain chromosome regions. Therefore, although the sequence of the genes on these chromosomes could be identical, they are not functionally equivalent.

Over 40 imprinted genes have now been characterized. They have been shown to influence embryonic growth and development, and are implicated in the inactivation of tumor-suppressor genes resulting in some childhood cancers, e.g. Wilms' tumor, embryonal rhabdomyosarcoma, osteosarcoma and bilateral retinoblastoma. These are thought to occur by the 'two-hit' hypothesis of cancer. The first inactivation of a

tumor-suppressor allele would occur by imprinting rather than mutation. Wilms' tumor appears to have two different tumor-precursor lesions. One type is thought to be due to an imprinting defect of the gene for insulin-like growth factor-II (IGF-II). The second subtype occurs after a mutation of the WT1 gene[43].

There is evidence that several syndromes are also caused by imprinting disorders, such as Prader–Willi, Angelman's, Russell–Silver, transient neonatal diabetes, Beckwith–Wiedemann, pseudohypoparathyroidism and McCune–Albright syndrome.

Two recent studies have suggested that there may be an increased incidence of Beckwith–Wiedemann syndrome after assisted conception[44,45]. Although small, these studies support previous findings. Olivennes and colleagues[46] reported a boy with Beckwith– Wiedemann in a cohort of 73 children conceived after IVF. An earlier study by Sutcliffe and coworkers in 1995[47,48] also reported a child with Beckwith– Wiedemann in a cohort of 91 children born after the replacement of frozen embryos[47,48].

Angelman's syndrome is caused by a loss of the maternal allele function secondary to uniparental disomy of the paternal allele, a mutation of the maternal allele or a sporadic genetic imprinting error causing a paternal imprint on a maternal chromosome[49]. A report of two children with Angelman's syndrome, conceived after ICSI, suggested that an inherited defect was unlikely in these cases, and therefore the defect was possibly caused at a postzygotic stage.

A study is currently being undertaken in the UK to investigate any epidemiological evidence for an association between ART and imprintable disorders. This study (ARTID, assisted reproductive therapies and intracytoplasmic sperm injection) will report in August 2004 and is population-based.

The clinician in fertility medicine should counsel subfertile couples about the following risks of ART:

(1) The highest risks are from prematurity (mainly from twins and higher-order births); therefore single embryo replacement, at least in the first cycle, is recommended.

(2) Mature babies are healthy generally and do not have long term health risks as a result of their mode of conception.

(3) There is probably a higher risk of congenital anomalies after ART, which is, at the most-double

that of the general population (i.e. still a small risk).

(4) It may be that in ICSI children there is specifically a higher risk of genitourinary anomalies, again only a little above that for the naturally conceived population.

(5) It is not possible to be sure that there are no longer-term risks from ART, as there are few children who have grown up and families are not always willing to agree to follow-up studies.

CONCLUSION

Generally, ART-conceived children who are born as singletons and at term are similar in most longer-term outcomes to naturally conceived children (with the exception of congenital anomalies). They do, however, appear to use more health-service resources. Some questions are unresolved concerning their progress into adult life. These are:

(1) What are the longer-term risks of imprintable disorders and cancer?

(2) Will these children be fertile when they are sexually mature?

ART-conceived children will be a significant client group as they grow up (at least 1% of the population in rich countries). If their ART conception has exposed them to undue risk because these factors were not studied when the techniques were first introduced, they may well take a very different view of the justifications for ART than the readers of this chapter. Further studies need to be performed. The ideal one has yet to be done.

REFERENCES

1. Sutcliffe AG. Health risks in babies born after assisted reproduction. Br Med J 2002; 325: 117–18

2. Jain T, Missmer SA, Hornstein MD. Trends in embryo-transfer practice and in outcomes of the use of assisted reproductive technology in the United States. N Engl J Med 2004; 350: 1639–45

3. Hansen M, Kurinczuk JJ, Bower C, Webb S. The risk of major birth defects after intracytoplasmic sperm injection and in vitro fertilization. N Engl J Med 2002; 346: 725–30

4. Bonduelle M, Liebaers I, Deketelaere V, et al. Neonatal data on a cohort of 2889 infants born after ICSI (1991–1999) and of 2995 infants born after IVF (1983–1999). Hum Reprod 2002; 17: 671–94

5. Katalinic A, Rosch C, Ludwig M. Pregnancy course and outcome after intracytoplasmic sperm injection (ICSI) – a controlled, prospective cohort study. Fertil Steril 2004; in press

6. Bergh T, Ericson A, Hillensjo T, et al. Deliveries and children born after in-vitro fertilisation in Sweden 1982–95: a retrospective cohort study. Lancet 1999; 354: 1579–85

7. Westergaard HB, Johansen AM, Erb K, Andersen AN. Danish National In-Vitro Fertilization Registry 1994 and 1995: a controlled study of births, malformations and cytogenetic findings. Hum Reprod 1999; 14: 1896–902

8. Ericson A, Kallen B. Congenital malformations in infants born after IVF: a population-based study. Hum Reprod 2001; 16: 504–9

9. Anthony S, Buitendijk SE, Dorrepaal CA, et al. Congenital malformations in 4224 children conceived after IVF. Hum Reprod 2002; 17: 2089–95

10. Wennerholm U-B, Bergh C, Hamberger L, et al. Obstetric outcome of pregnancies following ICSI, classified according to sperm origin and quality. Hum Reprod 2000; 15: 1189–94

11. Ericson A, Källen B. Congenital malformations in infants born after IVF: a population-based study. Hum Reprod 2001; 16: 504–9

12. Bonduelle M, Legein J, Buysse A, et al. Prospective follow-up study of 423 children born after intracytoplasmic sperm injection. Hum Reprod 1996; 11: 1558–64

13. Bonduelle M, Wilikens A, Buysse A, et al. Prospective follow-up study of 877 children born after intracytoplasmic sperm injection (ICSI), with ejaculated epididymal and testicular spermatozoa and after replacement of cryopreserved embryos obtained after ICSI. Hum Reprod 1996; 11 (Suppl 4): 131–55

14. Bonduelle M, Joris H, Hofmans K, et al. Mental development of 201 ICSI children at 2 years of age. Lancet 1998; 351: 1553

15. Bonduelle M, Wilikens A, Buysse A, et al. A follow-up study of children born after intracytoplasmic sperm injection (ICSI) with epididymal and testicular spermatozoa and after replacement of cryopreserved embryos obtained after ICSI. Hum Reprod 1998; 13 (Suppl 1): 196–207

16. D'Souza SW, Rivlin E, Cadman J, et al. Children conceived by in vitro fertilisation after fresh embryo

transfer. Arch Dis Child Fetal Neonatal Ed 1997; 76: F70–4

17. Cederblad M, Friberg B, Ploman F, et al. Intelligence and behaviour in children born after in-vitro fertilization treatment. Hum Reprod 1996; 11: 2052–7

18. Brandes JM, Scher A, Itzkovits J, et al. Growth and development of children conceived by in vitro fertilization. Pediatrics 1992; 90: 424–9

19. Morin NC, Wirth FH, Johnson DH, et al. Congenital malformations and psychosocial development in children conceived by in vitro fertilization. J Pediatr 1989; 115: 222–7

20. Mushin D, Spensley J, Barreda-Hanson M. Children of IVF. Clin Obstet Gynaecol 1985; 12: 865–76

21. Yovich JL, Parry TS, French NP, Grauaug AA. Developmental assessment of twenty in vitro fertilization (IVF) infants at their first birthday. J In Vitro Fertil Embryo Transf 1986; 3: 253–7

22. Barnes J, Sutcliffe AG, Kristoffersen I, et al. The influence of assisted reproduction on family functioning and children's socio-emotional development: results from a European study. Hum Reprod 2004; 19: 1480–7

23. Bowen JR, Gibson FL, Leslie GI, Saunders DM. Medical and developmental outcome at 1 year for children conceived by intracytoplasmic sperm injection. Lancet 1998; 351: 1529–34

24. Sutcliffe AG, Taylor B, Li J, et al. Children born after intracytoplasmic sperm injection: population control study. Br Med J 1999; 318: 704–5

25. Sutcliffe AG, Sebire NJ, Pigott AJ, et al. Outcome for children born after in utero laser ablation therapy for severe twin-to-twin transfusion syndrome. Br J Obstet Gynaecol 2001; 108: 1246–50

26. Sutcliffe AG, Taylor B, Saunders K, et al. Outcome in the second year of life after in-vitro fertilisation by intracytoplasmic sperm injection: a UK case–control study. Lancet 2001; 357: 2080–4

27. Leslie GI, Gibson FL, McMahon C, et al. Infants conceived using in-vitro fertilization do not over-utilize health care resources after the neonatal period. Hum Reprod 1998; 13: 2055–9

28. Saunders K, Spensley J, Munro J, Halasz G. Growth and physical outcome of children conceived by in vitro fertilization. Pediatrics 1996; 97: 688–92

29. McKibbin M, Dabbs TR. Assisted conception and retinopathy of prematurity. Eye 1996; 10: 476–8

30. Watts P, Adams GG. In vitro fertilisation and stage 3 retinopathy of prematurity. Eye 2000; 14: 330–3

31. Anteby I, Cohen E, Anteby E, BenEzra D. Ocular manifestations in children born after in vitro fertilization. Arch Ophthalmol 2001; 119: 1525–9

32. White L, Giri N, Vowels MR, Lancaster PA. Neuroectodermal tumours in children born after assisted conception. Lancet 1990; 336: 1577

33. Kobayashi N, Matsui I, Tanimura M, et al. Childhood neuroectodermal tumours and malignant lymphoma after maternal ovulation induction. Lancet 1991; 338: 955

34. Bruinsma F, Venn A, Lancaster P, et al. Incidence of cancer in children born after in-vitro fertilization. Hum Reprod 2000; 15: 604–7

35. Lerner-Geva L, Toren A, Chetrit A, et al. The risk for cancer among children of women who underwent in vitro fertilization. Cancer 2000; 88: 2845–7

36. Klip H, Burger CW, de Kraker J, van Leeuwen FE. Risk of cancer in the offspring of women who underwent ovarian stimulation for IVF. Hum Reprod 2001; 16: 2451–8

37. Ponjaert-Kristoffersen I, Bonduell M, Barnes J, et al. International collaborative study of intracytoplasmic sperm injection conceived, in vitro fertilization-conceived, and naturally conceived 5-year-old child outcomes: cognitive and motor assessments. Pediatrics 2005; 115: e283–9

38. Doyle P, Bunch KJ, Beral V, Draper GJ. Cancer incidence in children conceived with assisted reproduction technology. Lancet 1998; 352: 452–3

39. Stromberg B, Dahlquist G, Ericson A, et al. Neurological sequelae in children born after in-vitro fertilisation: a population-based study. Lancet 2002; 359: 461–5

40. Healy DL, Saunders K. Follow-up of children born after in-vitro fertilisation. Lancet 2002; 359: 459–60

41. Leviton A, Stewart JE, Allred EN, et al. Neurological sequelae in in-vitro fertilisation babies. Lancet 2002; 360: 718

42. Sutcliffe AG. Children conceived from IVF were more likely than naturally conceived children to have neurological disabilities. Evidence-based Obstet Gynecol 2002; 4: 193–4

43. Reeve AE, Becroft DM, Morison IM, Fukuzawa R. Insulin-like growth factor-II imprinting in cancer. Lancet 2002; 359: 2050–1

44. DeBaun MR, Niemitz EL, Feinberg AP. Association of in vitro fertilization with Beckwith–Wiedemann syndrome and epigenetic alterations of LIT1 and H19. Am J Hum Genet 2003; 72: 156–60

45. Maher ER, Brueton LA, Bowdin SC, et al. Beckwith–Wiedemann syndrome and assisted reproduction technology (ART). J Med Genet 2003; 40: 62–4

46. Olivennes F, Mannaerts B, Struijs M, et al. Perinatal outcome of pregnancy after GnRH antagonist (ganirelix) treatment during ovarian stimulation for

conventional IVF or ICSI: a preliminary report. Hum Reprod 2001; 16: 1588–91

47. Sutcliffe AG, D'Souza SW, Cadman J, et al. Outcome in children from cryopreserved embryos. Arch Dis Child 1995; 72: 290–3

48. Sutcliffe AG, D'Souza SW, Cadman J, et al. Minor congenital anomalies, major congenital malformations and development in children conceived from cryopreserved embryos. Hum Reprod 1995; 10: 3332–7

49. Cox GF, Burger J, Lip V, et al. Intracytoplasmic sperm injection may increase the risk of imprinting defects. Am J Hum Genet 2002; 71: 162–4

FURTHER READING

Sutcliffe AG. IVF Children the First Generation. Lancaster, UK: Parthenon Publishing, 2002

32

New family forms[*]

Susan Golombok

In July 2003, Louise Brown, the first 'test-tube' baby, celebrated her 25th birthday. In the years since her birth, *in vitro* fertilization (IVF) has made the transition from the realms of science fiction to a commonly accepted treatment for infertility. The 1970s was also a time when another new and controversial family type, lesbian mother families, came to the fore, and when families headed by single heterosexual mothers began to cast off the stigma associated with illegitimacy and divorce. Today, there exist a variety of new family forms made possible through advances in assisted reproduction technology. An example is the small but growing number of lesbian and single heterosexual women who are actively choosing assisted reproduction, particularly donor insemination, as a means of conceiving a child without the involvement of a male partner. In this chapter, I examine research on the psychological outcomes for parents and children in assisted-reproduction families with particular attention to the concerns and policy issues that have been raised by creating families in this way. The chapter is structured according to four major types of assisted reproduction:

(1) Those involving 'high-tech' procedures such as *in vitro* fertilization (IVF) and intracytoplasmic sperm injection (ICSI);

(2) Those involving gamete donation such as donor insemination (DI) and egg donation;

(3) Those resulting in non-traditional families such as single mother and lesbian mother families;

(4) Those involving surrogate mothers.

Although the four categories are not mutually exclusive, each raises a specific set of concerns regarding family functioning.

IVF involves the fertilization of an egg with sperm in the laboratory and the transfer of the resulting embryo to the mother's womb[1]. When the mother's egg and the father's sperm are used, both parents are genetically related to the child. With ICSI, a single sperm is injected directly into the egg to create an embryo. Donor insemination involves the insemination of a woman with the sperm of a man who is not her husband or partner, and the child is genetically related to the mother but not the father. Egg donation is like donor insemination in that the child is genetically related to only one parent, but in this case it is the mother with whom the child lacks a genetic link. Egg donation is a much more complex and intrusive procedure than donor insemination and involves IVF techniques. When both egg and sperm are donated, sometimes referred to as embryo adoption, the child is genetically unrelated to both parents, a situation that is like adoption except that the parents experience the pregnancy and the child's birth. With surrogacy, one woman bears a child for another

[*]Reprint of a chapter from Clarke-Stewart A, Dunn J, eds. 'Families Count: Effects on Child and Adolescent Development. Cambridge: Cambridge University Press, in press, with the permission of Cambridge University Press.

woman. There are two types of surrogacy: partial (genetic) surrogacy where conception occurs using the commissioning father's sperm and the surrogate mother's egg, and full (non-genetic) surrogacy where both the egg and sperm are those of the commissioning parents. As Einwohner[2] has pointed out, it is now possible for a child to have five parents: an egg donor, a sperm donor, a surrogate mother who hosts the pregnancy, and the two social parents whom the child knows as Mum and Dad. In the case of lesbian mother families, the two social parents are both mums, and in solo mother families, the dad is often an anonymous sperm donor whom the child will never meet.

'HIGH-TECH' FAMILIES

IVF families

Concerns about IVF families

Although it may seem that the only difference between IVF and natural conception is the conception itself, there are a number of reasons why having a child by IVF may result in a rather different experience for parents. One very important difference is the higher incidence of multiple births, preterm births and low-birth-weight infants following IVF[3,4]. Whereas only 1% of natural births involve twins, triplets or more[5], this is true of more than one-quarter of births resulting from IVF[6,7]. The problem is greatest in developing and newly industrialized regions, such as Latin America, where the multiple birth rate for assisted reproduction pregnancies in 2000 was 50%, with more than 13.5% of IVF and ICSI births involving triplets or quadruplets[8]. Parents who have multiple births have to cope not only with two or more infants born at once but also with infants who may have greater needs as a result of prematurity and low birth weight[4,9]. As the children grow older, twins have consistently been found to show delayed language development and to obtain lower scores on verbal intelligence and reading tests[10,11]. Although little is known about higher-order births, a small study of language development found triplets to show greater impairment than twins[12]. The impact of these factors on parenting and child development must be considered separately from the impact of IVF *per se*.

Most of the empirical investigations described below have focused on families with a singleton child born as a result of IVF, to avoid the confounding effect of a multiple birth.

It has also been suggested that the stress of infertility and its treatment may result in parenting difficulties when a long-awaited baby is eventually born. Burns[13] argued that parents who had difficulty in conceiving might become emotionally over-invested in their long-awaited child, and other authors have suggested that those who become parents after a period of infertility may be overprotective of their children, or may have unrealistic expectations of them, or of themselves as parents[14–17]. Additionally, it has been predicted that the stress of infertility and its treatment may lead to psychological disorder and marital dysfunction for those who become parents following IVF[15].

Research on parenting in IVF families

Investigations of parenting in IVF families have focused on three areas of functioning: the psychological well-being of parents, the quality of parent–child relationships and security in the parental role. Studies of IVF families with infants and toddlers have been conducted in Australia[18–21], The Netherlands[22,23], France[24] and the United Kingdom[25]. These investigations have generally found no evidence of psychological problems among IVF parents. However, in the only study to include fathers, fathers of 12-month-old IVF babies reported lower marital satisfaction than fathers whose babies had been naturally conceived[19]. The authors suggested that IVF mothers may have been more preoccupied with their baby and may have excluded the father more than natural-conception mothers, thereby contributing to the fathers' lower marital satisfaction. With respect to parent–child relationships, the few differences that have been identified between IVF and natural-conception families reflect more positive feelings towards the baby but also a tendency to view the baby as more vulnerable[19,23,25]. IVF mothers of infants were also found by Gibson and colleagues[19] to consider themselves less competent as parents than natural-conception mothers, which the authors attributed to the IVF mothers judging themselves too harshly. In contrast, van Balen[23] found that IVF mothers of 2–4-year-olds reported greater parental competence than did mothers with no history of infertility. This discrepancy may well reflect differences in the ages of the children between the two studies. It is conceivable that the lack of confidence reported by IVF mothers of infants diminishes over time.

IVF families with preschool and early-school-age children were the focus of the European Study of Assisted Reproduction Families conducted in the United Kingdom, The Netherlands, Spain and Italy[26,27]. With respect to parenting, we found IVF mothers to show greater warmth to their child, to be more emotionally involved, to interact more and to report less stress associated with parenting than natural-conception mothers. In addition, IVF fathers were reported by mothers to interact with their child more than natural-conception fathers, and the fathers themselves reported less parenting stress. In the first study to be conducted in a non-Western culture, Hahn and DiPietro[14] also examined IVF families with preschool and early-school-age children in Taiwan. The quality of parenting was generally found to be good, although IVF mothers showed greater protectiveness of their children. The children's teachers, who were unaware of the nature of the child's conception, rated the IVF mothers as more affectionate towards their children, but not more protective or intrusive in their parenting behavior, than the natural-conception parents.

When we followed up the families in the European study as the children approached adolescence, we generally found the IVF parents to have good relationships with their children characterized by a combination of affection and appropriate control[28,29]. The few differences identified between the IVF families and the other family types reflected more positive functioning among the IVF families, with the possible exception of the over-involvement with their children of a small proportion of IVF parents.

Research on children in IVF families

Cognitive development The early studies of the cognitive development of IVF children found no evidence that IVF resulted in impaired cognitive ability. However, these studies did not employ comparison groups and looked only at small samples of IVF children[16,30–32]. A number of controlled studies have now been reported. For example, the Bayley scale scores of 65 IVF infants were compared with a matched control group of 62 naturally conceived infants at age 12

months, and no significant differences were found[33]. Other studies with large samples of IVF infants and matched comparison groups have reported similar findings using the Bayley scales[34,35], the Brunet–Lezine test[36] and the General Cognitive Index[37].

With respect to school-age children, the cognitive development of a sample of IVF children in Israel did not differ from that of naturally conceived children as assessed by the Wechsler Intelligence Scale for Children[38]. Similarly, in France, educational attainment among children conceived by IVF was found to be within the normal range[39].

Socioemotional development In McMahon and colleagues' study[20], IVF mothers rated their infants as more temperamentally difficult at 4 months than did natural-conception mothers, and the IVF infants showed more negative behaviors in response to stress. Although at 1 year old, no differences between the two groups of infants were found for either social development or test-taking behavior[33], the IVF mothers rated their infants as having more behavioral difficulties, and more difficult temperaments, than the control group. The authors suggested that these findings may be related to IVF mothers' greater anxiety about their infants' well-being. The security of infant–mother attachment was assessed at 12 months of age using the Strange Situation procedure[40]. The IVF infants showed predominantly secure attachment relationships, and there was no difference between groups in the proportion classified as insecurely attached.

With respect to toddlers, no differences in the behavior of 24–30-month-old IVF and naturally conceived children as rated during an interaction task with the mother were found by Colpin and colleagues[22]. Similarly, two studies that used the Achenbach Child Behaviour Checklist found no indication of raised levels of psychological problems in children conceived by IVF compared to the general population[30,41]. In van Balen's study[23], IVF mothers, but not fathers, rated their 2–4-year-old children as more social and less obstinate than did the other mothers as assessed by a self-report questionnaire. The European Study of Assisted Reproduction Families assessed the socioemotional development of 4–8-year-old IVF children using standardized questionnaires of behavioral and emotional problems completed by mothers and teachers[27]. In addition, the children were administered tests of self-esteem and of feelings towards their parents. We found that the IVF children did not differ from their adoptive or naturally conceived counterparts with respect to these measures. In the UK, an assessment was also made of the children's security of attachment to their parents using the Separation Anxiety Test. In addition, interview transcripts relating to children's psychological functioning were rated by a child psychiatrist who was 'blind' to the child's family type. We found no group differences for either security of attachment or the incidence of psychological disorder[26]. When followed up at age 12, the IVF children were continuing to function well[28,29]. One study from Israel has reported a higher incidence of emotional problems among IVF children of middle-school age[38]. In comparison with naturally conceived children, the IVF children showed poorer adjustment to school as rated by teachers and reported themselves to be more aggressive, more anxious and more depressed. However, this finding may be explained by the older age of the IVF parents.

ICSI families

Concerns about ICSI families

The introduction of IVF has paved the way for increasingly 'high-tech' reproductive procedures such as ICSI. Specific concerns have been raised in relation to ICSI, including the use of abnormal sperm, the bypassing of the usual process of natural selection of sperm and the potential for physical damage to the egg or embryo, all of which may produce changes in genetic material[42,43] and may thus have implications for children's psychological development. As with IVF, multiple births are a common feature of ICSI[44].

Research on parenting in ICSI families

A five-center study conducted in Belgium, Denmark, Sweden, Greece and the United Kingdom compared 440 ICSI families with 541 IVF and 542 naturally conceived families. The family types did not differ on measures of parental psychological well-being, parenting stress or quality of the marital relationship. However, ICSI and IVF mothers reported greater commitment to their role as a parent and were less negative about their children[45]. Similarly, a study of a

Belgian sample found no differences between ICSI, IVF and natural-conception parents in anxiety, depression, marital satisfaction or parenting stress[46]. In contrast, an Australian investigation reported raised levels of marital distress in mothers and fathers of ICSI children[47].

Research on children in ICSI families

Cognitive development The Bayley scales were administered to 201 ICSI children at 2 years of age in Belgium[4,8] and no evidence was found of delayed mental development. A comparison between 439 ICSI children and 207 IVF children by the same research team found no difference in Bayley scale scores[49]. Similar findings were reported in the UK from the administration of the Griffiths scales to a representative sample of 1–2-year-old singleton ICSI children and a matched group of naturally conceived children[50,51], and in a small study of Greek infants using the Bayley scales[52]. In contrast, significantly lower Bayley scale scores were found among 89 1-year-old ICSI children when compared with 84 IVF and 80 naturally conceived children in Australia, particularly for boys[42]. Seventeen per cent of the ICSI children experienced mildly or significantly delayed development (mental development index, MDI < 85) compared with 2% of the IVF and 1% of the natural-conception children. However, when these children were followed up at age 5 and the sample size increased, there were no differences in intelligence quotient (IQ) scores between the ICSI children and the control groups, and no differences identified in the proportion of children who showed delayed development[53]. The five-center study of ICSI, IVF and natural-conception children at age 5 found no group differences for verbal or performance IQ scores[54].

Socioemotional development Again in the five-center study, Barnes and colleagues[45] found no differences in emotional or behavioral problems between ICSI children and either IVF or natural-conception children as assessed by the Achenbach Child Behaviour Checklist at age 5. In an investigation using the Strengths and Difficulties Questionnaire[55] completed by parents and teachers, Place and Englert[46] similarly found no evidence of raised levels of emotional or behavioral problems in ICSI children compared with IVF and naturally conceived comparison groups.

GAMETE DONATION FAMILIES

Donor-insemination families

Concerns about donor-insemination families

In recent years there has been growing unease about the secrecy that surrounds families created by DI. Although DI has been practiced for more than a century to enable couples with an infertile male partner to have children, the majority of adults and children conceived in this way remain unaware that the person they know as their father is not their genetic parent. It has been argued that secrecy will have an insidious and damaging effect on family relationships and, consequently, on the child.

Findings suggestive of an association between secrecy and negative outcomes for children have come from two major sources: adoption research, and the family therapy literature. It is now generally accepted that adopted children benefit from knowledge about their biological parents, and that children who are not given such information may become confused about their identity and at risk for emotional problems[56,57]. Parallels have been drawn to the DI situation, and it has been suggested that lack of information about the donor may be harmful for the child[58–61]. Family therapists have argued that secrecy can jeopardize communication between family members, and result in a distancing of some members of the family from others[62–64]. In relation to donor insemination, Clamar[65] has suggested that keeping the circumstances of conception secret will separate those who know the secret (the parents) from those who do not (the child). A further concern is that parents may feel or behave less positively towards a non-genetic child and that the child may not be fully accepted as part of the family, which may have an undermining effect on the child's identity and psychological development. Fathers, in particular, have been predicted to be to be more distant from their child[58].

Research on parenting in DI families

The majority of parents of children conceived by gamete donation have not told their children about the nature of their conception. In a review of studies of parents' disclosure of DI published between 1980 and 1995, Brewaeys[66] found that few parents (between 1 and 20%) intended to tell their child about his or her genetic origins, and in the majority of studies fewer

than 10% of parents intended to tell. In spite of their decision to opt for non-disclosure, almost half of the parents had told at least one other person that they had conceived as a result of DI treatment, thus creating a risk that the child would find out through someone else. Many parents regretted their earlier openness once the child had been born[67–69]. Although it might be expected that a higher proportion of parents in the more recent studies would be open with their children, this was not the case, a finding replicated by van Berkel and colleagues[70] in a comparison between recipients of DI in 1980 and 1996. In the European Study of Assisted Reproduction Families[27,71], which included a representative sample of more than 100 DI families in Italy, Spain, The Netherlands and the United Kingdom, we found that not one set of parents had told their child by early school age, and only 8.6% of parents had told their child by early adolescence. Recent studies in the United States have produced similar findings[72,73].

There are, however, some exceptions to this pattern. In New Zealand, the importance of knowledge about genetic origins to Maori culture has resulted in greater openness about donor conception[74]. In a study of a representative sample of 181 families, 30% of parents of children aged up to 8 years old had talked to them about the DI, and 77% of the remaining parents intended to do so[75]. In the United States, the Sperm Bank of California has instituted an identity-release program whereby donor offspring may obtain the identity of their donor on reaching age 18. Almost all of the parents who opted for identifiable donors informed their child about their donor conception[76]. The most recent information on the disclosure of donor insemination in the United Kingdom comes from a representative sample of 50 sets of DI parents with babies born between 1999 and 2001 in the UK, of whom 46% reported that they intended to be open with their child[77]. These figures suggest a marked rise in the proportion of parents who plan to tell their child about the donor conception. Nevertheless, the babies were only 1 year old at the time of study, and longitudinal research suggests that some parents who consider disclosure when their child is young change their mind as the child grows up[71]. Even in Sweden, where legislation gives individuals the right to obtain information about the donor and his identity, a recent survey found that only 11% of parents had informed their child about the DI, although a further 41%

intended to tell[78,79]. Parents who are most concerned about keeping the child's genetic origins secret are least likely to participate in research, and thus the figures relating to the proportion of parents who intend to be open with their children represent an over-estimate.

A number of studies have examined donor-insemination parents' reasons for their decision not to tell their child[60,80,81]. The predominant reason is parents' concern that disclosure would distress their child and would have an adverse effect on parent–child relationships. In particular, they fear that the child may feel less love for, or possibly reject, the father. Other considerations that are taken into account in parents' decision not to tell include a desire to protect the father from the stigma of infertility, concern about a negative reaction from paternal grandparents who may not accept the child as their grandchild, uncertainty about the best time and method of telling the child, and lack of information to give the child about the donor. In addition, some parents, emphasizing the greater importance of social than biological aspects of parenting for children's psychological adjustment, believe that there is simply no need to tell.

Brewaeys[66,82] also reviewed studies of the characteristics of DI parents. In the large majority of cases, DI was felt by parents to be a positive choice and, with few exceptions, fathers reported that DI did not influence their relationship with their child and that they felt themselves to be 'real' fathers. With respect to psychological adjustment and marital satisfaction, there was little indication of disorder in couples who opted for DI[69,83–87].

Regarding parent–child relationships, we found the outcomes for DI families with 4–8-year-old children in the European Study of Assisted Reproduction Families to be just as positive as for the IVF families, suggesting that genetic ties are less important for family functioning than a strong desire for parenthood[27]. When the families were followed up at adolescence, the findings pointed to stable and satisfying marriages, psychologically healthy parents and a high level of warmth between parents and their children accompanied by an appropriate level of discipline and control[29,71]. No differences were identified between the DI and the IVF families for any of the variables relating to the quality of relationships between parents and the child. Similar findings have been found with a new cohort of DI children born 15 years later than those in the original study[88].

Research on children in DI families

Cognitive development A small number of uncontrolled studies, reviewed by Brewaeys[66], have examined the cognitive development of children conceived by DI in comparison to general population norms. The results showed DI children to be more advanced than their same-age peers with respect to intellectual, psychomotor and language development[67,89–92]. One controlled study in France also found 3–36-month-old DI children to be more advanced in psychomotor and language development than a comparison group of naturally conceived children[93].

Socioemotional development The early studies found no evidence of emotional or behavioral problems in children conceived by DI[89,91]. One study did find a higher incidence of psychological problems among DI than naturally conceived children as assessed by an interview with parents[93], but other controlled studies that used standardized measures showed no evidence of raised levels of psychological disorder among children conceived by DI. For example, DI children aged 6–8 years old were studied in comparison with matched groups of adopted and naturally conceived children in Australia[94]. Also, we compared 4–8-year-old DI children with adopted, IVF and naturally conceived children in the UK[26] and Europe[27], and followed them up at age 11–12[29,71]. The children did not seem to experience negative consequences arising from the absence of a genetic link with their father, or from the secrecy surrounding the circumstances of their conception.

Little is known about children who are aware of their conception by DI, largely because the majority of children conceived in this way have not been told about their genetic origins. Rumball and Adair[75] reported that the majority of young children in their sample who had been told about their donor conception responded with interest, others appeared neutral or disinterested, and a small minority responded with disbelief. There are also qualitative studies of adults who are aware of their conception by DI, although the number of individuals for whom there are systematic data remains very small. Whereas some report good relationships with their parents[60], others report more negative feelings including hostility, distance and mistrust[95–97]. For example, the adults interviewed by

Turner and Coyle[97] expressed feelings of loss, abandonment and grief in relation to their lack of knowledge of their genetic origins, a need to find out about their donor father and, if possible, to have some kind of relationship with him in order to achieve a sense of genetic continuity. Some had felt that something was wrong since childhood and now attributed their poor relationship with their father to their DI origins. However, these adults were recruited from support groups, and it is not known how representative they are of the entire population of DI adults who are aware of their genetic origins.

Egg-donation families

Concerns about egg-donation families

Although the use of donor sperm to enable couples with an infertile male partner to have children has been practiced for many years, it is only since 1983, following advances in IVF, that infertile women have been able to conceive a child using a donated egg[98,99]. The concerns that have been expressed about egg donation are similar to those raised by DI. It is the absence of a genetic bond between the mother and the child, and the effect of secrecy about the child's conception that have been the topics of greatest debate. Unlike DI where the donor is usually anonymous, egg donors are more often relatives or friends of the parents and may remain in contact with the family as the child grows up. Contact with the genetic mother has been viewed by some as a positive experience for children in that they have the opportunity to develop a clearer understanding of their origins. However, it is not known what the impact of this contact will be on a child's social, emotional and identity development through childhood and into adult life, or how contact between the genetic mother and the child will affect the social mother's security as a parent and her relationship with her child.

Research on parenting in egg-donation families

The first study of parenting in families with a child conceived by egg donation was conducted in France[24]. The authors reported on 12 egg-donation families assessed at 9 months and 18 months, and nine of these families at 36 months. It was reported that all of the mother–infant relationships were excellent. However, no details were given of the way in which an 'excellent' mother–infant relationship had been defined. In a controlled study of families with 3–8-year-old children in the UK, we contrasted egg-donation families (where the child was genetically related to the father but not the mother) and DI families (where the child was genetically related to the mother but not the father)[100]. The only difference to emerge was that mothers and fathers of children conceived by egg donation reported lower levels of stress associated with parenting than parents of DI children. The egg-donation families, like the DI families, were functioning well. Interestingly, only one of the 21 sets of egg-donation parents had told their child about his genetic origins. The reasons for not telling are similar to those given by DI parents: a desire not to jeopardize the child's psychological well-being or the relationship between the parents and the child, and the view that there is no need to tell[101]. Similarly, a study conducted in Finland of 49 families with an egg-donation child aged between 6 months and 4 years found that none of the parents had told their child about the donor conception[102]. However, 38% of these parents intended to do so, a higher proportion than is generally reported for DI parents. As with the DI parents, many (73%) had told someone other than the child. In a recent study of egg-donation babies born in the UK between 1999 and 2001, 56% of parents intended to be open with their child, a higher proportion than that found for DI parents[88].

Research on children in egg-donation families

Cognitive development Data from Raoul-Duval and colleagues' study[24] of 12 egg-donation children showed no evidence of psychomotor retardation for any of the children investigated.

Socioemotional development Soderstrom-Antilla and associates[102] compared 59 egg-donation children to 126 IVF children, all aged between 6 months and 4 years. There were no group differences in the proportion of children with eating or sleeping difficulties, and the egg-donation parents were less likely than the IVF parents to express concern about their child's behavior. In the study of 3–8-year-old egg-donation children, we made assessments of the presence of emotional and behavioral problems by parental questionnaire, and the children were administered a standardized assessment of self-esteem[103]. There was no evidence of psychological difficulties among the egg-donation children.

NON-TRADITIONAL FAMILIES

Lesbian and solo mother DI families

Concerns about lesbian and solo mother DI families

There has been a great deal of controversy in recent years about whether lesbian couples and single heterosexual women should have access to assisted reproduction. With respect to lesbian mother families, there have been two main concerns: first, that the children of lesbian mothers would be teased and ostracized by peers due to the social stigma still associated with homosexuality, and would develop emotional and behavioral problems as a result; second, that the lack of a father figure alongside the presence of one or two mothers who are not following conventional sex-typed roles would affect children's gender development, i.e. that boys would be less masculine and girls less feminine than their counterparts from heterosexual homes. Although there is no evidence for either of these assumptions (see references 100 and 104 for reviews), the early body of research focused on families where the child had been born into a heterosexual family and then made the transition to a lesbian family after the parents' separation or divorce.

With respect to solo mothers, the concerns center around the effects of growing up in a fatherless family, and are based on research showing negative outcomes in terms of cognitive, social and emotional development for children raised by single mothers following parental separation or divorce[105–109]. However, factors such as economic hardship and the experience of parental conflict have been shown to play a major part in children's adjustment difficulties in single mother families. These outcomes cannot necessarily be generalized to children born to single mothers following assisted reproduction since these children have not experienced parental separation and generally are raised without financial hardship. It is possible, however, that other pressures on solo mothers, such as social stigma and lack of social support, may interfere with their parenting role, and leave their children vulnerable to emotional and behavioral problems.

Research on parenting in lesbian mother and solo mother DI families

In recent years, a number of controlled studies of lesbian couples with a child conceived by DI have been reported. In the United States, Flaks and colleagues[110] compared 15 lesbian DI families with 15 heterosexual DI families, and Chan and co-workers[111] studied 55 DI families headed by lesbian parents in comparison with 25 DI families headed by heterosexual parents. The sexual orientation of the parents was found to be unrelated to parental adjustment, parental self-esteem or relationship satisfaction. In the UK, we compared 30 lesbian DI families with 41 heterosexual two-parent DI families and 42 families headed by a single heterosexual mother[112]. We found the lesbian mother families to be functioning well in terms of maternal warmth and mother–child interaction. Similarly, in Belgium, Brewaeys and associates[113] studied 30 lesbian mother families with a 4–8-year-old child in comparison with 38 heterosexual families with a DI child and 30 heterosexual families with a naturally conceived child. No major differences were found between the lesbian couples and the other family types with respect to quality of parenting or the quality of the couples' relationship. The most striking finding to emerge from these investigations was that co-mothers in two-parent lesbian families were more involved with their children than were fathers in two-parent heterosexual homes. In the Belgian study, information was obtained from parents regarding the decision-making process about whether or not to tell the child about the method of their conception. All the lesbian mothers intended to tell their children that they had been conceived by DI, and 56% would have opted for an identifiable donor had that been possible[114]. Comparable findings regarding the openness of lesbian mothers have been reported in the United States[115–117]. The attitude of lesbian mothers toward this issue is in striking contrast to that of heterosexual parents who prefer not to tell.

Little research has yet been carried out on the quality of parenting of single women who opt for DI as a means of having a child. These mothers are referred to as 'solo' mothers to distinguish them from mothers who become single following separation or divorce[109]. A small, uncontrolled study of ten single women requesting DI (cited by Fidell and Marik[118]) found that an important reason for choosing this procedure was to avoid using a man to produce a child without his knowledge or consent. Donor insemination also meant that they did not have to share the rights and responsibilities for the child with a man to whom they were not emotionally committed. Similarly, in our investigation of 27 solo mothers of

1-year-old DI children, the main reason for opting for DI was to avoid the need to have casual sex in order to become pregnant[119]. There was a strong sense that time was running out to fulfill the lifelong dream of having a child, and that there was no choice but to have a child in this way due to the lack of a partner. Solo DI mothers appeared to be more open toward disclosing the donor conception to the child than were a comparison group of married DI mothers: 93% of solo mothers reported that they planned to tell their child compared with 46% of the married DI mothers. With respect to parent–child relationships, we found that solo DI mothers showed similar levels of warmth and bonding towards their infant to married DI mothers. However, solo mothers showed lower levels of interaction and sensitivity. A possible explanation for this finding is that the presence of a partner allowed married DI mothers more time with their child.

Research on children in lesbian and solo mother DI families

The evidence so far suggests that the DI children of lesbian mothers do not differ from their peers in terms of gender development[113]. Neither is there any indication of raised levels of emotional and behavioral problems as rated by mothers and teachers at age 4–8 years[110–113]. In addition, the children of lesbian mothers consider themselves to be just as accepted by peers as children of heterosexual parents[112]. In a follow-up of the children studied by Brewaeys[113] when they were aged between 7 and 17 years, 27% reported that they would like to know the identity of their donor, 19% wished to have non-identifying information about his appearance and personality, and the remaining 54% did not wish to have any information about him[120]. No detailed investigations have yet been conducted of the psychological adjustment of children born to single heterosexual mothers by DI. However, we found that DI infants born to single mothers were no more likely to experience eating or sleeping difficulties than DI children born to married mothers[119].

Surrogacy families

Concerns about surrogacy families

The practice of surrogacy remains highly controversial. As with known egg donors, surrogate mothers are often relatives or friends of the commissioning couple, and even when the surrogate mother was not known to the commissioning couple prior to the surrogacy arrangement, contact may continue after the child's birth. It is not known how this will impact on the child's psychological and identity development, and on the feelings and parenting behavior of the commissioning mother, particularly when the surrogate mother is also the genetic mother of the child. Neither is it known how children will feel when they discover that their gestational mother had conceived them with the specific intention of relinquishing them to the commissioning parents.

Research on parenting in surrogacy families

In interviews with 20 commissioning couples, Blyth[121] found that all believed that the child should be told the full truth about their origins. However, it is not known whether the parents followed through this intention. Similarly, MacCallum and colleagues[122] reported that 100% of a sample of 42 commissioning parents of 1-year-olds intended to be open with their child in the future. In the latter study, we found the commissioning parents to show higher levels of warmth and involvement with their child than a comparison group of natural-conception parents[88]. Interestingly, 95% of the surrogacy families had kept in touch with the surrogate mother to some extent, and the large majority reported that they maintained a good relationship with her.

Research on children in surrogacy families

In a study of cognitive development, no evidence of speech or motor impairment was found in singleton children born after IVF surrogacy[123]. Assessments of children's temperament using the Infant Characteristics Questionnaire[124] found no differences between children born through a surrogacy arrangement and either egg-donation children or natural-conception children for fussiness of mood, adaptability to new situations, general activity level or predictability of reaction[88].

CONCLUSIONS

Creating families by means of assisted reproduction has raised a number of concerns about potentially adverse consequences for parenting and child development. It seems, however, from the evidence available so far, that such concerns are unfounded. Parents of children conceived by assisted reproduction generally appear to have good relationships with their children, even in families where one parent lacks a genetic or gestational link with the child. With respect to the children themselves, children born at full term as a result of IVF or ICSI procedures do not appear to show raised levels of cognitive impairment, although research on ICSI children is still ongoing. The reports of superior cognitive functioning among DI children have not been supported by large-scale controlled studies but could conceivably result from the use of highly educated donors. In relation to socioemotional development, assisted-reproduction children appear to be functioning well. The greater difficulties of IVF infants are based on maternal reports and probably result from the higher anxiety levels of IVF mothers. Studies during the preschool and school-age years do not indicate a higher incidence of emotional or behavioral problems among assisted-reproduction children. Thus, new family forms do not appear to constitute a risk factor for children. Just because children are conceived in unusual ways, or live in unusual family circumstances, does not mean that they are more likely to grow up psychologically disturbed. Instead, the findings presented in this chapter suggest that family structure, in itself, makes little difference to children's psychological development. Instead, what seems to matter is the quality of family life.

Nevertheless, few studies have included children at adolescence or beyond, and little is known about the consequences of conception by assisted reproduction from the perspective of the individuals concerned. Moreover, the existing studies are of variable quality. Some investigations have been conducted with methodological rigor, for example, by matching the assisted reproduction families to the comparison groups with respect to the potentially confounding factors of maternal age, socioeconomic status and number of children in the family. However, research in this area is hampered by small, unrepresentative and poorly defined samples, the absence of appropriate control groups, and unreliable and poorly validated measures. In addition, there are some types of assisted-reproduction family, such as families created through embryo donation, about whom little is known at all[125].

POLICY IMPLICATIONS

As a result of growing concern about the escalating multiple birth rate arising from the increasing use of assisted reproduction procedures, a major policy issue in recent years has been the number of embryos that should be used in an IVF/ICSI cycle, and whether regulation should be introduced to limit the number of embryos that may be transferred. As the European Society of Human Reproduction and Embryology (ESHRE) Task Force[126] has pointed out, the decision about the number of embryos to be transferred in IVF or ICSI cycles can lead to conflict between the professional autonomy of the physician who has a responsibility towards the well-being of the prospective mother and her future children, and the reproductive autonomy of the prospective parents who may request the transfer of a high number of embryos due to a strong desire for a child, the inability to pay for repeated IVF/ICSI cycles and lack of information on the consequences of multiple births. A recent study in the United States has shown that the rate of multiple pregnancies following IVF has decreased as a result of fewer embryos being transferred[127]. However, this decrease reflects a reduction in the number of triplet and higher-order births rather than a decrease in the number of twins.

The other major policy issue at the present time is whether or not donor anonymity should be removed to allow offspring access to identifying information about their donor. The Ethics Committee of the American Society for Reproductive Medicine has recently come out in support of disclosure to offspring about the use of donor gametes, and the UK Government has recently announced a change in the law whereby children conceived by gamete donation from 2005 onwards will have access to identifying information about their donor on reaching age 18. Donor identification would allow offspring who so wish, providing they are aware of their donor conception, to find out about, and possibly have contact with, their genetic parent(s). They may also have the opportunity to meet half-siblings, and full siblings in the case of embryo donation. The psychological consequences of donor identification for offspring, parents, donors and their families are currently unknown. Light will be shed on this issue when offspring conceived with identifiable donors reach the age at which they become eligible for donor identification. At the Sperm

Bank of California, the first children to have been conceived through an identity-release program have just turned 18 and have begun to obtain the identity of their donor[76]. The impact on everyone concerned will be followed closely in the years to come.

FUTURE RESEARCH DIRECTIONS

Although existing knowledge about new family forms does not give undue cause for concern, there are many questions that warrant further investigation, for example: 'What are the long-term consequences of assisted reproduction, particularly of secrecy about the child's genetic origins?' and 'What is the effect on children conceived by gamete donation of finding out that one or both parents is genetically unrelated to them?' For children conceived through egg donation or surrogacy: 'What is the effect of ongoing contact with the egg donor or surrogate mother?' And with respect to lesbian or single mother families created through donor insemination: 'How will children respond as they grow up to the knowledge that their father is an anonymous sperm donor whom they will never meet?' These are just some of the questions that should be looked at more closely. Instead of uninformed opinion, systematic controlled studies of representative samples are needed so that the outcomes for both parents and children can be fully understood.

REFERENCES

1. Steptoe PC, Edwards RG. Birth after reimplantation of a human embryo. Lancet 1978; 2: 366
2. Einwohner J. Who becomes a surrogate: personality characteristics. In Offerman-Zuckerberg J, ed. Gender in Transition: A New Frontier. New York: Plenum, 1989: 123–49
3. Olivennes F, Fanchin R, Ledee N, et al. Perinatal outcome and developmental studies on children born after IVF. Hum Reprod Update 2002; 8: 117–28
4. Vayena E, Rowe PJ, Griffin PD, eds. Current Practices and Controversies in Assisted Reproduction: Report of a meeting on medical, Ethical and Social Aspects of Assisted Reproduction. Geneva: World Health Organization, 2002
5. Bergh T, Ericson A, Hillensjo T, et al. Deliveries and children born after in vitro fertilization in Sweden 1982–5: a retrospective cohort study. Lancet 1999; 354: 1579–85
6. Nygren KG, Andersen AN. Assisted reproductive technology in Europe, 1999. Results generated from European registers by ESHRE. Hum Reprod 2002; 17: 3260–74
7. Nyboe Andersen A, Gianaroli L, Nygren, K. Assisted reproductive technology in Europe, 2000. Results generated from European registers by ESHRE. Hum Reprod 2004; 19: 490–503
8. Zegers-Hochschild F. The Latin American Registry of Assisted Reproduction. In Vayena E, Rowe PJ, Griffin PD. eds. Current Practices and Controversies in Assisted Reproduction: Report of a Meeting on Medical, Ethical and Social Aspects of Assisted Reproduction. Geneva: World Health Organization, 2002: 355–62
9. Botting BJ, MacFarlane AJ, Price FV. Three, Four and More. A Study of Triplet and Higher Order Births. London: HMSO, 1990
10. Lytton H, Gallagher L. Parenting twins and the genetics of parenting. In Bornstein M, ed. Handbook of Parenting, 2nd edn. Hove, UK: Lawrence Erlbaum Associates, 2002; 1: 227–53
11. Rutter M, Thorpe K, Greenwood R, et al. Twins as a natural experiment to study the causes of mild language delay: 1: Design; twin–singleton differences in language, and obstetric risks. J Child Psychol Psychiatry 2003; 44: 326–41
12. McMahon S, Dodd B. A comparison of the expressive communication skills of triplet, twin and singleton children. Eur J Dis Commun 1997; 32: 328–45
13. Burns LH. An exploratory study of perceptions of parenting after infertility. Fam Sys Med 1990; 8: 177–89
14. Hahn C, DiPietro JA. In vitro fertilization and the family: quality of parenting, family functioning, and child psychosocial adjustment. Dev Psychol 2001; 37: 37–48
15. McMahon C, Ungerer J, Beaurepaire J, et al. Psychosocial outcomes for parents and children after in vitro fertilization: a review. J Reprod Infant Psychol 1995; 13: 1–16
16. Mushin D, Spensley J, Barreda-Hanson M. Children of IVF. Clin Obstet Gynecol 1985; 12: 865–75
17. van Balen F. Development of IVF children. Dev Rev 1998; 18: 30–46
18. Gibson FL, Ungerer JA, Leslie GI, et al. Maternal attitudes to parenting and mother–child relationship and interaction in IVF families: a prospective study. Hum Reprod 1999; 14 (Suppl 1): 131–2
19. Gibson FL, Ungerer JA, Tennant CC, Saunders DM. Parental adjustment and attitudes to parenting after in vitro fertilization. Fertil Steril 2000; 73: 565–74

20. McMahon CA, Ungerer JA, Tennant C, Saunders D. Psychosocial adjustment and the quality of the mother–child relationship at four months postpartum after conception by in vitro fertilization. Fertil Steril 1997; 68: 492–500

21. McMahon C, Gibson F, Leslie G, et al. Parents of 5-year-old in vitro fertilization children: psychological adjustment, parenting stress, and the influence of subsequent in vitro fertilization treatment. J Fam Psychol 2003; 17: 361–9

22. Colpin H, Demyttenaere K, Vandemeulebroecke L. New reproductive technology and the family: the parent–child relationship following in vitro fertilization. J Child Psychol Psychiatry 1995; 36: 1429–41

23. van Balen F. Child-rearing following in vitro fertilization. J Child Psychol Psychiatry 1996; 37: 687–93

24. Raoul-Duval A, Bertrand-Servais M, Letur-Konirsch H, Frydman R. Psychological follow-up of children born after in-vitro fertilization. Hum Reprod 1994; 9: 1097–101

25. Weaver SM, Clifford E, Gordon AG, et al. A follow-up study of 'successful' IVF/GIFT couples: social-emotional well-being and adjustment to parenthood. J Psychosom Obstet Gynecol 1993; 14: 5–16

26. Golombok S, Cook R, Bish A, Murray C. Families created by the new reproductive technologies: quality of parenting and social and emotional development of the children. Child Dev 1995; 66: 285–98

27. Golombok S, Brewaeys A, Cook R, et al. The European Study of Assisted Reproduction Families. Hum Reprod 1996; 11: 2324–31

28. Golombok S, MacCallum F, Goodman E. The 'test-tube' generation: parent–child relationships and the psychological well-being of IVF children at adolescence. Child Dev 2001; 72: 599–608

29. Golombok S, Brewaeys A, Giavazzi MT. The European Study of Assisted Reproduction Families: the transition to adolescence. Hum Reprod 2002; 17: 830–40

30. Cederblad M, Friberg B, Ploman F, et al. Intelligence and behaviour in children born after in-vitro fertilization treatment. Hum Reprod 1996; 11: 2052–7

31. Mushin DN, Barreda-Hanson MC, Spensley JC. In vitro fertilization children: early psychosocial development. J In Vitro Fertil Embryo Transf 1986; 3: 247–52

32. Yovich J, Parry T, French N, Grauaug A. Developmental assessment of 20 in vitro fertilization (IVF) infants at their first birthday. J In Vitro Fertil Embryo Transf 1986; 3: 225–37

33. Gibson FL, Ungerer JA, Leslie GI, et al. Development, behaviour and temperament: a prospective study of infants conceived through in-vitro fertilization. Hum Reprod 1998; 13: 1727–32

34. Brandes JM, Scher A, Itzkovits J, et al. Growth and development of children conceived by in vitro fertilization. Pediatrics 1992; 90: 424–9

35. Morin NC, Wirth FH, Johnson DH, et al. Congenital malformations and psychosocial development in children conceived by in vitro fertilization. J Pediatr 1989; 115: 222–7

36. Raoul-Duval A, Bertrand-Servais M, Frydman R. Comparative prospective study of the psychological development of children born by in vitro fertilization and their mothers. J Psychosomatic Obstet Gynecol 1993; 14: 117–26

37. Ron-El R, Lahat E, Golan A, et al. Development of children born after ovarian superovulation induced by long-acting gonadatrophin-releasing hormone antagonists and menotrophins, and by in vitro fertilization. J Pediatr 1994; 125: 734–7

38. Levy-Shiff R, Vakil E, Dimitrovsky L, et al. Medical, cognitive, emotional, and behavioural outcomes in school-age children conceived by in-vitro fertilization. J Clin Child Psychol 1998; 27: 320–9

39. Olivennes F, Kerbrat V, Rufat P, et al. Follow-up of a cohort of 422 children aged 6–13 years conceived by in vitro fertilization. Fertil Steril 1997; 67: 284–9

40. Gibson F, Ungerer J, McMahon C, et al. The mother-child relationship following in vitro fertilization (IVF): infant attachment, responsivity, and maternal sensitivity. J Child Psychol Psychiatry 2000; 41: 1015–23

41. Montgomery TR, Aiello F, Adelman RD, et al. The psychological status at school age of children conceived by in-vitro fertilization. Hum Reprod 1999; 14: 2162–5

42. Bowen JR, Gibson FL, Leslie GI, Saunders DM. Medical and developmental outcome at 1 year for children conceived by intracytoplasmic sperm injection. Lancet 1998; 351: 1529–34

43. te Velde ER, van Baar AL, van Kooij RJ. Concerns about assisted reproduction. Lancet 1998; 351: 1524–5

44. Van Steirteghem A, Bonduelle M, Devroey P, Liebaers I. Follow-up of children born after ICSI. Hum Reprod Update 2002; 8: 1–8

45. Barnes J, Sutcliffe A, Kristoffersen I, et al. The influence of assisted reproduction on family functioning and children's socio-emotional development: results from a European study. Hum Reprod 2004; 19: 1480–7

46. Place I, Englert Y. The emotional and behavioural development of ICSI children. How are the ICSI families coping in comparison with IVF and run-of-the-mill families? Presented at the 18th Annual Meeting of the European Society for Human Reproduction and Embryology, Vienna, 2002

47. Cohen J, McMahon F, Gibson F, et al. Marital adjustment in ICSI families: A controlled comparison. Presented at the 17th World Congress on Fertility and Sterility, Melbourne, Australia, 2001

48. Bonduelle M, Joris H, Hofmans K, et al. Mental development of 201 ICSI children at 2 years of age. Lancet 1998; 351: 1553

49. Bonduelle M, Ponjaert I, Van Steirteghem A, et al. Developmental outcome at 2 years of age for children born after ICSI compared with children born after IVF. Hum Reprod 2003; 18: 342–50

50. Sutcliffe AG, Taylor B, Li J, et al. Children born after intracytoplasmic sperm injection: a population control study. Br Med J 1999; 318: 704–5

51. Sutcliffe AG, Taylor B, Saunders K, et al. Outcome in the second year of life after in-vitro fertilization by intracytoplasmic sperm injection: a UK case–control study. Lancet 2001; 357: 2080–4

51. Papaligoura Z, Panopoulou-Maratou O, Solman M, et al. Cognitive development of 12 month old Greek infants conceived after ICSI and the effects of the method on their parents. Hum Reprod 2004; 19: 1488–93

53. Leslie GI, Cohen J, Gibson FL, et al. ICSI children have normal development at school age. Presented at the 18th Annual Meeting of the European Society of Human Reproduction and Embryology, Vienna, July 2002

54. Ponjaert-Kristoffersen I. Follow-up of ICSI children: cognitive and neurodevelopmental outcome. Presented at the 19th Annual Meeting of the European Society of Human Reproduction and Embryology, Madrid, June–July 2003

55. Goodman R. A modified version of the Rutter parent questionnaire including extra items on children's strength's: a research note. J Child Psychol Psychiatry 1994; 35: 1483–94

56. Brodzinsky DM, Smith DW, Brodzinsky AB. Children's Adjustment to Adoption. Developmental and Clinical Issues. London Sage Publications, 1998

57. Grotevant MD, McRoy RG. Openness in Adoption: Exploring Family Connections. New York: Sage, 1998

58. Baran A, Pannor R. Lethal Secrets. New York: Amistad, 1993

59. Daniels K, Taylor K. Secrecy and openness in DI. Politics Life Sci 1993; 12: 155–70

60. Snowden R, Mitchell GD, Snowden EM. Artificial Reproduction: A Social Investigation. London: George Allen & Unwin, 1983

61. Snowden R. The family and artificial reproduction. In Bromham EA, ed. Philosophical Ethics in Reproductive Medicine. Manchester: Manchester University Press, 1990: 70–185

62. Bok S. Secrets. New York: Pantheon, 1982

63. Karpel MA. Family secrets: I. Conceptual and ethical issues in the relational context. II. Ethical and practical considerations in therapeutic management. Fam Process 1980; 19: 295–306

64. Papp P. The worm in the bud: secrets between parents and children. In Imber-Black E, ed. Secrets in Families and Family Therapy. New York: Norton, 1993: 66–85

65. Clamar A. Psychological implications of the anonymous pregnancy. In Offerman-Zuckerberg J, ed. Gender in Transition: A New Frontier. New York: Plenum, 1989

66. Brewaeys A. DI, the impact on family and child development. J Psychosom Obstet Gynecol 1996; 17: 1–13

67. Amuzu B, Laxova R, Shapiro S. Pregnancy outcome, health of children and family adjustment of children after DI. Obstet Gynecol 1990; 75: 899–905

68. Back K, Snowden R. The anonymity of the gamete donor. J Psychosom Obstet Gynecol 1988; 9: 191–8

69. Klock S, Maier D. Psychological factors related to DI. Fertil Steril 1991; 56: 549–59

70. van Berkel D, van der Veen L, Kimmel I, te Velde ER. Differences in the attitudes of couples whose children were conceived through artificial insemination by donor in 1980 and in 1996. Fertil Steril 1999; 71: 226–31

71. Golombok S, MacCallum F, Goodman E, Rutter M. Families with children conceived by DI: a follow-up at age 12. Child Dev 2002; 73: 952–68

72. Leiblum S, Aviv A. Disclosure issues and decisions of couples who conceived via donor insemination. J Psychosomatic Obstet Gynecol 1997; 18: 292–300

73. Nachtigall R, Becker G, Szkupinski Quigora S, Tschann J. The disclosure decision: concerns and issues of parents and children conceived through donor insemination. Am J Obstet Gynecol 1998; 176: 1165–70

74. Daniels K, Lewis GM. Openness of information in the use of donor gametes: developments in New Zealand. J Reprod Infant Psychol 1996; 14: 57–68

75. Rumball A, Adair V. Telling the story: parents' scripts for donor offspring. Hum Reprod 1999; 14: 1392–9

76. Scheib J, Riordan M, Rubin S. Choosing identity-release sperm donors: the parents' perspective 13–18 years later. Hum Reprod 2003; 18: 1115–27

77. Golombok S, Murray C, Jadva V, et al. Families created through a surrogacy arrangement: parent–child relationships in the first year of life. Dev Psychol 2004; 400–11

78. Lindblad F, Gottlieb C, Lalos O. To tell or not to tell – what parents think about telling their children that they were born following DI. J Psychosom Obstet Gynecol 2000; 21: 193–203

79. Gottlieb C, Lalos O, Lindblad F. Disclosure of donor insemination to the child: the impact of Swedish legislation on couples' attitudes. Hum Reprod 2000; 15: 2052–6

80. Cook R, Golombok S, Bish A, Murray C. Keeping secrets: a study of parental attitudes toward telling about donor insemination. Am J Orthopsychiatry 1995; 65: 549–59

81. Nachtigall RD, Pitcher L, Tschann JM, et al. Stigma, disclosure and family functioning among parents of children concieved through DI. Fertil Steril 1997; 68: 83–9

82. Brewaeys A. Review: parent–child relationships and child development in donor insemination families. Hum Reprod Update 2001; 17: 38–46

83. Humphrey M, Humphrey H. Marital relationships in couples seeking DI. J Biosoc Sci 1987; 19: 209–19

84. Klock S, Jacob M, Maier D. A prospective study of DI recipients: secrecy, privacy and disclosure. Fertil Steril 1994; 62: 477–84

85. Owens D, Edelman R, Humphrey M. Male infertility and DI: couples' decisions, reactions, and counselling needs. Hum Reprod 1993; 8: 880–5

86. Reading A, Sledmere C, Cox D. A survey of patient attitudes towards artificial insemination by donor. J Psychosom Res 1982; 26: 429–33

87. Schover LR, Collins RL, Richards S. Psychological aspects of DI: evaluation and follow up of recipient couples. Fertil Steril 1992; 57: 583–90

88. Golombok S, Lycett E, MacCallum F, et al. Parenting infants conceived by gamete donation. J Fam Psychol 2004; 18: (3)

89. Clayton C, Kovacs G. AID offspring: initial follow up study of 50 couples. Med J Aust 1982; 1: 338–9

90. Izuka R, Yoshiaki S, Nobuhiro N, Michie O. The physical and mental development of children born following artificial insemination. Int J Fertil 1968; 13: 24–32

91. Leeton J, Backwell J. A preliminary psychosocial follow-up of parents and their children conceived by artificial insemination by donor (AID). Clin Reprod Fertil 1982; 1: 307–10

92. Milson I, Bergman P. A study of parental attitudes after DI. Acta Obstet Gynecol Scand 1982; 61: 125–8

93. Manuel C, Facy F, Choquet M, et al. Les risques psychologiques de la conception par IAD pour l'enfant. Neuropsychiatrie l'Enfance 1990; 38: 642–58

94. Kovacs GT, Mushin D, Kane H, Baker HWG. A controlled study of the psycho-social development of children conceived following insemination with donor semen. Hum Reprod 1993; 8: 788–90

95. Cordray B. Speaking for ourselves: quotes from men and women created by DI/remote father conception. Presented at the 11th World Congress on In Vitro Fertilization and Human Reproductive Genetics, Sydney, Australia, 1999

96. Donor Conception Support Group of Australia. Let the Offspring Speak: Discussions on Donor Conception. New South Wales: Georges Hall, 1997

97. Turner A, Coyle, A. What does it mean to be a donor offspring? The identity experiences of adults conceived by donor insemination and the implications for counselling and therapy. Hum Reprod 2000; 15: 2041–51

98. Lutjen P, Trounson A, Leeton J, et al. The establishment and maintenance of pregnancy using in vitro fertilization and embryo donation in a patient with primary ovarian failure. Nature (London) 1984; 307: 174

99. Trounson A, Leeton J, Besanka M, et al. Pregnancy established in an infertile patient after transfer of a donated embryo fertilized in vitro. Br Med J 1983; 286: 835–8

100. Golombok S. Lesbian mother families. In Bainham A, Sclater S, Richards M, eds. What is a Parent? A Socio-legal Analysis. Oxford: Hart, 1999: 161–80

101. Murray C, Golombok S. To tell or not to tell: the decision-making process of egg donation parents. Hum Fertil 2003; 6: 89–95

102. Soderstrom-Antilla V, Sajaniemi N, Tiitinen A, Hovatta O. Health and development of children born after oocyte donation compared with that of those born after in-vitro fertilization, and parents' attitudes regarding secrecy. Hum Reprod 1998; 13: 2009–15

103. Golombok S, Murray C, Brinsden P, Abdalla H. Social versus biological parenting: family functioning and the socioemotional development of children conceived by egg or sperm donation. J Child Psychol Psychiatry 1999; 40: 519–27

104. Patterson CJ. Children of lesbian and gay parents. Child Dev 1992; 63: 1025–42

105. Amato PR. Children's adjustment to divorce: theories, hypotheses and empirical support. J Marriage Fam 1993; 55: 23–38

106. Chase-Lansdale PL, Hetherington EM. The impact of divorce on life-span development: short and long-term effects. In Baltes PB, Featherman DL, Lerner RM. eds. Life-Span Development and Behavior. Hillsdale, NJ: Erlbaum, 1990: 105–50

107. Hetherington EM, Stanley-Hagan MM. Parenting in divorced and remarried families. In Bornstein M, ed. Handbook of Parenting. Hove, UK: Lawrence Erlbaum Associates, 1995; 3: 233–54

108. McLanahan S, Sandefur G. Growing up with a Single Parent: What Hurts, What Helps. Cambridge, MA: Harvard University Press, 1994

109. Weinraub M, Gringlas MB. (1995). Single parenthood. In Bornstein M, ed. Handbook of Parenting: Social Conditions of Parenting. Hove, UK: Lawrence Erlbaum Associates, 1995; 3: 65–87

110. Flaks DK, Ficher I, Masterpasqua F, Joseph G. Lesbians choosing motherhood: a comparative study of lesbian and heterosexual parents and their children. Dev Psychol 1995; 31: 105–14

111. Chan RW, Raboy B, Patterson CJ. Psychosocial adjustment among children conceived via DI by lesbian and heterosexual mothers. Child Dev 1998; 69: 443–57

112. Golombok S, Tasker F, Murray C. Children raised in fatherless families from infancy: family relationships and the socioemotional development of children of lesbian and single heterosexual mothers. J Child Psychol Psychiatry 1997; 38: 783–92

113. Brewaeys A, Ponjaert-Kristoffersen I, Van Hall EV, Golombok S. DI: child development and family functioning in lesbian mother families. Hum Reprod 1997; 12: 1349–59

114. Brewaeys A, Ponjaert-Kristoffersen I, van Hall EV, et al. Lesbian mothers who conceived after DI: a follow-up study. Hum Reprod 1995; 10: 2731–5

115. Leiblum S, Palmer M, Spector I. Non-traditional mothers: single heterosexual/lesbian women and lesbian couples electing motherhood via donor insemination. J Psychosom Obstet Gynecol 1985; 16: 11–20

116. Wendland C, Byrn, F, Hill C. Donor insemination: a comparison of lesbian couples, heterosexual couples and single women. Fertil Steril 1996; 65: 764–70

117. Jacob M, Klock S, Maier D. Lesbian mothers as therapeutic donor insemination recipients: do they differ from other patients? J Pychosom Obstet Gynecol 1999; 20: 203–15

118. Fidell L, Marik J. Paternity by proxy: artificial insemination by donor sperm. In Offerman-Zuckerberg J, ed. Gender in Transition: A New Frontier. New York: Plenum, 1989: 93–110

119. Murray C, Golombok S. Going it alone: solo mothers and their infants conceived by donor insemination. Am J Orthopsychiatry 2004; in press

120. Vanfraussen K, Ponjaert-Kristoffersen I, Brewaeys A. An attempt to reconstruct children's donor concept: a comparison between children's and lesbian parents' attitudes towards donor anonymity. Hum Reprod 2001; 16: 2019–25

121. Blyth E. Not a 'primrose path': commissioning parents' experiences of surrogacy arrangements in Britain. J Reprod Infant Psychol 1995; 13: 185–96

122. MacCallum F, Lycett E, Murray C, et al. Surrogacy: the experience of commissioning couples. Hum Reprod 2003; 18: 1334–42

123. Serafini P. Outcome and follow-up of children born after in vitro fertilization surrogacy (IVF surrogacy). Hum Reprod Update 2001; 17: 23–7

124. Bates JE, Freeland GA, Lounsbury ML. Measurement of infant difficulties. Child Dev 1979; 50: 794–803

125. MacCallum F. Families with a child concieved by embryo donation. Unpublished PhD thesis, 2004

126. ESHRE Task Force. Ethical Issues Related to Multiple Pregnancies in Medically Assisted Procreation. Brussels: European Society of Human Reproduction and Embryology, 2003

128. Jain T, Missmer S, Hornstein M. Trends in embryo-transfer practice and in outcomes of the use of assisted reproductive technology in the United States. N Eng J Med 2004; 350: 1639–45

33

Nursing care in an assisted conception unit

Margaret A. Muirhead and Janet Kirkland

INTRODUCTION

There are few issues that cause more anguish and heartache than infertility. To label a couple as infertile is fraught with problems, emotional and clinical. The role and expectations of the infertility nurse specialist encompass a wide spectrum of care, covering physical to psychological aspects far beyond the basic training of the registered general nurse. The holistic care of couples undergoing assisted conception demands a special kind of support, compassion, empathy and maturity.

Skills used vary from one center to another, often dependent on the number and types of treatment cycles undertaken. Over the past 24 years, infertility nurses have moved away from only carrying out nursing care under instruction from clinicians. They are now trained to carry out many procedures previously undertaken by medical staff. Nursing now includes planning evidence-based total patient care. Some nurses are taking full management responsibility in assisted conception treatment centers, including compliance with regulatory authorities, budget control and negotiation of contracts with health authorities. The large number of treatment cycles undertaken at Bourn Hall Clinic, in comparison with many other centers, has inevitably resulted in the refinement of nursing care around a specific model and philosophy

of care. Nurses have needed to develop specialist skills in response to rapid advances in technology and changing patients' needs, in order to deliver appropriate care of a high standard. Such required skills include the following.

Practical skills

In most centers, nurses perform venepuncture and ultrasound scans, and assist at oocyte collection. Some undertake intracervical and intrauterine inseminations and embryo transfers. In a few centers, nurses perform oocyte recovery and surgical sperm retrieval. Birch suggests that[1]:

> these are procedures within the capability of many nurse specialists should they wish to take the opportunity, but it should be left to each individual practitioner to decide for themselves if it is right for them. This allows for an even greater degree of continuity of care and patients appear to be happy about these procedures being performed by nurses.

Investigations undertaken by nurses may include hysteroscopy, hysterosalphingo-contrast sonography (HyCoSy), aqua scanning and ultrasound imaging Nurses with scientific backgrounds are performing yet more specialist tasks, such as semen preparation, and are being taught laboratory techniques such as intra-cytoplasmic sperm injection (ICSI).

Interpersonal skills

In the United Kingdom, the Human Fertilisation and Embryology Act (1990) requires that patients seeking licensed treatment must be given suitable opportunity to receive proper counseling about the implications of their treatment[2]. All patients attending are given the contact details of our independent counselors and are encouraged to use their services, which are at no extra cost; however, a natural extension of the nurse's role is to provide informal counseling as an ongoing process, but recognizing limitations and suggesting referral when appropriate.

Counseling may be:

(1) *Support counseling*: offered in recognition of emotional needs, especially during times of stress;

(2) *Information counseling*: because of the complex nature of treatment;

(3) *Implications counseling*: to enable couples to explore the relevance and importance of decisions taken now, and their subsequent effects;

(4) *Therapeutic counseling*: to help couples to develop strategies for coping, although this requires a higher level of skill and supervision, and is usually undertaken by an independent counselor.

Confidentiality in counseling is mandatory.

Communication skills

It is necessary to receive information from couples effectively, and to impart it appropriately, in order to:

(1) Program and co-ordinate treatment cycles;

(2) Liaise with other disciplines involved in treating infertile couples;

(3) Give bad news with sensitivity.

Teaching skills

(1) Explain treatments in anatomical terms understood by the patient;

(2) Give preconceptual health education;

(3) Show patients how to self-administer their prescribed medication.

Administration skills

The quality of total patient care relies on detailed planning, accurate documentation and communication. The effective management of complex treatment cycles, involving a number of different professions, demands special skills to ensure that the best use is made of valuable resources by:

(1) Maintaining accurate records of appointments in a diary used by the whole clinic community;

(2) Calculating treatment cycle dates, and making appointments in accordance with the prescribed protocol;

(3) Negotiating between the patient and other disciplines mutually agreeable dates and times for investigative procedures;

(4) Ensuring that letters are sent to couples following consultation, to confirm treatment dates and once the treatment cycle is completed;

(5) Arranging for prescriptions to be dispensed and drugs sent to couples at home and overseas, when requested;

(6) Planning arrangements for couples to have investigations undertaken locally, and for results and blood samples to be sent to Bourn Hall;

(7) Sending information to couples making an initial enquiry about treatment;

(8) Making sure that accurate documentation is maintained for patient records and for research;

(9) Processing information in compliance with the Human Fertilisation and Embryology Authority (HFEA), including:

   (a) Registration of new patients;

   (b) Treatment commenced and embryo creation;

   (c) Details of donor gametes used;

   (d) Treatment outcome, including pregnancy and delivery data;

(10) Achieving information technology (IT) proficiency in order to:

(a) Record and retrieve information on a database;

(b) Use email as a mode of communication;

(c) Add and retrieve information from an electronic diary;

(d) Access the Internet to update professional knowledge.

Combinations of these skills are used to a greater or lesser extent, according to the level or the stage of treatment. Nurses are involved with couples at 'grass-roots' level from the initial enquiry through to completion of their treatment cycle and follow-up. The stages include: information-giving, informal counseling and planning of the treatment cycle at the consultation visit; support and information during cycle monitoring, oocyte recovery and embryo transfer; and finally, at the completion of the cycle, pregnancy testing and the giving of results. The infertility nurse specialist must have a varied skill mix and the capacity to adapt to different roles at each stage of the treatment cycle. The roles can be described as: nurse co-ordinator, out-patient nurse, ward nurse and theater nurse.

THE NURSE CO-ORDINATOR

The fertility nurse's role as a co-ordinator is pivotal in forming the link between the clinic and the patient, by providing information and facilitating the passage of couples through all the varied treatments. This demands a high level of interpersonal, communication and administrative skills.

The daily routine includes seeing couples after consultation with the clinician, to discuss the practicalities of treatment, give preconceptual advice and initiate any investigations. The co-ordination of a treatment cycle is a challenging task, with the complexities of plotting dates and arranging baseline appointments, some carried out in different parts of the world with results sent by facsimile – often in foreign languages!

Day-case surgery and investigations, including semen assessments, blood tests for screening and scans, also need to be booked; the results need to be collated and information and advice must be disseminated to anxious couples. The nurse co-ordinator has

responsibility for arranging the many different specialized treatments and procedures carried out in clinics, such as:

(1) *In vitro* fertilization (IVF);

(2) Intracytoplasmic sperm injection (ICSI);

(3) Frozen embryo transfer;

(4) Monitored intrauterine artificial insemination (IUAI) cycles using partner/donor semen;

(5) Self-monitored IUAI cycles using partner/donor semen;

(6) Transport and satellite IVF;

(7) Egg donation (fresh and frozen cycles);

(8) Egg-share programs;

(9) IVF surrogacy (fresh and frozen cycles);

(10) Embryo donation;

(11) Rectal electroejaculation for ejaculatory dysfunction;

(12) Testicular and epididymal sperm aspiration (TESA/PESA);

(13) Cryopreservation of semen, and testicular tissue for men with conditions which may compromise their future fertility;

(14) Cryopreservation of eggs;

(15) Investigation including hysteroscopies, hysterosalpingograms, dilatation and curettage;

(16) Recruitment for infertility clinical trials.

The nurse co-ordinator's role is recognized as the most difficult for nurses, regardless of training or experience. The highly charged, emotionally stressed working environment is due to the amount of patient contact by telephone, an anonymous medium, which requires intuitive listening skills. The absence of visual body language demands skilled interpretation of verbal signals such as intonation, vocabulary and hesitation in a counseling situation.

It is accepted that the majority of patients will be unsuccessful with their treatment. This inevitably means that a high proportion of calls demand the giving of bad news. However, nurses in this position still report good levels of job satisfaction. This stems from knowing that couples have felt cared for and supported, that they were well informed, encouraged to appreciate small achievements and able to maintain a balance of positivity and realism. The opportunity to give a patient good news, an unequivocal positive pregnancy test, is a wonderful panacea for the stresses of this role.

THE OUT-PATIENT NURSE

This role is a continuation of the role of the nurse coordinator. It is essentially to act as a mediator from the beginning of the treatment cycle until the intervention stage. The out-patient department (OPD) nurse cares for couples primarily during the monitoring phase of treatment. The role demands practical, teaching, decision-making, communication and listening skills. Practical skills necessary for this role include venepuncture, undertaking routine screening tests and interpretation of ultrasound scans. The OPD nurse spends time teaching patients how to give their own injections and answers queries about the action, procurement and timing of the drugs used. Explanation is given about the reasons for blood tests and the implications of scan findings. The nurse ensures that informed and understood consent is obtained, that treatment instructions are made clear and that patients adhere to them and to protocols for any clinical trials.

Bourn Hall is working towards establishing a nurse-led center. This has already been achieved within the out-patient department. Nurses collate results of hormone assays and ultrasound scans to make decisions regarding the monitoring phase of the treatment in accordance with local protocols.

Reassurance and support counseling are required constantly by couples whose confidence is made fragile by anxieties about unfamiliar procedures, treatments and the invasion of sexual privacy. Stressful situations are often diffused by a sense of humor, sometimes by tears and by a comforting arm around their shoulders. Unreasonable behavior and anger are occasionally symptomatic of couples' frustration at their predicament.

The fertility nurse should endeavor to create an environment that makes it easier to release restrained and raw emotions, and to be aware that many couples are unable to confide in family or friends.

Less routine, although frequent, are emergency appointments for young men referred from oncology units, to attend for semen cryopreservation. These men will have been diagnosed recently with serious illnesses, requiring urgent chemotherapy or radiotherapy. Some are only teenagers and are accompanied by parents; all are shocked, frightened and anxious enough, but they face the tension and embarrassment of producing the semen specimen required, in an unfamiliar environment, while feeling unwell. Consent forms must be understood and signed, and screening blood samples taken for assessment of human immunodeficiency virus (HIV), hepatitis B virus (HBV) and hepatitis C virus (HCV) status, a prerequisite of storing gametes. Follow-up appointments are arranged at 3-day intervals if possible, before cancer treatment is begun. All this requires sensitive explanation and very special nursing skills provided on a named-nurse basis. There is very little opportunity to establish any professional relationship with these patients prior to discussing intimate and personal details, such as masturbation. Any discussion regarding use of stored semen after death is particularly difficult when these patients are already ill with potentially terminal conditions.

Cranshaw and colleagues[3] suggest that:

it is a concern for staff to refer to the fact that they had not received any specific training to equip them for carrying out this work. Infertility nurses frequently have no in depth knowledge of oncology as a speciality or of the conditions these young men are suffering.

It is recognized that the fertility center is a far from ideal environment for these young men to find themselves. The fertility nurse tends to adopt a protective role to shelter them from the attention of her fertility patients.

There are many other instances where the 'segregation' of patients is both important and essential in order to ensure confidentiality and to protect patients from difficult encounters. For example, an attempt is always made to shield a couple who have just received news of a blighted ovum from one with a healthy ongoing pregnancy, until this news is absorbed.

The HFEA requires that special care is also taken when treatments involve the use of donated gametes[4]:

In addition to the above, centres are expected to take extra care in respect of the separation of provider and recipient notes, facilities and procedures in treatment involving egg sharing and gamete and embryo donation. It is expected that particular care should be taken to ensure that confidentiality is not compromised, for example where the woman donating/sharing eggs and the woman receiving them are treated at the same centre at similar times.

Potentially stressful situations such as these need to be acknowledged and addressed for the emotional well-being of both patients and staff.

The restorative value of clinical supervision[5] as a form of support for the infertility nurse specialist must be appreciated to maintain the health of the practitioner working in this stressful environment.

Clinical supervision is a formal arrangement that enables nurses, midwives and health visitors to discuss their work regularly with another experienced professional. It involves reflecting on practice in order to learn from experience and improve competence. The functions of clinical supervision are described by Proctor[6] as:

(1) *Restorative*: supportive help for professionals working constantly with stress and distress;

(2) *Formative*: the educative process of developing skills;

(3) *Normative*: the managerial and quality control aspects of professional practice.

Butterworth and Faugier[7] specify that 'its purpose is to facilitate reflective practice and push forward a patient-centered focus'.

THE WARD NURSE

Nurses new to the field of infertility regard the ward as a 'safe haven' of conventional practice. How wrong they are! Almost akin to midwifery, our patients are fit and well, but, unusually, care is focused on the couple, not on the individual. Each are vulnerable, especially at this stage of treatment, and care of both partners is equally important.

The admission procedure is one of assessment. Both partners are anxious to produce gametes of the right quality on time, are frightened by the prospect of failure and of not being in control, and are embarrassed by the perceived indignity of the procedures. The ward nurse's objective is to provide a caring and friendly welcome and a good explanation of what is expected, ensuring respect, privacy and adequate time for them to get used to the conditions and feel comfortable.

Some couples may feel that all the treatment, drugs and monitoring to date, and all hope of a baby, is now dependent on the quality of the semen specimen produced in a clinical and impersonal environment, with the additional pressure of time constraints. The possible need for further semen specimens is a difficult request for the nurse to make, needing skills in diplomacy, tact and empathy to avoid feelings of inadequacy by the male partner.

The ward nurse undertakes routine preoperative and postoperative care, in accordance with the United Kingdom Central Council for Nursing, Midwifery and Health Visiting (UKCC) *Scope of Professional Practice*[8]. Clinic protocols and recommendations define care for patients undergoing day-case procedures under general anesthetic or sedation, ensuring safety and comfort. Intravenous fluids are administered on occasions, for example when there is evidence of ovarian hyperstimulation syndrome (OHSS).

The ward nurse must be acutely aware of the need for giving prompt information to allay all unnecessary anxiety. Constant liaison is required between the ward, the OPD, the embryology department, the doctor and the operating theater. The number of oocytes retrieved, the quality of a semen specimen, the signs of, or absence of, fertilization, the cleavage of embryos and the timing of embryo transfer are communicated to couples as soon as possible. All treatments are delivered on a day-care basis; therefore, information-giving is predominantly by telephone. Delivering bad news by telephone is always difficult, and an appointment for further discussion and explanation is always offered. Instructions following oocyte recovery and embryo transfer are given verbally and in writing, including postoperative advice, use of any medications prescribed, how to contact the doctor on call outside of clinic opening hours and general advice post-embryo transfer. It is important to check a patient's understanding of the advice and instructions given before discharge, as they may be experiencing a wealth of emotions, and it is therefore not always easy to absorb and retain information. How often we have heard the cry 'nobody told me'.

Contemporaneous records must be kept at all times.

THE THEATER NURSE

The role of the theater nurse is:

(1) To ensure safety, comfort and dignity for the patient;

(2) To provide support and reassurance;

(3) To maintain asepsis during surgical procedures and to prevent cross-infection.

In some units, nurses perform oocyte recovery, surgical sperm retrieval, embryo transfer and IUAI.

Procedures undertaken in the assisted conception unit operating theater can be categorized as investigative, diagnostic and therapeutic. These include hysteroscopy, dilatation of the cervix, polypectomy, rectal electroejaculation, surgical sperm retrieval, retrieval and transfer of gametes and transfer of embryos. The theater nurse is responsible for the assessment, planning and implementation of preoperative, perioperative and immediate postoperative care of all patients having any of these procedures. Good communication skills are vital to co-ordinate the diverse skill mix of people involved in patient care at this stage of treatment, and to make best use of resources. Skilled negotiation between embryologist, clinician and ward nurse is required in the timing of operating lists to ensure that couples' anxiety is not compounded by delay.

The theater nurse requires fine-tuned interpersonal skills to make an assessment of an individual patient's needs. When the patient is stressed before an operation, it is sometimes difficult to find the words to express these needs. The perceptive and intuitive ability to respond to body language is important in making this assessment. We all have our own 'personal space'. Recognizing this is important when assessing, for example, whether a patient wishes to have her hand held or not. Some patients prefer to be distracted by conversation or by background music; others prefer silence.

The theater nurse must be sensitive to individual patient needs, especially during procedures such as embryo transfer and IUAI. Many couples perceive this time as the moment of conception, so it is important that both partners share this experience if possible. For this reason, the patient's partner is permitted in theater, unless a general anesthetic is required. The presence of the partner at this critical stage can be an advantage. In most (but not all) cases, each partner will recognize in each other the need and level to which physical and emotional support and reassurance are required. Special consideration is given to couples receiving donated gametes. Even though counseling is an integral part of treatment, one or other partner may have previously had difficulty in accepting the use of donor sperm or oocytes. The presence of both partners at this emotional stage must be respected, as it can strengthen the bond between them, and with the potential child. To each couple this is a unique and intimate experience. The environment created by the theater nurse is important. Usually these procedures are carried out in a darkened, quiet space. If the environment is conducive and the patient relaxed, the procedure is more likely to be atraumatic. This may influence the potential of a successful outcome of treatment.

With the advances in the treatment of male factor infertility, the focus of surgical procedures is no longer primarily on the female partner. Therefore, consideration must be given to the different needs of men undergoing sperm retrieval.

Since 1989, spinal cord-injured men have been given the chance of biological fatherhood by a procedure known as rectal electroejaculation (REE) in combination with IVF. The procedure is also used, although less commonly, for able-bodied men with some types of ejaculatory dysfunction. For these men, the thought of this procedure can be distressing. The exposure of the most private and intimate body function, other than coitus itself, is perceived as degrading and humiliating, and as a further loss of control and dignity. The psychological effects on men with infertility problems is well documented. It must not be forgotten how difficult it must be for these men to cope with further invasion of their privacy, and every endeavor is made to respect this. The psychological and physical care before, during and immediately after REE is one of the most sensitive and demanding aspects of care by the theater nurse. REE can usually be tolerated by spinal cord-injured men without anesthesia or sedation. The patient is awake and alert. For this reason the priorities of care are:

(1) Provision of ongoing explanation and reassurance;

(2) Maintenance of privacy and dignity;

(3) Correct positioning of the patient (usually the right lateral position);

(4) Support and protection of limbs during the procedure, which often provokes violent muscle spasms;

(5) Monitoring of blood pressure before, during and immediately after the procedure. Stimulation of alpha receptors in the sympathetic nervous system can result in reflex hypertension, so it is important to monitor the blood pressure closely to detect signs of autonomic dysreflexia;

(6) Scheduling of the procedure at the end of an operating list, to eliminate the risk of cross-infection;

(7) Ensuring that equipment and instruments are adequately set up and maintained, to ensure safety and prevent dangerous complications such as burns.

The care of men before, during and after surgical sperm retrieval requires special skills and practical considerations. These patients are already anxious and embarrassed, and we must strive to avoid further distress to them caused by situations such as sharing a ward pre- and postoperatively with female patients. There must be adequate toilet facilities and a supply of theater gowns for male patients; these measures may seem to be incidental, but they can help to preserve dignity in what can appear to be an undignified procedure.

ESTABLISHING IDENTITY

The importance of checking the identity of our patients at each point of communication and treatment is stressed in the HFEA *Code of Practice*[9]:

> *Treatment centres have an obligation to take all reasonable steps to ensure the valid identity of all persons accepted for treatment, including male partners who might not often be seen at the centre during treatment. Where there is doubt about a patient's identity, this is expected to include the examination of photographic identification evidence such as photo-card driving licences and passports. Centres are expected to document this evidence in the patient's records.*

When patients attend for initial consultation at Bourn Hall, a photograph is taken to confirm identification at future visits. This helps to avoid the possibility of misidentification, or misrepresentation should a

patient present with a new partner. It is acknowledged that partners attending for treatment frequently have different surnames, and vigilance is imperative to ensure that gametes are used appropriately.

Local protocol dictates that at every point of communication the identification of the patient is cross-checked against the notes. At key points, such as embryo transfer, each professional involved in the procedure is required individually to check the identity of the patient and to document that they have done so. In addition, the patient confirms that the team are referring to the correct medical notes.

Telephone and electronic communication require the same degree of care to avoid misidentification and compromise of confidentiality.

CONSENTS

The consent forms required for fertility treatments are varied, complicated and many! A clear understanding of the implications is essential for the nursing, medical, scientific and counseling staff in order to explain them to the patients. The time of obtaining consent is also crucial, and consent forms need to be issued, considered and signed before treatment begins, in accordance with the HFEA code of practice[9]:

> *Treatment centres are expected to allow individuals seeking treatment, considering donation or storage sufficient time to reflect upon their decisions before obtaining their written consent. It is expected that a copy of the signed form will be provided for those who have given consent.*

We, as professionals, need to be aware of the possibility that these consents may be referred to at a later date, perhaps in difficult circumstances, and we must be confident that accurate information was provided, and the implications discussed, understood, agreed and documented. It could be argued that in no other field of medicine can consents have potentially such an influence on future generations.

COMMUNICATION

All aspects of effective nursing care rely on good communication. A reliable framework is essential to ensure meticulous and timely documentation of patient care during complicated treatments that involve many different processes.

An individualized patient Care Plan, jointly developed by medical and nursing staff at Bourn Hall, has revolutionized traditionally difficult communications between the different disciplines involved in infertility treatment. The development of the Care Plan was initiated in response to changing nursing regulatory requirements (UKCC, *Standards for Records and Record Keeping*[10]). A nursing philosophy emerged which focused upon individualized patient care. The need was quickly identified for all disciplines involved to have a common database that recorded treatment progression and actions, and which had the flexibility to travel with the patient throughout the treatment cycle. This flexible solution to a communication minefield also offered the added benefit of providing constantly updated information for the patient and ensured that key events in the treatment cycle were recorded in order to meet regulatory requirements. Two respected nursing models were adapted to form a nucleus of the Care Plan which was then expanded, specifically to consider the emotionally stressful nature of infertility and to include input from all disciplines in the care of patients from the beginning to the end of their treatment. This care plan was also adapted for patients attending through the Transport and Satellite programs to ensure continuity and accuracy of communication between units.

Peplau's model (from 1952)[11] is primarily concerned with mental health, and focuses on the personal interaction between nurse and patient. Communication and anxiety are seen as key factors. Consideration was given to this particular model, as the psychological issues that predominate in infertility were especially relevant. Such issues include recognizing and dealing with stress, bereavement and loss, gaining trust, building confidence and 'rehabilitation' or coming to terms with infertility. The Roper, Logan and Tierney[12] model was also used in an adapted form to include activities of daily living in terms of physical, psychological, environmental, sociocultural and politicoeconomic factors.

Development strategy for the Care Plan

There was a need to identify which different disciplines involved in infertility patient care would be contributors and users of the Care Plan and which

would be users only (Figure 1). The key events within each discipline which needed to be recorded were also identified. All these key events were then brought together on one multipage individualized Care Plan, which effectively travels with the couple as they progress through their treatment cycle. As each key event is reached, the relevant discipline updates the Care Plan, thereby providing a vital communication link and an up-to-the-minute overview of the patient's care, for the benefit of the whole user community and the patient. This document becomes a record of the treatment cycle and forms the basis of long-term data storage and analysis.

CONTINUITY OF CARE

Prior to May 1996, the majority of nurses at Bourn Hall Clinic worked in single, permanent designated areas and undertook roles as already described. The disadvantages of this working practice were:

(1) A lack of 'continuity of care' for couples;

(2) Little scope for individualized patient care;

(3) Task-focused nursing care;

(4) Development by practitioners of a specialty within a specialty, restricting continuing professional development;

(5) Evidence of low job satisfaction.

A fundamental change was brought about in direct response to patient demand for 'continuity of care' throughout their treatment cycles. Feedback surveys from patients who had completed treatment expressed their desire to see the same doctor and nurses throughout all phases of the treatment cycle, so that they would develop a closer rapport with those responsible for their total care.

Previously, nurses had worked as a single team. The total nursing establishment at Bourn Hall comprised: one nursing director, fulfilling a managerial role; two full-time registered nurses (RNs); nine part-time RNs (average 20–30 h each per week); bank staff (200–500 h each month); one full-time auxiliary nurse; and two part-time auxiliary nurses. In addition, there was a dedicated team of theater staff, comprising: one full-time RN; two part-time RNs; two part-time auxiliary nurses; and one full-time operating department assistant.

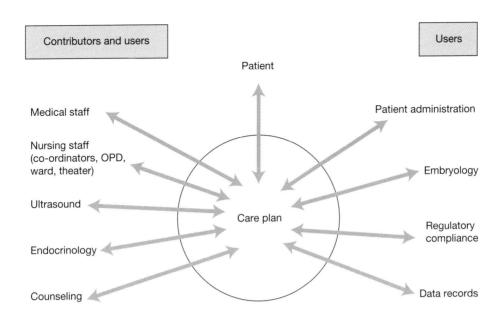

Figure 1 Structure of the Care Plan. OPD, out-patient department

Strategy for change

In order to fulfill patients' expressed wish for continuity of care, a working party from all disciplines was set up to review current practices and objectives, and to establish an action plan. It was important to have the involvement of personnel from all departments, as change was bound to impact on the way everyone worked and interfaced. It was clear that any new proposal in care management would have far-reaching effects on support services, such as security and catering, as well as those involved in direct patient care. Therefore, all current practices needed review and adaptation to accommodate changing patient requirements. The success of the project depended upon everyone's participation, and a desire to succeed.

Reorganization and planning

Medical and nursing staff (excluding theater nurses) were divided into two teams. Careful consideration was given to grouping people with an appropriate balance and mix of skills and experience, personalities and aspirations. The intention was that the teams would provide mutual support and encouragement, rather than create competition. The teams now comprise the staff shown in Table 1.

Table 1 Reorganized teams of medical and nursing staff

	Green team	Blue team
Full-time RN team leader	1	1
Full-time RH	1	1
Part-time RNs working a total of 70 h/week	3	4
Full-time team doctor	1	1
'Relief' doctor during the 'busy' week	1	1

RN, registered nurse

Nursing auxiliaries were not assigned to a team, but staffing hours were concentrated during week 1 and week 3 (see Figure 2), the busy weeks, when patients attend for their baseline appointments or others for operative procedures. Duties were diversified during week 2 and week 4 (see Figure 2), the quieter periods, when activity is concentrated away from the ward area. Theater, laboratory and ultrasound scanning staff were not divided into teams, but manpower was similarly concentrated into alternate weeks during the periods of higher demand.

Green Team

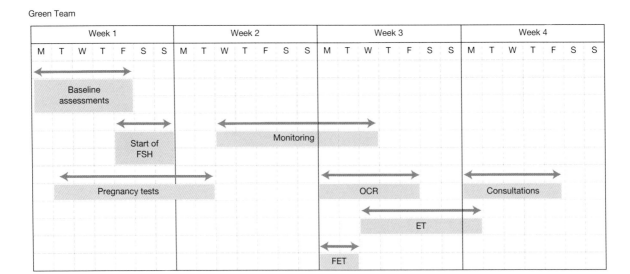

Blue Team

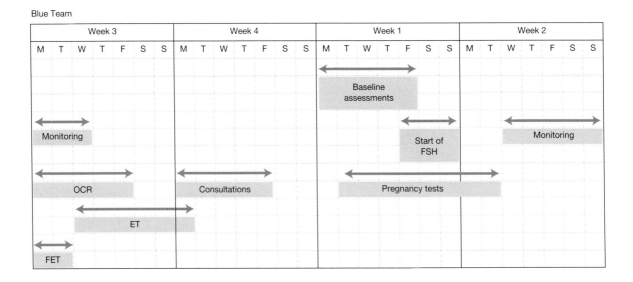

Figure 2 The treatment cycle, showing the 4-week treatment module and the working relationship between the two teams. FSH, follicle stimulating hormone drugs (Gonal-F®/Metrodin HP®; Serono Labboratories, UK); OCR, oocyte recovery; ET, embryo transfer; FET, frozen embryo transfer

Duty rosters were reviewed and reassessed to accommodate the need for rescheduled duty hours and shifts. In order to achieve continuity of care, it was necessary that the nurses became competent in all roles throughout the various phases of treatment. In so doing, the team would be able to provide a couple with seamless treatment and familiar faces throughout.

Training and development needs of individual nurses were identified and addressed by pairing one with high levels of experience with another learning new procedures and routines. Training sessions and workshops were set up to teach, revise and assess skills and build confidence. The team leaders were to adopt a unique role as participant/manager. Leadership skills and management training and development was introduced in preparation, and as an ongoing program.

The dynamics of the treatment cycle

In all appropriate cases, IVF treatment cycles were scheduled (Figure 2) by pituitary down-regulation with a gonadotropin releasing hormone agonist (GnRH-a), and a plan was devised such that groups of 40–45 couples started their treatment during the same 5-day period. Treatment cycles extended over a 4-week module. Couples commencing a treatment cycle were allocated to one of the teams and starting dates for each group were separated by 2-week intervals, allowing minimal overlap between teams in progress at any given time.

Monitoring the progress of the project

The process of monitoring the project was by evaluation of patient and staff feedback. Ongoing review was essential in order to redress problems and make modifications to keep pace with changes in practice.

Patient feedback

A key issue and priority during the transition stage from the old to the new system was that good customer care should be maintained. Couples were invited to complete questionnaires at different stages of treatment and the results were analyzed over a period of 3 months. Questions regarding care covered four phases of treatment: initial consultation, cycle monitoring, operating procedures and post-treatment. The questionnaires focused on a broad spectrum of care issues, including continuity of care. In response to the question 'how did you feel about continuity of care?' the following were reported: 73% felt that it was achieved, important and valuable; 23% felt it was satisfactory; and 4% regarded it as not important.

Couples remarked that they had greater confidence in staff and easier communication, which in turn helped to ensure optimum treatment. They also remarked that there was a better opportunity to select a particular doctor and nursing team. The improved treatment plan also provided greater flexibility for arranging clinic visits around their work and other commitments. Negative feedback from patients was minimal and far outweighed by the advantages of the new system.

Staff feedback

Questionnaires of a different design and orientation were issued to all staff of various disciplines, to measure how individuals felt about the changes made to the way in which they now worked. These were also used as a tool to assess positive and negative feedback from couples. The responses were anonymous and confidential. Constructive criticism was actively encouraged.

For the majority of staff, the change proved to be a positive experience. However, as the survey reflected, there was a reluctance by a minority to accept the fact that change was necessary. There was initially an increase in stress and anxiety experienced by some nurses induced by change and new or extra duties. Unsocial working hours and the need for extra 'bank' shifts were substantially reduced, with some inevitable loss of earnings, although there was no loss of jobs other than by natural wastage. Some concerns were expressed regarding new duty hours and the need for more advanced planning of annual leave and conference attendance.

Positive advantages to nurses were that job satisfaction and fulfillment were increased by caring for couples through an entire treatment cycle, and by developing a closer rapport with them. Other perceived benefits included a greater opportunity for research and training, and an increase in working skills and knowledge. The 'quiet' periods allowed time to analyze and assess results in detail.

There were also advantages of the new system to the clinic as a business unit. A realistic new working practice was necessary to keep pace with the changing workload and hence maintain the clinic's viability. It ensured more effective use of staff, better training and planning of activities, and ultimately a reduction in costs. Rationalization of costs was also a benefit to patients as savings made reduced the need to increase treatment fees.

A review of the project after 3 months identified a number of areas where further changes were felt to be necessary. The system was modified and adapted where appropriate. The immediate priority was to increase the number of nurses and doctors on duty during the 'busy' weeks to compensate for the increased workload. A second review after a further 10 weeks confirmed that the ground rules about the number of patients allowed into each treatment group must be observed so as to avoid excessive workloads, thus threatening the efficiency of the system. Patient feedback was generally positive. The most significant aspect of this feedback was that the majority of couples rated the quality of their care as 'excellent'.

It was, therefore, in direct response to patient demand for 'continuity of care' throughout their treatment cycles that this change in the management of their care was brought about.

The concept of a team approach evolved to address this desire, and, as a result, quality of care has been substantially improved. Care is more individualized and patient-focused. Job satisfaction has increased due to continuity of care. Costs have been rationalized by concentrating resources, which in turn will ultimately benefit couples having treatment.

The objectives of the working party set up to bring about the change to 'continuity of care' have now been successfully achieved. For further improvement of standards and continuity of care, constant review and quality assurance are required in order to fine-tune and modify the system in response to patient demand.

CONCLUSION

Historically the term 'nurse' was synonymous with the role of 'handmaiden'. Tasks were carried out under instruction of the clinician with little or no empowerment. In the 21st century, nursing as a profession has metamorphosed. The expectations of individual practitioners in many fields have changed, with a demand for greater responsibility, accountability and keenness to extend the boundaries.

The infertility nurse specialist is recognized as being the pivotal role player between all disciplines involved in the total care of couples having assisted conception treatment. Nurses are influential in care and enjoy the privilege of autonomy in their practice at Bourn Hall.

In the relatively new field of infertility, nurses have demonstrated that they are capable of holistic patient care. The contribution made by nurses to assessment, planning, implementation and evaluation of care is well respected. Research- and evidence-based care is the foundation of change. The introduction of the continuity of care program, for example, has fundamentally changed the way nursing at Bourn Hall

Clinic is implemented, with a greater focus on individualized care. This was a patient-driven initiative, brought about as a result of feedback, to improve the standard of care. The improvement of communications and documentation by the introduction of the medical/nursing Care Plan is further evidence of how nurses make an intelligent and valuable contribution to total patient care.

At Bourn Hall, nursing care has evolved over the past 24 years owing to the significant influences of new technology, politicoeconomic factors and changing sociocultural trends. Practice has also evolved as a result of the enthusiasm, imagination and creativity of the small, self-supporting group of nurses with a wide range of experience drawn from diverse areas of nursing care. Infertility nursing will continue to evolve and change as nurses, motivated by the potential to develop new skills, strive to be at the forefront in the pioneering sphere of assisted conception care.

Fertility treatments are becoming more readily available and ethically challenging.

The fertility nurse must address these issues and explore her own feelings with discussion and research. As the role continues to expand and her responsibilities and scope of practice broaden, she must ensure that she has proper training and support in the development of her role. The HFEA requires that the fertility nurse must be working towards nationally and/or locally set competencies, a higher-level award with a focus on women's reproductive health and, if involved in scanning, an accredited ultrasound course/qualification[13]. The Royal College of Nursing fertility nurse forum is developing a series of best-practice principles to support nurses, and is also developing infertility nurse training programs.

There are many educational opportunities, and nurses in the field should grasp them, not only to improve their knowledge, job satisfaction and ultimately patient care, but to allow them to meet with other nurses within the field and to share ideas and experiences.

REFERENCES

1. Birch H. The extended role of the nurse – opportunity or threat? Hum Fertil (Camb) 2001; 4: 138–44
2. Human Fertilisation and Embryology Authority. Code of Practice, 6th edn, part 7, Counselling. London: HFEA, 2003

3. Cranshaw M, Glaser A, Hale J, Sloper P. Professionals' views on the issues and challenges arising from providing a fertility preservation service through sperm banking to teenage males with cancer. Hum Fertil (Camb) 2004; 7: 23–30

4. Human Fertilisation and Embryology Authority. Code of Practice, 6th edition, part 12, Confidentiality. London: HFEA, 2003

5. Kohner N. Clinical Supervision: an Executive Summary. London: Kings' Fund Centre, Nursing Development Unit, 1994

6 Proctor B. Supervision: a co-operative exercise in accountability. In Marken M, Payne M, eds. Enabling and Ensuring. Leicester: National Youth Bureau, Council for Education and Training in Youth and Community Work, 1986

7. Butterworth CA, Faugier J. Clinical Supervision and Nursing Midwifery and Health Visiting. A Briefing Paper. Manchester: School of Nursing Studies, University of Manchester, 1994

8. UKCC. The Scope of Professional Practice. London: United Kingdom Central Council for Nursing, Midwifery and Health Visiting, 1992

9. Human Fertilisation and Embryology Authority Code of Practice, 6th edn, part 6, Consent. London: HFEA, 2003

10. UKCC. Standards for Records and Record Keeping. London: United Kingdom Central Council for Nursing, Midwifery and Health Visiting, 1993

11. Simpson H. Peplau's Model in Action. Basingstoke: Macmillan, 1991

12. Roper N, Logan W, Tierney A. The Elements of Nursing. London: Churchill Livingstone, 1980

13. Human Fertilisation and Embryology Authority. Code of Practice, 6th edn, part 1, Staff. London: HFEA, 2003

34

Transport and satellite assisted reproductive technology

Hazel Harrison

INTRODUCTION

By the early 1980s, *in vitro* fertilization (IVF) was an established treatment for infertility; however, it was out of reach to many couples. The cost of setting up specialist IVF centers[1–3], and the staff training required in such a specialized field, naturally limited the number of centers available. 'Satellite IVF' and 'transport IVF' evolved to help to overcome this problem, and to help to meet the demands of a public desperate for access to fertility services; it is still a program that is as necessary today as it was then.

This chapter describes the program as it is run at Bourn Hall and, similarly, by a few other clinics in the United Kingdom, where treatment can only be conducted by practitioners and in premises which are licensed by the Human Fertilisation and Embryology Authority (HFEA). Although the program described applies to UK clinics, the principles and practices will, essentially, be the same for clinics in other countries.

DEFINITION

The definition of satellite IVF (S-IVF), as stated by the Human Fertilisation and Embryology Authority (HFEA)[4], is any arrangement in which part of an IVF cycle takes place outside the primary or licensed center. More specifically, S-IVF may be defined as a secondary unit attached to a primary unit, which undertakes the responsibility of assessment, stimulation and monitoring of the patient, but the oocyte retrieval is carried out at the primary center, as is the culture and fertilization of oocytes, and the embryo transfer. In transport IVF (T-IVF), the assessment, stimulation, monitoring and oocyte retrieval takes place at the secondary unit, and the oocytes are then transported to the primary unit in a specially designed incubator for the embryology stage of the procedure. The overall medical management is by the secondary unit, with support at any time required from the primary unit.

HISTORY

In The Netherlands, where T-IVF started, the number of IVF laboratories was strictly limited by law, which gave rise to long waiting lists[5]. Therefore, in 1984, pilot studies of 'decentralized IVF' were carried out in Rotterdam by Jansen and colleagues[6]. This idea addressed several problems which had been identified, such as: covering large geographical areas[7]; reducing traveling times and therefore inconvenience to couples[8]; the loss of salary due to time away from the workplace; and the emotional upset of being separated from familiar surroundings[1–3]. At the University of Liverpool,

Kingsland and colleagues[2] developed the first transport IVF program in the UK, with the aim of assisting couples via their local gynecologists in the Mersey region. A different approach operates in Australia, where a team of experienced staff travel to remote provinces over several weeks to treat couples who have been carefully pre-programmed.

By the late 1990s, transport intracytoplasmic sperm injection (ICSI) was also an accepted form of treatment[3,9,10].

At Bourn Hall Clinic, a successful S-IVF program with Sandringham Private Hospital has been operating since 1992. By 1996 The James Paget Hospital in Gorleston, Great Yarmouth, and Ipswich General Hospital, had joined the program, but with National Health Service (NHS) funding. More recently, the Woodlands Private Hospital, and The Rosie Hospital at Addenbrooke's in Cambridge, and Jersey General Hospital have also joined the service, the latter two being satellite units (Figure 1).

SETTING UP THE LIAISON

Before any program of S-IVF can be put into place, much detail needs to be discussed and agreed between the secondary unit and the HFEA-licensed (in the UK) primary unit. A meeting between the units, including consultants, nurses and business managers, should take place to discuss and agree procedures and protocols[8,11], with a clear understanding and agreement of responsibilities[11]. The cost of treatments must be agreed to avoid any misunderstanding, especially the process for refunding the cost of incomplete treatments, so that they can be dealt with systematically and sympathetically. Changes to the cost of any treatment should be made only by agreement and after adequate notice has been given. The system for monitoring the T-IVF and S-IVF services requires the central licensed unit to apply to the HFEA for approval of each satellite unit and for them to be added to its license[11].

Ideally, the consent forms used at the primary unit should be used by the secondary units to achieve uniformity, which will avoid misinterpretation or misunderstanding by staff or patients. Any new or updated consent forms should be sent to the secondary units with the appropriate information and guidelines. Welfare of the child[12,13] issues and information, as required

by the HFEA, should be addressed by the staff at the secondary unit and consents must be in place before the patient begins treatment. Any queries raised on this sensitive subject should be referred to a senior consultant, and, if necessary, he/she can refer the query to the Ethics Committee.

Counseling is available to all couples undergoing or about to undergo treatment or part of their treatment at Bourn Hall Clinic, and couples are encouraged to use this facility[13].

It is a legal requirement for a contract to be in place between the primary and secondary units. All protocols and arrangements need to be agreed by the HFEA before the program can proceed. The overall responsibility for the program lies with the Person Responsible on the license at the primary unit, and it is their remit to ensure that the rules and guidelines, as set out in the *Code of Practice* of the HFEA, are adhered to by both parties. HFEA inspections at the primary unit can, at any time, include checks that the T-IVF and S-IVF programs are fulfilling their duties.

Transport IVF Guidelines (abstracted from reference 11)

Confidentiality

'Confidentiality as specified in the HFE Act and *Code of Practice* to be maintained'.

Welfare of the child assessment

'Assessing the welfare of any children born as a result of treatment and the effect on any existing children'.

Counseling

'The offer and availability of counseling before, during and after treatment'.

Patient information

'Availability of comprehensive verbal and written information'.

Consents for treatment and consent to communicate

'Informed consent to be given before commencing treatment'.

It is the policy at Bourn Hall Clinic that there is a protocol in place for each procedure. There are also process maps which are used to check that all stages of

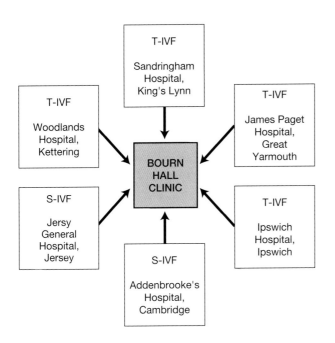

Figure 1 Relationship of satellite and transport units with Bourn Hall Clinic. T-IVF, transport *in vitro* fertilization; S-IVF, satellite IVF

the treatment are covered, to reduce the possibility of an adverse event occurring. The checking and updating of procedures and protocols is a continuous process, and any changes to the paperwork are sent to the secondary units, to be used with immediate effect. In addition, a copy of any protocols which are used independently at the secondary unit are kept at Bourn Hall Clinic for reference.

Changes in the *Code of Practice*, new 'directions' and any other items raised by the HFEA with the primary unit are immediately acted upon. Recent HFEA publications are discussed, actions implemented and all information is disseminated among the units.

The principal advantage of the satellite and transport arrangements is that the overall medical management of the patients rests with the consultant at the secondary unit. Generally, couples will have been under the care of this consultant for a period of time for investigations of their infertility, and it is this familiarity with staff and surroundings that helps couples with the stresses of the next stage of treatment[3]. In addition, the close proximity of their local hospital reduces stress and causes the least disruption to their lives and work[2]; however, counseling remains available to all.

The importance of good communication to the efficiency of the program cannot be overestimated[8].

Regular meetings[12] between Bourn Hall Clinic and the secondary units have been in place since this well-established T-IVF and S-IVF program began in 1992. These meetings are used to promote good relationships between the teams, and any members of staff connected with the program are encouraged to attend. It is an opportunity to identify any problems and act upon them accordingly, to review current practices and to update where appropriate, to advise on future financial changes, to discuss recent publications relating to IVF which may benefit staff or patients, and to exchange and to discuss results of their annual audits.

At these meetings the offer is reiterated to all staff of the secondary units that they are welcome to visit Bourn Hall for the purpose of updating their knowledge in all departments, particularly the embryology department to witness the embryo transfer procedures – the aim being to have a better understanding of the whole process when they are talking to their patients. Staff from Bourn Hall also visit the secondary units to obtain a better understanding of their workload and practices.

A constant review and update of procedures takes place, and patient satisfaction questionnaires are circulated and analyzed to obtain patient feedback. The regular audit of these surveys for quality-assurance purposes has led to the implementation of several changes to improve the service to patients.

To help with the transition of care from local consultant to Bourn Hall, couples are encouraged to visit the Clinic to familiarize themselves with the location and surroundings. Each month an 'Open Day' is held at Bourn Hall for couples considering IVF treatment, and satellite and transport IVF patients are encouraged to attend. This is an informal gathering, with a talk on assisted conception, followed by a question and answer session and an opportunity to talk with a member of the medical or nursing staff over tea.

THE BOURN HALL CLINIC TRANSPORT AND SATELLITE UNIT PROGRAM

Booking a treatment cycle

Before booking treatment, we ask the staff of each secondary unit to ensure that all relevant paperwork is sent to the Clinic. Following the correct procedure at the initial stage is crucial to the smooth running of the program.

At Bourn Hall we have extended a checklist (initially suggested by the HFEA) (Figure 2) to ensure that all the paperwork required for a patient's treatment is in order. This includes demographic details, a medical consultation checklist, male and female medical history, blood test results, all consent forms for treatment, and the consents to allow communication with their doctors, and that the 'welfare of the child' questionnaire has been signed by the patient's doctor. This enables us to prepare a completed file with a designated Bourn Hall medical number and to enter the details onto our database, preparatory to the forthcoming treatment.

The number of treatment cycles allocated to a unit each month will have been agreed between each unit and Bourn Hall. This is partly determined by demand and partly by the number of cycles that the embryology department at Bourn Hall can safely manage. Flexibility between units is encouraged, if spaces become available, to keep time on waiting lists to a minimum.

For each treatment, a new folliculargram is prepared (see Appendices on the CD-ROM that accompanies this book). This is a document which shows at a glance the patient's past treatment, proposed treatment and their medical and obstetric history. The rest of the document is used to record details of the current treatment, such as cycle monitoring, oocyte recovery and embryo transfer.

Each month, the secondary unit sends a form to Bourn Hall giving the name, baseline date and treatment plan of their patients. These details are used by the accounts department to prepare the appropriate account and to ensure that the Clinic is aware of who is having what treatment, and when. If surgical sperm retrieval, donor sperm, semen freezing or egg donation is required, liaison between staff at the onset (before booking) is essential. With good communication and a clear understanding of who is responsible for what, most treatments can be managed without problems arising. Patients requiring surgical sperm retrieval are seen by the specialist, and any investigations requested by him are carried out prior to treatment.

When donor sperm is required, the blood test results for human immunodeficiency virus (HIV), hepatitis B, hepatitis C and cytomegalovirus are sent to

Bourn Hall, followed by a completed characteristics form. This enables a donor to be assigned. Semen freezing may be necessary for different reasons: because the partner finds it difficult to provide a semen sample, illness, or prior to such treatment as chemotherapy. The initial semen assessment is carried out at the secondary unit. If the result is inconclusive, a second opinion will be given by a Bourn Hall embryologist and occasionally the male partner may be asked to produce a sample at Bourn Hall for a more detailed assessment.

When the treatment has begun, the secondary units are asked to keep Bourn Hall informed of their patients' progress[8,11]. As the day of human chorionic gonadotropin (hCG) approaches, this information is vital. The T-IVF units time the hCG to be given in accordance with the theater time available in their own hospital. The S-IVF patients are asked to have their hCG injection to fit in with the theater list times at Bourn Hall. This information, as well as the preoperative instructions, is given by Bourn Hall staff. It is also an opportunity to ensure that couples who are attending for treatment for the first time know where the Clinic is located.

To ensure that the program works efficiently, good, regular communication between the staff at the primary and secondary units is vital[8,11]. This may, if necessary, be on a daily basis by telephone, fax or e-mail. The important point to remember is to keep lines of communication open so that any change in a patient's progress is known to all staff involved. The Nurse Coordinator has a pivotal role to play between the primary and secondary units[1], to ensure the smooth running of the program.

The transport of gametes

The incubator used by the secondary units to transport oocytes to Bourn Hall is the Grant Incubator (Grant Instruments Ltd, Shepreth, Cambridge, UK) (Figure 3). It is widely used for the transport of samples and, when fully charged, maintains the correct temperature for several hours. It holds up to 18 tubes and measures $140 \times 65 \times 75$ mm, making it small enough to rest on the floor space of a car, where it can be plugged into the cigarette-lighter socket.

Each transport IVF unit is required to perform quality control tests on their portable incubators on a monthly basis, which include a 'test run' on the

Satellite and transport IVF check list

Patient name & address	Date of birth	Med No. (if known)

NOTE: THE FOLLOWING INFORMATION MUST ALL BE SENT TO BOURN HALL IN ONE PACKAGE, AS EARLY AS POSSIBLE BEFORE START OF TREATMENT

No	Details	Sent on	Received on *BHC use only*
1	Initial consultation questionnaire, demographic details		
2	Medical consultation checklist		
3	Female and male history sheet		
4	HIV, hepititis B & C, CMV, semen assessment, etc.		
5	Anesthetic/sedation questionnaire (*if required*)		
6	Completed consent for BHC to communicate directly with persons not covered by an HFEA		
7	Welfare of the child consent forms – completed by GP × 2		
8	Bourn Hall Clinic consent form (*pink*)		
9	HFEA (00) 6 and (00) 7 consents		
10	BHC embryo storage consent form		
11	ICSI consent form (*if required*)		
12	Consent for posthumous use		
13	Other consents (*if required*)		
14	Characteristic form (*if required*)		
15	Referral letter		

Key events	Date
Planned treatment	
Start down-regulation	
Baseline – week comencing	
Oocyte recovery – week comencing	
FET, transfer – week comencing	

Please forward to the Patient Liaison Officer at Bourn Hall Clinic, when all relevent information is available and the above list is completed

FOR BOURN HALL USE ONLY:			
Addressographs sent to unit		SA results sent to unit (if applicable)	

Figure 2 Satellite and transport *in vitro* fertilization (IVF) checklist as used at Bourn Hall Clinic (BHC). HIV, human immunodeficiency virus; CMV, cytomegalovirus; HFEA, Human Fertilisation and Embryology Authority; ICSI, intracytoplasmic sperm injection; FET, frozen embryo transfer

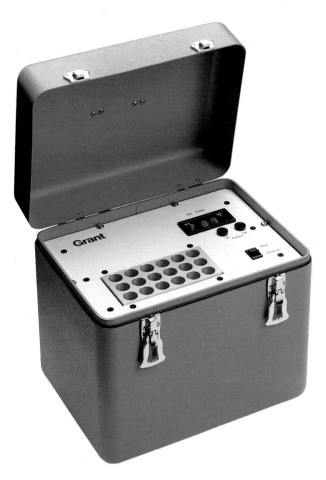

Figure 3 The Grant Incubator (Grant Instruments Ltd., Shepreth, Cambridge, UK)

incubator to ensure that any samples contained within it are maintained at the correct temperature throughout the duration of the journey. Every 6 months the incubators should be fully serviced and checked by the electrical and mechanical engineering department.

It is the T-IVF unit's responsibility to ensure that the male partner, who brings the incubator to Bourn Hall, is fully briefed with directions to the primary unit[12]. The furthest of the T-IVF centers is approximately 100 miles from Bourn Hall, no more than two and a half hours away. During the oocyte collection procedure, labeled tubes filled with follicular aspirates are transferred to warmed metal blocks and then placed in the portable incubator. Each tube in the incubator should be labeled with at least two points of identification, e.g. surname and medical number, and two members of staff should check these and sign the

form containing the egg collection details. Once the collection has finished, the male partner plugs the incubator into the cigarette-lighter point on their car dashboard and begins his journey. The Sister at the satellite unit telephones or faxes Bourn Hall with this information. On arrival at the Clinic, the incubator and patient medical records are passed to the embryologist, who checks with a nurse and the patient that the paperwork corresponds to that patient. At this point, the male partner is taken to a private room where he is expected to produce a semen sample. The incubator and medical notes are taken to the embryology laboratory where two embryologists are required to check the patient's notes for consents and viral screening before examining the contents of the tubes. The contents of the labeled tubes are examined and any oocytes found are placed in culture until the time of insemination. Upon receipt by the laboratory, the semen sample is examined and processed. The embryologist informs the nurse of the number of oocytes found and that, if the semen sample is suitable, the partner is free to leave the Clinic. He is given a telephone number and time to call for news of fertilization.

The day after oocyte recovery, all couples follow the same procedure. The patient or partner telephones the Clinic for news of fertilization. If appropriate, instructions are given regarding their attendance at the Clinic for embryo transfer on the following day. If the oocytes fail to fertilize, the information is relayed in a sensitive manner to the patient, allowing them time to ask any questions. The patient is then advised to contact the nurse at their own unit for further instructions and a follow-up consultation. The embryology information from the embryology department is faxed to the unit as soon as possible to enable the staff to advise the patient.

On the day of embryo transfer at Bourn Hall, each patient is given a sheet of instructions, as set out by their own unit, with guidelines to help them over the waiting time until the pregnancy test. The prescribed luteal support will have been discussed and supplied by their unit. The pregnancy test, either urine or blood, is performed at the secondary unit.

Each unit is responsible for relaying the outcome of the treatment to Bourn Hall Clinic by completing a monthly return form. This information is recorded in the notes and on the database, and the HFEA forms are then completed. If the pregnancy test is positive, the result of the scan is sent to Bourn Hall, and finally the information regarding the outcome of the pregnancy is returned with the required details.

CONCLUSIONS

The process of transporting aspirated oocytes from a satellite center to a central IVF laboratory is an accepted system for providing IVF services in many countries[1–3,5,7]. Studies have shown little difference in the fertilization and pregnancy rates between the primary and secondary units[3,8,9,14]. With the advent in the mid-1990s of more technically demanding procedures, such as ICSI, T-IVF and S-IVF have gained even more importance in this specialized field[3,9]. A transport IVF program requires the expertise of the laboratory staff[8], a fully committed team, and good communication and coordination between the primary and secondary units[8]. Patient surveys and in-house audits are essential to improving the program, as is the need regularly to reassess procedures and protocols. Patients generally are very enthusiastic about these programs, and appreciate the convenience of being able to use their local hospital and staff.

REFERENCES

1. Talbert LM, Hammond M, Baily L, et al. A satellite system for assisted reproductive technologies: an evaluation. Fertil Steril 1991; 55: 555–8
2. Kingsland CR, Aziz N, Taylor CT, et al. Transport in vitro fertilisation – a novel scheme for community-based treatment. Fertil Steril 1992; 58: 153–8
3. Alfonsin A, Amato A, Arrighi A, et al. Transport in vitro fertilisation and intracytoplasmic sperm injection: results of a collaborative trial. Fertil Steril 1998; 69: 466–70
4. Human Fertilisation and Embryology Authority. Direction Ref.D.2000/3 London: HFEA, 7 November 2000
5. Verhoeff A, Logmans A, Leerentveld RA, et al. Transport IVF and satellite transport IVF: one laboratory and several clinics, results of 860 ovum pick-ups. Hum Reprod 1992; 7: 160–1
6. Jansen CAM, Van Beek JJ, Verhoeff AATH, Zeilmaker GH. In vitro fertilisation and embryo transfer with transport of oocytes. Lancet 1986; 1: 676
7. Zarutskie PW, Kusan FB, More DE, et al. An in vitro fertilisation program using satellite physicians. Obstet Gynecol 1988; 72: 929–34
8. Roest J, Verhoeff A, van Lent M, et al. Results of decentralised in vitro fertilisation treatment with transport and satellite clinics. Hum Reprod 1995; 10: 563–7
9. De Sutter P, Dozortrsev D, Verhoeff A, et al. Transport ICSI: a cost-effective alternative to the 'ICSI-boom'. J Assist Reprod Genet 1996; 13: 234–7
10. Buckett WM, Fisch P, Dean NL, et al. In vitro fertilisation and ICSI pregnancies after successful transport of oocytes by air plane. Fertil Steril 1999; 71: 753–5
11. Royal College of Nursing. Transport IVF – guidelines for nurses working in units offering transport in vitro fertilisation. London: RCN, 1996
12. Milad M, Ball GD, Erickson LD, et al. A successful assisted reproductive technology satellite program. Fertil Steril 1993; 60: 716–19
13. Human Fertilisation and Embryology Authority. Code of Practice, 6th edn, 2003. Section 2.3;8.3;9.17. London: HFEA, 2003
14. Dorbohlav P, Huttelova R, Rezacova J, et al. Effect of oocyte transportation (IVF transport) program. Ceska Gynekol 1998; 63: 301–5

35

The distress of infertility: some thoughts after 22 years of infertility counseling

Tim Appleton

INTRODUCTION

Many couples postpone having a family for all sorts of reasons. Very often when they do decide that the time is right they discover that something is wrong. They see their friends becoming pregnant with the greatest of ease – but for them nothing happens! Others will postpone having a family for career, financial or social reasons. Then when the time seems right everything goes wrong. The friends, neighbors and other members of the family seem able to breed like rabbits and the childless couple is unable to share in their joy.

In this chapter I try and share some of my experiences over the years gained in the main from counseling at Bourn Hall Clinic from 1982 onwards. At that time treatment at Bourn Hall was on an in-patient basis, with the women staying in the wards for 14–21 days, and very often the husbands living in accommodation in the village. It was therefore very easy to spend two or three evenings each week talking with patients and listening to their anxieties and their hopes. Today, where treatment is on an out-patient basis, such regular and intense contact is not so easily possible, and counselors rely on referral by clinical staff, self-referral by patients or, in the case of donor-assisted treatments, as an integral part of the clinic protocol and required before treatment can proceed.

Coping with failure is difficult for everybody, patients, clinical staff and counselors alike. It is often difficult to face up to failure. We can be angry, confused, depressed and tearful. At other times tears are difficult to come when their presence, however embarrassing, may be therapeutic. I have often been guilty of inducing tears, either because of something I said (or Y did not say) or simply by passing the box of tissues when tears looked inevitable, and it is a humbling experience to be thanked when tears are flowing so freely. At the end of this chapter I offer some thoughts on 'coping with failure' by looking at a few cases.

THE PAIN OF INFERTILITY

Infertility is a major health-care problem which has very definite physiological, psychological, sociological and financial implications: in many countries state or insurance funding of infertility treatment is available on a limited basis, while other countries provide limited or even unlimited facilities. The World Health Organization defined infertility as 'a failure to conceive after unprotected intercourse for a period of one year'. A significant number of couples will still fail to conceive after 2 years, and it may be several years before a couple realizes that a problem exists. It has been estimated that between 5 and 9% of couples of child-bearing age in the UK have a problem in having a baby, with estimates of 50–80 million couples worldwide.

Very often the couple's general practitioner may have suggested that they 'keep on trying'. 'Try this...try that...' is the usual recommendation from doctor and well-meaning friends. What may have seemed 'convenient' in the early days of their relationship now becomes a nightmare. 'When are you two going to have a baby?' is a question they dread and try to avoid, to such an extent that they will avoid social events to protect themselves from distress. The prayers in the wedding service for the 'gift of children' and the injunction to 'be fruitful and multiply' are remembered with bitterness.

Couples suffering from infertility are continually reminded of their situation. Each month, when the woman menstruates, she experiences a sharp reminder that yet another month has gone by without any luck. The daily measurement of a woman's waking temperature, used as an indicator for the day of ovulation, becomes a sickening chore they dread. Our society is based on the family unit. Simple tasks that we take for granted become painful: almost every shop is stocked with goods for the baby or young family; the major stores proudly display their 'back to school' reminders, with displays of school uniforms, badges, satchels and useful kits for the classroom. The infertile couple is excluded from this ritual. They dodge the prams and pushchairs; they watch with envy the shopping trolley with the small child sitting at the back; they see the neighbor's washing line sagging under the weight of baby clothes; they watch their friends fill the car with all the paraphernalia that goes with a visit to the seaside or a day with grandma. The infertile couple is left out – they are on their own.

The stigma of infertility often leads to stress and tensions developing within the family[1].

Couples avoid their close friends. It can lead to mental disharmony, to marital and sexual problems, to divorce and, in some cultures, to ostracism from the wider family unit. The suffering is very real. A couple who experienced infertility and the eventual relief that successful treatment brought wrote in a letter to the *Daily Telegraph*[2]:

The sorrow of infertility for a happy couple can be compared with the sorrow of bereavement. The

'funeral' starts when a couple first learns the results of the tests which reveal that a problem exists. It continues with surges of hope that a miracle might happen. The sorrow is private, real, and often taboo; failure at any point is always painful.

The average general practitioner has little time or expertise to provide practical help to infertile couples. Advice 'to be patient' only prolongs the agony, until the time comes when they are too old to consider adoption and the likelihood of successful treatment at specialized clinics is becoming lower. The menopause seems just around the corner, and fears that the woman will 'run out of eggs' or that, if a pregnancy does occur, the child will be abnormal are only too common. Hopefully, society will be more aware of the scale of infertility and family doctors will refer couples for expert help earlier than in the past. It is not uncommon to meet couples who have been 'trying this and that' for 10–15 years – some even longer.

Some recent pages from *Child Chat*[3], the newsletter of the support group Child, had these comments from couples suffering from infertility:

Although it is mid-October, suddenly everybody is talking of Christmas, the shops are stocking up on and displaying their Christmas goods. For us Christmas is a very painful time and brings with it a feeling of dread. It only seems to heighten your childlessness. Although you enjoy buying and wrapping presents for the children of friends and relatives, a voice inside you is screaming – 'It's not fair . . . we should be doing this for our own children'.

Sometimes it is the reaction of society that shows a fundamental misunderstanding of some of the problems. We find it difficult to understand that someone who has had a child can be infertile. Infertility is a difficult subject to discuss at any time, but there is a certain understanding for those who never have had children.

When I tell people that I am infertile they cannot understand because I already have one child. When I explain the circumstances and that I am desperate to have another child, the usual reply is 'At least you do have a child – you should be thankful for that'. This gives me tremendous feelings of guilt for even wanting another, when some couples have none at all.

What we cannot tell from this letter is the reason for the woman's 'current' infertility. It is possible that there is now a failure to ovulate or that the condition of the Fallopian tubes has deteriorated. Perhaps she has developed antibodies to sperm or perhaps she was sterilized, but now regrets it because her husband has died and she has remarried. Perhaps the problem is not on her side at all but on her partner's side – poor sperm or perhaps none at all. Whatever the reason, it is clear that conception through intercourse appears impossible and her distress is very real. But, given the limited resources of a state-funded health service, someone must decide on priorities; that does not mean that we leave her without help: counseling is just as important for those who have reached the 'end of the road' as for those who do not know where to turn for help.

Other couples have expressed feelings of guilt for wanting a second child as a brother or sister to one born as a result of *in vitro* fertilization (IVF). Their guilt is not because they want a second child, but because they feel that they would be depriving the existing child if they bring it up as an 'only child'. They may have repeatedly tried further attempts at IVF without success. Their guilt about failing the existing child is in danger of being transferred onto that child. They are concentrating on their weakness rather than on their strengths. Infertility can dominate the lives of the infertile. One person confessed[3]:

> Sometimes, I just long to empty my head of all the feelings of hurt, resentment, shame, anger and bitterness that seems to build up inside me.

Many have found that their relationships with other couples are under strain; their friends have become pregnant when they themselves have failed. How can they continue with the friendship when there is awkwardness when they meet? Do they avoid each other, or skirt around the problems? Often the greater anxiety is with the lucky couple, and the unlucky ones cannot understand why they are being avoided. Some couples are able to cope with their infertility, come to terms with it, support each other and remain solidly together. Others have less strength in their relationship and find that they cannot be 'unified' in the absence of a child.

> Individuals, who during their younger years have seen their future selves not only as husbands or wives, but as parents, have to make tremendous psychological adjustments to their infertility. They face not only a loss of self as the kind of person they would have become, but loss of image as a family, and with it the kind of life they would have led.[4]

The new reproductive technologies that have resulted from the work which led to the birth of the first 'test-tube' baby on 25 July 1978 have raised new hopes for millions of infertile couples around the world. Throughout the world well over 1.3 million IVF babies have been born. In the UK alone it has been estimated that a million couples of child-bearing age suffer from infertility at any one time; the problem does not get smaller – it may even be getting larger. It is not just the 'high-tech' methods of treatment, such as IVF, which have benefited from this technology. A better understanding of the processes of human reproduction has meant that many of the simpler methods, such as timing of intercourse, artificial insemination and induction of ovulation using hormones and other drug therapies, have all improved.

Justice and equity suggest that all should have equal access to medical care, but this would stretch limited resources beyond what many find to be acceptable. Each new announcement in the press or on television brings hope to many, but for many others it will also potentiate their distress. The availability of treatment may have come too late for them: they have already reached the menopause, they may not be able to afford it or they may have doubts about whether such treatment is ethically or morally acceptable. The religious lobby frequently has a direct or indirect influence on their anxiety. Counseling can help individuals and couples to make adjustments to their life-styles, help them to maintain the strength in their relationships and equip them to make the choices that are right for them. It can also help them to empty out all those feelings of anxiety, hate, anger and dissatisfaction which can so easily build up in each of us. Sometimes it is enough that there is somebody who has the time and understanding and who is able to listen effectively – to allow the emotions to pour out. At other times, counseling in particular areas may need particular counseling skills, and we may need the humility to know when we should refer couples to somebody with more experience. A person who knows where to seek that help can be a very valuable member of any team treating the infertile. At the same time, if counselors have managed to develop a good relationship with a couple, it may be more effective for the counselor to seek advice than to refer the couple on to yet another person.

Counseling is a key element in the provision of any infertility service. Counseling should be distinct from discussions with a doctor of any treatment he proposes and should be carried out by somebody different, preferably by a qualified counselor[5].

The Warnock report[6] emphasized the need for counseling; it said:

> We recommend that counselling should be available to all infertile couples, and third parties, at any stage of the treatment, both as an integral part of the National Health Service provision and in the private sector. We recognize that there may not be sufficient counsellors trained in this field at present, but feel that it is possible for counsellors in other fields to adapt their skills to deal with infertility.

One of the main purposes of this chapter is to help those with experience in counseling methods to understand the clinical and scientific background to infertility and to help those who have a working knowledge of infertility to understand the role of counseling in this highly emotive area. The parish priest, teacher, social worker, family doctor and other community welfare workers are in a unique position to assist in the counseling role, particularly when a couple has to come to terms with their childlessness. At the same time, clinicians should not feel that their role is threatened by the involvement of the counselor. This chapter may help all who are concerned with infertility to understand the problems which infertile couples face and equip them with sufficient insight to join in that counseling role. We will often need to take on the care of those for whom treatment is not possible or for whom treatment has failed – failure is still more likely than success. They need support to help them to adjust to the realization that they have done everything in their power in exploring all the possibilities, and that perhaps the time has come to enable them to concentrate on other aspects of their lives.

A successful outcome does not necessarily imply successful clinical treatment. The role of counseling is to help people process their emotions and to arrive at a situation with which they feel comfortable and with which they can live a full life. We need continually to remind ourselves that we are treating 'people who are infertile' rather than just treating 'infertility'. That distinction should underline the point that care goes beyond clinical treatment. Often couples will bring with them other concerns, which may be a direct result of their infertility or be totally unrelated to it; these too must be our concern if and when they come to the surface. Counseling can be the means that will enable people to uncover those emotions which we all try to hide and which give rise to dissatisfaction and distress. At the same time, counselors must be aware that they could unintentionally add to the burdens by imposing on others anxieties which do not already exist.

Counseling must be informed to be effective, and can easily become a hindrance and a waste of time if it is uninformed or used without thorough experience in counseling skills and up-to-date knowledge of reproductive medicine. But what do we mean by counseling? The term is used in many different contexts. It is often taken as meaning 'I asked for their consent' or 'I told them the facts'.

Several important areas in infertility counseling have been identified:

(1) *Information counseling* is primarily the task of the clinical team, but experience has shown that patients do not always assimilate the information given at a clinical consultation or a chat with the nurse coordinator. Tension often erases much of the information which has been given, and, unless written explanations and instructions have been provided, many patients will not have fully digested what has been said. Infertility counselors need to be sensitive in detecting where the tensions shown by their patients are due to poor understanding of human reproduction. Many people will argue that coping with the flow of information is not the concern of counselors – yet a counselor who can fully understand the technology can swiftly remove many of the tensions by gentle explanation, which leads on naturally to some of the difficult stresses that need to be tackled.

(2) *Implications counseling* aims to enable people to understand the implications of taking proposed treatments, for themselves, their families and any children who might be born as a result. This will be particularly true of any donor-assisted treatments and with surrogacy. Implications counseling

will include the donor-related issues such as sperm, egg and embryo donation, egg sharing and surrogacy.

(3) *Support counseling* recognizes the emotional needs and the stress imposed by infertility treatment, drawing upon the patients' own resources. It does not seek to provide ready-made answers, but draws on the hidden strengths and resources of the patients.

(4) *Therapeutic counseling* seeks to help people cope with the consequences of treatment, helping them understand their expectations and resolving any problems, including the prospect of failure and adjusting to childlessness. It is doubtful whether any childless couple 'come to terms' with child-lessness – many dread the prospect. Counseling can, with time, help people adjust to that situation, with a gradual lowering of stress with time.

The Human Fertilisation and Embryology Authority (HFEA) requires clinics in the UK to take due regard of the future welfare and needs of any children resulting from licensed treatment. Some clinics ask the patients and family doctors to answer questions about any criminal records, problems with social services, psychiatric history, clinical depression, etc. before accepting them for treatment. Couples should also be aware that the *Code of Practice* of the HFEA requires that information about donors and those treated with those donors is recorded and kept by the Authority and that the child has a right to discover certain non-identifying information on reaching age 18, or on contemplating earlier marriage. From April 2005, in the UK, the child will have the right to know the identity of the donor. This might influence a couple's decision on whether to tell the child/children about the facts of their conception. There is a ground-swell of opinion throughout the world that this is the right approach. Time will tell whether it dissuades donors from coming forward.

These are certainly vital parts of a couple's rights, which certainly include education, support and infor-mation, and which are frequently well catered for by doctors, nurses, nurse counselors and other health-care professionals who come into contact with the patients. Those roles, while being important, are, I believe, quite different from the role of counselors. Many patients tell me that they miss a lot of information during

consultations; they are often confused and miss vital points of information through no fault of the doctor/nurse. So it is important that counselors ensure that these particular needs have been adequately catered for, since a considerable amount of distress is created by an inadequate understanding of the facts. Counselors also need to be independent, which may sometimes mean that they must pursue the 'cause of the patients', i.e. take their side in the pursuit of their 'peace of mind'.

Counseling does not ignore the obvious, but seeks to reach behind it. It requires the giving of sufficient time to help a person in distress to uncover and reach behind some of the less obvious and less acceptable feelings and thoughts which contribute to unhappi-ness and dissatisfaction. It is an approach which has isolated certain factors in caring relationships and stressed them, while at the same time played down other factors such as giving answers, expressing sym-pathy or actively trying to change the circumstances which appear to contribute towards that distress. It is above all an approach which tries to understand what goes on inside people, and how internal difficulties can stand in the way of change, rather than looking at external factors or external solutions[7].

We all have to learn to listen more carefully, so that we can help others more effectively. Counseling can only be really effective when we have heard the needs of each individual cry. There are no rigid formulae to follow: each cry will be different, each approach will be individual and a careful watch for body language may provide a valuable clue to the direction, or change of direction, which must be adopted. Counselors within a clinical situation must be a part of the team, so that they can listen to both patients and staff; they should be respected by that team, so that they can play their part in formulating new protocols as new advances are made. At the same time it is vital that the counselor keeps him/herself informed and up to date. It is only by informed counseling that we shall be able to 'seek behind the obvious'.

At one time, there was little that a childless couple could do to seek effective help; the new technologies have changed that. In the past the cause of infertility was always assumed to be the fault of the woman – that too has changed. We now know that male-factor infertility is the biggest single cause of infertility. Intra-cytoplasmic sperm injection (ICSI) has certainly revo-lutionized the treatment of male-factor infertility, but we should not lose sight of the simpler and often more accessible forms of treatment such as donor insemination. The additional 'interference factor' which micromanipulation imposes has led many couples to have to fight for what they feel is more realistic for them. IVF and ICSI is expensive and beyond the resources of many couples. Many men have expressed feelings of guilt because, although the problem lies with them, the suggested treatment imposes superovulation and egg collection on their partner. They have often reached a difficult point in coming to terms with the use of donor sperm, only to have that acceptance dashed by the understandable enthusiasm of the clinician to suggest a new 'solution' such as ICSI.

Childless women often share their problems with other women, but few men want to share their problems with other men, since infertility has been associated with impotence. In some cultures, childlessness is considered to be grounds for divorce. In many cultures it is the woman who is blamed, even when tests have clearly shown that there is a male 'factor' present.

Progress in the treatment of infertility has meant that we can tackle problems which seemed insurmountable just a decade ago. It has sounded alarm bells in our society and can add another level of decision-making for those who seek a family! Is technology moving ahead too fast, what does it all mean? Should we try yet another avenue when we were convinced we had explored every possibility? A couple searching the Internet will quickly find details of new advances: should we try blastocyst culture, is that the answer to our failure to succeed? Should we be considering preimplantation diagnosis and screening to sort out the good embryos from the bad, is aneuploidy screening raising its ugly head?

The introduction of embryo freezing in the early 1980s seemed to provide a solution to the creation of 'spare' embryos in IVF. Those who pioneered the new techniques predicted that the ability to freeze embryos would solve many problems; many couples would need all the embryos they could get; others might want to try for a sibling and 'space their family'. But reproductive medicine has advanced, and increasing success rates mean that the number of embryos going into the freezers exceeds the number being used after thawing. The embryo banks get bigger and bigger, and many couples have been faced with making desperate decisions about what to do with the embryos they no longer need. The law in the UK imposes a limit on the time that embryos can remain frozen. The first law that insisted on decisions was passed on 31 July 1996. Couples had to choose between:

(1) Using the embryos for themselves;

(2) Donating the embryos to another couple;

(3) Donating the embryos for research;

(4) Allowing the embryos to die;

(5) Continuing the storage for another 5 years, which was only possible with the consent of all parties and when the embryos were to be used for themselves.

In the absence of any of those decisions or loss of contact with couples, the embryos had to be destroyed after the storage interval of 5 years. For many the choices were too difficult, and many couples admitted to not being able to make a decision and hence left the decision to 'the law'. Those decisions are still no easier – they consider their embryos as potential babies.

We cannot ignore the concerns shown by different groups in our society about these issues, and we must be careful not to dismiss lightly the concerns of those which differ from our own; their concerns are often transferred to the couples who are seeking our help, and we may need to help them uncover those concerns. We need to use a pragmatic approach which puts modern technology into perspective, without forgetting the dreams of infertile couples. For some those dreams will be realized, but for many they will not come true. Our care and concerns must be for them all, not forgetting those for whom the treatment has been successful but who may still need support and counseling long into the future.

COPING WITH FAILURE: SOME EXPERIENCES FROM COUNSELING

We all have to cope with failure from time to time in our lives. Often failure is due to something we have done which results in things going wrong. At other times it is because we have failed to do something as effectively or thoroughly as we should have done. We may have failed our driving test, for example, because we pulled out in front of another driver who had the right of way, or we failed because we had not learnt the highway code. We can see where the fault lies and do something about it before the next attempt. Or it may have been plain bad luck because the examiner was in a bad mood. Whatever the cause it is probable that either we say it was bad luck, and that the chance of that happening again is slight, or we admit the fault and prepare for next time. Failure is transitory, and it is unlikely to dominate our lives. But there will be times when we may have to admit that we are not 'very good at some things'; we learn to be realistic in our expectations.

Patients who present themselves for treatment for subfertility do have very high expectations. Many clinics have found that patients' expectations of success are considerably higher than the success rates which were quoted at their initial consultation. There is a subconscious reluctance to admit that they might very well be among the unsuccessfully treated patients, although it is still clear that failure is more likely than success. Headlines which appear regularly in the press raise new expectations for those referred for treatment. A success rate of 25–40% means that the failure rate is still 60–75%.

No one likes to think about failure when embarking on a new venture. There can be very few medical programs where emotions are so highly charged and where the failure rate consistently exceeds the success rate. It is the duty of all concerned with assisted reproduction programs to be realistic with themselves and with their patients. Many couples will not be able to cope with the prospect of failure and we should help them to consider the alternatives, including adoption and coming to terms with childlessness. Treatment can fail at many stages: induction of ovulation, oocyte retrieval, fertilization, cleavage and implantation. Failure is potentiated by all that IVF demands of the person, financially and emotionally, and courage and determination. The Human Fertilisation and Embryology Authority recognizes a need for 'therapeutic counseling' to help couples through failure, including coming to terms with childlessness.

Failure is often easier to bear when we can pinpoint a reason for that failure, if we are expecting it or if we have been prepared for it. A couple's second reaction may be one of grief, shame, anger or other emotion which may not express itself in words. There is often a very real sense of grief surrounding failure. Something which was very much alive has died. In grieving, a person needs time to lick over their wounds, but within the confines of a crowded clinic

many will try to suppress their emotions. Anger is often suppressed but comes to the surface in other ways. Sometimes the anger is directed at others because they feel inadequate; often it is directed towards the self – a feeling that they have let somebody down. A man who had just heard that the eggs had not fertilized said:

I feel so angry at myself. My wife was the one who had to have all the injections, had to have the operation to recover the eggs – mine was the easy part – now I have let her down, I feel so angry.

It may be tempting to shrug off such emotions and to sympathize, when what is being asked for is help in resolving that anger, even perhaps by confronting them with it. Counselors will be tempted to hold back when we should speak, bringing the pain into the open.

A colleague asked me to see a couple who felt that they might not be able to cope with the stress of the IVF program. They had experienced a series of miscarriages. After listening to them for some time it became clear that both were 'putting on a brave face' for each other. Something I said brought floods of tears to the woman and a very obvious expression of hostility from the man, which nearly resulted in violence. It was the woman who restrained her husband and then both were able to admit that this was the first time they had allowed their grief to find expression, and that they needed to be able to mourn the loss of those pregnancies.

There will be many times when counselors feel completely helpless. What can they possibly do or say which will help a person in despair? One reaction is to talk too much in the hope that some 'solution' will present itself. It is at times like this when one is reminded of the saying: 'make sure that the brain is operating before engaging the mouth'. Just being there with a person in distress, waiting, being prepared to listen, sharing in that helplessness, may often be the best support we can give – waiting together for the anxiety to drop. One of the most effective ways of coping with stress is to talk about it.

We have already seen that it is much easier to cope with failure when we can see a definite reason for that failure, or when we see ways in which we can directly influence that situation by our own actions. It is much more difficult to turn failure into success either when circumstances are beyond our control or where there is no clearly definable reason why treatment is classed as a failure. Much will depend on our perception of the word failure. That perception may well be very different for those who are supplying the treatment to the patients and for those who are being treated. Those providing treatment in assisted reproduction must be careful not to transfer their perception of failure onto their patients. What may be a disappointment to the clinician/scientist (and which may clearly affect their statistics) may be the starting point where a couple is able to move forward in a positive way, even though the starting point is one of failure.

It may help to look at some actual cases.

Case 1

A couple treated by IVF in a private clinic could only afford one cycle of treatment. Three eggs were retrieved, all three fertilized and showed normal cleavage, and three embryos were replaced. Unfortunately a pregnancy did not result. They were obviously disappointed but some time later phoned to say that at least they knew that his sperm had successfully fertilized her eggs. They felt that they had done all within their limited financial resources, and they could now accept the situation and concentrate on their love for each other. They felt that they would have been unable to move forward if they had not 'given it a go'. They would always have regretted not having tried.

It would have been very easy to start discussing the 'next moves' with them on day 15 when they had heard the human chorionic gonadotropin (hCG) results: to talk with them about the statistical chances of success, that nature on its own achieves a success rate of only 25%, to suggest that it might be worth trying again and so on, when what they really needed was time to come to terms with the situation and to have someone who would listen and wish them well. I am sure that they would always retain some element of regret, but it was a decision which they could live with.

There is often considerable merit in delaying decisions after experiencing failure. This is particularly so when a couple have just heard the results of a drastic sperm count, or that fertilization has failed; they need time together, to recover from the shock, before even contemplating the next step, particularly if this is likely to involve the use of donor sperm. A deliberate break enables them to talk things through in the privacy of

their own surroundings so that they can approach counseling having discussed most of these issues themselves. Our task as counselors is one of reassurance and re-enforcement.

Case 2

A couple who had had six IVF treatment cycles, without any signs of success, had made a remark in passing: 'If we are to continue we shall have to sell the house, and buy something smaller, to raise the money for further treatment'. It was at this point when I felt that a thorough review of the situation was required, and invited them to meet on a Saturday away from the clinic, in either their home or mine. They chose to visit me, and in the event that was a 'lucky' choice. Very often the clinical environment can be intimidating.

After reviewing their previous cycles of treatment with them (and previously with a clinical colleague) it seemed to me that perhaps one partner was very much keener to continue with treatment than the other; I was still not sure who was the keener. After struggling for some time I put it to them quite bluntly: 'Are you really keen to continue? When was the last time you really talked this over between yourselves? It seems to me that the drive to continue is much stronger in one of you!'

I suggested that I should take our dogs for a walk and leave them together for a while - hence the 'lucky choice' of venue; the dogs played a vital part.

On returning I was met with a smiling couple who put my mind at rest. He had been pressing her to continue because he felt that it was his duty to provide the financial resources to make it possible, while she was acquiescing because she felt that she should support her husband's 'determination'. Both were relieved to know that the other was fed up with continuing and wanted to 'get on with the rest of their lives'.

It would have been very easy to persuade them that there was no reason why they might not eventually be successful, for there was no clinical reason which obviously precluded that option. We can all quote instances when the reverse would be true; when we have been tempted to suggest that 'enough is enough'; it is becoming an obsession; that surely ten attempts really was enough. Then something inside me (call it helplessness, intuition, a still small voice) made me keep my mouth shut and a healthy baby was born in the next cycle. It would have equally been easy to persuade that couple to give it all up. What was important was that they made the decision for themselves and were keen to move forward.

Case 3

A couple who had been through several IVF cycles without a pregnancy had asked to have an opportunity to review their situation with a senior clinician and a counselor. We both spent some time with the couple not knowing what their decision would be. After some months we received these comments from the woman:

> I have decided not to go ahead with treatment... since our meetings I have thought hard and long, talking with my husband, family and friends – frequently hopelessly muddled. I believe we have reached a resolution with which I can live... it is a positive and life-enhancing decision involving a recommitment to my work as a teacher, and a channeling of my energies towards a strength rather than a weakness.

This is a strong reminder that we often receive strength after having struggled through weakness. It is not often that I use biblical quotations, but St Paul in his Second Letter to the Corinthians said:

> I am content with my weakness, and with insults and hardships, persecutions and agonies I go through... For it is when I am weak that I am strong.

The role of counseling is not to tell patients what to do but to help them process their own emotions by providing them with the time, space and a suitable environment. There are no easy answers, no quick panaceas.

Case 4

A woman who had been through five IVF cycles without a pregnancy phoned to say that they were not pursuing further treatment. They had found that they would never regret having tried and the experience had brought them closer together. They did not want IVF to dominate their lives and felt that they would try to adopt a baby or toddler who could benefit from the stronger love they now experienced. They did not feel that they had failed at all.

No one can claim credit for decisions such as theirs, except to hope that somewhere and at some time during our contacts with them we may have been able to help them to make their own decisions, and it does not matter that we are unable positively to make that assertion or not.

On many occasions we may only discover that we have been of some assistance sometime later when a chance remark, 'I would never have continued if you had not helped me through that terrible time', encourages the counselor to continue. At other times we will never know. We cannot quantitate it, we cannot judge its cost-effectiveness; we will never be able to attach a 'productivity figure' against the time we spend in counseling. That should not matter. Common humanity suggests that we do everything in our power to help people in their distress.

COUNSELING GUIDELINES

ESHRE, the European Society of Human Reproduction and Embryology, have drawn up some useful guidelines in infertility counseling.

In September 1999, 15 delegates from seven countries came together to discuss counseling issues in infertility. Discussions in this and subsequent meetings produced a document entitled 'Guidelines for counselling in infertility', which aimed to describe key aspects of psychosocial care for individuals using assisted reproduction. The Guidelines were intended for both medical and mental-health professionals, and it was hoped that the information contained in the Guidelines would help maintain good practice with regard to psychosocial care among diverse professional groups. The Guidelines have been accepted by the Executive Committee of the European Society of Human Reproduction and Embryology as an official document, and have been published[8].

These Guidelines are headline suggestions which should form a framework for counseling. They are not and never were intended to be an authoritative definition of counseling in infertility.

REFERENCES

1. Appleton T. Counselling in Assisted Conception; An Analysis of Counselling 768 Patients between December 1988 and August 1991. Cambridge, UK: IFC Resource Centre, 1992

2. Henderson H. [Adapted from a letter to the] Daily Telegraph 6 June 1985

3. Child Chat, Issue No. 42, 1989. [The Magazine of CHILD, part of Infertility Network UK, 43 St Leonards Road, Bexhill on Sea, Sussex, UK

4. Brebner C. [Psychiatrist, quoted by Thomas Prentice, Science Correspondent of] The Times, 8 April 1986

5. UK Government White Paper, Human Fertilisation and Embryology; A Framework for Legislation. Presented by the Secretary of State for Social Services, Cm. 259. London: HM Stationery Office, November 1987

6. Warnock M (Chairman). Report of the Committee of Enquiry into Human Fertilization and Embryology. Presented by the Secretary of State for Social Services, Cm. 9314. London: HM Stationery Office, July 1984

7. Jacobs M. Still Small Voice. London: SPCK, 1982

8. Boivin J, Kentenich H. eds. Guidelines for counseling in infertility. ESHRE Monographs. Oxford, UK: Oxford University Press, 2002

36

Ethical aspects of assisted conception and the law

Françoise Shenfield

INTRODUCTION

As the first child from *in vitro* fertilization (IVF) is now over 25 years old, several ethical dilemmas linked to the field continue to be subjected to the world's scrutiny. The many questions raised can be split into two groups. The first may be described as encompassing 'essential' problems, because they pertain intrinsically to the essence of IVF (as in the status of the embryo *in vitro* and embryo research), or because they relate to techniques directly stemming from the ability to visualize and use the human embryo *in vitro* (such as the more recent preimplantation embryo manipulations, with all aspects of preimplantation genetic diagnosis (PGD) and therapeutic cloning). The second group relates to other dilemmas less directly linked to the nature of the embryo, but still in the realm of assistance to reproduction, such as gamete donation, reproductive tissue freezing or the avoidance of multiple pregnancy, which is the commonest complication of assisted reproductive treatments.

These 'microethical' issues should also be seen in the larger 'macroethical' context, with the problems of access to fertility treatment[1], unequal as it is worldwide, and the responsibility we owe to children from assisted conception. This includes their safety, a subject of relevance for instance in intracytoplasmic sperm injection (ICSI) with the possible transmission of sex

chromosome anomalies[2], which in particular might threaten the future fertility of the male child of an ICSI couple, and certainly the aforementioned problem of multiple pregnancies. Indeed, the notion of our responsibility to the future child is never far from our concerns, and could serve as a linking theme to all specific questions described here. Finally, we must note that the choice made here is necessarily somewhat eclectic, as even books dedicated to the issues cannot hope to be exhaustive[3,4].

THE DILEMMAS CENTERING AROUND THE STATUS OF THE EMBRYO

Embryo research

Embryo research is necessary for the continued improvement of assisted reproduction techniques, such as IVF, and was one of the most contentious fields when it began. Such were the emotions concerning the matter that a famous semantic debate took place, which, to many, seemed to obscure the matter further. The use of the term pre-embryo, or 'the stage of the conceptus for the interval from the completion of the process of fertilisation until the establishment of biologic individuation'[5], led to controversy and suspicion

589

that its human essence was deliberately being somewhat ignored or lessened by this prefix[6]. What status we feel a human embryo has, both in our psyche and for society in general, may or may not be reflected in national laws and international codes. Indeed, the *Convention for the Protection of Human Rights and Dignity of the Human Being with Regard to the Application of Biology and Medicine* (Convention on Human Rights and Biomedicine)[7], Article 18, concerns embryo research, and it is difficult to believe that anyone would object to the first part of the article (18.1: 'Where the law allows research on embryos *in vitro*, it should ensure adequate protection of the embryo'). However, debates abound about article 18.2, which states: 'The creation of embryos for research purposes is prohibited', the meaning of which has recently taken on a new dimension, with hopes about the possible therapeutic applications of stem cell research.

Only two examples of European legislation need to be recalled as symbolic of this potential disagreement. The first is the UK Human Fertilisation and Embryology Act (1990)[8], which allowed controlled embryo research within five specific categories (promoting advances in the treatment of infertility, increasing knowledge about the causes of congenital disease and causes of miscarriages, developing more effective techniques of contraception, or methods for detecting the presence of gene or chromosome abnormalities in embryos before implantation); new categories were added in 2001 in order to accommodate embryonic stem cell (ESC) research[9].

A contrasting example comes from France, where the 'bioethics' law of 1994[10] prohibited embryo research, unless it was 'therapeutic', and allowed undefined 'studies'. The latter was so difficult to interpret that it led to a standstill in research in France. A delayed revision, which was finally passed by the French Parliament in summer 2004, allows stem cell research as an exception to the same rule. However, an opposite example of this is the recent Italian legislation, passed in 2004[11], which totally forbids research, as well as cryopreservation and gamete donation. As far as the European bioethics convention is concerned, there is a clause that permits countries where legislation is already in place to be signatories of the convention, whilst claiming partial dissent to some specific points which are in contradiction with their national legislation, as would be the case for the UK, where it is not forbidden to create embryos for research.

Some have the view that the embryo has the same (symbolic) value as a child, indeed, that it is a person. This is one of the moral dilemmas that have led to many ethical and legal debates. The views of most scientists would be fairly represented by Professor Egozcue's qualification of the conceptus as an 'individual of a certain kind', whose protection, rather than nature, must be a matter for the state[12]. For many, however, the human embryo deserves respect because of its human 'potential' and kinship. Indeed, this very notion of respect is enshrined in both the French legislation of 1994 (law 94-654 concerns 'respect of the human body and its products'), and the Human Fertilisation and Embryology Act (1990). The British Act caused the Human Fertilisation and Embryology Authority (HFEA) to be set up, whose *Code of Practice* spells out that respect of the embryo is 'fundamental to the Act'[13], and sets a time limit of 14 days or the appearance of the neural plate for invited research, for which the consensus is internationally far-reaching. This does not reflect so much the principle of graduation and potentiality, but rather a compromise between varied interests, as in fact a 14-day embryo *in vitro* loses its potential to become a person, and thus could arguably be experimented upon (more easily) than a younger one[14].

If one accepts that embryo research is permissible, a further problem arises: the source of embryos for research. One might consider abandoned embryos, or those created for the purpose of study in IVF cycles. In the former case, by definition, there would not be any formal consent to research, as legally required, by the gamete donors. This path might be preferred by utilitarians who would consider the final aim to be a benefit in itself, but one that is impossible to contemplate if one respects consent as a paramount symbol of the autonomy of the donor of the gametes which society, in the form of the law, has deemed to be a superior interest.

The question of the nature of the embryo has also given rise to a complex debate in the United States, after the report of the National Institutes of Health (NIH) Embryo Research Panel endorsed preimplantation embryo research on the grounds that it offers potential benefits to infertile couples, and because the pre-embryo 'does not have the same moral status as infants or children'.

From 'therapeutic' to 'reproductive' cloning

Some of the issues concerning therapeutic cloning are similar to those of embryo research. The application to human reproduction, either theoretical or fantastic, of somatic cell cloning, which led to the birth of Dolly the sheep[15], has arguably been one of the biggest international media events, even in an area that has been replete with headlines in the past few years. All over the world, politicians and institutions have convened special meetings and asked august bodies to reflect on, or to pronounce on, the implications of this experiment in cloning, which was successful only to the extent that one of 277 embryos achieved a birth. As was made clear in the report of the British Science and Technology Parliamentary Commission, research on cloning may be a model for learning more about somatic cell differentiation or for obtaining targeted cell types of value in transplantation. However, what has recently shaken public opinion is the assertion from the USA that cloning is currently being performed to help sterile couples have their own genetic children. In the UK, the Human Fertilisation and Embryology Act (1990) clearly bans reproductive cloning, and the statutory instruments of 2001 make this a criminal offense. The very notion of reproductive cloning has led to an almost universal reaction of rejection. For instance, the report to the French President by the French National Ethics Committee (CCNE)[16] warns that personal (including psychological) identity and genetic identity are not to be confused, but stresses that cloning would totally disrupt their relationship and balance. Nevertheless, the notion of respect for the uniqueness of the person, whilst necessary, is not sufficient to justify the quasi-universal rejection of the planned replication of human beings. This is why we must add consideration of the social and psychological dimension of the individual, and where we return to the notion of responsibility towards the vulnerable party – the child-to-be. At the European level, the report of the Group of Advisers on the Ethical Implications of Biotechnology to the European Union (GAIEB)[17] is clear indeed: as there is no discrimination against identical twins *per se*, it follows that there can be no *per se* objection to genetically identical human beings. Human reproductive cloning is unacceptable on the grounds of risk (responsibility is underlined), instrumentalization and eugenics. Finally, a recent addendum to the Council of Europe Convention on Human Rights and Biomedicine banning reproductive cloning spells out a ban on 'any intervention seeking to produce genetically identical human individuals, in the sense of individuals sharing the same nuclear gene set' (Art 13-b)[18].

Overall, the strongest argument against cloning seems to be instrumentalization of the future child, and the burden of a narcissistic quest of an adult for self-reproduction, imposed on a new being who would have more than his/her share of predetermination.

Preimplantation genetic diagnosis

Preimplantation genetic diagnosis embryology triggers the fear of potential genetic manipulation, and is often considered, irrationally, to be on the slippery slope to all kinds of criminal eugenics[19]. Other fears concern phantasmagoric perversions of heredity, or at least poorly controlled intrusions into the genome of germ-line cells. The most complex ethical question is not so much the current practice of PGD, but rather what might be the consequences of its evolving techniques. Will couples demand, after PGD, the assurance of a 'perfect' baby? This question begs the definition of perfection, and its satisfactory integration into a society which may be richer from more variety. It was raised recently by Testard and Sele[20], who discuss the 'production of survivors of this choice, escapees and obligatory servants of an ideology of performance and exclusion', with the danger of exclusion of handicapped people, and 'a more and more restrictive definition of normality and humanity'. If eugenics is defined as a practice imposed on a population, and not individual couples' choice to achieve the potential for a healthy life of some of their embryos, this accusation can be contradicted[21].

A grave dilemma in the carer–patient relationship concerns the reluctance that most practitioners would feel when faced with a parental request to sort out, at the time of PGD for severe genetic disease, embryos also carrying genes associated with diseases which, although serious, are amenable to treatment, such as diabetes or cardiovascular disease. This semantic problem of the definition of a 'serious' (potential) handicap leads us to question further the gray area between prevention, avoidance and eradication of handicap, and also applies to prenatal diagnosis.

591

PGD and HLA matching

A new dilemma is that of choosing by PGD an embryo free of a disease which may also become a child who would be a human leukocyte antigen (HLA) match (European Society of Human Reproduction and Embryology (ESHRE) Ethics and Law Taskforce 9)[22]. The main argument against this kind of request is instrumentalization of the future child. But the endangered well-being of the existing sibling serves as the compelling reason to accept the technique. Even from the point of view of the future child, it may be seen as beneficial to be able to save its sibling as a matter of solidarity. Sensitive counseling may help the parents to foresee difficult events, for instance the failure of the initial aim: what if the planned child does not save the life of the elder sibling; how can the guilty feelings be assuaged in a situation where good will was assumed on behalf of a future person left necessarily with some grief feelings?

In practice, it must be emphasized, for instance, that cord blood donation is only possible if the affected child weighs less than 25 kg. In a recent publication[23], a series of 13 cycles was reported, where 199 embryos were created, with five singletons born after 28 embryos were replaced in 12 cycles.

Another problem is that of the acceptability of the motive for the selection of embryos; in this instance, the 'postnatal test' is useful, as it states that it is ethically acceptable to enable the birth of a child by PGD/HLA who can be used for a certain goal – if it is acceptable to use an existing child for the same goal, i.e. if it is acceptable to volunteer an existing child for stem cell donation to a sibling, it is acceptable to enable this birth by PGD/HLA. But adults' self-interest is not acceptable, i.e. not for parents themselves.

With the welfare of the future child and of 'any living child' in mind, one has to prove that the benefits to the receiving sibling whose life can be saved outweigh the disadvantages (if any) for the future child. It is felt that this solution is morally acceptable if the use of the child as a donor is not the only motive for the parents to have the child. This condition obviates the Kantian argument against using someone as a mere instrument, as it is the word 'mere' which is important. However, parental motivation is particularly difficult to assess[24], and thus the postnatal test is preferred, as long as the parents 'intend to love and care for this [future] child to the same extent as they love and care for the affected child' (Taskforce 5)[25]. This particularly applies to two different cases which may arise: the child conceived by PGD and embryo transfer (ET) is also at risk of the genetic disease affecting the older sibling, or this future child has no such risk and PGD is solely performed for HLA typing. This was illustrated in the UK by two cases, which were subjected to intense societal discussion via the media: those of the Hashmi and Whitaker families.

In the UK, each PGD case must be licensed by the HFEA. The Hashmis' request was accepted, as they wished for an embryo to be matched to their son, seriously ill with thalassemia, for whom all other treatment had become ineffective. However the Whitakers' request was refused, because their sick child suffered from Diamond–Blackfan anemia, a disease which is mostly non-genetic, and thus the future planned child was not at risk of this condition and would be planned perhaps 'merely' to save the older sibling. Another important criterion is the operation planned for the future child. The creation of a child for the purpose of harvesting non-regenerating organs seems extremely difficult to justify in view of the risks involved for the donor child. It seems acceptable if the future child's operation involves minimal risk (e.g. cord blood or bone marrow donation).

The benefits also include 'family welfare' in the wider sense, where the family at large is seen as an entity, which benefits from solidarity between its members.

OTHER DILEMMAS

Gamete donation and anonymity of donors

Sperm donation obviously antedates oocyte donation as a treatment option. Whilst there are undoubtedly differences between both the attitudes and the motivations of male and female gamete donors, and the latter are scarcer, they share several fundamental problems. In this field, the main ethical questions have centered around the question of paying for gametes, anonymity, secrecy and, more recently, the duties we owe to the (generous) donors. With the conviction that the human body and its parts and products should remain *res extra commercium*, as stated in the bioethics convention of the Council of Europe, an argument will be made against what some have held to be a pragmatic attitude in an environment of scarce supply (especially in the case of oocytes), thus allowing some type of financial inducement. It is easy to point out that a gift, by definition, implies no payment[26], but the argument is based mainly on the notion of respect for the person. Without entering the very complex debate regarding the meaning of 'personhood', the special quality of respect due to the person was most cogently articulated over 200 years ago by Immanuel Kant in formulation of the categorical imperative: 'to treat all humanity always at the same time as an end and never merely as a means', the symbol of the rational mind. Trading and buying persons (as in slavery) or 'products' (i.e. organs or gametes) entails treating the person or products as mere means and are thus demeaning, an affront to the respect due to human beings (and, for Kant, also to reason). This must also be placed in the context of another formulation, 'that one should only act according to principles which can be applied universally', and thus it allows no exception.

Furthermore, the utilitarian argument was also cogently refuted in the context of blood donation. In a scarce supply environment, Titmuss identified negative consequences in the context of blood donation, to be contrasted with the obvious positive side-effect of a probable increase of supply[27]. The problems encountered might be: the discouragement of voluntary donors, the increased risk of transmitting disease by donors motivated by gain only and willing to falsify information, and potential exploitation of the weakest socioeconomic groups of society. If one replaces the word 'blood' by 'gametes', the arguments obviously stand.

Exploitation can have many guises, and one is coercion, even if it is subtle. Currently, the 'benefits' in kind allowed by the HFEA for female donors in exchange for their gift of oocytes include 'treatment services' (sometimes in the form of a discount in IVF cost in the private sector) and 'sterilization': are these a form of coercion to donate, are they a form of payment or are they an acceptable 'exchange'? This arrangement stems from the fact that most oocyte donation and IVF procedures are not available in the UK within the National Health Service (NHS). The motivation of solidarity of subfertile patients might be a powerful incentive in the case of treatment services.

A very topical concern recently has been that of the traditional anonymity of gamete donors. The results of the Swedish experiment, which in 1985 recruited donors willing to identify themselves to the offspring, are up until now reassuring with regard to the supply of sperm donors, but uncertainty remains about whether the parents are more open with their offspring. Part of the basis for the Swedish stance stems from arguments in favor of 'the right of the child' to know about his/her 'origins' (the precise term used in the HFEA *Code of Practice*), and the potentially divisive effect of secrets in families. Plans now exist in Sweden to inform children thus conceived at their 'maturity', and we await with interest the findings of this social experiment. Finally, we must also allude to our duties towards gamete donors, a subject arguably long-neglected, and consider respect for their interests and confidentiality, which may clash with the desire for more knowledge of the recipient and future children. A possible solution may lie in the 'double track' policy suggested by Pennings[28], in which two groups of donors would be recruited – those willing to be identified and those wishing to stay anonymous. This path was effective in The Netherlands, but has now been relinquished there. In the UK it was announced in January 2004 that from April 2005 the same policy as in Sweden will be implemented. Transition times are always both fascinating and difficult, and it remains to be seen whether the number of gamete donors, especially egg 'sharers', is going to be affected. Needless to say, this change of policy shows the need for even more thorough and complex implications counseling of all concerned.

THE PREVENTION OF MULTIPLE PREGNANCIES

The need to consider this problem is the consequence of the progressive increase in incidence of multiple pregnancies of a high order (three or more) in all industrialized countries as a result of the increased use of ovulation induction and assisted reproduction techniques. The untoward effects of these multiple pregnancies stem from both the consequent prematurity of the babies born and the psychological upheaval for the parents. Embryo reduction has been accepted and recognized as a medical means of preventing these complications, but is not without its intrinsic problems, especially the high emotional cost to a couple to terminate (part of) a much wanted pregnancy. The rationale for the reduction stems from a 'consequentialist' approach – the lesser of two evils – where both parents and practitioner balance the benefits and risks from either keeping or reducing a high-order multiple pregnancy. If this cost–benefit analysis is clear in the case of triplets (and higher-order) pregnancies, in terms of both mortality and morbidity, it is still a grave ethical dilemma, with two main aspects. First, there are the intrinsic problems of termination of pregnancy, which have been discussed from time immemorial in all societies, and have been translated into legislation reflecting the more modern tolerance of the procedure in the last part of the 20th century. The second aspect, intrinsic to the reduction rather than the termination of pregnancy, revolves around the conflict of interest between the mother-to-be or the potential parents and the 'fetal siblings'[29]. The unease aroused by the procedure has been exemplified by the semantic arguments around its denomination. 'Selective birth' was the term used in 1981 to describe the outcome of a selective twin termination in a case of abnormality. Later, this procedure was called 'selective termination' in Anglo-Saxon countries, and 'selective abortion' or 'selective feticide' in France. As the choice of which fetus to reduce is purely technical, it is clear that no selection is involved in the process, and thus the terms 'embryo reduction' or 'multiple pregnancy reduction' are more accurate. This has been the subject matter of one of ESHRE's Taskforces in Ethics and Law: 'the aim of ART should be the birth of a live, as healthy as possible, singleton child, and all other results should be described as complications of the technique'[30].

GAMETES AND REPRODUCTIVE TISSUE STORING, AND THEIR USE IN SICKNESS AND HEALTH

Since the case of Diane Blood[31], it behoves all of us to reflect on a major problem, which can only loom larger and larger in the years to come, that is, posthumous assisted reproduction. This subject is especially fraught with psychological components, as it involves the cryopreservation of reproductive gametes or tissues in people often suffering from life-threatening disease (ESHRE Taskforce 7)[32]. It is especially complex and sensitive in the case of adolescents suffering from cancer, the treatment of which threatens their future reproductive capacity. Reproduction is not a matter

which they or their peers are accustomed to consider when they themselves are faced with the possibility of storing gametes or tissue. They are facing serious disease, if not possible death, and they are often under the age of consent to medical treatment, although often 'Gillick competent', but it is generally good practice to involve the parents in these sensitive decisions. The main problem, which may soon be resolved owing to swift progress in the field, revolves around the consent to be given by the child and/or the parents. Is this to therapy or to research? This may further be complicated by the fact that, in the case of ovarian biopsy, it may be a fairly risky procedure in a relatively sick adolescent girl, much more so than sperm donation or testicular biopsy is for a boy. We face a situation where the intent and the consent of the child or adolescent concerned may not be identical, where one could not be presumed to take place of the other. About 15% of treatments for childhood and adolescent cancer carry a substantial risk to future fertility. Until the advent of IVF and related techniques, the only alternative to forgoing one's future reproductive ability was, for the male, the cryopreservation of sperm prior to treatment. The first concern is of a psychological nature. Whilst the burden of the disease process is often reflected in the compliance problems many children and adolescents experience, children often assume that offers are prescriptive, and may view an offer to consider the possibility of storing gametes or gamete tissue as a 'must' rather than a 'may'. The more recent possibility of preserving the reproductive potential of women was followed with intense media exposure after presentation of the first successful follicular development in autografted previously cryopreserved ovarian tissue[33] and the first live delivery from the same techniques[34]. Testicular tissue freezing may be offered to young boys who do not produce sperm in their ejaculate, but in both cases there are risks, and the turning point between research and accepted practice may be exactly where we now stand.

Furthermore, there is, in the field of cryopreservation, an inherent inequality due to the unsatisfactory results and technical difficulties in freezing female gametes and ovarian tissue. Thus, whilst the treatment of males - or the repair, in the psychoanalytical sense, of a couple's infertility - by artificial insemination of frozen–thawed sperm is current practice, it may be argued that cryopreservation of prepubertal testicular and ovarian tissue is still research, whether later gametes are matured *in vitro* or *in vivo*, or tissues auto-grafted. The consent one needs to obtain from the patient is thus of a different kind[35], being further complicated by the distinction between therapeutic or non-therapeutic research. The definition of therapeutic research is one which would benefit the patient, which is the case in our dilemma. But this is usually understood as a more or less immediate benefit for a current condition, and not for possible applications in the future as a consequence of current treatment for a non-life-threatening disease.

The duty of care of staff involved is first to the child. What if the autonomy of the child and of the parents, caring adults, conflict, as they may, for instance, when the parents are keen for their child to undergo a procedure, implying either actual treatment of the present condition, or in order to protect future fertility, and the child refuses? Meanwhile, whilst it is still difficult to freeze oocytes[36], and there is no certainty that ovarian tissue may in the future be usable routinely to obtain gametes or as an autograft, adult women or parents have enquired whether oocytes could be stimulated and fertilized *in vitro* and frozen as embryos. Specific ethical dilemmas are linked to the freezing of embryos themselves, with regard especially to the duration of cryopreservation and their ultimate fate. This is complicated by the use of donor sperm, yet another complex decision, usually made within the context of a couple where the male sterility is absolute and incurable, although by no means exclusively. Here again, different legislative approaches to the treatment of single women reflect different ethical appraisals of the reproductive rights of women and the welfare or interest of the child-to-be, including the need for a father, as stated in the HFEA *Code of Practice*.

Finally, if the child eventually dies of the initial disease (as do 40% of total body irradiation patients), or suffers a recurrence or secondary cancer before even being in a relationship, provisions must be made to deal with the outcome of frozen gametes or tissue. Might the parents be allowed any access to the gametes, which represent the only life-potential of a dead child, in a time of overwhelming grief? One might argue that the concept of procreation totally outside a couple and decided by future grandparents, rather than parental figures, does not seem to be compatible with the need to consider the welfare of the child, as required both by the Human Fertilisation and Embryology Act (1990) and by the spirit of the Chil-

dren's Act (1989)[37], which places emphasis on parental responsibility rather than parental rights.

CONCLUSION

Among all the problems discussed, a true libertarian would argue that society and the professions involved are interfering with the autonomy of the future parents, informed consenting adults, by restricting their choice to have several embryos replaced, or to have oocyte donation at a very advanced age, for instance. However, if the notion of responsibility is as dear to us personally and to society as it is to Hans Jonas, who made it the key to his ethical theory by citing as a paradigm the case of parents' responsibility towards their children and future generations[38], we can find in this a common thread, which is indeed included in the British legislation as an injunction 'to take into account the welfare of the child' when offering licensed fertility treatment. This concept, together with concerns about exploitation, reflected by a purely 'market' approach to the means of treatment, outlines the common ground for the different dilemmas and also transcends national borders. Possible exploitation is illustrated in the case of surrogacy, for instance. Recent public controversy in response to allegations of large payments for 'expenses' to the surrogate mother have led the Department of Health to issue a public consultation document. The issues are similar to some discussed in relation to gamete donation (danger of coercion and exploitation), but the matter is further complicated by the fact that the surrogacy agreement is a contract which is unenforceable in law[39].

The common thread of responsibility also runs through the problem of sex selection for social reasons, which takes us back to our duty to future generations. Selection for gender is a good example of how the use of technology may be distorted; for example, ultrasound diagnosis for sex detection followed by termination of pregnancy has replaced infanticide in some parts of the world[40], and may in the future itself be replaced by the innocuous method of sperm sorting. When lack of discrimination on the grounds of sex is included in human rights declarations, it is worth wondering whether the acceptance of social sex selection does not reinforce the very attitudes one seeks to prevent. Discrimination still prevails under many guises, such as preferential education and medical treatments for sons rather than daughters in many poor societies, continuing the same vicious cycle. Equal respect of the sexes renders the means used for the purpose irrelevant.

Finally, the interests of future generations include the difficult dilemma presented by the need for surveillance of children resulting from the new techniques. This may give answers about the risk and possible long-term consequences of the newer procedures such as PGD, whilst trying to respect the confidentiality and privacy of the parents and avoid stigmatization of the children. This, in the end, may only be achieved by a sensitive approach to the solidarity between present and future generations.

At both personal and societal levels, nationally and internationally, the interests of the child-to-be (the aim desired in assisted conception, and a vulnerable future party to protect) must be the most important concern. To act responsibly is an ethical imperative.

REFERENCES

1. Shenfield F. Justice and access to fertility treatments. In Shenfield F, Sureau C, eds. Ethical Dilemmas in Assisted Reproduction. Carnforth, UK: Parthenon Publishing, 1997: 7–14
2. Morris RS, Gleicher N. Genetic abnormalities, male infertility, and ICSI. Lancet 1996; 347: 1277
3. Shenfield F, Sureau C, eds. Ethical Dilemmas in Assisted Reproduction. Carnforth, UK: Parthenon Publishing, 1997
4. Shenfield F, Sureau C, eds. Ethical Dilemmas in Reproduction. London: Parthenon Publishing, 2002
5. Jones HW, Schrader C. And just what is a pre-embryo? Fertil Steril 1992; 52: 189–91
6. Seve L. Pour une Critique de la Raison Bioéthique. Paris: Editions Odile Jacob, 1994
7. Council of Europe. Convention for the Protection of Human Rights and Dignity of the Human Being with Regard to the Application of Biology and Medicine. Strasbourg, November 1996: 2
8. Human Fertilisation and Embryology Act (1990). London: HMSO, 1990
9. Human Fertilisation and Embryology Act Research Purpose Regulations, 2000
10. Loi no 94-654 du 29 Juillet 1994, Relative au Don, Assistance Médicale la Procréation et Diagnostic Prenatal. Paris: Journal Officiel du 30 Juillet 1994 [law to be completed by loi 2004-800, relative a la biothique, Paris, Journal Officiel du 6 août 2004]
11. Italian ART legislation, 19-2-2004
12. Council of Europe. Medically Assisted Procreation and the Protection of the Human Embryo. Strasbourg, 1996
13. Human Fertilisation and Embryology Authority. 6th Code of Practice. London: HFEA, 2004
14. Baird P. Research on pre-embryos (zygotes). In Sureau C, Shenfield F, eds. Ethical Aspects of Human Reproduction. Paris: John Libbey Eurotext, 1995: 327–42
15. Wilmut I, Schnieke AE, McWhir J, et al. Viable offspring derived from fetal and adult mammalian cells. Nature (London) 1997; 385: 810–13
16. Réponse au Président de la République au sujet du clonage reproductif. Les cahiers du Comite Consultatif National d'Ethique pour les sciences de la vie et de la santé. Levallois-Perret: Biomedition, 1997
17. European Commission. Opinion of the Group of Advisors on the Ethical Implications of Biotechnology to the European Commission, 28 May 1997: ethical aspects of cloning techniques, rapporteur: Dr Anne McLaren, Brussels
18. Additional protocol on the prohibition of cloning human beings. Convention on Human Rights and Dignity of the Human Being with Regard to the Application of Biology and Medicine. Strasbourg: Council of Europe, 1998
19. Human Genetic Advisory Commission and Human Fertilisation and Embryology Authority. Cloning Issues in Reproduction, Science and Medicine, Consultation document. London: Office of Science and Technology, 1998
20. Testard J, Sele B. Towards an efficient medical eugenics: is the desirable always the feasible? Hum Reprod 1995; 11: 3086–90
21. Shulman JD, Edwards RG. Preimplantation diagnosis is disease control, not eugenics. Hum Reprod 1996; 11: 46–4
22. ESHRE Taskforce 9. The application of preimplantation genetic diagnosis for human leukocyte antigen typing of embryos. ESHRE Ethics and Law website, www.eshre.com 2004; 2005; in press
23. Verlinsky Y, Rechitsky S, Sharapova T, et al. Preimplantation HLA testing. J Am Med Assoc 2004; 291: 2079–85
24. Pennings G, Liebaers I. Creating a child to save another: HLA matching by means of PGD. In Shenfield F, Sureau C, eds. Ethical Dilemmas in Reproduction. London: Parthenon Publishing, 2002: 51–65
25. Shenfield F, Pennings G, Devroe P, et al., ESHRE Ethics Taskforce. Taskforce 5: preimplantation genetic diagnosis. Hum Reprod 2003; 18: 649–51
26. Shenfield F, Steele SJ. A gift is a gift is a gift or why gamete donors should not be paid. Hum Reprod 1995; 10; 253–5

27. Titmuss R. The Gift Relationship: from Human Blood to Social Policy. London: Allen and Unwin, 1971

28. Pennings G. The 'double track' policy for donor insemination. Hum Reprod 1997; 12: 2839–44

29. Rodeck CH. Selective feticide. In Chervenak FA, Isaacson GC, Campbell S, eds. Ultrasound in Obstetrics and Gynecology. Boston: Little, Brown, 1987: 1333–8

30. ESHRE Task Force on Ethics and Law. Taskforce 6. Ethical issues related to multiple pregnancies in medically assisted reproduction. Hum Reprod 2003; 18: 1976–9

31. Regina v Human Fertilisation and Embryology Authority ex parte Diane Blood [1997] 2 All ER 687

32. ESHRE Task Force on Ethics and Law. Taskforce 7: ethical considerations for the cryopreservation of gametes and reproductive tissues for self use. Hum Reprod 2004; 19: 460–2

33. Otkay R, Karlikaya G. Ovarian function after transplantation of frozen, banked autologous ovarian tissue. N Engl J Med 2000; 342:

34. Donnez J, Dolmans MM, Demylle, et al. Livebirth after orthotopic transplantation of cryopreserved ovarian tissue. Lancet 2004; 364: 1405–10, Eratum 2004; Dec

35. Kennedy I, Grubb A. Medical Law, 2nd edn. London: Butterworth, 1994: 1061–5

36. Dondorp WJ, Freezing the hands of time: fertility insurance for women? In Shenfeld F, Sureau C, eds. Ethical Dilemmas in Reproduction. London: Parthenon Publishing, 2002: 1–20

37. Children's Act. London: HMSO,(1989)

38. Fagot-Largeault A. Procréation responsable. In Sureau C, Shenfield F, eds. Ethical Aspects of Reproduction. Paris: John Libbey Eurotext, 1995: 3–18

39. Surrogacy Arrangement Act. London: HMSO,(1989)

40. Sen A. Missing women – revisited. Br Med J 2003; 327: 1297–8

37

The role of meta-analysis in clinical decision-making to optimize outcome

Salim Daya

INTRODUCTION

Developments are occurring at a rapid pace in the field of infertility, particularly in the area of assisted reproductive technologies (ART). The result has been a much welcomed increase in pregnancy rates worldwide. This observation has been confirmed in annual reports produced after analyzing the outcomes in treatment cycles collected in large databases such as those of the French national IVF registry (FIVNAT), the American Society for Reproductive Medicine (ASRM) and the UK Human Fertilisation and Embryology Authority (HFEA). Although much progress has occurred since *in vitro* fertilization (IVF) was first introduced, the increase in pregnancy rates from year to year has been modest, at best. In an effort to enhance the chances of success for patients, attention has focused on improvements in laboratory techniques and clinical protocols. Also, prognostic criteria are being sought whereby patients at high risk of failure (e.g. those with elevated levels of follicle stimulating hormone (FSH) on day 3) are dissuaded from persisting with therapy or are offered pre-IVF preparatory treatment (e.g. ablation or suppression of endometriosis, salpingectomy for hydrosalpinx, and so on).

In trying to provide optimal care for patients, clinicians regularly face questions about the efficacy of treatments, interventions or disease-preventive strategies, the accuracy and interpretation of diagnostic tests, the effect associated with exposure to putatively harmful agents, the course and prognosis of diseases and the cost-effectiveness of interventions. The standard approaches in trying to answer these questions include consulting colleagues who may be aware of recent advances in the areas of concern, or referring to textbooks and reviews. Unfortunately, textbooks are usually not up-to-date because of the time it takes to publish them. Similarly, reviews tend to be narrative summaries of the author's opinions about a particular subject and may be biased in their conclusions by selecting and reviewing only studies that support the author's beliefs. The problem is propagated by the rapid publication of such review articles as proceedings of scientific meetings, often at, or shortly after, the meeting. In the area of ART, the problem is further compounded by the constant change in treatment protocols, many of which have not been subjected to rigorous evaluation of their efficacy. Reports of such protocols contribute to the exponential growth in the body of medical information, the quality of which varies considerably from mostly poor to occasionally excellent. However, before such information can be used to assist clinicians in optimizing the care they provide to their patients, it should be evaluated to determine whether it is valid and relevant to clinical care.

THE IMPORTANCE OF RANDOMIZED CONTROLLED TRIALS

In the assessment of therapeutic efficacy, the gold standard is still the large, randomized controlled trial, because it is the most rigorous method of determining whether a cause-and-effect relationship exists between treatment and outcome. Although other study designs, including non-randomized controlled trials, have been used to identify an association between an intervention and an outcome, they cannot exclude the possibility that the association was caused by another factor that was linked to both intervention and outcome. One of the main purposes of randomization is to ensure that no systematic differences exist between the treated and the control groups with respect to factors that may affect outcome.

Despite its advantages, a good randomized controlled trial, with adequate sample size, is often difficult to undertake because it is time-consuming and costly, and may be fraught with difficulties in the commitment of patients. For example, with IVF treatment, to detect an improvement in clinical pregnancy per cycle of 5% from a control rate of 15% (a difference that represents a relative treatment effect of 33%) in a study with 80% power and a significance level of 5%, a sample size of 1800 patients would be required. Given that the average volume of activity in an IVF program is 200–300 cycles per year, accrual at a single center will take 6–9 years. At the conclusion of the study, it is likely that newer treatment options will have become available, rendering the results of the study less relevant. As a result, investigators resort to conducting smaller trials, which are less demanding and more feasible, in the hope of detecting large (but usually unrealistic) differences between the experimental and the control interventions. The growing numbers of such trials bear testimony to this fact and reflect the suboptimal peer-review process that currently exists with most journals in our specialty. Consequently, many of these trials are not sufficiently persuasive or have findings that are inconsistent in magnitude and/or direction of effect, leaving clinicians with increasing uncertainty about the appropriate management of particular disorders.

SYSTEMATIC REVIEW

In the absence of sufficiently large randomized controlled trials, the challenge facing clinicians, researchers and policy-makers is to develop an efficient method of synthesizing the accumulating information from smaller trials so that reliable inferences can be made about therapeutic interventions. The notion of systematically identifying, evaluating and combining the results of several independent studies has evolved in various research settings, including education, social science and health-care. Such reviews involve taking the large, and often unmanageable, amount of information from a complete search of the literature and reducing it to a concise summary that is easy to access.

A systematic review is a scientifically structured and rigorous process involving the assembly of original studies addressing a specific clinical question and subjecting them to critical appraisal so that bias and random error can be limited. The final common pathway for most systematic reviews is a quantitative summary of the data, or meta-analysis, which is a statistical procedure that integrates the results of several independent studies deemed eligible for pooling based on predefined criteria.

By combining the data from valid and eligible studies, the statistical power is increased, thereby reducing the probability of false-negative results. Meta-analyses provide treatment-effect estimates that are robust and with improved precision. In this manner they can help answer questions that single trials may have been unable to answer, because of insufficient power. The numbers of published meta-analyses in medical research have increased dramatically over the years; more than 500 appeared in 1996, compared with only 16 in the 1970s. This increase in popularity is testimony to the fact that meta-analyses have an important role to play in clinical decision-making.

There are several important and necessary steps in conducting a good systematic review. These steps include: clearly specifying a research question; outlining a search strategy to identify and select relevant studies; assessing the validity of each study; extracting and pooling the data; and summarizing the results so that appropriate inferences can be made.

There are two approaches to pooling data using meta-analysis. The first approach (i.e. meta-analysis by literature) utilizes published data from well-designed controlled trials. These data on subjects in each trial are extracted as summary data and then pooled. An alternative approach (i.e. meta-analysis by patient) is to obtain individual data for every subject enrolled in each controlled trial and pool them as if they had all been participants in one large trial.

SEARCH STRATEGY TO IDENTIFY POTENTIALLY RELEVANT STUDIES

The search for studies should be comprehensive and involve several sources. Searching computerized bibliographic databases of published research, such as the MEDLINE database, is a convenient first step. However, by focusing on only one database, it is likely that many studies will be missed. Therefore, the search should include other databases such as EMBASE, Citation Index and the Cochrane Controlled Clinical Trials register, as well as hand-searching relevant journals. Scanning the reference list of selected publications and review articles often yields useful papers not identified in the initial search. Another important source of relevant studies is the 'gray' literature, which includes dissertations, internal reports, non-peer-reviewed journals and pharmaceutical industry files. Abstracts and symposia of major scientific meetings should be scanned for trials that have been completed recently. Whenever possible, authors of primary studies should be contacted for more information and further clarification of the details of their studies. Finally, peer consultation should be sought for any remaining articles.

STUDY SELECTION

The method for selecting studies should be reliable and reproducible so that others wishing to confirm or update the findings can replicate it. The process requires that outlining the population being studied, the experimental and control interventions being compared and the outcome event that is of interest to the investigators develop the clinical question *a priori*. In this manner the clinical question is appropriately focused so that the selection criteria that provide direction for an efficient and comprehensive search of the literature can be established. The specificity of the retrieval process will depend on the explicit nature of the criteria established; any ambiguity will result in errors and, consequently, a reduction in the accuracy of this process.

Additionally, a decision must be made about whether the non-English-language literature should be accessed. Despite problems of retrieval and translation, much important information may be available from trial results published in non-English-language journals. However, contacting authors of these publications for more information poses a larger logistical problem, for which no immediate solution is available.

DATA EXTRACTION AND SUMMARY

To avoid errors in the extraction of outcome data from trials that have been selected for the systematic review, it is good practice to verify accuracy of the process by having a second investigator undertake the same exercise. Any discrepancies can be resolved by consensus after reviewing the publications in question.

The data to be combined can be classified as either categorical or continuous in type. Categorical data are usually in binary format involving a 'yes/no' response (e.g. pregnancy or no pregnancy). Continuous data are expressed over a range of values (e.g. serum estradiol levels on the day of human chorionic gonadotropin (hCG) administration). Binary data can be summarized using measures of treatment effect that describe either the relative efficacy of intervention, such as risk ratio (RR) and odds ratio (OR), or by the absolute benefit of the intervention such as the risk difference (RD).

Continuous data can be summarized by the raw mean difference between the two groups if measured on the same scale (e.g. estradiol level), by the standardized mean difference when different scales are used (e.g. pain scales) or by the correlation coefficient between two continuous variables[1].

DISPLAY OF SUMMARY DATA

The summarized results from each trial can be displayed graphically by the point estimates and their confidence intervals[1]. A hypothetical example, in which the summary measure is the OR with its 95% confidence interval (CI), is shown in Figure 1 for trials that met the inclusion criteria. The solid vertical line represents an OR of unity and indicates a null effect. If the 95% CI includes this value (i.e. the horizontal line representing the CI crosses the vertical line at

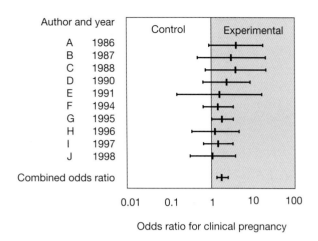

Figure 1 Odds ratio tree for clinical pregnancy per cycle started, comparing experimental and control interventions. Test for homogeneity of treatment effect: $\chi^2 = 4.02$; $p = 0.91$

OR = 1.0), then the observed effect of the experimental intervention is not statistically significantly different from the control intervention at the conventional level of significance (i.e. $p < 0.05$). In Figure 1, the CI in all ten studies crosses the vertical line, indicating that the estimate of treatment effect in each of these studies was not statistically significant.

Another advantage of the graphic display is that it allows one to visualize the direction and magnitude of the treatment effect easily. From Figure 1, it can be seen quite clearly that in all except one study, the OR for clinical pregnancy per cycle started was higher with experimental treatment. The magnitude of the OR varied from 1.16 to 3.79, showing the range of possible effect sizes that were observed.

HETEROGENEITY OF TREATMENT EFFECT

Variability in the effect of treatment is to be expected when trials are repeated. Even when the same population of subjects is used, a trial that is repeated using the same maneuver will be likely to yield different results. Therefore, before the data from the studies that have been selected for review can be combined, it is necessary to determine whether the effect of treatment is homogeneous across all studies. This assessment of homogeneity involves calculating the magnitude of

statistical diversity that exists in the effect of treatment among the different studies.

Statistical heterogeneity may be attributable to two sources. First, study results can differ because of random sampling error. In this situation, when the study is repeated several times, the size of the observed effect will vary randomly around the true (but unknown) effect, even if the same population was sampled. This variability is referred to as a within-study variance and is a fixed effect that occurs purely by chance. Second, each study sample may have been drawn from a different population, resulting in a variable size of the effect because of between-study variation. This type of variation is referred to as random effects variability.

The degree of variability in the treatment effect can be examined statistically using a test based on the χ^2 distribution. If the test indicates that significant variability (i.e. heterogeneity) is not present, then the differences among studies can be assumed to be a consequence of sampling variation and the data can be pooled using a fixed effects model.

The presence of heterogeneity is more problematic, even though the random effects model has been advocated for pooling data from such trials. It is important that a thorough search for possible causes of variability be undertaken when statistical heterogeneity is identified.

DATA POOLING

The purpose of pooling the data from studies that have been selected is to obtain an overall estimate of the effect of the experimental intervention. Such a summary estimate is likely to be a more reliable, generalizable and accurate estimate of the effect of treatment than one obtained from single studies, unless the latter are very large. This information is of relevance in guiding clinicians in the care of their patients.

A simple arithmetic average of the results from all the studies is easy to calculate but would give misleading information, depending on the relative contributions of small and large studies. The results of the smaller studies are likely to be more variable and should be given less weight in the pooled estimate. The methods employed in a meta-analysis take this fact into consideration by using a weighted average of the results such that the larger studies have more influence than the smaller studies.

In the fixed effects model, the variability (as reflected in the CI) is the result of random variation and is narrower than the random effects model, in which variability is the result of both within- and between-study variance. A useful method to assess the robustness of the pooled findings is to perform a sensitivity analysis whereby the combined effect, using both the fixed and the random effects models, is calculated. In situations in which there is little variation, the two combined effects will be virtually identical, although the CI will be slightly wider with the random effects model.

CUMULATIVE META-ANALYSIS

Evidence on treatment efficacy is gathered over time as reports become published. Cumulative meta-analysis is a method for evaluating the contribution of each study that is combined sequentially in a specified order (e.g. according to date of publication). It involves repeating the meta-analysis to calculate an updated pooled effect each time a new study becomes eligible for inclusion in the previously collected series of studies (Figure 2). This method is useful for determining whether the pooled estimate is robust over time. The precision of the pooled estimate improves with the accumulation of more studies. Consequently, the cumulative meta-analysis enables one to identify the point in time when the pooled estimate becomes statistically significant, so that a decision can be reached regarding the benefit (or harm) of the experimental intervention, or whether more trials are still necessary to produce convincing results.

Unfortunately, the standard cumulative meta-analysis does not have a predefined sample size, as is the case for efficacy trials. Consequently, reliance has been placed on interpreting the results based on the overall p value. The chosen p value is used to decide whether the observed effect could be a chance finding, but it gives no indication of the numbers of subjects included in the analysis. A larger data set provides a more reliable estimate of the effect of treatment, but this information is not conveyed by the p value alone; interpretation of the p value is the same whether the data set is small or large.

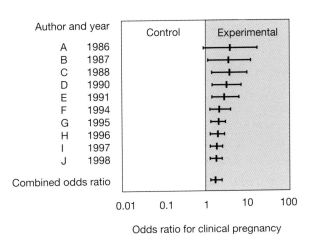

Figure 2 Cumulative meta-analysis of trials comparing experimental and control interventions

OPTIMAL INFORMATION SIZE

In any trial evaluating treatment efficacy, the subjects are enrolled sequentially until the sample size has been reached. By periodic interim analyses, the investigator can identify any unexpected benefits or potentially harmful effects as soon as the evidence becomes clear, thereby allowing the trial to be stopped early to avoid unnecessarily exposing additional subjects to an intervention that is inferior. In the context of meta-analysis, evidence is also gathered over time as more trials are completed. However, because there are no formal guidelines for weighing this accumulating evidence to identify a termination point to stop collecting more data, trials may continue to be undertaken, exposing future subjects unnecessarily to ineffective treatment or denying patients the benefit of effective treatment.

One method for dealing with this problem is to calculate the optimal information size (OIS) by outlining the conditions for a convincing meta-analysis[2]. The process requires first calculating the sample size necessary to conduct a single trial with sufficient power to test the research hypothesis. This entity is the minimal information size, and represents the smallest number of subjects needed for a reliable meta-analysis, and is based on the logical assumption that the amount of information required should not be less than that for an equivalent randomized controlled trial. However, more information will be required for a meta-analysis, because its reliance on evidence from several trials increases the potential for bias and heterogeneity compared with that expected with a single trial. This objective of obtaining more information can be achieved by taking a more conservative approach to selecting the levels for the components of a sample size calculation. The magnitude of the clinically important difference in outcome event rates can be reduced to that which is still biologically plausible and medically worthwhile. An observed pooled effect larger than this minimal value supports the claim of higher efficacy of the experimental intervention. The probabilities selected for the errors of hypothesis testing could be more stringent than the conventional values of 0.05 and 0.2 for type I and type II errors, respectively. The use of these more conservative levels would generate a much larger sample size. The result is an OIS that should be large enough to answer definitively the research question while minimizing the false-positive results, thereby enhancing the credibility of the effect size estimates obtained from the analysis.

The OIS can be used to establish monitoring boundaries which, when crossed, provide conclusive evidence of benefit (or harm) resulting from the intervention. Until this point is reached, further data from randomized trials would still be required.

PUBLICATION BIAS

In the search for evidence, it is possible that completed studies are unavailable for analysis; either they have been published in journals that are not readily accessible, or they have not been published at all, because the results were negative or demonstrated a null effect. There is now a sizeable body of evidence confirming the fact that a large number of studies, initially reported in summary format, are never published as complete manuscripts. Only a little more than half the abstracts of randomized trials presented at scientific meetings on human reproduction eventually reach full publication, the majority appearing within 3 years of presentation. The reasons for this publication deficit include methodological factors, such as inadequate sample size, and investigator-related factors, such as insufficient time, loss of interest and lack of enthusiasm. Availability of more detailed data from research findings, first presented in abstract form, is important for systematic reviews to be comprehensive.

Another type of publication bias results in 'positive' studies being reported more than once, thereby increasing the probability that they will be located in a search. There are two aspects to this problem. Disaggregation is the separate publication of selected results from a multicenter trial, and duplication involves repeated publication of the results of the same trial. Disaggregation is more likely to occur with multinational trials, because investigators are keen to publish data from their own countries in their national journals, to report on the treatment effect that represents their particular geographic, cultural and linguistic setting, even though the complete report from the multinational study has been published. Duplicate publication, in some cases, is overt, with clear cross-referencing to the original report. Such publications are seen when the data have to be reanalyzed to address questions that arise after the study findings are reported. More often, however, duplication is undertaken covertly, the intention not being to provide new information, but to further a personal or corporate agenda. The practice of using completely different authors or rotating the first authors for the same study when the findings are presented at different scientific meetings is not unusual. Multiple offerings of the same information violate the integrity of clinical research, place unnecessary pressure on the peer-review process and deliberately mislead the scientific community. These factors lead to the published literature becoming biased, with reports of 'positive' findings.

Although publication bias is difficult to eliminate, its presence can be suggested by two diagnostic methods. The first, called the 'Fail-Safe N' method, is a statistical calculation for estimating the number of negative unpublished studies that would have to exist to change the significance of the pooled results[3]. The judgment is then left to the meta-analyst to determine whether the number of such studies is sufficiently large to make it unlikely that this number of unpublished studies exists, or the number is so small that the pooled estimate of the effect size is unreliable.

The second method involves a visual exploration of the data using an inverted funnel plot[4]. In this method, a scatter plot is used to display the relationship between the precision of each study and the size of the treatment effect. The funnel plot is based on the fact that precision in estimating the underlying treatment effect will increase as the sample size of the study increases. By plotting the precision of the study (calculated as the inverse of the standard error) against the effect measure (e.g. OR, RR, etc.), as shown in Figure 3, it becomes apparent whether publication bias is present or not. An inverted, symmetrical funnel-shaped appearance of the data points suggests that no study has been omitted and publication bias is not a factor in the pooled estimate of the effect of the experimental intervention. In the presence of bias, the funnel plot will be skewed and asymmetrical, as shown in Figure 4. Although the funnel plot is a useful, simple visual test for the likelihood of publication bias, it is not very helpful when there are only a few small studies included in the meta-analysis.

META-ANALYSIS USING INDIVIDUAL PATIENT DATA

The more conventional approach to meta-analysis is based on combining summary data from trials published in the literature or presented at scientific meetings (i.e. meta-analysis by literature). A better, and more desirable, method involves collecting detailed outcomes and risk factors from the individual patients who participated in the trials (i.e. meta-analysis by patient) rather than the summarized results of the trials. The meta-analysis by patient method is more complicated, because it requires central collection, checking and analysis of individual patient data received from the investigators of the original trials, using comprehensive case-record forms designed for this purpose to obtain complete data on all variables of interest. Its biggest advantage is the opportunity to verify the accuracy of the data, confirm the integrity of the randomization process and ascertain the completeness of follow-up of the patients. The analysis is more thorough, permits multivariable evaluation and can be performed according to the intention-to-treat principle. Subgroup analyses are more reliable, and the consistency of the effect of treatment across well-defined groups can be assessed with more confidence. Another very important benefit is the possibility of calculating the time taken to reach a specific outcome event (e.g. time-to-pregnancy). This outcome measure not only is useful for comparing the efficacy of treatments but also provides information on prognosis.

The evidence obtained from a meta-analysis by patient is usually of such high quality that this approach is the gold standard in the hierarchy of

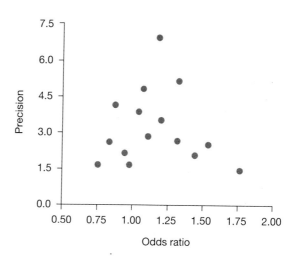

Figure 3 Symmetrical funnel plot of controlled trials

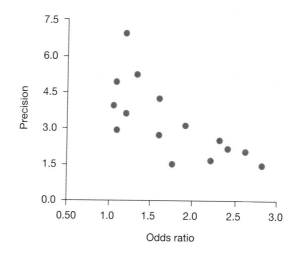

Figure 4 Asymmetrical funnel plot of controlled trials

evidence. However, despite its advantages, its use is relatively infrequent for a variety of reasons. It requires collaboration with the trialists who have to agree to share their data. Logistically, this is a difficult problem to overcome, because of time constraints, mobility among the researchers and staleness of the data making it difficult to retrieve them, especially if they were not recorded in an easy-to-access electronic format. The problem is magnified when the trials were initiated with pharmaceutical company support, because the case-record forms are often unavailable. The movement towards registration of all randomized trials and the call for the raw data to be made available on web sites in a manner that protects patient confidentiality will address some of the barriers to performing meta-analyses by patient.

EXAMPLE OF THE USE OF META-ANALYSIS

The case of the optimal GnRH-a protocol in IVF cycles

The inclusion of gonadotropin releasing hormone agonists (GnRH-a) in protocols of ovarian stimulation for the treatment of infertility with ART has resulted in a significant reduction in the cycle cancellation rate and an increase in the clinical pregnancy rate[5]. Different GnRH-a drugs, routes of administration and protocols have been used for ART cycles. There are four main protocols of GnRH-a administration. The ultrashort and short protocols make use of the initial stimulatory effect on gonadotropin secretion to promote follicle development. This phase is then followed by pituitary desensitization, whereby luteinizing hormone (LH) levels are suppressed later in the follicular phase. The agonist is administered from day 1, 2 or 3 of the cycle for 3 days in the ultrashort protocol or until hCG injection in the short protocol. Gonadotropin administration is usually commenced 2–3 days after initiating GnRH-a use. In contrast, the long protocol involves the administration of GnRH-a until suppression of ovarian activity has been confirmed, before commencing gonadotropin administration. There are two types of long protocol regimen: the long follicular protocol, which involves the administration of GnRH-a from day 1 of the cycle for approximately 14 days, and the long luteal protocol, in which GnRH-a is administered from the midluteal phase of the previous cycle.

Although several randomized trials comparing the long and short GnRH-a protocols have been undertaken, the lack of power in these small trials has made it difficult to draw definitive conclusions on which protocol is better. A systematic review was undertaken to determine whether the clinical pregnancy rate in infertile couples undergoing treatment with ART was better with the long protocol compared with the short or ultrashort protocols[6]. The review focused only on trials in which allocation to either group was random or quasi-random (e.g. alternate allocation, allocation by patient chart number and so on).

The search strategy involved scanning computerized databases of MEDLINE, EMBASE and the Cochrane Menstrual Disorders and Subfertility Groups specialized register. In addition, bibliographies of relevant publications and review articles were scanned, and abstracts of major scientific meetings were hand-searched. Finally, consultation was sought with colleagues and medical directors of the pharmaceutical industry marketing GnRH-a products regarding any remaining publications.

The methodological quality of each trial was assessed using a predetermined scoring system consisting of six criteria: type of randomized procedure; completeness of follow-up; study design; presence of co-intervention; inclusion of patients or cycles; and use of blinding[7]. Homogeneity of the treatment effect among trials was tested using the χ^2 test. There was no significant heterogeneity and the trial results were pooled using meta-analytical principles.

Of 40 potential trials, 14 were excluded because they did not meet the inclusion criteria[6]. In all trials, each patient contributed data from only one cycle of treatment. The sample size varied across the trials from 18 in the smallest trial to 320 in the largest, with a median sample size of 91.

Among the 26 trials that met the inclusion criteria, the common (pooled) OR for clinical pregnancy per cycle started was 1.32 (95% CI 1.10–1.57) in favor of the long GnRH-a protocol. The studies were subgrouped, depending on whether, in the long protocol, the GnRH-a was commenced in the follicular phase or the luteal phase. The respective ORs were 1.54 (95% CI 1.11–2.13) and 1.21 (95% CI 0.98–1.51). After excluding four trials in which the ultrashort protocol was used, the OR for long versus short protocols was 1.27 (95% CI 1.04–1.56). A comparison of long versus ultrashort protocols produced an OR of 1.47 (95% CI 1.02–2.12).

On the basis of this systematic review and meta-analysis, it can be concluded that the long protocol for GnRH-a administration for ART cycles results in a higher clinical pregnancy rate per cycle started, compared with the short and ultrashort protocols. Further analysis will be required to evaluate the effect on secondary outcomes, such as spontaneous abortion, ongoing and delivered pregnancy, amount of gonadotropin used, number of oocytes retrieved and the fertilization rate.

CONCLUSIONS

Although the randomized controlled trial is not entirely free from bias, its role in efficacy evaluation is unquestionable, particularly when it is well designed and rigorous. In the field of reproductive medicine, and in particular ART, the usual size of the treatment effect is likely to be moderate or small, rendering most trials incapable of detecting with certainty such clinically relevant differences. The net result is that inferences made from small trials often will be contradictory and will create confusion, because of the high degree of variability in effect size estimates. Consequently, it is necessary to conduct large trials. Unfortunately, because such a requirement is often not feasible in single centers, investigators resort to conducting smaller studies from which premature and often incorrect inferences are made. A solution to this problem of underpowered studies is to perform a systematic review with meta-analysis of the data, by combining the effect size from each trial into an overall pooled estimate that is more likely to represent the true effect in the population. In this way, the role of therapeutic interventions can be evaluated properly. Meta-analyses provide better and more robust estimates of treatment effect with enhanced precision, and can help to answer questions that single trials may have been unable to answer because of insufficient power.

However, it should be recognized that meta-analysis is a method of studying studies, and is not a substitute for a well-conducted randomized controlled trial. Its major strength lies in its ability to promote critical thinking and in exploring reasons for heterogeneity in the effect of treatment across trials. Its systematic approach and use of objective, quantitative methods emphasize the scientific rigor with which it is undertaken. The opportunity to perform meta-analyses by patient will significantly improve the generation of estimates of treatment effect, and will allow more comprehensive and exploratory analyses to be performed. The value that meta-analyses bring to assist clinicians in optimizing their care of their patients cannot be refuted. The challenge that remains is to improve clinical trials so that the problem of heterogeneity can be minimized.

REFERENCES

1. Lau J, Ioannidis JPA, Schmid CH. Quantitative synthesis in systematic reviews. Ann Intern Med 1997; 127: 820–6
2. Pogue JM, Yusuf S. Cumulating evidence from randomized trials: utilizing sequential monitoring boundaries for cumulative meta-analysis. Control Clin Trials 1997; 18: 580–93
3. Rosenthal R. The 'File Drawer Problem' and tolerance for null results. Psychol Bull 1979; 86: 638–41
4. Egger M, Smith GD, Schneider M, Minder C. Bias in meta-analysis detected by a simple, graphical test. Br Med J 1997; 315: 629–34
5. Hughes EG, Fedorkow DM, Daya S, et al. The routine use of gonadotropin-releasing hormone agonists prior to in vitro fertilization and gamete intrafallopian transfer: a meta-analysis of randomized trials. Fertil Steril 1992; 58: 888–96
6. Daya S. Comparison of gonadotropin releasing hormone agonist (GnRHa) protocols for pituitary desensitization in in vitro fertilization (IVF) and gamete intrafallopian transfer (GIFT) cycles. The Cochrane Library. Oxford: Update Software, 1998
7. Daya S, Gunby J, Hughes EG, et al. Follicle-stimulating hormone versus human menopausal gonadotropin for in vitro fertilization cycles: a meta-analysis. Fertil Steril 1995; 64: 347–54

38

The application of medical informatics to reproductive medicine

Julian Jenkins

INTRODUCTION

Since 1995 the ReproMED project has pioneered the application of medical informatics to reproductive medicine (Figure 1). After a brief overview of the

needs for informatics, this chapter mentions relevant technology followed by practical illustrations of applications mainly from the ReproMED project. Medical informatics has become a vital, rapidly developing and increasingly complex aspect of reproductive medicine

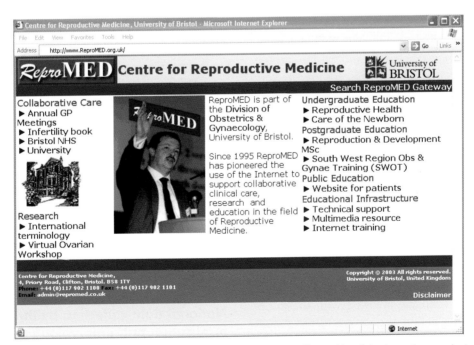

Figure 1 The principal homepage of ReproMED (http:// www.ReproMED.org.uk) provides links to various project websites such as Reproduction & Development MSc website (http://www. ReD-MSc.org.uk), ReproMED Electronic Multimedia Resource (http://www.REMR.org.uk) and South West Region Obstetrics & Gynaecology Training Website (http://www.SWOT.org.uk)

involving clinical practice, administration, audit, education, training and research. The field of medical informatics is concerned with the closely related problems of information and communication in health-care. Although computers play an important part in medical informatics, information management covers a much wider area and ideally the discipline should be needs-driven. A whole new vocabulary of jargon and acronyms of Communication and Information Technology (C&IT) has developed, at least as complex as that seen in reproductive medicine. Although this chapter focuses to some extent on reproductive medicine in the United Kingdom, the underlying principles and possible applications of medical informatics are relevant to many aspects of health-care throughout the world.

NEEDS

Clinical practice

When considering the information requirements of reproductive medicine, it is important to consider that there are many different groups involved with different priorities, different volumes of information and different budgets. Within any group, different individuals may have different information needs, which may change with time and place. Similarly, different communication needs exist between and within groups and an individual's communication needs may be very specific. Miscommunication between health-care professionals may lead to serious clinical problems[1], and many communications are event-driven and inefficient, commonly interrupting tasks, including patient consultations[2].

The patient record provides fundamental information to clinical management, and perhaps should be considered as the central point for managing patient care. Given the prime importance of the patient record it is worth considering a possible ideal patient record. Information should be easily and quickly added to the patient record as soon as it is generated by the person most directly involved with the information. Information held in the patient record should be easy to access and understand by all who have a legitimate right to this information, whereever needed, yet be secure from unauthorized access. The

patient record should be able to hold information as diverse as records of consultations, investigation results, treatments, correspondence, ultrasound pictures and photographs of babies. The patient record must be stored for many years, and patient information from any time period should be easily retrievable. Each entry in the patient record should be dated and attributable to an individual or other source, such as a pathology laboratory. The information may be required by a court of law; thus, although it may be necessary to change information in the patient record, the patient record must enforce that details of any such change are clearly recorded. It should be possible to communicate any information held in the patient record for central collation, identifying individual patients with internationally recognizable codes. It should be easy to pass from the clinical record to other related information for such uses as clinical decision support and administration. Both current paper folder systems and computer information systems fall short of this suggested ideal.

The smooth running of a reproductive medicine center is dependent on effective administration, which relies on accurate and efficient communication and information systems. Accurate and current information must pass between clinics, primary care and patients. Appointment systems are crucial to ensure optimal use is made of clinic time without keeping patients waiting, while accounting systems ensure that bills match services. Costs, including salaries, overheads and consumables, must be predicted to ensure that projected income will cover costs to assure the viability of a clinic.

To ensure that the highest standards of clinical care are maintained, it is important to audit practice to identify possible areas of weakness. Whereas differences in case-mix make it difficult usefully to compare pregnancy rates between clinics, this is less of a problem for internal audit. Many other measures of practice may usefully be audited, including completeness of patient records, including consent forms and accuracy of record keeping. Audit requires accurate, ongoing, efficient and detailed information collection.

National data collection by the human fertilisation and embryology authority

In response to an Act of Parliament, the Human Fertilisation and Embryology Authority (HFEA) was formed in 1991 to license and monitor UK clinics that carry out *in vitro* fertilization, donor insemination (DI) and embryo research[3]. The current system of notification is paper-based using a series of carbonated A4 sheets relevant to treatment and outcome, including sensitive details such as the treated couples' names and post-codes, their use of donated oocytes or sperm and whether pregnancy resulted from the cycle of treatment. This information is currently sent in envelopes by post. The accurate collation of such data is important, both for the HFEA and for the individual clinics, particularly as the results reported by licensed clinics are now available to the public and used by the media; hence, considerable efforts are under way to improve this system[4].

Evidence-based medicine

Evidence-based medicine requires the integration of individual clinical expertise with the best available external clinical evidence from systematic research. However, it is too expensive for even large teaching-hospital medical libraries to buy and store any more than a selection of the biomedical literature. The contents of a hospital library are not readily accessible when required to deal with a clinical situation or to refer to while studying at home. Even if the information was accessible, the sheer volume of information makes it extremely difficult to obtain the specific information that is required. In 1972 Archie Cochrane drew attention to the lack of evidence upon which health-care is based[5]. He suggested that randomized controlled trials could help to deploy resources more rationally, and systematic reviews of the evidence should be readily available to all those who need to make health-care decisions. Contributors in many countries and specialities now work together as part of the Cochrane Collaboration to prepare and maintain such reviews, which are disseminated using electronic media as the Cochrane Database of Systematic Reviews. Ultimately, clinical decisions are based on individual professional opinion, and even expert groups disagree on the interpretation of evidence, which is often incomplete. The logistics of producing and maintaining a comprehensive evidence base to support clinical decisions for reproductive medicine and making this available at the point of need is substantial, to say the least.

Education and training

The educational and training requirements of all those involved in the diverse and rapidly developing speciality of reproductive medicine provide particular challenges. Continuing professional development (CPD) is important to keep pace with developments, yet there are few established CPD schemes within the specialist fields constituting reproductive medicine, such as reproductive biology and assisted conception (e.g. Association of Clinical Embryologists). Obstetricians and gynecologists may find it difficult to obtain and maintain an appropriate level of training in reproductive medicine. Primary-care doctors may have received very little training in reproductive medicine, and they need to maintain competency in a broad area, including women's health[6]. Nurses and counselors both in specialist centers and in the community play an important role in the care of patients receiving reproductive medicine treatments. The educational needs of nurses in the community present particular challenges. A survey of nurses in the south west of England identified that the majority of nurses who wished to support patients undergoing assisted conception treatment felt inadequately informed to do so[7]. Similarly, counselors both in specialist centers and in the community need to have sufficient knowledge of reproductive medicine to counsel patients appropriately. Although reproductive medicine postgraduate education is a rapidly expanding area, often the inflexible study models of conventional university postgraduate courses do not fit with people's career paths or life-styles.

The importance of public education is increasingly recognized. If patients receive incorrect information this can sometimes be difficult to correct; thus, it is sensible for the profession to assist with public education. Further increasing the general awareness of infertility may decrease some of the problems. Couples may be encouraged to start trying for a family at an earlier stage, or make life-style modifications such as weight optimization and avoidance of smoking to improve their fertility.

Research

With the ever-increasing volume and subspecialization of biomedical research, it is difficult to keep up to date with current research and communicate with colleagues who may be dispersed around the world. The pressures on funding research make it difficult for researchers to attend conferences to exchange ideas. Access to the biomedical literature is expensive, and by the nature of the current publication process it always lags behind current research. The volume of research creates further problems in identifying relevant information amongst a constantly expanding information base. Technology may considerably aid the handling of research information and communication.

THE TECHNOLOGY

The pace of technological development has been unimaginable, transforming the ways in which we communicate and use information. An obvious example of progress is the increasingly functional desktop computers that are becoming steadily more compact, with such changes as compact flat screens replacing bulky monitors. The desktop computer may act as a network client, connecting via a network to resources that are held remotely on other computers termed servers. The available methods to capture and communicate information have become progressively more versatile and economic, as demonstrated by the fall in price and increased availability of digital storage media, digital cameras, color printers and electronic mail (e-mail). Perhaps the most significant change in the way we communicate relates to the Internet, and the technologies that this has spawned. Since the popularization of the Internet, networks have become more abundant, as illustrated by the many wireless networks now providing access to the Internet in public places to portable computers.

Although not immediately apparent but nevertheless of great importance are the embedded computer processors that control electronic devices. These embedded computer systems include medical monitoring equipment such as ultrasound machines, home appliances such as televisions, office systems such as photocopiers, building systems such as fire alarms, traffic systems such as traffic-lights, banking facilities such as credit-card systems, industry systems such as power-station safety controls and almost all communication systems including telephones. The programming and functionality within embedded process control systems is becoming remarkable, including wireless networking functionality. Modern society is now intimately dependent on technology that provides great benefits but also some disadvantages.

Databases

Whereas some reproductive medicine specialists may be unaware of the potential benefits of databases, others consider that computer databases provide a simple, inexpensive method of collecting and using large volumes of valid data. Providing that expectation matches investment, computer databases may be extremely useful in providing a simple, relatively inexpensive solution for simple tasks. Where expectation of a computer system does not match investment, this will inevitably lead to disappointment in the short or long term[8]. The situation is complicated in the absence of a cost–benefit analysis, where the values of benefits are not recognized and expenses to introduce a comprehensive system may be great. Substantial investment does not guarantee success, as is evident from some of the large United Kingdom National Health Service (NHS) database projects. Nevertheless, the potential benefits of high-quality clinical databases are so great that the NHS has invested over 6 billion pounds to develop an NHS clinical-care record service[9].

To explain basic terminology, a database can be considered as one or more structured sets of persistent data, usually used within a database management system (DBMS). A simple database might be a single file containing many records, each referring to an individual patient. In turn, each record contains the same set of fields, where each field contains discrete data about patients, such as age or name. This arrangement may be referred to as a flat-file database, which is simple to create and use, but too inflexible to solve complex tasks. A DBMS is a set of software programs that controls the entry, storage, security, integrity, functionality and retrieval of data in a database. Data security prevents unauthorized users from viewing or updating the database by such measures as passwords, which may further restrict access to the entire database or subsets of the database. The integrity of the database may be maintained, for instance, by not allowing duplicate records for the same patient in the database or preventing more than one user to update the same record at the same time. Other functions include query languages to interrogate the database, and automatic audit trails to record any changes to the database. All DBMSs provide some data validation, such as rejection of invalid dates entered into date fields, but more complex systems may reject incorrect spelling or coding of items.

The possible applications of databases become more apparent when considering some of the various methods of organizing data. A relational database management system (RDBMS) follows the relational database model[10]. Data and relationships between data are stored in tables. Each table stores a number of records, which each contain the same fields. Records held in different tables may be linked to each other where they have the same value in a particular field in each table. Certain important fields may be classified as key fields, for which a separate index will be generated, greatly speeding up searching for any value in a key field. Many variations of this model are in common use, such as Oracle and Microsoft Access. In contrast, an object-oriented database system provides DBMS functionality within an object oriented programming environment. The data are stored as objects with defined attributes, including references to and properties inherited from related objects. This option permits rapid retrieval of objects and correct interpretation of multimedia such as required by an interactive multimedia application. In a distributed database, what appears to the user to be a single database is in fact a collection of several different databases that may be located at different sites. This method of storing data has particular advantages on the Internet, such as storage of the addresses of all the computers connected to the Internet. This glimpse at three radically different methods of organizing data is an indication of the diversity of databases in current use, managing data on individual computers, small networks, larger networks and the Internet.

Before clinical information may be stored in a database, the diverse clinical information requires translation into a standard structured format, which requires a medical language of terms, codes and classifications[11]. Several terms may explain a specific concept such as a specific diagnosis, but only one code relates to one concept. Related codes may be grouped together and the groupings may be organized in a hierarchical structure to form a classification. A number of classification systems are in use with different functions. The tenth revision of the International Classification of Diseases (ICD-10) provides a mechanism to handle morbidity and mortality data from around the world. Diagnosis Related Groups (DRGs) aim to provide an indicator of cost of treatment to patient diagnosis[11]. The Systematized Nomenclature of Medicine (SNOMED) has been suggested as a method to classify all the events found in a medical record[12]. This has been combined with the Read codes as SNOMED-CT, which it has been hoped may code most relevant information in the NHS electronic patient record, although this has not been generally adopted in Europe[13]. Although coding sounds attractive, in practice the allocation of codes to the same information may be inconsistent between users, and data entry may take too long, particularly if it is cumbersome to look up codes. Regrettably, there is at present no perfect reproductive medicine classification system; thus, ReproMED is aiding the European Society of Human Reproduction and Embryology taskforce to develop a European Classification of Infertility (http://www.ecit.info).

Electronic data interchange

Electronic data interchange (EDI) has developed to allow direct transfer of information between computer systems, where information may be stored using very different database designs. Unlike e-mail, which uses unstructured messages and is primarily for human communication, EDI is designed for processing by computer systems without the need for humans to interpret and re-enter the information. This allows large volumes of electronic data to be transferred between different organizations' databases, reducing the amount of paper documents that are produced, improving the accuracy of the data recorded, increasing the speed with which it is processed and reducing the costs of the process. Of particular note is an international standard ideal for transferring information over the Internet, known as extensible markup language or XML (http://www.w3.org/XML/).

Security is an important consideration with EDI, particularly where sensitive clinical information is involved. It is possible through EDI to provide considerable degrees of security through data encryption, passwords and electronic keys, and a unique electronic signature may be added to the message to validate the source of the message. The recipient can even confirm receipt of the information before the sender releases electronic keys for decryption and subsequent use of the information. Although encrypted data are primarily intended to be sent through telecommunication lines they can be sent on digital storage media through the conventional post. If encrypted data are intercepted, the content of the message is meaningless to unauthorized persons without the necessary tools to access the information.

The Internet

The Internet (Net) is a worldwide computer network connecting millions of computers providing communication to health-care, education, governments, business and the public. On this network there are an ever-increasing number of services, the most popular of which are the World Wide Web, or Web (www, w3) for short, and e-mail. The Web is attractive in that it provides simple, consistent methods to find information on the Internet, and displays this information as web pages in an interactive format incorporating multimedia, when using an appropriate computer programme termed a web browser. A good place to start on the Web to learn about reproductive medicine is the ReproMED gateway (http://www.ReproMED .net).

The Internet owes its origins to the United States (US) Department of Defense, which recognized the strategic importance of communication in the event of war. The US Department of Defense funded the Advanced Research Projects Agency in 1969 to design a network which allowed computers on different types of networks to communicate with each other. Although there were many networking technologies which connected computers over short distances (local area networks), or even over large distances (wide area networks), these technologies generally did not allow connection between the different networks. The Internet addressed this problem using special computers called routers to connect between the different networks and a set of rules describing how to transmit data (networking protocol). The networking protocol has two components: Transfer Control Protocol (TCP) and the Internet Protocol (IP). Before information is sent along the Internet it is broken into small packets of data using the Internet Protocol. Once a remote computer receives these packets they are reassembled using the Internet Protocol. Each computer connects to the Internet by a unique numerical address (IP address), which routers use to guide the information packets from source to destination. A system also exists to register the numeric IP

address as a text address, such as 'http://www.nominet. org.uk'. In order to ensure that the packets go to the correct destination on the Internet, each packet contains the address of both the computer where it originated from and also the address of the computer to which it is being sent. The Transfer Control Protocol ensures that all these packets of data are reassembled correctly at the destination computer, and if necessary, automatically requests that any missing or incorrect packets are re-sent. An important feature of this arrangement is that there are many routes by which information may be sent from one computer to another on the Internet. The router computers will select the best route at any time. In the event of a nuclear strike wiping out a large part of the US network, communication would thus remain intact, as the router computers automatically redirected communication channels.

Intranets

An intranet provides a network connecting computers within an organization using similar technology to the Internet, but restricts access to the network to members of the organization. All the services available on the Internet, including web browsing, may be used on an intranet. An intranet may maintain security, yet connect to the Internet using a firewall. A firewall is essentially a computer system that blocks undesirable access to an intranet from the Internet while permitting desirable access, such as the passage of e-mails from the Internet and providing access to the Internet for users of the intranet.

In 1993, as part of wide sweeping communication strategy between organizations within the NHS, an NHS intranet was established – the NHSnet, which is being upgraded as part of a national program for information technology[9]. To link a patient to information held about the patient on different databases by different organizations within the NHS requires a unique identifier common to all the databases. The old NHS number had many formats that cannot be validated, and understandably many NHS organizations thus did not use it. This old number is gradually being replaced by a new ten-digit unique person-identifier number, with the last number acting as a check digit to guard against typographical error. Since July 1995, every newborn baby in the UK has been allocated a new NHS number, and there is a scheme already well advanced to replace everyone's old NHS number with the new number. As the new numbers permeate all existing databases of patient information, the ease with which patient information is transferred will greatly increase, particularly using EDI as explained above. The importance of this unique, identifiable, new NHS number cannot be understated, and the security of patient information linked to this number is of paramount importance to guard the confidentiality of the doctor–patient relationship.

Considering a network which spans the whole of the NHS, allows access to mobile phone users and links to the Internet presents many challenges for security. Connection between the NHSnet and the Internet is only through highly secure firewall gateways. Similarly, hospital trusts typically connect to the NHSnet through firewalls. Even within hospital trusts, networks may offer further levels of security down to individual password-protected access to sections of confidential databases.

Computer-assisted learning

Computer-assisted learning (CAL) has demonstrated great potential to aid learning, and with the advent of the Internet this potential is now being realized[14]. Although CAL has been with us for many years, it has had great difficulty competing with more conventional methods of education. In the past, educational media such as books have provided a much more convenient and less costly method of providing information than computers. It has been difficult to justify the costs of developing CAL for a limited audience, and difficult to fund expansion of infrastructure for the potential audience with a limited amount of CAL material available. The Internet now provides an extremely large potential audience, and the resources already on the Internet may be incorporated into educational programs.

There are both theoretical and practical benefits to the use of CAL. Educational modules using CAL may be designed according to good educational strategies[15]. Learning may be centered around the student, who may perform tasks which provide appropriate feedback leading to further tasks[16]. This goal–action–feedback cycle reinforces learning. The incorporation of multimedia elements such as images, sounds and video clips in CAL adds interest and enhances learning. Different individuals learn better in response to different media. It has been suggested that learning may be improved by providing information in more than one form simultaneously, such as animation with sound, so that the student has actively to process the presented information[17]. Student interaction with CAL may be automatically recorded, both to reduce administration of assessing students' performance and to identify weaknesses in CAL modules. A CAL package is digitally stored; thus, it may be reproduced without error as many times as required. By providing access to a CAL package over a network, many students may use a single resource. Further, if the CAL package is made accessible via an Internet browser, then it becomes potentially available to a very wide audience, using a diverse range of computers.

Communication and telemedicine

Communication is fundamental to health-care, and provides a method by which medical care may be provided from a distance. Telephone calls, letters and faxes are essential for everyday reproductive medicine practice, and new communication methods bring new possibilities. Communication may be asynchronous or synchronous, in either an unstructured (e.g. conversational) or structured format (e.g. EDI). E-mail is an attractive asynchronous method of communication, but should be used with caution. A survey commissioned by Novell revealed that over half of respondents had received abusive e-mails from colleagues and superiors[18]. It was suggested that: 'E-mail is completely void of the physical and tonal clues that face to face and voice communications provide to interpret meaning. Instead, e-mail is immediate, often impetuous and consequently wide open to misuse'. Further, the survey suggested that a substantial amount of time was wasted reading e-mail, and e-mails were even sent rather than speaking to colleagues at the next desk. Nevertheless, e-mail communication was extremely popular; thus, it is important for organizations to consider polices for e-mail use and for individuals to reconsider the content of their messages before sending e-mails. Perhaps one of the most exciting uses of synchronous communication is the option of video-conferencing. Tele-conferencing is a term that may be used when video-conferencing is combined with data-conferencing. Video-conferencing allows people at two or more sites to see live pictures with sound, whereas data-conferencing allows people at different sites to view and work on a common document or file.

Artificial intelligence, data mining, knowledge discovery

Computer systems may have a place to assist in decision-making and interpretation of large amounts of data. Artificial intelligence has been developed for many years, and is shown to be a useful aid to clinical management in a wide range of circumstances, including diagnostic systems, patient monitoring and decision support systems[11]. An interesting application of machine learning systems is to 'extract' knowledge from large collections of data by a technique referred to as knowledge discovery or data mining. These techniques have potential uses in many areas, such as analyzing large data sets arising from epidemiological research or bioinformatics. The Data Mining and Knowledge Discovery Resource Center provides a useful view of current progress in this dynamic field (http://www.kdnuggets.com).

HOW TECHNOLOGY MAY MEET THE NEEDS

It can be seen that medical informatics has much to offer to meet the communication and information needs of reproductive medicine. Where application does not meet potential there is room for improvement. However, technology is not without a price; thus, it is important to ensure that benefits will outweigh costs and that constantly changing technology is used most appropriately. This section considers how technology may meet some of the informatics needs of reproductive medicine. Many needs may be helped by common approaches, and it is likely that Internet/intranet technologies will become an increasingly important part of solutions to meet many informatics needs.

Internet library

The Internet is now starting to provide a workable solution to the library needs of reproductive medicine professionals. Although the Internet as a whole may be seen as a chaotic source of information, there is increasing order overlaid on the chaos. There are various search facilities (http://www.google.com) and

lists of approved sources of information on the Internet (http://www.hon.ch). A study of junior doctors in the south and west of England (http://www.swot.org.uk) clearly identified Internet access to MEDLINE as a major resource for the self-directed training of junior doctors. Although access to MEDLINE abstracts was freely available on the Internet (http://www.healthgate.com), it was concluded that full text with illustrations was required. Fortunately it is now possible to purchase access to complete articles of extensive areas of the medical literature on an individual or institutional level (http://www.ovid.com). This is particularly useful for organizations which do not have access to a large local medical library or have students working at a distance from the main campus.

Clearly, to benefit from Internet resources, users must have access to the Internet at the point of need. The fall in price of computer systems, with commercial Internet access and increased support to get started, makes it feasible for individuals to purchase systems for their home use. Similarly, hospitals could provide Internet access. However, the introduction of a secure network provided by the NHSnet makes it possible for hospitals to provide Internet access in the wards, clinics, operating theaters, offices, doctors' mess, etc., using the same system which may hold patient information. Further, once a user is taught how to use a web browser, this can provide access to a wide range of information systems both medical and non-medical.

Clinical record databases

The needs of different reproductive medicine centers differ, and, if expectations match investment, then computer database systems provide a very useful method to manage data[19]. At a very basic level, a flat-file database may be used to store only essential data, which are entered on only one computer. This database may be carried on a floppy disk or other movable data storage to be updated onto other computers, which can access a copy of the information, although they cannot enter new information. This 'sneaker net' provides a workable solution to the provision of simple audit, generation of standard forms and planned research. This system requires little maintenance, and, if the main data-entry computer were to fail, any of the other computers with a copy of the database could take on this role. Although such a system may be decried as primitive, it very confidently provides benefits in excess of its costs, which more complex systems may find difficult to match. The simple nature of the system makes it much more straightforward to create the database, export data into other software programs and ensure the data are accurate. Nevertheless, there tend to be higher expectations of what computers should deliver, and the information requirements are generally much greater than can be handled in this manner.

When producing a more sophisticated DBMS, key issues to consider are the consequences of the increased volume of data collected and the need for simultaneous access to the database by many individuals at different locations. It becomes important to involve a systems analyst to help identify needs, analyze the underlying issues, determine the indicators, formulate the problem and produce a solution. With the increasing volume of data entered, the chance of incorrect data entry increases substantially. Meticulous care must thus be taken to incorporate automatic checks of data entry into the system to ensure that duplicate records are not produced and that key information is always entered, and to minimize the entry of inaccurate data. In order to ensure accurate data entry, the data should be entered close to the point where the data are generated, whether this is in the outpatient clinic, the operating theater or anywhere else. Further, a person who understands the data and is responsible for the data should enter the data. As the volume of data increases, the way this is stored within the database becomes progressively more complex, and the technical problems of connecting many people simultaneously to one data source should not be underestimated. Information needs to change with changes in clinical practice and any system may develop faults; thus, the long-term support and development of the system is essential. Cost–benefit considerations and long-term reliability are clearly important aspects when developing or purchasing any sophisticated DBMS. Given the high costs of a comprehensive DBMS (including clinical records, accounts, laboratory results, clinical guidelines, laboratory guidelines, library resources and administration), the approach adopted by the ReproMED project has been to develop in small steps, closely focused on functionality, using separate commercial programs all viewed from a common desktop. Within the secure

clinical intranet, the separate programs gradually can be interfaced on a web server and accessed via a web browser, also further allowing views of remote data sources such as laboratory results, electronic libraries and even on-line learning environments (Figure 2).

National data collection

In the UK there is a statutory need for assisted conception clinics to provide information to the HFEA, and EDI is a proven secure, cost-efficient and reliable technology to transfer such information. In 1997 a survey was conducted of the 75 licensed in vitro fertilization (IVF) clinics in the UK to determine the number of databases in use and the views of clinics about sending information to the HFEA using EDI[20]. A questionnaire was sent by post to the clinical director or head of the IVF center. Where necessary a second questionnaire was sent. Of the 75 licensed IVF clinics approached, 60 clinics replied to the survey (80%). Of the responding clinics, 41 (69%) currently had a computer database for recording IVF-related information (Figure 3). Of the 41 computer databases for which information was collected, 20 were capable of generating the information required by the HFEA. Of the responding 60 clinics, 54 clinics (90%) stated an interest in EDI as an alternative means of information transfer, four clinics made no comment and only two clinics (3.3%) were not interested in this method (Figure 4). It is clear from both the high response rate (80%) and the individual responses that a majority of clinics with existing databases are interested in utilizing EDI. A similar level of interest was expressed by centers which did not have a database (many had intended to introduce one in the following 12 months; hence, by now the situation should be even more favorable).

For EDI to be effective would require reliable, accurate, well-supported databases, which may not universally be the case at present[8]. The 1997 survey revealed that a commercial computer software company provided only 21% of databases, and a trained programmer was involved in the design of a further 18% of the databases for EDI[20]. In the majority of cases an interested person in the department produced the databases or the origin of the database was unclear.

To store data related to reproductive medicine that may be meaningful for all databases requires commonly agreed codes. The HFEA statutory

Networks, Servers and Connections

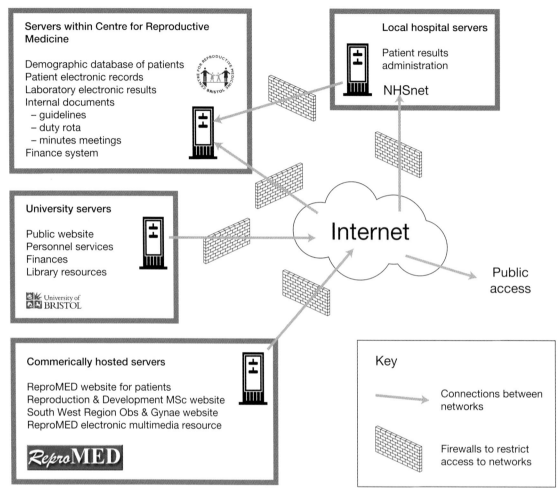

Figure 2 Diagrammatic representation illustrating some of the functions provided for the Centre for Reproductive Medicine by various servers on different networks. The diagram illustrates several networks and how they are connected. The use of firewalls and other security measures not only blocks unauthorized access to secure networks completely or partially, but also allows secure networks to connect to each other securely over the Internet

requirements could define a minimum set of codes, and a working group of the British Fertility Society has suggested an extended set of codes that could serve to facilitate more detailed communication between clinics that so wished[21]. Whether EDI should be adopted remains the decision of the HFEA, and pilot studies would be required to evaluate the logistics and optimal method of implementation. If EDI were to be implemented widely with a nationally agreed code set, beyond the obvious immediate advantages, there are significant long-term possibilities to improve infer-

tility management and target scarce resources to maximum effect based on sound audit and research.

Application of technology to education

The Internet provides a variety of methods to meet the diverse needs for reproductive medicine education. The wide availability of the Internet ideally lends itself to use as a vehicle to deliver and support education[22,23]. The use of distance learning models may widen participation by reducing geographical

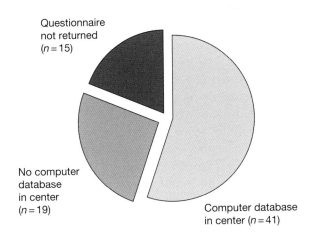

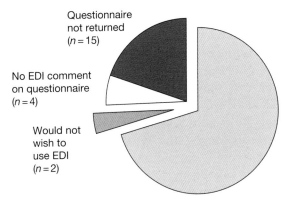

Figure 3 Response to questionnaire sent to all clinics licensed by the Human Fertilisation and Embryology Authority (HFEA) to perform *in vitro* fertilization (IVF) in 1997 enquiring whether centers currently used a computer database

Figure 4 Response to questionnaire sent to all clinics licensed by the Human Fertilisation and Embryology Authority (HFEA) to perform *in vitro* fertilization (IVF) in 1997 enquiring whether centers would wish to use electronic data interchange (EDI) to send statutory information to the HFEA

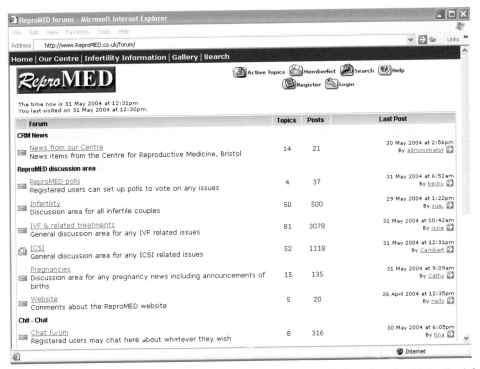

Figure 5 ReproMED provides extensive on-line support for patients including general information about infertility, infertility treatments, interactive information, multimedia gallery and a patient support forum to enable patients to support each other (http://www.ReproMED.co.uk)

restrictions, while part-time options allow students to remain in full-time employment. Although asynchronous communication between students using an electronic bulletin board has been suggested to be an effective complement to learn reproductive endocrinology[24], integration of on-line conferencing within a comprehensive on-line learning environment is more challenging[25]. As part of the ReproMED project, a critical review was performed on the place of technology to support postgraduate education[26], leading to a pilot training program delivering reproductive medicine education over the Internet by the Centre for Reproductive Medicine, University of Bristol[27]. At this time, many doctors, scientists and others requested training at the Centre that was not possible to grant, mainly due to limitations of space, staff and accommodation. When the pilot RepoMED program proved very successful it was only logical to develop it to a comprehensive Masters training program delivered over the Internet (http://www.ReD-MSc.org.uk). This program has proved extremely popular, attracting doctors, scientists and nurses from as far afield as the Phillipines, Sudan, China, Saudi Arabia, India, North America and throughout Europe[28]. Illustrating the economies of scale of computer-supported learning, this same infrastructure has been used to support undergraduate medical education (http://www.rhcn.org.uk), junior doctor training (http://www.swot.org.uk) and multiprofessional health-care education including primary care (http://health.mattersonline.net).

Supporting clinical decisions

MacDougall and Brittain[29] commented that the NHS reforms placed a demand for 'extensive, comprehensive, accurate and up-to-the minute information of all types to support the work of NHS staff at all levels, and to provide information for health care consumers'. Analysis of the information needs of general practitioners showed that they required a fast, flexible and very user-friendly system to deliver information at the point of decision[30], and it is likely that reproductive medicine specialists would require similar systems. Access to information using a web browser on the NHSnet or Internet could provide a viable solution if there was sufficient authoritative information available, professionals had adequate access to the network and there were effective methods for rapid retrieval of required information. Attention has to be given to the logistics of providing simple access to the most effective, valid resources to support clinical decision at the time of need. Integration of clinical decision support into monitoring systems and patient database systems may be a useful method to help deliver information at the point of need. Authoritative websites may provide pointers to resources maintained by appropriate

bodies, e.g. http://www.rcog.org.uk/guidelines.asp? PageID=105 and http://www.cochrane.org. Further, ReproMED illustrates how extensive local guidelines may be provided on a restricted website confined to a clinic's network, and public websites with information tailored to patients needs (http://www.ReproMED.co.uk). The patient support can extend beyond simple information and even interactive multimedia to include peer support in the form of on-line patient support groups (Figure 5)[31]. This is an exciting area for medical Informatics research, with clear benefits for implementation into clinical practice.

CONCLUSION

As with all areas of health-care, medical informatics is now an integral part of reproductive medicine. The constantly expanding volume of increasingly complex information necessitates efficient and effective methods of handling and communicating information. The methods to achieve this are largely common to clinical practice, administration, audit, education, training and research. As advancing technology provides new opportunities, it is vital that health-care professionals including doctors, nurses and scientists help to shape the changes. It is important through awareness to take appropriate advantage of technology and not to fall victim to inappropriate investment, inappropriate use, inappropriate design or short-term cost savings, leading to long-term costs. Computer-assisted learning, clinical decision support systems and clinical information systems could, in time, merge together within a sophisticated communication infrastructure based on the Internet to improve the standards of patient care. In a small way the ReproMED project illustrates this convergence today.

REFERENCES

1. Gosbee J. Communication among health professionals. Br Med J 1998; 316: 642
2. Coiera EW, Tombs V. Communication behaviours in a hospital setting: an observational study. Br Med J 1998; 316: 673–6
3. Human Embryology and Fertilisation Act. London: HMSO, 1990
4. Human Fertilisation and Embryology Authority. Twelfth Annual Report, 2002/2003. London: HFEA, 2003: 16–17

5. Cochrane AL. Effectiveness and Efficiency. Random Reflections on Health Services. London: Nuffield Provincial Hospitals Trust, 1972, (reprinted in 1989 in association with Br Med J)

6. Chambers R, Wakley G, Jenkins J. Appraisal and Revalidation: Demonstrating your Clinical Competence, Book two: Women's Health. Oxford, UK: Radcliffe Medical Press Ltd, 2004

7. Ashcroft SA, Meadowcroft J, Corrigan L, et al. A fertility network for nurses. Presented at the British Fertility Society, Sheffield, UK, April 1998

8. Keay SD, Rennie A, Liversedge NH, et al. Reliability of IVF databases – suggestions for improvement. J Br Fertil Soc 1, No 2; 14B. Hum Reprod 1996; 11 (Suppl): 7

9. Humber M. National programme for information technology. Br Med J 2004; 328: 1145–6

10. Codd EF. A relational model for large shared data banks. Commun of ACM 1970; 13: 377–87

11. Coiera E. Guide to Medical Informatics, The Internet and Telemedicine. London: Chapman & Hall Medical, 1997: 139–90

12. Côté RA, Rothwell JL, Palotay RS, et al. Systematized Nomenclature of Human and Veterinary Medicine SNOMED International. Washington DC: College of American Pathologists, 1993

13. De Lusignan S, Minmagh C, Kennedy C, et al. A survey to identify the clinical coding and classification systems currently in use across the European Community. Medinfo 2001; 10: 86–9

14. Jenkins JM. Computer assisted learning. Curr Obstet Gynaecol 1997; 7: 139–44

15. Laurillard D. Rethinking University Education: A Framework for the Effective Use of Educational Technology. London: Routledge, 1993

16. Jelovsek FR, Adebonojo L. Learning principles as applied to computer assisted instruction. MD Computing 1993; 10: 165–72

17. Penney CG. Modality effects and the structure of short-term verbal memory. Memory Cognition 1989; 17: 398–422

18. Fisher PJ. Shot down in flames. Personal Computer World August 1997: 45

19. Mason RD, Jenkins JM, Anthony FW. Computers in assisted conception. In Brinsden PR. Rainsbury PA. eds A Textbook of In Vitro Fertilization and Assisted Reproduction. Carnforth, UK: Parthenon Publishing, 1992: 405–6

20. Keay SD, Corrigan E, Wardle PG, et al. Electronic transfer of mandatory infertility information: survey of option of licensed treatment centre. Hum Fertil 2000; 3: 11–12

21. Rutherford AJ, Jenkins JM. Hull and Rutherford classification of infertility. Hum Fertil 2002; 5 (Suppl 1): 41–5

22. Jenkins JM. The Internet, intranets and reproductive medicine. Hum Reprod 1999, 14: 586–9

23. Conole G, Hall M, Smith S. An evaluation of an online course for medical practitioners. J Education Technol Soc 2002; 5: 66–75. http://www.ifets.info

24. Letterie G, Salminen ER, McClure GB. An electronic bulletin board for instruction in reproductive endocrinology in a residency in obstetrics and gynaecology. Fertil Steril 1996; 65: 883–5

25. Cahill DJ, Cook J, Jenkins J. How useful are world wide web discussion boards and email in delivering a case study course in reproductive medicine? In Ghaoui C, ed. Usability Evaluation of Online Learning Programs. London: Information Science Publishing, 2003; 360–70

26. Draycott TJ, Cook J, Fox R, Jenkins J. Information technology for postgraduate education; a survey of facilities and skills in the South West Deanery. Br J Obstet Gynaecol 1999; 106: 731–5

27. Jenkins J, Cook J, Edwards J, et al. A pilot Internet training programme in reproductive medicine. Br J Obstet Gynaecol 2001; 108: 114–16

28. Whittington K, Cook J, Barratt C, Jenkins J. Can the Internet widen participation in reproductive medicine education for professionals? Hum Reprod 2004; 19: 1800–5

29. MacDougall J, Brittain JM. Use of Information in the NHS. Library and Information Research Report 92. London: British Library, 1992

30. Taylor TR. The computer and clinical decision-support systems in primary care. J Fam Pract 1990; 30: 137–40

31. Hinks JA, Gosmore JP, Jenkins JM, Corrigan E. Is the Internet replacing local patient support groups? Hum Reprod 2004; (Suppl 1): O–047: i17

39.1

Regulation of assisted reproductive technology: the UK experience – themes and trends

Suzi Leather and Peter Mills

Assisted reproduction has now touched the lives of a significant proportion of people, with *in vitro* fertilization (IVF) now accounting for about one in every 100 children born in the UK[1]. Despite this familiarity, its capacity to excite strong and contradictory responses among the public remains undiminished. It is against this background, indeed partly because of the capacity of assisted reproduction to generate strong, conflicting responses, that the Human Fertilisation and Embryology Authority (HFEA) was set up by Parliament under legislation passed in 1990[2].

ORIGINS AND FUNCTIONS OF THE HFEA

The Warnock Report, voluntary regulation and the 1990 Act

Legislation on assisted conception and human embryo research was preceded by considerable debate and deliberation beginning, in July 1982, with the establishment of a Committee of Enquiry chaired by Dame Mary (now Baroness) Warnock. Even at that time, only 4 years after the first IVF birth, public enthusiasm for, and suspicion of, the new techniques of assisted conception had become well developed. As the Committee's 1984 report, subsequently known as the 'Warnock Report', observed:

Society's views on the new techniques were divided between pride in the technological achievement, pleasure at the new-found means to relieve, at least for some, the unhappiness of infertility, and unease at the apparently uncontrolled advance of science, bringing with it new possibilities for manipulating the early stages of human development[3].

Sensitive to this unease, the Committee's terms of reference extended beyond purely scientific and clinical considerations to include, in particular, the ethical and social implications of the techniques.

One of the Committee's key recommendations was 'the establishment of a new Statutory Licensing Authority to regulate both research and those infertility services which we have recommended should be subject to control'[4]. While the Government consulted over how to enshrine these recommendations in legislation, the Medical Research Council and Royal College of Obstetricians and Gynaecologists (RCOG) acted, in 1985, to establish a Voluntary Licensing Authority (VLA) giving guidance on appropriate conduct and good practice. When a White Paper was introduced in 1989, broadly reflecting the recommendations made in the Warnock Report, the VLA changed its name to the Interim Licensing Authority in anticipation of the establishment of a statutory regulator. The experience and information accumulated

623

by the VLA and its successor proved invaluable to the HFEA when, following a gestation of – appropriately – just 9 months, it had to put into place a regulatory structure, produce its first code of practice and assume its licensing and regulatory responsibilities in August 1991. The recognition by clinicians of the value of public confidence and close collaboration with regulators, and by regulators of the need for informed understanding of clinical practice, has been a major theme of regulation since 1991, and has helped to ensure the good public reputation enjoyed by reproductive medicine in the UK.

Pillars of the Act

The framework legislation, the Human Fertilisation and Embryology Act 1990, which became law on November 1, 1990, passed through Parliament following a very well-informed debate. In both houses of Parliament members were given free votes by their political parties, allowing them to vote according to their consciences.

Some of the concerns identified in the Warnock Report were embedded in the 1990 Act as a series of absolute prohibitions. Activities absolutely prohibited under the Act or incapable of being licensed and, accordingly, subject to criminal sanction are: placing live gametes or a live embryo other than a human embryo in a woman, keeping an embryo beyond the appearance of the primitive streak (or in any case beyond 14 days), placing a human embryo in an animal, or replacing a nucleus of a cell of any embryo with a nucleus taken from a cell of any person, embryo or subsequent development of an embryo. Other activities, which would otherwise be prohibited, are permitted subject to license from the HFEA; these are: creating or using human embryos outside the body, providing assisted conception treatment using donated gametes and mixing human gametes with the live gametes of any animal. Placing in a woman an embryo created other than by fertilization (i.e. human reproductive cloning) was banned under separate legislation in 2001[5].

While some have found the architecture of the Act confusing, the basic approach (that, within a circumscribed area, everything is prohibited unless it is permitted) has meant that the Act has proved, at the time of writing, to be sufficiently flexible and robust to withstand the challenges of more than a decade of rapid scientific and technological advance.

The 1990 Act is supported by the twin pillars of informed consent and concern for the welfare of any child who may be born as a result of treatment services. In all cases, those whose gametes are stored or used outside their bodies retain non-transferable rights of disposal over their genetic material, including embryos produced from those gametes, up until such time as they are transferred to a woman. But in addition to this the legislation ensures that the unique feature of assisted conception – that the consequences of a treatment provided to one person are the conditions of existence of another – is properly addressed by clinicians who are required to take account of the consequences of treatment, social as well as medical, for the children resulting from it as well as for the adults undergoing it.

Constitution of the HFEA

The Act formally established the HFEA as a non-departmental public body (NDPB). This means that the Authority, a type of body unique in medicine and, until comparatively recently, unique in the world, is accountable to Parliament through the Secretary of State for Health, but independent from Government and party-political interest.

The HFEA's members are appointed by the Secretary of State following open public advertisement for a term of 3 years, with a possible option of extension for a further 3 years. Members do not represent constituencies or interests but are appointed for their individual expertise and come from a wide variety of disciplines. Typical membership includes those with an expertise in clinical and research medicine, nursing, science, law, ethics, religion, psychology, counseling, regulation and the media. It is noteworthy, in view of its explicitly social and ethical responsibilities, that the HFEA must comprise a membership the majority of which are lay-persons, and that neither the Chair nor the Deputy Chair may be clinicians or scientists working in the area of assisted conception or human embryo research. The Authority usually meets in full about ten times a year. It retains a part-time inspectorate of about 60 clinicians, scientists, ethicists, nurses and counselors[6], and can draw on an internationally respected pool of peer reviewers to advise on license applications and policy matters. The Authority is supported by a permanent executive staff based in London.

Functions and powers of the HFEA

Regulation is achieved through a system of licensing, inspection and monitoring. The activities for which the Authority may issue licenses are set out in Schedule 2 to the 1990 Act, and are divided into licenses for treatment, licenses for storage and licenses for research. Licenses are granted following the approval of an application from a center by a license committee comprising more than three and up to five members of the Authority. Licenses are issued to a 'Person Responsible' at the clinic who must oversee and take responsibility for activities conducted in pursuance of the license. All licensed activities must be carried out on premises designated in the license. Licenses are generally issued for a term of 3 years, although in certain circumstances shorter licenses may be issued. Before a license is issued, and every year during which the license is held, centers are inspected by the HFEA and inspection reports are submitted to a license committee for review. More recently, in addition to its program of regular inspections, the HFEA has started to carry out unannounced inspections.

Licenses are issued subject to conditions, some of which – general conditions applicable to all licenses of a certain sort – are specified in the 1990 Act itself (for example, the condition that a woman may not be provided with treatment services unless account has been taken of the welfare of any child who may be born as a result[7]). Other conditions may be imposed by the Authority, either as general conditions reflecting a matter of policy or as conditions applicable to an individual center as determined by a license committee. Centers may appeal a decision of a license committee to a panel comprising members of the Authority who did not sit on that committee. If an appeal is unsuccessful, decisions of the Authority are susceptible to judicial review on matters of law.

Other powers of the Authority are exercised through Directions, which tend to relate not to clinical practice but to administrative matters. Directions, which have the same force as license conditions, may be either general, applying equally to all licensed centers, or special, applying to individual centers, and have the same force as license conditions. General directions typically concern matters such as the recording and reporting of information, and money that may be paid in respect of the supply of gametes or embryos; special directions apply to matters such as the continued discharge of the functions of the Person Responsible where a center ceases activity, or the import of gametes and embryos from abroad.

Code of Practice and license committees

The Authority is required by the 1990 Act to produce a *Code of Practice* 'giving guidance on the proper conduct of activities carried on in pursuance of a license [...] and the proper discharge of the functions of the person responsible and other persons to whom the license applies'[8]. The content of the *Code* is informed by principles implicit in the legislation which are adumbrated in its introduction:

(1) The respect which is due to human life at all stages in its development;

(2) The right of people who are or may be infertile to the proper consideration of their request for treatment;

(3) A concern for the welfare of children, which cannot always be adequately protected by concern for the interests of the adults involved;

(4) A recognition of the benefits, both to individuals and to society which can flow from the responsible pursuit of medical and scientific knowledge[9].

The *Code of Practice* is arranged in sections which reflect the different aspects of the provision of treatment services: the staff and facilities of a licensed center, consultation and assessment of patients and donors, the information with which they should be provided, consent, counseling, the storage and use of gametes and embryos, the use of reproductive material in research, records that must be kept, and procedures that must be in place for handling complaints. Whilst the layout of the *Code* has remained relatively similar throughout consecutive editions, the content has evolved substantially as a result of increasing knowledge and experience and changes in the legislative context. The considerably expanded sixth edition of the *Code*, published in 2003, contains dedicated sections giving guidance on preimplantation genetic testing and intracytoplasmic sperm injection, and on witnessing clinical and laboratory procedures[10]. This edition also, for the first time, sets out in the main text the legal provisions underlying the *Code* in order to help ART professionals to distinguish between legal requirements (what they 'must' do) and guidance on proper procedure (which they 'are expected' to observe). Thus, whilst the Act draws the parameters of what is permissible in the abstract, regardless of whether it is appropriate or even possible in any particular circumstances, it is left to the Authority to determine, within these parameters, what is permitted at any particular time, in the light of current knowledge and experience and, through its licensing system, to whom.

The guidance contained in the *Code* is designed to assist licensed centers to comply with the mandatory requirements of the Act, in particular giving guidance on the interpretation of the words 'proper' and 'suitable' where they occur in the Act (for example, the requirement that before people consent to treatment they are given 'proper information'). Whilst it is acknowledged that what is 'suitable' and 'proper' may vary in relation to particular circumstances, and that in exceptional circumstances good clinical judgment may demand a justifiable departure from the guidance given by the *Code*, compliance with the *Code* may be taken into account by a license committee as a guide to determining whether a license should be varied or revoked, or whether an application should be approved.

In framing the *Code of Practice* it is therefore important that the guidance given is appropriate, reasonable and proportionate, and that it commands a high degree of acceptance within the professions. In developing the *Code*, as well as taking the advice of its clinical, scientific and legal members, the HFEA seeks advice from professional bodies such as the RCOG, the British Fertility Society, the British Andrology Society, the Association of Clinical Embryologists, the British Infertility Counselling Association and the Fertility Nurses Group, among others. On particular measures, and on the *Code* as a whole, the Authority consults with the professions and, especially on matters of public interest, with the public, other government and advisory bodies and foreign and international organizations.

The *Code of Practice* is not only, however, an interpretative tool for clinicians and a yardstick for inspectors and HFEA license committees. It is also of value to patients and those seeking treatment, informing them of what to expect when they undergo licensed treatment and reassuring them about the standards that should be maintained by those treating them.

Policy and advisory functions

The *Code* is a statutory document, the whole of which must be approved by the Secretary of State and laid before Parliament before it can be brought into force. For this reason it is revised only every 2–3 years. Developments in assisted reproduction do not, however, occur in such convenient cycles. The growth in treatment from a small initial base, the increasing technical complexity of treatment services and innovations which raise complex social and ethical issues all make continuous and comprehensive review of the field essential. It is a core function of the HFEA to monitor and review these developments and knowledge about them, and continuously to provide advice and guidance to those seeking and providing treatment services.

In order to support these functions the HFEA maintains a number of subcommittees comprising members of the Authority and other co-opted members. Whilst the arrangement of these committees has altered over time in response to the Authority's changing requirements, they have generally included a committee with responsibility for considering social and ethical issues[11], a committee with responsibility for reviewing scientific and clinical developments[12], and a committee to oversee regulatory practice[13]. These committees report on a regular basis to the full Authority, where recommendations are discussed and implementation decisions taken.

For clearly delimitable projects the HFEA sometimes establishes *ad hoc* working groups to develop a particular policy or to advise on specific matters[14]. These committees typically draw on the assistance of acknowledged experts in the relevant fields, assemble and consider evidence from the UK and other jurisdictions, consult with those on whom their recommendations will impact and, particularly on matters of social and ethical significance, with the public at large. The work of these committees usually comes to an end with the submission of advice or recommendations to the Authority or to the Secretary of State and, where appropriate, with the publication of a report[15].

The results of these policy reviews are published and disseminated through *ad hoc* communications such as Chair's and Chief Executive's letters, published reports on specific matters and periodic publications such as the Patients' Guides[16]. In addition to these, the HFEA publishes a number of information leaflets for patients and those seeking treatment which relate to specific issues and a regular newsletter, the *HFEA Update*. More recently the HFEA's website, which now has a dedicated section for licensed centers, is another important and regularly updated source of information.

The Register

In addition to human embryo research and the treatment and storage services it regulates, the HFEA is also required to maintain a Register of licensed treatment services and of donors whose gametes are used. The conditions under which information may be disclosed from the Register are highly restrictive, the confidentiality provisions of the Act, for instance, prevent data linkage between the Register and any other medical databases. However, in its own right the Register is capable of providing a valuable source of information for research into assisted conception[17]. In addition to its value as a research tool, the Register's other primary function is to safeguard information that may be disclosed to donor-conceived people when they reach the age of 18 (or beforehand, if they intend to marry before their 18th birthday)[18].

THEMES AND TRENDS IN REGULATION IN THE UK

The interests of offspring

For a large number of infertile men whose wives or partners have undergone treatment using donor sperm since August 1991, the 1990 Act performed a significant service by making them irrefutably the legal fathers of the resulting children. This measure also gave donors the confidence that it was not merely their anonymity that protected them from any legal relationship to children conceived using their gametes. It also helped to formalize legally the social bond between infertile fathers and their children. In fact, the number of patients receiving donor insemination treatment has declined from a peak of about 7000 in the mid-1990s to a level of just over 4000 by the year 2000. This has been attributed to the introduction of micromanipulation techniques such as intracytoplasmic sperm injection (ICSI) to circumvent male-factor infertility and perhaps also preimplantation

genetic diagnosis (PGD) for genetic disease. It is doubtful, however, that this downward trend will continue indefinitely. Donor conception remains the only available assisted conception treatment for the partners of azoospermic males and for those women, steadily increasing in number, who wish to begin a family without a male partner.

In the years since the 1990 Act, increasing numbers of pre-Act donor-conceived people have reached adulthood, constituting a large and important stakeholder group whose unique perspective and interests are coming to be voiced and understood. In particular, the interest of donor-conceived people in access to information about the donors used in their conception has prompted a significant reappraisal of the law protecting the anonymity of donors. The HFEA has been active in this debate and, following a lengthy consultation by the Department of Health, Regulations were passed by Parliament to remove statutory guarantees of anonymity from those who register as donors of gametes or embryos after April 1, 2005. The Authority continues to work with the Department of Health and others to encourage a 'culture change' which it is hoped will have the effect of making the value and benefits of gamete donation more widely recognized.

The use of evidence in reducing risk

Developments and innovations in IVF have undoubtedly contributed to an improvement in the overall live birth rate. Improvements in cryopreservation have also increased the success from frozen embryo transfers, meaning that women are less likely to undergo repeated stimulated egg collections, thereby reducing the risks to their health. Despite these advances, however, the incidence of multiple births resulting from IVF remains disproportionately high.

From its first *Code of Practice*, the Authority recommended that no more than three eggs or three embryos should be transferred to a woman in any one cycle. As techniques have improved and as evidence has accumulated, information about IVF treatments from the HFEA's Register and other sources has come to show that a maximum of two embryos transferred to women under age 40 will significantly reduce the multiple pregnancy rate without significantly affecting the likelihood of a healthy live birth. On the strength of this evidence, in its sixth *Code of Practice* the HFEA recommended for the first time that no more than two eggs or embryos should be transferred to a woman under 40 or to any woman where donated eggs or embryos are used.

The growth in experience and evidence relating to assisted conception has been one of the most significant developments since 1990. The comprehensive collection of data about assisted reproduction and the regular publication of this information from the HFEA register has gone a long way to addressing many of the concerns that surrounded IVF in the early years, and continues to be an important means of evaluation, particularly for newer techniques. This growing evidence base, supported by information obtained from licensed embryo research, and sometimes from other jurisdictions too, has meant that the HFEA has been increasingly able to found policy developments on more realistic estimations of risk and benefit.

The involvement of the HFEA with research groups and the more recent establishment of an international horizon scanning group, comprising those at the cutting edge of infertility research and treatment, has contributed to the HFEA's ability to anticipate and evaluate new technologies. As the introduction of these technologies into clinical practice requires a license from the HFEA, the licensing process in turn presents an opportunity to evaluate the latest evidence and allows the techniques to be introduced in a controlled manner, ensuring that results are monitored, and that knowledge is shared as quickly and widely as possible. Additionally, the introduction by the HFEA of a formal alert system in 2003 has greatly facilitated the rapid communication of emerging knowledge about risks and risk management between the HFEA and licensed centers.

Transparency, communication and patient involvement

The careful assessment and use of evidence is, however, only one element in the development of better regulatory processes and decisions. As availability of, and demand for, assisted conception treatment has grown, so has the expectation that treatment and regulation will be carried out with greater transparency and accountability. Measures such as making available inspection reports and license committee decisions have contributed to this transparency. Although

demanding on inevitably scarce resources, the accurate and balanced communication of information to patients, stakeholders and the wider public about assisted conception practice, embryo research and the work of the HFEA has helped to inform the decisions of those seeking treatment, create a more informed public debate and build confidence in the sector.

The involvement of patients and patient groups in policy development (e.g. through stakeholder consultation) and the regulatory cycle (e.g. through participation in inspections) has also been invaluable in developing an understanding of the values, expectations and experiences of those receiving treatment and their families.

Reproductive rights

Debates in bioethics and jurisprudence about reproductive rights have inevitably affected the field of assisted conception since 1990. A focus of these debates, particularly since the passage of the Human Rights Act 1998, which imported into UK law the rights guaranteed by the European Convention on Human Rights[19], has increasingly been the extent of the legitimate interference by the State and public authorities with the freedoms of individuals. The articles of the Convention most relevant to assisted conception are, generally, Articles 8 ('right to respect for private and family life') and 12 ('right to marry and found a family'), combined with Article 14 ('prohibition of discrimination'). Interference by public authorities with the exercise of these rights may only be justified, generally, where it can be shown to be lawful, necessary, proportionate to the aim to be achieved, and applied equitably and without unfair discrimination[20]. However, it is established that restrictions applied by a public authority may have regard to the values of the society in which it acts, as shown by the 'margin of appreciation' allowed to individual States by the European Court of Human Rights on matters of public morality. The effect of human rights legislation has so far, however, been not to shift the balance between individual freedom and state regulation, but rather to multiply the forces holding that balance in place.

Regard to the rights of individuals and societal values is particularly important for the HFEA as a public authority with responsibility for setting, through its guidance and licensing decisions, the contingent limits of what is permitted at any one time. It is noteworthy, however, that in providing a service to the public, or a section of the public[21], fertility clinics are themselves capable of being regarded as 'public authorities' for the purposes of the 1998 Act and are consequently also open to claims under that Act. The guidance provided by the HFEA in its *Code of Practice* provides some protection to clinics and may thereby minimize their exposure to such claims. On the other hand, the 1998 Act also gives clinicians an additional strand to appeals against unjustified interference by the HFEA in their legitimate activities, helping to ensure, if this were necessary, that regulation remains proportionate, accountable, consistent, transparent and targeted.

An international perspective

In addition to applications for judicial review of decisions made by the HFEA, the years since 2000 have also seen claims that the law governing assisted conception itself is incompatible with European law and Convention rights[22]. An early indication of this trend was the invocation of the EC Treaty to demonstrate that the opportunity to receive treatment abroad should not be inhibited, as this would interfere with the free movement of goods and services within the European Community (EC)[23].

The years since then have seen a growth of what has since become known as 'procreative tourism': traveling abroad to obtain treatments that would be prohibited under domestic law. The lack of consistency or harmonization in assisted conception regulation across the European Union (EU), indeed worldwide, has increased the difficulties of regulation. Developments such as the EU Tissues and Cells Directive may provide a higher level of harmonization of standards, but even so it is likely that differences in what is permitted or prohibited within national jurisdictions will continue to exist even within the EU. Procreative tourism may therefore continue to provide an attractive option for a number of people in the UK and other countries. Partly in recognition of this, the HFEA increasingly takes an international perspective, building and consolidating links with the growing number of government agencies, voluntary regulators, professional societies, patient groups and individuals across the EU and beyond.

Reprogenetics and new ethical challenges

Finally, a development which has affected assisted conception dramatically since the HFEA was established, is the convergence between ART on the one hand and advances in genetic knowledge and genetic testing on the other. Improvements in micromanipulation (blastomere biopsy) and genetic testing have led to increased reproductive options for those with known genetic conditions in their families. As well as reliable methods of sexing preimplantation embryos for the avoidance of X-linked conditions, the discovery of increasing numbers of markers for monogenic diseases has allowed more and more people who choose to do so to exclude affected embryos at the preimplantation stage rather than risking an affected pregnancy or opting to have a child who is not genetically related to them. Cytogenetic testing of embryos to identify aneuploidies has also become possible, and, although the evidence of reproductive benefit has been slow to emerge, this too has increased the reproductive options available to those who have difficulty conceiving or carrying a pregnancy.

The challenges that these developments raise are not strictly about assisted reproduction but about the uses to which the techniques of assisted reproduction may be put over and above the project of producing a healthy child. In reviewing these questions the Authority has found it useful to carry out stakeholder and public consultation, for example on preimplantation genetic diagnosis, sex selection and preimplantation tissue typing, using a variety of qualitative and quantitative methods. It has also found it indispensable to draw on the advice and expertise of other bodies such as the Human Genetics Commission. However, as exercising reproductive choice in this way involves the use of licensed ART, it is the HFEA, as the statutory licensing authority for these technologies, that must give a determination on their permissibility.

Conclusion: evolving regulation

When the HFEA came into existence as a statutory regulator it was the first body of its type in the world, and the field it regulated was comparatively new. At that time both clinicians and regulators were pioneers in their respective fields. With the growth and development of ART, and the consolidation of knowledge and experience, much of this pioneering work has evolved into well-established practice. Fears have been laid to rest, business has boomed, and expectations – of both clinicians and regulators – have grown. A measure of the establishment of this practice is the provision of National Health Service (NHS)-funded fertility treatment which is set to increase significantly as the recommendations of the National Institute of Clinical Excellence, the independent organization responsible for providing national guidance on treatments and care for people using the NHS in England and Wales, are implemented.

But despite the bridgehead that ART has established in medicine and in the public mind, the advance of science and technology continues apace, and the social, ethical and legal context in which it takes place continues to evolve. In these circumstances the need for and demands on a modern, professional regulator, like the capacity of ART to excite strong public reactions, seem set to continue undiminished and may, in the future, be all the greater.

NOTES AND REFERENCES

1. Between July 1978, when the first birth following IVF treatment was recorded, and August 1991, when the Human Fertilisation and Embryology Authority assumed its statutory responsibilities as the regulator of assisted conception treatment and human embryo research in the UK, IVF had helped nearly 6000 families in the UK to have children. By mid-1995 that figure had doubled. By 1998 it had doubled again and by 2002 yet again, with the number of IVF babies passing the 50 000 mark
2. The Human Fertilisation and Embryology Act 1990 (c 37)
3. Report of the Committee of Inquiry into Human Fertilisation and Embryology. London: HMSO, 1984. Cmnd 9314 ('Warnock'), Ch 1, 'The General Approach'
4. Warnock, op. cit., 75
5. The Human Reproductive Cloning Act 2001 (c 23)
6. The HFEA provides training for inspectors and is committed to continuing professional development of its inspectors and staff. It now provides regular inspector training events to update inspectors on regulatory procedures and to ensure consistency
7. HFE Act 1990, s 13(5)
8. HFE Act 1990, s 25
9. Code of Practice, 6th edn. HFEA, 2003

10. 1991–93 the Committee on Social and Ethical Issues; from 1993 to 1999 social and ethical issues were considered by the Authority as a whole and ad hoc working groups which reported on individual areas of work; in 1999 a standing Ethics Committee was established, which became the Ethics & Law Committee in 2003
11. From 1995 to 2003 the Working Group on New Developments in Reproductive Technology; from 2003 the Scientific and Clinical Advances Group
12. From 1990 to 2003 the Licensing and Fees Committee supported by a dedicated Code of Practice Committee; from 2003 the Regulation Committee. In addition to these advisory committees the Authority also maintains internal committees to consider operational matters of fees and finance, audit, information and communications
13. Examples of these are the Working Group on Embryo Freezing (1993–94), the Working Group on Information (1993), the Working Group on Training in Infertility Counselling (1993), the Working Group on Payment of Donors (1994–98), the Advisory Group on Safe Cryopreservation (1995–98), the PGD (Special Issues) Working Group (2001), the Tissue Directive Implementation Working Group (2003–), the Review of the Act Working Group (2003–), the Sperm, Egg and Embryo Donation Review Steering Group (2004–) and the Welfare of the Child Advisory Group (2004–)
14. Examples of matters on which the HFEA has published large-scale public consultation papers and reports include Sex Selection (1993, 2003), Use of Fetal Ovarian Tissue (1994), Cloning Issues in Science and Medicine (with the Human Genetics Advisory Committee, 1998), the Withdrawal of Payments to Gamete Donors (1998) and Preimplantation Genetic Diagnosis (with the Advisory Committee on Genetic Testing, 1999). The Authority has also consulted with stakeholders on clinical and operational issues such as the Safe Cryopreservation of Gametes and Embryos (1998) and HFEA Modernisation of Regulation and New Fee Strategy (2002)
15. The HFEA produces guides for patients on all aspects of assisted conception treatment, including information and outcome data from all licensed centers
16. Some relaxation of restrictions on disclosure of information by licensed centers was provided for by the Human Fertilisation and Embryology (Disclosure of Information) Act 1992 (c 54), but the confidentiality provisions relating to assisted conception remain more restrictive than in other areas of medicine
17. Those over age 18 may apply to the Authority to be given notice stating whether the information

contained in the Register shows that they were born as a result of donor-assisted conception and, if so, to be given certain non-identifying information about the donor used (Human Fertilisation and Embryology Authority (Disclosure of Donor Information) Regulations 2004 (S I 2004 No. 1511)). Those conceived using gametes or embryos from donors who register after March 31, 2005, may, in addition, apply to receive identifying information about the donor used. Those who intend to marry before their 18th birthday, and applicants over 18, may apply to discover whether the information contained on the Authority's Register shows that they are or might be related to a person they intend to marry

18. Convention for the Protection of Human Rights and Fundamental Freedoms, Council of Europe (Rome, 1950), ETS No 005

19. For example, Article 8 is qualified as follows: 'There shall be no interference by a public authority with the exercise of this right except such as is in accordance with the law and is necessary in a democratic society in the interests of national security, public safety or the economic well-being of the country, for the prevention of disorder or crime, for the protection of health or morals, or for the protection of the rights and freedoms of others'. ECHR, Art 8

20. In section 2 of the 1990 Act 'treatment services' are defined as 'medical, surgical or obstetric services provided to the public or a section of the public for the purpose of assisting women to carry children'

21. For example, in 2004 a judicial review application citing Articles of the Convention was followed by an amendment to the 1990 Act to permit a deceased man being recorded as the father of a child born as a result of treatment services provided after his death (The Human Fertilisation and Embryology (Deceased Fathers) Act 2003 (c 24))

22. R. v. HFEA ex p. Blood [1997] 2 F.L.R. 742

39.2

Regulation of assisted reproductive technologies: the Australian experience

Geoffrey Driscoll and Sandra K. Dill

INTRODUCTION

Australia is a commonwealth of just over 20 million people, and nearly 2% of births in the year 2003 were classified as being 'assisted' in their conception. Australia is the only country in the world with unrestricted access to public reimbursement for assisted reproductive technologies (ART) treatment. Crucial to securing this coverage has been the genuine and continuing involvement of consumers in all aspects of regulation, legislation, accreditation and policy development. It is therefore appropriate that this chapter is coauthored by the medical director of one of the country's largest clinics and by the Chief Executive Officer of the national infertility network, ACCESS.

A COALITION OF THE COMMITTED

When the Fertility Society of Australia (FSA) was established in 1982, consumers were invited and included in the membership. This co-operation seemed natural and appropriate to those of us well used to a collaborative approach to health-care, although it was at that time quite unusual in many other areas of medicine. The membership of the FSA includes clinicians, scientists, nurses, counselors, administrators and lay-people such as consumers and

even journalists. This cross-sectional involvement appears to be unique, but it works, and should provide a model for those countries where conflict – pressure groups – exerts inordinate control over research, clinical practice and, most importantly, peoples' life-changing decisions. These partnerships are also appropriate as they particularly recognize that consumers of ART services must live with the consequences of policy and treatment decisions.

The challenge then for consumers is to ensure that all other stakeholders have confidence in their integrity and professionalism. They must exhibit an ability to work effectively with: the medical profession, allied health professionals, government ministers and senior public officials.

This may not always be an easy task, particularly in environments where such relationships have not existed, but the very real suffering of those who come to all of us for treatment and/or support compels us to commit to nothing less.

A significant factor in the success of negotiations with the Government in relation to regulation and reimbursement issues in Australia has been the commitment of consumers and providers to work in such a partnership to achieve common, well-established, clear goals.

The inclusion of a consumer representative on the Federal Council of the Fertility Society of Australia

(FSA), the Reproductive Technology Accreditation Committee (RTAC) and the IVF Directors' Group ensures that consumers have access to reliable information about treatment outcomes, possible drug side-effects and the quality of service provided by individual clinics.

This paradigm shift, from consumers as passive participants to partners, has been difficult for *in vitro* fertilization (IVF) clinicians in some countries to embrace, but the political benefits for consumers and providers can be significant, and an increasing number of international bodies are now beginning to see the benefits.

THE AUSTRALIAN HEALTH SYSTEM

Australia has a 'universal' centrally funded health system, known as Medicare, providing financial subsidy for most medical procedures including, particularly since 1990, infertility treatment.

The objective of a health system is to deliver health-care to all those in need. However, in most countries the seemingly limitless demand for health-care cannot be met due to the scarcity of resources. This has been exacerbated in Western countries by an aging population and costly advances in technology, which have exceeded the system's ability to pay. Therefore, the need for rationing or microallocation of health resources becomes apparent, even in the so-called wealthy countries. No system of allocating limited resources at the level of the individual patient can work without resorting to notions of utility. While rationing is a necessity, it is important that the system used to decide who gets health-care is one that promotes equity of access.

In 1986 the Australian Federal Department of Health released a discussion paper entitled 'Commonwealth Perspectives on IVF Funding'. As there was no coverage for IVF, and related procedures, in Medicare, the Government had difficulty in determining the real costs and outcomes of IVF treatment and they needed this information. Negotiations commenced about the possible reimbursement for such procedures, and, consistent with the inclusive approach, consumers accompanied clinicians to negotiations. We represented our respective interest-groups, but met before each meeting to discuss any issues we thought would arise, to avoid being in conflict in front of Departmental officers. It became apparent that decisions about medical treatment were going to be politically motivated and not necessarily based on rational discussion about health-care needs. It was suggested that it was not only women undergoing treatment who would be concerned about the Government's attitude, but also their partners, families and friends.

Governments have argued that the costs of providing reimbursement for infertility treatment are too high, but it has been argued that the financial costs are less significant than the real costs of infertility, such as the industrial, social and emotional costs[1].

Thus, this coalition of consumers and providers successfully lobbied the Australian Federal Government for recognition of infertility as a medical condition, and for reimbursement for ART treatment. In 1990 the Prime Minister announced the provision of reimbursement of ART procedures through Australia's national health plan. This has helped to provide equity of access to health-care for infertile people in Australia. A variation on the rebate procedures, virtually removing constraints on fees charged, was introduced in 2004, an election year in Australia, but no one expects the largess to continue given the reality of the finite 'health dollar'. The continuing participation of consumers in public policy and the regulation of IVF clinics is a reassuring demonstration by health ministers, bureaucrats and physicians in ensuring transparency and quality in the delivery of infertility services.

Methods of rationing the limited 'health dollar' can use medical or social criteria. The use of social criteria is necessarily subjective and arguably immoral. However, it is difficult to see how those making decisions about rationing resources can avoid such judgments. Value judgments can be made based on an individual's past and potential contribution to society or, in the case of ART, on old-fashioned prejudices masquerading as new ethical dilemmas[2].

Examples of social criteria influencing decision-making include discussion about whether it is ethical to allow single women, lesbian or homosexual couples access to ART. Many believe that this is morally wrong, arguing that it is preferable for a child to be raised within a stable, heterosexual relationship.

Whatever our personal views, those who argue that the traditional concepts of family must be maintained fail to recognize a different reality. An Australian Government statistical report found that 69% of households had no children, 32% of households comprised two persons, 19% had two or more children and that

13% of households had one child. Marriage rates continue to fall, divorce occurs in more than 40% of marriages and 27% of births were to single women[3]. These figures demonstrate the diversity of family arrangements.

Thus, the need to have access to health-care is balanced against the need for governments to manage scarce resources responsibly and to distribute them justly and equitably for the good of the whole community. The challenge for health-care professionals and consumers of infertility services is to persuade governments that infertility is a medical disability which causes suffering, and as such, is worthy of inclusion in their national health plan.

AUSTRALIAN LAW

We now have the anomaly whereby centralized funding assistance is offered but delivered into different jurisdictions. With six states and two territories all having different regulatory or indeed in some cases few, if any, legislative guidelines, centralized objectives and approaches are often confused by local constraints and restraints. Under our constitution, federal law supersedes most state laws, so those who prepare state legislation are required to avoid conflict with parallel federal laws. In particular we have seen legal activity surrounding concepts embracing issues covered in the Commonwealth Sex Discrimination Act (SDA 1984), particularly involving *de facto* and same-sex relationships. ART programs which may be in breach of the SDA may seek exemption from this Act by application to the Human Rights and Equal Opportunity Commission. At the time of printing, legislation dealing with ART has only been enacted in Victoria, South Australia and Western Australia. The intermittent attempts to achieve a uniform country-wide approach have met with opposition predominantly from those state legislatures defending their constitutional rights, and also by those who, perhaps also quite rightly, fear that such an approach would inevitably be that of compromise and the achievement of a least-common-denominator effect. The quandary remains, but fortunately common sense reigns in most areas, and in most states (the notable exception being Victoria) ethical research and development continue unimpeded. Other inappropriate anomalies still exist, such as the Western Australian legislation, gazetted in 1992 but still in force,

that prohibits preimplantation genetic diagnosis (fortunately allowed in other states, but the equity of access issue remains). In Australian states free from restrictive legislation, there has been no evidence that consumers or society have been disadvantaged. It can be argued that where genuine informed decision-making occurs and there is a process for legitimate ethical review, restrictive laws make little sense, and in some cases deny access to appropriate treatment for some couples who have no other means of forming their families. History has demonstrated that governments can often make ill-informed, politically expedient decisions, which are not necessarily in the best interests of those they represent. Furthermore, legislation is difficult to repeal. Even the most well-intentioned legislation in a high-tech, rapidly evolving area such as ART can quickly prove to be obsolete.

The questions are whether particular legislation will necessarily protect citizens from harm, and, where it is considered necessary, what degree of protection the law should impose in a society where most citizens are free to make a multitude of choices about their lives and health-care, including their options involving reproduction.

Once promulgated, the relevant laws need to be constantly reviewed to accommodate not only evolving technology but also community attitudes and expectations. Detailed discussion of current laws, particularly on a state by state basis, is therefore inappropriate, but it is important to mention some of the more significant decisions that have shaped the current situation.

As the first IVF baby in Australia (second in the world) was born in the southern state of Victoria, it was the Victorian Government that first developed a legislative framework. As Ian Johnston stated in an earlier edition of this textbook, the Victorian community started pressing the 'panic button', as IVF presented a challenge to the whole understanding of human reproduction. In 1984 the Infertility Treatment Act was passed, comprising some 23 pages. Its subsequent revision added a further 200 pages. Ironically, the feminist movement saw IVF as an attack on women, not something to help them.

In 1987, the Human Embryo Experimentation Bill was introduced into the Federal Parliament. It deemed all IVF procedures to be experimental, and, if passed, it would have threatened the closure of all IVF clinics in

Australia. Once again, the coalition of stakeholders successfully blocked that repressive bill.

When governments consider whether infertile people should have a right to equity of access to infertility treatment, they need to be mindful of the United Nations Declaration of Human Rights which recognizes that: 'Men and women of full age, without any limitation due to race, nationality or religion, have the right to marry and found a family'[4]. This right is supported by the European Convention on Human Rights, which guarantees respect for family life and the right to found a family[5].

It can be argued that these provisions create a positive right to access ART to achieve this goal, one taken for granted by fertile people in the community.

Adherence to the 'best interests of the child' principle, while laudable, can be difficult to apply in practice. It would be difficult to argue that it would be in the best interests of a child not to be born at all. In South Australia, the Reproductive Technology Act requires that a couple seeking assisted conception must demonstrate that they have no outstanding criminal charges or a history of an offence that was sexual or violent in nature. It also states that a couple must have no disease or disability which could interfere with their capacity to parent a child.

This is challenged by Douglas who argues that instituting a 'fitness to parent' code is 'difficult enough to apply in cases concerning children who are in existence, let alone those who are only a twinkle in the doctors' eye and it is open to many different assessments, depending on the person making the judgment'[6].

Judgments are being made about a child who does not exist, when patients who do exist and to whom the practitioner owes a fiduciary duty are being refused treatment, which may not be in their best interests, leaving a practitioner vulnerable to an accusation that he/she may have acted in an ethically questionable manner.

Surrogacy, outlawed in most states, has been permitted since the Australian Capital Territory (ACT) introduced the Substitute Parent Agreements Act 1994, making it the only jurisdiction where specific legislation has been enacted to allow non-commercial (altruistic) IVF surrogacy. The Act prohibits commercial surrogacy but does not prohibit the facilitation of pregnancy where there is a non-commercial agreement. Children have been born through ART surrogacy in the ACT since 1994, with full knowledge and contact between the children and the women who gave birth to them. There has been no evidence of harm done to any party, except by inadequate legislation with unintended consequences, which left the children being raised by their biological parents but not recognized as such in law.

In 2000, an amendment was passed to the Artificial Conception Act (1985), since replaced by the Parentage Act 2004. Section 25 provides for biological parents living in the ACT to obtain, through the Supreme Court, legal parentage of a child born to another woman as the result of a surrogacy arrangement. Conditions of an application for a parentage order include that it be made when the child is between 6 weeks and 6 months old and that the birth parents have agreed freely and with full understanding of what is involved in issuing the order. Primarily, it provides certainty to any children born as permitted under the Substitute Parents Agreement Act (1994) as to his/her parentage, thus allowing their best interests to be served. It also humanely provides closure for the biological parents who may have undergone many years of medical treatment in order to have a child.

In those states without laws specifically permitting surrogacy, another very significant barrier to treatment is that insurers are reluctant to indemnify clinics that may wish to offer this service, even when the law is silent.

Since 2002, the stem-cell debate that has been raging around the world has inevitably involved stakeholders in Australia, as people have argued the morality of using surplus IVF embryos for stem-cell research.

Consumers and providers of ART services were concerned about the implications of the proposed Research on Human Embryos Bill, which went beyond banning human cloning to involve stem-cell research and impact on routine IVF clinical and laboratory practice, already governed by several layers of regulation in Australia.

During the parliamentary debate and subsequent Senate inquiry, infertile people heard inaccurate and misguided assumptions being made about their attitudes to their embryos[7]. These included that they:

(1) Stored them like frozen vegetables;

(2) Treated them without respect;

(3) Allowed them to be used as fodder for scientists;

(4) Considered them not 'surplus' but 'unwanted';

(5) Treated their embryos as a commodity and that the guardianship of them should be transferred.

The degree of paranoia of some senators was evident when one suggested: 'if I were to sneak back into a lab at night somewhere, I could get away with it and you would never know'[8].

When invited to give evidence to the Senate inquiry, representatives of ACCESS emphasized their care about the fate of the embryos that once had the potential to be their children. They rejected the suggestion that anyone else valued or respected frozen embryos more, saying: 'We value life and we value children, which is why we have been prepared to go through extensive investigations and treatment in order to try to create a family'[9].

The contentious nature of this debate provided clear evidence of sincerely held but different moral views, whether faith-based or otherwise. It was argued that this diversity of views should be respected, citing C. Everett Koop, former US Surgeon General and a Christian, who argued that personal moral beliefs should not automatically be enacted into laws enforced by the state[10].

Senators were asked to treat infertile people with the same respect as enjoyed by fertile people in the community to enable them to act in their children's best interests, by ensuring them corresponding rights to make decisions about embryos that once had the potential to be their children.

This debate has highlighted the need for infertile people and their carers to remain vigilant and involved in public debate to ensure that their voice is heard. There can be little argument that there are many daunting ethical challenges facing the researchers and the community concerning the use of stem cells, but it is important that the debate remains focused on the issues, rather than being hijacked by those with repressive anti-ART views who see the debate as an opportunity to undermine the whole technology.

REGULATORY MECHANISMS

ART is arguably the most scrutinized area of medicine in Australia. There are the formal controls and numerous indirect, informal controls such as the media and insurers (Figure 1). The most important formal controls are the legislations, where present, the Reproductive Technology, Accreditation Committee (RTAC) and the National Health and Medical Research Council (NHMRC).

Despite the confused legislative situation, the NHMRC established by the Federal Government, provides guidelines in the areas of ethical human research, and these guidelines control most research, except where they conflict with laws – laws always prevail over guidelines. A recent addition to the NHMRC has been a Licensing Committee for research involving human embryos, which came about from the Research Involving Human Embryos Act 2002, following the stem-cell debate. While the purpose was to monitor research on human embryos, a consequence of this new layer of legislative control has been that most training of laboratory personnel requires a specific license.

Clinics must demonstrate compliance with NHMRC guidelines, together with those of the Australian Health Ethics Committee, a code of practice and relevant statutes in some states. To gain approval to conduct research or undertake new treatment with ethical implications, individual clinics must also apply to their local Institutional Ethics Committee, constituted under NHMRC guidelines. This ensures that the concerns of the local community are addressed and that the interests of consumers are protected. As adherence to NHMRC guidelines is a requirement for clinic accreditation, this confers a form of *de facto* centralized control which, not surprisingly, works well.

The Reproductive Technology Accreditation Committee (RTAC) is a subcommittee of the Fertility Society of Australia, and its role is to inspect and accredit (or otherwise) all clinics involved in ART. Access to government-funded drugs used in treatment, which make up a substantial proportion of the costs involved, is provided only to RTAC-accredited clinics. Whilst not absolute in its power, this indirect financial control means in effect that it is not practicable to have a clinic that is not accredited, and the loss of accreditation would necessitate closure.

The availability of counseling is a requirement of accreditation, as is provision of detailed, written information on treatment, prior to its commencement. This is crucial to ensure that genuine, informed decision-making occurs.

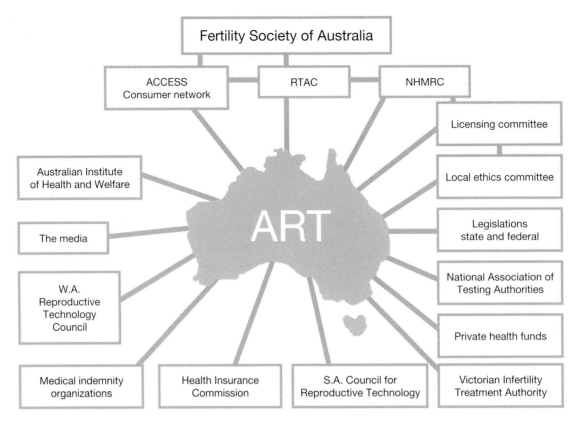

Figure 1 Controls of assisted reproduction technologies (ART). RTAC, Reproductive Technology Accreditation Committee; NHMRC, National Health and Medical Research Council: W.A., Western Australia; S.A., South Australia

RTAC also ensures clinical and laboratory adequacy in terms of standardized, measurable outcomes and advice and guidance where needed. Clinics inspected by RTAC can receive full accreditation for 3 years, preliminary accreditation for 12 or 18 months or have their accreditation withdrawn. Therefore, mechanisms for initial and periodic review of all aspects of ART centers exist.

RTAC is composed of independent nominees appointed by professional associations representing gynecologists, nurses, counselors, scientists and consumers. Once again the active participation of consumers in such accreditation of ART centers has helped to ensure transparency and quality in the delivery of infertility services.

The terms of reference and guidelines of RTAC can be viewed at www.fsa.au.com/rtac/index.

It has been argued that the self-regulation model is weak, as the locus of control lies with 'the doctors'. However, a strength of the RTAC model in Australia is that providers and consumers participate as equal

partners. Any successful attempt inappropriately to manipulate the process would quickly destroy the credibility and effectiveness of RTAC.

Benefits of self-regulation include its flexibility, as it is more able to respond to emerging medical evidence, and as Jansen argues, 'enable delegation of the making of decisions to those who are to be the most personally affected by the consequences'[11].

Despite the initial skepticism of the Government, RTAC has demonstrated that self-regulation can work.

Further protection is also embodied in the common law. The High Court of Australia, challenging the acceptance of the Bolam principle[12], has made it clear that it is for the courts to determine what is a reasonable standard of professional care in relation to information giving. The landmark case of *Rogers v Whitaker* provides the definitive guide. The Justices of the High Court found that the patient's consent to treatment was valid after he or she had been informed about the proposed procedure to be undertaken and stated that[13]:

the choice is, in reality, meaningless unless it is made on the basis of relevant information and advice. The law should recognise that a doctor has a duty to warn a patient of a material risk inherent in the proposed treatment; a risk is material if, in the circumstances of the particular case, a reasonable person in the patient's position, if warned of the risk, would be likely to attach significance to it or if the medical practitioner is or should reasonably be aware that the particular patient, if warned of the risk, would be likely to attach significance to it. This duty is subject to the therapeutic privilege.

In 1998, the Australian High Court case of *Chappel v Hart*[14] reinforced the obligation to supply patients with all information, regardless of whether the doctor may feel it necessary.

SUCCESS

Success, like happiness, can be different things to different people. For some, success in IVF is a confirmed pregnancy, for others it is a healthy baby 9 months later and some have suggested that success is a few years down the track when your child is enrolled in medical or law school.

League tables are vulnerable to a simplistic ranking of clinics, particularly by the media, and can drive clinics to limit access to treatments and selectively to treat patients most likely to succeed.

The conflict of clinics to provide the best information for their patients while presenting their clinics in a positive light has been discussed, as has the problem of how best to present that information[15]. The inadequacies of the simplistic scenario of dividing the number of pregnancies by the number of patients who have undergone treatment were highlighted, and a suggestion made for improvement by a method of identifying a monthly pregnancy rate and cumulating the outcome many years ago[16]. This was further developed by expressing results as a 'life table analysis', which has become an accepted method of reporting results for donor insemination[17], ovulation induction[18] and *in vitro* fertilization[19]. This provides information to couples about the prospects of success over a specified number of treatment cycles, but the debate continues as to the best way to present data, particularly with the heartening trend towards single embryo transfer. However, many variables remain, including questions about what

a pregnancy is. Should success be regarded as a positive β-human chorionic gonadotropin (β-hCG) test 14 (or 15 or 16) days after embryo transfer? Or could it be when a sac or a fetus is visible on ultrasound scan (but this will exclude ectopic pregnancies and early miscarriages)? Is success determined when a normal fetal heartbeat can be detected? Is it more realistic to express success as a live birth, often referred to by consumers as the THB or 'take home baby' rate? Success rates can seem better if expressed 'per transfer' rather than 'per oocyte retrieval' or 'per cycle commenced'. Other variables include:

(1) That the probability of success is higher in the first few cycles, so programs with new patients will have higher success rates;

(2) Younger women are more fertile;

(3) Multiple pregnancies can increase THB rates (but at what price?);

(4) Cancellation rates (during stimulation) can have a negative (or positive depending on the denominator) effect on success rates;

(5) The number of embryos transferred will have a major impact on reported results, but that most important issue is beyond the scope of this chapter.

An integral function of accrediting bodies and licensing authorities is to collect results for a specific group of patients who have a similar likelihood of having a live-birth pregnancy, in order to compare success rates at different clinics. The use of these data to measure performance for accreditation purposes is a useful means of identifying ways to improve practice, while maintaining confidentiality. However, publishing success rates that identify clinics in league tables can weaken the quality of the information available for consumers, as has happened in the UK.

In Australia, figures are centrally collected and collated, and, although scrutinized by RTAC, the clinics remain anonymous when the annual report is published.

A major strength of the annual Australian Institute of Health and Welfare (AIHW) report, compiled by ANZARD (The Australian and New Zealand Assisted Reproduction Database), is its anonymity. Confidentiality is ensured by the AIHW Act of 1987. There is no incentive to manipulate data, so stakeholders can be confident of its reliability. Patient associations encourage consumers to approach individual clinics, perhaps more than one, to discuss the options available for their individual needs and the clinic's ability to meet them. Because there are wide differences between individuals, specific information about a couple's chances of success should be obtained from the clinicians. Consumers can be confident when seeking treatment at an accredited clinic that the clinic has been thoroughly evaluated. This approach seems preferable to selecting a clinic based on statistics that do not reveal the full picture.

The uniqueness of the regulation of ART in Australia has been the proven effectiveness of the continuing co-operation between all stakeholders: health professionals, Government and, most significantly, consumers.

REFERENCES

1. Kon A. Infertility: The Real Costs, ISSUE, CHILD for National Fertility Week, 1993
2. Tizzard J. The deserving and the undeserving. In Tizzard J, ed. Progress in Reproduction. London: Progress Educational Trust, November 1996
3. Madden R. Women's Health. Australian Bureau of Statistics Cat No 4365.0; Marriages and Divorces. Australian Bureau of Statistics Cat No 3310.0, Canberra, 1994, 1995
4. Universal Declaration of Human Rights, Article 16.1, United Nations, 1948
5. Charter of Fundimental Rights of the European Union, Articles 7 and 9, 2000/C 364/01
6. Douglas G. Law, fertility and reproduction. In Kennedy, Grubb, eds. Medical Law, 2nd edn. London: Butterworths, 1994: 119–22
7. Tighe M. Senate Hansard 17 September 2002, CA 64
8. Senator Heffernan. Senate Hansard 29 August 2002, CA 2
9. Dill SK. Senate Hansard 26 September 2002, CA 270
10. Yancey P. Soul Survivor, How my Faith Survived the Church. London: Hodder & Stoughton, 2001
11. Jansen R. Evidence-based ethics and the regulation of reproduction. Hum Reprod 1997; 12: 2068–75
12. Bolam v Friern Barnet Hospital Management committee 1 WLR 582 (1957)
13. 175 CLR 489–90 (1992)
14. HCA 55 (1998)
15. Driscoll GL, Tyler JPP. What is the best strategy for presenting ART results? A controversial comment. J Assist Reprod Genet 1999; 16: 463–7
16. Chong AP, Taymor ML. Sixteen years' experience with therapeutic donor insemination. Fertil Steril 1975; 26: 791–5
17. Kovacs GT, Lording DW. Artificial insemination with donor semen. A review of 252 patients. Med J Aust 1980; 2: 609–12
18. Kovacs GT, Dennis PM, Shelton RJ, et al. Induction of ovulation with human pituitary gonadotrophins: 12 years experience. Med J Aust 1984; 140: 575–9
19. Kovacs GT, Rogers P, Leeton JF, et al. In vitro fertilisation and embryo transfer. Prospects of pregnancy by life-table analysis. Med J Aust 1986; 144: 682–3

39.3

Regulation of assisted conception treatment: Germany

Michael Ludwig, Ricardo E. Felberbaum and Klaus Diedrich

INTRODUCTION

The introduction of *in vitro* fertilization (IVF) and subsequent techniques such as intracytoplasmic sperm injection (ICSI) and cryopreservation of embryos or fertilized oocytes in the field of assisted reproductive technology caused enormous public interest in Germany. Modern reproductive medicine in humans focuses on the biological roots of mankind, and therefore leads to conflicting ethical, philosophical and religious areas. From the beginning there was fear within German society that misuse of these techniques was possible, as well as the risk of increased morbidity and mortality of offspring conceived by assisted reproductive technologies (ART). To avoid these drawbacks several laws and regulations have been implemented in Germany, which deal with topics related to assisted conception treatment. These are:

(1) Law for the protection of the embryo (Gesetz zum Schutz von Embryonen: Embryonenschutzgesetz (EschG))[1];

(2) Guidelines for IVF and embryo transfer and intrafallopian gamete and embryo transfer for the treatment of human infertility (actual version 1998).

(3) Several regulations concerning payment for assisted conception treatment by public health insurance[2].

Some of these regulations have been applicable since the early 1960s. As early as 1959 at the Annual Meeting of German Physicians, where topical general guidelines are ratified, homologous insemination was accepted only in special cases, while heterologous insemination was principally rejected (Table 1).

In 1998, the 'Guidelines for IVF and embryo transfer and intrafallopian gamete and embryo transfer for the treatment of human infertility' were brought up to date, including mainly intracytoplasmic sperm injection, but also the obligation to participate in the national German IVF registry (Deutsches IVF Register, DIR). Other related techniques, such as preimplantation genetic diagnosis (PGD) or embryo selection and embryo freezing, are not allowed, and are still a subject of intense public debate.

EMBRYONIC STEM CELL RESEARCH

Regarding research on embryonic stem (ES) cells, in June 2002 the law on 'Reassurance of embryo protection in the context of import and use of human embryonic stem cells (Stammzellgesetz, StZG)' became valid[4]. According to this law, the importing of ES cells is rejected. However, the exception is made that ES cells may be imported and used if the embryos were produced and ES cells harvested according to the

Table 1   History of regulation regarding assisted conception treatment. Modified from reference 3

Year	Regulation	Purpose
1959	62. Deutscher Ärztetag*	homologous insemination only in special cases acceptable; heterologous imsemination principally rejected
1970	73. Deutscher Ärztetag*	homologous insemination principally acceptable
1985	88. Deutscher Ärztetag*	IVF and ET acceptable for treatment especially of tubal infertility proposals for the generation of an embryo protection law (e.g. regulation of sperm and oocyte donation, prohibition of embryo donation, surrogate motherhood, generation of hybrids and chimeras, generation of research embryos, germ-line therapy)
1985	Bender Commission	proposals for the regulation of genetic research
1987	Enquete Commission	proposals for the legal regulations of reproductive medicine
1988	Commission 'Reproductive Medicine'	
1991	Embryo protection law	
1998	Revision of the 'Guidelines for IVF and embryo transfer and intrafallopian gamete and embryo transfer for the treatment of human infertility'	
2002	Law on 'Reassurance of embryo protection in the context of import and use of human embryonic stem cells (Stammzellgesetz, StZG)'	

*Annual meeting of German Physicans, among other things to ratify topical general guidelines; IVF, *in vitro* fertilization; ET, embryo transfer

legal regulations of the respective country of origin before 1 January 2002. Scientific projects must be presented for approval to the Central Ethical Committee located at the Federal Center of Disease Control in Berlin (Robert Koch Institut). To date, six projects using ES cells have been approved.

THE GERMAN EMBRYO PROTECTION LAW

The ESchG deals mainly with problems of IVF and embryos *in. vitro*. Other techniques, such as intrauterine insemination (IUI), ovulation induction or assisted fertilization, including ICSI, are not directly mentioned within the text of the law. However, whenever an embryo may be accessible to laboratory approaches the law has to be respected anyhow.

The main intention of this law was to avoid misuse of embryos and the problem of high-order multiple pregnancies. The law became valid in January 1991.

Definition of the term 'embryo'

The law defines an 'embryo' as a fertilized oocyte after the pronuclei have disappeared, with an obvious potential to develop into a human being. This even applies to each totipotent blastomere taken from an embryo, as it has the theoretical potential to develop into a human-being[1].

Regulations to avoid multiple pregnancies

A maximum of three embryos is allowed to be transferred to a patient in each IVF cycle[1]. No surplus oocytes at the pronuclear stage are allowed to be cultured *in vitro*[1]. In some parts of Germany (Hamburg) the transfer of only two embryos is permitted in women below 35 years of age. However, cryopreservation of these cells is allowed, and this is successfully performed in Germany[5]. Cryopreservation of embryos at the cleavage stage is possible only when transfer cannot be performed if the patient is unwell on the day of embryo transfer, or is suffering from severe ovarian hyperstimulation syndrome, or if the patient refuses to have the embryos transferred[1]. Although these regulations were intended to avoid a high incidence of multiples in Germany, this goal was clearly missed, as about 40% of all children born in Germany after ART are multiples.

Results of the German IVF registry regarding the incidence of multiples

Since 1997, data collection in Germany has been performed 'cycle by cycle', using nationwide implemented computer software. The catalog of items covers all aspects of ART treatment which can be completed in a retrospective or prospective manner. In the latter case the treatment file has to be created within 8 days after starting patients' stimulation. Data are forwarded to the registry's headquarters, where all files are checked for completeness and plausibility. Data are analyzed for every year and officially published. In 2001[6], 108 centers participated in the data collection, forwarding files on 75 086 treatment cycles. Some 84.4% (62 305) of the cycles were documented in a prospective manner, reflecting the high data quality. Of 9648 children born in 2001 after ART, 61.9% (5969) were singletons, 34.5% (3326) were twins and 3.7% (353) were triplets. No quadruplets were born. There was a strong correlation between the number of embryos replaced and the incidence of multiple pregnancies. In women < 35 years of age, after replacement of two embryos, an incidence of 23.9% twin pregnancies and 0.2% triplet pregnancies was observed, while replacement of three embryos led to an incidence of twins and triplets of 28% and 5.4%, respectively. On the other hand, replacement of two high-quality embryos led to an overall pregnancy rate of 32.5%, while after replacement of two non-high-quality embryos, this was only 13.35%. The mean birth weight of triplets born was 1810 g. In spite of restrictive legal regulations in Germany, about 40% of all children born after ART are multiples, some 4% of which are triplets. A reduction of this incidence and in particular the avoidance of triplets and the corresponding neonatal morbidity can only be achieved if embryo selection is allowed in the future, and a maximum of only two embryos are transferred in patients < 35 years of age. At present, legal regulations in Germany reduce patients' prognosis regarding pregnancy, while they do not prevent multiple pregnancies, pathology and morbidity. These results should be taken into account by politicians in other countries when discussing new and more restrictive legal regulations for ART.

Heterologous IVF

Oocyte donation, embryo donation and surrogate motherhood in IVF and related techniques are forbidden by law[1]. IVF using donated sperm is not forbidden, but is not covered by health insurance[7]. Posthumous sperm use is not permitted in IVF[1]. In every case, both partners must give consent for the use of their gametes in an IVF cycle[1].

Preimplantation genetic diagnosis

The term 'preimplantation genetic diagnosis' (PGD) is not mentioned in the law. However, it is permissible to sort X-bearing sperm for gender selection in cases of severe inherited disorders. As an example, Duchenne's muscular dystrophy is mentioned[1]. Sorting of X- or Y-bearing sperm purely for sex selection is forbidden by law[1].

Three regulations would seem to prevent the performance of PGD in Germany:

(1) If totipotent cells are taken by biopsy for diagnostic testing, embryos are wasted, which is not allowed[1]. A literature review shows that, in animals[8] as well as in humans[9], the blastomeres lose their totipotency after the eight-cell stage. Therefore, this paragraph (§8, EschG) cannot be applied to PGD.

(2) No procedures are allowed which harm the further development of embryos in vitro. Since it has been shown that the biopsy procedure does not harm the embryo[10–13], this paragraph (§2 (1) EschG) should not be a problem.

(3) Only embryos that are planned to be transferred may be created in vitro (§1 (1) 2, EschG)[1] and allowed to be cultured. It is a matter of interpretation whether these paragraphs are violated by PGD or not, as all embryos are planned to be transferred. If patients are told of the diagnosis, they have the right to select the embryos considered for transfer, since patients cannot be forced to undergo an embryo transfer (§4 (1) 2, EschG)[1].

However, the term PGD is not mentioned in the embryo protection law. Because other interpretations of the law are possible, PGD is not yet performed in Germany. An alternative procedure polar body biopsy, can be performed in Germany at least to rule out genetic disorders or aneuploidy of the oocytes to be used for assisted reproduction. As polar body biopsy is performed before syngamy of the pronuclei, this is in accordance with the German embryo protection law.

It is still uncertain whether new legislation will be passed in the future which could specifically allow the performance of PGD in certain cases.

Other problems

Cloning, the creation of hybrids or chimeras and germ-line therapy are forbidden by the embryo protection law.

REGULATIONS OF THE ÄRZTLICHE BERUFSORDNUNG

The 'Ärztliche Berufsordnung' has the status of a professional law for physicians. In a special section, aspects of the organization of IVF centers, their performance and other aspects of IVF are covered[14].

Each IVF center has to be registered by the local chamber of doctors (Ärztekammer), the German professional organization of physicians, and only these centers are allowed to perform IVF. They must have at least three physicians who are specialists in gynecological endocrinology and reproductive medicine, gynecological sonography, operative gynecology, reproductive biology and andrology. Each of these persons can cover a maximum of only two of these fields. On each occasion, hormone diagnostics, ultrasound, sperm analysis and IVF must be available for use.

PUBLIC HEALTH INSURANCE REGULATIONS

The social law[2] principally regulates payment for treatment procedures by public health insurance. Private health insurance normally pays for the same procedures; sometimes the more specialized treatments are also paid for. Other regulations, which do not have the same status of law, propose the amount of money for each procedure, and the situations in which the procedure has to be paid for.

The regulations for IVF and IUI contain the following points:

(1) An indication for the procedure must be made by a specialist physician who must counsel the couple about principles, risks and success rates of the various treatments.

(2) Until December 2003, three procedures were fully covered by insurance. Due to changes in the laws regarding public health since 1 January 2004, only three treatment cycles of IVF or IVF–ICSI are covered by public health insurance, with 50% of the costs including medical treatment, laboratory work and medication; 50% of the costs have to be paid by the patients themselves. Obviously this has had a tremendous impact on reproductive medicine in Germany. For 2004, it was expected that only about 70% of cycles, compared with previous years, would be carried out.

(3) Only homologous IVF and IUI in married couples is covered by insurance. However, the performance of heterologous IVF is not forbidden, if couples pay privately. In these cases, the local ethical committee has to be asked their opinion whether it is reasonable to perform the treatment or not.

(4) The woman must be above 25 and below 40 years old, and her husband must be above 25 and below 50 years old to be eligible for the 50% supplementation by the public health insurance company. The lower age limit has been set by politicians without any medical reason or explanation. Obviously, this has been done to reduce costs for public health insurance.

CONCLUSION

In Germany, comprehensive regulation has been established which guarantees maximum protection for the human embryo. The various regulations are summarized in Table 2. However, the treatment possibilities are not always optimum for patients, and the aim of preventing high-order multiples has not been realised. There is also no possibility for research on human embryos, since no surplus embryos are available and research on embryos is absolutely prohibited. The possibility to carry out research using embryonic stem cells is available only in a very restricted manner.

It seems somewhat of a paradox that the results of research on human embryos as carried out elsewhere are used in daily practice in reproductive medicine in Germany, but that such research is forbidden here.

The German legislature has tried to provide the best possible protection for the embryo, and this has in fact worked. However, in some respects, less forceful regulation and more scientific freedom would be most useful and would allow progress in this field.

Table 2 Summary of regulations regarding assisted conception treatment in Germany			
	Allowed	Not allowed	Not regulated
IVF	√		
GIFT/ZIFT	√		
ICSI	√		
IUI/IVF in unmarried couples	√‡		
Sperm selection	√*		
PGD			√
Oocyte donation		√	
Sperm donation	√		
Embryo donation		√	
Heterologous IVF (sperm)	√		
Heterologous IVF (oocytes)		√	
Surrogate motherhood		√	
Cryopreservation of embryos		√†	
Cryopreservation of pronuclear oocytes	√		
Cryopreservation of gametes	√		
Transfer of more than three embryos	√		
Cloning/creation of chimeras or hybrids		√	
Germ-line therapy		√	

*Only in cases of severe X-linked diseases such as Duchenne's muscular dystrophy; †only in cases in which no transfer can be performed; ‡allowed but not covered by health insurance; IVF, *in vitro* fertilization; GIFT/ZIFT, gamete/zygote intrafallopian transfer; ICSI, intracytoplasmic sperm injection; IUI, intrauterine insemination; PGD, preimplantation genetic diagnosis

REFERENCES

1. Bundesgesetzblatt. 13 December 1990; 1: 2746
2. Bundesgesetzblatt. 26 June 1990; 1: 1211
3. Keller R, Günther H-L, Kaiser P. Embryonenschutzgesetz. Stuttgart: Verlag W Kohlhammer, 1992
4. Bundesgesetzblatt Jahrgang 2002, Teil I, Nr. 42, ausgegeben zu Bonn, 29th Juni 2002
5. Al Hasani S, Ludwig M, Gagsteiger F. Comparison of cryopreservation of supernumerary pronuclear human oocytes obtained after conventional in-vitro fertilization. Hum Reprod 1996; 11: 604–7
6. Deutsches IVF Register, yearbook 2001 and yearbook 2002. Bundesgeschäftsstelle Ärztekammer Schleswig–Holstein, Bismarckallee 8–12, 23795 Bad Segeberg
7. Bundesausschuß der Ärzte und Krankenkassen über Maßnahmen zur küstlichen Befruchtung (1991)
8. Willadsen SM. The developmental capacity of blastomeres from 4- and 8-cell sheep embryos. J Embryol Exp Morphol 1981; 65: 165–72
9. Gerber S, Winston RML, Handyside A. Proliferation of blastomeres from biopsied cleavage stage human embryos in vitro: an alternative to blastocyst biopsy for preimplantation diagnosis. Hum Reprod 1995; 10: 1492–6
10. Krzyminska UB, Lutjen J, O'Neill C. Assessment of the viability and pregnancy potential of mouse embryos biopsied at different preimplantation stages of development. Hum Reprod 1990; 5: 203–8
11. Tarin JJ, Handyside AH. Embryo biopsy strategies for preimplantation diagnosis. Fertil Steril 1993; 59: 943–52
12. Cui K-H, Barua R, Matthews CD. Histopathological analysis of mice born following single cell embryo biopsy. Hum Reprod 1994; 9: 1146–52
13. Harper JC. Preimplantation diagnosis of inherited disease by embryo biopsy: an update of the world figures. J Assist Reprod Genet 1996; 13: 90–5
14. 100. Dutscher Ärztetag. Musterberufsordnung. Abschnitt D Nr. 15. 100. Deutsches Ärzteblatt 1997; A-2354

39.4

Legislation and regulation of assisted reproductive technology in the Nordic countries

Johan Hazekamp and Lars Hamberger

INTRODUCTION

More than twenty-five years have passed since the birth of Louise Brown in 1978, over a quarter of a century. Few areas in medicine have received as much attention from the media and put as much pressure on politicians and legislators to scrutinize, understand and control this boundary-breaking new medical technology. The Nordic experience is an excellent arena for studying the effects and value of self-regulation by treatment providers themselves, in both the private and national sectors, or by regulation through legislature.

The ethical and socioeconomic aspects of assisted reproductive technologies (ART) are very intricate. Politicians and legislators face considerable and continuous difficulties in their attempts to produce laws suitable for their own political environment. The result is a curious difference between laws of different countries. This is also true for the three Scandinavian countries. Denmark, Norway and Sweden – geographically, historically and linguistically closely related and with similar cultural, religious, social and political make-up – serve to confirm the ethical difficulties. A few of these differences have major effects on the availability of infertility treatment.

In the Nordic countries, initial laws on *in vitro* fertilization (IVF) were passed in 1987 (Norway), 1991 (Sweden), 1996 (Iceland) and 1997 (Denmark). Finland has yet to pass a law, which places this country in a unique position for the evaluation of over 25 years of responsible self-regulation.

GENERAL FEATURES

The Nordic laws or health regulations for ART cover a good deal of common ground. ART centers must be licensed, and there are demands on minimum qualifications for persons bearing the responsibility for these clinics. Regulations require the securing of informed consent and demand availability of a psychosocial support system. Furthermore, clinics have to provide a minimum of annual summary reports to the health authorities on treatment details, including the number of cycles and outcome. Couples seeking treatment need not be married, but it is required that they officially live together in a stable 'marriage-like' state. The treatment decisions and selection of couples for treatment are the sole responsibility of the treating physician.

Nordic laws are clear on paternity and maternity issues related to IVF.

NORWAY

Being the first nation in the world to legislate on such a difficult issue as *in vitro* fertilization may in itself be an achievement, although not necessarily without creating major problems. Despite several amendments (1994, 2003), Norwegian legislation on ART remains one of the most restrictive in the world. Very few restrictions have been removed since the initial law of 1986, and not all legislative conclusions are easily understood in a logical, medical and ethical context today.

Forbidden are all forms of embryo research, including simple methodological research, making Norway totally dependent on other countries for simple developments in embryo culture and handling techniques.

In contrast to sperm donation, which is allowed, oocyte (egg) donation is still strictly forbidden. Sperm donation was, until recently, not allowed in combination with IVF, similar to the ruling in Sweden. The argument forwarded by politicians and legislators in both countries at the time was that, whereas IVF on its own, or donor insemination on its own, was an acceptable manipulation of human reproduction, the combination of the two passed beyond this acceptable limit. These questionable rulings have now been repealed.

Oocyte freezing was forbidden in earlier legislation but is now permitted, but the law stipulates that the method may not be used to preserve reproductive capacity in order to delay reproduction.

The embryo cryopreservation period has steadily been extended in each amendment from 1 year to 3 years and now recently to 5 years.

An excellent example of the dilemma related to legislation based on party politics rather than sound science is the latest restriction in Norway on preimplantation genetic diagnosis (PGD), which is now allowed only in the case of severe sex-linked genetic conditions. Only a few months after passing this very restrictive law, the responsible political parties are at loggerheads about interpretation of the law, and there is a demand for a new amendment, in order to provide

the benefits of PGD also to other families troubled by severe familial genetic disorders.

Human embryonic stem-cell research is totally forbidden. Not only does this prohibit development in an important and exciting field of medicine, but it also excludes Norway from the scientific arena where decisions are made on the direction and uses of such developments.

A new restriction in Norway (2003) is the prohibition of anonymous sperm donation. Here Norway joins the Swedish experiment on non-anonymous sperm donation together with Austria, Switzerland and the state of Victoria in Australia. Whether this ruling shifts the emphasis to nature (biology) at the expense of nurture (social relationships), time must tell.

The initial Norwegian law permitted IVF only for female indications. As a result of this, Norway was the last Nordic country to introduce intracytoplasmic sperm injection (ICSI) (1994) when the indication spectrum was widened to include also the male. But governmental health authorities were evidently not ready for this development and stopped all ICSI treatment by decree for a period of 1 year, to gain time to assess and regulate this new technology. Nonetheless, the first child resulting from ICSI performed in Norway was born in 1995 (Volvat Medical Center in Oslo).

The fundament of the Norwegian restrictions lies in the principle of 'better safe than sorry', and in giving the early human embryo an exceptionally high status. The latter stands in sharp contrast to the legal restrictions demanding destruction of frozen embryos after 5 years of cryopreservation, the forbidding of embryo donation and the longstanding liberal Norwegian abortion laws.

SWEDEN

Sweden was the first Nordic country to produce a child through IVF (Sahlgrenska Sjukhuset in Gothenburg 1982) and second to pass IVF legislation (1991). This initial Swedish law also included a few restrictions similar to those in the Norwegian law. This includes forbidding the combination of donor insemination with IVF, and forbidding oocyte donation.

The forbidding of oocyte donation in Sweden and Norway was based on the argument that maternity is subject to the uninterrupted alliance between ovary and uterus. The ovary (oocyte) and the uterus (implantation and pregnancy) should not be separated in order to preserve the traditional concept of a mother. This was seen to contrast sharply with donor insemination where such a separation does not occur. Sweden amended this law as of 1 January 2003, and egg donation is now permitted. Perhaps, unnecessarily, this treatment may only be provided by the National Health Service. Private ART centers which are and have always been an integral part of infertility treatment in Sweden, and forerunners in ART quality assurance, have so far been excluded from providing this treatment. Sweden allows a wide variety of oocyte donor candidates, including donation by a relative or close friend.

Sweden was the first country in the world to pass a law prohibiting anonymous donor insemination as early as 1984. Several other countries have followed the Swedish example including Austria and Switzerland, and currently a similar law has been passed in the British Parliament and is awaiting approval in the House of Lords. The law provides children with the right to know the identity of the sperm donor from the age of 18, which means that the first revelations are now due and the assessment of the effects and an evaluation of this law can now begin. However, in a recent follow-up study performed by the Government, it was reported that only 11% of the parents had informed their children about the sperm donation procedure.

Current central discussions in Sweden may open the way for ART treatment of lesbian women in the near future, and give them access to sperm donation.

The Swedish law of 1991 was farsighted in its liberal attitude to embryo research (14 days), which has made it possible to develop human embryonic stem-cell research. Sweden is now among the leading countries in the world in this research area.

Genetic manipulation of embryos, in the Nordic countries, is only permitted in Sweden, provided that the resulting embryos are not used in infertility treatment. This research is restricted to donated ART surplus embryos.

Also, Sweden has seen attempts at political regulation of ART. The high incidence of multiple pregnancy after ART has increased political scrutiny of treatment policy, making clear demands on a reduction of twin births. Failure to achieve this may activate a standing law proposal demanding single embryo transfer in all treatment cycles.

ICELAND

The Icelandic laws (1996 and 1997), coming 5 years after the Swedish law, are more liberal, and do not include the earlier restrictions imposed in Norway and Sweden. Sperm donation is practiced both anonymously and non-anonymously according to the stated wishes of the sperm donor and those of the sperm-accepting parents. This provides a unique possibility to assess societal attitudes over time, without the pressure of restrictive legislation.

Oocyte donation is permitted in Iceland, while embryo donation and surrogacy are not.

DENMARK

The last to legislate on ART in the Nordic countries was Denmark (1997). The basis for Danish legislation is the concept that once a treatment modality is permitted, improvement of the technique should be encouraged.

Danish law allows oocyte donation, but in contrast to practice in Sweden and Finland this is restricted to the donation of surplus oocytes related to ART treatment.

Before the introduction of the law, Danish IVF was regulated by governmental decrees. Introduction of the law introduced a new restriction forbidding the treatment of single women, which was possible earlier. Anonymous sperm donation, but not embryo donation, is permitted.

Denmark is the first Nordic country to initiate and currently to develop *in vitro* maturation (IVM)[1].

A scheduled amendment of the Danish law in 2005 will extend the allowed period for cryopreservation of embryos to 5 years.

The more liberal Danish law makes Denmark a welcome provider of ART to many Norwegian and Swedish couples seeking anonymous donor insemination in Denmark to bypass local waiting-lists and the non-anonymity regulations. No other country apart from Israel has a higher IVF availability, last year accounting for 3.4% of all children born in Denmark.

FINLAND

Finland has yet to pass a law on ART. Until the present, ART in Finland has been regulated by the Finnish infertility clinics themselves, with consensus guidelines and the assistance of local and national ethical committees. It is interesting to note that Finland has shown no signs of departure into commercialism or controversialism. Oocyte donation[2], embryo donation, surrogacy and the treatment of single women and lesbian women are all done on the basis of altruism, with no or minimal economic reimbursement to donors. Counseling plays a major role in all these treatment modalities.

Finland has been in the frontline in the Nordic countries to combine single embryo transfer and an excellent embryo cryopreservation program to reduce the multiple pregnancy rates to the lowest of the Nordic countries. *In vitro* maturation is an ART research area successfully practiced clinically in Finland.

Different Finnish governments have already presented several proposals to Parliament for a law put together by the Departments of Health and Justice and experts in the field of ART, but as yet no law has been passed. There are some controversial issues that need to be resolved especially related to the treatment of single women and lesbian women, and surrogacy.

Embryo donation is practiced on a small scale, and the Finnish legislative proposals indicate that embryo donation will also be possible in the future.

Gestational surrogacy is practiced in Finland on strictly medical indications[3]. Surrogate mothers are often selected relatives and do not receive payment for the gestational service. Surrogacy under careful regulation and with extensive counseling is likely to be permitted in future law as well.

As Finland is the last Nordic country to legislate, there are strong reasons to believe that it will benefit from the lessons learned from its Nordic neighbors. Finland is likely to have the most liberal of the Nordic laws (personal communication, Professor Outi Hovatta).

Finland is a haven for Nordic couples needing treatment forbidden in their own countries. Today Finland is the only Nordic country that can offer ART to single women. Extensive counseling plays a key role in such treatment. Also, lesbian women have access to treatment. The age limits applied to acceptance for treatment in Finland are similar to those in other Nordic countries, and there is little evidence that postmenopausal women are being treated to prolong fertility.

INTRACYTOPLASMIC SPERM INJECTION

Microinsemination (ICSI) is available in all Nordic countries today. Epididymal or testicular sperm retrieval is available in all the countries.

DONATION OF GAMETES AND EMBRYOS

Artificial insemination by donor sperm is allowed in all the Nordic countries.

The human immunodeficiency virus (HIV) problem has to a large extent phased out the use of fresh sperm. This has resulted in the establishment of a professional anonymous sperm bank in Denmark that supplies much of the sperm used in anonymous donor insemination for couples from most of the Nordic countries.

Anonymous donor insemination is not allowed in Sweden and Norway. Children born as a result of donor insemination will be supplied with the identity of the donor on request at the age of 18 years.

Oocyte donation is allowed in all Nordic countries except Norway. Denmark is exceptional in that only surplus oocytes from ART treatment may be donated.

Embryo donation is forbidden in all the Nordic countries except Finland.

Surrogacy is forbidden in all Nordic countries except in Finland.

Reproductive cloning is forbidden in all the Nordic countries.

CRYOPRESERVATION OF GAMETES, EMBRYOS AND OVARIAN TISSUE

Sperm freezing is allowed in all countries without any limitation to the cryopreservation period.

Oocyte freezing is now permitted in all the Nordic countries. No limitation has been specified for the cryopreservation period, except in Denmark (2 years).

Embryo freezing is allowed in all Nordic countries, with permitted cryopreservation periods from 2 to 5 years. In Finland the cryopreservation period for donated embryos is 10 years.

TREATMENT OF SINGLE WOMEN

Single women and lesbian woman may currently be treated only in Finland.

Lifting of the restriction on the treatment of lesbian woman is at present being considered in Sweden.

EMBRYO TRANSFER

There is no legislation today on the maximum number of embryos to be transferred. Elective single embryo transfer (eSET) is now very common in Nordic IVF units, both in private and national-health clinics[4]. There seems to be little problem in motivating both couples and physicians to rely on eSET or eDET (elective double embryo transfer), and replacement of more than two embryos is now very rare. Embryo or fetal reduction is allowed and practiced in all Nordic countries except in Norway, where this is forbidden. Low-number embryo transfer policies have grossly reduced the need for fetal reduction.

PREIMPLANTATION GENETIC DIAGNOSIS

PGD is permitted in all Nordic countries and it is available in several countries. A variety of severe genetic conditions can be diagnosed in Sweden (Sahlgrenska hospital in Gothenburg and Huddinge hospital in Stockholm). Strict restriction of PGD in Norway has been relaxed in a recent amendment of the law. A clinical ethics committee is being set up to judge individual applications for PGD, including investigation of tissue compatibility to already-born children. PGD is currently not practically available in Norway.

RESEARCH

Embryo research with a 14-day culture limit is permitted in all Nordic countries with the exception of Norway.

Genetic manipulation of embryos is permitted in Sweden only. Such embryos may not be transferred back to the uterus for fertility purposes. Only donated ART embryos may be used in this research. Gene therapy on embryos is not a current Nordic research area.

Human embryonic stem-cell research is currently performed in Sweden and Denmark. All forms of reproductive cloning are forbidden in the Nordic countries. A new law was recently passed in Sweden which will permit formation of research embryos and will also accept therapeutic cloning procedures.

All embryo research is subject to government approval, as are all new ART procedures (Table 1).

THE EFFECTS OF LEGISLATIVE DIFFERENCES

Scrutiny of legislation and regulation of ART in the five Nordic countries shows some surprising differences that have profound effects on accessibility of treatment. Infertile couples do not waver to seek necessary treatment across the national borders. Many Swedish couples still seek anonymous sperm donation in Denmark and Finland, and many Norwegian couples will follow suit as the new Norwegian law forbidding anonymity comes into effect. Norwegian couples seek PGD mainly in Sweden, and women with Turner's syndrome and others dependent on egg donation travel to Finland, and now also to Sweden, and even as far as the USA at exorbitant cost, to achieve their greatest wish to have a child of their own. Demands for oocyte donation and the limited supply of oocytes for donation have resulted in long waiting-lists in Finland, Denmark and Sweden.

Single women and lesbian women seek treatment in Finland, or in some of the other European countries (especially Belgium and England). The occasional Nordic couples requiring gestational surrogacy on sound medical grounds seek treatment in Finland and England.

In our opinion, the export of one country's ethical dilemmas to a neighboring country is not worthy of a Western democratic society. It also creates a difficult situation for couples, who may feel guilty for disobeying the laws of their own country, and it is all too convenient for local politicians to wash their hands and be saved from paying the bills. Language problems and costs for the couples may also be considerable.

After more than 25 years it seems that the goal of synchronization of Nordic laws and regulations on ART is still quite remote.

An obvious mission for the European Union in the future should be to synchronize the availability of ART procedures better, to avoid export and import of ethical problems in the field of human reproduction.

Table 1 Nordic legislation as per April 2004: legislation (L) and practice (P)

Assisted reproduction	Denmark	Finland	Iceland	Norway	Sweden
In vitro fertilization (IVF)	L: allowed P: practiced	L: no legislation P: practiced	L: allowed P: practiced	L: allowed P: practiced	L: allowed P: practiced
IVF with sperm donation	L: allowed P: practiced	L: no legislation P: practiced	L: allowed P: practiced	L: allowed P: practiced	L: allowed P: practiced
Micromanipulation					
ICSI	L: allowed P: practiced	L: no legislation P: practiced	L: allowed P: practiced	L: allowed P: practiced	L: allowed P: practiced
MESA	L: allowed P: practiced	L: no legislation P: practiced	L: allowed P: practiced	L: subject to approval P: not yet practiced*	L: allowed P: practiced
TESE	L: allowed P: practiced	L: no legislation P: practiced	L: allowed P: practiced	L: subject to approval P: not yet practiced*	L: allowed P: practiced
Assisted hatching	L: allowed P: practiced	L: no legislation P: practiced	L: allowed P: practiced	L: allowed P: practiced	L: allowed P: practiced
Cryopreservation					
Sperm	L: allowed P: practiced	L: no legislation P: practiced	L: allowed P: practiced	L: allowed P: practiced	L: allowed P: practiced
Oocytes	L: allowed (2 years) P: not practiced	L: no legislation P: practiced	L: allowed P: practiced	L: allowed P: not yet practiced	L: allowed P: practiced
Embryos	L: allowed P: practiced	L: no legislation P: practiced	L: allowed P: practiced	L: allowed P: practiced	L: allowed P: practiced
Cryopreservation period					
Gametes	unlimited (oocytes 2 years)	unlimited	unlimited	unlimited	unlimited
Embryos	5 years	lifetime: 10 years for donation	5 years	5 years	5 years
Donation					
Sperm	L: allowed P: practiced	L: no legislation P: practiced	L: allowed P: practiced	L: allowed P: practiced	L: allowed P: practiced
Oocytes	L: allowed (restricted) P: practiced	L: no legislation P: practiced	L: allowed P: practiced	L: forbidden P: not practiced	L: allowed P: practiced
Embryos	L: forbidden P: not practiced	L: no legislation P: practiced	L: not allowed P: not practiced	L: forbidden P: not practiced	L: forbidden P: not practiced
Donor anonymity	anonymous*	anonymous*	free choice*	non-anonymous	non-anonymous
Other					
Surrogate motherhood	L: forbidden P: not practiced	L: no legislation P: practiced*	L: not allowed P: not practiced	L: forbidden P: not practiced	L: forbidden P: not practiced
Treatment of single women	L: forbidden P: not practiced	L: no legislation P: practiced*	L: forbidden P: not practiced	L: forbidden P: not practiced	L: forbidden P: not practiced

Continued...

Table 1 Continued

Assisted reproduction	Denmark	Finland	Iceland	Norway	Sweden
Other					
Treatment of lesbian women	L: forbidden P: not practiced	L: no legislation P: practiced*	L: forbidden P: not practiced	L: forbidden P: not practiced	L: allowed P: practiced
Preimplantation diagnosis	L: allowed P: practiced*	L: no legislation P: practiced*	L: allowed P: not practiced	L: allowed (restricted) P: not practiced	L: allowed P: practiced*
Introduction of new procedures	L: subject to approval	L: no legislation	L: subject to approval	L: subject to approval	L: no legislation
Research					
Method research	L: subject to approval P: practiced	L: no legislation P: practiced	L: allowed P: practiced	L: forbidden P: not practiced	L: allowed P: practiced
Embryo research	L: subject to approval P: practiced	L: no legislation P: practiced	L: subject to approval P: not practiced	L: forbidden P: not practiced	L: allowed (restricted) P: practiced
Maximum culture period	14 days		14 days		14 days
In vitro maturation (IVM)	L: allowed P: practiced	L: no legislation P: practiced	L: allowed P: practiced	L: subject to approval P: not yet practiced	L: allowed P: practiced
Genetic manipulation					
gametes	L: forbidden P: not practiced	L: no legislation P: not practiced	L:allowed P: not practiced	L: no legislation P: not practiced	L: allowed P: not practiced
embryos	L: forbidden P: not practiced	 P: not practiced	L: forbidden P: not practiced	L: forbidden (restricted) P: not practiced	L:allowed P: practiced
Stem-cell research					
somatic stem cells	L: allowed P: practiced	L: no legislation P: practiced	L: allowed P: practiced	L: allowed P: practiced	L: allowed P: practiced
embryonic stem cells	L: allowed P: practiced	L: no legislation P: practiced	L: allowed P: not practiced	L: forbidden P: not practiced	L: allowed P: practiced

*Export ART (reproductive tourism); Not allowed, forbidden but not legislated; restricted: see text; ICSI, intracytoplasmic sperm injection; MESA, microsurgical epididymal sperm aspiration; TESE, testicular sperm extraction

REFERENCES

1. Mikkelsen AI, Smith SD, Lindenber S. In-vitro maturation of human oocytes from regularly menstruating women may be successful without follicle stimulating hormone priming. Hum Reprod 1999; 14: 1847–51
2. Söderström-Anttila V, Blomqvist T, Foudila T, et al. Experience of in vitro fertilization surrogacy in Finland. Acta Obstet Gynecol Scand 2002; 81: 747–52
3. Söderström-Anttila V, Vilska S, Makinen S, et al. Elective single embryo transfer yields good delivery rates in oocyte donation. Hum Reprod 2003; 18: 1858–63
4. Hazekamp J, Bergh C, Wennerholm U-B, et al. Avoiding multiple pregnancies in ART. Consideration of new strategies. Hum Reprod 2000; 15: 1217–19

FURTHER READING

Hamberger L, Hazekamp J. Regulation of assisted reproductive technology: the Nordic Experience. In Brinsden P, ed. A textbook of In Vitro Fertilization and Assisted Reproduction, 2nd edn. Carnforth, UK: Parthenon Publishing, 1999. 435–40

Hamberger L, Svalander P, Wikland M. The Future: Toward Single Embryo Transfer. Serono Symposium, Norwell, MA, USA. New York: Springer-Verlag, 2001

Gardner DK, Lane M. ART and the Human Blastocyst. Serono. Symposium Norwell, MA, USA, New York: Springer-Verlag, 2001

39.5

Regulating *in vitro* fertilization – the risks of over-regulation: Italy

Guiseppe Benagiano and Luca Gianaroli

INTRODUCTION

Within all advanced civil societies there is a widely acknowledged requirement to protect the couple, as well as the new human-being to be conceived and eventually born from any successful application of assisted reproduction[1]. This is the reason why, over the past quarter of a century, all major industrialized countries – with the exception of the United States, where the political climate favors self-regulation by medical bodies – have enacted legislation aimed at regulating assisted reproductive technologies (ART) and, almost without exception, at banning techniques or modalities unacceptable to the majority of their citizens. This, of course, raises the issue of the right of majorities to impose restrictions to *reproductive freedom*, an issue that is not likely to be resolved in the foreseeable future.

Given this reality, public health policy and any ensuing legislation can only result from a synergistic interaction between specialists (scientists, physicians, economists, etc.), lawmakers and the public. Thus, creating health legislation cannot mean simply applying scientific knowledge, or following political considerations; rather, it implies a constructive dialog between the public, the media, scientists and policy-makers[2].

When this dialog fails to materialize and policy-makers use their power to impose rules that go against prevailing medical practice and public feeling, the results can only be divisive and, in the final analysis, doomed.

Italy represents a typical example of a situation where the extreme sensitivity of the matter to be regulated should have promoted an ample and detailed debate within Parliament and outside, with the aim of 'fine-tuning' the provisions of the law, even within an overall philosophy of protection for the beginning of human life. What happened was the exact opposite: the debate within civil society was ample and detailed, but the proposed text went through the Health Commissions and the main floors of the two Houses without modification; in other words, the text remained totally 'locked' and 'impenetrable' to change throughout the entire procedure, which took 2 years. Those promoting the legislation have defended this 'locked-in' approach on the grounds that opening up the text to modification would have meant postponing indefinitely its approval[2].

What happened in the months that followed the coming into effect of the new legislation has clearly proved this position wrong: groups opposed to the new law have promoted a national referendum to abolish each of four specific points in the text, and even a referendum to abolish the law in its entirety. In addition, since the text is clearly imprecise and confused even within the confines of its inspiring principles, litigation started within 3 months of publication of the law. Proponents have collected almost one million signatures for each of the five referenda (the minimum being 500 000); for this reason it is likely that the referenda will pass the scrutiny of the Italian Constitutional Court.

REGULATING ASSISTED REPRODUCTION TECHNOLOGIES

The need for some form of guidance and regulation in the work leading to the creation of new human-beings was recognized very early; already in 1972, Edwards and Sharpe wrote in *Nature*[3]:

> *Does anything need to be done to regulate the application of new scientific and clinical advances? – Why not* laissez-faire? *Almost any scientific advance can be used for good or harm and free and open discussion of emerging issues – an invaluable safeguard – is readily available nowadays. …Forms of regulations or consultation intermediate between* laissez-faire *and state pre-emption might be useful…If some form of regulation is required, perhaps what is needed is not heavy handed public statute, or rule-making committees, or the conscience of individual doctors, but a simple organization easily approached and consulted to advise and assist biologists and others to reach their decisions.*

From a health policy perspective, three main areas must be considered: *first* and foremost, the technical excellence of the services rendered; *second*, a licensing and monitoring system to control all practitioners and the premises in which they work[4]; and *third*, legislation to avoid abuse, prevent possible damage to the mother and the child and outlaw techniques unacceptable in a given cultural setting, including mechanisms to ensure the adherence by all to ethical and deontological principles.

Whereas the usefulness of enforcing the first two principles is thoroughly acknowledged and accepted by all concerned, when it comes to legislating on ART two types of issues are debated: and on the one hand the tendency to limit or exclude the use of certain techniques, and on the other the tendency to prevent by law access to existing technology by certain individuals. On these two issues, not only is the debate open, but views are often totally divergent.

Legislation, regulations, guidelines, monitoring and licensing are all necessary ingredients in a field where science, technology and ethics are so closely interwoven. For this reason, it seems useful to enact legislation to place human interventions aimed at creating a new human-being within clear boundaries. Unfortunately, a law is a rigid instrument that, once issued, remains unaltered, often for years, in spite of scientific progress or practical experience pointing to its flaws. This is why policy-makers must themselves abide to certain general principles, first and foremost to avoid placing the specialist in the position of practicing 'bad medicine'. Problems therefore arise when legislators over-regulate ART, imposing not only restrictive social norms, but also rules that limit the ability of health personnel to apply existing methods correctly. Italy represents an excellent example of this situation, and, as such, some features of the Italian law are briefly described to show how they impact negatively upon the proper application of medical technology.

THE RISKS OF OVER-REGULATION

The law that came into effect in Italy on 19 February 2004 follows one overarching philosophy: the sanctity of human life from its inception. This is a position shared in principle by the majority of Italians; at the same time, not only does Italy have a liberal abortion law, but this was subjected to and withstood a popular referendum over 20 years ago. Because of this reality, the 'IVF Law'[5] had to be harmonized with the 'Abortion Law'[6], and this was done in Article 14, comma 1, that specifically states: 'Embryo cryoconservation and suppression are forbidden; however the provisions of the Law of 22 May 1978, no. 194 stand valid'. Now, Law 194/78 gives a pregnant woman the power to request termination of her pregnancy within 90 days since her last menstrual period for a whole series of reasons, and, in more than 25 years, this law has been interpreted in such a way as to enable people to say that – for all practical purposes – first-trimester pregnancy termination in Italy is *on demand*. As a consequence, today we have a law that protects every early, preimplantation embryo, and another law that allows the 'suppression' of practically every postimplantation one.

There are three orders of problems with the new Italian law: they involve *social issues*, *human rights* and the *application of technology*. Here, discussion concentrates on one aspect: that the new rules infringe upon basic human rights and the proper application of *in vitro* fertilization (IVF) technology.

As already stressed, the new legislation aims at preventing the loss of *any* early human embryo, although it says nothing about the status of a fertilized ovum. The fundamental objection to this philosophy is of theoretical nature: human fecundability rarely exceeds 0.3[7–9]; this means that nature 'wastes' – in the very early stages – the large majority of all fertilized human ova[10]. Since at least 60% of human embryos never reach the stage of a 'recognized' pregnancy, how can ART be applied without 'wasting' a single one?

Thus, Italian legislators have refused to draw the sole logical conclusion that stems from their ideological premise, namely to ban IVF altogether as has been done in Costa Rica[11]; this has resulted in a major challenge to the law.

The following are the main inconsistencies in the new law: Article 6, subheading 3, of the law is entitled 'Informed consent', and deals with procedures to be utilized to ensure that both partners express their will to undergo the procedure 'jointly, in writing to the physician in charge'. This subheading continues by stating: 'the decision can be revoked by each of the subjects indicated in the present, up to the moment of ovum fertilization'. This means that Law 40/2004 strips the woman (and, indeed, both partners) of the right to change her mind after the time of ovum pick-up, with a major infringement of a basic human right: freedom of treatment, while contemporaneously, Law 194/78 gives the same woman every right to abort the pregnancy later on.

Another apparent violation of a basic human right, that to privacy, is contained in Article 11, which, in subheading 1, states: 'With a decree by the Minister of Health, a national registry is created at the Higher Institute of Health [the National Institute of Health] of the structures authorized to apply techniques of medically assisted procreation, of embryos formed and of those born out of the application of said techniques'. The entire article says nothing about protection of the identity of those born from IVF, who apparently have no right to anonymity, since their names must be included in a national register. Similarly, nothing is said about protection of the identity of women submitting to IVF, in contrast to the UK Human Fertilisation and Embryology Act of 1990,

which mandates that disclosure of information that identifies anybody given treatment in an IVF clinic may only be done with the specific consent of the patient.

Article 16, named 'Conscientious objection', specifically exonerates 'health personnel and those exercising auxiliary health activities' from participating 'in the procedures for the application of techniques for medically assisted procreation'; in other words, it authorizes any medical or paramedical person to refuse to take part in any ART procedure that he/she may object to on ethical grounds. This provision has been included to 'protect' individuals who – on ethical grounds – object to IVF as a whole; an identical clause also exists in the law that instituted legal termination of pregnancy in 1978. In the case of induced abortion, however, the procedure is simple enough for any gynecologist to perform. Therefore, at the time, it was argued that, without the right to conscientious objection, physicians might be forced by hospital administrations to perform an act they could not ethically carry out. When dealing with ART, however, the provision may be theoretically valid in the case of paramedical personnel. For specialists involved in IVF, nevertheless, this clause is clearly redundant, since IVF is definitely a technology that requires specific training: it is highly unlikely that those totally opposed to it would become so competent in its practice to be 'forced' to perform the procedures. Therefore, ironically, the only specialists who might avail themselves of the conscientious objection clause are those who believe that, by applying the law, they may harm the patient! Many such specialists are now finding themselves in an impossible situation. They trained in techniques that cannot be properly applied; therefore, ethically, they may be forced to refrain from performing IVF in certain circumstances, and to refer couples for whom the restrictions placed by the new legislation pose a medical problem to centers outside Italy. Article 16, however, does not allow 'selective conscientious objection': either you accept the law as it is and apply it to all couples, or you cannot practice IVF.

The difference between exercising conscientious objection in the cases of voluntary abortion and IVF is underlined by one fact: in 1978, some 80% of all gynecologists availed themselves of the right to object, whereas, as far as is known, no one has exercised the right to conscientious objection with regard to IVF!

Article 14, commas 1 and 2, forbids: (a) 'embryo cryoconservation', (b) 'embryo suppression' and (c) 'to create a number of embryos exceeding that strictly necessary to a unique and contemporary implant [transfer], at any rate, never to exceed three'. Such a policy is clearly the result of assigning a higher value to protection of the embryo than to the interest of fertile women and couples[12]. To anyone even vaguely familiar with IVF technology, the inescapable conclusion is that – in all cases – the Italian law permits the fertilization of only three oocytes and mandates the transfer of all three possible embryos. This is unacceptable on medical grounds; on the one hand, fertilizing only three oocytes will impair the chances of success of an older woman, since fertilization rates decline with age[13], and the best results are obtained when there is retrieval of between 6 and 10 oocytes[14]; on the other, transferring three embryos may be excessive in the case of a young woman[15]. In this connection, Robertson[12] argues that if a country places high value on the status of an embryo:

> it may certainly ban freezing, research on, or discarding of embryos. But it should be aware of the costs and burdens that such a policy imposes on women and children through increased multiples, more failed repeated cycles, and possible resort to highly experimental and unreliable options such as oocyte freezing.

Robertson[12] also suggests a way out of this impasse:

> it would be possible to improve the situation of women undergoing IVF in Italy, while maintaining respect for embryos, by explicitly recognizing that embryos exist only when the two haploid pronuclei merge at syngamy into the new unique genome of the zygote.

In reality, the new Italian law does not mention zygotes (whether pronucleate or completely formed), possibly because those writing the text presumed that 'a zygote is an embryo', when obviously this is not the case. Indeed, as pointed out by Ford[16], a well-known and respected Catholic theologian, even in philosophical terms, there is hardly an ontological continuity between a zygote and an embryo. Therefore, it is difficult to argue that the clause in the law that forbids embryo cryopreservation automatically applies to freezing of zygotes, a procedure allowed even in restrictive legislations, such as the German one; as a result, Germany has reasonably high success rates for IVF[17].

Indeed, freezing pronuclear zygotes yields such good results as to warrant a comparison with cryopreservation of embryos. In a recently published theoretical model[18], a case was simulated in which ten oocytes per woman are retrieved from ten women and are inseminated; in the model, half of the resulting embryos are immediately transferred and the remaining five are cryopreserved. This situation is then compared with the alternative, in which, after inseminating all the oocytes, an average of 3.5 per cycle are kept in culture, whereas the remaining ones are cryopreserved at the pronuclear stage. Calculations indicate that, in the case of embryo freezing, the resulting cumulative percentage of babies born would be 33.6%, a figure significantly lower than that obtainable when freezing pronuclear zygotes; in this scenario, representing the situation permitted under German law, the cumulative percentage of babies to be born is an excellent 55%.

In conclusion, Italy is today confronted with new legislation which not only severely compromises the ability of physicians to apply ART correctly, but is so confused that – depending on the interpretation – anyone may try to nullify the main ideological premise upon which the entire law has been structured.

REFERENCES

1. Brinsden PR. Reproductive health care policies around the world. The effect of the Human Fertilisation and Embryology Act 1990 upon the practice of assisted reproduction techniques in the United Kingdom. J Assist Reprod Genet 1993; 10: 493–9
2. Benagiano G, Farris M. Public health policy and infertility. Reprod Biomed Online 2003; 7: 606–14
3. Edwards RG, Sharpe DJ. Social values and research in human embryology. Nature (London) 1972; 231: 87–91
4. Lunenfeld B, Van Steirteghem A, on behalf of all participants. Infertility in the third millennium: implications for the individual, family and society. Condensed Meeting Report from the Bertarelli Foundation's Second Global Conference. Hum Reprod Update 2004; 10: 317–26
5. Repubblica Italiana, Legge 19 febbraio 2004, no. 40. Norme in materia di procreazione assistita. Gazzetta Ufficiale della Repubblica Italiana. Serie generale 2004; 45: 5–12
6. Repubblica Italiana, Legge 22 maggio 1978, no. 194. Norme per la tutela sociale della maternità e

sull'interruzione volontaria della gravidanza. Gazzetta Ufficiale della Repubblica Italiana. Serie generale 1978; 140: 22

7. Balakrishnan TR. Probability of conception, conception delay and estimates of fecundability in rural and semi-urban areas of certain Latin-American countries. Soc Biol 1979; 26: 226–36

8. Vessey M, Doll R, Peto R, et al. A long-term follow-up study of women using different methods of contraception. An interim report. J Biosoc Sci 1976; 8: 373–427

9. Wang X, Chen C, Wang L, et al. Conception, early pregnancy loss, and time to clinical pregnancy: a population-based prospective study. Fertil Steril 2003; 79: 1517–21

10. Benagiano G, Pera A. Il destino dell'uovo umano fecondato nei primi giorni del suo sviluppo. In Mori M. ed. Quale statuto per l'embrione umano: problemi e prospettive. Milan: Biblioteche, 1992: 45–51

11. Republica de Costa Rica, Decreto de la Reproduccion assistida 24029–S 1995 Gazeta Oficial 45, 3 March 1995

12. Robertson JA. Protecting embryos and burdening women: assisted reproduction in Italy. Hum Reprod 2004; 19: 1693–6

13. Lim AS, Tsakok MF. Age-related decline in fertility: a link to degenerative oocytes? Fertil Steril 1997; 68: 265–71

14. Melie NA, Adeniyi OA, Igbineweka OM, Ajayi RA. Predictive value of the number of oocytes at ultrasound-directed follicular aspiration with regard to fertilization rates and pregnancy outcome in intracytoplasmic sperm injection treatment cycles. Fertil Steril 2003; 80: 1376–9

15. Jones HW. Multiple births: how are we doing? Fertil Steril 2003; 79: 17–21

16. Ford NM. When Did I Begin? Conception of the Human Individual in History, Philosophy and Science. Cambridge: Cambridge University Press, 1988

17. European Society of Human Reproduction and Embryology. Assisted reproductive technology in Europe, 1998. Results generated by European registers by ESHRE. Hum Reprod 2001; 16: 2459–71

18. Benagiano G, Gianaroli L. The new Italian IVF legislation. Reprod Biomed Online 2004; 9: 117–25

39.6

Regulation of assisted reproductive technology: the USA experience

Howard W. Jones, Jr

INTRODUCTION

Surveillance and regulation in the USA are greatly influenced by the United States Constitution, which provides no niche for national regulation. The only circumstances under which there can be direct federal regulation applicable to all 50 states of the Union is if federal funds are involved, or if some aspect of interstate commerce is involved. The following discussion reflects the impact of this constitutional issue on surveillance in the USA.

ETHICS ADVISORY BOARD, 1977

Following a series of questionable practices involving research on humans, Congress passed the National Research Award Act of 1974 (PL 93-348) establishing a National Commission for the Protection of Human Subjects of Biomedical and Behavioral Research. The Commission specified that all federally funded research be reviewed and approved by a local review group called an Institutional Review Board (IRB). Interestingly, for research involving humans, from a legal point of view, IRB approval is required only for federally funded research; in practice, many institutions in which research takes place require IRB approval regardless of funding.

During the Commission's 4-year tenure, it issued a number of regulations concerning fetuses, pregnant women and *in vitro* fertilization (IVF). The Commission also recommended to Congress the establishment of an Ethics Advisory Board (EAB) to render advice to the Secretary of Health, Education and Welfare, and to review specific proposals to fund IVF research. A further recommendation stated, 'no application or proposal involving human *in vitro* fertilization may be funded by the Department, or any component thereof, until the application or proposal has been reviewed by the Ethics Advisory Board (EAB), and the Board has rendered advice as to its acceptability from an ethical standpoint'. Congress approved the recommendation of the Commission to appoint an EAB in 1977. However, the appointment of members to the EAB by the Secretary of Health, Education and Welfare was delayed, so that the Board first met only in 1978. In 1979, after extensive public hearings, the EAB issued a report which found in a generic sense that research in IVF was ethically acceptable. The Board was among the first bodies, if not the first, to promulgate the 14-day rule, wherein it pointed out that the early conceptus, i.e. up to 14 days, deserved respect, but not the respect of full personhood. It did not comment on the status of the conceptus after 14 days.

In 1980, the Secretary of Health, Education and Welfare allowed the authorization of the EAB to expire, and it has not been in existence since. Therefore, it became impossible for any grant request for research in any aspects of IVF to be fully processed by the granting mechanism of the National Institutes of Health (NIH). There therefore existed in the USA a *de facto* ban, at least insofar as federal funding was concerned, on the investigation of any aspect of IVF. All research and clinical activity were carried out by private funding. To complete this aspect of the story, it can be noted that the overturn of this *de facto* ban was achieved on 10 June 1993, when President Clinton signed the National Institutes of Health Revitalization Amendments into law. This law specifically provided that the provisions of the Commission's 1975 regulation with respect to the review of proposals for research in IVF by the EAB were no longer operational. This lifting of the ban on using federal funds for IVF was, of course, welcome news to those in the field. However, it must be realized that funds for research at the disposal of the NIH were in no way increased by this Bill. Responding to pressure from special interest groups, President Clinton in 1996 issued an executive order banning federal funding. Nevertheless, the NIH has initiated requests for proposals for reproductive research that could result in the creation of fertilized eggs, i.e. early pre-embryos. Such research must conform to NIH guidelines.

In July 2001, President George W. Bush issued an executive order providing for federal funding for stem-cell research provided that the stem cells were derived from cryopreserved spare pre-embryos created before a certain date. Pre-embryos created after this date, and pre-embryos created expressly for research, were excluded.

ETHICAL CONSIDERATIONS OF THE NEW REPRODUCTIVE TECHNOLOGIES (AMERICAN FERTILITY SOCIETY, 1986)

The action of the executive branch of the federal government, in failing to continue the EAB, effectively removed the federal government from offering ethical opinions with respect to assisted reproductive technologies (ART). This had a major role in prompting the President of the American Fertility Society (AFS), now the American Society for Reproductive Medicine (ASRM), in November 1984 to activate a special ethics committee of the Society to address the ethical issues in reproduction and provide guidelines concerning all of the various ramifications of IVF. The committee consisted of four gynecologists, one andrologist, two lawyers, two theologians, one scientist and one professor of public policy. Six of the 11 were members of the American Fertility Society.

This committee worked for several months and utilized several consultants in specialized areas. In the 1986 AFS report[1], the committee divided the various procedures of assisted reproductive technology into three groups:

(1) Those that were ethically acceptable;

(2) Those that were tentatively acceptable, but should be carried out as a clinical trial. A clinical trial was defined as a systematic effort to improve an existing clinical procedure. The committee furthermore pointed out that procedures carried out under this rubric required institutional review board authority;

(3) Procedures that were classified as clinical experiments, a clinical experiment being defined as an innovative procedure with no historical record. As such, it required institutional review board authority, and was labeled as inappropriate and premature for general application and use.

In the 1990 revision of the AFS ethical guidelines[2], it is interesting that there were no procedures still remaining in the clinical trial category. In 1990, the ethically acceptable procedures were listed as IVF, gamete intrafallopian transfer (GIFT), donor insemination, donor eggs, donor embryos and cryopreservation. In the clinical experiment group was listed items such as zygote intrafallopian transfer (ZIFT), all micromanipulative procedures on the egg and/or embryo, such as microinsemination, preimplantation genetic diagnosis and assisted hatching. Furthermore, IVF surrogacy was listed in the clinical experiment group.

In the 1994 revision[3], there were still no procedures listed as clinical trials. ZIFT was transferred from a clinical experiment to being ethically acceptable. Still listed as a clinical experiment was oocyte cryopreservation. Furthermore, microtechniques remained classified as clinical experiments. Surrogacy was considered to be highly problematic, and was continued to be classified as a clinical experiment.

For the first time, in the 1994 revision, the question of the number of eggs or embryos to transfer was addressed. Rather than rigidly suggesting a number, the guidelines specified that, owing to the multiple variations involved, individual programs needed to adjust the number transferred to eliminate quadruplet births and reduce triplet continuing pregnancies to a level of 1–2% of all pregnancies. The committee condemned the practice of transferring an uncontrolled large number of pre-embryos with the intention of using selective reduction to achieve reasonable multiple pregnancy rates.

Following the comprehensive reports of 1986–1990–1994, the *ad hoc* committee responsible for them was dissolved. In its place was established a permanent ethics committee by the ASRM. This committee now issues periodic reports on specific problematic ethical issues and issues of practice. For example, those involving the number of pre-embryos to transfer, the source of donor gametes, etc. These interim reports are easily available on the worldwide web at www.asrm.org/media/ethicsmain.html.

In early 2004 several subjects were in the process of revision, such as, 'family members as gamete donors and surrogates', or, 'donor spare embryos for embryonic stem cell research', or, 'preconception gender selection for non-medical reasons', or, 'human somatic cell nuclear transfer-cloning'.

The availability of these reports on the worldwide web makes them instantly and widely available to practitioners and others who have an interest in the ethical aspects of reproductive medicine.

There is, of course, no way to determine whether the guidelines are rigidly followed.

CLINICAL AND EMBRYOLOGY LABORATORY CERTIFICATION (CLINICAL LABORATORY IMPROVEMENT AMENDMENTS, 1988)

There are three laboratories involved in ART. Two of these, in andrology and endocrinology, are clearly clinical laboratories in the accepted use of that definition. As such, in all states, they are subject to state quality-assurance regulations, as all states have such regulations. Most states have minimal requirements at least up to those specified by the Clinical Laboratory Improvement Amendments (CLIA) of 1988.

The situation with embryology laboratories is different. The Health Care Financing Administration charged with implementing CLIA-88 in effect, up to the time of writing, has apparently accepted the concept that embryology laboratories are not clinical diagnostic laboratories, but are laboratories in which medical procedures are carried out, and therefore are outside the CLIA mandate.

The ASRM and the College of American Pathologists (CAP) developed a program to provide embryology laboratory accreditation. This is an entirely voluntary process.

In 1997, the Society for Assisted Reproductive Technology (SART) altered its by-laws to require embryology laboratories to be accredited by an outside agency approved by SART, in order to continue as members of SART. The only agencies available to do this are CAP and the laboratory section of the Joint Commission on Hospital Accreditation (JCHA). In spite of these movements, there is at this time no federal mandatory surveillance of embryology laboratories in the USA.

FERTILITY CLINIC SUCCESS RATE AND CERTIFICATION ACT (PUBLIC LAW NO. 102-493, 1992)

From the middle and later part of the 1980s and continuing to the present day, there have been large numbers of reports in audio, video and print media about this method of reproduction. On many occasions, pieces have alleged that many programs have issued inadequate and misleading information about pregnancy rates, or were involved in procedures thought to be problematic from an ethical or even legal point of view. This resulted in considerable consumer disquiet in an era when consumerism is rather rampant in the USA. This phenomenon was picked up by the political process, and Representative Ron Wyden of Oregon held hearings on the matter before the Subcommittee on Regulations and Business Opportunities, of which he was Chairman. There were a number of consequences of these hearings.

One was to stimulate SART, an affiliate society of the AFS, to certain activities, described below. Another consequence of the public hearings was that Public Law 102-493, called the Fertility Clinic

Success Rate and Certification Act, became law when signed by President Bush on 24 October 1992. During the course of the Wyden hearings, it became evident that the members of the committee, and Representative Wyden in particular, correctly or incorrectly were impressed by the fact that program success was very much related to quality control in human embryo laboratories. As a result, Representative Wyden was successful in having the General Accounting Office (GAO) survey certain standards which were being observed by embryology laboratories. This resulted in a publication: *Human Embryo Laboratories – Standards Favored to Ensure Quality*, in December 1989 (GAO/HRD-90-24 Human Embryology Laboratories). On the basis of the information developed by that survey, as well as other aspects of the hearing, Congress passed and President Bush signed, on 24 October 1992, the Certification Act referred to above. There are two significant aspects of this Act.

First, the Centers for Disease Control (CDC) was charged with promulgating model embryology laboratory standards. In conformity with the constitutional situation referred to at the beginning, the Act provides that the model standards promulgated by the CDC be distributed to the states for their consideration. There is no mandate that the states adopt these guidelines, whatever they might be. It is uncertain at this point how many states will adopt these regulations, which may duplicate the joint AFS/CAP effort at voluntary laboratory certification.

Second, the Act provided that the CDC publish nation- and clinic-specific data. The deadline for the implementation of this was also October 1994.

To implement the clinic-specific reporting portion of the Wyden Act, the CDC joined with ASRM, SART and RESOLVE and published clinic-specific data for 1995 in December 1997. This presentation made only minor adjustments to the annual data as had already been published by SART since 1990. It can therefore be open to concern about the same misrepresentation of clinic performance as applied to the SART reports[4].

The CDC–SART–RESOLVE reports have been published annually and are available in print or on the worldwide web at www.cdc.gov/reproductive-health/art.html.

There is usually a lag of 2 or more years before the publication of the data for a given year. Thus, the data

for 2001 did not become available until the latter part of 2003.

In 2001 there were 384 clinics that submitted data. However, it was estimated that there were 37 more clinics that existed that did not submit data. In all, there were 107 587 ART cycles during 2001 which resulted in 29 304 live births giving rise to 40 687 live babies. This gives a gross live birth delivery rate of 27% for the entire nation with all sorts of procedures combined.

During 2001, 80 864 cycles, or 75.2% of the total, involved fresh non-donor eggs. There were 14 705 cycles, or 13.7%, with frozen non-donor eggs, and 8592 cycles, or 8%, with fresh donor eggs, and 3426 cycles, or 3.2%, with frozen donor eggs.

There has been some criticism of the method of reporting in the United States in that the report is a cycle-based report rather than a patient-based report. It is anticipated that with time there will be some revision in the present method of reporting, although this may take a few years.

THE FOOD AND DRUG ADMINISTRATION (FDA)

The FDA has long been concerned with approving and regulating pharmaceutical products and medical devices. It has not regulated the practice of medicine, which is a function of each state. During the 1980s and early 1990s, the FDA seemed to take no notice of assisted reproductive technology. However, the FDA became concerned with disease transmission through tissue transplantation. In 1993, the FDA became involved in human cellular and tissue based products (HCT/Ps)[5].

In 1997, the FDA published proposed regulations on all HCT/Ps and included for the first time semen and reproductive tissue. The FDA claimed authority with this under Section 361 of the Public Health Service (PHS) Act which authorized regulations to prevent the transmission of communicable diseases. Since HCT/Ps are of human origin and are transferred from one individual to another, they pose such a risk.

As of 2003–04, a registration requirement has been imposed on all ART and sperm bank programs. This is in anticipation that there will follow a good tissue practice (GTP) rule and donor suitability rule. These latter rules have been proposed but the finalized versions have not been promulgated at the time of this writing. The initial registration and annual re-registration aspect requires the filing of all establishments practicing use of HCT/Ps.

The FDA has indicated that facilities which have been registered can expect unannounced FDA inspections about once every 2 years.

As the good tissue practice and donor suitability rules have not been finalized, it can only be roughly indicated what they may contain.

It is thought that the donor suitability rule will require specific communicable disease testing for a variety of things, such as human immunodeficiency virus (HIV), hepatitis, chlamydia, gonorrhea and so forth. The proposed good tissue practice rule will likely contain provisions on personnel, procedures, facilities and environmental controls, storage, distribution, labeling, tracking and reporting adverse reactions.

When these various rules were in the proposal stage, the FDA received many comments from various organizations, including the ASRM. They, for example, indicated that there was a lack of known disease transmission from oocytes and embryos and that the GTPs go beyond the risk–benefit approach initially proposed by the FDA. Such protests did not deter the FDA's intention to proceed. The FDA stated, 'We are not attempting to govern practitioners' use of HCT/Ps, but rather to ensure that HCT/Ps would be used by practitioners in their treatment of patients which are in compliance with the applicable regulations, including regulations designed to prevent the transmission or spread of communicable diseases'[6].

Over and above the regulations referred to above, the FDA has already claimed jurisdiction in certain procedures in ART. On July 6, 2001, letters were sent to six ART programs informing them that the use of ooplasm-containing mitochondrial genetic material constituted a clinical investigation, and that the submission of an Investigational New Drug (IND) would be required before they could proceed with ooplasm transfer procedures. This has effectively resulted in the discontinuation of the heterologous ooplasm transfer. While the FDA's intention has not been fully implemented, there is no reason to think that it will not be, in spite of the fact that this will be expensive to the patient, with little anticipated prevention.

STATE REGULATIONS

From what was said at the beginning, it might be expected that there would be a number of states that have regulations explicitly covering ART. This is true of only a few states. However, about half of the states do have statutes covering some aspects of donor insemination. For the most part, these statutes provide that the rearing parents are, in fact, the legal parents, and that the donor has no claim on or responsibility for the child. A very few states, for example Ohio, have in their legislation some requirements for the screening of donors. A few states have now extended the same concept to donor eggs, that the legal parents are the rearing parents.

In a law adopted in 1993, Florida defined paternity and maternity for users of donor eggs and sperm, as well as specifying contractual arrangements for surrogacy. There are three other states that have regulations that might be considered to be aimed at ART. In 1986, Louisiana passed a law that impinges on IVF. It defined what an embryo was, the definition excluding a pronuclear egg; it prohibited the sale of embryos, and prohibited the culture of embryos solely for research. It stipulated the qualifications of facilities and physicians, and prohibited the intentional destruction of an embryo. It indemnified clinics and physicians from acts done in good faith during IVF. This law seems effectively to prevent research on pre-embryos in the state of Louisiana. In 1988, Pennsylvania adopted a law to enable monitoring of IVF. The law provides that anyone conducting IVF must file quarterly reports with the Department of Health concerning certain details of the IVF program, but without reporting the names of patients, donors or recipients. The effectiveness of this statute does not seem to have been evaluated.

There is a very curious law on the books in the state of Virginia. To understand this, it should be explained that private insurance companies, for the most part in the states, do not cover ART. This has resulted in several states adopting mandated coverage, that is, passing laws which provide that if insurance companies cover health in other aspects, they must include infertility and IVF services in the coverage they offer. There is no such mandated coverage in Virginia, but a Bill was introduced into the legislature in 1992 which provided for mandated coverage. There was a companion Bill that provided that, before a physician began treatment, the patient must execute a document stating that they had been informed of the success rates for the particular procedure at the clinic or hospital where the procedure was to be performed. In actuality, this companion law was passed, and became effective on 1 July 1992, but the mandated insurance coverage failed. Virginia is, therefore, the only state in the Union that has a law which requires that the patients be informed in writing, and sign a document that they have been so informed, of the results of the program they are attending.

ACCOUNTABILITY IN THE USA

From this account of the multiple and often overlapping efforts at certification, surveillance and the like, it is evident that the surveillance issue has not been resolved in the USA at this point. For those who live in countries other than the USA, where national regulation is the rule, it may be difficult to understand the absence of federal surveillance. It can only be said that this happens to be the way the USA works. Whether it is good or bad remains uncertain at this moment.

REFERENCES

1. The Ethics Committee of the American Fertility Society. Ethical considerations of the new reproductive technologies. Fertil Steril 1986; 46 (Suppl 1): 1S–94S
2. The Ethics Committee of the American Fertility Society. Ethical considerations of the new reproductive technologies. Fertil Steril 1990; 53 (Suppl 2): 1S–107S
3. The Ethics Committee of the American Fertility Society. Ethical considerations of the new reproductive technologies. Feril Steril 1994; 62 (Suppl 5): 1S–125S
4. Jones HW, Veeck LL, Muasher SJ, Gibbons WE. On reporting pregnancies by ART. Fertil Steril 1993; 60: 759–61
5. Application of Current Statutory Authorities to Human Somatic Cell Products, and Gene Therapy Products, 58 Fed Reg 53248 (October 14, 1993)
6. A Proposed Approach to the Regulation of Cellular and Tissue-Based Products, 62 Fed Reg 9271 (March 4, 1977)

39.7

Regulation of assisted reproductive technology: the French experience

Jean Cohen

INTRODUCTION

France was one of the first countries to take part in the development of *in vitro* fertilization (IVF) and medically assisted procreation. Two French teams participated in the meeting of pioneers at Bourn Hall in 1983 (Jean Cohen, René Frydman, Jacqueline Mandelbaum, Michèle Plachot and Jacques Testart).

FRENCH BIOETHICAL LAW

Since 29 July 1994, France has had a law concerning medically assisted procreation. The important points are:

(1) The law covers insemination with husband or donor semen, IVF (including intracytoplasmic sperm injection (ICSI)), research on embryos and antenatal diagnosis;

(2) With the exception of insemination, treatments may be performed only in licensed centers under the responsibility of an agreed practitioner. Licensing is granted for 5 years by the Ministry of Health after notification from a National Committee of Reproduction Medicine, Biology and Antenatal Diagnosis (NCRMBPD). This committee is composed of practitioners proposed by

their representative organizations, experts, lawyers and representatives of relevant administrative and professional bodies and family associations. All accredited infertility clinics are required to present an annual report of activities to the Minister of Health. The French Social Security reimburses all types of protocol without control.

Medically assisted procreation is intented to remedy medical infertility. The men and women in the couples must both be alive, of reproductive age, married or able to prove 2 years of living together, and give written consent after receiving precise counseling. Single mothers and homosexual couples are excluded. Unmarried couples must produce a certificate showing 2 years of living together, which must be kept in their file. The couple must seek counseling from a multidisciplinary team. Practitioners must provide guidance documents and there must be 1 month between giving the information and the decision to proceed.

IVF, ICSI and embryo freezing are permitted. The number of embryos that can be transferred is not specified. Selective reduction of pregnancy is not mentioned, but is practiced. Embryo freezing may be requested by the couple for a period of 5 years.

When considering gamete or embryo donation, recipient couples must obtain consent by a joint declaration before a judge or solicitor. Both members of the couple are legally responsible for the child. Couples who donate gametes must have had children, and no payment is allowed. Anonymity is mandatory and advertising is forbidden. Gametes may be obtained only through an agreed center. Negative biological analysis for human immunodeficiency virus (HIV), hepatitis, cytomegalovirus and syphilis must be obtained and quarantine for 6 months is observed before the donor gametes are used. Embryo donation is very rare, because of how complicated the procedures are (anonymity, consent forms, biological analysis, quarantine, etc.) and the lack of donors, as they cannot be IVF patients and cannot receive any money. IVF surrogacy is not allowed. Laws decree and encompass precisely assisted reproductive technologies (ART), including preimplantation genetic diagnosis (PGD). Authorizations are given to clinics and to doctors after inspection and advice of the NCRMBPD. For PGD, three authorizations are required: one for the clinical embryologist who performs the embryo biopsy, one for the cytogeneticist who performs fluorescent *in situ* hybridization (FISH) analysis and one for the molecular geneticist who searches for single gene defects by polymerase chain reaction (PCR). To be authorized, doctors must demonstrate that they have relevant formations, diplomas, and experience in animal models and/or human cells.

The disease to be diagnosed must be particularly severe and incurable at the time of diagnosis. Defining such severe diseases is difficult because of the variable expression of many of them. Moreover, which severity are we talking about: for the child, for the parents or for society? Does the disease concern the newborn, the child or the adult? It is generally accepted that genetic diseases that can be diagnosed by PGD are the same as those in the framework of prenatal diagnosis, on the understanding that diagnosis on a single cell (or two cells) is available. But in contrast to prenatal diagnosis, only abnormalities responsible for a disease previously and precisely identified in one of the parents can be searched for. This means that aneuploidy screening of embryos of women of advanced aged is not allowed. Recently, selection of an embryo in order to treat a diseased brother or sister has been accepted. However, preconception genetic diagnosis performed on the first polar body of the oocyte is not forbidden because, by law, only biological diagnosis based on cells taken from an embryo *in vitro* is regulated.

At present, although about 100 IVF centers are authorized to perform ART in France, only three teams with an IVF center and a genetic laboratory combined are allowed to perform PGD and only two are really active. Because of the small number of authorized centers, 1–2 years' delay is observed before inclusion of couples and their first PGD cycle.

The law was subjected to further examination by Parliament within a maximum of 5 years from its publication, i.e. in 1999. Only in July 2004 was the law re-examined.

The new law:

(1) Creates an agency of biomedicine and vigilance in order to control the results of ART;

(2) Agrees on embryo research for a period of 5 years;

(3) Refuses the right of a widow to be impregnated with an embryo conceived while her husband was still alive;

(4) Allows stem-cell research for a period of 5 years;

(5) Declares that cloning is a crime punishable by 20 years in prison;

(6) Will be re-examined in 5 years.

THE FRENCH RESULTS

There are approximately 150 centers of medically assisted procreation in France. They perform more than 40 000 attempts per year. Most of the centers participate in a national IVF registry (FIVNAT). In the 17th survey of FIVNAT, published in 2003, 59 centers registered their results. Table 1 shows the evolution since 1998. Not all the French attempts are included, because registration is on a voluntary basis, but FIVNAT registers approximately 80% of national attempts. In 2002, ICSI represented 53.4% of all attempts. Tables 2 and 3 show the evolution of frequency rates for IVF and for ICSI. There is a small decrease of the pregnancy rates, probably due to a diminution of the number of transferred embryos. On average, 25% of cycles involve embryo freezing and thawing.

Table 4 presents a comparison between gonadotropin releasing hormone (GnRH) agonists (long protocol) and GnRH antagonists. According to this

Table 1 French national data 1998–2002[1]

	1998	1999	2000	2001	2002
French centers (n)	94	94	93	92	92
Centers in FIVNAT (n)	78	82	79	79	59
Forms received (n)	36 590	37 946	38 731	41 308	28 212
Cancellation (%)	4.9	3.7	3.7	2.7	2.5
Punctures: total France (n)	40 379	41 503	43 092	45 701	
Punctures: total FIVNAT (n)	35 017	36 379	37 298	40 131	27 507
Conventional IVF (%)	54.4	53.4	47.3	48.1	46.0
Microinjection (%)	44.4	46.1	52.5	50.4	53.4
IVF + microinjection (%)	1.1	0.5	0.2	1.4	0.6
GIFT, ZIFT, TET (%)	0.1	0.02	0.04	0.01	0.0
No oocytes collected (%)	1.4	3.0	1.6	3.4	3.0
Thawed cycles (n)	7188	8126	8640		
Thawed cycles in FIVNAT (n)	4797	6863	7377	7202	5761
Clinical pregnancies in France (n)	9966	10 744	11 344		
Clinical pregnancies in FIVNAT (n)	6027	6960	7003	5472	

IVF, in vitro fertilization; GIFT, gamete intrafallopian transfer; ZIFT, zygote intrafallopian transfer; TET, tubal embryo transfer

Table 2 Evolution of success rates: in vitro fertilization (IVF)[1]

	1998	1999	2000	2001	2002
Transfers/punctures (%)	81.0	81.4	83.5	79.6	78.4
with frozen–thawed embryos (%)	18.8	22.7	26.3	23.7	23.2
Clinical pregnancy rate (%)					
per puncture	20.8	21.4	21.7	20.0	19.9
per transfer	25.7	26.5	26.2	25.1	25.4
Birth of at least one normal live baby/puncture (%)	17.0	17.1	17.2	16.5	

Table 3 Evolution of success rates: intracytoplasmic sperm injection (ICSI)[1]

	1998	1999	2000	2001	2002
Transfers/punctures (%)	92.3	92.8	91.9	92.2	91.9
with frozen–thawed embryos (%)	21.4	24.5	30.8	25.2	25.5
Clinical pregnancy rate (%)					
per puncture	23.7	25.1	24.3	23.0	23.8
per transfer	25.7	27.5	26.6	25.0	25.9
Birth of at least one normal live baby/puncture (%)	19.7	21.1	19.5	18.5	

Table 4 *In vitro* fertilization: comparison of gonadotropin releasing hormone (GnRH) antagonists and GnRH agonists (long protocol). Values are given as mean ± SD[1]

	Analog type	
	Agonist	*Antagonist*
n	60 787	4983
Age (years)	34.0 ± 4.4	34.7 ± 4.5
Gonadotropins (IU)	2546 ± 1203	2465 ± 1240
Estradiol (pg/ml)	1972 ± 1090	1806 ± 1530
Stimulation duration (days)	12.1 ± 2.3	11.6 ± 2.2
Oocytes collected (*n*)	9.2 ± 5.7	8.1 ± 5.7
Fertilization rate (%)	55.7 ± 31.8	59.4 ± 31.2
Total embryos (*n*)	4.94 ± 4.20	4.67 ± 3.92
Transferred embryos (*n*)	2.33 ± 0.81	2.23 ± 0.78
Pregnancy rate/puncture (%)	22.8	18.7
Pregnancy rate/transfer (%)	27.4	22.8

Table 6 Outcome of pregnancies: *in vitro* fertilization (IVF) and intracytoplasmic sperm injection (ICSI) (1997–2001)[1]

	IVF	ICSI	p Value
Pregnancies (*n*)	10 688	9642	
Spontaneous abortions (%)	17.8	17.6	NS (0.65)
Ectopic pregnancies (%)	3.5	1.8	0.001
Medical terminations (%)	0.66	0.71	NS (0.73)
Deliveries (*n* (%))	8357 (78.2)	7711 (80.0)	0.01
Singletons (% delivery) (%/babies)	72.5 56.6	74.7 59.4	0.01
Twins (%/delivery) (%/babies)	26.2 40.0	24.1 37.7	0.01
Triplets (%/delivery) (%/babies)	1.54 3.4	1.25 2.9	NS (0.11)
Quadruplets + (*n*)	1	0	
Embryo reduction (%)	2.07	1.44	0.01

NS, not significant

Table 5 Use of gonadotropins: annual rate per puncture. Other results are given as mean (SD)[1]

Gonadotropins	1998	1999	2000	2001	2002	p Value
Recombinant FSH (%)	64.8	84.7	87.0	87.2	85.4	
Urinary FSH (%)	11.5	2.3	0.2	0.2	0.1	
Rec-FSH + hMG (%)	2.9	2.2	2.3	3.6	3.6	0.001
Urinary FSH + hMG (%)	2.6	0.2	0.0	0.0	0.0	
hMG alone (%)	18.2	10.5	10.6	9.1	10.9	
Total given (IU)	2572 (1236)	2517 (1240)	2525 (1246)	2496 (1253)	2549 (1218)	0.001
Stimulation duration (days)	12.1 (2.4)	12.1 (2.3)	12.0 (2.2)	11.9 (2.3)	11.9 (2.1)	0.001
Estradiol (pg/ml)	1910 (1076)	1926 (1192)	1941 (1080)	1947 (1134)	2020 (1135)	0.001

FSH, follicle stimulating hormone; Rec-FSH, recombinant FSH; hMG, human menopausal gonadotropin

table, 10% of patients are treated with antagonists. Recent data show an increase of antagonist use. Results are better with GnRH agonists (long protocol).

Table 5 shows the use of gonadotropins. Recombinant follicle stimulating hormone (rec-FSH) represents 80–90% of cycles.

Table 6 indicates the outcome of IVF pregnancies: 26.2% were twins and 1.54% were triplets (after embryo reduction of 2.07%).

In France, one-half of the medically assisted procreation centers are publicly funded and the other half are private. French Social Security reimburses all attempts, including ovulation stimulation, follicle puncture, laboratory techniques, etc. If a couple are treated in a public center, they do not pay anything, except for special procedures such as freezing. If a couple are treated in a private center, they may have to pay the difference between the doctor's fees and the Social Security reimbursement. Waiting-lists do not generally exceed 2–3 months in public hospitals. The most recent list of French centers has been published[2].

REFERENCES

1. FIVNAT. Dossier FIVNAT 2003. France: Organon, 2003
2. Cohen J, Ramogida C, eds. Nous Voulons un Bébé. Paris: Seuil, 1997

USEFUL CONTACT

FIVNAT France, c/o J. De Mouzon, INSERM Hôpital de Bicêtre, 94276 Kremlin Bicêtre Cedex, France. Tel: +33 1 45 21 22 80 or +33 1 45 21 22 96. Fax: +33 1 45 21 20 75.

Index